Ambulatory
Pediatric Care

Ambulatory Pediatric Care

Edited by
ROBERT A. DERSHEWITZ, M.D., Sc. M., F.A.A.P.

Chief of Pediatrics
Harvard Community Health Plan
Braintree Center;
Clinical Instructor in Pediatrics
Harvard Medical School;
Clinical Associate in Pediatrics
Massachusetts General Hospital;
Courtesy Staff (Medicine)
Children's Hospital;
Associate Pediatrician
Brigham and Women's Hospital
Boston, Massachusetts

WITH 127 CONTRIBUTORS

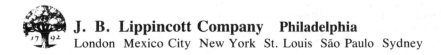

J. B. Lippincott Company   Philadelphia
London Mexico City New York St. Louis São Paulo Sydney

Developmental Editor: Delois Patterson
Manuscript Editor: Marjory I. Fraser
Indexer: Julia Schwager
Senior Design Coordinator: Anita R. Curry
Production Manager: Kathleen P. Dunn
Production Coordinator: Fred D. Wood IV
Compositor: Maryland Composition Company, Inc.
Printer/Binder: Murray Printing Company

6 5 4 3 2 1

Library of Congress Cataloging-in-Publication Data
Ambulatory pediatric care.

  Includes bibliographies and index.
  1. Pediatrics. 2. Ambulatory medical care for
children. I. Dershewitz, Robert A. [DNLM: 1. Ambulatory Care. 2. Pediatrics. WS 200 A4965]
RJ47.A42 1988   618.92   87-22525
ISBN 0-397-50758-5

The authors and publisher have exerted every effort to ensure that drug selection and dosage
set forth in this text are in accord with current recommendations and practice at the time of
publication. However, in view of ongoing research, changes in government regulations, and
the constant flow of information relating to drug therapy and drug reactions, the reader is
urged to check the package insert for each drug for any change in indications and dosage
and for added warnings and precautions. This is particularly important when the
recommended agent is a new or infrequently employed drug.

By convention of J. B. Lippincott Company and for ease of readability, only the
masculine pronoun, rather than both "he/she," is used. Thus, "he" is intended to refer to
either male or female and should not be interpreted as a sexist bias.

To my parents, Dr. Irving and Bess Dershewitz for
their influence; to my children, Naomi and Dana, for their understanding;
and to my wife Lydia, who knows why.

Contributors

RUSSELL ASNES, M.D.
Clinical Professor of Pediatrics
College of Physicians and Surgeons
Columbia University
New York, New York

IRVING W. BAILIT, M.D.
Clinical Instructor in Pediatrics
Harvard Medical School;
Associate in Allergy
Children's Hospital
Boston, Massachusetts

VICTOR C. BAUM, M.D.
Director of Pediatric Intensive Care Unit
Michael Reese Hospital and Medical Center;
Assistant Professor of Pediatrics
Pritzker School of Medicine
University of Chicago
Chicago, Illinois

MARGARET L. BAUMAN, M.D.
Assistant Professor of Neurology
Harvard Medical School;
Assistant Neurologist and Pediatrician
Massachusetts General Hospital
Boston, Massachusetts

JAY E. BERKELHAMER, M.D.
Professor and Associate Chairman
Department of Pediatrics
Wyler Children's Hospital
University of Chicago
Pritzker School of Medicine
Chicago, Illinois

JAMES H. BERMAN, M.D.
Research Fellow, Harvard Medical School;
Fellow, Combined Program in Pediatric
  Gastroenterology and Nutrition
Children's Hospital and
Massachusetts General Hospital
Boston, Massachusetts

DONALD M. BERWICK, M.D., M.P.P.
Associate Professor of Pediatrics
Harvard Medical School;
Associate in Pediatrics
Children's Hospital Medical Center;
Vice-President for Quality-of-Care
  Measurements
Harvard Community Health Plan
Boston, Massachusetts

HERBERT BOERSTLING, M.D.
Pediatrician
Harvard Community Health Plan;
Clinical Instructor in Pediatrics
Harvard Medical School
Boston, Massachusetts

WILLIAM P. BOGER, III, M.D.
  Associate in Ophthalmology
  Children's Hospital
  Boston, Massachusetts;
  Active Staff, Emerson Hospital
  Concord, Massachusetts

KENNETH M. BOYER, M.D.
  Director, Section of Infectious Diseases
  Department of Pediatrics
  Rush–Presbyterian–St. Luke's Medical
    Center;
  Associate Professor of Pediatrics
  Rush Medical College
  Chicago, Illinois

JEAN BRODNAX, M.D.
  Pediatrician, Harvard Community Health
    Plan
  Clinical Instructor in Pediatrics
  Harvard Medical School
  Boston, Massachusetts

DAVID I. BROMBERG, M.D.
  Clinical Assistant Professor of Pediatrics
  University of Maryland Medical School
  Baltimore, Maryland

LORIN M. BROWN, M.D., F.A.A.O.S.,
F.A.C.S., F.A.A.P.
  Director of Pediatric Orthopedic Surgery
  Michael Reese Hospital and Medical Center
  Chicago, Illinois

THOMAS R. BROWNE, M.D.
  Professor of Neurology and
  Associate Professor of Pharmacology
  Boston University School of Medicine
  Boston, Massachusetts

PAUL K. BRUCHEZ, PsyD
  Psychologist
  Child Mental Health
  Harvard Community Health Plan—
    Wellesley Center
  Boston, Massachusetts

HUGH A. CARITHERS, M.D.
  Clinical Professor of Pediatrics
  Jacksonville Health Education Programs
  Division of the Health Center
  University of Florida
  Jacksonville, Florida

ROBERT A. CATALANO, M.D.
  Pediatric Ophthalmology Service
  Wills Eye Hospital
  Philadelphia, Pennsylvania

VERNE S. CAVINESS, Jr., M.D., D.Phil.
  Joseph & Rose Kennedy Professor of Child
    Neurology and Mental Retardation
  Harvard Medical School;
  Chief, Division of Child Neurology
  Massachusetts General Hospital
  Boston, Massachusetts

TIEN–LAN CHANG, M.D.
  Combined Program in Pediatric
    Gastroenterology and Nutrition
  Massachusetts General Hospital and
    Children's Hospital
  Department of Pediatrics
  Harvard Medical School
  Boston, Massachusetts

PAUL H. CHAPMAN, M.D.
  Associate Professor
  Harvard Medical School;
  Chief of Pediatric Neurosurgery
  Massachusetts General Hospital
  Boston, Massachusetts

EVAN CHARNEY, M.D.
  Professor and Chairman
  Department of Pediatrics
  University of Massachusetts Medical School
  Worcester, Massachusetts

KATHERINE K. CHRISTOFFEL, M.D., M.P.H.
  Associate Professor of Pediatrics and
    Community Health and Preventive
    Medicine
  Northwestern University School of
    Medicine
  Chicago, Illinois

EDWARD R. CHRISTOPHERSEN, Ph.D.
  Professor of Pediatrics,
  Chief of Behavioral Sciences Section
  The University of Kansas Medical Center
  Kansas City, Kansas

WILLIAM D. COCHRAN, M.D.
  Clinical Associate Professor of Pediatrics
  Harvard Medical School;
  Physician in Charge
  Newborn Service
  The Beth Israel Hospital
  Boston, Massachusetts

HERBERT E. COHN, M.D.
  Clinical Instructor in Pediatrics
  Harvard Medical School;
  Consultant in Pediatric Cardiology
  Harvard Community Health Plan
  Boston, Massachusetts

EDWARD M. CONNOR, M.D.
  Assistant Professor of Pediatrics
  University of Medicine and Dentistry of
    New Jersey
  New Jersey Medical School
  Newark, New Jersey

JOHN F. CRIGLER, Jr., M.D.
  Divisions of Endocrinology and Adolescent
    and Young Adult Medicine
  The Children's Hospital
  Department of Pediatrics
  Harvard Medical School
  Boston, Massachusetts

BARRY DASHEFSKY, M.D.
  Assistant Professor of Pediatrics
  University of Pittsburgh School of
    Medicine;
  Division of Ambulatory Care and Pediatric
    Infectious Diseases
  Children's Hospital of Pittsburgh
  Pittsburgh, Pennsylvania

G. ROBERT DELONG, M.D.
  Assistant Professor of Neurology
  Harvard Medical School;
  Associate Neurologist
  Associate Pediatrician
  Massachusetts General Hospital
  Boston, Massachusetts

ROBERT A. DERSHEWITZ, M.D., Sc.M.
  Chief of Pediatrics
  Harvard Community Health Plan
  Braintree Center;
  Clinical Instructor in Pediatrics
  Harvard Medical School
  Boston, Massachusetts

COLETTE DESLANDRES–LEDUC, M.D.
  Combined Program in Pediatric
    Gastroenterology and Nutrition
  Massachusetts General Hospital and
    Children's Hospital
  Department of Pediatrics
  Harvard Medical School
  Boston, Massachusetts

THOMAS G. DEWITT, M.D.
  Director of General Pediatrics Division
  Assistant Professor of Pediatrics
  University of Massachusetts Medical Center
  Worcester, Massachusetts

ELIZABETH C. DOOLING, M.D.
  Assistant Professor of Neurology
  Harvard Medical School;
  Associate Neurologist and Associate
    Pediatrician
  Massachusetts General Hospital
  Boston, Massachusetts

HENRY L. DORKIN, M.D.
  Assistant Professor of Pediatrics
  Tufts University School of Medicine;
  Chief of Service
  Pediatric Pulmonary and Allergy Division
  New England Medical Center
  Boston, Massachusetts

A. STEPHEN DUBANSKY, M.D.
  Assistant Professor of Pediatrics
  Division of Hematology–Oncology
  State University of New York at Syracuse
  Health Science Center
  Syracuse, New York

PAUL G. DYMENT, M.D.
  Professor of Pediatrics
  University of Vermont;
  Chief of Pediatrics
  Maine Medical Center
  Portland, Maine

ARTHUR ELSTER, M.D.
  Associate Professor of Pediatrics
  University of Utah Health Science Center
  Salt Lake City, Utah

HELEN M. EMERY, M.D.
  Associate Professor of Pediatrics
  University of Chicago
  Pritzker School of Medicine;
  Co-Director, Section of Rheumatology
  La Rabida Children's Hospital and Research
    Center
  Chicago, Illinois

ROBERT P. FOGLIA, M.D.
  Assistant Professor in Surgery
  University of California at Los Angeles
    School of Medicine;
  Attending Surgeon
  University of California Center for the
    Health Sciences
  Los Angeles, California

VICTOR L. FOX, M.D.
  Combined Program in Pediatric
    Gastroenterology and Nutrition
  Massachusetts General Hospital and
    Children's Hospital
  Department of Pediatrics
  Harvard Medical School
  Boston, Massachusetts

ELLEN M. FRIEDMAN, M.D.
  Assistant Professor of Otolaryngology
  Harvard Medical School;
  Adjunct Assistant Professor of
    Otolaryngology
  Boston University School of Medicine;
  Associate in Otolaryngology
  The Children's Hospital
  Boston, Massachusetts

PIERRE GAUDREAULT, M.D.
  Clinical Assistant Professor of Pediatrics
  University of Montreal;
  Scientific Director
  Poison Centre
  Sainte-Justine Hospital
  Quebec, Canada

DANIEL A. GOLDSTEIN, M.D., A.B.M.T.
  Clinical and Research Fellow in Clinical
    Pharmacology
  The Hospital for Sick Children
    and University of Toronto
  Toronto, Ontario
  Canada

SAMUEL P. GOTOFF, M.D.
  Professor and Chairman of Pediatrics
  Rush Medical College;
  Chairman of Pediatrics Department
  Rush–Presbyterian–St. Luke's Medical
    Center
  Chicago, Illinois

KENNETH E. GRANT, M.D.
  Pediatric Gastroenterology and Nutrition
  Memorial Medical Center
  Long Beach, California

EDWARD S. GROSS, M.D.
  Instructor in Pediatrics
  Boston University School of Medicine and
    Harvard Medical School;
  Pediatrician
  Harvard Community Health Plan
  West Roxbury Center
  Boston, Massachusetts

ROBERT GROSS, M.D.
  Assistant in Ophthalmology
  Children's Hospital and Harvard Medical
    School
  Boston, Massachusetts

ROOPA S. HASHIMOTO, M.S., M.D.
  Postdoctoral Fellow in Ambulatory
    Pediatrics

University of Iowa;
Staff Pediatrician
Nightime Pediatric Clinic
Salt Lake City, Utah

THOMAS J. HATHAWAY, M.D.
  Pediatrician
  Harvard Community Health Plan
  Boston, Massachusetts

PETER B. H'DOUBLER, Jr., M.D.
  Assistant Professor of Surgery
  Emory University School of Medicine
  Atlanta, Georgia

PETER T. HEYDEMANN, M.D.
  Director, Section of Neurology
  Department of Pediatrics
  Rush Medical College;
  Attending Child Neurologist
  Rush–Presbyterian–St. Luke's Medical
    Center
  Chicago, Illinois

MARGARET HIGHAM, M.D.
  Pediatrician, Harvard Community Health
    Plan
  Boston, Massachusetts

MARTIN I. HOROWITZ, M.D.
  Clinical Instructor in Pediatrics
  Harvard Medical School;
  Health Center Director
  Peabody Center
  Boston, Massachusetts

JULIE R. INGELFINGER, M.D.
  Assistant Professor of Pediatrics
  Harvard Medical School;
  Director of Hypertension Clinic
  The Children's Hospital;
  Associate in Medicine
  The Children's Hospital;
  Associate in Medicine
  Brigham & Women's Hospital
  Boston, Massachusetts

JOSEPH J. JANKOWSKI, M.D.
  Associate Chief of Ambulatory and
    Community Services
  Division of Child Psychiatry
  New England Medical Center Hospitals;
  Associate Clinical Professor of Psychiatry
  Tufts University School of Medicine
  Boston, Massachusetts

PAULA KIENBERGER JAUDES, M.D.
  Associate Professor of Clinical Pediatrics
  University of Chicago

Pritzker School of Medicine;
Chief of Medical Staff
Section Chief of Chronic Disease
La Rabida Children's Hospital and Research
  Center
Chicago, Illinois

MICHAEL S. JELLINEK, M.D.
Associate Professor of Psychiatry
  (Pediatrics)
Harvard Medical School;
Psychiatrist and Pediatrician
Massachusetts General Hospital
Chief of Child Psychiatry Service
Massachusetts General Hospital;
Director of Outpatient Psychiatry
Massachusetts General Hospital
Boston, Massachusetts

MURRAY M. KAPPELMAN, M.D.
Professor of Pediatrics
Director of Behavioral and Developmental
  Pediatrics Division
University of Maryland
Baltimore, Maryland

HARVEY P. KATZ, M.D.
Associate Professor of Pediatrics
Harvard Medical School;
Health Center Director
Braintree Center
Boston, Massachusetts

LUCINDA LEE KATZ, M.D.
Professor, Erikson Institute
Clinical Assistant Professor
University of Chicago
Wyler Children's Hospital
Chicago, Illinois

CONSTANCE H. KEEFER, M.D.
Instructor in Pediatrics
Harvard Medical School
Pediatrician, Harvard Community Health
  Plan
Boston, Massachusetts

DOROTHY H. KELLY, M.D.
Assistant Professor of Pediatrics
Harvard Medical School;
Associate Pediatrician
Massachusetts General Hospital
Boston, Massachusetts

JANICE D. KEY, M.D.
Clinical Assistant Professor of Pediatrics
University of North Carolina School of
  Medicine;
Pediatric Teaching Staff

Moses Cone Memorial Hospital Pediatric
  Teaching Service
Greensboro, North Carolina

SAMUEL H. KIM, M.D.
Associate Clinical Professor of Surgery
Harvard Medical School;
Visiting Surgeon
Massachusetts General Hospital
Boston, Massachusetts

ROBERT Z. KLEIN, M.D.
Professor of Pediatrics
Dartmouth Medical School;
Coordinator of New England Congenital
  Hypothyroidism Collaborative
Hanover, New Hampshire

RONALD E. KLEINMAN, M.D.
Assistant Professor of Pediatrics
Harvard Medical School
Combined Program in Pediatric
  Gastroenterology and Nutrition
Massachusetts General Hospital and
  Children's Hospital
Boston, Massachusetts

ILANA KRAUS, M.D.
Chief of Pediatrics
Harvard Community Health Plan
West Roxbury Center
Boston, Massachusetts

KALPATHY S. KRISHNAMOORTHY, M.D.
Assistant Professor of Pediatrics
  (Neurology)
Harvard Medical School;
Assistant Neurologist
Assistant Pediatrician
Massachusetts General Hospital
Boston, Massachusetts

CRAIG B. LANGMAN, M.D.
Associate Professor of Pediatrics
Northwestern University School of
  Medicine
Nephrologist, The Children's Memorial
  Hospital
Chicago, Illinois

ALLEN LAPEY, M.D.
Clinical Instructor of Pediatrics
Harvard Medical School;
Assistant Pediatrician
Director of Cystic Fibrosis Center
Massachusetts General Hospital
Boston, Massachusetts

LAURIE A. LATCHAW, M.D.
Assistant Professor of Surgery
Tufts University School of Medicine;
Lecturer in Surgery
Boston University School of Medicine;
Attending Surgeon
New England Medical Center;
Chief of Pediatric Surgery
Boston City Hospital
Boston, Massachusetts

WAYNE I. LENCER, M.D.
Research Fellow in Pediatrics
    (Gastroenterology and Nutrition)
Harvard Medical School;
Children's Hospital
Boston, Massachusetts

LYNNE L. LEVITSKY, M.D.
Professor of Pediatrics
Pritzker School of Medicine
University of Chicago
Director of Pediatric Endocrinology and
    Metabolism
Michael Reese Medical Center
Chicago, Illinois

JACOB A. LOHR, M.D.
Professor of Pediatrics
University of Virginia Children's Medical
    Center
Charlottesville, Virginia

MICHAEL L. MACKNIN, M.D.
Head of General Pediatric Section
The Cleveland Clinic Foundation
Cleveland, Ohio

WILLIAM C. MACLEAN, Jr., M.D.
Clinical Professor of Pediatrics
The Ohio State University;
Medical Director of Pediatric Nutrition
Ross Laboratories
Columbus, Ohio

M. JOAN MANSFIELD, M.D.
Instructor, Harvard Medical School;
Assistant in Medicine
Children's Hospital
Boston, Massachusetts

STEVEN M. MARCUS, M.D.
Associate Professor of Pediatrics and
Environmental and Community Health
University of Medicine and Dentistry of
    New Jersey
New Jersey Medical School;
Assistant Director of Pediatrics

Newark Beth Israel Medical Center
Newark, New Jersey

STEVEN M. MATLOFF, M.D.
Allergy Department
Harvard Community Health Plan
Boston, Massachusetts

JACK L. MAYER, M.D.
Clinical Instructor in Pediatrics
University of Vermont
Burlington, Vermont

PAUL L. MCCARTHY, M.D.
Professor of Pediatrics
Yale University School of Medicine
Chief of General Pediatrics Division
Yale–New Haven Medical Center
New Haven, Connecticut

MICHAEL A. MCGUIGAN, M.D.
Assistant Professor of Pediatrics and
    Pharmacology
Faculty of Medicine
University of Toronto;
Medical Director
Poison Information Centre
The Hospital for Sick Children
Toronto, Ontario
Canada

HENRY S. METZ, M.D.
Professor and Chairman of Ophthalmology
University of Rochester
School of Medicine and Dentistry
Rochester, New York

MOHAMAD MIKATI, M.D.
Assistant Professor of Neurology
Harvard Medical School;
Assistant in Neurology
Children's Hospital
Boston, Massachusetts

ANTHONY B. MINNEFOR, M.D.
Chief, Divison of Infectious Diseases
Associate Chairman
Department of Pediatrics
St. Joseph's Hospital & Medical Center
Paterson, New Jersey;
Clinical Associate Professor
University of Medicine & Dentistry of New
    Jersey
New Jersey Medical School
Newark, New Jersey

ANNE MUNCK, M.D.
Hopital Bretonneau
Paris, France

JODY R. MURPH, M.D.
Assistant Professor of Pediatrics
University of Iowa
University of Iowa Hospitals & Clinics
Iowa City, Iowa

LEONARD B. NELSON, M.D.
Pediatric Ophthalmology Service
Wills Eye Hospital
Philadelphia, Pennsylvania

L. GERARD NIEDERMAN, M.D., M.P.H.
Clinical Assistant Professor of Pediatrics
Pritzker School of Medicine
University of Chicago;
Attending Physician
Michael Reese Hospital
Chicago, Illinois

SAMUEL NURKO, M.D.
Research Fellow, Harvard Medical School;
Fellow in Pediatric Gastroenterology
Children's Hospital
Boston, Massachusetts

JOAN M. O'CONNOR, D.M.D.
Winchester, Massachusetts

JAMES M. OLESKE, M.D., M.P.H.
Professor of Pediatrics
University of Medicine and Dentistry of
New Jersey
New Jersey Medical School
Newark, New Jersey

EILEEN M. OUELLETTE, M.D.
Assistant Professor of Neurology
Harvard Medical School;
Assistant Neurologist
Assistant Pediatrician
Massachusetts General Hospital
Boston, Massachusetts

AMY PALLER, M.D.
Assistant Professor of Dermatology and
Pediatrics
Rush Medical College;
Assistant Attending in Dermatology and
Pediatrics
Rush–Presbyterian–St. Luke's Medical
Center
Chicago, Illinois

STEPHEN I. PELTON, M.D.
Associate Professor of Pediatrics
Boston University School of Medicine;
Associate Director of Pediatrics
Boston City Hospital
Boston, Massachusetts

ODETTE PINSONNEAULT, M.D.
Assistant Professor of Obstetrics and
Gynecology
University of Sherbrooke
Sherbrooke, Quebec
Canada

ORAH S. PLATT, M.D.
Associate Professor of Pediatrics
Harvard Medical School
Children's Hospital and Dana-Farber Cancer
Center
Boston, Massachusetts

MARGARET B. RENNELS, M.D.
Associate Professor of Pediatrics
Chief, Clinical Studies Section
Center for Vaccine Development
University of Maryland School of Medicine
Baltimore, Maryland

PETER B. ROSENBERGER, M.D.
Assistant Professor of Neurology
Harvard Medical School;
Associate Neurologist
Associate Pediatrician and Director of
Learning Disorders Unit
Massachusetts General Hospital
Boston, Massachusetts

LINDA V. ROSS, R.N., Ph.D.
Adjunct Professor
University of Missouri—Kansas City
School of Nursing;
Behavioral Sciences Section
Children's Mercy Hospital
Kansas City, Missouri;
Director of Well Child Project
University of Kansas Medical Center
Kansas City, Kansas

CHARLES F. SANZONE, M.D., Ph.D.
Assistant Professor of Orthopaedic Surgery
Boston University;
Director of Pediatric Orthopaedics
Associate Director of Orthopaedics
Boston City Hospital
Boston, Massachusetts

RICHARD M. SARLES, M.D.
Clinical Professor of Psychiatry and
Pediatrics
University of Maryland School of Medicine;
Director of Child and Adolescent Psychiatry
Division
The Sheppard and Enoch Pratt Hospital
Baltimore, Maryland

EDWARD L. SCHOR, M.D.
  Henry J. Kaiser Foundation
  Menlo Park, California

JANET L. SCHWANER, M.D.
  Department of Pediatrics
  Harvard Community Health Plan
  Boston, Massachusetts

JONATHAN SCHWARTZ, M.D.
  Clinical Fellow, Harvard Medical School;
  Child Psychiatry Service and Consultant to
    the Language Disorders Unit
  Massachusetts General Hospital
  Boston, Massachusetts

DAVID J. SEIDMAN, M.D.
  Department of Pediatric Ophthalmology
  Wills Eye Hospital
  Philadelphia, Pennsylvania

BRUCE K. SHAPIRO, M.D.
  Associate Professor of Pediatrics
  The Johns Hopkins University School of
    Medicine;
  Developmental Pediatrician
  The Kennedy Institute for Handicapped
    Children
  Baltimore, Maryland

EDWARD SILLS, M.D.
  Associate Professor of Pediatrics
  The Johns Hopkins University School of
    Medicine;
  Director of Pediatric and Adolescent
    Collagen Vascular Service
  Johns Hopkins Hospital
  Baltimore, Maryland

DEBORAH E. SMITH, B.M., B.Ch.
  Assistant Professor of Pediatrics
  University of Virginia Medical School
  Charlottesville, Virginia

HOWARD G. SMITH, M.D.
  General and Medical Coordinator
  Boston Children's Deafness Network
  Boston, Massachusetts

BROOK SWEARINGEN, M.D.
  Neurosurgical Service
  Massachusetts General Hospital
  Harvard Medical School
  Boston, Massachusetts

CHARLES N. SWISHER, M.D.
  Associate Professor of Clinical Pediatrics
    and Clinical Neurology

University of Chicago;
  Director of Pediatric Neurology Division
  Michael Reese Hospital and Medical Center
  Chicago, Illinois

KATHERINE C. TEETS GRIMM, M.D.
  Director of Ambulatory Pediatrics Division
  The Mount Sinai Medical Center
  New York, New York

KENNETH H. TELLERMAN, M.D.
  Behavioral/General Pediatrician
  Director of Pediatrics
  Central Maryland Medical Group
  Baltimore, Maryland

MILTON TENENBEIN, M.D.
  Associate Professor of Pediatrics
  University of Manitoba;
  Director of Emergency Department
  Children's Hospital, Winnipeg;
  Director of Manitoba Poison Control Centre
  Winnipeg, Manitoba
  Canada

JOHN UDALL, M.D., Ph.D.
  Combined Program in Pediatric
    Gastroenterology and Nutrition
  Massachusetts General Hospital and
    Children's Hospital
  Department of Pediatrics
  Harvard Medical School
  Boston, Massachusetts

DAVID VAN BUSKIRK, M.D.
  Clinical Assistant Professor of Psychiatry
  Harvard Medical School
  Boston, Massachusetts

ELLEN R. WALD, M.D.
  Associate Professor of Pediatrics
  University of Pittsburgh School of
    Medicine;
  Division of Infectious Disease and
    Ambulatory Care
  Children's Hospital of Pittsburgh
  Pittsburgh, Pennsylvania

W. ALLAN WALKER, M.D.
  Professor of Pediatrics
  Harvard Medical School;
  Chief, Combined Program in Pediatric
    Gastroenterology and Nutrition
  Massachusetts General Hospital and
    Children's Hospital
  Boston, Massachusetts

MARILYN WARREN, Ph.D.
   Coordinator of Audiology Services
   Children's Hospital
   Boston, Massachusetts

MARC WEISSBLUTH, M.D.
   Associate Professor of Pediatrics
   Northwestern University School of
      Medicine;
   Director of Sleep Disorders Center
   Children's Memorial Hospital
   Chicago, Illinois

HARLAND S. WINTER, M.D.
   Assistant Professor of Pediatrics
   Harvard Medical School
   Assistant in Gastroenterology
   Children's Hospital;
   Clinical Associate in Pediatrics
   Massachusetts General Hospital
   Boston, Massachusetts

RAOUL L. WOLF, M.D.
   Associate Professor of Pediatrics
   Pritzker School of Medicine
   University of Chicago;
   Director of Allergy/Immunology
   Department of Pediatrics
   Michael Reese Hospital & Medical Center
   Chicago, Illinois

JEROLD C. WOODHEAD, M.D.
   Assistant Professor of Pediatrics
   University of Iowa College of Medicine
   University of Iowa Hospitals & Clinics
   Iowa City, Iowa

BASIL J. ZITELLI, M.D.
   Associate Professor of Pediatrics
   University of Pittsburgh School of
      Medicine;
   Pediatrician, Diagnostic Referral Service
   Children's Hospital of Pittsburgh
   Pittsburgh, Pennsylvania

JOHAN ZWAAN, M.D., Ph.D.
   Associate Professor of Ophthalmology
   Harvard Medical School
   Director of Pediatric Eye Service
   Massachusetts Eye and Ear Infirmary
   Boston, Massachusetts

ROBERT G. ZWERDLING, M.D.
   Associate Professor of Pediatrics
   University of Massachusetts Medical School
   Director of Pediatric Pulmonary Diseases
   Director of In-Patient Pediatrics
   University of Massachusetts Medical Center
   Worcester, Massachusetts

Preface

Most children who visit a physician in an office-based or primary care setting are fundamentally well; they are usually seen for preventive health care, relatively minor illnesses, needs' assessment, or reassurance. The diversity of a pediatric practice, however, requires that the primary care provider must have a broad-based knowledge of all of pediatric medicine. He must know when to seek immediate secondary and tertiary care, and when *not* to refer. *Ambulatory Pediatric Care* is directed both to the physician (pediatrician, family or general practitioner) and to the mid-level health worker (nurse practitioner or physician's assistant) who must examine, accurately diagnose, and expeditiously treat such children. On the basis of the National Ambulatory Care Survey data, we know that concerns responsible for almost all (>99%) pediatric visits are included in this text.

The organization of this book and the topics emphasized are designed to meet the demands of pediatric practitioners. Parts 2 and 3 (The Well-Child and Environmental Influences on Children) include concepts, principles, and applications that are widely recognized as cornerstones of child health maintenance. The chapter on the Well-Child Visit (Chap. 8) is deliberately the largest in the book. The content of each scheduled well-child visit and the common issues raised by parents at these visits are discussed. Most psychosocial issues and problems facing the clinician are included in Part 4, Behavioral Pediatrics, and Part 5, Developmental Pediatrics and School Health. The remainder of the book is devoted to the most common childhood symptoms and illnesses seen in the primary care setting.

All chapters are oriented toward primary care: They include guidelines for hospitalization or referral to other specialists and conclude with an annotated bibliography to facilitate further reading and study. The reader should consult either general or specialty pediatric textbooks for the esoteric or rarely encountered conditions and for detailed management of the hospitalized child.

Robert A. Dershewitz, M.D., Sc.M., F.A.A.P.

Acknowledgments

It is a truism, and I hope not banal, to say that many people are needed to bring a book to fruition. The contributors, who have all written so well and in the required format, have played a main role in this book. I extend a warm "thank you" to them.

I am greatly indebted to the Harvard Community Health Plan for its encouragement and support throughout this project. Drs. Roger Platt, Harvey P. Katz, and Martin I. Horowitz were particularly helpful by enabling me to arrange or facilitate many of the practical aspects needed for this book. Dr. Gordon Moore, Director of Teaching Programs, Harvard Community Health Plan, provided me with both guidance and support. The entire Pediatrics Department, Harvard Community Health Plan, Braintree Center was wonderfully supportive and tolerant of my involvement with this, my "other job." It is a privilege and a pleasure to be part of that group.

Drs. Doris Bennett, Katherine Christoffel, Jonathan Cronin, A. Stephen Dubansky, Gary R. Fleisher, and Robert Peterson provided valuable consultation. Dr. Allan Goroll not only offered advice, but also created the framework for this book with *Primary Care Medicine*, edited by Drs. Goroll, May, and Mulley.

Mr. William Burgower, formerly at J. B. Lippincott Company, recruited me for this project. I would also like to thank J. Stuart Freeman, Jr., Medical Editor, Delois Patterson, Developmental Editor, and Marjory I. Fraser, Copy Editor, of the J. B. Lippincott Company, who were instrumental in converting first the prospectus and then the stack of chapters into a coherent book.

To those whom I have not acknowledged, I ask your pardon and express my gratitude.

Contents

1
The Office

1
Models of Office Practice
JAY E. BERKELHAMER

Physicians often complete their training in pediatrics with little idea about the type or style of clinical practice that they will pursue. In the past, although the choices were relatively few they were readily available. Today, there is not only a bewildering array of practice arrangements but also a much more competitive environment for the more desirable locations and subspecialty areas. The physician-in-training who carefully considers the various practice options and prepares for one or another will have more opportunity to obtain the best position and to enter a practice enthusiastically. The basic practice arrangements and their relative merits are introduced in the following discussion.

GENERAL VERSUS SUBSPECIALTY PRACTICE

One of the first choices that pediatricians entering practice must make is between general and subspecialty care. Although it is possible to combine part-time subspecialty work and general pediatrics, the physician who chooses to be only a subspecialist has narrowed his options. The general pediatrician who practices primary care has maximized the number of possible arrangements and locations. Of course, the concepts and responsibilities of a primary care practice are not suited or do not have appeal for all who enter pediatrics. The general pediatrician is a primary care doctor who coordinates the child's medical care and is responsible for assisting the family in obtaining the necessary pediatric subspecialty or surgical care. The

management of certain chronic problems such as asthma, obesity, rheumatoid arthritis, or diabetes have become increasingly important to the responsibilities of general practice. Behavioral and developmental problems have been characterized as the *new morbidity* and should be areas of interest and expertise for the new general pediatrician. The generalist will also need to be available to direct the care of acute episodic and emergency problems that may occur at any time of the day or night and that must be considered in establishing a practice.

Subspecialty practice has its own advantages and disadvantages. Many find the greater sophistication of providing expert knowledge in a specific area of medicine more intellectually satisfying than general practice. Certain subspecialty areas tend to be procedure-oriented and are, therefore, generally more remunerative. However, since fellowship training is required for most subspecialty areas, there is a 2- or 3-year delay after training in general pediatrics before entering practice. Start-up costs may be greater than in primary care because specialized equipment may be required. There is also less flexibility in practice locations because a community must be large enough to support a referral base. A mixed subspecialty and general practice may be politically difficult because new patients often come from general pediatricians and family practitioners. Referring physicians will want to be sure their patients will return to them for future primary care. Some pediatricians have solved the dilemma of combining a part-time subspecialty practice with general pediatrics by joining a large group practice in which each member provides subspe-

1

cialty coverage in a different area. These considerations make a subspecialty practice in larger physician groups or medical centers more attractive than traditional small private office settings.

The distribution of physicians by specialty and location has been a major concern in the United States for several years. The National Health Service Corps and training grants for general medicine and pediatrics in primary care are examples of government programs that encourage physicians to enter primary care practice and locate in underserved areas. Although we have now entered an era in which physicians are in surplus supply in the United States, opportunities should continue for pediatricians who are interested in general practice in underserved communities. Inner city locations populated by the urban poor and small towns in many parts of the country present the most opportunities for new physicians. Primary care doctors are also sought by newly organized systems of care such as health maintenance organizations and for-profit health care corporations.

SOLO VERSUS GROUP PRACTICE MODELS

An American Medical Association study in 1983 showed that almost half of all practicing physicians in the United States are in solo practices. Considerably fewer physicians who enter practice today consider solo practices. The advantages of a solo practice relate primarily to issues of independence and location. The solo practitioner is relatively free to set up his office and style of practice. Decisions on space utilization, medical records, fee schedules, office hours, and choice of treatment can be individualized. Rural practice settings that cannot support the activities of a group practice usually work well for the doctor willing to assume the responsibilities of a solo practice. Such communities are grateful to have new pediatricians and local banks are generally willing to create favorable loan and credit lines. Some communities and local hospitals will even underwrite the start-up costs of practice and guarantee initial income. A major difficulty with a solo practice is the necessity of providing continuous care to patients. Unless other solo physicians are available to share weekend and off-hours coverage, the solo practitioner may feel trapped by a practice with little time off. Practice obligations may constrain opportunities for continuing medical education. Starting a solo practice also has significant financial ramifications because earnings may be delayed during the early years. One option is the purchase of an established practice

that would provide an immediate income to the new physician and gradual payments to the older pediatrician for his practice.

It is imperative that the physician should understand the mental and emotional requirements of a solo practice because failure to consider these facts could be devastating. Although no other practice model is more conducive to a close physician–patient relationship, the inherent responsibilities can be enormous. A solo practice in a relatively isolated area may have limited support facilities and personnel. The physician must have the mental capability to function away from the academic and protective environment under which he received his training. Nevertheless, many pediatricians want the satisfactions related to solo practice and will continue to choose that option.

Group practice formats have become more common for several reasons. Many pediatricians who enter a practice want the security of sharing patient care and financial matters with others. A group practice has the obvious advantage of allowing physicians more flexibility in planning work schedules and the business aspects of practice. In addition, colleagues can provide immediate consultation and greater intellectual stimulation. The two general categories of group practices are *single specialty* and *multispecialty*. A group that consists of only pediatricians is referred to as a single specialty whereas a multispecialty group may consist of pediatricians, internists, gynecologists, surgeons, and others. The multispecialty group has the advantage of referrals from within the group. The more inclusive the group, the better it is positioned to contract with insurance companies seeking preferred provider relationships and outlets for prepaid medical care. As the medical "industry" becomes increasingly organized, group practice formats will continue to expand at the expense of solo practice.

PRACTICE LOCATIONS AND FACILITIES

Although not immediately obvious to the pediatrician entering practice, the office site and location often have a major impact on the practice style and satisfaction. Office settings are so varied that any imaginable situation can be included. Doctors who practiced out of their home with kitchen table bookkeeping systems and a living room that served for examinations and treatments are nostalgically remembered. Today, pediatricians who desire a strong personal identity with their office will likely locate in a general purpose office building near their patients or the hospital where they admit their patients. Professional office buildings are frequently built in commercial districts or adjacent to hospitals. Initially most physicians rent space but once their practice is well established, the physician or group commonly purchase their office space. Free-standing space can be developed and often includes parking for parents and a separate entrance for sick-child visits. Facilities without laboratory or radiology capability are best suited for the solo practitioner or smaller group practice. If a physician group expands to more than three or four full-time doctors, the facility will likely develop to include ancillary services. Radiology and laboratory services may also be adjacent facilities operated by other independent practitioners.

Ambulatory Care Facility

The term *ambulatory care facility* has become increasingly common as the complexity of office-based activities has increased. The group practice format lends itself to much more extensive facilities than the relatively simple solo practitioner's office. Ambulatory care facilities will often include radiology, laboratory, and physician-related functions such as a pharmacy or optometry and even ambulatory surgery and obstetrical units. The community health centers that were developed in the 1960s as part of the model cities' programs have been the nidus for development of these more comprehensive ambulatory care centers. The notion of comprehensive health care services within a single setting has gained considerable acceptance by consumers and health care providers. Pediatricians who enter a practice today may be as attracted to this style of practice facility as to its financial stability. Whereas an ambulatory care facility may be free standing and independent, some are integrated into or affiliated with a hospital (hospital-based) or other type of health care facility, for example a municipal or county public health department.

Thus, a decision to enter office practice must be viewed within a broad context. The pediatrician should assess the physical surroundings where his practice will be located, the type of patients attracted to a facility, and the opportunities for collaborative work with other health care professionals.

FINANCIAL ARRANGEMENTS

Physicians entering practice will find the opportunities for financial arrangements as varied as practice types and facilities. Remuneration (direct and fringe benefits) should be considered an integral factor and these benefits will be determined largely by the delivery mode and the marketplace factors. Patient payment mechanisms (cash at the time of service, credit cards, prepayment systems, and so forth) are basic to the nature of the practice. Most families also have several options for their medical insurance coverage that will need to be understood by the practicing pediatrician.

Indemnity Insurance

Typically, *traditional indemnity insurance* provides parents with protection against the high cost of inpatient or catastrophic medical care but assumes that primary care visits will be paid by the parents without reimbursement from the insurance company. This arrangement fits well with the professional role of the physician as a private practitioner with a fee-for-service relationship with his patients. Most pediatricians have felt most comfortable with this system until recently.

Alternative Delivery Systems

An *alternative delivery system (ADS)* provides insurance through the delivery of services for prenegotiated rates. The system may provide medical care with or without a co-payment by the patient's family. The key difference from traditional insurance is that ADSs combine the delivery of medical care with an insurance function and a financing arrangement. They may preserve fee-for-service reimbursement to the physician but not without utilization review to monitor and thereby ultimately control medical care costs. These plans typically cover preventive care and discourage the use of more expensive hospital-based and acute care services. One major but unsubstantiated criticism of ADSs is that, in accomplishing one of their major goals (reducing costs), the quality of medical care may suffer. In the traditional fee-for-service system, there is a tendency to err on the side of overutilization of laboratory tests and subspecialty care because the reimbursement mechanism supports this approach. ADSs, on the other hand, emphasize controlling these services and may result in underutilization of needed medical care. Nevertheless, alternative health care delivery and reimbursement systems have now become part of the American mainstream. The word "alternative" is no longer appropriate because almost 10% of all insured patients choose such an option. It is projected that more than one third of all patients will participate in an ADS by the 1990s.

Health Maintenance Organization

The best known of the various alternative delivery systems is the *health maintenance organization* (HMO). An HMO is an organized group of physician and hospital care facilities that contracts to provide comprehensive health care services for a fixed prenegotiated *per capita* payment (capitation) to a defined population of voluntarily enrolled members. HMO pediatricians provide primary care services to children. They attempt to be efficient by controlling referrals and restricting outside utilization. HMOs function as umbrella organizations mediating financial arrangements for different types of physician practices. The parent HMO corporation receives a premium or capitated payment, but may contract (straight salary, capitation agreement, or fee-for-service payments) with physicians. There are four principle types of HMOs, which consist of the *staff model*, the *group model*, the *independent practice association*, and the *network independent practice association*.

Staff Model. In the *staff model*, physicians are employees of the HMO and receive a salary. Some portion of earnings may be linked to productivity, which is defined, for example, by the number of patients served. Salary scales, however, are usually related to years of experience and specialty training. Physicians typically see their patients in an ambulatory care facility using a group practice format.

Group Model. Group model HMOs differ from the staff model in that the physicians are a separate group, often a separate corporate entity, that contracts with the HMO to provide medical services. Although the practice settings are similar to the staff model HMO, issues related to physician's earnings are determined by the group practice. Legally, the physicians form a corporation that may or may not have an exclusive arrangement with the HMO.

Independent Practice Association. An *independent practice association* (IPA) refers to an arrangement whereby physicians participate in an HMO using their own private offices. This model also preserves fee-for-service–type reimbursement. The IPA reimburses physicians according to a predetermined formula. After the physician renders services, he bills the plan, not the patient's

family. The IPA may enlist a large number of physicians who do not actually practice together.

Network Independent Practice Association. In a *network IPA*, the HMO contracts with groups of physicians allowing them to develop their own scheme for reimbursement. IPAs are attractive to pediatricians with established practices because they provide a means to serve families who want prepaid medical care with minimal disruption to their style or location of practice.

Preferred Provider Organization

A *preferred provider organization* (PPO) is still another alternative available to help patients budget their health care costs. The character of a PPO is influenced by the organization's sponsor. If, for example, the plan is organized and funded by a large employer who owns a hospital or clinic, the employee's family may be given strong financial incentives to use those facilities. Entrepreneurs who market insurance programs to unions and self-insured employers, insurance companies, hospitals, and physicians have all established PPOs. PPOs share an economic incentive for having patients utilize the preferred providers. Patients maintain a limited freedom of choice in selecting their child's doctor. Payments made by the PPO to the preferred-provider physicians are on a fee-for-service basis, but at a rate generally lower than the customary fee. A strong program of utilization review to control overall PPO expenses is critical to the success of this system. PPOs establish criteria to determine the eligibility of the practicing physician to join the program. These criteria may include prudent practice patterns or staff privileges at a "preferred" (lower cost) hospital. This approach to health care will gain acceptance by physicians and hospitals who are willing to discount their services in order to attract new patients.

As described above, demands for cost controls have affected the traditional fee-for-service physician–patient relationship. Increases in the number of practicing physicians and lower birth rates resulting in fewer children per doctor have also resulted in more competition for patients. Prepaid comprehensive medical care systems have become attractive options because they limit the family's total expenditures for health care and encourage earlier utilization. Under traditional insurance coverage families with limited budgets have often delayed important routine visits to limit out-of-pocket expenses. Since many state Medicaid programs have developed fee schedules so far below the actual costs of office operation, physicians cannot afford to serve these children on a fee-for-service basis. For these reasons, younger physicians entering practice are more receptive to the various alternative delivery systems. They are generally willing to modify the traditional fee-for-service physician–patient relationship. Salaried positions in organized systems of care and larger multispecialty groups are becoming the norm for physicians, especially pediatricians.

Societal concern for the cost of health care has caused major changes in reimbursement mechanisms. Pediatric practice in the future will reflect these changes. The 1980s will be remembered as the decade when a revolution occurred in medical care financing and, therefore, health care delivery. Medical care has become a part of big business. Physicians are likely to become employees in large organized systems of care. The challenge for pediatricians will be to assure high-quality medical care in a setting that preserves the time-honored and respected physician–patient relationship, but at a cost that society is willing to pay.

TEACHING AND RESEARCH

Participation in the educational and academic programs of a medical school or teaching hospital may be essential to a pediatrician's personal satisfaction in an office-based practice. Many find the role of teacher to physicians-in-training enjoyable and will look for practice opportunities that include supervision of medical students or residents in their office. Some practicing pediatricians will join the voluntary faculty of a nearby medical school. Others will want more intensive involvement and will choose to work as a part-time salaried practicing clinician on an academic faculty. Many academic medical centers have established ambulatory programs that combine clinical practice with teaching and clinical research for full-time faculty members.

Research in the ambulatory setting can also be exciting for the general pediatrician. Clinical problems can be studied in collaboration with those working in the laboratory. Protocols can be developed to appeal to various funding agencies with no

increased cost of medical care to the patient. Epidemiological problems also lend themselves to study in the office setting. Health services research on issues relating to organization and finance are often the result of office-based physicians working with experts in the social sciences. Most pediatricians, however, will not choose a practice setting based on research opportunities.

ANNOTATED BIBLIOGRAPHY

Freund DA, Allen KS: Factors affecting physicians' choice to practice in a fee-for-service setting versus an individual practice association. Med Care 23:799, 1985 (IPAs must be able to recruit physicians from the community to be successful in the future. Physicians with lower incomes and fewer physician visits and those who are newly established in the community are more likely to join.)

Gerber PG: Fee-for-service: Is it really dying? Physician's Management 25:232, 1985 (More than 15 million people around the country belong to over 320 HMOs. Physicians are concerned about being paid a reasonable amount for their services; it will not be important to them whether they are paid as contractors with a hospital or directly as fee-for-service private entrepreneurs.)

Malach M: Medicine in the 1980s: Cognitive vs procedural. Physician's Management 25:101, 1985 (Need to recognize the importance of visits to the physician that do not result in a procedure. By improving the reimbursements to physicians who are more likely to treat the patient in this manner, the overall costs of medical care can be better controlled.)

Martin JT: What you should have in your group contract. Physician's Management 24:290, 1984 (Fairness to the established group should be the overriding factor for each individual physician who enters into a group contract. This article gives tips on how a physician can protect his interests.)

Miller LJ: Forms of Medical Practice. Chicago, IL, AMA, 1983 (Defines the various forms of medical practice from a legal point of view. Discusses the advantages and disadvantages of these forms of practice.)

Starr P: The Social Transformation of American Medicine. New York, Basic Books, 1982 (A social history of medicine that describes the development of the American system with particular attention given to the relationship of physicians, the State, and the growth of corporations.)

2
Planning an Office
MARTIN I. HOROWITZ

When a pediatrician considers establishing an office, it is assumed that prior to this decision, long-range considerations were made, including personal goals and the strategies and the systems needed to attain them. It would be imprudent to select an office site without forethought and research, because without this planning, the chosen facility would dictate to a large degree the style of the practice rather than *vice versa*.

Many factors enter into the decision of where to locate an office. The usual central issues focus on desirability and compatibility. Is an attractive residential community important? What kind of schools are available (an important consideration for the pediatrician with a family)? Is your philosophy similar to that of the community's? What are the community's prejudices, if any? Are there existing organizations? What are the recreational, cultural, and other nonmedical opportunities in the area? There are, however, several disadvantages to living in the same community as the practice, such as intrusions on privacy, restrictions on involvement in local political activity for fear of offending a segment of the practice, and family members' feelings that they are living in a "fishbowl." These disadvantages (or advantages) often vary depending on whether the community selected is urban, suburban, or rural.

A good way to evaluate the potential of the community for establishing a practice is to examine the demographics of the population, such as wealth, growth, birth rate, and age distribution (a vital consideration for a new pediatrician). It is, at best, risky to establish a pediatric practice in an area with an aging and declining population. United States census data from the local Chamber of Commerce are usually readily available. Personal surveys may also be helpful.

The best way to learn first-hand about a community is to visit and talk to several people including pediatricians with established practices. One must evaluate whether a "potential competitor" is being open and honest or is trying to discourage the start of another pediatric practice in the community. One approach is to speak with other medical colleagues, especially the obstetricians whose new-born referrals would be critical, and the staff at the hospital where you would practice. Discussions with the clergy of one's faith and realtors for both professional and personal opportunities are recommended to further assess the community.

After choosing the appropriate community, the next step is to find the site for the practice. The cost and location are prime considerations. The location should ideally be as near to a hospital as possible, and easily accessible to patients. Pediatricians with a practice near a hospital have an improved quality of life because their rounds, practice, and emergency care can be more efficiently regulated. This convenience minimizes office disruption and allows the pediatrician to monitor more seriously ill children with greater ease, even allowing multiple visits to the hospital each day.

When planning an office, visit other practices to study their layouts. Permission could be sought to take photographs, although some physicians may object due to competition in business. The competition factor should not be underestimated, because the pediatrician is faced with an increasing number of well-trained colleagues and organized health care delivery systems, all seeking relatively fewer patients.

The nature and style of one's practice largely determine the office design, particularly as it relates to the need for special facility requirements. For example, an allergy testing area would be needed if this were to be a significant part of one's practice. Will other ancillary services, for example, roentgenograms or electrocardiograms (ECG) be performed? Will the office have a laboratory and, if so, which tests (*e.g.*, hematology, bacteriology, or urinalyses) will be performed? Special planning must also be given to areas for visual and hearing screening, an integral part of well-child care. The type of testing may be determined by office space. For example, a Titmus vision screen requires only a small area as opposed to a 20-ft lane for Snellen eye chart testing.

One must also think of the employees one will hire and whether they might have specific facility requirements as in the case of x-ray or laboratory technicians. Another important consideration is to plan for growth. Might partners be added at a later date and how might their needs be incorporated in the design of "expandability" of the facility to save future expense, rather than remodeling or relocation? The biggest error that can occur in designing an office is to fail to plan for practice growth and ample file space. Present and future computer needs should also be considered.

Space requirement recommendations for a pediatric office vary from 1000 sq ft to 1200 sq ft per doctor. Additionally, it is recommended that parking for six to ten cars be available per doctor. In planning the outside of one's office, landscaping should be attractive with an open space design at least one half the total inner space plus the parking area. Future expansion will require at least one half of the aforementioned total space.

When planning the layout of any medical office, it is important not to underestimate the required size of the business area, hallways, and storage areas. Many medical supply houses offer the services of office designers or architects at nominal or no fee to advise the new physician. In return, it is expected that the office furniture and equipment be bought from the supply house. These designers can be extremely helpful; however, one must know what budget, style, and system of practice one will have so that overly expensive or unnecessary purchases will be avoided.

The ideal internal space of an office is functional, free flowing, yet tightly controlled, and is a balance between public (*i.e.*, patient) and medical space. The waiting room requires about three to four chairs per doctor in a general office. This conforms well to a suggested space need for two children and two adults for each pediatric patient scheduled, since almost all these youngsters are accompanied by one or several family members or even friends. The waiting room should be about 40 sq ft plus 10 sq ft for each individual (adults and children included) using a room; this does not include a children's play area. The adult chairs in the waiting room should allow an adult to sit comfortably and be able to hold an infant in her arms. Current magazines and books relating to family, child rearing, and other contemporary issues should be available in the waiting area. In addition, a bulletin board with *timely* articles, pictures, or patient artwork is an interesting and personal touch.

Although one study concluded that there is not an increased crossover of illness to well children when sick children share the same waiting area, many pediatricians and parents still believe that a second waiting room for ill children is desirable. Most parents are pleased by such an arrangement; thus, if space is available, separate waiting rooms and examining rooms for sick and well children should be considered.

In a pediatric office a special children's play area is essential. It should be furnished with solid, sturdy chairs that can be stood upon and not easily tipped over, and it should have durable and attractive toys. It is important that all toys be easy to thoroughly clean and store. A small table in this children's area for play, with perhaps blackboards and maps, will make a child's waiting time seem much faster.

An area where employees may take a break or eat their lunch is a worthwhile office amenity. This area need not be large and would also allow the entire staff to meet to discuss office problems or issues. Moreover, this room can provide additional storage space. One can furnish this area with enough chairs for everyone to be comfortable (or have stackable chairs available) as well as a coffee pot or other amenities that one can afford to give the staff. In addition, staff and patient restrooms are required. A special area may be needed if smoking is permitted. Areas for drinking water and a public telephone should be considered.

The business aspects of the practice should be contained in the receptionist/bookkeeping area. A practical guideline is for the receptionist's area to have twice the square footage as the number of patients at the busiest hour. It is suggested that in a solo practice, the combined waiting room/receptionist area be between 150 sq ft and 200 sq ft. Space requirements in a group practice are dependent on the number of people required to do bookkeeping, telephone, reception, and computer chores. In some large offices, the billing area is placed away from the reception area. The advantages of this arrangement are noise control and privacy in discussing a patient's financial status. The receptionist/bookkeeping area should have enough space for at least two desks and file space for both the medical and financial records. Security and privacy considerations should be kept in mind while designing this space. One might wish this area to have two exits for these purposes. The extensive use of safety glass is encouraged so that the staff may see the entire waiting area.

It is suggested that the most efficient office requires three examining rooms per physician. The most commonly recommended size for these rooms is about 8 ft by 10 ft if they are used exclusively for examination purposes. If the physician's office is combined with an examination room, then the room should be at least 9 ft by 13 ft. However, for many reasons including the need for privacy and contemplation, combination rooms should be avoided wherever possible. Each examining room should be able to comfortably accommodate three adults and two children including the patient's clothing, since it is not uncommon to have an entire family come in while a youngster is being examined. The placement of chairs in an area to keep the adults out of the way of the examiner is important.

If there is not a combination room, each physician must have a consultation room. This room should be about 100 sq ft and should contain a desk, two or three chairs, bookcases, and a telephone. The consultation room's decor should be tasteful and appropriate. Adequate filing space is an important consideration.

All examining rooms should contain a sink and a table large enough to hold a large adolescent. Although some pediatricians set aside a special examining room for the adolescent patients, this may not always be possible. If a separate room is available, an adult-sized table which folds and on which pelvic examinations may be performed offers most flexibility. Equipment and supplies in an adolescent room are generally similar to other examining rooms, but should also include appropriate lighting, screens for privacy, and supplies necessary for gynecological examinations. Many pediatricians decorate this room in a manner appropriate for the adolescent.

An infant scale and adult scale should be placed in the other examining rooms, although the third room may not be as well-equipped and used only for brief visits. All rooms should contain equipment for complete examinations including otoscope, ophthalmoscope, sphygmomanometer, hammer, syringes, bandages, rubber gloves, water-soluble gel, and immunization materials. They should also have tissues, paper goods such as gowns, table paper, cups, and simple first aid equipment such as splints and bandages. It is essential that the supplies in these rooms be checked daily.

In some offices, an additional room may be set aside for special procedures such as suturing, blood drawing, minor surgical procedures, débridement, and perhaps even lumbar punctures. This room might be equipped with an overhead operating light or at least a spotlight and surgical equipment including suture kits. Bandages and casting material can be kept here as well. The table in this room may be an operating type, so that a child can be

positioned in various ways depending on the procedure. The cost of such a table, however, may be prohibitively expensive.

Each examining room should be laid out identically so that the clinician knows where all the equipment is kept. One of the most commonly seen layouts is the mirror-image room that is constructed because common walls hold common utilities. Although it may decrease expense, this arrangement may prove confusing.

A laboratory and a nurse's station may be desirable in a busy practice. Many offices efficiently combine the nurse's station and laboratory into one area. The laboratory itself should be approximately 8 ft by 4 ft and include a refrigerator, incubator, small sink, microscope, autoclave, and a centrifuge. Space for supplies to keep the laboratory well-stocked must be provided.

The base price of running each laboratory test should be considered as well as the fixed overhead costs in the utilization of the allotted space. The established charge must also be based on reasonable charges for the same or similar tests in the community.

Quality assurance is an important issue in running a laboratory even in a small practice. Duplicate unknowns can be sent to other laboratories or commercially prepared standards may be used. Many states have regulations and even license requirements for operating a laboratory (Table 2-1).

Laboratory tests other than those listed in Table 2-1 are often ordered by a pediatrician. However, for reasons of quality and volume, it is more convenient to either send a patient or a specimen to an outside laboratory.

The nurse's station should have a 5-ft counter wall or base cabinets. The nurse may give allergy injections or immunizations and also answer the phone in this area. It is important that adequate space is provided for writing in patients' records.

As previously mentioned, it is useful to consult an architect or office designer after assessing one's space needs. It is best to find one who is familiar with the unique needs of a pediatric office for advice on total layout so that the patient flow is kept efficient and that security and safety needs are assured. Other areas where professional assistance may be useful is in regard to soundproofing, lighting, and telecommunications, which also includes interoffice communications. Lighting is critical and most recommend 100-ft candles of light at table height. Lighting also plays a large role in office decor and must not be addressed casually. Attention to windows for privacy as well as soundproof-

Table 2-1. Commonly Performed Office Laboratory Tests

TEST	SUPPLIES NEEDED	COMMENTS
Blood glucose determination	B-G Chem Strips or Dextrostix	Rapid, easy to teach procedure to staff
Cultures		
Throat	Sheep's blood agar plates; sterile swabs; bacitracin disks	Need incubator; skilled reader; takes 24 to 48 hours
Urine	Commercial kit	Takes 24 to 48 hours; many kits, e.g., Abbott's UTI–Tect, give specific organism; positive screening tests may be sent to outside laboratory for identification and sensitivities.
Gram stain	Dyes; alcohol; flame for fixing specimen; slides	Skill needed to read and stain properly
Hemogram	Wright's stain; slides, cover slips; immersion oil; white cell chamber; pipettes	Skilled reader; white cell counter; Coulter counter may be too expensive for small volume to justify; platelet estimated and red cells evaluated from Wright stain
Hematocrit	Heparinized capillary tubes; centrifuge; hematocrit gauge	Rapid
Hemoglobin	Dilution sticks or fluid; hemoglobinometer	
KOH preparation	Slides; cover slips; KOH	Skill needed to interpret
Mono spot	Commercial kit	Convenient for patient and physician
Pregnancy	Commercial kit	Too expensive if done infrequently
Rapid strep	Commercial kit	Advantage in a pediatric office, but, unless tests are batched, each requires at least 10 minutes of technician time.
Stool guaiac	Commercially available cards	Easy to do; helpful; inexpensive
Urinalysis	Slides, cover slips; centrifuge, dip sticks	Rapid; easy to teach procedure to staff

ing is especially important in dealing with adolescents.

Planning telecommunications should include the placement of instruments and the number of incoming and private outgoing lines. For efficiency, many authorities recommend a telephone in each examining room. The system should be equipped with a private intercommunication system so that the doctor may be quickly interrupted for emergencies; however, the use of this system for routine problems should be avoided.

A safe milieu is necessary in any office, especially in a pediatric one. Indeed, the entire office should be a model for good safety practices.

With regard to decor and ambience, the pediatrician's office must be easy to clean, well-decorated, and bright. The colors and designs should evoke a feeling of warmth and friendliness. The decorator should consider how the practical requirements can be blended into the general decor in order to enhance the effect desired. The office must be a pleasant environment for the pediatrician who often spends more of his waking hours in his office than anywhere else, and also for his patients and staff.

ANNOTATED BIBLIOGRAPHY

Bank of America National Trust & Savings Association: Establishing a Medical Practice. San Francisco, Bank of America, 1970 (Good rundown of essentials of practice start-up advice, though not specific to pediatric practice.)

Beck LC: The Physician's Office. Amsterdam, Excerptica Medica, 1977 (Descriptive book of layout and design.)

Farber L (ed): Medical Economics Encyclopedia of Practice and Financial Management. Oradell, NJ, Medical Economics Books, 1985 (Exhaustive text on all aspects of the management of a medical practice from an economic point of view.)

Lobovits AM, Freeman, J, Goldman, D, McIntosh FIN: Risk of Illness After Exposure to a Pediatric Office. N Engl J Med 313 (7), 1985 (Study of the risk of cross-infection in a pediatric office.)

McCormick J, Rusting RL, Davis WG: The Management of Medical Practice. Cambridge, MA, Ballinger Publishing Co, 1978 (Advice on start-up style.)

Saltzman EJ, Shea DW: Management of Pediatric Practice. Elk Grove, IL, American Academy of Pediatrics, 1986 (Essential for the pediatrician in private practice whether new or experienced.)

3

Ancillary Personnel

MARTIN I. HOROWITZ

Hiring is one of the most important decisions a new pediatrician makes when opening an office. How many employees does one need to run an efficient practice and how can the physician evaluate his needs? What special skills are needed? When should employees be phased into an expanding practice? How does one go about finding well-qualified people who would interact well in the office setting?

The importance of having the right kind of ancillary staff in any office cannot be overemphasized. For example, the receptionist is usually the patient's or parent's first exposure with your office and the climate created in this initial contact will affect how the physician–patient relationship develops. Ideally, the physician should only employ as many assistants as it takes to enable that he do virtually nothing in the office except practice medicine, and do that as efficiently as possible. Trained office personnel are important to assure maximum office harmony and efficiency. Staffing ratios have not been defined, and they depend mainly on variables such as style of practice, patient volume, and time in the office. Twenty percent of pediatric offices have one medical assistant, 27% have two, 12% have three, and 20% have four or more medical assistants. It would seem wise, therefore, to start with one or two assistants and periodically evaluate one's needs. The need for receptionists, bookkeepers, and other kinds of staff will reflect personal needs and practice requirements. Changes in one's style of practice or the addition of clinicians to the group will change the staffing requirements.

The delegation of certain office tasks must be weighed against greater contact between patient and physician. However, additional staff may increase productivity. Physicians with three office assistants see one and one half times as many patients as physicians with only one assistant. This must be balanced by the fact that overstaffing is not only inefficient but can lead to inadequate training.

The ancillary personnel that a pediatrician may consider hiring are administrator(s), registered or licensed practical nurse(s), physician assistant(s) or nurse practitioner(s), laboratory or x-ray technician(s), and secretarial (clerical) employees.

Before hiring ancillary personnel, it is prudent to have carefully written job descriptions for the positions one wishes to fill. All personnel policies should be carefully detailed. The offered salary should be competitive with a merit plan integrated with regular cost of living adjustments. Fringe benefits should also be competitive.

There are many ways to find excellent staff. Usual sources include private employment agencies, other medical offices, advertisements, and appropriate vocational and technical schools and colleges. Recommendations from present staff or from families of patients already in the practice may be helpful. Written advertisements or postings should be as explicit as possible.

Options for screening applicants are varied, including an agency or a trusted employee such as the office manager. The physician must interview the applicants if he is just beginning to create a staff. Some applicants can be eliminated by questioning the candidates about their availability, salary requirements, typing skills, and background (*e.g.*, if they have worked in a medical office before). Ascertain the academic credentials and experience of the applicant. If the initial screening is favorable, consider if the candidate should be tested for typing or other skills needed for the job. This is usually done in the pediatrician's office.

The interviewing process must be carefully arranged. The same person should interview all the candidates who have passed the initial screening. In addition, the candidates should be asked to provide a list of personal references, including previous employers.

The interviewer should ask open-ended questions such as: Why would you like to work in a pediatrician's office? How did you acquire your skills? In which jobs did you use them? How do you react when you must occasionally stay late at work? How do you feel about pressing people to pay the medical bill? Have you handled money for anyone before? Are you willing to be bonded? Would you like to ask me anything? The health of the applicant is important, although it is illegal to ask about health status specifically if it is unrelated to the qualifications for the position.

These questions are intended to provide an overall insight about the person. The personal interview can also create impressions about the candidate's appearance, personality, alertness, poise, ability to express ideas, sensitivity, voice, and diction. If any problems are uncovered, these should be discussed openly. The applicant's work history should be reviewed; it is important that it be stable, since few offices have the luxury of on-the-job training.

An important aspect of hiring personnel is checking references. It is prudent to speak directly with the applicant's references, usually by telephone. The most important question to ask is, "Would you hire this applicant again?" It is not necessary to ask specifically if one may speak personally with these references since they were originally supplied by the candidate.

After this careful screening process, the top candidates should be asked to return for a second interview. If the applicant had initially been screened by someone else, the physician should personally interview these top candidates and choose (with staff input) the person who will be offered the position.

Sensitivity should be shown to those not selected. A fair explanation should be given and mention should be made that they will be considered for future openings. Frequently, one may wish to employ one of these applicants in the future.

After hiring a new employee it is important to orient him to the job and its responsibilities. The job description and an office manual can make the orientation process easier. Larger offices usually offer more formal training programs. Subjects include communications, patient flow, human relations, and medical records. The idiosyncrasies of a pediatrician's office and its systems should be taught. Phone training and the office systems training are important aspects of this program, even in the small office. The standards of excellence expected of the office personnel should be emphasized: this includes spelling, giving precise phone information, and making appointments.

The first employee usually hired is the receptionist, who at first may also function as a secretary, bookkeeper, and even as a limited medical assistant. It is important that he be punctual, neat, and reliable, and that his telephone voice be pleasant, reassuring, and intelligible. One may actually test an applicant for this position by having him use the phone with the interviewer on the other end.

When one's practice enlarges (or even at the beginning) a clinical assistant should be hired, if financial circumstances allow. This person usually places patients in the examining room, obtains a basic history that includes the reason for the visit, takes the vital signs, does hearing and visual screening, and may also give injections as directed by the physician. The assistant also prepares the room and the patient appropriately. Because these tasks increase the efficiency of the pediatrician's practice, he can see more patients in a given time.

Clinical assistants should be trained to give telephone advice on commonly occurring pediatric illnesses such as vomiting, diarrhea, fever control, and respiratory infections. They should also be able to perform tuberculosis screening and common laboratory tests such as hematocrits and urinalyses. They should also be able to make appointments, accept money, give receipts, telephone prescriptions to a pharmacy and keep a record of them, file, do secretarial work, and even remind the pediatrician of his appointments or commitments. This ability to perform several common office functions keeps the staff flexible and allows for both clinician and ancillary staff absences without total disruption of the normal office routine.

A pediatric office may run quite efficiently with only a receptionist and a clinical assistant. As the practice grows one may wish to run a larger laboratory service, and a laboratory technician may become necessary, at least on a part-time basis. If the billing or numerous third party forms become voluminous, the addition of a bookkeeper to handle this aspect of the practice should be considered.

At some point the question, "When should I hire a registered or practical nurse versus a midlevel practitioner (*i.e.*, a physician's assistant or nurse practitioner)?" is likely to be raised. The answer is based on personal and fiscal considerations. The RN/LPN can augment the clinical assistant's role by developing a more extensive telephone triage system and by performing procedures (*e.g.*, giving allergy shots that require minimal supervision from the physician). One can also use this individual to act as an office manager in the supervision of the other staff and in the distribution of office work. The distinction between the RN and the LPN is one of degree of education and often "bedside" experience, thus the selection may again be based on personal preference and the applicant selection pool.

On the other hand, in an area where it may be difficult to attract an additional physician or to increase practice volume (*i.e.*, the work is more than one pediatrician can handle, but not enough for two), a nurse practitioner or physician's assistant may be ideal. If one wishes to distinguish the qualifications of these two mid-level clinicians, it would be worthwhile to consult with the appropriate boards in your state and nearby academic institutions who train such clinicians.

A mid-level clinician can perform routine well-child care and treat most illnesses. He usually sees fewer patients in a given time period than the pediatrician. This usually allows the mid-level clinician to do more health education or be involved with health issues such as sex education, discipline, or even in the long-term management of certain chronic illnesses such as diabetes mellitus.

After the training period, a period of probation not exceeding 6 months should follow. The employee should be aware of this probation period. At its conclusion the physician or his designee (usually the office manager or senior mid-level clinician) should conduct a formal review. The review process should be appropriate for the level of the position (*e.g.*, a clinical review for the mid-level provider and a task-oriented review for other members of the staff). The new employee should be gradually delegated increasing responsibility during the probation period and review process.

The ability to run a successful office and to be fair to one's staff depends on regular staff evaluation. In order to do this properly one must keep a personnel folder on each employee. The folder should include notes and the written review of the employee signed by the physician and employee. Support and encouragement are important ingredients in keeping a happy, efficient staff.

Skilled ancillary personnel operate the office, maximize the pediatrician's patient contact by making the best use of his time, and serve as both facilitators and ombudsmen for the patients. Patients perceive this as personalized service and they feel both comfortable and welcome in the office.

ANNOTATED BIBLIOGRAPHY

American Academy of General Practice, Committee on Medical Economics: Organization and Management of Family Practice: An Advisory Manual for the Family Physician in Private Practice. Kansas City, MO, Brookside, 1968 (General guide but not very specific.)

Bass LW, Wolfson JH: The Style and Management of a Pediatric Practice. Pittsburgh, University of Pittsburgh Press, 1977 (Helpful guide for training ancillary personnel to fit the practice style of the clinician.)

Farber L (ed): Medical Economics Encyclopedia of Practice and Financial Management. Oradell, NJ, Medical Economics Books, 1985 (Exhaustive resource for all aspects of medical practice.)

Mattera MD (ed): How to Hire, Train, and Manage Your Employees. Oradell, NJ, Medical Economics Books, 1982 (Good reference for all practitioners, although not specific to pediatric practice.)

McCormick J, Rusting RL, Davis WG: The Management of Medical Practice. Cambridge, MA, Ballinger Publishing Co, 1978 (Assistance on style and philosophy, especially about interviewing and reviewing personnel.)

McCue J: Private Practice: Surviving the First Year. Lexington, MA, Collamore Press, 1982 (Interesting reading, though not specific for the pediatrician.)

Pressman RM, Siegler R: The Independent Practitioner—Practice Management for the Allied Health Professional. Homewood, IL, Dow Jones–Irwin, 1983 (Useful guide for the pediatrician integrating mid-level practitioners into the practice.)

Wingate MB et al (eds): Management for Physicians. New Hyde Park, NY, Medical Examination Publishers, 1983 (General reference book but not specific to pediatrics.)

4
Medical Records
EDWARD S. GROSS

Accurate and efficient records are essential for the provision of health care, especially in a primary care or office setting. A patient file or record contains several different kinds of information, with most of it changing over time, but at differing rates of change. For example, medications for the treatment of minor acute illnesses may change rapidly while a patient's name is less likely to do so. The following listing is one possible outline of areas into which a patient record may be divided. A practical recording system must be able to absorb information in these areas and provide ready access to the information as it changes.

HEALTH HISTORY: including birth, prior illnesses, and prior care provided elsewhere as well as areas of continuing care for illness, preventive care, and immunizations

FAMILY HISTORY: including illness in family members and exposures, subject to continuing updates. *Genetic history* is usually contained in this section; this must be updated as problems of potential concern are discovered in family members

HEALTH CARE PROVIDED: including well care, management of problems, medications prescribed or renewed, counseling, anticipatory guidance, recommendations, and referrals. Care received elsewhere concurrently, including the responses from consultants and the results of tests performed, should also be included

GROWTH AND DEVELOPMENT: measurements of growth and their relationship to previous measurements and to the population in general (percentiles); achievement of developmental milestones

HEALTH CARE ANTICIPATED: including recommended well care and follow up, unanswered questions, and related plans for investigation or referral

SOCIAL AND ENVIRONMENTAL: including family constellation, living arrangements, sources of support, and school and work information with special reference to hazards

FISCAL: including insurance coverage, guarantors, charges incurred, and payments made

PREPAID CARE PROGRAM FEATURES: including membership or coverage status, special limitations or other features of coverage, referrals made, care authorized elsewhere, utilization information according to program needs.

CHOOSING A RECORD SYSTEM

At its best, a patient record permits the physician to "model" or understand the patient in the context of his or her health and illness-related needs: What problems does the patient have? How much is known about these problems? What plans for further investigation or treatment have been made? What home, school, or job-related factors might affect the plans or other aspects of the patient's health? What screening or other health maintenance activities are due or overdue? The ideal record permits efficient focusing of relevant information for reliable and prompt responses to new situations without loss of past knowledge or of current needs (*e.g.*, incomplete immunizations or abnormal blood pressure). Although the solo practitioner can sometimes rely on memory to note important needs in a small patient population, he cannot do this in a large practice. Moreover, public health agencies, schools, and hospitals (the larger societal context of health care) cannot afford to lose or loosely store key health information.

Several systems have been designed to capture, store, and permit access to these data. There is a wide variability in the amount of organizing effort demanded of those who record entries in the system, the difficulty of reading the chart, the requirements for forms and storage, and the cost. In larger groups, portability, durability, and legibility become more important considerations. Over the past several years, considerable effort has been made to try to use computers to accomplish many, if not all, of these tasks.

TYPES OF RECORDING SYSTEMS

File Folder Systems

File folder systems are the most loosely structured arrangements, but they can be sufficient for a generally healthy patient group in a small office.

	1 mo	2 mo	3 mo	4½ mo	6 mo	8 mo	10 mo	1 yr	15 mo	18 mo	21 mo	2 yr	2½ yr	3 yr	4 yr	5 yr	6 yr
HISTORY — AGE																	
DATE																	
HEIGHT																	
WEIGHT																	
HEAD CIRC.																	
HEALTH																	
EATING																	
SLEEPING																	
ELIMINATION																	
BEHAVIOR/HABITS																	
MAT-CHILD REL																	
TOILET TRNG.										Start		Bow aim complete	Bladder during day	Total control			
DEVEL. & MARKS — GROSS MOTOR	Prone lifts head		Head to 90°	Rolls over	No head lag	Sits W/O support	Pulls to stand	Cruises	Walks/stoops		Walks upstairs	Kicks ball	Throws Overhand	Jumps in place		Hops one foot	Copy ☐
FINE MOTOR ADAPTIVE	Symm. movements			Grasps rattle	Reaches	Transfers	Pincer grasp	Bangs blocks	Drink from cup	Piles 2 blocks	Scribbles	Piles 4 blocks		Imitates vertical line	Copies + and 0		
LANGUAGE	Responds to bell	Coos		Squeals		Turns to voice	Dada/Mama	Imitates sounds	Dada/Mama specific		3-10 words	Knows 1 body part	2-3 word sentence	Plurals	1st & last names	Knows 3 colors	
PERSONAL SOCIAL	Regards face	Smiles responsively	Laughs		Smiles spon	Feeds self cracker	Peek-a-boo	Pat-a-cake, waves bye-bye	Indicates wants	Mimics chores	Feeds with spoon	Simple tasks		Washes/dries hands	Dresses with help	Dresses W/O help	
GUIDANCE — DIET	Fluoride 5 gtt/d	Cereal/fruit	Vegs	Meats	Yolk	Jr. foods								Fluoride tabs 1mg'd			
HEARING																Audio meter	
VISION	M-L		Follow past M-L	Follows 180°		Looks after objects		Cover test	Cover test						Snellen		
ACCIDENT PREV.	Falls-car	ASA		Playpen, toys		Stairs, sunburn	Poisons	Burns			Pica		Pets				
FEEDING TECH.	Demand/schedule			Schedule family				Wean	Finger foods	Spoon							

AGE	1 mo.	2 mo.	3 mo.	4½ mo.	6 mo.	8 mo.	10 mo.	1 yr.	15 mo.	18 mo.	21 mo.	2 yr.	2½ yr.	3 yr.	4 yr.	5 yr.	6 yr.
GUIDANCE																	
STIMULATION	Mobile	Infant seat	Rocking		Touch	Body contact			Music	Talk	Pencil & paper	Pull toy		Trike			
HABITS	Pacifier	Sleep alone	Thumb sucking			Cup						Brush teeth			Use of money		
DISCIPLINE							Punishment		Temper tantr			Negative					Praise
APPETITE							Normal →				Normal →						
SOCIAL ADJUSTMENT	Spoiling				Teething	Stranger anxiety		Separation anxiety		Stranger anxiety		Unable to share		Sex educ	Nursery head start	Separates easily	Allow
DATA																	
URINE	PKU/obtain bag	Screen					Obtain bag				Urine bag						
HGB.																	
IMMUNIZATIONS		DPT/OPV	DPT	DPT/OPV	OPV	Tine		Measles	Mumps	DPV/OPV	SPV, tine	Rubella		Tine, DPT	Tine	Tine	Tine, DT (Ad) OPV
PHYS. EXAM.														Dental exam	DOST next visit		
OTHER							Ipecac										

KEY:
A - Abnormal
N - Normal
X - Achieved
O - Problem
Not Achieved
To be Evaluated

COMMENTS

Figure 4-1. Pediatric data sheet. (Gross E, St Denis M, MacFarlane A: The Child Health Manual. Boston, Blackwell Scientific Pub, 1984)

Use of a *problem list* or *summary sheet* at the front of a folder can enhance its value for the care of the patient. For a patient with complications, considerable shuffling of loose papers may be repeatedly necessary to find important information such as current medications and consultants' recommendations. File folders containing loose papers are poor travelers and are thus unsuitable for multisite use.

An unusual enhancement of the file folder approach is the recording of an entire family's health care summaries in a single file folder. If not maintained properly, the chart may be confusing, and in some states it may violate patients' confidentiality rights.

Structured note forms are provided gratis by several pharmaceutical companies for use in this and the following format.

Bound Charts

Bound charts are the familiar hospital-style record used in most large clinics and group practices. An important drawback is the clerical labor required to place notes and other materials into their appropriate locations in the chart. There is also a greater cost (albeit relatively small) than for file folders. The busy clinician finds that the most important deficit of the bound chart is its structure. Being organized in temporal order, it is difficult to capture the essence of the patient's prior care and ongoing problems unless the physician is either familiar with the patient or has the benefit of legible and well-structured notes from previous physicians. The time lost in reading past and illegible notes can substantially reduce the time available for patient care or other more productive activities.

The use of *problem lists* and *problem-oriented notes* provides an important organizational enhancement in a bound chart format but obviously cannot solve the problems of illegibility, misfiling, and that of the occasional clinician whose important contributions are not similarly structured and so must be translated by another user of the record. Despite these drawbacks, the bound chart is the most commonly used and accepted record system. A color-coding arrangement is widely used to permit rapid location of charts in record rooms. In multisite practices, it has often been necessary to install computer systems to monitor these charts as patients go from appointment to appointment so that their charts meet them in appropriate places; success with such schemes is rarely above 70%.

In both of the paper-based systems described, the fiscal component is usually separate and is not determined by the method of record keeping.

Shingled or Staggered Note Systems

Shingled or staggered note systems are an innovative method of organizing care notes by types. Paper sheets about half the standard letter size ($\sim 8\frac{1}{2} \times 5$ in.) are used and may be preformatted to allow easy entry of the chief complaint, physical findings, and other notes. Along the bottom edge of the sheet a small field is ruled off for a summary of the visit (*e.g.*, diagnosis, medications, date, immunizations, and so forth) and the sheets are then inserted on a page in a file folder so that the summary along the bottom edge is visible. Sheets may be coded (*e.g.*, by color to indicate visit types). In the course of inserting the sheets into the patient record, office staff are able to use the code or visit type to generate billing or utilization information. The summary lines along the bottom margins of the individual visit sheets provide a quick overview of the patient record. As with other paper-based record files, the organization of information is temporal and not related to the significance of problems. However, by use of color or other coding devices, it is relatively easy to highlight important entries. This system represents a distinct advantage over other paper chart systems in its ease of use and comprehensibility, although information generated outside the office must still be handled either by producing a note or by filing separately from the record pages. Home-grown versions of this idea are fairly common, though a copyright on this system exists.

Grid Devices

Grid or graph record devices can be helpful in quickly surveying a patient record for completeness and problems (Fig. 4–1). These are essentially expanded problem lists with the well-child and pediatric anticipatory guidance items inserted; they serve to remind the clinician to provide age-appropriate screening. Supplementary notes will generally be necessary for each record in addition to the care chart.

Computer-Based Systems

Computer-based medical records systems are currently of great interest. An ideal system combines the various records activities, including the fiscal portions, into a single mass of data for each patient, allowing for required reports, automated billing, and other mailings (*e.g.*, reminders of necessary immunizations and appointments). Several obstacles must be overcome to permit this to happen. Although computers are capable of these integrated automatic activities, the language used by physicians is not standardized. In order to capture information as it usually flows, the computer system must be powerful and thus costly. Some clinical data are readily definable, such as test results, measurements, and diagnoses coded according to standard schemes. However, observations, variations, plans, and many other clinical notes are not standardized.

One highly effective computer-based system is the one in use at the Harvard Community Health Plan, where a fully computer-dependent medical record has been in use since the early 1970s. This system uses preformatted Encounter Forms for patient visits; these permit entry of coded diagnoses and several lines of text for each problem noted at a visit or other patient activity. Dictation is available as a way of creating lengthier notes where needed. The system has obvious advantages: legibility, availability in multiple sites at the same time, a certain degree of standardization leading to somewhat easier reading for the unacquainted. Results of laboratory tests and other procedures are grouped together, as are medications. Several disadvantages have also been discovered: growth charts cannot be in the familiar graphic format, owing to the complexity and the cost of printing out graphics at patient visits; frequent need to abbreviate if dictation is not desired, occasionally leading to inadequate descriptions; delays in inputting caused by notes illegible to inputters as well as difficulties in training and retaining inputters and transcription personnel. However, the system has allowed centralization of emergency services with full records available to emergency personnel; referral services at multiple centers; and easy generation of reports and management and research information.

To be useful as the summary grid or shingled note systems, a computer-based system must summarize the well-child or preventive care component of the pediatric record. This has required considerable design and programming effort but has resulted in a reasonably efficient and highly legible system with good report-generating ability (*e.g.*, for schools and camps) and rapid access at multiple locations.

COSTAR is a commercial system closely allied to the Harvard Community Health Plan Automated Medical Record. This system is marketed nationwide through vendors of computer systems for health care and management and is extensively supported by research in many institutions.

For most pediatric practitioners, computers are most useful in accounting and other financial functions. Comprehensive and fast computer-based record systems will come into being as the current difficulties in capturing descriptions of care are overcome.

ANNOTATED BIBLIOGRAPHY

Gross E, St Denis M, Macfarlane A: The Child Health Manual. Boston, Blackwell Scientific Publications, 1984 (Concise outline.)

POMR: The Problem-oriented Medical Record. Chicago, IL, American Medical Record Association, 1971 (Collection of articles on the record-keeping method originated by Weed, with practical applications to hospital and clinic settings. Written with the record-room in mind but useful to the clinician.)

Weed LI: Medical records that guide and teach. N Engl J Med 278:593, 1968 (This article began the "SOAP" style of progress note writing, now fairly common in medical schools and hospital programs. A valuable discussion of the limitations of traditional discursive style.)

Sources of Record Materials

COSTAR Automated Systems: For information contact COSTAR Users' Group, North County Health Services, 348 Rancheros Drive, San Marcos, CA 92069 (For information about vendors for the COSTAR Automated Systems and the systems' capabilities.)

Formedic Communications Ltd, 12D Worlds Fair Drive, Somerset, NJ 08873–1345 (Suppliers of free forms [with advertising] of various types for pediatric office use; minimal but acceptable degree of organization.)

"Shingles System" from Orion Systems, Inc, 3350 Scott Blvd. #34, Santa Clara, CA 95051 (Proprietary, highly formatted and specialized sheets. Catalogue available.)

Standards of Child Health Care, 3rd ed. Evanston, IL, American Academy of Pediatrics, 1977 (General outline of care by age, recommendations for recording, especially routine maintenance.)

5
Medical Care by Telephone*

HARVEY P. KATZ

In 1977, 17% of all medical contacts were by phone. The volume of calls can be staggering—in one HMO health center there were 38,000 telephone daytime calls monthly representing one call per member per month in the 38,000 member plan. At one Kaiser Health Plan Center, there were 650 calls per 1000 patients less than 18 years old. Approximately 60% of calls are for immediate problem care; 45% of these result in a same day visit, 30% of calls result in home management advice and 25% are referred elsewhere. The huge volume of calls dictates that the doctor's telephone system be efficient and effective. More importantly, the dependence, trust, and confidence placed in the system by our patients and families are compelling reasons for it to be as good as all the other components of practice. Unfortunately, it frequently is not.

There are many reasons for suboptimal service: Some relate to hardware, some to systems, and some to people. The reality is that the responsibility for managing most calls needs to be delegated to someone other than a pediatrician. Appointments need to be made, and questions need to be answered about bills and insurance, illness, injury triage, and emergencies. These, and an endless array of other telephone calls need to be handled, at least initially, by the office staff. This telephone person is key and how he practices his "specialty" can make or break the practice.

Care by telephone is both a stress and a true specialty of pediatric practice. Many factors determine which way the pendulum will swing. The most important factors are the degree of training in telephone medicine for physicians prior to practice; how well office personnel are trained, supervised, and evaluated by their physician employer; and the operation of the various systems that are necessary for a smoothly functioning office telephone. Too often the telephone specialty is either neglected or left to chance. Yet a patient's satisfaction with med-

ical care may be judged on the basis of telephone encounters.

Common patient complaints about the office telephone include being placed "on hold" too long and without being given a chance to speak; encountering repeated busy signals that make it impossible to "get through," and even more difficulty in getting to speak directly to the doctor; and rude receptionists. For physicians, too many calls for minor complaints in the middle of the night, too many calls in general, and the lack of compensation for telephone time are the usual frustrations. In a survey of Baltimore and Denver pediatricians, over two thirds of pediatricians rated the telephone as the most frustrating part of their practice; 42% expressed dissatisfaction with the role of the telephone in their practice.

In 1985, only half of residency training programs had formalized a system for managing telephone calls, and less than half incorporated specific training in telephone medicine. It is surprising that the telephone is viewed as something less than a "specialty" by our pediatric program directors, since this facet of pediatric practice accounts for 30% of a pediatrician's total time.

TELEPHONE PERSONNEL

The personnel selected for telephone-care responsibility represent the vital link between families and the physician. How well this responsibility is performed will have a profound influence on the quality of care, patient and physician satisfaction, and the growth and vitality of the practice. Individuals selected for telephone responsibility must be properly recruited and oriented. They are, in effect, the image and voice of the practice. Care must be taken, however, to avoid telephone "burn out," for even the right person is at high risk for this "occupational hazard." The extent of training and supervision necessary depends on the degree of responsibility the physician wishes to delegate, the knowledge, experience, and motivation of the person answering the telephone, and the characteristics of the population served.

---

* Parts of this chapter have been adapted from the *Management of Pediatric Practice*, published by the American Academy of Pediatrics, copyright 1986.

GUIDELINES FOR STAFF USING THE TELEPHONE

1. Be alert and always express interest in the caller.
2. Convey a friendly greeting with your message, and refer to patients by their names.
3. Speak clearly, distinctly, and confidently.
4. Be polite, warm, and businesslike at all times.
5. Be very helpful; put yourself in the patient's position.
6. Express yourself well.
7. Talk naturally. Use a normal tone of voice and a moderate rate of speech. Avoid slang, technical language, and irrelevant, personal chitchat. Other patients are waiting. Make every effort to be efficient and relevant so you can answer the other calls quickly.
8. Answer the telephone promptly. Ringing telephones are a source of irritation to everyone. Set a goal of picking up the telephone after no more than three rings, and make every effort to meet that standard (the telephone usually rings 10 times per minute).
9. Never be argumentative. Always be helpful.
10. If you cannot provide information, offer to find someone who can. When you are overloaded, take the number and call back as soon as possible.
11. Be discreet, confidential, and sensitive to the problem. A caller may be upset and anxious for reasons that are not obvious. For example, there may have been a recent death in the family, or the parent may have been up all night with an ill child.
12. Avoid the "May I put you on hold?" habit. Don't put a patient on hold before they have a chance to respond. When you return to the line after a hold, thank the caller for waiting. If you must put the caller on hold for a moment, explain, "Mrs. _____, will you hold the line please while I check that information" . . . or "while I answer another telephone" . . . or "while I get the doctor." If you anticipate a long hold, offer to call back.

Those who answer the telephone in a pediatrician's office should hear themselves speaking with patients. This can be accomplished by using a tape recorder for training purposes. The staff should be reminded that when they use the telephone their voice creates an image of the practice.

ORGANIZATION OF A TELEPHONE-CARE SYSTEM

Both conceptually (for purposes of training new personnel) and functionally, it may be helpful to view the telephone-care system in two components:

1. Nonmedical or administrative information, including future appointments
2. Medical or problem care

All staff should be trained to schedule appointments relative to the nature of the presenting complaint and to know when an immediate or same-day appointment versus a future appointment (within 2 weeks at most) is indicated. The person who receives a request to make an appointment for a problem needs to make one of three basic decisions: (1) to proceed to schedule an appointment, (2) to give home management advice, or (3) to refer the call elsewhere. The management of emergency situations needs to be reviewed carefully. Each person answering the telephone must know the exact procedure to follow if there is a life-threatening emergency, especially when the pediatrician is not immediately available.

Other situations that require referral to the physician for management may arise: the caller is anxious; the caller is unable to understand the questions asked or to comprehend the answers; the medical problem appears to be complicated or the complaints are unusual; the caller provides too little information or shows questionable competence (*e.g.*, a babysitter or a young child).

Registered nurses, licensed practical nurses, and on-the-job-trained non-nursing pediatric personnel are all capable of telephone health care management if properly trained and supervised. The choice of how much responsibility to delegate and which kind of personnel to use is entirely that of the supervising physician.

TELEPHONE ENCOUNTER RECORD

A record should be made of each telephone encounter. Methods and formats of encounter systems differ widely. Some offices use a telephone encounter form, others use a spiral notebook. Portable, pocket-sized pads adapt nicely for after-hours use and for later placement into the patient's chart. Portable, in-office dictation equipment can be used to record after-hours telephone encounters.

The telephone encounter form may, at first glance, appear cumbersome; however, as the person answering the telephone becomes familiar with the format, recording of the relevant information during the conversation becomes second nature. The encounter form can be ordered with a self-sticking adhesive back so that a record of the telephone contact can be easily inserted into the patient's chart, or the encounter form can be printed on both sides for economy reasons.

There are several reasons for written documentation of phone conversations and for retaining records. Salient details of past conversations, as well as the date and name of the office staff member who received the call, can be quickly retrieved. This information is invaluable if the patient subsequently registers a complaint and past history must be separated from intervening events to objectively evaluate the problem. Also, in a group practice, it is helpful for a pediatrician to be able to review details of prior telephone instructions when the patient's regular physician is absent. If follow-up information needs to be conveyed to a patient or if instructions must be modified, it is helpful to have the patient's telephone number and details of the earlier call readily available. The tabulation of telephone data also provides useful management information about the number and type of calls received.

OUT-OF-OFFICE NEEDS

Rapid on-call accessibility to the pediatrician is crucial for the quality of care and patient satisfaction. An answering service, where available, is literally a necessity. It increases accessibility for the pediatrician on call and, when not on call, forestalls unnecessary interruptions for the pediatrician and family. Telephone calls after hours or on weekends can be managed by a direct line switch to an answering service or to a hospital switchboard if an answering service is not available. Either the answering service or switchboard then contacts the pediatrician on call. Telephone answering services should be monitored for efficiency and accuracy.

The radio paging system ("beeper") enhances accessibility and should be considered a necessity. Two home telephone lines are desirable if personal and family telephone use compromise on-call accessibility. Telephone answering machines that only record messages are not appropriate for the physician on call, and many patients dislike these devices. An answering machine, however, may be useful if the message provides an emergency number and is easily understood by even a distressed parent. For example, the message may say, "Office hours are 9 AM to 5 PM Monday through Friday. In case of an emergency, call _____." The use of the terminology "in case of an emergency" may defer nonurgent calls until regular office hours, yet a patient who has an emergency is told how to obtain an immediate, personal response.

BASIC EQUIPMENT FOR A NEW PRACTICE

Two or three telephone lines generally are required for solo pediatric practice. But it is wise to ask the telephone company about the need to reserve additional sequential telephone numbers for later service expansion. Placement of telephones within the office is determined by staff needs. A base unit in the appointment–reception area, an extension at the back office station, and a readily accessible, privately located telephone are minimum needs. Telephones in examining rooms are a matter of personal taste. However, telephone calls concerning patients made in the presence of other patients may compromise patient confidentiality, as may intercom or speaker-phone equipment.

EQUIPMENT FOR THE EXPANDING PRACTICE

Three pediatricians generally require five telephone lines; five pediatricians may require eight lines. The ratio of phones per pediatrician diminishes in a large practice. If requested, the telephone company will monitor the office service and provide a printout that will identify busy signals at peak periods; this is one way to know if additional lines are needed. Reserved sequential phone numbers prevent the inconvenience of having to change the office number later. As more staff members are added, more extension phones may be needed. Appointment, business office, insurance, and laboratory staff all generally require telephone access, as do the pediatricians' offices, consultation rooms, and a library or lounge.

Investigate needs thoroughly. It may be necessary to talk with a professional management consultant periodically as well as with representatives of the telephone company and some of the private telephone system vendors. Too little equipment sacrifices efficiency and too much wastes money.

Microprocessing has revolutionized telephone equipment. Previously unknown features are now commonly available and affordable. Formerly only available by rental, these systems may now be purchased. Many other "own-your-own" systems (called interconnects) are widely available from private companies. Remember that, when purchasing

Five-Step Approach to Telephone-Care Training

STEP 1

Task
Survey of the existing telephone system

Method

1. Use a specialized encounter form to collect important telephone data.
2. Invite a representative of the local telephone company to observe the telephone style of office personnel and the organization of the present system and to make practical recommendations regarding telecommunication systems best suited for the practice.

Objective

1. Analyze the current telephone system in a detailed, descriptive fashion (*e.g.*, the number of calls for advice versus administrative or appointment information, the total number of calls and peak times, the number of referrals, and the inquiries for health education information).
2. Evaluate the telephone manner of all office or clinical personnel who answer the telephone, and document the number of callers unable to make contact because of busy or limited trunk or search lines.

STEP 2

Task
Study of written materials by staff under supervision of a pediatrician or nurse

Method

1. Staff should study available telephone-care literature, algorithms, and decision guidelines in a concentrated time frame with special emphasis on taking a medical history, making appointments in relation to types of problems, telephone style, common presenting symptoms, prescribing over-the-counter medication, and avoiding potential errors.
2. The use of live tape recordings of actual telephone encounters, for example fever, hysterical parents, and emergencies, is becoming increasingly invaluable for educational purposes and is strongly encouraged.

Objective

1. Learn how to obtain a relevant medical history and how to present home management advice accurately, safely, and efficiently.
2. Learn to distinguish between a true emergency, and future versus same-day appointments.
3. Become aware of the potential pitfalls and errors that should be avoided in telephone care.
4. Learn to distinguish between problems that can safely be managed at home and those that require an appointment.

STEP 3

Task
Observation of experienced senior staff on the job

Method

New staff should spend approximately 24 hours of direct observation over a 3-month period (8 hours per month) listening in to conversations on a separate phone. Informal discussions with senior staff are important as time permits.

Objective

1. Reinforce techniques in history taking that permit rapid differentiation of and response to problems that need appointments from those that can be managed effectively at home.
2. Learn the time factors involved in appointment scheduling and how to keep pace with heavy volume.
3. Become familiar with the management of administrative matters and how to respond to patient requests for prescription refills, laboratory results, and such health education information as immunization schedules and proper automobile safety seats or belts.
4. Learn how to respond to acute emergencies.
5. Learn how to deal effectively with difficult or upset patients.

STEP 4

Task
Interviews with pediatricians and other health care staff

Method

Set up 1-hour appointments with each health care team member. Topics and the audit forms should be distributed well in advance.

Objective

1. Evaluate objectively the telephone assistant's knowledge.
2. Improve knowledge by constructive criticism.
3. Encourage more outside reading or listening to tapes in the areas recommended by the supervising pediatrician or nurse.

STEP 5

Do this concurrently with steps two and three, and then independently.

Task
Conferences and mock telephone role playing

Method

Regular meetings of the team of pediatrician, nurse, and office staff are an excellent way to integrate telephone training into business and staff meetings.

(continued)

Five-Step Approach
to Telephone-Care Training (*continued*)

STEP 5

Objective

1. Provide a forum for updating and refinement of information.
2. Stimulate group discussions after role playing so all benefit from the educational experience.

AVAILABLE TRAINING MANUALS AND TELEPHONE CARE PUBLICATIONS

Brown JL: Telephone Medicine: A Practical Guide to Pediatric Telephone Advice. St. Louis, CV Mosby, 1980 (Reference tool that can supplement other manuals.)

Katz HP: Telephone Manual of Pediatric Care. New York, John Wiley & Sons, 1982 (Useful, practical training method particularly suitable for office staff who answer the phone in any medical setting.)

Rosenkraus J et al: Pediatric Telephone Protocols. Darien, CT, Patient Care Publications, 1979 (Detailed protocols that are useful but somewhat more complex.)

Schmitt BD: Pediatric Telephone Advice. Boston, Little, Brown, 1980 (Detailed resource material especially suited for pediatric housestaff.)

equipment, the local telephone company's responsibility ends at the point of access. The decision about what to buy depends on four factors: reliability, service, features, and cost.

All systems have both standard and optional features. A careful investigation will reveal the advantages and disadvantages of each. A preliminary survey of needs will help determine what is important and avoid costly overequipping. Some features to consider are one-direction lines, digital switching, speed dialing, call forwarding, line privacy, call paging, speaker-phone, and intercom. Optional software may be added such as an electronic sequencer that holds calls sequentially and provides digital readouts of the total number of calls, the number placed on hold and for how long, and the number of abandoned calls. The use and advantages of these and other features are best demonstrated by a sales representative.

TRAINING OFFICE PERSONNEL

A common question parents ask is, "When should my sick child see the pediatrician?" There are no firm rules, but a child should be seen whenever parents are worried about how the child is acting in response to a particular illness. These decisions are usually made independently at home. For example, if a mother decides her child is playful and not too ill, she usually does not call the pediatrician. Medical attention should be sought immediately if the child is listless and irritable. Decisions in the gray zone, and sometimes even in the extremes, vary tremendously from parent to parent. It is especially true in this area that telephone advice may be valuable. An appropriate balance between the benefits versus the risks of home management for a particular medical situation and sound, informed judgment are required.

Telephone decision guidelines are directed toward helping parents decide when it is safe not to bring a child to the office and what to do and look for while the child is being observed at home. These guidelines also provide information about when it is important to see the pediatrician. The objective of this approach is to help promote a more informed decision-making process. For this purpose, a five-step training approach to handling telephone calls is suggested (see the box, Five-Step Approach to Telephone Care Training). It must be emphasized that this training can only be done under the most careful supervision by the pediatrician.

ANNOTATED BIBLIOGRAPHY

Caplan S: The Telephone in Pediatric Practice. Pediatrics Update. (Moss AJ[ed]) Amsterdam, Elsevier Biomedical Press, 1983 (Comprehensive literature review of the role of the telephone in pediatric care.)

Katz HP, Mushlin A, Posen J: Quality assessment of a telephone system utilizing non-physician personnel. Am J Pub Health 68:31, 1978 (Assessment of quality that stresses outcome rather than process.)

Wood PR: Pediatric resident training in telephone management: A survey of training programs in the United States. Pediatrics 77:822–825, 1986 (Survey that describes the extent of training in telephone medicine.)

2

The Well Child

6

Normal Growth and Development: An Overview

CONSTANCE H. KEEFER

Issues of growth and development are fundamental in pediatrics. All of our patients grow and develop in various ways, and the resulting changes provide a constant challenge to parents, forcing new stages in their relationships to their children. A child's adequacy, in the general sense, is played out in many areas such as physical growth, language, cognition, and social and motor skills, and is as fundamentally important to parents as the child's survival. Delay in any of these areas produces a serious blow to a parent's sense of competence; not being able to adequately nurture a child is very threatening to a parent's self-confidence.

The pediatrician has a broad responsibility to promote normal growth and development. Within the office, the first responsibility is awareness, which may be operationalized in several ways. The following scheme is helpful in organizing an approach for overseeing the process of growth and development during well-child visits.

For routine visits

Screen with a physical examination; measurements of growth, plotted against standards; and developmental items. Review these with parents for indication of risk or evidence of delayed growth or development.

Anticipate by helping parents understand and prepare for changes in the child's behavior.

Educate and *empower* parents.

When deviations are noted

Monitor indices of improvement or worsening.

Problem-solve or explore with parents for diagnosis as well as intervention.

If developmental issues are addressed in this way with the cooperation of parents, the child's future development can be influenced. The well-child visit is an opportune time for detecting problems in behavior and development because parents come with two important expectations: to have their child examined, and to seek help and advice.

Although the sequence of normal growth is usually uncomplicated and orderly, variations exist and individual growth patterns may be confused with problems of hormonal regulation. Plotting height and weight on standard curves provides a useful and objective assessment of the adequacy of growth. Parents can understand visually the concept of following a particular percentile curve as opposed to achieving a specific height or weight. Convenient "rules of thumb" to remember growth norms are listed in the box, Growth Guidelines.

When deviations occur, they may reflect problems in other areas, ranging from the child's temperament, endocrine, or nutritional status to the family or community. It is important that the pediatrician is aware of this signal value of growth and that he uses it as a diagnostic point.

Responsibility for growth and development goes beyond the office. The pediatrician must be an advocate for the child in the home and the community. The only insight into life in the home that most pediatricians get is the representation of it in the office by the mother. This is important information for the

Growth Guidelines

WEIGHT

Birth weight is regained by the 14th day.

During the first 3 months, the average gain is about 1 kg/month (abut ½ to 1 oz/day).

Birth weight doubles at about 4 months; triples at 12 months; quadruples at 24 months.

By the sixth month, the average gain per month is 0.5 kg.

During the second year, the average gain per month is 0.25 kg.

After age 2, the average annual increment is 2.3 kg (5 lb) until the adolescent growth spurt.

HEIGHT

Average birth length is 50 cm (20 in.)

By the end of the first year, birth length increases by 50%.

Birth length doubles by 4 years.

Birth length triples by 13 years.

Average annual growth is 5 cm (2 in.) or better per year.

pediatrician to gather, but caution must be exercised in acting on that information alone as it may be subjective, spotty, or inaccurate. Similarly, the view of the child's behavior and development provided in a short (even 20- or 30-minute) visit, occurring once every several months, may also be flawed. Even when efficient and reliable assessment tools are used, one can get only a narrow and shallow view of the real child. Teachers and parents may often have a more complete, if less sophisticated, assessment; thus, communication with school and community observers (both professional and family) is essential.

However, there are limitations to what can be done in solving developmental and growth problems in primary care. The most significant limitation that pediatricians should be aware of is their own desire not to find anything wrong with a child. This is only compounded by (and perhaps directly related to) not knowing what to do or whom to turn to if a problem is discovered. One example is that of making the diagnosis of spasticity in early infancy. When referred by their parents, children with cerebral palsy are seen in specialty clinics at an average age of 8 months; when referred by pediatricians, the average age is 16 months. Accurate, current information on what services are available to families with a child with developmental problems, even if only the phone number of an early

intervention program, helps overcome the difficulty in initiating a referral.

Three theoretical dimensions that underlie the pediatrician's responsibility regarding growth and development will now follow. These dimensions consist of timing, perspective (e.g., through cultural determinants of behavior; how problems are approached; theoretical and scientific bases of the practice of pediatrics; temperament, or the child's style of behavior), and the role of the parents. The timing of encounters with parents is of some theoretical interest. The spacing of well-child visits in the first 2 years of life is determined primarily by a set of standard immunization and screening procedures (e.g., diphtheria, pertussis, tetanus (DPT), oral poliovirus vaccine (OPV), measles, mumps, rubella (MMR), *Hemophilus influenzae* type B (HIB), free erythrocyte protoporphyrin/hemoglobin (FEP/Hgb). These procedures happen to come frequently enough and at ages when many developmental, growth, and behavioral issues can be dealt with concurrently. The American Academy of Pediatrics published *Guidelines for Health Supervision* which are excellent in their coverage of age-related issues. As economic pressures on medical caregivers lead to fewer and shorter visits, it is important for primary care pediatricians to visualize what it is that they are doing in well-child visits and the value of those visits. However, not all well-child visits coincide with important changes and thus timely help either for the avoidance or resolution of problems may be missed. Table 6-1 presents events in which preventive intervention is particularly critical.

In dealing with growth and development, perspective or attitude is important and must transcend the framework of "traditional" medicine. The first of these perspectives is cultural. It is essential to have a sense of the cultural determinants of behavior, of the relationship between values and beliefs, and the practices that support those values. A culture, which is a shared system of practices, beliefs, and values, may be specific to an individual, a family, or a whole community. Helping parents discover their own, sometimes hidden, beliefs and values is often useful in solving behavior problems.

There is also a cultural dimension for parents to the meaning of illness and symptoms in the child. A scientifically based medical explanation may not completely satisfy them if it does not fit in with their own theories.

Much advice given about the management of illness and child rearing is derived from the pediatrician's own background or culture, often without his

Table 6-1. Normal and Non-Normal Developmental Crises in Which Intervention is Most Helpful and Necessary

NORMAL CRISES	NON-NORMAL CRISES
Pregnancy	Miscarriage
Birth or adoption	Birth of premature, defective, or stillborn infant
Intensity and lack of boundaries of infancy	
Aggression and autonomy of the toddler	Diagnosis of a significant illness or handicap
Developmental milestones that change the parent-child relationship	Divorce
	Emergence of problematic behavior
Regression prior to developmental progress	Abuse or neglect
Adjustment to secondary care	
Preparation for a well-child visit	

being aware of it. It is important in our continuing re-education of ourselves to recognize these cultural biases.

The second dimension of attitude relates to how problems are approached. When dealing with issues of behavior and development, the medical model for care, characterized by action and authority, has to be replaced with an approach that includes negotiation with the patient, problem-solving rather than answer-giving, and an acceptance of and willingness to deal with, rather than deny, a high degree of uncertainty.

A third attitudinal dimension pertains to the theoretical and scientific bases of the practice of pediatrics. The pediatric medical model is excellent for the pursuit and treatment of physical pathology, but it is inadequate in the area of growth and development, where the scientific bases are in the areas of developmental biology and developmental psychology. Four appropriate models emerge from these two fields: development, temperament, mastery, and interaction.

A developmental model explains how change occurs in growth and behavior. One can view development as linear or staged. Whichever pattern is most appropriate may depend on the phenomenon in question. Linear development usually refers to the gradual accretion of size, skill, or knowledge. Stages imply more uneven development with short periods of rapid change followed by plateaus or long periods in which change is not as obvious.

Stage theories, like Erik Erikson's theory of psychosocial development, are often epigenetic (*i.e.*, each new stage relies on or carries remnants of the old stage[s]). In a linear development model, currently acquired skills are not dependent on previous change.

A paradoxical phenomenon accompanying staged development is regression. In periods prior to a major advance or developmental change, in moving from one plateau to another (*e.g.*, crawling to walking), one often sees regression either in the skill area involved or in areas of state regulation or dependency. These periods of regression are often easier for parents to tolerate when the clinician can help them to be understood as fueling the emergency of the next, more mature state of development.

A similar phenomenon, occurring when skills are being acquired, is that of the suppression of other areas of development in favor of the skill being practiced (*e.g.*, the child at 13 months who stops talking during a few weeks of intense practice in pulling to stand or taking first steps).

Self-motivation is also relevant to the developmental model. The child's own desire to be skillful, to create, or to act on his own sense of what might be possible, is a powerful force in development. This will lead the child to seek out and use whatever the environment has to offer. It may explain why there is often normal development in unnatural or nonoptimal environments, for example, those children who were hospitalized for a long time as infants and whose cognitive development remains normal.

In addition to these processes, a developmental model indicates areas in which change or remediation is recommended. The most basic of these changes include gross and fine motor development, cognitive development, affective development (attachment and autonomy), language development, perceptive/adaptive functioning, social/peer relations, and bodily functions (*e.g.*, feeding, sleeping, and toilet habits).

A temperamental/constitutional model is drawn largely from the work of Chess and Thomas, and is second only to the developmental model. Together, these two models (one addressing what children do, the other addressing how they do it) form a matrix from which the pediatrician (and parent) can more fully understand developmental and behavioral phenomena.

Temperament, or the child's style of behavior that has a permanence over time, often explains apparent deviations in development and is an essential area to assess when the complaint is a behavior problem. The temperamental dimensions provide a nonjudgmental way of describing the child and his behavior, capturing the child's interactive qualities.

A mastery and coping model, drawn from the work of Lois Murphy and her colleagues, is helpful in understanding behaviors of children in regard to their reactions to new and challenging situations. For example, oppositional behavior on the part of a 4- or 5-year-old is often just a manifestation of coping.

An interactional model is best suited to address the age-old question of nature versus nurture as a determinant of growth and development. This model acknowledges both the major role that the force of the organism's "nature" plays as well as the importance of the shaping that the environmental constraints and facilitators ("nurture") provide. The outcome is therefore not predictable from knowledge of either the environment or the child alone, but rather from both and from the interaction between them. For parents who are burdened by the belief that their every move has an impact on their child's future, the fact that much of that outcome will be a result of the child's own self can be freeing, enabling them to more fully enjoy the child and their parenting role.

The general categories of growth, behavior, and development presented in this chapter give the practitioner a framework on which to hang the "milestone" data. Table 6-2 lists standard developmental tests and the areas that each measures. Details of specific milestones of development are given in Chapter 36.

Even if these assessment techniques are not formally utilized, knowledge of them is helpful and makes working on developmental issues possible in a time-limited setting. For example, it is rarely necessary to do a full Brazelton assessment on a newborn, but knowledge of the categories of behavior and the ways in which they are manifested in the scale is most helpful for sorting out questions of subtle deviation from normal behavior or development in the first 3 months of life. When a parent of a 10-month old describes new night wakening, the child's stage of attachment, stage of motor development, temperament, and the meaning to the parents of crying and their beliefs about their responsibility to the child should be explored. Usually just mentioning these areas and helping parents start to explore them solves most problems, even without a formal analysis. Another common ex-

Table 6-2. Assessing Development

ASSESSMENT	FUNCTIONS STUDIED
Dubowitz Gestational Development Examination	Gestational age
Brazelton Neonatal Behavioral Assessment Scale	Newborn behavior of motor, state-control, and sensory orientation Newborn neurologic function
Carey Temperament Questionnaire	Temperamental style of behaving
Denver Developmental Screening Test and Gesell Scales of Development	Fine and gross motor, perceptual, cognitive, language, and social skills
Anna Freud's Lines of Development	Development of play, body functions, and social relations
Hunt and Uzgiris' Cognitive Scales	Development of thought
Margaret Mahler's Stages of Attachment	Development of attachment to others and sense of identity

ample is a 5-year-old's difficulty adjusting to kindergarten. To identify the proper locus of difficulty and help parents focus their efforts in understanding and managing this situation, several factors must be considered. These include parental concerns such as the mother's view of her child and her own role, and depression in the mother; and factors directly related to the child, such as school readiness skills, temperament (especially adaptability to or "fit" with a particular type of teacher or a particular educational philosophy), and level of development in self- to other-centered activities or even bodily function.

The last important dimension to the pediatrician is the role of the parents. Awareness of the parents' role in the child's development is important in guiding the pediatrician's own responses, interactions, and expectations of them. The parent is a separate adult ego, an ally in the care for the child. But the parent is also inextricably linked with the child. Personality issues of the parent and the age and personality of the child are often part of the developmental problem to be solved. An example is nonorganic failure to thrive, where maternal factors are intermingled with nutrition and growth. Even in organic failure to thrive, the parents' confidence and competence come into question at least by themselves if not by others, and this invariably affects the child.

One must always work between reliance on the parent as a partner in the diagnostic and therapeutic work and assessment of the parent as a potential part of the problem. The pediatrician who states, "I'm only treating the parents," should take this problem seriously; it is an opportunity to re-examine the situation and address seriously the parents' needs.

A conceptualization of the parental role may help to determine when to intervene directly with the parent as a parent. The basic functions of love, nurturance, protection, limit setting, and education are easy to remember. There are other, more sophisticated ways to conceptualize parent functions and to judge them according to variables such as the stages of the parents' life and the stresses and supports present for the parent. As with child assessments, knowledge of these other standards can be used in the time-limited primary care setting without performing formal assessments. The normative models for parental behavior are not intended to judge parents, but rather to enhance their performance in their roles as parents.

ANNOTATED BIBLIOGRAPHY

Brazelton TB: Toddlers and Parents. New York, Delacorte, 1974 (Realistic description of autonomy in the second and third years of life, with helpful suggestions for management of the tantrums and negative behavior.)

Erickson ML: Assessment and Management of Developmental Changes in Children. St. Louis, CV Mosby, 1976 (Concise, practical descriptions of the administration and interpretation of many developmental assessment instruments, including Dubowitz Gestational, Brazelton Neonatal Behavior, Denver Developmental, and Carey Temperamental.)

Erikson E: Identity and the life cycle. In Psychological Issues (1) New York, International Universities Press, 1959 (Defines eight stages of psychosocial development, five of which apply from birth through adolescence. The integration of biological, psychological, and social forces on development and the relationship of emerging stage to previous stages are particularly helpful.)

Fraiberg S: The Magic Years. New York, Charles Scribner's, 1959 (Childhood blossoms before your eyes as the psychological issues of development from 2 years to 5 years are described in realistic and practical detail.)

Hunt JM, Uzgiris I: Assessment in Infancy. Urbana, University of Illinois Press, 1976 (Systematic and detailed look at cognitive development from birth through 2 years, based on the work of Piaget. Particularly helpful when language is delayed or when physical problems make an accurate assessment of "intelligence" difficult.)

Knoblock H, Pasamanick B (eds): Gesell and Amatruda's Developmental Diagnosis: The Evaluation and Management of Normal and Abnormal Neuropsychologic Development in Infancy and Early Childhood. Hagerstown, MD, Harper & Row, 1974 (Highly detailed description of what children do in gross and fine motor, cognitive, perceptual, language, and social skills from infancy through age 3 years.)

Mahler M: The Psychological Birth of the Human Infant. New York, Basic Books, 1975 (Detailed look at the stages of development of attachment in the first 2 years of life.)

Murphy LB: The Widening World of Childhood: Paths Toward Mastery. New York, Basic Books, 1962 (Rich clinical examples of coping and mastery and their influence on the child's negotiation of new situations and new stages of development.)

7

Nutrition and Nutritional Status: An Overview

WILLIAM C. MACLEAN

Parents are increasingly concerned about nutrition, both as it affects their children's immediate growth and development and as it affects later health. Misinformation abounds, and most parents have no means of distinguishing reliable information. Pediatricians have a major role to play in guiding parents through the changing nutritional needs of their children and in calculating sound nutritional practices that will persist throughout life. To do so requires a basic understanding of nutrient requirements, how they are estimated and how they can be met at different ages, and an appreciation of what a good diet can and cannot be expected to accomplish.

NUTRIENT REQUIREMENTS AND DIETARY ALLOWANCES

The requirement for any nutrient is related to the age, size, growth rate, and later the gender of the individual. It represents the amount needed to replace obligatory losses (fecal, urinary, integumentary, and so forth) and to support synthesis of new tissue. Requirements of specific nutrients at different ages are known with variable degrees of precision. For example, the protein requirement of the growing low-birth-weight infant is still subject to considerable debate, whereas the iron requirement of the adolescent is known with greater certainty.

Recommended Dietary Allowances* (RDAs) are published periodically and are an attempt to translate estimates of requirements of nutrients into the amounts that should be consumed to meet the requirements. RDAs are determined for groups of people (populations) rather than individuals. RDAs virtually always exceed a given individual's requirements. The RDA for all nutrients except energy (calories) is defined as the amount needed to meet the needs of "nearly all healthy individuals," that is, ~97% of the population. (The RDA for energy is given as a range of intakes.) The RDAs are useful in assessing the nutrient intakes of population groups but are less useful in evaluating the diet of an individual. Because of the way RDAs are defined, most children can and will consume less than the RDA for most nutrients and remain nutritionally healthy. However, the lower the intake relative to the RDA and the longer low intake persists, the greater is the risk of nutrient deficiency.

The dietary choices that provide appropriate amounts of nutrients broaden progressively as an infant develops the capacity to tolerate solid foods. In the typical American family, parents frequently express concern that children may not be eating enough. Parents seem especially preoccupied about protein and vitamins. In fact, most nutrients are consumed in excess; the only serious concern for undernutrition in most children is iron.

---

* The Recommended *Dietary* Allowances of the Food and Nutrition Board, National Research Council, of the National Academy of Sciences should not be confused with the United States Recommended *Daily* Allowances (US-RDAs) of the Food and Drug Administration. Although derived from the RDAs, the USRDAs group children under 4 years together and children 4 years and over and adults together. These USRDAs are the values used for consumer labelling of nutrient contents of food products and are the "goals" some parents try to meet.

Widely divergent diets are capable of meeting a child's nutrient needs. The concept of "a proper diet" must be broadly interpreted in the cultural and social context of the family. Most parents and pediatricians would do well to relax a bit and to recognize that as long as the child is growing normally and maintaining a normal hemoglobin concentration, the diet is most likely adequate.

Infancy

The normal infant will gain approximately 165 grams (about 6 oz) per week for the first 6 months of life. Based on data from the National Center for Health Statistics (NCHS), birth weight is expected to double by about 4 months of age and to triple by about 12 months of age. The normal diet of the infant (human milk) is low in protein (about 6% of calories) and high in fat (about 52% of calories), specifically saturated fat and cholesterol. Mineral intakes of the full-term breast-fed infant are relatively low but are sufficient to meet requirements. Infant formula provides slightly more protein (~ 9% of calories) than human milk. The distribution of protein, fat, and carbohydrate in standard infant formulas approximates that found in human milk. Both human milk (possibly with vitamin D supplementation) and infant formula are sufficient to meet the full-term infant's nutrient needs for at least the first 4 to 6 months.

Solid foods are generally withheld for the first 4 to 6 months. This delay is dictated less by concerns about the digestibility of solids than by concerns that the infant's head control and oromotor coordination are not sufficiently developed before that age to allow the infant to participate appropriately in the feeding process. As long as the protrusion reflex persists, the infant given solids will essentially need to be force-fed. Although a specific weight is often suggested as the guideline for timing the introduction of solid foods, developmental readiness is more important and a better criterion. The possible exception to this is the breast-fed infant whose growth rate has begun to falter after lactation is well established. Some infants may outgrow their milk supply as early as 3 months of age. In these instances, earlier introduction of solids may be considered, although it may be preferable to supplement with formula.

The order in which solid foods are usually introduced into the diet is based primarily on tradition. Typically, cereals are begun first, followed by fruits, vegetables, and meats. This order is not followed in many countries, and departures from it are of no particular nutritional concern. A good case could be made for starting meats initially in breast-fed infants, to provide additional protein and iron, both of which reach low levels in human milk as lactation continues. Nevertheless, most mothers in the United States probably expect cereal to be their infant's first solid food, and there is no compelling reason to try to change this. High-protein cereals specifically should be avoided, however; they supply more protein than needed and consequently increase the renal solute load. Initial baby foods are purées. The term *junior food* usually implies a coarser texture or the presence of small chunks of fruit, vegetable, or meat in the product. (Some junior foods, applesauce for example, may be the same purée in a larger jar.) The age at which the infant will accept these coarser foods is highly variable. It is wise to obtain product information from the major manufacturers, because the contents of protein and energy (and other nutrients) vary among cereals, fruits, vegetables, and so forth, and among corresponding products of different manufacturers.

The older infant, 8 to 10 months of age, is usually ready for a cup. Some infants can be weaned directly to a cup at an earlier age; some prefer a bottle even at meal time beyond this age. There seems no reason to force the issue either way. Older infants should not be put to bed with a bottle because of the danger of nursing-bottle caries. At the same age, finger foods can begin to be introduced. Care should be taken not to offer chunks of food (*e.g.*, cheese or small hot dogs) that can easily be aspirated.

Breast-feeding with appropriate supplementation after 4 to 6 months is desirable for at least the first year of life. When breast-feeding is not adopted or is stopped earlier, infant formula provides the most appropriate alternative. The age at which whole cow's milk should be introduced is still debated. Analysis of dietary data from the second National Health and Nutrition Examination Survey (NHANES II) indicates that mothers who introduce cow's milk at an early age are also more likely to introduce table foods inappropriately. Their infants tend to be fed excessive amounts of protein and sodium and inadequate amounts of iron. Low-fat milks should never be introduced in the first year of life because of the potential for inadequate energy intake and essential fatty acid deficiency, particularly when skim milk is fed.

Toddler and Older Child

The nutrition of the toddler is characterized by a decrease in appetite and the emergence of iron deficiency in a sizeable percentage of children. Growth rate slows toward the end of the first year of life. During the second year the child will gain only 50 grams (1.7 oz) per week, about 30% of the rate early in infancy. Appetite decreases in parallel. Parents need anticipatory guidance to alert them to this change. The major goal is to prevent meal times from becoming periods of daily conflict and coaxing. The child's appetite should be respected, and parents should be urged to be less concerned about undernutrition and more concerned with the risk of establishing a life-long pattern of overconsumption.

There is a valid concern about emerging iron deficiency between 12 and 18 months of age. Most full-term infants are born with adequate iron stores. Depending on the diet consumed during the first year, iron stores are drawn upon to meet iron needs. As the diet shifts from iron-fortified foods (*e.g.*, infant formula, infant cereals) to whole cow's milk and table foods, iron intake decreases. Iron deficiency becomes clinically apparent when the stores are exhausted and the intake continues to be suboptimal. This occurs most commonly between 12 and 18 months of age.

Two groups of infants are particularly at risk of iron deficiency, the former low-birth-weight infant and the breast-fed infant. The low-birth-weight infant is born without adequate iron stores. Iron supplementation is delayed in some infants. The requirement for dietary iron is higher in these infants throughout the first year of life and probably well into the second year. The breast-fed infant receives small amounts of iron in human milk ($\leq$0.5 mg/L). The low concentration of iron in human milk is largely offset by high bioavailability. The addition of solid foods to the diet of the breast-fed infant, however, adversely affects iron absorption. Breast-fed infants probably rely to a large extent on their iron stores to meet iron needs during the second 6 months of life. Careful attention must be paid to the iron content of the diet of former low-birth-weight infants and breast-fed infants.

There is a transition from the diet of infancy to an adult diet during the toddler years. Eating habits that may persist throughout life are established. The introduction of table foods is accompanied by a marked increase in salt intake in most households. Fiber intake also increases. Depending on the family there may be a shift toward lower fat intake and from saturated to polyunsaturated fats. Extreme modifications of the diet of young children in an attempt to prevent later development of diseases such as atherosclerosis, cancer, or hypertension are not warranted. For example, authorities advise against any significant changes in the high-fat diet of the infant before the age of 2 years. The low-fat diet (<35% of dietary energy from fat) recommended for adults as part of a prudent diet to reduce serum lipid concentrations implies increased intake of complex carbohydrates. Foods meeting this goal are bulkier in the stomach (*i.e.*, they tend to be more filling and they are often less digestible). It becomes difficult for many young children to meet energy needs on such a diet.

There are generally few nutritional concerns between the ages of 2 or 3 years and the onset of adolescence. Growth rate is modest and nutrient requirements are easily met by most diets. Strong food preferences and dislikes are established during this time. The child develops progressively more control, direct or indirect, over what is eaten.

Adolescence

During no time other than infancy are growth rates as fast or nutrient requirements as high as during the pubertal growth spurt. Rapid linear growth imposes particularly high requirements for energy, protein, calcium, and phosphorus. Iron requirements are high in both sexes. Muscle mass and hemoglobin mass increase, especially in boys. Once the growth spurt is complete, however, the need for iron in the male decreases. Because of menstruation, the iron requirement for girls remains high (about twice that of the male) throughout adolescence and beyond.

Meeting the iron requirements of adolescent girls can be difficult. Iron intake relates directly to energy intake. The typical American diet provides about 5.5 mg to 6.0 mg iron per 1000 kcal. Adolescent boys tend to eat "everything in sight." Studies of body image suggest that most teenage boys would like to be bigger and more muscular than they are. Adolescent girls, on the other hand, tend to feel they are overweight. They are often weight watchers. Their attempts to limit calorie intake effectively reduce iron intake during a period of high iron requirement. This situation is not unique to the teenaged girl and often persists into adulthood. Screening for iron deficiency in adolescent girls is an important part of their medical care.

Adolescents participating in athletics require careful nutritional monitoring. Strenuous exercise imposes nutritional stresses during a period of rapid growth. Certain sports, such as wrestling, may foster attempts to lose weight, which is undesirable at this time. Athletes may espouse inappropriate dietary regimens that promise improved performance. Excessive training, as in long-distance running, may induce amenorrhea in girls and has been associated with iron deficiency anemia, the exact cause of which is unknown.

"Junk food" and teenagers seem inseparably linked. The appropriate role of "junk food" in the diet is hotly debated. Much of this debate derives from the lack of any reasonable definition of what "junk food" truly is. One man's hamburger is another man's junk food. Fast food seems to have become synonymous with junk food, an unfortunate link. Fast foods often parallel what is served at home and can be quite nutritious. A quarter-pound hamburger, an order of French fries, and a chocolate shake provide the growing adolescent male with about 33% of the RDA for energy, 70% of that for protein, and more than 35% of the RDAs of calcium, phosphorus, and iron. Similarly, pizza comes as close to being well-balanced as most single-dish items can. Parental concerns often center on the fear that the diet will be deficient in some nutrient. This is rarely the problem except for iron, as noted previously. If there is a valid nutritional concern for fast food other than the apparent monotony of the diet, it is the potential for high intakes of sodium and fat and, in some instances, low intakes of vitamin A. "Junk foods" do have a place in the teenager's diet. Parents have little control over this in any case and should direct their nutritional concerns to what is available at home for snacks and what is served at meal times.

ASSESSMENT OF NUTRITIONAL STATUS

The main use of screening of nutritional status in office-based pediatric practice is the early detection of illness or inappropriate dietary patterns. The assessment of nutritional status in the well child is essentially the assessment of growth. Iron nutriture is also a concern at the end of infancy and during adolescence. Chronic illnesses can have devastating effects on nutritional status. There is a high prevalence of malnutrition and of specific nutrient deficiencies in those conditions. More complex situations will not be discussed here.

The assessment of growth involves three steps: (1) accurate measurement of length, weight, and head circumference, (2) careful plotting of *serial* measurements on appropriate growth charts, (3) correct interpretation of the data. The measurement of weight is done accurately in most offices. Nevertheless, it is important to standardize scales periodically with known reference weights and to weigh children consistently with minimal clothing. Measurement of length is often not done and when it is, it is frequently done poorly. Recumbent length should be measured for children less than 2 years of age and standing height (stature) for those over 3 years of age. Either measurement may be used for the 2- to 3-year-old child, depending on the child's cooperation, provided that it is plotted on the appropriate growth chart (recumbent length 0 to 36 months, standing height 2 to 18 years). Good equipment for measuring recumbent length and standing height is as important as any equipment in the office. The height bar attached to most scales, for example, is unacceptable. Errors of several centimeters in height are easily made. Differences of this magnitude can change the percentile ranking of a 4-year-old child from the 25th percentile to approximately the 10th percentile or *vice versa* (both directions can be a problem). Ancillary staff must understand the need for accurate measurements and must be trained to make them reproducibly.

A single value for stature or weight is of little value except when a child is already obviously under- or overnourished. Serial measurements of stature, weight, height, and in younger children head circumference should be plotted on standard growth charts (NCHS reference data). Because growth charts are a statistical representation of the growth of a population of children, the place on the chart of a single child cannot be equated with health or illness. For example, we instinctively worry more about the 4-year-old child whose height falls at the 10th percentile and whose weight falls at the 5th percentile than we do about a child of similar age with height and weight at the 50th and 25th percentiles, respectively. Height, however, is within the normal range, and both have a weight-for-height at approximately the same percentile within the normal range. On the other hand, if one of these children had a rapid decrease in percentile rank, concern about undernutrition or disease might be warranted.

A different problem arises in the interpretation of adolescent growth data. The commonly used growth charts mask the growth spurt because the pubertal growth spurt occurs in different children at widely different ages. Children with early growth spurts appear to accelerate on the chart and then appear to fall back. The reverse is true of children whose growth spurt occurs later. In some instances

charts that permit the plotting of growth velocity (increments), rather than height or weight attained, may be useful.

There are two patterns of growth aside from frank cessation of increases in weight and stature that should alert the pediatrician to impending problems: continuing linear growth with stable weight, and proportionately slow growth in both stature and weight. The child whose length (height) continues to increase, perhaps more slowly, while weight gain ceases or weight loss ensues will become *wasted*, a state characterized by low weight-for-height. The child who grows slowly in both stature and weight is termed *stunted*. Wasting (acute nutritional insult) may be superimposed on stunting (chronic nutritional insult) in some instances. Both wasting and stunting can be associated with marginal nutrient intakes, mild to moderate malabsorption, or chronic illness.

Measurement of triceps or subscapular skinfold (fatfold) thickness can be useful in assessing body fatness. Inexpensive plastic calipers and good reference data (percentile charts) are available for these measurements. Skinfold measurements are likely to prove useful in separating the overweight child from the overfat child and in following fat loss in an obese child who is growing. In the latter situation, frank weight loss may be undesirable. Slower weight gain with normal linear growth can be used to achieve fat loss, which is most easily monitored by skinfold measurements. Such measurements should be reserved for specific children and need not be routine.

Screening for specific nutrient deficiencies is rarely required in the office situation. Protein status should be assessed in children with either wasting or stunting. This is most easily accomplished by measurement of serum total protein and albumin concentrations. Proteins with shorter half-lives, for example, prealbumin, are more sensitive indicators, especially of response to recovery, but they are not needed routinely. Low serum albumin concentration is rarely the result of low protein intake in the United States but may point to pathologic conditions in which protein requirements are elevated or protein is being malabsorbed or lost. Screening for iron deficiency is routine in most offices, usually by measuring hematocrit or hemoglobin concentration. A therapeutic trial of iron may be preferred over extensive laboratory testing in office practice. Screening for other specific nutrients should be done on an individual basis. For example, children who are raised as vegetarians are known to have low intakes of vitamins D and B_{12}; thus the screening of vitamins D and B_{12} status is indicated (see Chap. 12). Consultation with someone knowledgeable in laboratory diagnosis of nutrient deficiencies is advisable, because the plasma concentration of many nutrients is less indicative of body stores than are other indirect measures related to metabolic functions of the nutrient.

ANNOTATED BIBLIOGRAPHY

Dallman RP, Siimes MA, Stekel A: Iron deficiency in infancy and childhood. Am J Clin Nutr 33:86–118, 1980 (Probably the best review of iron from the nutritional and clinical perspectives.)

Harper AE: Dietary goals—a skeptical view. Am J Clin Nutr 31:310–321, 1978 (A respected nutritionist suggests that we may be expecting too much from dietary modification.)

Holliday HL, Lappin TRJ, McClure GM: Iron status of the preterm infant during the first year of life. Biol Neonate 45:228–235, 1984 (Report on iron status of 49 preterm infants, a high percentage of whom became iron-deficient.)

Jung E, Czajka–Nasius DM: Birth weight doubling and tripling times: An updated look at the effects of birth weight, sex, race, and type of feeding. Am J Clin Nutr 42:182–189, 1985 (Reality for many infants differs from the NCHS growth charts.)

Kerr CM Jr, Reisinger KS, Plankey FW: Sodium concentration of homemade baby foods. Pediatrics 62:331–335, 1978 (When mothers cook for their infants, salt intake increases dramatically.)

MacLean WC Jr, Graham GG: Vegetarianism in children. Am J Dis Child 134:513–519, 1980 (Review of nutritional and non-nutritional effects of being raised as a vegetarian.)

Montalto MB, Benson JD, Martinez GA: Nutrient intakes of formula-fed infants and infants fed cow's milk. Pediatrics 75:343–351, 1985 (Differences in nutrient intakes were due not only to different concentrations of nutrients in each of the milk feedings but also to the different amounts and types of solid foods fed to the two groups of infants.)

Moore WM, Roche AF: Pediatric Anthropometry, 2nd ed. Columbus, OH, Ross Laboratories, 1983 (Describes how to perform anthropometric measurements properly and provides guidelines for interpretation of values obtained.)

8
The Well-Child Visit
KATHERINE C. TEETS GRIMM

The prenatal visit and subsequent well-child visits provide the physician with an excellent opportunity to acquaint himself with the child and his family, to develop a data base on the child, and to practice preventive pediatrics. Such visits are helpful when the physician treats the same child for an acute illness. Knowledge of what the child is like when he is well and knowledge of the family, their ability to cope with illness, their judgment during crises, and their compliance with past medical regimens, helps the physician to determine how sick the child is and what the treatment plan should be.

SOME GOALS OF THE WELL-CHILD VISIT

Every physician should determine the goals for each well-child encounter. Such goals guide the content of the visit. Examples of goals might, and indeed often, include the following:

- To establish a relationship of trust and open communication with the patient and the patient's family.

- To gain an understanding of the child's cultural, ethnic, religious, and socioeconomic background. (Do culturally influenced ideas strongly affect how the family deals with illness?)
- To observe and inquire about the child's relationship to the parents and to other family members and to know the attitudes and expectations that they have toward each other. (Is the child considered to be a "bad" child? Is the child a "vulnerable" child? Is the child the only reason why the parents are still together? Do the parents have realistic expectations given the child's developmental level?)
- To detect stresses that affect the family and anxieties that the family or the child are experiencing (Does the mother feel overwhelmed or incompetent with her child care responsibilities? Are there financial pressures?)
- To inquire about the child's environment. (Are there environmental hazards such as lead-based paint in the child's home or in the babysitter's home? Is either parent involved in an occupation

that might bring hazardous materials into the home? Have proper precautions been taken in the home and the babysitter's home to prevent accidents?)

- To determine the risk for genetically transmitted diseases (*e.g.*, Is there a history of early cardiovascular disease?)
- To detect early developmental and behavioral problems and to monitor their remediation
- To detect early disease processes by an interview, a physical examination, and screening tests
- To provide health maintenance (*e.g.*, immunizations)
- To provide appropriate counseling and anticipatory guidance
- To communicate to the family that the physician is there to help and provide support

GENERAL PRINCIPLES OF THE WELL-CHILD VISIT

Frequency of the Visits

The American Academy of Pediatrics (AAP) recommends a *minimum* of five health supervision visits from birth to 2 years of age, three visits from 2 to 6 years of age, and four visits from 6 to 18 years of age. The AAP also recommends that the frequency of the visits should be increased for the following situations:

a. First-born or adopted children or those who do not have natural parents
b. Parents with a particular need for education and guidance
c. Disadvantaged social or economic environment
d. The presence or possibility of perinatal disorders, congenital defects, or familial disease
e. Acquired illness or previously identified disease or problems

It is apparent that each child and family must be treated individually and that the number of visits should be adjusted accordingly.

Organization of the Visits

The average initial well-child visit during which a complete family history is obtained will generally take at least 30 minutes. The typical follow-up well-child visit will normally take 15 to 30 minutes. The physician frequently faces the dilemma of how to provide full services to a family and yet conserve time. The counseling and anticipatory guidance portion of the visit are often short-changed. Several suggestions on how to deal with this dilemma follow:

- For the initial visit parents can fill out a data base form while waiting to be examined by the physician.
- If more intensive counseling is necessary, a separate visit with the family should be arranged.
- The physician or his nursing assistant can hold periodic parent group conferences during which topics of common concern are discussed. The topics conducive to group discussion include: the advantages and disadvantages of old and new vaccines, toilet training, sleep disorders, feeding problems, discipline, and limit setting.
- The physician can use written patient education materials, either commercially or personally formulated, to reinforce guidance provided during the counseling and anticipatory guidance portion of the well-child visit. The physician can also give the parent materials to read *in preparation* for the next well-child visit.
- The physician can use audiovisual materials appropriate for both the child and the parent in the waiting room. Many excellent materials are available.
- The physician can use a nursing assistant to do exit interviewing with the child and family to ensure that all the instructions are clear and to do any further teaching.

Content of the Visits

Interview. The physician should gain a sense of how the child and the family are doing. Are there any stresses? What activities does the parent enjoy doing with the child? Is parenting an overall positive experience? Do the parents have time by themselves? What are the overall supports? The physician should also ask a sufficient number of open-ended questions in order to unearth "hidden complaints." For example, "Is there anything that you are worried or concerned about today?", "Is there anything else that you would like to discuss?", or "Do you have any other questions?" The initial interview should explore the family history, the perinatal history, hospitalizations, accidents, medications, allergies, dietary history, growth and development, habits, behavioral problems, discipline, living conditions, environmental hazards, and a review of systems. Subsequent interviews build on this initial base. Once the child has started to talk,

AGE	INFANCY						EARLY CHILDHOOD					LATE CHILDHOOD					ADOLESCENCE			
	By 1 mo	2 mos	4 mos	6 mos	9 mos	12 mos	15 mos	18 mos	24 mos	3 yrs	4 yrs	5 yrs	6 yrs	8 yrs	10 yrs	12 yrs	14 yrs	16 yrs	18 yrs	20+ yrs
HISTORY Initial/Interval	•	•	•	•	•	•	•	•	•	•	•	•	•	•	•	•	•	•	•	•
MEASUREMENTS Height and Weight	•	•	•	•	•	•	•	•	•	•	•	•	•	•	•	•	•	•	•	•
Head Circumference	•	•	•	•	•	•														
Blood Pressure										•	•	•	•	•	•	•	•	•	•	•
SENSORY SCREENING Vision	S	S	S	S	S	S	S	S	S	O	O	O	O	O	S	O	O	S	O	O
Hearing	S	S	S	S	S	S	S	S	S	S	O	O	S	S	S	O	S	S	O	S
DEVELOPMENT BEHAVIOR ASSESSMENT	•	•	•	•	•	•	•	•	•	•	•	•	•	•	•	•	•	•	•	•
PHYSICAL EXAMINATION	•	•	•	•	•	•	•	•	•	•	•	•	•	•	•	•	•	•	•	•
PROCEDURES Hereditary Metabolic Screening	•																			
Immunization		•	•	•			•	†												
Tuberculin Test						•						•					•			
Hematocrit or Hemoglobin					•				•					•					•	
Urinalysis				•					•					•					•	
ANTICIPATORY GUIDANCE	•	•	•	•	•	•	•	•	•	•	•	•	•	•	•	•	•	•	•	•
INITIAL DENTAL REFERRAL										•										

Key: • = to be performed; S = subjective, by history; O = objective, by standard testing method; † = DPT-4 and OPV-3 if not given at 15 mo.

Figure 8-1. Guidelines for health supervision. (Reprinted with permission from the American Academy of Pediatrics, News and Comment May, 1982)

the physician should interview the child as well as the parent. When the child is in early puberty, the physician should not only interview the patient alone but also the patient and parent together.

Physical Examination. The physical examination should be *complete* and should include the appropriate measurements (Fig. 8-1) and *developmental assessment.* With younger children it is good to initiate the examination by observation and then to proceed with the least threatening part of the examination. The physician can do a good part of the respiratory and neurological examination by observation, and then proceed to examine the chest and abdomen. It is sometimes wise to begin the examination with the child in the mother's lap and to solicit the child's involvement as much as possible. An examination of first the child's doll or teddy bear often helps to dispel anxiety. An older child should be allowed to undress and dress in privacy and to use a gown. Children who are in puberty should be examined without the parent in the room unless the patient wishes otherwise. Female patients who are being examined by a male physician may prefer to have the mother stay in the examining room. Detailed guidelines for the age-appropriate physical examination can be found in several books (Gundy, 1981; Athreya, 1986).

Preventive Care and Periodic Health Screening. The content of the well-child visit recommended by the AAP at various ages is described in Figure 8-1.

Counseling and Anticipatory Guidance. A well-child visit is incomplete without adequate time spent on this topic. In fact, this subject is generally considered the cornerstone of the visit. Specific guidelines for counseling and anticipatory guidance now follow.

SPECIFIC GUIDELINES FOR THE WELL-CHILD VISIT AT DIFFERENT AGES

The American Academy of Pediatrics issued two companion manuals in 1985, *Guidelines for Health Supervision* and *Health Supervision Visit.* These manuals address in good detail the interview, developmental assessment, physical examination, preventive care, and anticipatory guidance for each well-child visit. More abbreviated comments for each well-child visit follow and also a collection of common parental questions with suggested answers that the physician can give.

Prenatal Visit

During this visit, the parents and the physician become acquainted and the parents decide if they want this physician for their expected child. Practice arrangements and philosophy of care should be discussed. Concerns and questions should be solicited from the parents. Generally, feeding should be discussed (breast-feeding versus bottle feeding versus both). Some anticipatory guidance such as the need for a car seat, circumcision if the baby is a boy, and help for the mother, should be provided. Appropriate patient education pamphlets might be given.

Newborn Visit

This is a time of euphoria, exhaustion, and sometimes postpartum blues. A complete physical examination with a close follow-up to detect problems early is important. Parents need to be informed of all procedures and tests, including "nonconsequential" ones. Most families, but especially first-time parents, need repeated reassurance and encouragement. Feeding is discussed, particularly with breast-feeding mothers who may need help with the mechanics (see Chap. 11). Arrangements after discharge should be addressed.

2- to 4-Week Visit

At this visit, various concerns are usually raised by the parents, but they are most often reassured that everything is fine. This is especially important for the breast-feeding mother who may fear that her child is not gaining weight properly. In addition to the interview and the physical examination, common topics to discuss include the parent's exhaustion and how to deal with it, the reaction of siblings to the new baby and how to handle them, the baby's sleep and feeding patterns, and what to do when the baby is fussy. The physician might prescribe vitamins A, D, and C with fluoride and iron for the baby who is being exclusively breast-fed and fluoride for the formula-fed baby who receives no fluoridated water.

2-Month Visit

By this visit, the family is generally more adjusted to the new baby. If the mother is returning to work, child care arrangements need to be discussed. Remind the parents that the babysitter's home needs to be accident-proofed as well as their own. Development is assessed: Is there a social smile, does the child regard the parent's face, does the child respond to sound, does the child coo? Immunizations are normally initiated with oral poliovirus vaccine (OPV) and diphtheria, pertussis, tetanus (DPT). Anticipatory guidance includes safety advice such as not leaving the child on the bed unattended and not drinking a hot beverage while holding the baby. Parents need to be encouraged to start having time "alone." Guidance concerning choosing a babysitter, even if the mother is not returning to work, should be given.

4-Month Visit

By this visit, the baby is generally more responsive to his environment and is happy most of the time. The infant generally sleeps through the night; if not, the parents are often concerned and ask what to do. There are also questions about the addition of solids to the diet. Depending on the philosophy of the physician, solids are slowly introduced at this age or their addition is deferred until 5 or 6 months of age. If the baby is being fed with formula, it should be iron-fortified. Development is assessed: Does the baby laugh or squeal? Does the baby follow objects around the room? Is the baby alert to the human voice? Does the baby hold his head high when put on his stomach? Does the baby try to roll over? Anticipatory guidance should reinforce previous counseling on the necessity of car seats and other pertinent aspects of home safety (see Chap. 18).

Parents may want suggestions on how to play with their baby. Several excellent books are available on this subject (Eden, 1980). DPT and OPV No. 2 are given.

6-Month Visit

A baby at this age is normally highly engaging and a joy to be with. If the parent shows signs of ambivalence, the physician should carefully explore the stresses in the parent's life and determine if supportive intervention, perhaps by a social worker or by an infant stimulation program, is indicated. The parent may possibly only need more time by herself. Development is assessed: Does the baby babble (use vowel sounds)? Is the baby happy most of the time? Does the baby roll over? Does the baby sit with or without support? Does the baby pick up toys? Does the baby transfer toys? Has the baby started showing anxiety toward strangers?

Anticipatory guidance includes a discussion on the need for iron-fortified foods and fluoride in the diet. The parent should avoid using the bottle as a pacifier and not put the child asleep with the bottle because such an action might predispose to "milk caries." Safety instructions are reinforced. Teething and footwear might also be discussed. DPT No. 3 and OPV No. 3 (optional) are given. If the child was premature, a complete blood count (CBC) should be done.

9-Month Visit

By this visit the child will probably show great gains in motor skills. Generally, at this age children are sitting up by themselves, picking up small objects, and playing well with toys. It is common for children this age to pull to stand and crawl: Some are cruising or walking. The child is entering his "dangerous" developmental stage. The parent needs to understand that a child at this age and for the next year will not understand dangers, and thus all hazardous or breakable items should be inaccessible. When this is not possible, rooms should be cordoned off by gates or locks, and closets that contain hazards should be locked. These precautions also make parenting much easier. Language and social interactions are considerably more important developmental milestones to assess than motor skills. Is the child babbling with monosyllables and polysyllables? Does the child respond to his name, "No," or "Where is mama?" Does the child enjoy interactive games? If the child's babbling is decreasing rather than increasing, a hearing evaluation is necessary. Anticipatory guidance will include counseling on "accident-proofing" the home such as the need for window gates for windows on the second floor and higher, and the avoidance of foods that could be aspirated. A *tuberculin test* may be administered and a *hemoglobin/hematocrit* taken at this visit (or at the next one). Many pediatricians obtain a free erythrocyte protoporphyrin (FEP) test at the same time. If it is done separately, a routine FEP screening is usually at 12 months of age. A sickledex is also done when indicated.

12-Month Visit

A baby at this age is usually highly social and interested in exploring his environment. His motor skills make him adept at getting around. He is also developing strong likes and dislikes. Some parents find this developmental stage exciting and others find it highly stressful. Difficulty may arise because parents are no longer completely in control; they are at a loss to manage an active toddler who gets into "trouble" and who does not respond to the word "no." Such parents need kind, supportive intervention. Developmental achievements that should be noted are language and communication: Does the child say one to three meaningful words or sounds? Does he point to what he needs? Anticipatory guidance may address nutrition, accident prevention, and parent–child interactions: Should the baby be switched to whole cow's milk? Should the bottle be stopped? The telephone number of a poison control center should be readily available. What should the parent do about stranger and separation anxiety? The parent should try to spend at least 10 minutes each day reading, playing games, and cuddling with the infant. The parent should also start praising the child for desired behavior. FEP screening is done if the child is at risk of lead exposure.

15-Month Visit

The 15-month-old is usually walking quite well and on the verge of rapid language acquisition. He usually uses much jargon and gestures. The toddler can often understand simple commands such as "Go and get your book" and he is usually more proficient at receptive, rather than expressive, language. The child may also be adept at self-feeding with his fingers and with a spoon. He may know one or two body parts. Anticipatory guidance might include phasing out the bottle and pacifier by 18 months, avoiding a bottle in bed, reinforcing accident-proofing the home including a reminder of the dangers of dangling cords, electrical sockets, plastic bags, unattended water, and small objects that could be aspirated. The child's readiness for bowel and bladder training at 18 or 24 months can be discussed. The topic of discipline can also be raised. The measles–mumps–rubella immunization is generally given at this visit along with the DPT and OPV (as according to the 1986 guidelines).

18-Month Visit

The 18-month-old child is entering the "problem-solving" stage of development. He can make rapid intellectual advances if he is given the proper stimulation. The child can often say four to ten words and frequently more. He can usually express

two or more wants. Motor skills are more refined: he may walk up the stairs with one hand held and he may kick and throw a ball. He will also tend to have a low frustration threshold and may sometimes behave negatively. He is unlikely to share and when he plays with other children, it will probably not be interactive play. Parents who are aware that this is normal development will better be able to cope when their child "misbehaves." Parents should avoid situations in which temper tantrums may be embarrassing and a major source of frustration. For example, taking a child this age to a grocery store or a restaurant is a gamble. Parents also need to know that even though their child seems to understand much more, he still cannot fully understand danger and he is still at high risk of ingesting something poisonous or otherwise harmful such as a small object. The house must therefore be safety-proofed. The physician might also reassure the parents that toilet training can be deferred and that they should have fun with the child. The value of play groups both for the child and the mother might be mentioned. The first DPT and OPV boosters are given at this visit if they were not given with the MMR at the 15-month visit. If an FEP was done at the 9- or 12-month visit, some pediatricians repeat one at this age.

24-Month Visit

At 2 years of age, some of the child's negative behavior may be decreasing. However, the child will have good days and bad days. Language should be well established with a vocabulary of more than 50 words and some two-word phrases. Words may include some pronouns and will be intelligible to parents. A hearing and speech evaluation should be considered if language has not developed to this degree. Anticipatory guidance should re-emphasize accident prevention. Also, it is a good idea to discuss the importance of routines, such as a regular bedtime preceded by reading a story, prayers, and so forth. Toilet training is another topic. If the child is not yet toilet trained, which is common at this age, the parents should not feel frustrated. An explanation about physiologic readiness is helpful. Parents should continue to try to praise the child for good behavior and they should be good role models. Children at this age are great imitators and they are beginning to develop attitudes and habits. Urinalysis may be appropriate at this visit. Some pediatricians would also do a tympanogram and repeat a hematocrit/hemoglobin, tuberculin test, and FEP.

3-Year Visit

The 3-year-old is no longer a toddler. He is very communicative; he thoroughly enjoys being with other children; and he is skilled at pretend play. The 3-year-old can also be defiant at times, which may be a source of frustration. Because of the child's communicative abilities, the parents may have greater expectations than what is developmentally appropriate. Parents should observe and then try to avoid conditions that are most likely to cause the child to decompensate. For example, fatigue is a common precipitant of misbehavior. Parents also need to learn the importance of setting realistic limits and avoiding overindulgence. Limit setting, however, must be balanced by praise for good behavior and by a good deal of love, affection, and "special" times together. Injuries continue to be problematic and continue to need emphasis. This is also the age in which sexual molestation can begin. The child needs to be taught about strangers and the rights that he has in as sensitive a manner as possible. Several children's books, including coloring books, can help in this educational endeavor. The topic of nursery school or play groups should be raised again. At this age, the child usually has his first dental visit and has vision and hearing screening. The physician should also start taking the child's blood pressure and if not previously obtained, do a blood count, administer a tuberculin test, and obtain a urine culture (if the patient is a girl).

4-Year Visit

A 4-year-old is generally self-sufficient. Motor skills are such that the child can walk up and down stairs alternating feet, hop, jump forward, and ride a tricycle well. Fine motor skills are developed so that the child can cut and paste, begin drawing a person with face and arms or face and legs, and copy a cross, circle, and possibly a square. The child can dress and undress with supervision. Parents can begin giving the child more responsibilities, such as setting and clearing the table. They should remember to give praise when deserved. The parent and child can jointly get involved with special projects, such as going together to the museum or to a movie. If there are other siblings in the house, some of these special projects should be done alone with the child if possible. At this visit,

a dental screening is advised and if indicated, a blood count and vision screening done, a tuberculin administered, and a urine culture done in girls. Between 4 and 6 years of age, the second and last DPT and OPV boosters are administered.

5-Year Visit

The 5-year-old is generally in kindergarten or preschool. The child's development should include such tasks as naming four or five colors, knowing his age, defining at least one word, and drawing a person with head, body, arms, and legs. If the child is in school, the physician should seek feedback on how the child is progressing and, if there are problems, evaluate the situation more thoroughly. Since there is a great variability in development from one child to another, sometimes school "readiness" and placement need to be addressed (see Chap. 37). Educational consultants can assist in this task. Parents should again be counseled about safety; the need for the child to know his name, telephone, and address; how to approach strangers (and *vice versa*); and discipline. The child at this age will have sexual curiosities. Parents need to answer questions at the child's level and not answer more than what the child actually asks. If parents feel uncomfortable about a particular question, they can defer an answer until the child is older and better able to understand. Pejorative explanations and accusations of "dirtiness" must be avoided. Screening procedures vary from one physician to another but they may include a tuberculin test, a blood count, urinalysis, vision, and audiometry. The child should be advised to have a dental check-up.

6-Year Visit

The 6-year-old may be in the first grade. The same issues that relate to school readiness in the 5-year-old are also important for the 6-year-old. In terms of developmental achievements, the 6-year-old may be able to ride a bicycle, tie his shoelaces, count to ten, print his first name and numbers up to ten, know right from left, and draw a person with six parts including clothes. The physician should inquire about the child's social interactions with his family and peers. Good health habits need to be reinforced, such as avoiding junk food, eating a balanced diet, the need for adequate exercise and sleep, and good dental care. The importance of special times with the parents, the use of appropriate praise, and the importance of responsibilities in the home are reiterated. If the physician sees that the child needs adult role models other than those available at home and in school, the physician can recommend a good after-school program or other programs such as the Big Brother Program.

8-Year Visit

The 8-year-old is generally in third grade and is beginning to read reasonably well. He can also tell the time, take care of himself and his belongings, and participate more fully in household activities and chores. The physician should ask about school—attitudes, academic performance, and social interaction. Good health habits are again discussed.

Television viewing should be included in the discussion. Television viewing should be limited and the child not allowed to watch violent or sexually provocative programs. Parents should have fair rules in the house and try to avoid being too harsh. Praise and affection are still important and will continue to be so as long as the child is in the home. The parents should become involved in the school and they should actively seek feedback from the teacher for means by which they can help their child. Any academic problems should be vigorously addressed. Office screening tests done at this visit are variable but they may include a tuberculin test and vision screening. Dental screening should be done at least yearly.

10-Year Visit

A 10-year-old is usually sophisticated. Some 10-year-old girls are pubertal. It is wise to do a substantial portion of the interview with the child as well as with the parent. If the physician senses tension, it is prudent to speak to the child and parent separately. The physician should get a sense for how the child is doing in general, what sorts of things he likes to do, how he is progressing at school, what kind of feelings he has, whether he has friends, and what activities he and his friends do together. Health habits and safety issues should be discussed. The physician should explore the level of communication between the parents and the child. If there is not open, supportive communication, then counseling is indicated. Screening procedures done at this visit may include a blood count, urinalysis, vision screening, audiometry, and a tuberculin test.

12-Year Visit

This young adolescent should not only be examined alone but also with the parents and he should be asked questions similar to those asked of the 10-year-old. The physician should also explore sexuality issues and drug or alcohol experimentation. Since these are delicate subjects and since it may take several visits before the teenager can trust the physician, the physician might say to the patient, "I'm going to ask you some questions about your personal life and your social life and if you would rather not answer them, that's okay. The reason I'm asking them is so that I can be of help to you and I will not tell your parents what you say to me unless you give me permission." The physician should also explore school issues, hobbies, the family life-style, and the level of communication between the patient and his family. Guidance should be given on good health habits, safety, and issues related to rapid physical and sexual changes. Parents need to be reminded to respect the patient's privacy, to have rules in the home but not overly harsh ones, to continue to have special times together, and to foster open communication. Parents may also need counseling on "danger signs" to look for in terms of drug and alcohol abuse and depression.

14-Year Visit

Children in this age range are still variable in terms of development and maturity. Some behave like prepubescent children and others behave like adults. Despite these differences in behavior, most teenagers at this age are somewhat insecure about relationships with others. They are also concerned about their body images and they are strongly influenced by peer pressure. Such issues are important for the physician to discuss alone with the patient and reassure him that these feelings are normal and that they will pass with time. Parents need to be aware that "acting out" behavior is often a reflection of insecurity underneath the surface and that they should deal with unacceptable behavior not only with consistent rules, but also with love, affection, time, and sympathetic listening. A response of anger tends only to increase the schism that frequently develops between parents and teenagers. The parents should remind themselves when they are upset of the basic worth of their teenager as a human being. Parents should also strive to be excellent role models and they should not have double standards. The physician should ask about school, likes, dislikes, performance, extracurricular activities, and hobbies. Whenever possible, the physician should try to encourage and praise the teenager. Either at this visit or the next one, girls should be instructed in breast self-examination and boys in testicular self-examination. Screening tests done at this visit might include a blood count, vision screen, tuberculin test, and rubella titer. A tetanus and diphtheria (Td) booster should be given if 10 years have elapsed since the last DPT. Female adolescents should be referred for gynecologic care if the primary physician does not provide it himself.

16-Year Visit

All teenagers should be in puberty by this age. Once again it is good to interview the parents and the teenager separately. The physician should specifically discuss with the teenager alone sexuality issues including birth control because this is often an area of conflict. Many issues previously raised should be raised again. It is also appropriate for the physician to discuss plans after high school graduation. Office screening tests are the same as for the 14-year-old except for rubella titer and Td.

18-Year Visit

The 18-year-old is legally an adult. He can now vote, enlist in the military, and drive. The process of emotional maturation, however, will continue for many years. The patient continues to require understanding, support, and encouragement from his family, friends, and physician. The physician should discuss many of the previous issues: school, work, home situation, social outlets, sexuality, and habits including drugs or alcohol. A discussion on communication (and if necessary how to improve it) is appropriate. A discussion on future plans and aspirations should also be held. The patient needs to be counseled concerning good ongoing health maintenance, including gynecologic care. If the patient is being seen by a pediatrician and will be transferred to an internist, this transition should be discussed and made as smoothly and as easily as possible.

COMMON PROBLEMS ENCOUNTERED BY THE PARENT OF THE INFANT

Crying

In infants less than 3 months, it is normal for the child to cry 1 to 3 hours a day. Infants will usually cry for physiologic reasons such as hunger, tiredness, excessive gas, wet or dirty diapers, and loneliness. The crying usually stops when the needs are met. It is common for a baby to have a "fussy" period, which often occurs in the evening. If the baby is not responsive to the usual comforting measures, the physician should make sure there are no underlying causes. (For a more extensive discussion on crying and colic, see Chap. 204.)

Colic

Many physicians do not like the term "colic" because of the connotations it has for many parents. Colic basically refers to paroxysms of irritability. These paroxysms occur in healthy, well-fed infants, and they are often associated with the infant drawing up his legs as though in pain, often for more than 3 hours a day. Classically, colic begins at about 2 weeks of age and lasts until about 16 weeks of age. It is frequently worse in the evening and it is often attributed to an immature digestive system.

Colic is frustrating to manage. Various therapies have been used, none of which is consistently successful. The first two modalities are often helpful, whereas the other ones are usually ineffective.

- Picking up the infant and carrying him around
- Rocking the infant; exposing the infant to other motion such as car rides
- Placing a small hot water bottle on the abdomen
- Using small doses of antacids or antiflatulents
- Using GRIP Water
- Removing all dairy products from the mother's diet if she is breast-feeding on the chance that the child has a milk allergy
- Changing formula from cow's milk to soy on the chance that the child has a milk allergy

In the past, many physicians used antispasmodics combined with barbiturates, but these are generally not used today because of side effects and possible overdosage.

Parents with a "colicky" baby need a great deal of support and empathy. Since a screaming child can be a major stress, they should be encouraged to have some time by themselves if at all possible. They should also be reminded that the condition is only temporary (see also Chap. 204).

Sleep

It is normal for a baby to get up in the middle of the night for the first few months of life. Some babies develop a pattern of sleeping during the day and keeping awake most of the night. Parents can slowly reverse this pattern of sleep by awakening the child earlier and earlier during his lengthy daytime naps (see Chap. 29 for a more detailed discussion on sleep disturbances).

As the child gets older, parents can also develop

routines that will promote good sleep habits, such as the following:

• A regular bedtime
• Avoiding excessive stimulation to the child while the child is sleeping (*e.g.*, the room should be dark, there should be little noise, the child should sleep alone)
• Not responding to the first cry. Occasionally, children will cry in their sleep and then stop.

Diet

Every physician has his own style of giving dietary advice. Some guidelines, however, are generally accepted. Breast milk or formula should be the major source of nutrition for the first 5 to 6 months of life. If the mother is breast-feeding exclusively, the child should receive a vitamin D (400 U) and fluoride (0.25 mg) supplementation daily. If the child is fed on formula, the child should use an iron-fortified formula and should receive a fluoride supplementation unless the formula is reconstituted with fluoridated water. When the child is drinking more than 32 oz of formula a day, many physicians would start the child on cereal and then add fruits or vegetables, one at a time. Meats are generally introduced into the diet at 6 to 8 months of age. Parents may use a mill to grind table foods but they should avoid foods with added salt or simple sugars.

COMMON PROBLEMS ENCOUNTERED BY THE PARENT OF THE TODDLER

Sleep

It is normal for a child to have periodic wakening during the night. If a child awakens and cries or calls for the parent, the child should be reassured of his parent's presence and love. The parent should make sure the child is not sick, and then leave the room. The parent should not stimulate the child further by playing with him or feeding him. After being comforted, the child may cry himself to sleep. When the child realizes that night time is sleeping time both for himself and his parents, his night-time awakening will lessen (see Chap. 29).

Tantrums, Including Breath-holding Spells

During a tantrum, the parent should make sure the child is safe and then ignore the act. When the child is not having a tantrum, the parent should be generous with love and attention.

Behavior and Discipline

As a child's verbal skills progress, many parents overestimate their toddler's ability to control his behavior. Thus, the "terrible twos" evolve. Some hints to decrease the stress include the following:

• Decrease the number of temptations to which the toddler is exposed. If the toddler continually hears the word "no" from his parents, he will learn how to say "no" very well; furthermore, if the toddler continually has his hand slapped he will learn how to hit very well. Examples of temptations are leaving breakable items in easy reach of the toddler or taking the toddler to the grocery store.
• Try to anticipate misbehavior on the part of the toddler and distract him before it happens (Brenner, 1983).

Toilet Training

Toilet training requires patience on the part of the parent. It is common even for a precocious child not to be toilet trained until 3 years of age, but it happens sooner or later. Toilet training should be viewed as any other developmental task: It should be regarded as a skill for the child to acquire, such as walking or climbing the stairs, rather than as a task for parents to accomplish.

Most children are not ready to be introduced to the potty or toilet until they are 24 months old. At that time, the parent may choose to purchase a small potty that the child can play with, sit on, or have his doll sit on. When the child expresses a need to urinate, the child should be put on the potty. The child should not be coerced to sit on the potty if he shows no interest whatsoever, nor should the child be overly praised for success on the potty; praise should be consistent with praise given for other accomplishments.

Some authorities advocate gradually guiding a child to the use of the potty starting at age 2. During the first week the child is brought to sit on the potty fully clothed for as long as he likes. During the second week he sits on the potty without a diaper and, as before, he is not coerced. No attempt is made to catch urine. During the third or fourth week he is brought to the potty after he has wet his diaper. The dirty diaper is placed in the potty to show the child where eventually the urine or stool should go. Subsequent to these introductory weeks, the child is periodically put on the potty and encouraged to urinate or defecate. In the case of boys, it is advisable to teach them to urinate standing up. They can learn this behavior from their fathers.

Diet

Any child who is not destined to be obese as a child will demonstrate a decreased appetite. This decrease in appetite frustrates almost every parent. The physician can reassure the parents by showing them the child's normal growth curve. The physician should encourage the parent to feed the child the wholesome foods that he likes. Most children in this age range like cheese, pasta, juice, and fruit (see Chap. 30).

Preparing for the New Sibling and Sibling Rivalry

Preparing a child for a new sibling may help decrease some of the trauma of the arrival of the new sibling. Since a toddler and preschooler both have a distorted sense of time, it is probably appropriate to begin the process when the mother is in her last trimester and "showing." Parents will have different ways to introduce the topic. They may want to use one or more of the excellent books written for children who are expecting a new brother or sister or who already have one. The parents should generally make the child feel a part of the team that is expecting the new baby and they should emphasize to the older child how important he is in their lives. Many hospitals now also have a special tour of the delivery room and postpartum floor for children prior to their mothers' deliveries. The same hospitals also allow sibling visitation after delivery. Such programs allow the older sibling to understand his mother's absence from the home and to see "his" baby very early on. It is conceivable that some sibling "bonding" may occur. Nevertheless, in spite of these measures, the older child may still regress in his behavior. Parents should try to tolerate this regression and not pay much attention to it. Other ways to help the older child cope are:

- Parents should remove the child from the baby should he strike out against the baby. The parents should also allow the child to hold and cuddle the baby under close supervision when the older child is in a nonaggressive mood.
- The parents should take turns spending special times with the older child.
- The older child should be made to feel important in his new role as the older sibling. Parents can solicit the older child's opinion: such as, "Why

do you think—is crying? What do you think we can do?" Parents can also ask the older child to help with some small tasks.
- Parents should make a concerted effort not to show favoritism.

Biting, Kicking, and Sharing

Biting and kicking are behaviors that are common between the ages of 15 months and 36 months. Frequently, they are signs that social demands, such as sharing and waiting a turn, are being placed on a child who is not mature enough to handle these demands.

Parents need to be advised that biting is a "normal" response to a stressful situation. They should try to provide play situations that are less stressful (e.g., ones that do not require ongoing sharing). They should try to anticipate biting and direct the child's attention or have him bite on something inanimate such as a wet washrag. They should *not* bite back.

With regard to sharing and interactive play, parents need to be aware that this does not occur easily until the child is about 3 years old. If the child has a temper tantrum about sharing, it is best to remove the child or the object from the situation.

COMMON PROBLEMS ENCOUNTERED BY THE PARENT OF THE PRESCHOOLER

Diet

The problem is the same as for the toddler, if not worse, and the same principles of management apply. If the child has totally eliminated all calcium-containing foods from his diet, the physician might recommend children's chewable calcium tablets. Otherwise, dietary sources of calcium other than milk should be encouraged, such as cheese or yogurt.

Behavior and Discipline

The "terrible twos" are sometimes replaced by the "defiant" threes. One can often reason with children this age and make "deals." Occasionally, "time out" is required for misbehavior. "Time out" can mean sitting on a chair in the corner for a few minutes until the child has gained control of himself. Corporal punishment should be reserved for the most serious offenses. Frequent spankings become meaningless and just convey to the child that hitting is okay. Parents should also try to evaluate underlying causes for misbehavior and make appropriate interventions. For example, is the child misbehaving because he is tired, or because he is bored, or because he needs more time with his parents?

Lying and Stealing

Preschoolers have big imaginations and they have difficulty distinguishing between truth and nontruth, their own possessions and those belonging to others. Parents of preschoolers who "lie" or "steal" should not be harsh with them; they should instead gently correct and be good role models.

School

Children at about 2½ or 3 years become highly social and enjoy interactive play. Parents should be encouraged to provide their child with opportunities to interact with other children of the same age. This can be done in nursery school or in play groups supervised by parents.

Nightmares or Night Terrors

Nightmares occur commonly in children. A child with a nightmare wakes up fully; he is anxious; and he has excellent recall of the bad dream. Nightmares are generally infrequent and require no intervention except reassurance and affection from the parents. Occasionally, however, nightmares will be frequent, in which case they may indicate some environmental stress in the child's life. The content of the bad dream may be a clue.

Nightmares should be distinguished from night terrors. Night terrors occur in 5% or less of children and are characterized by a child who is out of control but still "asleep." There is no recall of the event on the child's part. Night terrors are generally infrequent and require no therapy. In those rare cases in which they are frequent, a more thorough social, psychiatric, and sleep evaluation are appropriate with an option for pharmacologic therapy (see Chap. 29).

Imaginary Playmates

Approximately 10% to 30% of children between the ages of 3 years and 5 years have imaginary companions. It is more common in first-born children and in girls. Parents need to know that this play is normal and they should not be worried about it. Rarely, a child may be so involved in his imaginary world that he appears to have difficulty distinguishing the real from the unreal. In such a situation, the parents should encourage more activities with real persons and less time alone.

COMMON PROBLEMS ENCOUNTERED BY THE PARENT OF THE SCHOOL-AGED CHILD

School Problems

It is good to gain some assessment as to how a child is doing the first few years in school. If a problem becomes apparent, active intervention is required. This may include a conference with the child's teacher, perhaps a psychometric evaluation, and if a learning disability is suspected, an evaluation by a learning disability consultant or clinic (see Chap. 41 for a more complete discussion).

Crying

Some school-aged children cry easily. This reflects their sensitivity. They should not be criticized and called "cry-baby," but rather told that it is okay for even boys and adults to cry. If the child is embarrassed about crying easily, the parents and physician can offer suggestions on how he can control his emotions.

Lying and Stealing

When these activities occur in the child aged 6 and older, the physician and parents should carefully look for reasons for this behavior. Does the child feel too much pressure so that he is forced into lying? Is the child fearful that the punishment will be too harsh? Is the child needy? Is the child being strongly influenced by a group of friends?

Parents should show love and attention while setting limits. Parents must also set good examples by being truthful and honest. Children who lie or steal should be corrected and, where appropriate, the misdeed should be rectified without undue embarrassment and humiliation.

COMMON PROBLEMS ENCOUNTERED BY THE PARENT OF THE ADOLESCENT

Drugs

In our present society, it is almost impossible for a teenager to escape exposure to drugs. It is important for both the physician and parent to recognize the danger signs. An excellent review on the subject is given in an article by George D. Comerci and the warning signs that he enumerates are quoted *verbatum*:

1. Poor school performance and attendance
2. Mood swings more pronounced than those usually experienced by teenagers
3. Recent change from age-appropriate "acceptable" friends to older, unacceptable associates
4. Increased interest in the drug culture, manifested by possession of drug literature, paraphernalia, and clothing such as belt buckles and T-shirts with a drug theme
5. A change to sloppy dress and poor grooming and hygiene
6. A rebellious and paranoid flavor to all interpersonal relationships with adults, siblings, and authority figures

Immediate intervention is indicated if a physician feels that a patient has a high potential for drug abuse or that he has already started experimentation. This will include counseling both of the teenager and the parents and may include referral to a drug treatment program. It is not uncommon for the parents of a drug-using teenager to be overindulgent, permissive, and uninvolved in the teenager's life. These issues need to be included in any counseling program (see Chap. 177).

Suicide

Suicide is considered to be of epidemic proportions in the 15- to 24-year-old age range. Individuals who attempt suicide often feel an overwhelming sense of hopelessness and loneliness and they feel that their lives are not worth anything. These individuals frequently have such high expectations for themselves that they are almost "destined" to feel like chronic failures. Physicians and parents need to be sensitive to these personality traits and they should intervene when such traits are seen. Healthy, open communication between the parents or another adult role model and the teenager are critical in detecting early signs and also in the prevention of suicide (see Chap. 35).

Pregnancy

Many teenagers are sexually active. By the age of 15 to 19, 50% of women in metropolitan areas have had sexual intercourse. It is important for the physician to develop a trusting relationship with the teenage girl and to frankly ask her in private what her sexual activities are. Birth control may be indicated (see Chap. 42).

ANNOTATED BIBLIOGRAPHY

American Academy of Pediatrics: Guidelines for Health Supervision. Elk Grove Village, IL, 1985 (Another more expanded presentation of guidelines for conducting well-child care.)

American Academy of Pediatrics: Report of the Committee on Infectious Diseases. Elk Grove Village, IL, 1986 (Comprehensive reference book that covers all aspects of immunizations, recommendations for care of children in special circumstances (*e.g.*, day care, isolation, and sexually transmitted diseases), summaries of infectious diseases, and information on antimicrobials and antimicrobial prophylaxis.)

American Academy of Pediatrics: Standards of Child Health Care. Evanston IL, American Academy of Pediatrics, 1977 (Manual that outlines delivery of perinatal care, preventive child health care, and care of the child during illness. It also contains guidelines for equipment, procedures, and office facilities needed for child health care. It includes a chapter on the use of nonphysician health personnel. It is complemented by a large appendix of clinically useful information.)

Athreya BH, Silverman BK: Pediatric Physical Diagnosis. E. Norwalk, CT, Appleton–Century–Crofts, 1986

Block RW, Rash FC: Handbook of Behavioral Pediatrics. Chicago, Searle Book Medical Publishers, 1981 (Excellent, easily read manual that addresses such topics as anticipatory guidance, behavior modification, antisocial behaviors, "He's driving me crazy" behaviors, eating problems, depression and suicide, sleep problems and school problems, among other topics.)

Brenner B: Love and Discipline. New York, Ballantine, 1983 (Excellent book on the topic of discipline.)

Comerci GD: Recognizing the five stages of substance abuse. Contemp Pediatr August, 1985, pp 57–66.

Eden N: Positive Parenting. New York, Signet, 1980 (Useful paperback for parents of children up to the age of 3 years. Each chapter addresses a specific age range and includes information on growth and development, nutrition, exercise and play, safety, toys, and other practical topics.)

Gundy JH: Assessment of the Child in Primary Health Care. New York, McGraw–Hill, 1981

Illingsworth RS: The Normal Child—Some Problems of the Early Years and Their Treatment. London, Churchill Livingstone, 1979 (More lengthy book that addresses most issues related to the normal child. Its chapter on development and the evaluation of development is noteworthy.)

9
Genetic Risk Factors
JANICE D. KEY

Genetics plays an important role in general pediatrics. Genetic histories are obtained at every initial pediatric visit when a complete family history is taken to help determine which diseases a child is at risk of developing and to evaluate the child with multiple birth defects. Birth defects are present in 2% to 4% of newborns and are the major cause of morbity and mortality in the neonatal period. This chapter is concerned with general topics important in the prenatal and family history of the patient as well as an evaluation of the newborn. A detailed discussion of the hundreds of genetics conditions will not be attempted. Further information can be found in the excellent references listed in the annotated bibliography.

FAMILY HISTORY

Usually at the initial visit, regardless of the age of the patient, a complete family history is obtained, often by having the patient or parent answer a questionnaire listing numerous conditions such as hypertension, stroke, atopia, mental illness as well as more classic mendelian conditions such as sickle cell disease. In general, little information is available regarding what exact risk their presence imparts to the patient. For most, all that can be said is that there is an increased risk, the exact value of which is not known.

Atopic Disease

Atopic disease is a common finding in the family history. It is not a strict mendelian condition, meaning that it does not follow the inheritance pattern of an autosomal dominant or recessive or sex-linked condition. However, as all practitioners know, there appear to be increased numbers of family members with various forms of atopic disease in an affected patient's family. A single family may have members with different expressions of atopic disease including asthma, eczema, allergic rhinitis, and other allergies. In retrospective analysis of family histories of patients with atopic disease, there are positive family histories in 80% as opposed to

20% among control families. There is also an increased concordance of 50% in monozygotic twins.

Diabetes Mellitus

Diabetes mellitus is another example of a condition with a strong genetic component. Diabetes is caused by a heterogeneous group of etiologies. The most common cause is "idiopathic" but diabetes may also be associated with specific genetic syndromes, most of which are rare. Both type I, insulin-dependent diabetes mellitus (DM), and type II, adult-onset or noninsulin-dependent DM have some evidence of a genetic component. There is an increased family history of diabetes in families of diabetics (25% to 50% compared to 15% of controls). Glucose tolerance tests are more likely to be abnormal in relatives of diabetics. There is an increase concordance in monozygotic twins, especially for type II. An association of type I diabetes mellitus with certain HLA types (specifically B8, B15, Dw3, and Dw4) has been found. In practical terms, this indicates that there may be a general genetic tendency to develop diabetes but that other factors besides genetics are important. The empiric risk is 4% to 6% for siblings of an affected patient and 1% to 2% for offspring.

Ethnic Origin

Ethnic origin is important in determining what conditions the child will be at increased risk of having and whether screening tests should be done. Some of the various ethnic groups and the more common conditions within those groups are outlined.

American Black Population. The American black population has a increased incidence of several hemoglobinopathies, the most common of which is sickle cell (SS) disease. Sickle cell trait has a incidence of 1:12 and SS disease of 1:600 newborn black infants. Although the trait has no medical significance, patients with SS disease have numerous serious medical problems (see Chap. 125). Black children should be screened as soon as possible for sickle cell disease. Some hospitals screen cord blood. Newborns with positive tests are identified before their first febrile illness and hopefully penicillin prophylaxis will have already begun. If it has not been performed, screening can be done at about 6 weeks, when the fetal hemoglobin has usually decreased. Regardless of age, if a patient has not had SS screening, it should still be done. Other fairly common hemoglobinopathies of the B hemoglobin gene in the black population are Hb C and β-thalassemia. Hb C trait is found in 3% of blacks and therefore the incidence of SC disease (the combination of one sickle cell gene and one Hb C gene) is 1:800 black newborns. A patient with SC disease has similar clinical findings and course as does a patient with sickle cell disease, but usually milder. β-Thalassemia results from inheriting the β-thalassemia gene either on one chromosome 11 resulting in β-thalassemia trait or on both chromosomes resulting in β-thalassemia. The course of β-thalassemia in blacks is milder than that seen in the Mediterranian form and is referred to as β-thalassemia intermedia.

The black population has also a high incidence of α-thalassemia trait. There is a total of four genes for the α-hemoglobin chain (two on each chromosome 16). Two abnormal genes will result in α-thalassemia trait. In the form carried by the black population, these two mutated genes are always on the opposite chromosomes (one is abnormal on each chromosome and is referred to as the "trans"configuration). A child cannot have more than two abnormal genes and therefore clinically has the trait even if both parents carry the α-thalassemia trait. This form of α-thalassemia is designated α-thal$_2$. 2% to 5% of black newborns are α-thal$_2$ homozygotes and an estimate 28% are α-thal$_2$ carriers. Clinically, α-thal$_2$ homozygotes have microcytosis with a normal electrophoresis but no other symptoms.

Glucose-6-phosphate dehydrogenase (G6PD) deficiency is the most common abnormal genetic trait in humans and has a high incidence in the black population. It is an x-linked recessive condition affecting 10% of black males. The specific mutation found in the black population is G6PD A- which has 10% to 20% of normal activity. Therefore, affected patients usually only have hemolysis when they are exposed to specific drugs.

White Population

The white population has specific diseases in increased frequency in each subpopulation. Overall, cystic fibrosis is the most common genetic disease in the white population. It is an autosomal recessive disease with a carrier rate in whites of 1:50 and an incidence of 1:2000 (see Chap. 205). There is currently no reliable method of carrier detection. The *Irish* population have an increased risk of neural tube defects including spina bifida and anencephaly. Whereas the incidence of neural tube defects overall in the United States is about 1:2000, the incidence in babies of Irish descent is estimated to be 1:400. Other diseases with an increased incidence are Tay–Sachs disease in both the Jewish and French-Canadian populations and tyrosinemia in French Canadians. Both these conditions are autosomal recessive. Carrier detection and prenatal diagnosis are available in Tay–Sachs disease.

The Mediterranian-descent population has an increased risk for both G6PD deficiency and β-thalassemia. As mentioned before, the Mediterranian forms of both these diseases are more severe than in the black population. The Mediterranian variant of G6PD has only 0.5% of normal activity and may clinically result in chronic hemolysis exacerbated by any stress or medication causing increased hemolysis. The β-thalassemia major in the Mediterranian population is the classical Cooley's anemia with severe anemia and extramedullary hematopoeisis.

Oriental Population

The oriental population has an increased incidence of α-thalassemia; however, it differs from that seen in the black population in that the deleted α-hemoglobin genes are both missing from the same chromosome 16 (the cis configuration). Therefore, when both parents carry the α-thalassemia trait, there is a 25% risk that the child will inherit these two abnormal chromosomes and will have no α-hemoglobin genes. The affected infant will have hydrops fetalis and severe disease. Prenatal diagnosis is available for this form of α-thalassemia.

PRENATAL HISTORY

Teratogens

Exposure to teratogens is an important aspect of the prenatal history. A positive history of exposure to a particular teratogen should be noted even if the infant is unaffected at birth, because many subtle effects such as learning defects and hyperactivity will be come apparent with time. Only some of the more common or the most severe teratogens are discussed here. More information about specific drugs taken prenatally can be obtained from teratology hotlines, texts, and from the drug company that manufactures the drug.

In the general category of *anticonvulsants*, dilantin and valproic acid are proven teratogens. *Fetal hydantoin syndrome* has been well described and may include multiple birth defects such as congenital heart disease, dysmorphic facial features (*e.g.*, hypertelorism, flattened nasal bridge, epicanthal folds), and hypoplastic nails as well as central nervous system effects such as microcephaly and mental retardation. Of all exposed infants, about 1:10 will have one or more of these serious birth defects. More subtle effects not recognized at birth may been seen in more exposed infants, perhaps up to 1:3. These effects may include learning disorders and hyperactivity. *Valproic acid* has only recently been recognized as a teratogen and therefore the full spectrum of its effects is not clearly described. There is an increased risk of neural tube defects if the developing fetus was exposed to valproic acid during the closure of the neural tube. This risk is then increased from the baseline 1:2000 overall risk to about 1:200 (a ten-fold increase). Other associated birth defects such as mental retardation, congenital heart disease, and dysmorphic facial features have been reported, but the exact risk of these defects is unknown.

Isoretinoic acid has been a recently recognized and highly publicized severe teratogen. The infant, if exposed prenatally, has a high risk of multiple birth defects that may include mental retardation, congenital heart disease, and dysmorphic features. Structural central nervous system defects such as hydrocephalus may also occur.

Another severe teratogen (not commonly used during pregnancy) is *warfarin*. One third of exposed infants will suffer serious effects such as growth deficiency, developmental delays, microcephaly, and dysmorphic features (especially a hypoplastic nose).

Probably the most common teratogen is *alcohol*. *Fetal alcohol syndrome* was first recognized in the offspring of chronic alcoholics where it affects at least one third of exposed newborns. Its features include mental retardation which is usually mild, growth deficiency, congenital heart disease, joint abnormalities, and dysmorphic facial features (*e.g.*, a long, flattened philtrum with thin upper vermillion, hypertelorism, and narrow palpebral fissures). There may also be a risk of these birth defects as well as less obvious effects such as hyperactivity and learning problems with less alcohol exposure. The absolutely safe dose of alcohol below which

there is no risk is unknown. The amount and timing (trimester) of alcohol exposure should always be noted in a prenatal history even if there is no obvious defect at the time of birth because it may be important information several years later if the child is having problems in school.

Other Medications

There are many other medications commonly used during pregnancy that patients often ask about, especially if their usage is elicited during the interview. *Aspirin* is usually taken at some point in the pregnancy. Although massive doses of aspirin, especially in the third trimester, have been associated with fetal hemorrhage and perhaps with patent ductus arteriosus, there is no increased risk of birth defects from occasional use. *Valium* was thought to be associated with cleft lip and palate, but more recent controlled studies indicate that there is no increased risk with use of valium. *Acetaminophen*, like aspirin, has not been proven to be a teratogen. Use of *marijuana* and *cocaine* has not been shown to cause birth defects. *Smoking* does have a well known negative effect on fetal growth, which is dose dependent. It also increases the risk for spontaneous abortions, miscarriage, prematurity, and neonatal deaths. It is not associated with structural birth defects. *Caffeine* use, when separated from concomitant smoking, does not have a proven negative effect.

Maternal Medical Conditions

Maternal medical conditions can influence the outcome of the pregnancy and the possibility that the baby will have neonatal problems or congenital defects. *Diabetes mellitus* is a common condition that may cause an increased risk of both. The exact risk for each pregnancy depends on the classification of the mother's diabetes and her control during pregnancy. As expected, the worse the classification and the poorer the control, the higher the risk to the pregnancy. Transient neonatal effects seen in infants of diabetic mothers include large size at birth, hypoglycemia, hypocalcemia, and polycythemia. There is also a risk to the fetus of having congenital defects such as congenital heart disease, neural tube defect, and syringomyelia.

Maternal *epilepsy* causes an increased risk of defects independent of medication. Patients who do not take anticonvulsants have only a slightly higher risk of defects and patients who do take anticonvulsants have about a 10% overall risk. The exact risk depends on the anticonvulsant.

Maternal *infection* can cause specific neonatal problems when the infection is transmitted to the fetus. The TORCH infections are the classic example. However, in other types of infections where the fetus is not directly infected by the pathogen, there may be a teratogenic effect from the fever alone. Hot tubs, saunas, or any other extreme heat may result in a rise in internal body temperature and should be avoided during pregnancy. Sustained *fever* of 102° to 104°C for several days can cause severe defects, the exact nature of which depends on the stage of embryogenesis. Most of the defects that have been described affect the central nervous system. The most severe cases have occurred from first-trimester exposure, but second-trimester exposure may also cause severe mental retardation.

Maternal *age* is related directly to some specific risks for the fetus. With advancing maternal age, there is an increased risk of an autosomal aneuploidy in the fetus, with trisomy 21 being the most common in live-born infants. The risk does not rise at a rapid rate with each year until after age 35, and it rises at an even faster rate after age 40. There is not an increased risk for other nonchromosomal birth defects in offspring of older healthy mothers. Although in 15% to 20% of cases of trisomy 21, the extra chromosome 21 can be identified as paternal in origin, there does not seem to be the increased risk of aneuploidy with increasing paternal age.

Paternal Conditions

Paternal conditions and drug exposure have not been associated with increased risk to the fetus in most cases. The exception to this is the direct genetic risk of inheriting a condition. Even paternal exposure to such powerful agents as dioxin and Agent Orange has not been proven to cause an increased overall risk of birth defects or be associated with specific defects.

PRENATAL TESTING

Maternal Serum Alphafetoprotein

Increasingly, a common screening test performed in all pregnancies is maternal serum alphafetoprotein (MSAFP). AFP normally increases in the maternal serum with the advancing pregnancy until it reaches a peak in the second trimester. Conditions that are associated with an abnormally high MSAFP (greater than 2.5 standard

deviations from the median) are multiple gestations, neural tube defects, ventral wall defects (*e.g.*, omphalocele or gastroschisis), congenital nephrotic syndrome, cystic hygroma, and nonspecific problems such as small-for-gestational-age infants, and prematurity. If MSAFP is low, there is an increased risk of trisomy 21. The exact value that is defined as low is dependent on the maternal age.

Ultrasound

Ultrasound is the second most commonly performed prenatal screening test. There are numerous indications for its use, most of which are obstetrical. Ultrasound can visualize gross birth defects; for example, it may detect a large ventricular septal defect (VSD) but not an atrial septal defect (ASD). It can also give important information about fetal size. The defects detected by ultrasound are often not lethal and will not result in abortion, but they will have medical implications in the care of the newborn.

Amniocentesis

Amniocentesis is a prenatal test that is performed on many otherwise normal pregnancies because of the mother's age. The test is offered currently to all women who are, or will be, 35 years or older at their due date. This is because of the increased risk of autosomal trisomies (most commonly trisomy 21), but any chromosomal abnormality will be detected. Some of these conditions may not result in an abortion such as Turner syndrome or Klinefelter syndrome, but they may cause the child to be at increased risk for certain abnormalities and learning problems. In addition to advanced maternal age, an amniocentesis may be indicated because the couple had a previous child with a chromosomal defect and have, therefore, an increased chance of recurrence (*e.g.*, when they have had a child with trisomy 21 the risk of having another child with trisomy 21 increases to about 1% despite a young maternal age). Amniocentesis may also be done when a parent is known to carry a chromosomal abnormality such as a balanced translocation.

Aside from chromosomal analysis, amniocentesis is used for enzyme analysis and DNA analysis for certain specific defects. This would only occur when the parents are known to carry a certain inherited condition either by carrier detection or by their already having an affected child. Tay–Sachs disease is an autosomal-recessive condition for which there is a widely used screening test to detect carriers. If both parents are carriers, then amniocentesis can be performed to detect Tay–Sachs disease in the fetus. In some cases, however, the enzyme or protein defective in the disease is not produced in fibroblasts, and direct deoxyribonucleic acid (DNA) analysis may be done to detect the gene for the disease. One example is sickle cell disease which can now be diagnosed using DNA restriction analysis; whereas until recently a sample of fetal blood was necessary.

A new technique that may become widely used in the future is *chorionic villus sampling* (CVS). It also involves collecting a sample of fetal tissue through suctioning a piece of the chorion surrounding the fetus, which can then be used for chromosomal, enzyme, or DNA analysis. It has the advantage of being done at an earlier gestation (at 10 weeks compared to an amniocentesis which is done at 16 weeks). The risk to the fetus of miscarriage or birth defects due to the procedure is not well established but appears to be higher than the risk of amniocentesis.

EVALUATION OF THE NEWBORN

Phenylketonuria

Phenylketonuria (PKU) and elevated blood phenylalanine may be caused by several different conditions. Classical PKU is an autosomal recessive caused by a deficiency of hepatic phenylalanine hydroxylase. It results in a very elevated phenylalanine (at least above 12 mg/dl in the newborn) that remains elevated unless the patient is treated with a low phenylalanine diet. If the patient is not treated, he will have severe mental retardation and often seizures and autism. The patient will be normal if treatment is begun in the newborn period and continues throughout at least childhood. Other hyperphenylalaninemias result in a positive screen. Transient hyperphenylalaninemia is one and, as its name implies, requires no treatment. Persistent mild hyperphenylalaninemia will cause a chronically elevated phenylalanine level but not cause mental retardation and therefore doe not require treatment. The third much more serious condition is dihydropteridine reductase deficiency, which is an autosomal recessive like PKU but causes severe neurologic deficits despite dietary treatment.

PKU may be important not only in childhood when dietary treatment is necessary but also in adolescence and adulthood because of the teratogenic effect of maternal PKU on the fetus. If not treated during pregnancy, maternal PKU may cause birth defects such as microcephaly and congenital heart disease in offspring. Therefore, as a patient with PKU enters adolescence, this information and contraception should be available to her.

Hypothyroidism

Hypothyroidism is usually the second screening test done. Although strictly speaking not a genetic condition, early detection and treatment will prevent mental retardation. Hypothyroidism may have various etiologies, from agenesis of the thyroid to ectopic hypoplastic thyroid. Screening is done by measuring T_4 and, if low, measuring thyroid-stimulating hormone (TSH). Hypothyroidism is found in one of 4000 to 5000 newborns. If left untreated, it will result in poor growth and mental retardation (see Chap. 73).

Galactosemia

Galactosemia may be included in neonatal screening. Elevated serum galactose may be caused by several conditions. Classical galactosemia is caused by a deficiency of galactose-1-phosphate uridyl transferase. If not treated with a galactose-free diet, failure to thrive, hepatomegaly and liver failure, and an increased risk of sepsis will occur. Long-term sequelae include mental retardation and cataracts. It is autosomal recessive and is detected by enzyme measurement. Galactokinase deficiency may also cause an elevated galactose but is different clinically from classical galactosemia. It will cause late onset (in early adulthood) cataracts if it is left untreated. Finally, uridine diphosphate galactose-4-epimerase deficiency will cause an elevated galactose but no clinical effects.

Other conditions that may be included in neonatal screening vary. Homocystinuria due to a deficiency of cystathionine β-synthetase results in mental retardation, ectopia lentis, vascular obstruction, and musculoskeletal problems and can be treated with a low methionine and pyridoxine diet. Maple syrup urine disease is caused by a deficiency of any one of several enzymes involved in decarboxylation of derivatives of leucine, isoleucine, and valine. It results in neurologic abnormalities and may be improved by dietary treatment.

APPROACH TO A CHILD WITH A BIRTH DEFECT

Approximately 2% to 4% of liveborn infants have a major birth defect requiring medical attention. Many defects will be isolated in an otherwise normal child but others will be found in conjunction with several other defects. Each newborn with a defect should be fully evaluated to ascertain if other associated defects are present; if there is an overall unifying diagnosis; and to inform the family of the prognosis for the child and the risk of a recurrence in future children. Besides a careful physical examination, several approaches will be helpful in this evaluation, including analysis of each defect, family history, and a differential diagnosis of each defect.

Analysis of each birth defect includes careful measurement to document that feature. The eyes, for example, appear close set both in hypertelorism (where there is a true increase in distance between orbits) and in telecanthus (where there is an increase in distance between the two inner canthi but the orbits are normally placed).

Family history should be detailed with particular emphasis on teratogenic exposures during pregnancy and history in the family of any related findings. An examination should also be made of the parents for any similar features. For example, familial megalencephaly may be a benign trait, or a child with a cleft lip may have a parent with small pits in his lips indicating an autosomal-dominant condition (van der Woude syndrome).

After each finding is fully characterized, a differential diagnosis for each should be made using texts of birth defects as a reference source. Most of the differential can be eliminated because of essential features for each syndrome that the patient does not have. The remaining differential for each birth defect can be compared for common diagnoses.

A correct diagnosis should be obtained as soon as possible for several reasons. The most immediate reason is the impact it will have in the medical management of that child. Once a particular diagnosis has been made, the patient should be further evaluated for other associated defects that have not already been diagnosed. The prognosis and treatment can then be determined.

The genetic risk factors in a patient's history can be used throughout his life to improve his medical care. These may include diagnosis of a condition prenatally, preventive care for a known condition, or better diagnosis and treatment of a condition that occurs later in life (*e.g.*, an evaluation of hyperactivity in a child exposed to alcohol prenatally). Thus, knowledge about genetic risk factors improves the care that a general pediatrician can provide.

ANNOTATED BIBLIOGRAPHY

Emery AEH, Rimoin DL (eds): Principles and Practice of Medical Genetics. New York, Churchill Livingstone, 1983 (Exhaustive text on most genetic disorders including their biochemistry or pathophysiology when applicable. An excellent resource for reading about any particular disorder.)

McKusick VA: Mendelian Inheritance in Man, 5th ed. Baltimore, The Johns Hopkins University Press, 1978 (Computerized catalog of thousands of disorders that are proven to be, or are hypothesized to be, mendelianly inherited. It includes recent references for each disorder and a short discussion.)

Smith DW: Recognizable Patterns of Human Malformation, 3rd ed. Philadelphia, WB Saunders, 1982 (Very readable, brief description with accompanying photographs of numerous dysmorphic syndromes. The last chapter contains tables of normal standards for anthropomorphic measurements and facial feature measurements. The appendix is helpful and has a differential diagnosis for many dysmorphic features and birth defects.)

10
Immunizations

MARGARET B. RENNELS

There are currently eight infectious diseases for which routine immunizations in childhood are recommended. Vaccine development is an active field leading to continual additions and refinements in the arsenal of vaccines. There has also been a marked improvement in the delivery of vaccines to almost all segments of our population of children. When, in 1977, it was estimated that one third of the children in the United States between 1 and 4 years of age were not fully immunized, the Department of Health and Human Services launched a Childhood Immunization Initiative. Over 90% of children entering school in 1980 received the recommended immunizations as a result of increased federal support for immunization programs and the enactment of laws in all 50 states requiring documentation of immunity as a condition of a child's first entry into school. All physicians are responsible for providing child health supervision to maintain and improve this record, because immunization levels in the United States are still inferior to those of many other developed countries.

GENERAL ISSUES

Informed Consent

Parents should be told of the benefits and risks of each of the vaccines that their child is to receive. The Center for Disease Control has developed for each of the recommended routine vaccines "Important Information Statements" which are useful aids for educating parents and can also be used for written informed consent. These statements are continually updated as new information becomes available. They can be obtained through local health departments.

Record Keeping

All 50 states have now developed a standard immunization record that is to be kept by the parents. Because evaluation of the safety and efficacy of a vaccine is an ongoing process, optimally, the following data should also be entered into the child's medical record: date, vaccine, manufacturer, batch number, expiration date, site, and route. Physicians are obligated to report unexpected reactions occurring within 1 month of vaccination and vaccine failures to the manufacturer and local health department which will then forward the information to federal agencies.

Logistics of Injection

Refer to the package insert for the route and dose, which may vary with the manufacturer, or even the batch, of the same vaccine. It is preferable to use disposable syringes and needles and discard them after one use. Each vaccine should be given in a separate site. After insertion of the needle, draw back on the plunger; if blood appears in the syringe, remove and change the needle and use a new site. Intramuscular injections are given in the anterolateral thigh of infants or the deltoid of older children with a 1 to 1¼-inch long, 20- or 22-gauge needle. Subcutaneous or intradermal injections should be given using a ⅝-inch-long, 25-gauge needle.

Scheduling

Postpone the vaccination if the child is experiencing a febrile illness; a mild afebrile upper respiratory illness does not contraindicate vaccination. If a child's immunization status cannot be determined, he should be considered susceptible and should be vaccinated. A lapse in the routine schedule of immunizations does not interfere with the immune response; therefore, it is unnecessary to reinstate or repeat doses. Reduced doses or multiple small doses are not recommended because they may not induce an adequate immune response.

Update Information

Recommendations regarding vaccinations are constantly changing; therefore, textbook chapters such as this should not be one's sole source of information. Vaccination updates appear periodically in the *Morbidity and Mortality Weekly Report* and *Pediatrics*. An additional valuable and recommended resource is the American Academy of Pediatrics' Report of the Committee on Infectious Diseases, or *Redbook*.

SPECIAL CIRCUMSTANCES

Premature Infants

It is common practice to begin immunization of premature infants at 2 months' chronologic age, if they are clinically stable. Limited data suggest an adequate immune response and no increase in reactions at that age. Oral polio vaccine should not be administered to hospitalized infants because of the possibility of transmission of the vaccine virus to an immunosuppressed infant.

Immunosuppression

No live viral vaccines should be given to individuals who have immunodeficiency diseases or who are undergoing immunosuppressive therapy. Topical steroid therapy should not contraindicate immunization unless it results in systemic immunosuppression.

Immunoglobulin

Live viral vaccines should generally not be given within 3 months of receipt of an immunoglobulin preparation because immunoglobulins may interfere with the replication of the vaccine virus and the immune response. If it is is necessary to give immunoglobulin within 14 days after immunization with a live viral vaccine, repeat the vaccination in 3 months.

Table 10-1.   Recommended Schedule for Active Immunization
of Normal Infants and Children

RECOMMENDED AGE*	VACCINE(S)†	COMMENTS
2 mo	DPT-1, OPV-1	Can be given earlier in areas of high endemicity
4 mo	DPT-2, OPV-2	A 6-wk to 2-mo interval is desired between OPV doses to avoid interference.
6 mo	DPT-3	An additional dose of OPV at this time is optional for use in areas with a high risk of polio exposure.
15 mo	MMR, DPT-4, OPV-3	Completion of primary series
18 mo	DPT-4, OPV-3	DPT-4 and OPV-3 may be given if not administered with MMR at 15 mo‡
24 mo	Hib§	High-risk groups‖ may be immunized at 18 mo and then reimmunized at ≥24 mo.
4–6 yr#	DPT-5. OPV-4	Preferably at or before school entry
14–16 yr	Td	Repeated every 10 years throughout life

* These recommended ages should not be construed as absolute (*i.e.*, 2 mo can be 6–10 weeks, and so forth).
† Consult manufacturer's package for instructions for storage, handling, and administration of all products used.
‡ This alternative is especially for patients who are compliant with health care recommendations.
§ *Hemophilus influenzae* type b polysaccharide vaccine.
‖ Children with anatomic or functional asplenia, malignancies associated with immunosuppression or in day-care.
# Up to the seventh birthday.
DPT = diphtheria and tetanus toxoids and pertussis vaccine; MMR = live measles, mumps, and rubella viruses in a combined vaccine; OPV = oral, attenuated polivirus vaccine contains poliovirus types 1, 2, and 3; Td = adult tetanus toxoid and diphtheria toxoid in combination, which contains the same dose of tetanus toxoid as DPT or DT and a reduced dose of diphtheria toxoid. (Adapted from the Centers for Disease Control: New recommended schedule for active immunization of normal infants and children. Morbidity and Mortality Weekly Report 35:577, 1986

DIPHTHERIA, TETANUS, AND PERTUSSIS VACCINES

Formulations

The diphtheria (D) and tetanus (T) vaccines are formaldehyde-inactivated toxins of the respective bacteria; pertussis (P) vaccine, currently licensed in the United States, consists of whole inactivated *Bordetella pertussis* cells. These three vaccines are each available separately and in the following combinations: DPT, DT, and Td.

Vaccine Usage

The recommended schedules of vaccinations are shown in Tables 10-1, 10-2, and 10-3. Children between 6 *weeks through 6 years* should receive a primary series of four immunizations with DPT beginning at 6 to 8 weeks of age. The first three doses are given at 4- to 8-week intervals and the fourth

administered 6 to 12 months after the third. A booster DPT is then given at age 4 to 6 years, before school entry; this booster is unnecessary if the fourth DPT was given after the fourth birthday. *After 7 years of age* the dose of diphtheria vaccine is lowered and routine pertussis immunization is not recommended because side effects are more common in older children. Individuals in whom vaccination is initiated after age 7 years should receive a primary series of three doses of Td; given the second dose 4 to 8 weeks after the first and the third dose 6 to 12 months after the second. Booster doses of Td are recommended every 10 years.

Special Circumstances

When pertussis vaccination is contraindicated for a child under 7 years (see the following precautions and contraindications) the DT combination is substituted for DPT. If immunization is initiated

Table 10-2. Recommended Immunization Schedule for Infants and Children Up to 7th Birthday Not Immunized at the Recommended Time in Early Infancy*

TIMING	VACCINE(S)	COMMENTS
First visit	DPT-1, OPV-1, (if child is ≥15 mo of age, MMR)	DPT, OPV, and MMR can be administered simultaneously to children ≥15 mo of age.
2 mo after first DPT, OPV	DPT-2, OPV-2	
2 mo after second DPT	DPT-3	An additional dose of OPV at this time is optional for use in areas with a high risk of polio exposure.
6–12 mo after third DPT	DPT-4, OPV-3	
24 mo (up to 60 mo)	Hib†	
Preschool† (4–6 yr)	DPT-5, OPV-4	Preferably at or before school entry
14–16 yr	Td	Repeat every 10 years throughout life.

* If initiated in the first year of life, give DPT-1, 2, and 3, OPV-1 and 2 according to this schedule and give MMR when the child is 15 months old.
† *Hemophilus influenzae* type b polysaccharide vaccine.
‡ The preschool dose is not necessary if the fourth dose of DPT and the third dose of OPV are administered after the fourth birthday.
DPT = diphtheria and tetanus toxoids with pertussis vaccine (DPT may be used up to the seventh birthday); MMR = live measles, mumps, and rubella viruses in a combined vaccine; OPV = oral, attenuated poliovirus vaccine contains poliovirus types 1, 2, and 3; Td = adult tetanus toxoid and diphtheria toxoid in combination, which contains the same dose of tetanus toxoid as DPT or DT and a reduced dose of diphtheria toxoid. (Adapted from the Centers for Disease Control: General recommendations on immunization. Morbidity and Mortality Weekly Report 32:5, 1983.)

prior to 1 year of age simply follow the schedule as for DPT in Table 10-1. Children who received their first vaccination after the first birthday need to be given only three primary doses of DT (the second 4 to 8 weeks after the first and the third 6 to 12 months later). *Infections with diphtheria or tetanus* may not confer protection; therefore, vaccination should be performed. *Pertussis infection* is gener-

ally followed by lifelong immunity; children who have had disease confirmed by culture to be due to *B. pertussis* need not receive further immunization. *Tetanus prophylaxis for wounds* varies depending on the nature of the wound and the person's immunization history. Patients with minor, uncontaminated wounds who have already received a primary series of three tetanus immunizations require a

Table 10-3. Recommended Immunization Schedule for Persons 7 Years of Age or Older

TIMING	VACCINE(S)	COMMENTS
First visit	Td-1,* OPV-1,† and MMR‡	OPV is not routinely administered to those ≥18 years of age.
2 mo after first Td, OPV	Td-2, OPV-2	
6–12 mo after second Td, OPV	Td-3, OPV-3	OPV-3 may be given as soon as 6 weeks after OPV-2.
10 years after Td-3	Td	Repeat every 10 years throughout life.

* Td—Tetanus and diphtheria toxoids (adult type) are used after the seventh birthday. The DPT doses given to children under age 7 who remain incompletely immunized at age 7 or older should be counted as prior exposure to tetanus and diphtheria toxoids (*e.g.*, a child who previously received 2 doses of DPT, needs only 1 dose of Td to complete a primary series).
† OPV—Oral, attenuated poliovirus vaccine contains poliovirus types 1, 2, and 3. When polio vaccine is to be given to individuals 18 years or older, IPV is preferred.
‡ MMR—Live measles, mumps, and rubella viruses in a combined vaccine.
(Adapted from the Centers for Disease Control: General recommendations on immunization. Morbidity and Mortality Weekly Report 32:6, 1983.)

Table 10-4. Adverse Events Occurring Within 48 Hours of DPT Immunizations

EVENT	FREQUENCY*
Local	
Redness	1:3 doses
Swelling	2:5 doses
Pain	1:2 doses
Mild/moderate systemic	
Fever ≥38 C (100.4°F)	1:2 doses
Drowsiness	1:3 doses
Fretfulness	1:2 doses
Vomiting	1:15 doses
Anorexia	1:5 doses
More serious systemic	
Persistent, inconsolable crying (duration ≥3 hours)	1:100 doses
High-pitched, unusual cry	1:900 doses
Fever ≥40.5°C (≥105°F)	1:330 doses
Collapse (hypotonic-hyporesponsive episode)	1:1,750 doses
Convulsions (with or without fever)	1:1,750 doses
Acute encephalopathy	1:110,000 doses
Permanent neurologic deficit	1:310,000 doses

* Frequency of adverse events, regardless of dose number in DPT series, occurring within 7 days of DPT immunization. (Adapted from Centers for Disease Control: Diphtheria, tetanus and pertussis: Guidelines for vaccine prophylaxis and other preventive measures. Morbidity and Mortality Weekly Report 34:411, 1985)

booster only if the last tetanus injection was given over 10 years ago. Administer a tetanus booster if the patient with a clean, minor wound has not received the primary series or if the vaccination history is unknown. The management of all other wounds is as follows: (1) if the patient has received three tetanus immunizations in the past, give a booster if more than 5 years has elapsed since the last dose; (2) a person whose primary series was incomplete or immunization history unclear should be given both a tetanus booster and tetanus immune globulin (250U, IM) at separate sites. In all of these situations, DPT (DT, if pertussis vaccine is contraindicated) is preferred to tetanus toxoid alone for children under 7 years of age and Td is preferred to tetanus toxoid alone in those children older than 7 years.

Side Effects and Adverse Reactions

Local erythema, induration, or tenderness occur commonly following immunization with DPT (Table 10-4); occasionally, a nodule and rarely an abscess will form at the injection site. Mild to moderate systemic reactions are also frequently seen

(e.g., fever, drowsiness, fretfulness, or anorexia); these symptoms are significantly more common following immunization with DPT than DT. More serious systemic events occur infrequently; these include fever ≥40.5°C, persistent, inconsolable crying (crying for 3 or more hours), unusual high-pitched crying, collapse (hypotonic-hyporesponsive episode), and convulsions. Catastrophic adverse reactions including prolonged seizures, encephalopathy, permanent neurologic deficits, and anaphylactic reactions have rarely been reported associated with DPT administration. The local reactions and fever are encountered with increasing doses in the series, whereas the other mild to moderate systemic events are more common following the early doses.

Precautions and Contraindications

Further immunization with pertussis vaccine is absolutely contraindicated if any of the following have occurred after receipt of DPT or P: (1) allergic hypersensitivity, (2) fever ≥40.5°C within 48 hours, (3) persistent, inconsolable crying for ≥3 hours, (4) high-pitched, unusual crying occurring within 48 hours, (5) convulsions (febrile or afebrile) within 3 days, or (6) encephalopathy within 7 days. The question of whether or not to vaccinate a child who has, or is suspected of having, a neurologic disorder or who has experienced one or more seizures should be made on an individual basis. It is prudent to delay initiating or repeating immunization with DT or DPT until the child's neurologic status is clarified. Pertussis vaccination is contraindicated in conditions that are characterized by changing neurologic or acquired findings (i.e., uncontrolled epilepsy, infantile spasms, or progressive encephalopathy), because further immunizations may coincide with or even exacerbate symptoms. Immunization with DPT may be given to children with stable or resolved neurologic conditions such as well-controlled seizures, cerebral palsy, and shunted hydrocephalus without seizures. The occurrence of a single seizure, unassociated with DPT administration, need not necessarily contraindicate vaccination, particularly if the cause is determined. Children who have experienced seizures (febrile or afebrile) may have a slightly increased risk of post-immunization convulsions. Parents should be informed of this risk and consideration should be given to administering anticonvulsant prophylaxis if these children are vaccinated. The Immunization Practices Advisory Committee of the Public Health Service (ACIP) and the Committee on Infectious

Diseases of the American Academy of Pediatrics (AAP) do not presently consider a family history of convulsions or other central nervous system disorders a contraindication to pertussis vaccination. It may be reasonable to administer an antipyretic for 2 to 3 days following DPT vaccination to children with personal or family histories of seizures. The decision whether to vaccinate a child with a neurologic disorder should be made by 12 months of age, taking into consideration the underlying disorder, the risk of exposure to infection, and the risk of vaccination.

The only contraindication to diphtheria or tetanus toxoid is a history of a neurologic reaction or a severe hypersensitivity reaction following a previous dose. Individuals who have experienced an Arthus–type hypersensitivity reaction or a temperature of $\geq 39.4°C$ following tetanus vaccination should not receive tetanus toxoid more frequently than one time every 10 years, even if they suffer a wound that is neither minor nor clean.

Conclusions

Fear of a rare serious side effect from pertussis vaccination must not deter routine immunization. The benefits of the current vaccine clearly outweigh the risks. Pertussis is not a rare or benign infection. When immunization levels fell in Japan and Great Britain, large epidemics with significant morbidity and mortality occurred. A less reactogenic vaccine against pertussis may become available in several years. An acellular product has been developed in Japan that consists of a toxoid (formalin-treated, lymphocytosis-promoting factor) and a possible attachment factor (filamentous hemagglutinin) derived from the bacterium. This vaccine has been used in Japan since 1981 and, although vigorously controlled studies are not available, it appears to produce far fewer side effects and to be as protective as the whole cell vaccine. Preliminary safety and immunogenicity testing of a similar vaccine is underway in the United States (see Chap. 196).

POLIOVIRUS VACCINES

Formulations

Oral polio vaccine (OPV) and inactivated polio vaccine (IPV) are licensed in the United States; both contain all three strains of poliovirus. OPV consists of live attenuated poliovirus and is given by mouth, whereas IPV is killed virus that is administered parenterally. OPV is currently recommended as the preferred vaccine for primary immunization of immunocompetent children in the United States. The advantages of OPV over IPV are that it is simple to administer, fewer doses are required, it induces intestinal immunity, and the excretion of vaccine virus in the stools results in vaccination of some contacts. The disadvantage of the OPV is that there is a rare association with paralytic disease in vaccine recipients or their contacts (1 case : 2.64 million doses distributed). Parents should be informed of the option of IPV and the benefits and risks of both vaccines.

Vaccine Usage

OPV is given as a primary series of three doses integrated with DPT (see Tables 10-1, 10-2, and 10-3); in high risk areas it is recommended that an additional dose be given in the first 6 months of life. A booster dose of OPV is then given before the child starts school, at 4 to 6 years of age. IPV is given integrated with DPT as four primary doses. The first three injections of IPV should be divided by 4- to 8-week intervals and the fourth is administered 6 to 12 months after the third. A fifth supplementary dose of IPV is required between 4 and 6 years of age; this injection is omitted if the fourth dose was given after 4 years of age. Thereafter, a booster dose of IPV should be administered every 5 years until the individual is 18 years old. It is preferable to immunize with only OPV or IPV; if a combination of the two is used, a 4-dose primary regimen should be given, followed by a supplementary dose when the child starts school.

Special Circumstances

Because OPV is shed in the stools, *inadequately immunized adult contacts* have a small risk (~4 cases/year) of developing OPV-associated paralytic disease. The routine procedure in the United States is to inform the parent of this small risk and administer OPV to the child, regardless of the vaccination status of the adults in the household. If prompt immunization of the child can be assured, adult contacts may be given a series of IPV prior to administering OPV to the child. Under no circumstances should OPV be given to *immunosuppressed persons or their household contacts*; IPV should be used to vaccinate these individuals. If OPV has been given inadvertently to a household-type contact of a person who is immunosuppressed, the two people should avoid contact for 1 month.

Adverse Reactions

IPV contains trace amounts of streptomycin and neomycin; individuals allergic to these antibiotics may experience a hypersensitivity reaction. There is a rare occurrence of paralytic poliomyelitis associated with OPV administration.

MEASLES, MUMPS, AND RUBELLA VACCINES

Vaccines consisting of live, attenuated strains of measles, mumps, and rubella were licensed in the United States in the 1960s. Routine immunization of young children has resulted in a greater than 95% reduction in the incidence of each of these infections and has prevented major epidemics. Very few cases of congenital rubella (~2 cases/year) are now reported. A change in the epidemiology of measles and rubella has occurred as a result of vaccination programs. Whereas mumps is still primarily a disease of young children, the age incidence of measles and rubella has shifted upward. Outbreaks of rubella and measles in adolescent and young adult populations continue to be a problem that requires attention.

Vaccine Usage

These vaccines are available as the following preparations: measles, mumps, rubella, measles–rubella, mumps–rubella, measles–mumps–rubella (MMR). All of these preparations must be stored at 2°C to 8°C or colder and protected from light. Because optimal seroresponse to measles vaccination may not occur until 15 months of age, it is recommended that children be routinely immunized with the combined MMR at age 15 months. The MMR is now recommended to be given at the same time as the DPT and OPV. Data indicate that immunogenicity and reactogenicity are similar to when the vaccines are administered separately. Additionally, increased efforts on the part of all physicians should be directed to vaccinating or revaccinating susceptible adolescents and young adults against measles and rubella. A person should be considered susceptible and should be vaccinated unless he has proof of adequate immunization with live vaccine on or after the first birthday, laboratory evidence of immunity (any antibody titer) or, in the case of measles, a history of infection diagnosed by a physician. A person who previously received killed measles vaccine has a small risk of experiencing an extensive local reaction and prolonged fever following receipt of live measles vaccine. It is the consensus of the ACIP that this risk of revaccination is outweighed by the risk of severe atypical measles which individuals who received killed measles vaccine may develop when exposed to the wild measles virus.

Precautions and Contraindications

Pregnant women should not be vaccinated with measles, mumps, or rubella vaccine because there is a theoretical possibility of risk to a fetus. It is sufficient to ask women of child-bearing age if they are pregnant; to exclude from vaccination those who say they are; and to explain to the others that they should not conceive for 3 months after vaccination. Measles and mumps vaccines are grown in chick embryo cell cultures; anyone who has a history of an *anaphylactoid reaction to egg ingestion* (*e.g.*, hives, swelling of the mouth or throat, difficulty in breathing, or hypotension) should be vaccinated with extreme caution. Because trace amounts of neomycin are contained in the measles, mumps, and rubella vaccines, persons who have experienced an *anaphylactoid reaction to neomycin* should not be given these vaccines. Unlike OPV, MMR vaccine virus is not transmitted; close contacts of immunosuppressed persons should be vaccinated. Skin testing for *tuberculosis* is not a prerequisite for measles vaccination; however, vaccination may suppress the reaction to tuberculin skin tests. If tuberculosis testing is to be done, it should be performed on the day of vaccination or 4 to 6 weeks after measles immunization.

Side Effects and Adverse Reactions

Following *measles* vaccinations, approximately 5% of children will experience a transient rash and 5% to 10% will have a high fever (≥39.4°C) beginning around the sixth day and lasting up to 5 days. There have been reports of subacute sclerosing panencephalitis occurring in vaccine recipients who have no history of wild measles virus infection. These cases may be either a consequence of unrecognized natural measles in the first year of life or from the vaccine virus. It is reassuring that the incidence of subacute sclerosing panencephalitis has declined since the introduction of the measles vaccine. Temporally associated reactions that are uncommonly to rarely associated with *mumps* vaccination are allergic reactions and central nervous system abnormalities (*e.g.*, febrile seizures, unilateral nerve deafness, or encephalitis). It is not known whether the association is causal or simply temporal; the background incidence of nervous system dysfunction in the normal population exceeds that observed the month following mumps immunization. Children vaccinated against *rubella* sometimes experience a low-grade fever, rash, and lymphadenopathy. Uncommonly (~3%), children will develop arthralgia. Arthritis is rare in children but up to 15% of adult women will develop it. The other side effect that is rarely associated with the rubella vaccine is transient neuritic complaints, including parasthesias and pain in the extremities.

HEMOPHILUS INFLUENZAE TYPE B VACCINE

Formulation

A vaccine composed of the purified, capsular polysaccharide of *H. influenzae* type b was licensed in 1985. Unfortunately, this vaccine is poorly immunogenic in young children. Levels of anticapsular antibody thought to correlate with protection are achieved in approximately 75% of children 18 to 24 months and 90% of children 24 to 35 months of age. Field trials in Finland demonstrated 90% protective efficacy in 18- to 71-month-olds. The currently available vaccine is not efficacious in children less than 18 months of age. In spite of lack of effectiveness in the age group at greatest risk for invasive *H. influenzae* type b (Hib) disease, licensure of the vaccine is justified because 40% of invasive infections occur in children over 18 months and 25% occur in those older than 24 months of age.

Vaccine Usage

Immunization of the general childhood population is recommended at 24 months of age; children who did not receive vaccine at that time should be immunized up to 5 years of age (60 months). Children who have had invasive *H. influenzae* type b infection when they were under 2 years of age should receive the vaccine because they may not have developed an immune response. The ACIP states that immunization of children in high-risk groups for *H. influenzae* type b disease should be considered at 18 months of age. High-risk groups include children in group day care, individuals with functional or anatomic asplenia, and persons with malignancies associated with immunosuppression. Because response to the vaccine in children between 18 and 24 months is not consistent, the ACIP suggests reimmunization 2 to 12 months after the initial dose, but not before 24 months of age. The

AAP has deferred making a recommendation regarding early vaccination of these high-risk children until more data are available. Factors that should be considered when deciding at what age to vaccinate children include the child's risk of disease; the probable lower efficacy of vaccination at 18 months; and whether the child will be brought back for immunization at 24 months of age. If a child is vaccinated at 18 to 23 months, the parents should be informed that protection may not result. Older children with chronic conditions associated with enhanced risk of *H. influenzae* type b disease (*e.g.*, asplenia, Hodgkin's disease) may benefit from vaccination. The AAP recommends that they receive one dose of vaccine; the ACIP has chosen to postpone making a recommendation until more information is available. Simultaneous administration of Hib and DPT may be performed at separate sites. There is also no known contraindication to administering Hib and pneumococcal vaccine at the same time at separate sites.

Side Effects, Adverse Reactions, and Contraindications

Hib appears to be a safe, well-tolerated vaccine. Approximately 2% of recipients develop a local reaction, and fever (>101.3°F) is seen in less than 1% of patients vaccinated. One serious systemic reaction has been reported; a child experienced a possible anaphylactoid reaction that responded promptly to epinephrine. Individuals with known hypersensitivity to any components of the vaccine, including thimerosal, should not be immunized.

Conclusion

The present vaccine is a first step in the control of *H. influenzae* type b disease through immunoprophylaxis. Second generation vaccines, in which the Hib polysaccharide is conjugated to a protein antigen such as diphtheria toxoid, have been developed. Preliminary evidence suggests that conjugated vaccines are substantially more immunogenic in young infants. Field trials of conjugate vaccines are currently underway in infants less than 1 year of age.

VACCINATIONS FOR SELECTED POPULATIONS

Several vaccines that are not part of the routine childhood immunization program are required for children with certain chronic medical conditions.

Table 10-5. Recommended Vaccinations for Selected Populations

VACCINE	FORMULATION	TARGET POPULATION	USAGE*
Pneumococcal	23-valent polysaccharide vaccine	Children ≥2 yr with anatomic or functional asplenia; nephrotic syndrome; CSF leaks; conditions associated with immunosuppression	0.5 ml SQ or IM
Meningococcal	Quadrivalent A, C, Y, W-135 polysaccharide vaccine	Children† with anatomic or functional asplenia; terminal C' component deficiencies	0.5 ml SQ
Influenza	Killed influenza strains, generally 2A and 1B strains	Highest priority are individuals with chronic cardiovascular or pulmonary disorders severe enough to require regular medical follow-up or hospitalization in the preceding year or persons who reside in a chronic care facility.	≥12 years of age‡ 0.5 ml of whole or split virus 1 dose
		High priority are those children on long-term aspirin therapy or with chronic metabolic diseases (including diabetes mellitus), renal dysfunction, anemia, immunosuppression, or asthma severe enough to require regular medical follow-up or hospitalization in the preceding year. Vaccination is recommended for providers of care to and household contacts of high-risk people.	3–12 yr‡ 0.5 ml of split virus 2 doses separated by ≥4 weeks 6–35 mo‡ 0.25 ml of split virus 2 doses§ separated by ≥4 weeks

* Check package insert for manufacturer's recommended dose and route.
† The C, Y, and W-135 polysaccharides are immunogenic in children over 2 yr; serogroup A induces antibody in some children as young as 3 mo.
‡ Based on recommendations for 1987–1988.
§ One dose is usually sufficient if vaccinated against influenza during last 6 years.

Indications for and details of administration of pneumococcal, meningococcal, and influenza vaccines are listed in Table 10-5. (Refer to the bibliography for more information on these vaccines and to Chap. 110 for a discussion of the hepatitis B vaccine.)

FUTURE

In the next several years, improved vaccines may become available against *B. pertussis* and *H. influenzae* type b infection. A live attenuated varicella vaccine, which was developed in Japan in 1974, has been tested both in Japan and the United States and has been found to be highly effective and acceptably safe, even in children with leukemia. This varicella vaccine may be licensed in the future. Promising advances toward the development of a vaccine against rotavirus diarrhea are occurring. Attenuated animal strains of rotavirus administered orally are being evaluated in field trials; preliminary results indicate that they are safe and efficacious. As these accomplishments have been achieved, serious problems threaten the vaccination program in this country. The number of lawsuits and the magnitude of the claims being made against vaccine manufacturers are jeopardizing the continuing production of vaccines and the development of new vaccines. A partial solution to the problem may be the recently passed Federal vaccine injury compensation legislation.

BIBLIOGRAPHY

Centers for Disease Control: Diphtheria, tetanus, and pertussis: Guidelines for vaccine prophylaxis and other preventive measures. Morbidity Mortality Weekly Report 34:405–426, 1985

Centers for Disease Control: General recommendations on immunization. Morbidity Mortality Weekly Report 32:1–17, 1983

Centers for Disease Control: Measles prevention. Morbidity Mortality Weekly Report 31:217–231, 1982

Centers for Disease Control: Meningococcal vaccines. Morbidity Mortality Weekly Report 34:255–259, 1985

Centers for Disease Control: Mumps vaccine. Morbidity Mortality Weekly Report 31:617–625, 1982

Centers for Disease Control: New recommended schedule for active immunization of normal infants and children. Morbidity Mortality Weekly Report 35:577–579, 1986.

Centers for Disease Control: Poliomyelitis prevention. Morbidity Mortality Weekly Report 31:22–34, 1982

Centers for Disease Control: Polysaccharide vaccine for prevention of *Haemophilus influenzae* type b disease. Morbidity Mortality Weekly Report 34:202–205, 1985

Centers for Disease Control: Prevention and control of influenza. Morbidity Mortality Weekly Report 34:261–275, 1985

Centers for Disease Control: Rubella prevention. Morbidity Mortality Weekly Report 33:301–318, 1984

Centers for Disease Control: Update: Pneumococcal polysaccharide vaccine usage—United States. Morbidity Mortality Weekly Report 33:273–281, 1984

Centers for Disease Control: Update: Prevention of *Hemophilus influenzae* type b disease. Morbidity Mortality Weekly Report 35:170-180, 1986

Committee on Infectious Diseases: *Hemophilus* type b polysaccharide vaccine. Pediatrics 76:322–324, 1985

Committee on Infectious Diseases: Pertussis vaccine. Pediatrics 74:303–305, 1984

Committee on Infectious Diseases: Report: 1986 Red Book, 20th ed. Elk Grove Village, IL, Committee on Infectious Diseases, 1986

11

Breast-Feeding

KATHERINE C. TEETS GRIMM

Women have breast-fed since the beginning of time. Breast-feeding is a subject that is often made needlessly complicated. As a result, many women who are breast-feeding for the first time are anxious as to whether they can be "successful" at it. Most women can be, but some may require much counseling, because it is a skill that may not "come naturally." Many books have been written about breast-feeding, including several books specifically for the medical profession: these books should be referred to for more detail.

ADVANTAGES

The advantages of breast-feeding include the following:

- *Promotion of maternal–infant bonding*: Breast-feeding not only encourages eye-to-eye contact but also close body contact and touch. Such closeness fosters the bonding process.
- *Excellent nutrition with good digestibility*: Breast milk contains all the essential nutrients required for good growth with the possible exception of vitamin D. It is high in fat and lactose and low in casein and sodium. The low casein promotes good digestibility. The stools of breast-fed infants tend to be soft and easier to evacuate than those of formula-fed infants.
- *Allergen free*: The proteins of breast milk are species-specific and are therefore nonallergenic. Occasionally, foreign proteins that the mother ingests, such as from cow's milk, pass through the breast milk and sensitize the infant. "Colic" in a breast-fed baby can sometimes be relieved by the elimination of cow's milk products from the mother's diet.
- *Soluble and cellular immune protection*: This includes secretory IgA as well as other immunoglobulins, macrophages, lymphocytes, other cellular elements, chemotactic factors, and antibacterial factors. There is a lower incidence of enteric and respiratory infections in breast-fed infants. Of interest, the predominant intestinal flora in breast-fed infants is the nonpathogenic *L. bifus*. In contrast, the intestinal flora of bottle-fed babies is enterobacteria.
- *Convenience*: The nursing mother does not need to prepare bottles of formula or get up in the middle of the night to heat a bottle. If she wears a proper dress, she can easily feed the baby anytime and in any place without any preparation.
- *Low cost*: The nursing mother requires an additional 500 calories and 20 g of protein a

day. The cost for these additional calories is a few dollars a week. The cost for formula will depend on whether the mother buys ready-to-feed, concentrate or formula by the case. However, formula is more expensive than breast-feeding.

DISADVANTAGES

A woman who is trying to decide whether to breast-feed or not should know that breast-fed babies tend to feed more frequently. It is also difficult to breast-feed exclusively if the mother returns to work. Working mothers, however, can easily breast-feed part-time and formula feed part-time.

CONTRAINDICATIONS

The contraindications include the baby with an inborn error of metabolism (*e.g.*, phenylketonuria [PKU], galactosemia) who requires a special formula, the baby born to a mother who has a highly contagious disease such as AIDS, and the baby born to a mother who is on certain medications (see Appendix 1).

BREAST-FEEDING MANAGEMENT

Pregnancy

The topic of breast-feeding is best introduced during the third trimester. The pediatrician can discuss feeding during the prenatal visit. The advantages and disadvantages have already been mentioned. A woman who does not find breast-feeding appealing should be supported in her decision. A woman who desires to breast-feed should be counseled on what to expect in the immediate postpartum period (*e.g.*, colostrum, breast engorgement) and how to prepare her nipples. Although there is a controversy about the need for nipple preparation in women with normal nipples, women with flat or inverted nipples will benefit from preparation. Preparation includes avoiding soap to the breast area to allow for the build-up of body lipids, rubbing the nipples with a wet wash cloth ten times a day, and pulling at the nipple (Hoffman maneuver) ten times a day. (For more detail, one of the breast-feeding manuals listed in the bibliography should be consulted.)

Postpartum Care

The mother needs to be instructed in the proper mechanics of breast-feeding; for example, the whole areola goes into the baby's mouth and the nares should not be obstructed by the breast. The baby should feed at least every 3 hours unless the mother is sick or utterly exhausted. At first, nursing should be for 3 to 5 minutes on each side and gradually increased to 10 or 15 minutes on each side. The mother should alternate which breast is offered first. The mother may want to try several positions, such as lying down and sitting up. These changes in position may decrease breast soreness. In addition, the mother needs to know how to break the suction of the baby's sucking by gently inserting her finger into the baby's mouth. The mother should also expect a loose-watery stooling pattern.

The mother needs to know that colostrum is present before the milk comes in. The baby does not require extra fluid supplementation since the baby is born with an excess of body fluid. If water is offered, it should be *after* each feed.

The mother should be aware that at about the third day postpartum she will experience engorgement that can be quite painful. This may be more of a problem for primiparas, whose milk takes longer to come in than multiparas. The best treatment is frequent feeding. The engorgement is sometimes so tense that pumping some milk prior to breast-feeding may be necessary for the baby to insert the areola and nipple properly into his mouth. The use of hot pads before feeding may also relieve some discomfort.

If the mother develops sore nipples, she should limit the time the baby breast feeds on each nipple. She should try different positions and she should air-dry her nipples, taking care to avoid breast pads that retain heat and moisture. She may find using a breast shield helpful if her nipples are very sore.

Since the mother's milk often does not come in until after she is discharged from the hospital, she will need a great deal of support. This help can be given by the physician or the postpartum floor nurse by telephone or a visiting nurse.

Discharge Instructions

These instructions should be simple and brief. Ideally, she should feed on demand but generally not more often than every 1½ to 2 hours. It is common for a baby to feed eight to twelve times in 24 hours. Frequent short feeds are preferable to prolonged infrequent feeds. She should drink approximately 64 oz of fluids per day, be well-rested, and take her prenatal vitamins with iron. Her major occupation will be to feed the baby. If the baby has six wet diapers a day without water supplementation, she should feel confident that the baby is getting enough breast milk. The mother need not avoid certain foods unless she observes consistent increased fussiness in the baby in association with the mother ingesting particular foods. Foods commonly incriminated are garlic, onions, cabbage, chocolate, and great quantities of caffeine. Excessive colic has been attributed occasionally to the baby developing an allergy to cow's milk proteins which can be excreted in the mother's milk. The mother should not take any medications without first talking to her physician. She may drink small amounts of alcohol; in fact, a glass of sherry or wine may be beneficial in the late afternoon if she is having let-down reflex problems.

The mother's clothing should be comfortable. A brassiere is not essential although she may find that it gives her support. A tight brassiere, however, should be avoided.

The mother and father need to be counseled that the father has a major role even if the baby is exclusively breast-fed. The baby still needs much holding and cuddling which the father can do. Furthermore, the father may wish to give the baby his regular bath, which can be a special time together. The father can also feed the baby a bottle of expressed milk or a bottle of water on a daily basis. This allows the mother to have a rest and also introduces the baby to a bottle.

2-Week Check

This is an important visit since most mothers need to be reassured that their babies are getting enough milk. If the baby has gained weight, the mother will be reassured and encouraged. If breast-feeding is going well, the physician may recommend a periodic relief bottle or regular breast pumping so that the mother has milk stored for those times when she will be away from the baby. The baby should take 400 U of vitamin D daily. Some pediatricians also prescribe iron and fluoride supplementation although there is a controversy as to the necessity and age of starting such supplementation.

COMMON PROBLEMS ENCOUNTERED WITH BREAST-FEEDING

Poor Let-Down (Milk Ejection Reflex)

The let-down is characterized by tingling or fullness in the breast. The milk will often spray from the nipple in a stream. Let-down is often precipitated by seeing the baby, hearing the baby cry, or by the baby's sucking. When the let-down is active, one may hear a gulping sound when the baby is sucking. A poor let-down is characterized by the absence of these findings. The best way to condition the let-down is to have the mother relax prior to feeding, drink plenty of liquids, and rest.

Poor Weight Gain

Poor weight gain is usually caused by infrequent feeds (*e.g.*, less than 7 times a day) or an inadequate let-down. Infrequent feeds are easy to rectify. Some babies are quite placid in spite of inadequate caloric intake and need to be awakened during the day to be fed every 2 to 3 hours. If the weight is of concern, the mother can also give one or two supplementary bottles while she is increasing feeds. She should offer these relief bottles during the most stressful part of the day.

Mastitis

Infection in the breast is often characterized by fever, local redness, and soreness. It is usually precipitated by infrequent feeds. Treatment consists of rest, hot compresses, frequent feeds, and an antibiotic such as dicloxacillin or a cephalosporin.

Cracked Nipples

A sore nipple may result in a cracked or fissured nipple if the sore nipple problem is not immediately addressed. Once the nipple is cracked, the mother should use a nursing position that places the point of stress away from the fissure. She should begin each feeding on the uninvolved breast. Applying expressed milk to the fissure and allowing it to dry has been shown to be effective. Ointments should be avoided. The baby should be fed frequently but briefly. Occasionally, the fissures bleed and can result in the baby vomiting blood or having dark stools.

Jaundice from Breast-Feeding

This generally occurs with the onset of the milk coming in and peaks at about 10 to 14 days of age. All other causes of jaundice should be excluded. If the bilirubin level gets dangerously high, the mother should stop breast-feeding for 12 to 48 hours. If the etiology of the jaundice is the milk, the bilirubin level will fall, even as much as 2 mg/dl in 12 hours. Breast-feeding can then be reinstituted. Generally, the bilirubin does not rise to its previous high point. The mother should pump her breasts during the observation period so that breast-feeding is not compromised when reinstituted.

OTHER CONSIDERATIONS

Working Mother

The mother who goes back to work can usually continue breast-feeding without problems. The milk supply adjusts itself to the demand. If the mother is working at least 8 hours, it is sometimes prudent to pump the breasts once during her work day in order to stay comfortable and maintain a good milk supply. Each woman is different in what is required to maintain a supply. Some women can work for a long time without pumping and without compromising the supply. Others have a supply that is more responsive to decreased feeds. A woman will rarely "dry up" because she has returned to work.

Logistics of Nursing Twins

A mother of twins can produce a large milk supply so that she can adequately breast-feed both babies. It is customary for the mother to breast-feed twins simultaneously; in so doing, she is breast-feeding by using a modified demand approach. Thus, if one twin wakes up and is hungry, she may awaken the other twin in order to feed him as well. The mother of twins who breast-feeds may be more likely to get mastitis, and she should be aware of the early symptoms.

Weaning

Weaning is an individual decision. Some women stop when the baby is young, and others wait until the baby is a toddler. The physician should avoid making judgments as to the "right" time. The physician should, however, advise slow weaning if possible, which involves cutting back on one feeding a day every few days. Slow weaning makes the woman's physiologic adjustment less painful.

Breast Pumps and Storage of Milk

Hand expression is superior if the woman can learn the technique. Generally, the nurse on the postpartum floor will be able to teach it. Several pumps are available if the woman is unable to express by hand. The pump that works best will depend on the woman (e.g., the inexpensive hand-held type and the electric pump that can often be rented from a pharmacy). It is good if the woman can borrow a pump from a friend before she decides which pump to purchase.

Milk should be stored in clean containers and immediately refrigerated or frozen. If refrigerated, it will stay good for 48 hours. If frozen at 0°F, it will keep for months.

ANNOTATED BIBLIOGRAPHY

Eiger US, Olds S: The Complete Book of Breast-feeding. New York, Workman Publishing Co, 1972 (Excellent guide for the breast-feeding mother. A new edition is forthcoming.)

Goldfarb J, Tibbetts E: Breastfeeding Handbook. Hillside, NJ, Enslow Publishers, 1980 (Excellent handbook for health care professionals. It contains a number of summary tables, some of which can be copied for patient use. There are also useful appendices on resources for professionals and mothers, and on breast-pump suppliers.)

Kelts DG, Jones EG: Manual of Pediatric Nutrition. Boston, Little, Brown, 1984

Lawrence RA: Breastfeeding, a Guide for the Medical Profession. St. Louis, CV Mosby, 1985 (Written expressly for health professionals with many diagrams and illustrations.)

Report of the Surgeon General's Workshop on Breast-feeding and Human Lactation. Publication No. HRS-D-MC-84-2. Rockville, MD, US Department of Health and Human Services, 1984 (Report that highlights the advantages of breast-feeding and successful approaches to promote breast-feeding.)

Follow-up Report: The Surgeon General's Workshop on Breast-feeding and Human Lactation. Publication No. HRS-MC-85-2. Rockville, MD: US Department of Health and Human Services, 1985 (Valuable to health professionals who wish to promote breast-feeding in their institutions or communities.)

Riordan J: A Practical Guide to Breast-feeding. St. Louis, CV Mosby, 1983 (Has several excellent photographs and illustrations as well as an extensive chapter on breast-feeding education programs and an appendix on audiovisuals for such programs.)

12
Vegetarianism
KATHERINE K. CHRISTOFFEL

All pediatricians are likely to have some patients who are vegetarians. The number of vegetarian children in a practice may be substantial in some areas, due to clustering of families who share ethnic origins, religion, or beliefs that promote vegetarianism. The practicing pediatrician needs to be familiar with various types of vegetarian diets and their dietary strengths and weaknesses in order to be able to evaluate if there are possible advantages or disadvantages of a particular diet for a particular patient, and when to enlist a dietitian's help in dietary assessment.

The pediatrician may become aware from several indications that a child is on a vegetarian diet. The parent may sometimes volunteer the information. More often, the pediatrician learns of the atypical diet while taking a dietary history to assess a problem that may be related to diet, such as iron-deficiency anemia. It is preferable to know about a child's diet before problems arise, so that likely problems can be anticipated; thus, a brief dietary history should be a routine part of office practice. Anticipatory guidance based on the composition of the diet can then be tailored to prevent or minimize growth disturbances and dietary deficiencies.

MOTIVATIONS OF VEGETARIAN FAMILIES

Vegetarian diets may be less expensive than omnivorous diets, but economics is not a common reason for the adoption of a vegetarian diet. The diet is chosen most often because the mother or father believes that the family will benefit from it, either in terms of health or spirituality. Because a family's motives are likely to affect specific food choices, it is essential that they be identified and understood by the pediatrician (Table 12-1).

TYPES OF VEGETARIANISM

Parents' meanings differ when they classify themselves as vegetarians. It is, therefore, necessary to make inquiries regarding which specific food categories they avoid. Although many intermediate types of vegetarian diets exist, there are four dominant ones. *Ovolactovegetarians* consume eggs and milk as well as vegetable foods; they are the largest group of vegetarians worldwide and within the United States. *Ovovegetarians* not only consume eggs but also vegetable foods, however they avoid milk. *Lactovegetarians* consume milk as well as vegetable foods, but they avoid eggs. *Vegans* eat only foods of vegetable origin, avoiding both milk and eggs as well as flesh foods. In addition, a large and possibly growing number of Americans may be described as *semivegetarians*: They eat flesh foods sparingly (often only fish and fowl) and thus they have a diet that in many ways resembles that of ovolactovegetarians. Followers of *macrobiotic* diets restrict their diets in various ways and to varying degrees: Some macrobiotic diets are comparable to omnivorous American diets, others are severely restricted vegan diets.

Adults who adopt vegetarianism (not because it is their cultural heritage but rather because they choose it) may lack familiarity with traditional ways of maximizing the nutritional value of vegetarian meals by combining foods with complementary nutrients. An assessment of the adequacy of a family's vegetarian diet therefore requires information about meal planning as well as about categories of foods used and avoided. Particular attention should be given to the protein content of meals, which may be low in vegan diets if the family does not follow the principles of protein complementarity (which assure appropriate balance of the eight essential amino acids).

VEGETARIANISM AT DIFFERENT AGES

Because a child's growth and activity vary with maturation, so do dietary needs. Consequently, likely positive and negative effects of vegetarian diets on children vary at different stages of development.

During *prenatal* life, fetal well-being depends mainly on the maternal nutritional status. The caretaking physician's usual attentiveness is warranted to assure that the mother consumes the necessary calories, calcium, and iron. Extra attention is required to assure that vegetarian mothers receive ad-

Table 12-1. Motivations for Vegetarianism

MOTIVE	ANTICIPATED BENEFIT
Health/Nutrition	
Lower calories	Less obesity, hypertension
Lower fat (especially saturated)	Less atherosclerosis
Less pesticides/hormones	Less cancer
More fiber/bulk	Less constipation, cancer
Spiritual	
Religious tenets	Obedience/conformity/blessedness
Respect animal life	Ecologic awareness
Economic	
Lower family food costs	Budget stretching
Lower world food costs	Famine relief
Food Preference	Enjoying meals more
Cultural/Social	Following familiar or favored customs

equate vitamin B_{12} and vitamin D, because mothers deficient in these vitamins put their infants at risk of abnormal postnatal growth. The motives of some individuals in following vegetarianism also favor the use of megavitamins or other unusual nutritional supplements. The possibility of toxicity or of a postnatal withdrawal state must be explored if a pregnant mother uses any such supplements.

In *infancy*, nutrition depends on breast milk or infant formula. If a vegetarian mother is deficient in a nutrient (*e.g.*, vitamin B_{12} in a vegan mother), her baby may also suffer from a deficiency. Most nutritional considerations are not different for infants of well-nourished vegetarian mothers than for other infants, but some are unique. As in prenatal life, if a nursing mother takes megadoses of vitamins or other atypical nutritional supplements, the possibility of risk to the infant must be considered as it would be for a prescribed medication. Some vegetarian mothers prefer to prepare their own formulas, usually based on soy beans or almonds, with added oils, vitamins, or other ingredients. The nutritional adequacy of such formulas varies and must be specifically assessed if deficiencies are to be avoided. Some vegetarian infants are fed the usual commercial formulas and thus they do not have any special dietary problems.

During *childhood*, vegetarian diets can readily meet the child's needs if properly balanced or ap-

propriately supplemented. Children who grow up in vegetarian households become accustomed to the family diet, just as other children do. However, unless they live in a self-contained vegetarian community, children from vegetarian families face the social/cultural conflicts that arise for all children whose families differ from the mainstream culture. The degree of conflict faced by vegetarian children is likely to be proportional to the degree to which the families are atypical (*i.e.*, least for semivegetarians and most for vegan macrobiotics). The pediatrician can help children and parents find ways to deal with these conflicts that respect both the values that underlie the choice of the vegetarian diet and also the child's inevitable drive to conform to societal norms. Such conflicts are predictably accentuated during *adolescence*. At the same time, nutritional requirements increase (*e.g.*, for calories, protein, calcium, and iron). The adolescent's physical and emotional needs must be assessed and the diet evaluated and adjusted if necessary to meet those needs.

Although it is possible to become (or remain) obese on a vegetarian diet, individuals on vegetarian diets are generally leaner than those on omnivorous diets. This may sometimes be an advantage and thus the pediatrician may suggest that some families with obese children explore vegetarian ways of eating.

Although nutrient deficiencies do occur, particularly on severely restricted diets, the benefits of sound life-long vegetarian nutrition for most adherents are substantial. When compared to their omnivorous counterparts, *adult* vegetarians tend to be leaner, to have lower cholesterol and blood pressure levels and less constipation and osteoporosis. Internationally, lower levels of intake of food from animal sources are associated with reduced mortality from coronary heart disease and breast cancer, and possibly also from colon cancer.

AREAS TO MONITOR

Because vegetarian diets are often defined by food avoidances, monitoring of vegetarian children for dietary deficiencies and growth disturbances should be even more thorough than similar monitoring of omnivorous children (Table 12-2). There is good evidence that vegetarian diets have no adverse effect on intelligence; thus, special monitoring of this aspect of child development is not required.

Table 12-2. Most Likely Dietary Deficiencies

DIET	CALORIES	PROTEIN	ZINC	CALCIUM	VITAMIN D	VITAMIN B$_{12}$	IRON
Semivegetarian			None				
Ovolactovegetarian			None				
Lactovegetarian			X				X
Ovovegetarian			X	X	X	*	†
Vegan	X	X	X	X	X	X	X
Macrobiotic	?‡	?	?	?	?	?	?

* Vitamin B$_{12}$ is in the yolk; a deficiency is possible if the yolk is discarded or rarely eaten.
† Iron in egg yolk is poorly absorbed.
‡ Depends on the degree of dietary restriction.

Growth

Linear growth of vegetarian children is slower than that of omnivorous children, particularly after weaning. As a result, vegetarian children cluster in the lower growth percentiles. Growth velocity, however, is not likely to be obviously impaired unless dietary restrictions are severe.

If a child on any diet is severely malnourished, as evidenced by wasting or growth arrest, anthropometry and measurements of albumin are indicated. As for any child, if growth is poor, the diet must be examined for adequacy.

Caloric intake may be inadequate if the diet is excessively rich in vegetable bulk, which can induce early satiety. Caloric deficiency is also likely if there is a marked avoidance of dietary fat.

Protein intake may be low as a result of the quantity or quality of dietary protein. Compared to the proteins in meat, milk, and egg white, all other proteins are less than completely usable by the human body. This occurs because in order for protein to be fully used, the essential amino acids must occur in a fixed ratio, and all vegetable proteins are relatively lacking in one or another of those amino acids. However, since the nature and degree of these amino acid "deficiencies" vary, different vegetable proteins can be combined in a meal so that they complement each other. This protein complementarity is embodied in many traditional food combinations (*e.g.*, beans and rice), and is both readily learned and available.

Inadequate *calcium* intake can contribute to rickets, with associated growth arrest. In most diets, calcium is primarily obtained from milk and milk products. Other foods also contain calcium, but (with the exception of soy bean products) generally in small amounts. Common nonanimal sources of calcium are listed in Table 12-3. Even though increased need results in increased absorption, growing children on milk-free diets are likely to require calcium supplements to assure adequate intake.

Vitamin D deficiency may occur, either alone or with calcium deficiency, resulting in rickets. It is most likely in a child who is dark-skinned and breast-fed by a mother who was herself vitamin D depleted during pregnancy (as a result of diet, limited sun exposure, and lack of supplements). Since most vitamin D metabolites in breast milk are inactive, absence of rickets in breast-fed infants generally depends on prenatal repletion, exposure to the sun, or dietary or medicinal supplementation. Supplementation is mandatory for dark-skinned babies who are born in winter and who are breast-fed by vegan mothers who did not take vitamin D supplements during pregnancy. In other situations, the need for supplementation can be assessed by a review of maternal diet before and during pregnancy.

Vitamin B$_{12}$ is present in flesh foods, the

Table 12-3. Nonanimal Sources of Minerals

CALCIUM	ZINC	IRON
Soybean products: tofu, formula/milk	Beans	Beans
	Whole grains	Whole grains
Some green vegetables: mustard greens, broccoli	Some green vegetables	Most green and yellow vegetables
		Some dried fruits: prunes, peaches
Other: blackstrap molasses, medicinal supplements		Other: blackstrap molasses

aqueous portion of milk, egg yolks, and some sea vegetables and cultured soy products (most common in Asian diets, *e.g.*, tempeh). Generally, vegan and ovovegetarian diets require supplementation. Vitamin B_{12} deficiency in a nursing vegan mother can cause a deficiency in her baby, with resulting reversible aberrations in growth and development, and in hematologic and biochemical measures.

Zinc, which is most plentiful in foods of animal origin, has a positive effect on appetite and growth of muscle. Zinc balance may sometimes be adversely affected by dietary excess of phytic acid, a substance present in fibrous plants (*e.g.*, green leafy vegetables) that forms unabsorbed phytates with several minerals. The possibility of a zinc deficiency should be considered when growth is deficient and associated with poor appetite, marginal dietary intake of zinc, or a diet rich in phytate-containing foods. A trial of zinc supplementation (5 mg/day) may be beneficial and is benign. Some non-animal sources of dietary zinc are listed in Table 12-3.

Laboratory Tests

Although vegetarianism does not predispose to iron-deficiency anemia, the most common laboratory abnormality in vegetarian children is microcytic anemia due to iron deficiency, just as it is in omnivorous children. Evaluation and treatment of microcytic anemia is the same as for an omnivorous child except that meat consumption cannot be relied on as a means of iron repletion. Anemia may sometimes be macrocytic and due to vitamin B_{12} deficiency in vegan children (or nursing infants of unsupplemented vegan mothers); folate is plentiful in vegetarian diets (due to inclusion of foliage), and is not a likely cause of macrocytosis in this context.

Although heme iron (in meat) is much more available than nonheme iron (in vegetables), iron deficiency is not a common consequence of vegetarianism. This is probably due to the coincidence of several dietary and metabolic factors that promote iron homeostasis: nonheme iron absorption is increased by simultaneous consumption of ascorbic acid, which is generally plentiful in vegetarian meals; iron absorption is increased by increased need; nonheme iron is ample in many vegetable foods (see Table 12-2). Despite these facts, severe dietary restriction (as in some macrobiotic diets) or huge phytic acid intakes can result in iron deficiency. Recommendations to avoid excess phytate intake and to have a vitamin-C-rich food in most meals are practical and readily followed.

If a child has rickets, this is likely to be reflected in abnormalities of serum calcium (low), phosphorous (variable), or alkaline phosphatase (high). The alkaline phosphatase becomes abnormal first and returns to normal last. X-ray films will show richitic changes of the epiphyses unless the process is mild or of recent onset, or is virtually healed. When a diagnosis of rickets is made, it is prudent to rule out renal, liver, and parathyroid pathology by means of a careful history and physical examination, and with appropriate laboratory tests. The possibility of other etiologies (*e.g.*, familial hypophosphatemic rickets, vitamin D dependency) should be further explored if the child fails to respond to the usual therapy for vitamin D deficiencies.

PRINCIPLES AND PRACTICALITIES IN MANAGING THE VEGETARIAN CHILD

It is essential that the pediatrician develop and convey the same attitude of respect for vegetarian parents as for omnivorous parents. It should be explicitly acknowledged that the physician recognizes that parents adhere to a vegetarian diet with the intention of improving their children's lives. This positive posture not only reflects reality, but it is also an essential basis for recommendations concerning necessary dietary changes. The physician who displays ignorance—or worse, contempt—for vegetarianism will be ineffective in assessing or modifying the diet and growth of a vegetarian child. It is useful to have appropriate books available for consultation.

Many pediatricians do not have the experience or interest necessary to assess and manage the most unusual or restricted vegetarian diets. In such instances, it is most appropriate to work with a dietitian or to refer the patient to a pediatrician with special expertise (as one might for a child on a special diet because of a metabolic error).

ANNOTATED BIBLIOGRAPHY

Adams SF: Use of vegetables in infant feeding through the ages. J Am Diet Assoc 35:692–703, 1959 (Historical perspective.)

Anderson JJB (ed): Nutrition and Vegetarianism. Proceedings of Public Health Nutrition Update. Chapel Hill, Health Sciences Consortium, May 1981 (Wide-ranging review, including specific guidelines for pregnancy and childhood.)

Christoffel KK: A pediatric perspective on vegetarian nutrition. Clin Pediatr 20:632–641, 1981 (Review of the literature through 1980; tables listing nutrient sources; management guidelines.)

Ewald EB: Recipes for a Small Planet. New York, Ballantine Books, 1973 (Sequel to *Diet for a Small Planet*, with usable recipes exemplifying protein complementarity.)

Lappe FM: Diet for a Small Planet. New York, Ballantine Books, 1971 (Essential background concerning recent growth of interest in vegetarianism, with excellent figures.)

Nutritional aspects of vegetarianism, health foods and fad diets. In American Academy of Pediatrics: Pediatric

Nutrition Handbook, Chap. 33. Elk Grove Village, IL, American Academy of Pediatrics (Includes specific information on megavitamin toxicity.)

Robertson L, Flinders C, Godfrey B: Laurel's Kitchen: A Handbook for Vegetarian Cookery and Nutrition. Petaluma, CA, Nilgiri Press, 1976 (Nutrition text-cum-cookbook. Highly readable, usable recipes, and fine tables of nutrient contents.)

Shinwell ED, Gorodischer R: Totally vegetarian diets and infant nutrition. Pediatrics 70:582–586, 1982 (Report on a religious sect with severe dietary restrictions and resistance to change: The most difficult situation.)

13

Special Needs of the Premature Infant

WILLIAM D. COCHRAN

Premature infants have been going home from hospitals for over 100 years and home birthed "prematures" survived before that. However, premature infants have only recently been sent home while still weighing under 5½ lb and even more recently some of the tiniest prematures have been sent home "normal" with perhaps a few lingering problems. The special needs of these premature infants and the special concerns of their parents are dealt with in this chapter. Generally, premature infants are assessed as ready-for-discharge when they can take all their feedings by mouth, maintain their temperature while sleeping in a crib, no longer need an incubator, and gain weight consistently (10 to 20 g/day) over a 2- to 3-day span. It is often helpful to explain to parents that their infant, until 40 weeks' gestation, is still prematurely born and that much of his fetal physiology continues.

TEMPERATURE CONTROL

Because the temperature control of prematures under 40 weeks' gestation may not be well developed, both chilling and more commonly overheating assume greater importance than in full-term babies. Questions about either can most easily be assessed by the parents taking the baby's rectal temperature; thus, this might be a technique taught before discharge. Generally, a rectal temperature between 97.5°F to 100°F is within the normal range, with the lower temperature more common in the morning. A temperature below 97.5°F probably means the baby is too cold. Besides the usual sweaters and booties, hats are helpful in stabilizing a baby's low temperature.

NUTRITIONAL NEEDS

The nutritional needs of premature infants differ from those of full-term babies. Most "premies" will be sent home from the hospital on a 20 cal/oz formula or, hopefully, on breast milk—or at least bottle feeding their mother's pumped breast milk. Generally, such premature infants will gain weight if they are getting 120 to 140 cal/kg/day, though occasional ones (especially those with continuing bronchopulmonary dysplasia [BPD]) may require 160 to 180 cal/kg/day because of their increased caloric needs. There are a number of healthy prematures who consume an inordinate amount of formula each day "catching up" to their probable genetically set growth curve. They take as much as 200 to 220 ml/kg/day of formula at 140 to 150 cal/kg/day. As long as no obvious untoward reaction occurs, such infants may continue their large intake; their appetite will be satiated eventually. Other infants will be going home on milk fortifiers such as polycose, MCT, or Human Milk Fortifier (HMF) to increase their formula to 24 cal/oz or more in order to get sufficient calories without becoming overloaded with fluid (Table 13-1).

In most cases, (the most common exception is infants with significant lingering BPD) by 5 lb weight, if not before, the infant should be on a 20 cal/oz formula. The desired weight gain of 15 to 20 g/day is used as a rough guide. In fact, most infants

Table 13-1. Common Formula Supplements

MILK FORTIFIERS	PROTEIN	FAT	CARBOHYDRATE	CALORIES (per oz or ml)
HMF* (4 packets to 100 ml breast milk)	0.7 g	–	2.8 g	4/oz
Polycose	–	–	+	4/ml
MCT	–	+	–	9/ml

* HMF is a product of Mead Johnson. It can usually only be purchased through the distributor. Polycose and MCT can be purchased over the counter from a pharmacy.

will not be discharged home before they are on a 20 cal/oz formula. A reasonable guide to parents concerning *frequency* and timing of feedings is that 7 feedings/day may be necessary for the first week or two at home in order to maintain a minimum weight gain. The infant should generally consume 2.5 oz/lb baby wt/day of formula. Premature infants should also not go longer between their feedings in hours than they weigh in pounds (*e.g.*, a 5-lb baby should not wait more than 5 hours between any feeding) and he will have to make up feedings during the day, hopefully to get in the usual six or more feedings. As the weight and the oz/feeding increase, however, the number of feedings per day can be decreased.

Whether to give added *vitamins* is controversial. All prepared formulas are supplemented with vitamins but many parents (and some physicians) wonder if it is enough. Although the answer is not available, the added vitamins are probably adequate. Large doses of vitamin E are now usually no longer necessary. Fluoride supplementation (0.25 mg/day) is recommended for breast-feeding mothers, where the community water supply is deficient or when using commercial ready-made formulas with an unknown fluoride content.

Iron supplementation has proven beneficial. Premature infants tend to become more anemic in the first few months after birth than full-term babies. In the nursery, it is customary to transfuse prematures in order to maintain their hematocrits around 40% until they weigh about 1500 g (3 lb 5 oz). This is usually done to help abort or to treat "apnea of prematurity." After this weight is attained and no medical condition—such as continuing apnea or BPD—is present, the hematocrit is allowed to fall. It is not unusual to have it drop as low as 24%, occasionally even lower. A transfusion is not necessary if the baby continues to do well and the reticulocyte count rises to greater than 1%.

However, because of the known poor iron stores of premature infants, it is recommended to start iron supplementation (2 to 3 mg/kg/day) 8 to 12 weeks after the last transfusion done in the hospital.

THEOPHYLLINE AND APNEA MONITORING

The subjects of theophylline and apnea monitoring are controversial and highly charged (see Chap. 202). Parents are desperate for good advice but, depending on the expert, that advice varies. At present, it is suggested to let the parents know of the conflicting recommendations, tell them your opinion (my opinion is that the monitor is for their peace of mind only) and then support them in their decision. The report by Southall of pneumograms on more than 2000 prematures showed that they had no predictive value in regard to subsequent sudden infant death syndrome (SIDS).

An occasional premature infant is sent home still on theophylline for apnea or its potentially beneficial effect on residual BPD. It is generally true that some infants will have a tendency for continuing central apnea and therefore a need for theophylline up to their 34th or even 35th week of gestation. However, many have proven that they have no need for it as early as the 30th week of gestation and that they are no longer taking it (or never needed it). If they are taking theophylline when discharged, it is usually given 3 to 4 times/day. To achieve a desired serum level of around 12, the dose is around 9 to 12 mg/kg/day. With 2 weeks at home of continuing apnea-free behavior (and the infant being now at least 36 weeks' gestation), the general consensus is to allow the infant "outgrow" the dose (*i.e.*, continuing the same dose in the face of the usual weight gain). The medication can be discontinued either around 40 weeks' gestation or at a serum theophylline level of less than 6.

IMMUNIZATION

Immunization of premature infants has been shown to be worthwhile. It may even be started for some of the smaller ones still in the hospital growing for discharge. The current advice is to start immunizations at the routine time (around 2 months of actual age) and at the normal dosage level. Fewer severe reactions seem to occur among premature infants although their immune response is almost equal to that of normal full-term infants.

SPECIAL PHYSICAL PARAMETERS

Special physical parameters of prematures are noteworthy. For instance, almost all normally growing prematures have a head circumference (HC) that grows at a considerably faster rate than the infant's height or even weight. In fact, the sagittal suture may be split to a small degree for some time. Most small prematures will have had a cranial ultrasound in their first week of life. A normal result is assuring that such a rapidly growing head is normal. This extra rapid growth will usually slow down as the higher percentiles are reached. As long as the percentile of HC is not over 50% higher than the weight or it remains under the 95%, expectant care is reasonable, especially in the presence of normal neurologic behavior.

Because of changing signs and findings, the neurologic examination of all "normal" term infants as well as prematures may be difficult to interpret. Since many prematures have an increased incidence of diplegia (with its tiptoe posture and hyperactive knee jerk), one may look for it—and then find it! Then one must decide whether to inform the parents of such a worrisome finding or monitor it to see if it persists or worsens. I would strongly advocate the latter, especially if it is an otherwise isolated neurologic finding. If, on the other hand, there are such findings as continued fisting of the hands, excessive spitting or vomiting, or a marked "setting sun sign," then further investigation might be worthwhile sooner.

Non-neurologic physical findings of prematures that one should be aware of are hernias, more flattened heads (mostly from positioning the baby on its back), and the characteristic high forehead that often persists for a year or so.

Special attention needs to be paid to the premature infant's ability to see and hear and that these two senses are working and developing properly. Many physicians advise that otologic and opthalmologic consultation or tests be routinely carried out. My opinion is that this can be done on an individual basis. An involved parent watching and observing carefully can usually see responses to natural faint visual or auditory stimuli in her child. The pediatrician should ask about such responses at routine well-child visits. If there is any question, further investigation is warranted.

COUNSELING

Counseling parents of a premature is especially important and they will most likely need and should get special instructions, special help, extra "routine" visits, and extra time per visit. A premature birth often shatters the parents' expectation that their baby is perfect; it allows among other fears all sorts of worries about cerebral palsy, mental retardation, and so forth to surface. Thus, the parents of a premature, especially the mother, feel guilty ("that she had a premature delivery") and are often ambivalent about the increased care involved and the increased needs of such an infant. Parents often do not know how to deal with this problem. In addition to consideration and understanding on the part of the physician (allowing the parents time to ask all their questions), a worthwhile suggestion is to encourage parents of prematures to form a group, or at least talk to another set of parents of a premature. The discussion of similar problems with parents of other premature babies is generally beneficial.

ANNOTATED BIBLIOGRAPHY

Ronnholm KAR, Siimes MA: Haemoglobin concentration depends on protein intake in small preterm infants fed human milk. Arch Dis Child 60:99–104, 1985 (Evidence that, at least when solely receiving breast milk, premature infants are more anemic by 12 weeks of age than when fed a protein-fortified formula.)

Southall DP, Richards JM, de Swiet M et al: Identification of infants destined to die unexpectedly during infancy: Evaluation of predictive importance of prolonged apnoea and disorders of cardiac rhythm or conduction. Br Med J 286:1092–1096, 1983 (Subsequent data support these findings that the pneumogram fails to predict SIDS.)

14
Sexuality Education
EDWARD L. SCHOR

Sexuality is central to the personality and daily life of every individual. It has its beginning in the intimacy and love of the mother–child relationship, and it is developed through the child's continuing interaction with his culture and society, especially as these are represented and interpreted by his family. Sexual development, like other aspects of child development, is a continuing process, susceptible to errant experience that can lead to a poor self-image and aberrant sexuality and sexual behavior. It is an area of preventive pediatrics in which the pediatrician can play a valuable role as an educator of children and their parents and as a facilitator of open and honest communication among them.

Pediatricians are uniquely able to follow a child's and his family's development over an extended period of time. Sexuality is an integral part of that development. By making sexuality education a regular part of child health care, pediatricians are able to normalize and legitimize it as an aspect of child development that should be considered and discussed. The primary goal of sexuality education is to enhance normal social and psychological development, including developing a positive self-image and the capacity for intimate, mutually supportive, and satisfying relationships. Successful sexuality education may also help to prevent sexual abuse, teenage and unwanted pregnancies, sexually transmitted diseases, and adult sexual dysfunction.

Pediatricians who omit sexuality education from their child care visits convey a strong message to the parents that such topics are uncomfortable or off-limits. Parents who avoid discussing these topics with their children give a similar message. However, although pediatricians should consciously include sexuality education as a normal and comfortable part of their interactions with parents and children, a certain amount of discretion is advisable. All families have boundaries beyond which some topics or conversations become uncomfortable if not taboo. On one hand, pediatricians should not restrict their entry into the family's value system to the extent that normal sexual development is not discussed. Cultural and societal attitudes, especially as played out within some families, may

feel repressive to a developing child who is responding to inherent biologic and cognitive imperatives. A tactful professional intervention can be helpful. On the other hand, the pediatrician must sufficiently assess the family's boundaries so that he does not offend them, thus limiting his effectiveness as an educator and child advocate.

The biologic determinants of sexuality begin at conception when the genetic gender of the child is determined. At birth, or following amniocentesis, the gender of the child becomes known to his parents and others. Based on gender, the child (boy or girl) begins to be exposed to differential societal expectations. The child, influenced by attitudes about his sex role, begins to actively identify with others of his own gender. Learning gender identity, whether by a boy or a girl, is established by 3 years of age. The child develops the foundation for his gender role by perceiving differences in social roles based on gender and by valuing things that are like himself. Gender identity is a fixed characteristic. On the other hand, gender roles, masculine or feminine, may be transcended, and children and adults are able to base their behavior on personally meaningful experiences, interests, and abilities.

PRENATAL STAGE

Many of the topics routinely discussed during a prenatal pediatric visit are issues of sexuality. The decision to breast-feed is partly a decision in favor of maximum intimacy between mother and child. It also provokes questions about the intended role of the father in the care of the child, and thus addresses aspects of sexuality and gender roles of both parents. Circumcision is a decision on the part of the parents that is linked to the child's body image and sexuality. Even the choice of possible names for the child and their connotation to the parents and others have implications for the child's sexual development. By raising questions about these topics and discussing them in a relaxed and open dialogue, the pediatrician can establish a relationship with the family that includes consideration of all aspects of the child's development. By creating an atmosphere that encourages discussion of sexual matters, the pediatrician is modeling for the parents how to help their child feel safe to ask questions, show concerns, and express feelings. These parenting skills are fundamental to normal, healthy development, sexual and otherwise.

NEONATAL STAGE

Sexuality education occurs as the neonatal examination is performed in the presence of the parents. As in every subsequent examination of the child, examination of the genitalia should be included as a matter of course. During the first examination, the pediatrician should, using the correct terminology, comment on the genital anatomy. Penile and clitoral erections, the former reported to occur as early as the second trimester, or vaginal secretions and bleeding should be discussed, as should the presence of breast tissue. The contribution that nestling, suckling, rocking, and other such behaviors make to the child's sense of intimacy and trust should be discussed and encouraged.

INFANCY

During infancy, children begin to learn that it is good or pleasant to be touched. If holding is absent or associated with unpleasant feelings, the infant may fail to learn pleasure and to be comfortable with physical contact. Infants will normally find and explore their genitals and will take pleasure in touching themselves. Masturbation is natural and inevitable, and infants appear to be capable of having an orgasm. Parental reactions to children touching their genitals will influence the formation of attitudes associated with self-pleasure and with genital parts of the body. The pediatrician may inquire whether the infant has developed the motor skills and sense of his own body necessary to play with his genitals. Sexuality is normalized when placed in such a developmental context.

TODDLER STAGE

The development of expressive language, which progresses rapidly between 18 and 36 months, is a period of extensive sexual learning. The child names body parts and learns of their functions along with the affect attached to the words. Toilet training also occurs during this stage. Children find pleasure in urinating or having a bowel movement, and thus toilet training, including exploring their feces, urine, or the toilet bowl is a part of discovering their

bodies. Parents' reactions to these explorations can influence children's attitudes toward bodily functions.

Children now begin to engage in mutual exploration, usually with siblings and peers, although they take careful note of their parents' anatomy and behavior. They question the reason for genitalia and other mysteries such as their umbilicus. Social sexual issues begin to arise within families. Much early parent–child communication deals with sexuality, because many of the child's first interests are with his own body parts and functions. Parents will find it necessary to address questions about nudity and when clothing is necessary, separate sleeping areas, and sexual privacy for themselves.

PRESCHOOL STAGE

Active psychosexual development occurs at this stage. The child now becomes aware of the physical boundaries between "me" and "somebody else." He should learn that his body belongs to himself. A child who has a positive view of his own physical anatomy and control of his own body is less likely to be an object of sexual misuse. Parents need to learn to listen to their children, especially if the child tells them that something happened that made them feel uncomfortable.

Although children need to understand when to say "no" and to respect their bodies, it is also important for them to understand that sexual behavior can and should be good. Children need experiences that reinforce a positive self-image. Sexual development includes a period of experimentation and exploration. Sex play, cuddling, touching, kissing, playing "doctor" or "mommy and daddy" are normal. They are ways of acting out situations to test their ideas of how things happen, to discover how things look, and to learn what feels good. This may be seen as a form of sexual rehearsal play that will help them develop a sense of sexual competence. Children are also likely to be intensely attached to the parent of the opposite sex during this stage of development. They may harbor jealous feelings toward the same-sex parent. This is an affirmation of their own gender identity and an unconscious testing of their sex role.

Instead of asking for labels, at this time children ask questions about body functions. They are unable to conceive of any reason for having a baby and they believe that it has always existed somewhere. Thus the question, "Where do babies come from?" is a quite literal one. Children, as they get a little older, begin to attribute babies to some cause, although their thinking is "magical" and filled with illogical connections. Their questions may then be mechanistic, such as "How are babies made?", "How does it feel to be born?", or "Can I watch you and daddy make a baby?"

The innocent, naive, and embarrassing questions and behavior of children between 3 to 5 years should be handled graciously and respectfully. Parents should be encouraged to address such situations not as good or bad, right or wrong, but rather as appropriate or inappropriate depending on the time, place, or person. Masturbation, for example, may be permissible at home or in the car, but not in public—the place is inappropriate. Similarly being naked with your family might be permissible, whereas with a friend's family it may be frowned on—the person is inappropriate. Although a child's behaviors and questions at this age may be embarrassing for the parents, sexual topics do not have the same emotional significance for children. The quality of this dialogue, the ability of the parent to allow the child to broach any subject without fear of judgment or censorship, can establish future patterns of sharing and relating to others.

Parents can also be guided to recognize the sexuality in the everyday life of their child. Much sexual learning can take place gradually, informally, and incidentally. Parents should take advantage of family events such as pregnancies, weddings, and birthdays to discuss sexual topics. Picture books offer examples of gender roles; discussions about family relationships can be introduced by looking at photo albums; and reproduction can be discussed when dealing with pets.

ELEMENTARY SCHOOL STAGE

When a child starts going to school he is exposed to a world in which new information and attitudes abound, and rewards are given for understanding how things work. At this age, children offer explanations for phenomena that seem technically feasible, albeit less than convincing, and ascribe will and purpose to all things in nature. Thus, their questions about sex and reproduction increase as they try to find reason in conflicting "facts"; as a part of their developing sexuality, they are fascinated by what they perceive as deviant, such as twins or profanity. Their interest in the fantastic and bizarre extends to their choice of toys, games, and television viewing. Parents should be encouraged to actively participate in the selection of these activities.

By 8 or 9 years of age, most of the basic facts of sexual life may have been learned, but children will not yet be able to weave them into a consistent whole with which they are comfortable. Consequently, they begin showing embarrassment when discussing sexual topics such as pregnancy and childbirth, and they may be reluctant to ask questions that might clarify their misconceptions. "Dirty jokes" appear at this time and reflect both their confusion and reluctance; such behaviors test the receptivity of their parents to discussing these topics.

During this and subsequent stages, the sexuality of single parents is a topic that pediatricians are increasingly required to address. There are no easy answers to parents' questions, and, as always, their values and circumstances must be respected. As is true for couples, single parents need to honestly confront their own sexuality and be clear concerning how they wish to convey their values to their children. Divorced parents may have different sexual values; they may need to agree to disagree. Parents should be reassured that the formation of normal gender identity and roles seem to take place without the presence of a same-sex parent, and under various child-rearing conditions.

Later during this stage, the pediatrician can begin to see the child alone for part of the examination, offering this option directly to the child. In this way, the pediatrician acknowledges that an advance in maturation of the child has occurred and he introduces the concept of responsibility for ones own body and health. The communication between the parents and the child should be observed; it is the key to a good family relationship and healthy psychosocial development. When communication is not adequate—when open discussions do not occur; when children's opinions are not solicited before judgments are made; or when their decisions are not respected—intervention in the office or referral for brief counseling is appropriate.

The wide variation in the age of onset of puberty makes the timing of pubertal counseling difficult to determine. Since an examination of the genitalia should occur at each well-child visit, the pediatrician will be able to identify the first changes of secondary sexual characteristic development—testicular enlargement in boys and breast buds in girls. By or at this time, discussion of secondary sexual characteristic changes should begin, including genital and breast development and gynecomastia, linear growth, voice changes, muscular development, hair pattern differences, and menstruation. Controversy exists concerning the role of the parents, schools, and physician in sexuality education. Most would agree that the family's values should be respected. This question has led to a hesitancy on the part of many school systems to incorporate sexuality education into their curricula. The pediatrician should ascertain what the parents' values are with regard to sexuality, and he should offer pubertal counseling congruent with them. It should, however, be emphasized that this is an integral part of health care. It is useful to include the parents in the process of sexuality education. This reduces their anxiety about what is being discussed and increases the potential for continued discussion in the home.

PUBERTY

The physical changes associated with puberty are significant factors in self-image, and they are best managed by the young adolescent whose self-esteem, comfort with his body, and ability to communicate with significant others is well developed. Previous sexuality education should have prepared him for the more visible changes. Other changes may be more problematic. Young adolescents are concerned with how they appear to others and with how they feel about themselves. Their principal concern is with normality, and thus with peer acceptance. Conventional role conformity is evident in their spoken beliefs, their dress, and their behavior. Their development is described by their ability to form intimate, interpersonal relationships outside of their families as they move toward families they may form in the future. Their behavior displays a stepwise progression of sexual behavior from kissing to intercourse.

In some ways, pubertal sexuality is undifferentiated; this can lead to concerns both about homosexuality and "adequacy" for heterosexual roles. Other topics of interest at this age and later in adolescence include menstruation, masturbation, intercourse, birth control, pregnancy, and venereal diseases. Theses subjects invoke a considerable number of questions. The pediatrician should encourage the adolescent to raise questions of his own rather than depend entirely on a preplanned teaching agenda.

When the pediatrician perceives that he will be the primary source of sexuality education for a young adolescent, an increase in the usual number of health maintenance visits is necessary so as to allow adequate opportunity for discussions. During each visit, most of the time should be spent with the adolescent alone. Privacy and confidentiality are important for adolescents, especially when sexual histories are taken; homosexuality, sexual ac-

tivity, or an ignorance of sexual knowledge may be revealed. Parents and other adults who enjoy teenagers' confidence are those who respect their privacy, who do not expect to be told everything, and who do not push for more information than they are offered. Another reason for seeing the adolescent alone is to encourage a sense of responsibility for himself that hopefully will also extend to others. The physical examination of young adolescents should be performed in a way that helps them learn about their changing bodies and that reinforces a sense of normality. Some pediatricians find it useful to guide adolescents through a self-Tanner staging. It is also a time to consider teaching self-breast and testicular examinations.

ADOLESCENCE

Whereas early adolescence is a time to experience changes, midadolescence is a time to manage and incorporate them into a functional life-style. Teenagers are physiologically ready for sexual activity before our society makes it possible for them to cope with its consequences; however, it is a part of reality for most adolescents. Sexuality should be cast in the context of relationships, a framework that is usually welcomed by adolescents and their parents.

The pediatrician can initiate a discussion about sex by taking a sexual history as a part of the general history. Aspects of physical and physiologic maturation can be explored as appropriate to the age of the adolescent. Questions may be asked about sexual feelings, concerns, and, perhaps with more difficulty, behaviors. Finally, the issues of responsibilities and consequences can be addressed. Such discussions can help adolescents to explore sexuality and sexual life-styles that serve to increase their sense of self-mastery and good decision-making. The pediatrician should support and encourage good communication between parents and their children throughout the span of sexuality education. Teenagers who believe that they are basically good and competent people and that they are loved and respected, will be better able to cope with the pressures their sexuality creates and to develop loving and lasting relationships.

PATIENT EDUCATION

Pediatricians should present sexuality education as part of the professional services they offer and as an integral part of health care. The education of patients and parents in sexuality requires a combination of teaching (*e.g.*, providing facts) and counseling (*e.g.*, providing emotional support and reassurance). It also requires that the pediatrician first assess his own beliefs, values, and experiences regarding sexuality. Thus prepared, he will be better able to engage in effective and empathetic communication, and he will more likely succeed as an educator.

When introducing education regarding sensitive topics such as sexuality, it is essential to understand the family's value system and to map out its boundaries. Similarly, the knowledge that patients and their families already possess should be assessed and used as a foundation for discussion. Problem-based learning with active participation of the patient is most effective. Concerns and questions expressed by the parent or child should be used to direct the educational process. The pediatrician should also be sensitive to unspoken messages and indirect questions and he should tactfully address these covert communications. The number of issues discussed during any single visit and the amount of factual material presented should be limited. Sequential visits allow the organized presentation of information and provides the opportunity for reinforcement of previous discussions. During patient education, it is essential to evaluate as the process occurs. The pediatrician should not assume that what is being presented is being understood.

The practice of pediatrics naturally lends itself to the inclusion of the family in the educational process. This is an important advantage. Family involvement allows a more complete understanding of what knowledge, attitudes, and behaviors form the context for the sexual development of the child. During childhood and early adolescence the parents are the primary participants in sexuality education, because they can either apply advice being offered by the pediatrician or undermine its message to the child. Parents should be made to feel competent as educators themselves, since the most successful sexuality education occurs when the parent–child

communication is good. Finally, the role of the pediatrician as a health educator should extend beyond the patient and his family. Pediatricians can become more effective in promoting child health care by participating in educational programs in schools and communities.

ANNOTATED BIBLIOGRAPHY

Bartlett EE: Effective approaches to patient education for the busy pediatrician. Pediatrics 74(suppl):920–923, 1984 (Brief, but one of the few practical references on health education for pediatricians.)

Bernstein AC: How children learn about sex and birth. Psychology Today pp 73–78, Jan. 1976 (Succinct and interesting article outlining children's understanding of sexuality based on a Piagetian formulation.)

Calderone MS, Johnson EW: The Family Book About Sexuality. New York, Harper & Row, 1981 (Comprehensive, well-illustrated book that promotes open discussion within the family of all aspects of sexuality.)

Litt IF, Martin JA: Development of sexuality and its problems. In Levine M, Carey WB, Crocker AC, Gross RT (eds): Developmental-Behavioral Pediatrics, pp 633–649. Philadelphia, WB Saunders, 1983 (Useful chapter that provides an overview of several theories and concepts about childhood sexuality. Discusses sexuality during adolescence in detail.)

Parcel GS, Finkelstein JW: Adolescent sexuality. In Buchanan N (ed): Pediatric Issues for General Practitioners. Sydney, ADIS Health Science Press, 1987 (Excellent chapter on adolescent sexual development covering most of the important considerations for pediatricians providing sexuality education for this age group.)

Planned Parenthood: How to Talk with Your Child About Sexuality. Garden City, NY, Doubleday, 1986 (One of the best sexuality education resources for parents and professionals; provides sound advice and information on promoting effective parent–child communication.)

Rutter M: Psychosexual development. In Rutter M (ed): Scientific Foundations of Developmental Psychiatry, pp 322–339. London, Heinemann Medical Books, 1980 (Thorough, scholarly review of biologic and psychosocial aspects of the development of sexuality.)

15
Sports Medicine
PAUL G. DYMENT

The subject of pediatric sports medicine is vast; in fact, there have been three recent monographs on this specific subject. It has long been considered the domain of the orthopedic surgeon alone, but most sports injuries are minor and can be handled by a primary-care physician. A physician who has an interest in preventive medicine has an important role in sports medicine performing preparticipation physical examinations, being a team physician, and working to make athletics safe as well as enjoyable.

This chapter focuses on two areas of common concern to the nonorthopedist physician interested in sports medicine: how to make the preparticipation physical examination worthwhile and the team physician's responsibilities.

PREPARTICIPATION PHYSICAL EXAMINATION

Sports preparticipation physical examinations are common reasons for adolescents to visit their doctors. The physician may only see them at these visits because half of the high-school athletes undergoing such examinations will have no other contact with a physician during that year. The number of such examinations that are performed annually in the United States is striking. Seven million high-school students are involved in interscholastic sports, and most state high-school athletic associations still require an annual physical examination. In the experience of most physicians, such examinations are not very productive in detecting conditions that might affect athletic participation, and the effectiveness of sports preparticipation examinations as usually performed is arguable. Most adolescents are generally healthy and the mere fact that they are trying out for a sport further diminishes the likelihood of their having a significant disease. The fact that only 1% of such patients have a disqualifying condition revealed by the traditional examination underscores why this type of examination is widely believed to be not very cost-effective.

If, however, the physician is aware that most sports injuries are reinjuries and thus focuses the physical examination toward the musculoskeletal system, abnormalities will be detected in 10% of patients. Most of these abnormalities will be easily treated musculoskeletal conditions such as tight hamstring muscles, patellofemoral syndrome (chondromalacia patella), and ligamentous ankle instabilities that generally only require some rehabilitative exercises using training equipment available in most schools. Such a musculoskeletal examination is not only good practice, but one that also makes the physical examination much more productive and therefore more interesting.

The sports preparticipation examination can occur during a "locker-room" type of mass screening, but this is not ideal. It is much better to incorporate this examination into the health maintenance examination that all youths should undergo every 2 years. It would then occur in a physician's office where preventive health care and counseling, some of it sport-specific, can be offered.

Purposes

A sports preparticipation physical examination should be performed not only to detect physical abnormalities, which would predispose the athlete to injury or death or which could affect the athlete's ability to compete effectively, but also to evaluate the size and maturity of younger athletes in order to counsel whether collision or contact sports with their peer group would be safe. Another major reason is to identify residual disabilities from previous injuries, because this will allow the physician to recommend rehabilitative exercises that will decrease the probability of a reinjury.

Frequency

Most schools still insist on an annual examination, even though the American Academy of Pediatrics has recommended this need only be done every 2 years. Presumably the schools do this because of a vague belief that this will be legally advantageous to the school in case of litigation over an injury, or it may be because the physical educator believes that annual examinations represent optimal medical practice. Regardless of the frequency, an interval history should be obtained before each sports season so that illnesses or injuries that have occurred since the last examination can be considered and decisions made as to whether an athlete requires to have another physical examination done by a physician.

Laboratory Tests

A determination of the hemoglobin or hematocrit and a urinalysis are not considered essential for this kind of examination. In one study of 701 children undergoing a sports physical examination, 40 had abnormal urinary protein on screening, but *none* of these were found to have any significant abnormality after further work-up. Iron-deficiency anemia has to be severe before the body's compensatory mechanisms, such as increased stroke volume and heart rate, fail to maintain appropriate oxygen flow to the tissues. However, iron depletion that is not severe enough to cause anemia may limit endurance and ability to exercise and it is certainly much more common than frank anemia. Since serum assays of ferritin or iron are expensive, it is recommended that they only be obtained on highly competitive state, national, and world-class female athletes and on male distance runners, many of whom can be shown to be hypoferremic.

Medical History

In addition to the usual questions asked during a medical review of systems, the athlete should be asked the following six questions:

1. Have any members of your family under age 50 had a "heart attack" or "heart problem"?
2. Have you ever been told you have a heart murmur, high blood pressure, an extra heart beat, or a heart abnormality?
3. Do you have to stop while running around a one-quarter mile track twice?
4. Are you taking any medications?
5. Have you ever "passed out" while exercising or been "knocked out"?
6. Have you ever had any illness, condition, or injury that:
   a. Required you to go to the hospital either as a patient overnight or in the emergency room or for x-rays?
   b. Required an operation?
   c. Lasted longer than a week?
   d. Caused you to miss a game or practice?
   e. Was caused by allergies (*e.g.*, hay fever, hives, asthma, or medicine)?

Examination

If this examination takes place in the physician's office in the context of a health maintenance examination, then a complete physical examination should be performed. In the mass-screening form, it is acceptable to concentrate on examining the chest, abdomen, inguinal canals in the male, and the musculoskeletal system. Even then the examination should be sport-specific; thus, swimmers would also have their tympanic membranes observed, and wrestlers would have their levels of body fat determined using skinfold calipers so that advice can be given on how to "make weight" in a medically sound manner.

Cardiopulmonary. Most sudden, unexpected deaths in adolescent athletes are from abnormalities of the heart, and few of them would have had their abnormality detected even during a carefully performed physical examination. The aberrant left coronary artery syndrome has been associated with sudden death in young persons. Although there is

Table 15-1. 2-Minute Orthopedic Examination

INSTRUCTIONS	OBSERVATION
Stand facing the examiner.	Acromioclavicular joints, general habitus
Look at the ceiling, floor, over both shoulders; touch ears to shoulders.	Cervical spine motion
Shrug shoulders (examiner resists).	Trapezius strength
Abduct shoulders 90° (examiner resists at 90°).	Deltoid strength
Do a full external rotation of arms.	Shoulder motion
Flex and extend elbows.	Elbow motion
Arms at sides, elbows 90° flexed; pronate and supinate wrists	Elbow and wrist motion
Spread your fingers; make a fist.	Hand or finger motion and deformities
Tighten (contract) quadriceps; relax quadriceps.	Symmetry and knee effusion; ankle effusion
"Duck walk" four steps (away from examiner with buttocks on heels).	Hip, knee, and ankle motion
Keep back to the examiner.	Shoulder symmetry, scoliosis
Keep knees straight, touch toes.	Scoliosis, hip motion, hamstring tightness
Raise up on toes, raise heels.	Calf symmetry, leg strength

(Committee on Sports Medicine: Sports Medicine: Health Care for Young Athletes, Evanston, IL, American Academy of Pediatrics, 1983)

no heart murmur, in most instances they have had a history of fainting during exercise. Hypertrophic obstructive cardiomyopathy (idiopathic hypertrophic subaortic stenosis [IHSS]), although uncommon, is a potentially lethal defect associated with exercise. It may be associated with an apical systolic murmur that increases when the patient performs a Valsalva maneuver, and there may be a hyperdynamic left ventricular impulse. Particular attention should be paid to blood pressure, even though mild forms of hypertension are not a reason for a disqualification from sports (in fact, exercise generally lowers the blood pressure), and levels greater than 140/90 in adolescents need rcpeated determinations before deciding that hypertension is present.

Abdomen and Genitalia. The athlete should lie

Table 15-2. Classification of Sports

COLLISION	LIMITED CONTACT/IMPACT	NONCONTACT STRENUOUS	MODERATELY STRENUOUS	NONSTRENUOUS
Boxing	Baseball	Aerobic dancing	Badminton	Archery
Field hockey	Basketball	Crew	Curling	Golf
Football	Bicycling	Fencing	Table tennis	Riflery
Ice hockey	Diving	Field*		
Lacrosse	Equestrian	Running		
Martial arts	Gymnastics	Skiing (cross-country)		
Rodeo	Raquetball	Swimming		
Wrestling	Skating, ice and roller	Tennis		
Soccer	Skiing (downhill, cross-country, and water)	Track		
	Softball	Weight-lifting		
	Squash, handball			
	Volleyball			

* Field events: Jumping events such as pole vaulting and high jump are "limited-contact" sports.

down while a careful palpation for intraabdominal masses and hepatosplenomegaly is performed. Males should then have their testicles palpated and inguinal canals examined, and both sexes should have their Tanner pubic hair staging assessed.

Musculoskeletal. This component of the examination can be performed in less than 2 minutes, and the emphasis should be on detecting the residua of previous injuries so that the athlete can undergo rehabilitative exercises which may prevent a reinjury. The athlete, wearing only underwear, should stand in front of the examiner, and the physician should call out the commands listed in Table 15-1. The physician should look for the listed abnormalities.

Disqualification

Unfortunately, the most widely used list of reasons for disqualifications from athletic events is now obsolete. It was first compiled by the American Medical Association (AMA) in 1966 and was last revised in 1976. An example of one of its guidelines that perhaps is not now applicable is its proscription from playing even non-contact sports for the boy with an inguinal hernia, whereas many pediatric surgeons would currently advise elective herniorrhaphy after the sports season. Those guidelines also forbid athletes with the absence or loss of function of one eye from all contact or collision sports, but the availability now of American Society for Testing and Materials (ASTM)-approved safety eye-guards might make these risks more acceptable. The AMA list is being revised by the American Academy of Pediatrics, but until that is published the practitioner could consider the guidelines in Tables 15-2 and 15-3, which represent my views.

SCHOOL TEAM PHYSICIAN

A physician is often asked to be the school's team doctor for the team in which his child is a member. If he agrees, then he cannot merely sit in the stands waiting to be called in the case of an injury. The physician should only agree to do the job if a total team–physician program is instituted. The physician should also obtain in writing the school's agreement to this program with their recognition that the team physician has the ultimate authority to keep a player off the field. The tasks and responsibilities of the team physician include the following:

1. Know the general factors that contribute to injuries: conditioning, coaching techniques, rules, equipment.
2. Educate self, parents, coaches, and students as to the risk factors of the involved sport and what procedures are needed to reduce these risks.

(*Text continues on p. 80*)

Table 15-3. Qualifying Conditions for Competitive Sports Participation

CONDITIONS	COLLISION	LIMITED CONTACT	NONCONTACT STRENUOUS	MODERATELY STRENUOUS	NONSTRENUOUS
Atlanto-axial Instability	No	No	Yes (no butterfly, breast stroke, or diving starts in swimming)	Yes	Yes
Acute Illnesses	Need individual assessment (*i.e.*, contagious to others, risk of worsening illness, and so forth)				
Cardiovascular Carditis	No	No	No	No	No
Hypertension Mild	Yes	Yes	Yes	Yes	Yes
Moderate		Needs individual assessment	Needs individual assessment		Yes
Severe		Needs individual assessment	Needs individual assessment		Yes
Congenital heart disease	Patients with mild forms of congenital heart disease can be allowed a full range of physical activities. Patients with moderate or severe forms of cardiac disease, or who are postoperative, should be evaluated by a cardiologist before athletic participation.				Yes
Eyes Absence or loss of function of one eye	The availability of ASTM-approved eye guards may allow the competitor to compete in most sports, but this must be judged on an individual basis.				
Detached retina			Consult ophthalmologist		
Hernia Inguinal	Yes	Yes	Yes	Yes	Yes
Kidney Absence of one	No	Yes	Yes	Yes	Yes

Condition					
Liver					
Enlarged	No	No	Yes	Yes	Yes
Neurologic					
History of previous serious head or spine trauma, repeated concussions, or craniotomy	Needs more assessment		Yes	Yes	Yes
Convulsive disorder					
Well controlled	Yes	Yes	Yes	Yes	Yes
Poorly controlled	No	No	Yes (no swimming or weight lifting)	Yes	Yes (no archery or riflery)
Ovary					
Absence of one	Yes	Yes	Yes	Yes	Yes
Respiratory					
Pulmonary insufficiency	May be allowed to compete if oxygenation remains satisfactory during a graded stress test			Yes	Yes
Asthma	Yes	Yes	Yes	Yes	Yes
Skin					
Boils, impetigo, scabies, herpes	No wrestling, martial arts, gymnastics with mats, or skin-to-skin contact until not contagious	Yes	Yes	Yes	Yes
Spleen					
Enlarged	No	No	No	Yes	Yes
Testicle					
Absence or undescended	Yes Certain sports will require protective cup	Yes	Yes	Yes	Yes

("No" = Should not participate)

3. Evaluate the playing surface and the equipment for dangerous conditions.
4. Evaluate all injuries and establish a system for the management and follow-up of these problems.
5. Evaluate the conditioning and training procedures for safety factors.
6. Establish criteria for disqualification from participation in competitive sports and for returning to competition after an illness or injury.
7. Review all histories and physical examinations done by other physicians. Re-evaluate the student or contact the physician if any questions arise from this review, and do the examination if no primary physician is available.
8. Establish a record system for all injuries.
9. Establish rehabilitation procedures for injuries.
10. Establish a transportation and referral system for all serious injuries.
11. Learn the rules of the sport and evaluate the officials' adherence to enforcing the rules that pertain to player safety.
12. Observe the techniques used by the coaches in teaching the sport and advise them of those techniques that contribute to injuries or excessive stress.

The question of compensation for the team physician is complicated by the fact that some state "good Samaritan" statutes protecting physicians from medical liability when responding to emergencies specifically include the rendering of care at school athletic events, but this protection ceases if a fee is rendered for the service. This is generally an academic discussion, however, as schools only rarely have any funds available for this service, and by and large the physician should accept the fact that this activity will be a service to the community.

ANNOTATED BIBLIOGRAPHY

American Academy of Orthopedic Surgeons: Athletic Training and Sports Medicine. Chicago, IL, American Academy of Orthopedic Surgeons, 1984 (Covers the important and practical aspects of caring for and preventing soft-tissue injuries such as taping, elastic bandaging, recognition of injuries, and rehabilitative exercises.)

Committee on Sports Medicine: Sports Medicine: Health Care for Young Athletes. Elk Grove Village, IL, American Academy of Pediatrics, 1983 (Consists of chapters covering the entire field of pediatric sports medicine. It is directed toward the primary care physician.)

Goldberg B, Saraniti A, Wiltman P et al: Preparticipation sports assessment—an objective evaluation. Pediatrics 66:736–745, 1980 (One half of the high-school athletes in this series had no other contact with a physician during the school year. Only about 1% of those undergoing the traditional medical examination had physical abnormalities detected that might affect safety or performance.)

Micheli LD (ed): Pediatric and Adolescent Sports Medicine. Boston, Little, Brown, 1984 (Directed toward the primary-care physician rather than the orthopedist and covers many of the same subjects as the aforementioned handbook by the American Academy of Pediatrics.)

Thompson TR, Andrish JT, Bergfeld JA: A prospective study of preparticipation sports examinations of 2670 young athletes: Method and results. Cleve Clin Q 49:225–233, 1982 (In this series of adolescents the focus of the examination was on the musculoskeletal system; 10% had abnormalities detected, usually residua of previous injuries.)

3

Environmental Influences on Children

16
Common Environmental Concerns

JACK L. MAYER

Parents often express concerns about environmental hazards that may adversely affect their children. Environmental toxins can and do produce morbidity and mortality that we can prevent with anticipatory guidance. The most common environmental concerns are discussed in this chapter with the dual purpose of informing health professionals and helping them counsel families on actual risks, risk abatement, and prevention. Linking exposure to illness requires a high index of suspicion, documentation of exposure, and temporal relation to illness. Queries and clinical observations may be referred to the American Academy of Pediatrics Committee on Environmental Hazards.

AIR POLLUTION

Outdoor

The sources of air pollution are unbiquitous in our industrial society. Combustion in industrial, domestic, and transportation activities are the primary sources. The Clean Air Act of 1970 and its subsequent revisions have improved outdoor air quality significantly. Health effects of such pollution depend on the length of time of exposure and the concentration of pollutants. Well-controlled studies have linked air pollution, including acid rain, mist, and fog, with recurrent respiratory disease. The Environmental Protection Agency (EPA) sets air quality standards (permitted levels of contamination) for six major or "criteria pollutants": sulfur dioxide, nitrogen dioxide, carbon monoxide, ozone, total suspended particles, and lead.

Pollutants will be regulated in the next decade. Benzene, added to gasoline after lead is removed, is a prime example, with ambient levels in urban areas sometimes exceeding EPA guidelines. Wood stoves are another example. The toxic gases released into the environment are distributed almost at ground level in residential neighborhoods. Wood-burning stoves may contribute to more health effects than any other outdoor pollution in northern latitudes. Air-tight stoves produce the most pollution. The EPA has still not established standards and regulations. Since this is a community problem that can be corrected by the installment of catalytic combustors in stoves, its amelioration depends on regulation of the sale or use of stoves.

Indoor

Indoor air pollution, more so than outdoor air pollution, causes and contributes to respiratory disease in infants and children with sensitive airways. Second-hand smoke, kerosene space heaters, gas stoves with pilot lights, improperly drafted wood stoves, and leaks in stove pipes allow odorless combustion products (e.g., CO, NO_2, SO_2, Ozone) to attain high concentrations in households. Weatherization and tight home construction further increase concentrations.

The role of the practitioner is to identify susceptible children and inform them or their parents of the hazard. When outdoor air quality is poor, prophylactic medication and avoidance of exposure to the outdoors may be indicated. Inquire about sources of indoor air pollution. On the community level, health care professionals can support efforts to enforce and strengthen the Clean Air Act.

WATER POLLUTION

Water pollution may be natural (siltation in a river during flooding) or created by humans. Human sources are the most troublesome and include logging, mining, grazing, irrigation, feedlots, sewage discharges, urban storm drainage, refuse disposal, and toxic waste dumps.

Water quality is evaluated on the basis of four characteristics: physical, chemical, biologic, and radiologic. Physical characteristics (*e.g.*, taste, odor, color, temperature, turbidity, suspended solids, and dissolved mineral content) are of ancillary concern with the exception of dissolved minerals such as sodium. High mineral content has a laxative effect and in extreme situations may represent an unacceptable solute load for formula-fed infants.

Water softening is a process that removes calcium and magnesium. Epidemiologic evidence links the softness of drinking water with increased morbidity and mortality from cardiovascular disease. Some community water systems have a softening process in line but it is inadvisable for individuals to add a softener under usual circumstances.

Chemical characteristics are of more concern. Inorganic substances such as metals and salts are often regulated but, in residential situations, not monitored. Lead leaches out of soldered joints in pipes, especially in hot or acidic water, and may contribute to the lead problem. Organic substances (oil, grease, pesticides, organochlorides, and organic salts) are becoming a major concern. Some pesticides and chemicals are regulated, but most are not, and they may pose serious public health risks.

Risks must often be balanced by benefits. Chlorine, as a disinfectant routinely added to residential and community water systems, reacts with trace organic sustances producing trihalomethanes that may be carcinogenic. However, since chlorination protects the public from lethal infectious disease, the risk from trihalomethane ingestion is considered "acceptable." Alternatives to chlorination are being investigated.

The usual biologic monitoring of water is accomplished by coliform counts that are reliable indicators of fecal contamination from grazing, manure spreading, or sewage. Routine surveillance of community water systems is the responsibility of the health department, but residential water supplies unassociated with a community system may be a source of illness. A simple coliform count, usually free of charge, will rule out this possibility.

Radiologic characteristics depend on the soil and rock through which the water percolates. The EPA standard of annual exposure from water is 4 mrem/year. Many natural springs are more radioactive in orders of magnitude than the EPA standards allow. A concerned parent can obtain a radiologic sampling from the health department. It is best for the physician to facilitate such testing, thereby allaying anxiety and suspicion.

TOXIC WASTE DISPOSAL

The EPA has estimated that as little as 10% of all hazardous wastes are properly disposed. Love Canal has dramatized the problem of toxic wastes and their health effects. Pesticides, toxic organic and inorganic chemicals, and radioactive wastes are discarded in landfills, virtually all of which leak. The Senate Health and Scientific Research Committee estimates that 1.2 million Americans are exposed to highly and moderately serious health hazards from dumping sites. Ground water contamination is the chief concern. Almost half of the nation's drinking water is ground water—a fragile and easily polluted resource.

Breast milk may be contaminated with such toxins as DDT, PCBs, Chlordane, dioxin, dieldrin, and Heptachlor from ambient as well as occupational exposure. Risk assessment depends on expensive and often inaccessibile laboratory studies. The actual hazards are unknown but some chemicals, like dioxin, are ubiquitous and are often found in concentrations higher than those permitted for formula or whole milk. Breast-feeding should still be encouraged, but pregnant and lactating women should avoid eating freshwater fish from contaminated waters (notably the Great Lakes), should not use pesticides or herbicides, and should be advised against excessive weight reduction that mobilizes these chemicals from fat stores. Testing of breast milk is recommended after known exposure or heavy consumption of contaminated sport fish; concerned parents may request such analysis regardless of exposure. Interpretation of the results in terms of risk is controversial.

Brought-home toxins are a major source of childhood exposure. Work clothes, including footwear, can carry significant quantities of dusts, metals, and solvents into the home. A parent occupationally exposed to solvents may also bring these home on hair, skin, and through respiratory excretion. Part of the environmental database should include the occupations of household members and an inquiry regarding the presence of unusual odors in the home after work days.

The impact on health of this large number of contaminants is difficult to discern. Synergistic action of various chemicals and individual sensitivity or allergy play confounding roles in trying to determine health effects. In 1980 the Surgeon General concluded, "We believe that toxic chemicals are adding to the disease burden on the U.S. in a significant, although as yet ill-defined way." Because of long latency periods, the long-term health effects of low-dose exposure are still not conclusively documented.

Exposures are certainly occurring and health professionals should be alert to unknown health effects. Toxic dumps have compounded the problem of waste isolation. Waste reduction, chemical and biologic treatment of waste, incineration, and recycling are all possible alternatives that should be fostered. Pediatricians should influence environmental legislation to curb exposures to toxic wastes.

PESTICIDES AND HERBICIDES

Control of pests and weeds on lawns, houseplants, in gardens, and in homes are a major source of exposure. Chlordane, the most frequently applied termite control chemical, achieves toxic levels in homes and often causes illness. Its use has been banned in New York, Massachusetts, and Japan. Aerial spraying of agricultural land and ground water contamination expose many other people. Most ground water in the United States has measurable levels of pesticides.

HOUSEHOLD TOXICS

Proper disposal of household toxics should be advised as part of routine anticipatory guidance. The average American home has 3 to 10 gallons of hazardous chemicals in the garage, basement, shed, and kitchen. Routine housecleaning with aerosols, oven cleaners, polishes, and volatile liquid cleaners may pose a toxic threat. Ventilation should be encouraged. These products are hazardous because they are poisonous, flammable, corrosive, reactive, explosive, or carcinogenic.

ASBESTOS

Many practitioners will face the dilemma of asbestos abatement. Asbestos is a potent carcinogen and there may be no safe level of exposure. Asbestos, however, is ubiquitous in the environment. It is a remarkable synthetic fiber that strengthens, insulates, and fireproofs and it is both easy and economical to work with. When inhaled, the long, thin fibers of asbestos are the most likely to cause harm. Of the various fiber types *Crocidolite* and *Amosite* fibers are more hazardous than *Chrysotile*.

Among the products that contain asbestos are pipe coverings, brake linings, plaster, plaster board, thermal and acoustic insulation, roofing and flooring products (including vinyl asbestos floor tiles), textiles, cements, paper, and felt. Until 1978, fireproofing materials containing asbestos were sprayed onto the structural components of buildings. School children are exposed to asbestos in walls, ceilings, and other exposed surfaces. Sources of asbestos in the home include old spackling compound, paper-maché (containing up to 50% asbestos), asbestos gloves or cement board, hand-held hair dryers, and furnace air ducts insulated with asbestos in homes and schools built in the 1940s and 1950s. The EPA estimates that 5,000 to 10,000 excess cancer deaths occur each year as a result of industrial exposure to asbestos. Spouses and children of asbestos workers appear to be at risk of contracting mesothelioma and lung cancer secondary to "brought home" asbestos on workers' clothing.

There is no acute illness associated with asbestos exposure. The question of a dose–response relationship between asbestos inhalation and cancer is still controversial. Such a dose–response relationship seems to exist for bronchogenic carcinoma and asbestosis but has not been established for mesothelioma. Thus, the risk for lung cancer and asbestosis is low in nonoccupational settings but it is unknown for mesothelioma. The latency period for the development of mesothelioma is 20 to 40 years, creating a dilemma for epidemiologists and regulators.

In the school setting, risk assessment must be based on current and potential exposure. Low dose implies low risk except for questions about mesothelioma. The Asbestos Hazard Emergency Response Act of 1986 now requires that all public and private schools should be inspected for asbestos-containing material and requires abatement of the exposure.

Local physicians should address the health issues and allay anxiety. The risks are low. Depending on the circumstances, asbestos abatement is best accomplished over the summer when school is closed. If friable sources are present, they can be temporarily sealed. Hasty abatement is often worse than no abatement at all. Aggressive removal programs carried out by uncertified contractors create high levels of asbestos in the air while the material is torn out of the building, accentuating existing low levels of fibers in the air.

FORMALDEHYDE

The chief sources of formaldehyde in the home are particle board, plywood, carpets, urea–formaldehyde (UF) foam insulation, combustion appliances, tobacco smoke, cosmetics, deodorants, solvents, disinfectants, and fumigants. Urea–formaldehyde foam was approved for use as insulation in the early 1970s and an estimated 500,000 homes in the United States are insulated with it. Exposure sources of most importance are UF foam insulation, particle board, and plywood in mobile homes. In the United States alone there are in excess of 4 million mobile homes, most of which are tightly constructed allowing for little air exchange with the outside. Floors and furniture are often made of particle board and plywood.

The health effects are related to the concentration in the environment and the individual's sensitivity. Levels of formaldehyde increase and decrease as much as 20-fold depending on heat and humidity, which may account for markedly different measurements in the same home. Even at low levels infants, asthmatics, allergic children, and sensitized individuals may suffer dermatitis and recurrent bronchospasm. Formaldehyde is considered an animal, and possibly a human, carcinogen. As the ambient concentration increases, the effects include neurophysiologic effects (including EEG changes, ataxia, headache, dizziness), eye, nose, and throat irritation, persistent cough, nausea and vomiting, respiratory distress, and frequent respiratory infections. Infants are especially susceptible with symptoms including vomiting, diarrhea, watery eyes, restlessness, excessive crying, and anorexia.

A National Academy of Science study suggests that as many as 20% of healthy adults experience reactions to formaldehyde at less than 0.25 ppm, which is half the usual standard.

Homes built before 1970 in the United States probably do not contain UF insulation. If the insulation was not blown in, it is not UF. Sampling of insulation material is the most accurate way to determine composition. If the material definitely is UF foam or if the family resides in a mobile home, the next question is what are the levels? Local or state health departments may be equipped to conduct formaldehyde testing. If not, many commercial laboratories can perform the analysis (see the Yellow Pages under "laboratories"). Levels less than 0.1ppm are probably safe, although some individuals are sensitive. If levels are greater than 0.1ppm as an average over 24 hours, additional measurements are required to determine how the levels change with time, temperature, and humidity.

Substitution and encapsulation are two methods of formaldehyde reduction that can be recommended. UF foam can be replaced with other insulation at great cost. Some states and Canada provide financial aid to homeowners faced with this problem. Encapsulation (covering particle board with shellac, varnish, polymeric coating, or other diffusion barriers) is cheaper but its effectiveness has not been proven.

MERCURY

Mercury dental fillings have been suggested as a source of mercury contamination because of releases of mercury vapor. No signs or symptoms of mercury toxicity have been found in dentists. Removing amalgam fillings to replace them with non-mercury fillings creates significant exposure to mercury during the procedure. Most dental authorities do not suggest wholesale replacement of mercury fillings. Rarely, an individual is allergic to mercury and appropriate allergy testing can confirm this.

Alternatives to mercury include gold castings (caps or inlays) and plastics or composite resins that may have untoward health effects not yet appreciated.

HEAVY METALS

Lead, mercury, and cadmium are found everywhere in the environment. Industrial pollution and "brought-home" dust from occupational settings are sources of childhood toxicity. Lead, mercury, arsenic, chromium, and manganese are associated with the use of glazes, paints, and inks in such hobbies as ceramics and stained glass. Strengthening the Clean Air Act is essential to reduce industrial emissions of these toxins.

HOBBIES

Children using art materials are routinely exposed to solvents and heavy metals including benzene, carbon tetrachloride, toluene, lead, hexane, cadmium, and so forth. Artists, craftsmen, and their children are exposed to such known toxins and carcinogens as solvents (in paints, inks, thinners, and paint removers), heavy metals (in pigments, glazes, enamels, and solders), and dusts (silica and asbestos in clays, talcs, and glazes). Children who build models are exposed to solvents. Artists' materials are not always adequately labelled to indicate their potential toxicity.

Anticipatory guidance consists of adequate ventilation, avoidance of skin contact, and full knowledge of the toxicity of materials and methods. Pregnant and breast-feeding women should avoid using solvents. Information can be obtained from the *Center for Occupational Hazards* listed with the Poisindex. *The Arts and Crafts Materials Institute* established a voluntary program to ensure the safety of children's art material. Products bearing the approved product (AP) seal have been certified by a toxicologist to be safe, even if ingested. Those with the certified product (CP) seal have also been certified safe.

RADIATION

Natural sources of radiation account for half of all exposures. This does not imply that such exposure is benign.

Radon

As many as 20% of homes in the United States have radon levels above the EPA action standard. Radon, a colorless, odorless gas produced naturally in the ground from uranium, seeps into homes and may cause 5 to 20,000 lung cancer deaths each year. Regulatory programs will probably be administered by each state. The EPA has released consumer guides on radon and radon reduction methods which are available on request.

Cosmic rays, minerals, food, water, air, and other natural sources may be responsible for as many as 45,000 cancer deaths per year. Radioactive fallout persists in the form of ^{90}Sr and plutonium. France and China still test nuclear weapons in the atmosphere. The effect on health of low-level radiation is controversial.

X-Rays

With the notable exception of radon, a practitioner can do little about natural exposures, but the medical and dental professions add to this burden with x-rays. Forty percent of the total radiation exposure of individuals and 90% of man-made radiation exposure results from medical and dental x-rays. A high percentage of x-rays are ordered because of repeated examinations due to poor technique, patient demand, concern over litigation, institutional requirements (routine preoperative and admission films), and inappropriate use in tuberculosis screening.

In May 1984 the American Dental Association (ADA) approved recommendations for radiographic practices that stressed individualized assessment of the need, type, and frequency of dental x-rays. The ADA rejected the concept of routine radiography as a part of periodic examinations of all patients. Leaded aprons and collars should be used to minimize unnecessary radiation exposure.

Food Irradiation

In 1985 the Secretary of the Department of Health and Human Services authorized gamma irradiation of fruits and vegetables. Because of anxiety generated by radiation, practitioners are likely to be asked about eating irradiated food. The food itself poses no radiologic threat. Irradiation will reduce spoilage (which wastes 25% to 30% of the world's food). The food has a longer shelf life and can be transported better. There is a sharply decreased need for chemical adulteration with nitrates, nitrites, preservatives, and fumigants. Irradiation does not deplete nutrients as drastically as canning.

However, there may be serious problems. Irradiation of food generates unique radiolytic products (URP) that are uncharacterized and untested for toxicity. Furthermore, food irradiation will not replace pesticides because it is used post-harvest. Widespread food irradiation will greatly expand the nuclear economy exposing more workers and the public to radiation hazards, multiplying the transport (and accidental release) of radioactive material, and raising concern about the eventual disposition of ^{60}Co and ^{137}Cs when they lose effectiveness as food irradiators, but still emit radiation. A major concern is that current regulations do not call for adequate labelling of irradiated food.

NOISE

Acoustic trauma is damage to the ear from a sharply rising wave front such as an explosion. This type of injury is often painless and the damage and subsequent hearing loss is insidious. Continuous exposure of adults to 85 dB (the sound energy of heavy traffic) is capable of causing hearing loss. A significant hearing loss may also arise from sounds associated with communication (headphones, cordless telephones), transportation (living near an airport), mechanization in the home (power tools), and children's toys (capguns, infant squeak toys).

In addition to the obvious concern of noise exposure causing hearing loss, the extra-auditory effects of noise, such as increased blood pressure, heart rate, respiratory rate, and general contraction of muscles are now being documented.

STRESS

Stress can be defined as a dysequilibrium between environmental demands and the person's coping resources that disrupts that person's physical or psychological well-being. Stress can be normative or exceptional. All children experience some form of normative stress. Eighteen percent of children move each year. Sibling rivalry, separation anxiety, new schools, and so forth, are some examples of the wide array of common stresses that children endure. Exceptional stress represents a subjectively heavier burden of distress for the child. 1.1 million children were involved in divorce in 1982. By 1990, one third of children in the United States will have experienced the effects of divorce.

The adult literature strongly suggests a link between levels of stress and illness such as hypertension, myocardial infarction, ulcers, asthma, and colitis. The pediatric literature relates stress to an increasing frequency and duration of minor illness and injuries as well as perinatal complications. Recurrent abdominal pain, headaches, school failure, and acting-out behavior are often related to stress and anxiety.

The pediatrician's role is to identify and reduce stress and promote coping. Identification of support factors such as social network availability, family ties and values, and social connections for adults and children should be included in the data base. An excess of sick visits should prompt further investigation of particular stressors. Certain questions facilitate such communication: "What is it about your child's illness or symptoms that concerns you?"; "What else is going on in your family that might be upsetting your child?"; "What do you do when you're angry, sad, isolated?"

NUCLEAR WAR

Awareness of nuclear weapons and anxiety about nuclear war develops early in childhood, chiefly through the media. The American Psychiatric Association's Task Force on Nuclear Developments reported that "thoughts of nuclear annihilation had penetrated deeply into the consciousness of children and adolescents."

A growing world-wide literature, increasingly quantitative, finds young people's concerns about nuclear war to be part of the broader context of other issues traditionally important to youth. The remarkable consistency of these studies' findings strongly suggests that nuclear concerns transcend class and ethnic lines. Large numbers of children and adolescents (consistently more than 30%) think often about the risk of nuclear war and worry that it may, or believe that it will, take place in their lifetime.

In communicating with young people about our nuclear dilemma, we should foster thoughtful, age-appropriate discussion taking into account developmental stage, individual vulnerabilities, and young people's need to know. Most children, by age 9, are ready to talk about nuclear issues. In June 1985, the National Parent–Teacher Association adopted a second resolution at their national conference supporting nuclear age education.

Since we all share in the nuclear dilemma, pediatricians have a personal as well as a professional role to play. It is unnecessary to burden children with adult concerns that exceed their questions and concerns. However, it is appropriate to validate young people's concerns and share with them how difficult it is to talk about nuclear war. This means we have to listen, reassure them that many people are working to end the threat of nuclear war, and that we expect to be successful.

ANNOTATED BIBLIOGRAPHY

Boyce WT (ed). Stress and Child Health. Pediatr Ann 14(8), 1985 (Collection of articles reviewing the evidence for a relationship between stress and illness in children.)

Eisenbud MM, Van Hoorn JL, Gould BB: Children, adolescents and the threat of nuclear war: An international perspective. Adv Internat Maternal and Child Health 6:1–23, 1986 (Complete review of the international literature with a comprehensive bibliography.

This article will be valuable for school boards and administrators trying to document the need for a nuclear education curriculum.)

Imperato PJ, Mitchell G: Acceptable Risks. New York, Viking, 1985 (Very readable book that explores the complexity of risk assessment by detailing conflicting views on such issues as radiation, formaldehyde, and air pollution.)

Jones S, Thompson G, Berman S: "Mom, What *Is* Nuclear War?" Boston, WBZ-TV and Boston Area Educators for Social Responsibility, 1985 (This 13-page pamphlet is a guide for parents, teachers, and other concerned adults to answering children's questions about nuclear issues. Physicians may want to order this pamphlet in bulk for distribution to parents.)

Rom WN (ed): Environmental and Occupational Medicine. Boston, Little, Brown, 1983 (One of the standard textbooks detailing physical, biological and chemical hazards and controversies.)

Turiel I: Indoor Air Quality and Human Health. Stanford, Stanford University Press, 1985 (Intended for readers outside the research community and conveys public health information in a thorough, concise fashion.)

17
Lead Poisoning
STEVEN M. MARCUS

Interest in lead as a poison dates back many centuries. Within the last 15 years, renewed interest has developed in lead poisoning both as an industrial and environmental problem. The realization that childhood lead poisoning may have lasting effects on child development has kindled increased interest. Lead poisoning in adults occurs primarily in those involved in industries utilizing lead. Over 900 occupations are considered at risk; some are obvious such as smelter workers, others are less obvious such as policemen, and still others are quite cryptic, such as roofers and utility meter readers. Other adults become exposed to lead through their hobbies: stained glass workers, sport shooters, or automotive restorers. Children may be subjected to exposure through close contact with parents with such occupations or hobbies.

DEFINITION. Lead poisoning is defined by the United States Centers for Disease Control (CDC), as a blood lead level over 25 μg/dl and free erythrocyte protoporphyrin (FEP) of over 35 μg/dl.

Children usually develop lead poisoning through the ingestion of lead-containing substances, principally lead-based paint. A significant portion of the housing stock was painted at least once with lead-based paint. When this paint peels or flakes it becomes an inviting hazard for a toddler who tends to test his environment with his mouth. Nearly 5% of all children tested for lead poisoning are found to have excessive amounts of lead in their blood.

Children living in inner-city residences appear particularly prone to develop lead poisoning, with a significantly increased incidence found in the black population. Gentrification of inner-city dwellings by affluent people who sand, burn, or otherwise remove layers of lead-laden paint may expose entire families to excessive amounts of lead.

The greatest number of cases and the severest cases of lead poisoning appear to occur from the late spring to the early fall months. This apparent seasonal variation is not well understood.

PATHOPHYSIOLOGY

Lead is a protean poison; it has been shown to disturb the cellular metabolism of every tissue and organ in the body. Perhaps its best known effect is on the hematopoietic system in which it interferes with the biosynthesis of heme. This produces an anemia that mimics that of iron deficiency, with a rise in heme precursors, particularly erythrocyte protoporphyrin (EP), also known as free erythrocyte protoporphyrin (FEP), or zinc protoporphyrin (ZPP).

A more serious concern is the effect of lead on the central nervous system (CNS), particularly on the developing brain of the child. Lead has been reported to produce a syndrome that ranges in severity from no defects to learning disabilities, frank retardation, and seizure disorders. Lead has also been implicated in the etiology of chronic renal disease, hypertension, and gout.

CLINICAL PRESENTATION

Most patients with lead poisoning present with *little* or *no overt symptomatology*. When symptoms do occur, they imply serious poisoning. Among the common symptoms referable to the gastrointestinal tract are vomiting, abdominal pain, constipation, and loss of appetite. The common CNS symptoms include projectile vomiting, lethargy, irritability, and lack of attention span; there may be an arrest or a regression in developmental stages. There may also be signs of a peripheral neuropathy, such as hypoesthesias and paresthesias.

It is imperative that a careful parent, occupational, and environmental history be obtained from any patient or parent of a patient presenting with complaints such as these, especially during the summer months.

LABORATORY TESTS

The laboratory evaluation of a patient for lead poisoning is relatively simple. The definitive tests are determinations of *blood lead* and *FEP* values. This can be done in most proprietary and in some hospital laboratories. A sample must be obtained in a lead-free container that contains an anticoagulant. Both the lead and FEP values are subject to a 10% to 15% laboratory error. Of the two tests, the FEP test is perhaps the more reliable. Lead levels tend to vary more widely than FEPs both physiologically and because of laboratory factors. FEP reflects aberrations in hemoglobin synthesis; it may reflect the presence of iron deficiency anemia as well as lead poisoning. FEP closely reflects *biologic* effects of lead poisoning.

Hemoglobin (Hgb), hematocrit (Hct), or mean corpuscular volume (MCV) should not be used as the only screen for lead poisoning because mild to moderate degrees of lead poisoning may exist in small children in the absence of these hematologic abnormalities.

A *peripheral smear* may reveal a hypochromic, microcytic anemia. Microcytic hypochromic anemia, in adolescence, indicates a need for further evaluation. If such an adolescent is occupationally exposed to lead, then he should be considered to have lead poisoning until proven otherwise. Iron deficiency anemia is not uncommon in menstruating females. Basophilic stippling of the red blood cells occurs in chronic lead poisoning of a significant nature. Basophilic stippling also occurs in certain hemoglobinopathies, but it is of a different character and can be differentiated by a good technologist or hematologist. Urinalysis may reveal the presence of glucose or protein secondary to the renal tubular dysfunction caused by lead. X-rays may reveal the presence of radio-opaque foreign material in the gastrointestinal tract in children who ingest lead-containing substances. Further, growth arrest lines in the distal metaphyses of the growing

bones of children may be seen in individuals with chronic lead poisoning.

The *EDTA mobilization* test may be useful in determining which patients will excrete significant quantities of lead in response to chelation therapy. This test is not advised if lead levels are elevated. The CDC recommends that an EDTA mobilization test be performed on every child with a lead level of over 25 μg/dl and a corresponding FEP over 35 μg/dl. Lead levels over 55 μg/dl are universally associated with a prompt postchelation plumburesis. Any delay in therapy waiting for the results of the mobilization would, therefore, not be indicated. Children with lead levels between 25 μg/dl and 60 μg/dl who are *symptomatic* should be placed on chelation therapy without any further evaluation. Children with blood lead levels between 25 μg/dl and 60 μg/dl who are *asymptomatic* and who have no overt signs of biologic damage from lead may benefit from a mobilization test in an attempt to determine if chelation therapy will successfully lower the body burden of lead. After the patient empties his bladder, a dose of 50 mg/kg of calcium disodium EDTA is administered either intravenously over a 1-hour period or intramuscularly. All urine produced during the next 24 hours is collected in a lead-free container and is analyzed for total lead excretion. This test must be performed and interpreted with the awareness of the difficulties in collecting 24-hour urine specimens. Lead excretion over 24 hours in excess of 1 μg of lead for 1 mg of EDTA administered is considered an indication that a good response will occur from a full course of chelation. Some studies suggest that an 8-hour collection in children is adequate. A modification is then made: A urine excretion greater than 0.5 μg Pb/mg EDTA suggests a good result from full chelation.

TREATMENT

Treatment of patients with lead poisoning depends on the presence or absence of symptoms and the degree of lead burden. *Patients should be removed from their lead exposed environment.* Patients who are *symptomatic* should have chelation therapy initiated as soon as possible. Asymptomatic children with positive EDTA mobilization tests will probably benefit from chelation therapy. Since data concerning the long-term effects of lead poisoning on development relate effects to lead levels and not FEP, it is the lead level that determines the need for therapy.

Available lead chelation therapy regimens include BAL and EDTA, EDTA alone, and d-penicillamine. Animal data suggest that of the chelators available, only dimercaprol (BAL) crosses the blood–brain barrier in any appreciable concentration. Patients presenting with lead encephalopathy should, therefore, be treated with an initial dose of BAL followed by both BAL and EDTA. BAL is not water soluble and must be administered intramuscularly in a dose of 3 to 4.5 mg/kg per dose administered every 4 hours. Its administration carries with it a significant risk of local problems such as sterile abscesses, febrile responses, and hepatic inflammation.

Nonencephalopathic patients with lead levels above 80 µg/dl require large amounts of chelator to be administered to assure an appropriate chelator to lead ratio. Administration of sufficient amounts of either BAL or EDTA alone in such circumstances is limited by their inherent toxicity. The use of concurrent administration of both EDTA and BAL is thus recommended in such cases.

EDTA is a water-soluble chelator that is essentially nonmetabolized. EDTA can be used alone when patients have no signs or symptoms of CNS involvement or when lead levels are below 80 mg/dl. When used intravenously, it has been shown to have few toxic effects. Five hundred milligrams of EDTA is added to 1000 ml of IV solution and is administered at a rate of delivery to provide a dose of 50 mg/kg/day. When used intramuscularly, side effects such as local irritation at the injection site and renal impairment have been common. Pain at the injection site may require that either xylocaine or procaine be incorporated into the injection solution. Creatine phosphokinase (CPK) levels may be elevated because of the large amount of tissue damage caused by the injection. EDTA may also produce significant renal impairment, thus careful attention must be paid to urinalysis. Oral EDTA is contraindicated because it increases lead absorption from the GI tract.

It is unclear whether EDTA itself has any local effects on the kidney or whether it is the chelated lead that impairs renal function. The lead–EDTA complex is water soluble and stable at physiologic pH; however, free lead may be released in acid environments. There may be justification for the alkalinization of the urine to protect against the effects of the lead–EDTA complex on the renal tubule. Incorporation of EDTA into a continuous intravenous infusion appears to decrease the incidence of renal toxicity and hence is preferable to bolus injection. Some physicians use intramuscular EDTA in outpatient chelation when lead levels are low. Considering the need to separate children from lead sources and toxicity found with IM EDTA, this technique should be restricted to selected patients for which hospitalization is impossible.

D-penicillamine is an orally effective chelating agent. Although shown to be an effective chelator of lead, it has not yet been approved by the Food and Drug Administration for such use. However, it is used commonly in a dose of 20 to 40 mg/kg/day and appears to produce a prompt plumburesis. D-penicillamine should be used only in the *chronic* phase of treatment; there is no role for its use in the acute treatment of lead poisoning, especially when encephalopathy is present.

A close follow-up of all patients treated for lead poisoning is mandatory. All patients chelated should be retested no later than 2 weeks after completion of the therapy. The lead levels of many patients treated for lead poisoning may "rebound" due to the re-equilibration of lead from bone and soft tissue or from re-exposure. If lead levels rise too high, chelation may have to be repeated.

It is still unclear whether treatment after the lead level has reached the highly toxic range is effective in reversing or preventing long-term effects. Until this point is settled, it is the physician's responsibility to attempt to keep lead levels within the low, acceptable ranges.

All children who have lead poisoning deserve nutritional counseling. A diet rich in calcium, protein, and iron is beneficial whereas excess salt and fat should be avoided. A correlation has been found between dust-lead content, dust-control measures, and lead poisoning. Thus, attention must be paid to careful housekeeping methods. Such measures as wet-mopping and moist dusting must be implemented.

Close follow-up, removal of sources of lead, and early chelation are imperative.

CHELATING REGIMENS

Several chelating regimens accepted for treatment of lead poisoning are outlined below. They were developed by the New Jersey Lead Consortium as an adaptation of the CDC guidelines for therapy after successful treatment of over 1000 lead-poisoned children. These regimens have now been used to treat over 10,000 children.

1. Dual Chelation Therapy: BAL–EDTA combination
   Dosages
   BAL = 18 mg/kg/day (375 mg/m²/day); a dosage range of 3 to 4.5 mg/kg/dose Q4h is acceptable. Divide daily dose into 6 parts, give Q 4 hours

EDTA = 50 mg/kg/day (1000 mg/m^2/day); a dosage range of 40 to 50 mg/kg/day is acceptable. See (3) below for specifics concerning EDTA administration.

Schedule

Divide total daily BAL dosage into 6 parts. Give an *initial dose of BAL alone* (3 to 4.5 mg/kg/dose Q4h) by deep IM injection. Four hours later and continuing Q4h thereafter BAL and EDTA are given simultaneously. BAL is given by deep IM injection. EDTA is given at the same time Q4h at a separate IM site, or may be given intravenously. *See (3) for specifics concerning EDTA administration.*

The usual course of treatment is 5 days.

Note

On completion of this course, further chelation should be considered, as outlined under chelating regimens (3) or (4). Alternatively, further chelation therapy may be withheld until results of postchelation rebound Pb values are available. Based on laboratory studies and the patient's medical and social conditions, a regimen for further chelation therapy can be selected.

2. Modified Dual Therapy: BAL–EDTA combination for 3 days followed by EDTA alone for 2 days

Dosage

BAL: As described under (1) dual chelation therapy.

EDTA: See (3) for specifics of EDTA administration.

Schedule

For the first 3 days of chelation, proceed as described under (1) dual chelation therapy. Beginning with day 4 when EDTA is given alone, the total daily dosage of 50 mg/kg/day may be divided into 2 to 4 portions as best suits the patient's circumstances to be given IM Q 12 to 6 hours, respectively or may be given by continuous IV infusion.

Again, various schedules for giving EDTA are acceptable: Q4h, Q6h, Q8h, Q12h, OD.

Note

On completion of this course, further chelation should be considered, as outlined in chelating regimens (3) or (4). Alternatively, further chelation therapy may be withheld until results of postchelation rebound Pb values are available. Based on laboratory studies and the patient's medical and social conditions, a regimen for further chelation therapy can be selected.

3. EDTA Alone

Dosage

50 mg/kg/day (1000 mg/m^2/day) A dosage range of 40 to 50 mg/kg/day is acceptable either as IV (preferably as a slow drip) or as a divided IM dose.

Schedule

a. Inpatient Chelation— calculate the dose at 100 ml/kg/24 hr of this solution that will give the recommended EDTA dose of 50 mg/kg/day. Alternatively, 1.0 g (5 ml) of EDTA in 250 ml to 500 ml of 5% D/W or isotonic saline can be administered slowly by intravenous drip (in not less than 1 hour). Two such courses per day for 3 to 5 days can be administered.

b. Ambulatory Chelation—a single daily dose of 50 mg/kg/day is given by deep IM injection for 5 consecutive days. It is irritative to veins and may produce thrombophlebitis. IV bolus should thus be avoided. Calculate the dose at 100 ml/kg/24 hr of this solution that will give the recommended EDTA dose of 50 mg/kg/day. Alternatively, 1.0 g (5 ml) of EDTA in 250 ml to 500 ml of 5% D/W or isotonic saline can be administered slowly by intravenous drip (in not less than 1 hour). Two such courses per day for 3 to 5 days can be administered.

4. Penicillamine

Note

This drug has not been approved for use in treating lead poisoning. Penicillamine should be used in compliance with approved FDA policy.

Dosage

30 mg/kg/day. Maximum dose = 750 mg/day. Usual course of therapy is 1 to 3 months.

Schedule

Daily dose may be administered in 1 to 3 doses. Given on an empty stomach, at least ½ hour before feeding. Contents of capsule may be emptied into a small amount of fruit sauce, fruit slush, or chilled fruit juice. Continue therapy until Pb < 30 and EP is < 50.

At this point, stop therapy but follow patient until EP returns to normal range.

ANNOTATED BIBLIOGRAPHY

Centers for Disease Control: Preventing Lead Poisoning in Young Children. US Govt Printing Office, 1985 (Guidelines are as set forth by CDC.)

Needleman HL et al: Deficits in psychologic and classroom performance of children with elevated dentine lead levels. N Engl J Med 30:689,1979 (Probably the most widely cited reference to lead's effects on neurodevelopment. It compares the school performance and intellectual function of children who had elevated dentine levels of lead compared to those with normal leads.)

18
Injury Control
ROBERT A. DERSHEWITZ

No area in child health is more important than injury control (formerly called, and often used interchangeably with, *accident prevention*). Almost half of all deaths in children result from injuries. Motor vehicle-related injuries are the leading causes of accidental death, followed by drowning, fires and burns, firearms, aspiration and asphyxiation, and falls. Each year, approximately 19 million children receive medical care for injuries, and over 100,000 children become permanently disabled. Governmental regulations and legislation have proven beneficial in reducing childhood injuries. Health education is not as effective because altering behavior is considerably more difficult. Nonetheless, health education is the primary intervention strategy employed during well-child visits.

The educational impact may be improved by limiting the content of the education, explaining its relevance, repeating the message, and having the recommendations practical and easy to implement. Most importantly, the message must be targeted to the group being taught and must be appropriate to the developmental level of the child.

The practitioner can rely on several programs in providing safety counseling. The most widely used program is The Injury Prevention Program (TIPP) sponsored by the American Academy of Pediatrics. Parents complete a safety survey, which the provider uses to identify areas in which the parents are in need of safety education. Injury fact sheets are available to parents as a reinforcement. A checklist is also provided to remind the clinician of the most relevant safety topics that should be covered at each well-child visit. These topics constitute the minimum injury prevention topics that should be discussed at each visit, and they are listed in Table 18-1 with other important injury categories.

The magnitude of car-related injuries is so great and prevention is so effective that car safety should be discussed at each well-child visit.

Since ultimate success at safety counselling cannot be measured directly, clinician gratification must come from heightened parental awareness and compliance. The remainder of this chapter offers relevant safety suggestions for each injury category listed in Table 18-1.

AUTOMOTIVE SAFETY

The focus of education must be on parents consistently using infant car restraints. This message should start either at the prenatal or the newborn hospital visit. Ideally, infants ride semireclined and facing backward in the back seat of the car. Parents must read the manufacturer's directions to ensure that the car seat is used properly. At 17 to 20 lb, the baby is too large to remain in an infant carrier and will need to use a toddler seat, which should face forward. When the child reaches 40 to 44 lb, he may use either an approved booster seat or a seat belt (which is not as safe as a booster seat). The shoulder harness should not be worn if the child is under 4½ ft tall. Remind parents also that car doors should be locked.

Parents may be confused by the variety of models and whether to buy one that converts to a toddler seat. All new car seats must pass rigorous dynamic testing, and hence are "safe." The choice depends on parental preference, whether it fits on the car, and ease of installation because some seats do not require the use of a tethering strap. All models are probably equally comfortable. Although a convertible car seat is more expensive than an infant carrier, it is cheaper in the long run because there is no need to purchase a separate toddler seat. Parents must not mistake the flimsy infant seats, which are not intended to be used in cars, with car seats.

The most unsafe place in a car for a child is on an adult's lap in the front seat. At 20 miles an hour, a 20-lb child will be propelled forward at a force of 400 lb. Since virtually no parent can contain this force, the child is thrown against the dashboard, followed by the adult's body, crushing the child and causing further injury.

Some children object to riding in car seats, especially if they have not always been required to ride in one. If the child protests, explain why it is important and be insistent. Tell parents to set an example by wearing a seat belt themselves. Bring toys in the car for the child to play with, if necessary. Reward the child for his good behavior. If he still objects, be adamant, because the potential risk is too great.

Table 18-1. Injury-Prevention Topics That Should Be Discussed with Parents

VISIT	TIPP (Minimal Topics to Cover)	OTHER RELEVANT TOPICS
Prenatal/ Hospital	Infant car seat* Smoke detector Crib safety	
2–4 wk	Falls*	Car seats
2 mo	Burns: hot liquids	
4 mo	Choking	Toy safety
6 mo	Poisonings Burns: hot surfaces	Poisonous plants
9 mo	Water safely Toddler car seat	Aspiration
12 mo		Poisons
15 mo		Guns Cuts
18 mo		Appropriateness of toys
24 mo	Playgrounds Tricycles Pedestrian safety	Yard safety
3 yr		Appropriateness of toys How to approach strange animals
4 yr		Fire prevention Fire drills
5–6 yr		Bicycle safety
Adolescents		Car safety Risk taking Firearms Power tools (*e.g.*, lawn mowers) Sports injuries

* Counsel at every well-child visit.

PEDESTRIAN INJURIES

Pedestrian deaths account for most of all motor vehicle-related deaths in children between 4 to 8 years of age, and for one half of all traffic-related deaths in children 1 to 9 years of age. Most of the 2000 child pedestrian fatalities each year occur while the child is crossing a street. The seriousness of this danger is underscored by the fact that pedestrian injuries have the highest death-to-injury ratio of any type of motor-vehicle-related injury. Thus, parents must be warned to exercise proper caution and supervision when children play outside. Children should not be allowed to play near or in traffic, and parents must teach their children how (and where) to cross streets. Regrettably, parents sometimes run over children in their own driveways.

FALLS

Falls are the fifth leading cause of death in children and result in enormous morbidity. For example, in 1978, 147,000 children were injured from falling down stairs. Although falls can never be entirely prevented, those with the greatest potential for harm can be greatly reduced with relatively little effort.

Infants should never be left unattended on an elevated surface such as a changing table or a bed, and the crib railing should be raised. Infants often attempt to squirm out of their high chairs and baby carriers, thus proper supervision is important. Gates on staircases should be used when children first learn to walk. This will also prevent falls from walkers, an occurrence resulting in about 24,000 visits to emergency rooms per year in the United States. Window sills and bunk beds must be forbidden play areas. Until children can be completely trusted, use sensible additional precautions to prevent children from falling out of windows (*e.g.*, screens) and use window locks to limit how high windows may be raised. Avoid situations that greatly increase the likelihood of falls such as overwaxing floors, storing objects on stairs, scatter rugs, and leaving spills on floors.

Each year, many children require medical attention from falls involving playground equipment. Forty to fifty percent occur at home, rather than in parks or school playgrounds. Falls from swings, slides, play houses, and monkey bars are most common, and the head, neck, and face are most frequently injured. Many falls occur outdoors during play. Those activities in which the child is more likely to be injured from falls (*e.g.*, roller-skating) warrant close supervision until the child gains proficiency.

Preventive measures that should be emphasized include having all equipment in good working order; having parents try to teach their children to minimize risk-taking behavior, and, if the gross motor activity is too advanced developmentally for the child, either supervising the child more closely or preventing that activity. Skate boards and trampolines are dangerous. Children should be discouraged from playing with the former, and they should be banned from the latter, because trampolines often cause spinal cord injuries.

BURNS

Hot Liquids

About 75% of all burns to children are scalds, and most occur in the kitchen. Infants are often scalded when sitting on the lap of a person drinking a hot beverage. As an additional precaution directed at toddlers, coffee and tea pots should not be left on the table, and pot handles should face the back of the stove. Parents should be advised to buy cool mist, rather than a steam vaporizer. The hot water should be set no higher than 125° F as both an energy-saving and injury prevention measure.

Hot Surfaces

Most environmental hazards in this category are obvious. Young children should not be allowed to play near hot ovens and barbecues. Wire screens around fireplaces prevent children (especially their hair and clothing) from catching fire. Sleepware should be flame-resistant or retardant, and children should not be allowed to play with toys that can hurt them. Place guards in front of heaters and caution parents to unplug an iron when it is not being used. The insertion of plugs in unused outlets, and the removal or taping of extension cords to the plug prevent many electrical burns.

FIRE PREVENTION AND DRILLS

One out of every 17 homes in the United States has a fire, and house fires cause 75% of all deaths related to fires and burns. Smoke detectors have the greatest potential of saving lives from fires, and all three types (heat, photoelectric, and ionization) are effective. Parents must be encouraged to install them and they must be reminded to check the batteries monthly. Matches and lighters must not be accessible, and parents ought to be warned, especially if a grandparent lives at home, never to smoke in bed.

Each household should conduct periodic fire drills and should have a clearly delineated escape plan if a fire occurs. Although it would appear sensible to recommend purchasing a fire extinguisher and leaving it in the kitchen (because most fires begin there), some firefighters disagree. They would advise leaving the house as quickly as possible because the fire may spread rapidly.

CHOKING

Accidental choking is the most common cause of indoor deaths in young children and it may occur from either food or nonfood products. Parents should be taught how to perform the Heimlich maneuver, and, if unsuccessful, how to deliver back blows. They should also be told not to attempt the Heimlich maneuver if the child is speaking, breathing, or coughing, because it is both unnecessary and dangerous.

Because hot dogs, nuts, grapes, and raisins are the foods most commonly aspirated, they should not be fed to infants. Furthermore, toddlers should not be allowed to run with food in their mouths or to chew gum. Small objects are also commonly aspirated, particularly balloons, pacifiers, and jacks, and thus these items should be kept away from young children.

TOY SAFETY

Children need to play with toys, but their toys should be safe and age-appropriate. For example, a 2-year-old riding on "big wheels" or an 8-year-old child on a mini-bike are clearly at a high risk of injury. Common sense and awareness of potential injuries are best guides for parents. Although well-constructed toys from reputable manufacturers provide one safeguard, parents should inspect the toys that their children play with. Worn and broken toys are likely to be dangerous. Darts, trampolines, and BB guns are dangerous at any age. Objects not intended to be used as toys such as refrigerator boxes may also be dangerous because children may suffocate in them. Even "cuddly" toys may be lethal. For example, a stuffed animal with small parts that an infant can easily pull off are highly dangerous because they might be aspirated.

POISONS

Toddlers are at greatest risk of accidental ingestions. The rate of poison fatalities has declined, largely as a result of legislative measures. However, poisonings remain a major pediatric problem.

Safety proofing should usually start when the child is 6 months old, before the crawling stage. The most dangerous household items are cleaning agents, especially furniture polish and products containing caustic agents. Therefore, they should all be stored high in cabinets with locks. Safe items such as flour may be kept at ground level, a reversal of the usual situation. Medicines must be kept in locked cabinets or boxes, and parents reminded that pocket books containing medications should be left out of the reach of youngsters. Substances found commonly in most households such as insecticides and alcohol should also be inaccessible to children.

A parent with a young child should keep syrup of Ipecac at home. The telephone number of the poison control center should be written on the label. Parents must be instructed never to give syrup of Ipecac to their child without medical authorization because inducing vomiting is contraindicated for certain types of ingestions.

Five to ten percent of calls to poison control centers involve plant ingestions. Most households have plants, and it is unrealistic to expect parents to know the names of more than 700 plants that have been identified as poisonous. The severity of toxicity from each plant may vary (*e.g.*, depending on which part of the plant is ingested) and fortunately, relatively few plants are considered highly dangerous. If unsure, parents are strongly advised to make certain that their indoor and outdoor plants are not toxic. Lists of the names of poisonous plants are widely available. Regional poison control centers are useful sources of information (see Chap. 172 for further discussion on this topic).

WATER SAFETY

Drowning is the second leading cause of death in children between 5 to 14 years of age. Most children are drowned in pools and bath tubs because they are poorly supervised. Boating injuries are another major cause of drowning. Infants can drown in less common ways at homes (*e.g.*, pail immersions and toilet bowls). Since supervision is the key to prevention, parents must vigilantly watch their young children when they are in water. Other parental responsibilities include teaching their children to swim, teaching them proper conduct around water, and following other water safety precautions (*e.g.*, having life preservers on boats).

GUNS

It has been estimated that three quarters of homeowners in the United States have guns and that unintentional shootings are a major cause of death in children. A little more than half of these fatalities occur at home. Guns other than firearms such as BB guns, pellet guns, spring-operated guns, and air guns are widely marketed as toys; thus, many people mistakenly think they are harmless.

Any type of gun is a dangerous weapon that is capable of causing severe injuries such as blindness. Prevention is straight-forward: Lock up all firearms and do not let children play with *any* type of gun.

CUTS

Most cuts to children are relatively minor, but account for thousands of emergency room visits each year. Kitchen knives and scissors may cause serious cuts. The most dangerous type of cut results from falls through non-safety glass (*e.g.*, patio doors). The glass may break into razor sharp pieces, causing severe lacerations. Children should be told not to play near glass. If high-risk glass doors cannot be replaced by safety glass, easily visible decals must be placed on them.

Many children are cut in their yards. Parents should inspect the grounds and remove dangerous objects such as broken glass. Bushes with thorns should also be avoided.

BICYCLE AND TRICYCLE SAFETY

There are approximately one million bicycle injuries each year with injuries peaking between the ages of 5 to 14 years. More than 600 children die annually in this age group, mostly by colliding with an automobile. Injuries from tricycles usually occur at an earlier age. Although the resultant mortality is uncommon, serious injury may occur. Children should not ride bicycles unless they are developmentally ready. Parents must teach the following safety rules to their children to minimize injuries: observe traffic lights; ride along safe routes; slow down at intersections; walk with the bicycle in heavy traffic; use proper hand signals for turning; and never ride when it is dark. It is risky to have passengers on bicycles. Children should be discouraged from riding double, and infants who ride with their parents should wear helmets. A prudent precaution is to encourage all bicycle riders to wear protective helmets.

ANIMALS

Each year, nearly one million children are bitten by animals, many of which are domestic pets. Children must be taught how to interact with and approach animals. Young children who mistreat their pets often get bitten by them. Pets, especially if accustomed to a household without children, may become jealous and therefore must prove themselves (it cannot be assumed) safe to be around children. It is uncommon for children less than 4 years old to obey safety rules around animals. Nonetheless, teaching must start earlier. Instruct children to avoid strange animals and not to tease or hit animals. Children should also be warned not to awaken or take food away from an animal or to feed strange dogs or be licked by one.

ADOLESCENT CONCERNS

Adolescents are at particular risk of vehicle-related injuries. Adolescents who are novice drivers have a tendency for risk-taking behavior (especially males). When they experiment with drugs and alcohol the risk of injuries is increased. Motorcycles are even more dangerous. Mile for mile, the death rate from motorcycles is 15 times greater than from cars. For each year an adolescent rides a motorcycle, he has a 2% chance of being killed or seriously injured. Helmets greatly reduce the severity of injury, but unfortunately, many riders choose not to wear them. Several states have even repealed their mandatory use. Unfortunately, there are no effective measures of reducing risk-taking behavior and driving without the influence of alcohol or drugs.

PEDIATRICIAN AS ADVOCATE

Although potentially time-consuming, the advocacy of safety practices outside the office (*e.g.*, in the political arena) can be very beneficial and worthwhile. As an example, the enactment of the law by all 50 states relating to car safety restraints for children was mainly due to practitioners who persuaded elected officials that such legislation was in the public interest. Any government (local, state, or federal) would be an appropriate forum to lobby for the passage of prudent regulation. At the very least, safety issues would be debated, thus heightening the awareness of the danger. Governed by one's time commitment and interest, there are different levels of involvement, ranging from telephoning legislators to writing letters or to testifying for the passage of safety standards. In addition, if dangerous toys or situations (*e.g.*, unsafe playgrounds) are noted, the pediatrician has an ethical responsibility to try to correct the situation (*e.g.*, by notifying the toy manufacturer or school officials).

ANNOTATED BIBLIOGRAPHY

Alpert JJ, Guyer B (eds): Injuries and Injury Prevention. Pediatr Clin North Am. Philadelphia, WB Saunders, 32(1), 1985 (Relevant and concise presentation of the major areas in injury control.)

Baker SP, O'Neill B, Karpf RS: The Injury Fact Book. Lexington, MA, Lexington Books, 1984 (All the facts you would ever want to know about injuries.)

Moriarty RW: Poisonous plants. Drug Therapy pp 101–109, July 1978 (Summarizes the experience of one poison control center and presents a concise compilation of clinically relevant information regarding poisonous plants.)

Public Health Service, FDA, Bureau of Drugs, Division of Poison Control: Common Poisonous and Injurious Plants, HHS, Pub No (FDA) 81–7006. (Beautiful pictures to facilitate identification. Try to get a copy!)

19
Impact of Poverty on the Child
KATHERINE K. CHRISTOFFEL

Most pediatricians at one time or another have indigent patients: during training, in a clinic, in an emergency department, or on an inpatient service. In addition, private patients of longstanding may come on hard times and become poor, (*e.g.*, as a result of divorce or devastating illness) and may turn to their trusted provider for care and guidance. All pediatricians, therefore, need to be familiar with the health and psychosocial correlates and the effects of poverty. Poverty makes dealing with any type of illness more difficult because of the limitations it imposes. An understanding of the implications of poverty can improve the physician's ability to assist the sick child and his family in coping with illness and to navigate the bureaucracy that manages social welfare programs.

Physician advocacy for improved social welfare programs for indigent children is likely to be the most beneficial intervention for such children. Because poor families are usually unable to mobilize policy makers and legislators to meet their children's needs, this responsibility falls to child advocates. Pediatricians, working as individuals or through professional and other organizations, can

Table 19-1. Child Advocacy Resources

ORGANIZATION	ADDRESS
American Academy of Pediatrics	141 Northwest Point Road P.O. Box 927 Elk Grove Village, IL 60007
Children's Defense Fund	122 C Street, NW Washington, DC 20001
Food Research and Action Center	1319 F Street, NW, Suite 500 Washington, DC 20004
Physicians Hunger Task Force	Harvard University School of Public Health 677 Huntington Avenue, L-7 Boston, MA 02115

play a critical role when decisions are made concerning the scope and level of funding of public assistance grants and other such programs. Advocacy is needed at local, state, and national levels. National organizations that have been vocal advocates for poor children and that may provide information or other assistance to pediatricians engaged in such advocacy are listed in Table 19-1.

DEFINITION OF POVERTY

The Random House Dictionary defines poverty as "a serious lack of the means for proper existence. . . ." The United States government defines poverty as income below the official poverty level. That level, which varies with family size and is adjusted for inflation, is very low. For example, in 1985 for a family of four, the poverty level was a cash income of less than $10,650. The median income in the United States in 1985 was $26,433.

Degree of poverty is used to determine eligibility for specific government programs, including Aid to Families of Dependent Children (AFDC), Food Stamps, Services for Crippled Children, Aid for the Aged, Blind, and Disabled (AABD), and Medicaid. These programs are underwritten both by federal and state funds, but most specific eligibility criteria and grant levels are set by the states. As a result, benefit levels vary substantially, although all are low. In some states at some times, individuals may be eligible for partial poverty benefits. For example families with income above the poverty line may, if faced with catastrophic or chronic illness, sometimes be eligible for Medicaid but not for cash income (*i.e.*, for Medical Assistance, No Grant

[MANG]). On the other hand, most states deny AFDC benefits to impoverished families if the father remains in the home. In 1983, approximately half of all officially poor children received AFDC benefits, reduced from 80% in 1973.

CAUSES OF POVERTY AND ITS CORRELATES

In the United States, as in other societies, poverty affects a part of the population and thus indicates unequal distribution of the nation's wealth. The extent and nature of that inequality reflect the nature and cycles of the nation's economy and also government policies. Policies that affect the occurrence of poverty include not only those related to direct funding of social welfare programs but also those related to taxation of individuals and institutions, control of inflation and the national debt, and military spending. The existence and prevalence of specific correlates of poverty must be recognized as effects of existing policies. For example, a study of 141 countries documented that infant mortality rates are negatively correlated with economic development, health resources, and social spending, and positively correlated with the percentage of the gross national product spent on the military. In the United States, cutbacks in spending on social programs during the military buildup of the early 1980s have been associated with reduced prenatal care to uninsured women, less frequent visits to neighborhood health centers, increased incidence of low-birth-weight births, increased hospital admissions for malnutrition ("failure to thrive") and diarrhea, and increased incidence of measles. It has been argued that these are not simply effects of the recession of the early 1980s, as the recession a decade earlier, during which social spending was not cut and was not characterized by the same range of indices of worsening health.

PREVALENCE AND SEVERITY OF POVERTY

The number of people who are poor in the United States varies over time, as does the composition of the subpopulation of poor people. The proportion of poor children rose rapidly in the early 1980s to levels not recorded since the mid-1960s. Three million children joined the ranks of the poor from 1980 to 1985.

Children are over-represented among the poor, accounting for 27% of the population but for 39% of the poor; in some states the proportion is even higher. Minority children are further overrepresented: in 1983, one of every five American children was poor, including one of every two black children. The likelihood of living in poverty is greatest for those living in female-headed households, particularly if the mother is black, young, and poorly educated. However, in 1983, one of every six poor children lived in a family with at least one full-time worker, and child poverty rates rose most quickly for two-parent families in the years 1978 to 1983.

The severity of poverty has also increased in recent years. In 1968 the poorest families had an average of 91% of the income considered necessary for basic needs, whereas in 1983 their income was only 60% of that level. This reflects the net effect of changes that have led to the increased prevalence of poverty, reduced public assistance (in real dollars), and increased taxes paid by the working poor.

DIRECT EFFECTS OF FAMILY POVERTY

The many aspects of life that depend on the availability of cash are directly affected by poverty. Regular family expenses include housing, utilities, food, clothing, and transportation. Poor families experience intense competition among these basic needs.

Appropriate housing is often unavailable to families whose sole income consists of public assistance benefits. Even inappropriate housing may require more than the monthly public assistance cash grant. This situation causes many families entirely supported by such grants to sell some of their food stamps so that part of the value of the food stamps can be shifted to housing and utilities. The remaining food stamps are used for food, but often do not last throughout the month. As a result, emergency food resource distribution points (including private food pantries, soup kitchens, and government commodity distribution centers) are more heavily used at the end of each month. In 1985, families accounted for approximately one third of all people using emergency food resources in 25 cities in the United States.

When the competition between food and shelter for available cash cannot be "solved" as described, families put their available resources toward food and become homeless. Families accounted for approximately one quarter of all homeless people in the 25 cities in 1985. Homeless children live with their families in various settings: on the street, in cars, in abandoned buildings, in emergency shelters, with relatives, or with acquaintances.

For families whose sole income is from public assistance, there may be little or no cash left for needs other than food and shelter, especially in winter (when utility costs are highest). The range of potentially unmet needs is wide. *Hygiene* may suffer directly because food stamps cannot be used for soap. Laundromats, which require cash, may be inaccessible to those least likely to have access to washing machines in their homes, or even to plumbing adequate for handwashing of *laundry*. New *clothing* and a *telephone* may become luxuries.

Transportation also requires cash, which therefore limits a family's ability to obtain medical care, to take advantage of poverty benefits that must be applied for or obtained at a distance from home, or to pursue opportunities for education or employment that might lead to a route out of poverty.

Child care of good quality is usually costly. The lack of cash therefore may restrict a mother's ability to go to school or to become gainfully employed. The absence of alternative child care often requires mothers to bring all their children to the Public Aid Office, WIC distribution center, or hospital emergency room. Difficulty in simultaneously supervising the children and taking care of business often adversely affects both tasks.

Higher education poses direct costs (*e.g.*, tuition, transportation, reduced work time), which is one of the reasons that access to higher education is restricted for poor youths.

Health services have always been less accessible to the poor. During the 1960s and 1970s, with the growth of Medicaid, medical expenditures for the poor grew to the point that *per capita* expenditure exceeded that of the nonpoor. When the prevalence and severity of illness are taken into account, health care expenditures for the poor remained relatively low, but the increased care was followed by improvement in various measures of health status. But problems with access persist. In 1980, one third of poor children (but only one seventh of nonpoor children) were uninsured for at least part of the year.

In the 1980s health services are becoming progressively difficult for uninsured people to obtain. During the recession of the early 1980s, while the number of poor children increased, government programs enabling the poor to have access to care were curtailed. The many impoverished families that are not covered by Medicaid often forego nonemergency child health services. For those covered by Medicaid, specific needed services and medications may not be covered without prior approval, a lengthy appeal process, or a physician's written prescription (which usually requires the costs associated with a medical visit). Dental care, eyeglass, and prosthesis coverage are restricted; their absence may result in functional and cosmetic problems that reduce ultimate employability as well as quality of life. The consequences of this rationing of health care, medication, and appliances for the poor are unclear, but they are not likely to be salutory.

Even when access is assured, the medical care of poor children is usually not equivalent to that of children who are not poor. Institutional care and the lack of a regular physician are prominent features of care available to poor children, due mainly to the extreme lack of private physicians in poor neighborhoods. Impersonal and institutional care are associated with reduced use of preventive services and increased use of episodic sickness care (*e.g.*, in emergency rooms). Neighborhood health centers have been shown to increase use of preventive services and to decrease episodic care. The problems of uninsured, episodic, and discontinuous care are probably the greatest and the least readily addressed for children of migrant workers.

INDIRECT EFFECTS OF POVERTY ON CHILDREN

Although these effects are not due directly to a shortage of cash, there are well documented associations between poverty and various aspects of family life, health, illness, and survival.

Mortality

The relatively high infant mortality rate in the United States reflects high rates among poor and minority infants. The infant mortality rate for black infants is approximately double that for whites: 19.6 per 1000 versus 10 per 1000 in 1982, the widest black:white gap since 1966. The low birth weight rate, which is closely related to the neonatal infant mortality rate, is also approximately twice as high among black births as compared to white births: 12.6% versus 5.7% in 1983, the largest gap since 1970. The relative contributions to infant mortality of various interrelated factors remain to be clarified. The factors under study include social class, income, nutritional status, race/ethnicity, maternal age, and prenatal care.

The longstanding downward trend in postneonatal infant mortality rates is slowing; in some areas, rates have begun to rise. These rates are believed to reflect environmental conditions and are generally higher among poor and minority children. Deaths caused by respiratory and other illnesses contribute to this, as do deaths caused by injuries. The association is strongest and most consistent for homicide and deaths by fire but has also been observed for other deaths by injury.

Nutrition

The association between poverty and adverse nutrition has been documented repeatedly. The Special Supplemental Nutrition Program for Woman, Infants, and Children (WIC), which fortifies the nutrition of indigent pregnant women and their young children, has repeatedly been shown to improve pregnancy outcome, particularly as measured by the percentage of low birth weight. Because low-birth-weight rates are closely correlated with infant mortality rates, this nutrition program is believed to be a key to improving infant mortality rates in the poor and minority segments of the American population. Severe protein calorie malnutrition, often believed to be confined to developing countries, has been observed in indigent American infants; its prevalence is unknown. Severe malnutrition can impair growth and development and increase incidence and severity of infection; the possibility that such effects may also result from mild or moderate malnutrition has not been well studied. Vitamin deficiencies (particularly vitamins A, C, B_1, and B_6) have been shown to exist in poor communities. Surveillance programs in public health clinics have documented high prevalences of iron deficiency, short stature, and obesity among the poor children served by the clinics. The short stature is believed to represent stunting, and adaptation to chronically inadequate nutrition. The obesity is not yet explained, but is likely to reflect various factors, including poor nutritional knowledge and habits and the inadequate exercise that is common among children whose activity is restricted to avoid street crime in poverty neighborhoods. Poor adolescents evidence excessive obesity and anemia.

Illness, Injury, and Disability

Illness, injury, and disability are increased among poor children. The association of increased morbidity with poverty begins before birth and is consistent throughout childhood and adolescence. It has been demonstrated for conditions both acute and chronic. The types of child and adolescent morbidity that have been shown to be associated with poverty are summarized in Table 19-2.

Mechanisms of Adverse Effects

Adverse social and health outcomes flow from the direct and indirect effects of poverty. Adverse outcomes are not evenly distributed among poor people. Rather, the occurrence and distribution of the consequences of poverty depend on the individuals involved, the environment in which they find themselves, the interaction of people with one another and with their environment, and the degree to which stress and sense of defeat have generated these. *Individual attributes* that may affect the severity of the damage resulting from poverty include genetic factors (*e.g.*, caloric requirements, inherited disease), learned behaviors (*e.g.*, coping skills, interaction style); and preexisting handicaps (*e.g.*, those due to inadequately treated chronic illness). *Environmental* factors include the accessibility of food, hygiene, and proper housing; a lack of these factors breeds infection and injury. In addition, poor neighborhoods are characterized by disturbing noise, unhealthy air pollution, and heavy traffic.

Poverty thwarts child development at every stage. Marginal prenatal care, health, and nutrition endanger birth weight and perinatal brain devel-

Table 19-2. Childhood and Adolescent Conditions Associated with Poverty

CONDITIONS	AVAILABLE APPROACHES FOR PREVENTION AND EARLY INTERVENTION
1. Acute conditions	
a. Venereal disease	a. Screening
b. Tuberculosis	b. Screening
c. Poisoning	c. Ipecac, other guidance
d. H. flu meningitis	d. *Hemophilus influenzae* vaccine
e. Rheumatic fever	e. Diagnosis and treatment of streptococcal infection
f. Pneumonia	f. ?‡
g. Diarrhea/gastroenteritis	g. ?
h. Otitis media	h. ?
i. Scarlet fever	i. ?
j. Parasitic disease	j. ?
k. Hospitalization	k. ?
l. Long hospitalization	l. ?
m. Restricted activity from acute illness	m. ?
2. Chronic conditions	
a. Iron deficiency and anemia	a. Diet assessment, screening
b. Lead poisoning	b. Screening
c. Poor vision	c. Screening
d. Hearing disorders	d. Screening
e. Severe asthma	e. ?
f. Assorted chronic conditions	f. ?
3. Other	
a. Prematurity	a–c. Nutrition supplements for mothers, prenatal care
b. Small for gestational age	
c. Low birth weight	
d. Protein–calorie malnutrition	d. Food supplementation, monitoring
e. Vitamin deficiency (A, C, B_1, B_6)	e. Food supplementation, diet assessment
f. Adolescent pregnancy	f. School-based contraception
g. Cytomegalic inclusion disease	g. ?
h. Psychosocial* and psychosomatic† conditions	h. ?

* Includes psychiatric diagnoses, learning disorders, behavior problems; substance problems.
† Includes insomnia, headache, asthma, colitis, constipation, irritable bowel, abdominal pain, dysmenorrhea, speech disorders, chest pain, dyspepsia, and flatulence.
‡ Clearly effective approaches have not been identified.

opment. Young mothers and mothers in charge of households often lack the support systems they need in order to provide optimal nurturing of infants and young children. The physical dangers of delapidated housing are likely to result in injury or restricted mobility for the toddler, who is disadvantaged either way. Poor nutrition may reduce spontaneity and attentiveness, and thus impair social interactions and school performance as well as physical well-being. Children in poverty may not have the opportunity to learn skills that are necessary for success in school (*e.g.*, scheduling or the habit of reading). A lack of success is likely to make school a frustrating experience. Children's behavioral responses to frustration may promote their being labelled as problem children, which serves as a further obstacle to success. Although some strong, exceptionally bright children overcome these problems, many more experience poor self-images and other potentially disabling consequences of impeded psychosocial development.

The *stress* of living in poverty itself promotes illness, social disorganization, and child abuse/neglect, which all adversely affect child development and other aspects of family function. Poor urban neighborhoods breed the desperation that supports substance abuse and gang violence, with epidemic health effects related to drug and gun use. Illness, injury, drugs, and violence can affect both the quantity and quality of education, further limiting employability and future income, and thus perpetuating poverty.

MANAGEMENT

The physician caring for an impoverished child must maintain *awareness of the likely adverse health effects of poverty* discussed. Alertness to the possible presence of such effects is particularly needed in episodic care settings to which acutely ill children may be brought for acute problems that may be less serious than other associated conditions (*e.g.*, malnutrition). Appropriate evaluation and treatment are of course needed when a specific medical problem is detected. In addition, when feasible, attention must be given to screening for other conditions and to anticipatory guidance directed to prevention. Applicable screening and anticipatory guidance approaches are listed in Table 19-2.

Some of the effects of poverty may make it tempting to judge harshly the families of poor children. Such effects include, but are not limited to, impaired hygiene and late arrival for appointments. The temptation to judge—and to blame—the victims must be resisted. When problems arise, they

should be openly discussed. Solutions can often be found which improve the child's situation by making the physician–family interaction smoother. For example, if the problem is recurrent missed appointments, it may be possible to arrange referral to a closer facility, to identify alternative transportation, or to provide visiting nurse visits to the home to allow longer intervals between office visits. The physician can set the office's tone for interactions with indigent families by providing *dignified and respectful care* for all patients, regardless of their financial status.

Because so many health problems relate to or are compounded by the social effects of poverty, thorough care of indigent children requires *coordination of medical and social services*. This is facilitated by access to a medical social worker, who can assist the family with the many tasks involved in being poor, such as applications for and clarification of types of available public assistance. In the physician's office, the staff person who handles the Medicaid billing will often be in the best position to provide this help. Others in the office who know the community's resources can share the role filled by the social worker in the hospital or clinic setting. Because of their status, education, and skills, physicians, nurses, and social workers can often be articulate and effective advocates for individual families confronting unsympathetic or complex bureaucracies.

ANNOTATED BIBLIOGRAPHY

Committee on Ways and Means, US House of Representatives: Children in Poverty. Washington, DC, Congressional Research Service, May 22, 1985 (Thorough analysis of interrelationships among poverty, race, and family structure and how these affect children. Policy options are discussed.)

Egbuonu L, Starfield B: Child health and social status. Pediatrics 69:550–557, 1982 (Thorough review of published studies and data from national surveys.)

Listernick R, Christoffel KK, Pace J, Chiaramonte J: Severe primary malnutrition in U.S. children. Am J Dis Child 139:1157–1160, 1985 (Evidence of severe illness due to underfeeding in the United States in the current era.)

Morse AE, Hyde JN, Newberger EH, Reed RB: Environmental correlates of pediatric social illness: Preventive implications of an advocacy approach. Am J Public Health 67:612–615, 1977 (Evidence is presented that achievable environmental improvements make things better for children in poverty.)

Mundinger MO: Health service funding cuts and the declining health of the poor. N Engl J Med 313:44–47, 1985 (Concise summary of the negative health effects of funding reductions in social programs, including health care expenditures, in the early 1980s.)

Oberg CN: Health care and the corridor poor. Pediatrics 76:461–463, 1985 (Concise discussion of the problem of uninsured children and the possible legislative solutions.)

Starfield B: Motherhood and apple pie: Effectiveness of medical care for children. Milbank Mem Fund Q 63(3):523–546, 1985 (Summary of available information, which indicates benefits of access to medical care, particularly for poor children.)

Wise PH, Kotelchuck M, Wilson ML, Mills M: Racial and socioeconomic disparities in childhood mortality in Boston. N Engl J Med 313:360–366, 1985 (City-wide study in a multiracial urban center, showing a strong correlation between poverty and mortality.)

Zee P, DeLeon M, Roberson P, Chen C-H: Nutritional improvement of poor urban preschool children: A 1983–1977 comparison. JAMA 253:3269–3272, 1985 (Demonstrates the efficacy of food supplementation for poor children.)

20
Child Abuse
PAULA KIENBERGER JAUDES

Child abuse and neglect have existed throughout the history of man. Both are written about in the Old and the New Testament. Child abuse and neglect (*e.g.*, infanticide) were a means of population control by the ancient Greeks and other societies in which the child was considered the property of the parents and had no rights of its own. In more recent times, Charles Dickens depicted the problem of child abuse as it existed in England during the Industrial Revolution. Scattered reports in the medical literature described abuse, but it was not until 1962 that Dr. Henry Kempe first described and named the *battered child syndrome*.

Child abuse and neglect are a major pediatric problem in the 20th century. In the United States it is estimated that approximately 4000 children die annually after battery or gross neglect. One million children are maltreated by their parents each year, and more than 200,000 children are sexually abused annually.

On the average, the practicing physician will see 4 to 6 patients with child abuse each year. Child abuse and neglect exist across social, racial, geographic, and economic boundaries. The spectrum of child abuse is broad and includes physical abuse, sexual abuse, and emotional abuse. Forms of neglect include medical, supervisional, educational, physical, and failure to thrive. The physician must be aware of all these manifestations.

ABUSE

The key to the diagnosis of child abuse is the *suspicion* of the examining physician. The physician must have an open mind concerning the potential of abuse in every pediatric patient. Clues

that may arouse suspicion begin with the case history of an injured child. The following clues are helpful for the diagnosis of child abuse:

1. The parent's or caretaker's story does not explain the child's injuries. An important aspect that should be considered is normal child development (*e.g.*, a 5-month-old infant cannot climb into a tub of hot water).
2. The story told by the parent or caretaker may be inconsistent or contradictory. Does the story change? Does one parent give one explanation and the other parent give another? What does the child say?
3. There is an unnecessarily long time interval between the injury and seeking of medical treatment.
4. The parent's reaction to the seriousness of the injury is inappropriate.
5. The parent's interaction with the child is inappropriate.

In addition to the history, the physical examination of the child helps the physician to determine whether to suspect abuse. The physical examination should begin with observation of the behavioral pattern of the child. Is the child afraid, is he withdrawn, and does he have a frozen stare? The whole body should be examined, with documentation of injuries and the stages of their resolution. Injuries on several areas of the body, in various stages of healing, indicate physical abuse.

Physical Abuse

Bruises. The skin is the most common site where physical abuse is diagnosed. Therefore, it is important to examine the skin of the entire body.

The physician must distinguish between inflicted and accidental trauma. Accidental injuries usually occur on the knees, shins, and elbows. Suspicion of abuse should be aroused by signs of trauma on the face, buttocks, neck, back, genitalia, and chest.

The shape of the lesion is also important. An electric extension cord is perhaps the most common "weapon" used on a child. An extension cord, rope, or belt, when folded back on itself, can leave a characteristic loop mark on the body. These objects may also leave linear marks. A hand slap can leave red linear marks the size of the hand on any part of the body. A human bite causes a crescent-shaped crushing injury. One can distinguish the difference between a child's bite and an adult bite by the size of the arch. A dog's bite characteristically causes a puncture, rip, or tear injury. If a child has been tied down, a linear circumferential burn or abrasion is usually seen around the wrists or ankles. Pinpricks cause petechiae, usually found on the palms and soles.

In documenting bruises and correlating them with the patient history, the physician needs to estimate the age of the skin lesion. A bruise is initially red to purple. Within the first week, the color changes to dark purple, and during the second week, to yellow. By the third to fourth week, the bruise has usually resolved.

Burns. Approximately 10% of all injuries inflicted on children are burns, including cigarette burns and immersion burns. A cigarette burn initially leaves a characteristic circular ulcerative lesion that may resemble bullous impetigo or an infected insect bite. On a pigmented child, it may leave a hypopigmented circular lesion after healing has occurred. Typically, cigarette burns are found on the hands, feet, or buttocks. If a child has been burned by another object (*e.g.*, if the child has been placed on a radiator, hot plate, or iron), the burn will resemble the outline of the object. These types of burns could be accidental however, thus a history is important to help determine accidental from inflicted burns. Splash burns are commonly accidental burns. Typically, such a burn is unilateral and is not well defined, and there are satellite burn lesions that are caused by the splashes. On the other hand, an immersion burn is an inflicted injury, in many cases as a form of punishment related to issues of toilet training. The child is dunked into hot water, with the buttocks and perineum making contact with the water first. The burn leaves characteristic water level marks around the buttocks and feet where these were immersed.

Fractures. In the diagnosis of accidental versus inflicted fractures, the location and the type of fracture are important. Accidental rib fractures are rare in children; they are found most often in adolescents who participate in contact sports. Rib fractures are usually caused by a fist, foot, or blunt object that strikes the front or back of the chest. Skull fractures can be caused accidentally; however, a thorough history and physical examination should be obtained in cases of skull fractures so that the possibility of abuse can be explored. A spiral fracture is caused by the twisting of a bone. Children who are not ambulatory and thus do not bear weight are unlikely to have this type of fracture by accident. A metaphyseal chip fracture is the result of the wrenching, forcing, or pulling of an extremity. Blunt trauma to a bone may cause subperiosteal hemorrhage, with subsequent periosteal thickening and elevation. Beginning calcification and remodeling of the bone will be seen on radiographs approximately 7 to 10 days after the trauma has been inflicted. The presence of multiple fractures of the same or various ages should be considered a sign of abuse, unless the clinical history provides another explanation for the pattern of the fractures.

Visceral Trauma. When visceral trauma is inflicted deliberately, there is often no visible evidence of injury except for bruises on the abdomen. Forceful blows to the abdomen may cause a ruptured viscus, tears of organs, and hematomas. Any abdominal structure may be damaged. The child may have a distended abdomen as well as bowel obstruction, coma, shock, or death.

Central Nervous System Trauma. Physical abuse is recognized as a leading cause of subdural hematomas in infants. The whiplash shaken infant syndrome is caused by a severe shaking of an infant, usually under 1 year of age, which may cause subdural hematomas, cerebral injury, and retinal hemorrhages. The child may be lethargic or in a coma, with bruising around the arms or the chest in a pattern that fits the offender's hands. Infants who have been shaken usually do not have skull fractures or signs of scalp injury. Accidents such as a fall from a couch or a bed rarely cause serious bleeding in the brain, including subdural hematomas. Therefore, all children with major head trauma, including epidural, subdural, and subarachnoid hematomas and depressed skull fractures, should be investigated for abuse.

Poisoning. Accidental poisonings are common in children under 3 years of age. Intentional poisoning is difficult to prove but should be considered in poisoning of children especially if they are over 3 years of age. Substances that have been identified in cases of intentional poisoning include tranquilizers, hypnotics, alcohol, diuretics, and all forms of street drugs. More commonly, however, small children have been poisoned by having water withheld and by being fed salt.

Munchhausen Syndrome by Proxy. Munchhausen syndrome by proxy is a syndrome in which parents give a fictitious history and lie about symptoms in their children, causing the children to undergo multiple hospitalizations with unnecessary diagnostic and therapeutic procedures. Parents may actually poison the child in order to cause symptoms of disease or to manipulate signs and symptoms that simulate disease.

Sexual Abuse

Sexual abuse is probably the least reported and most underdiagnosed of all types of child abuse. A conservative estimate is that one in ten children will be exposed to this form of abuse. Kempe defined sexual abuse as "involvement of dependent, developmentally immature children and adolescents in sexual activities that they do not fully comprehend, or are unable to give informed consent, and that violate the social taboos of family roles." Sexual abuse of children includes incest, sexual assaults, and exposure to sexual assaults. Incest is best defined as any sexual relation or activity between various combinations of "legal relatives," including step-parents. Sexual assaults include rape, molestation, and fondling of the genitalia, anal or oral region, and fellatio or cunnilingus, and sodomy. Sexual abuse also includes the child's presence during sexual acts of others and exhibitionism.

The offenders are predominantly male. In approximately 80% of the cases involving a child, the offender is previously known to the child (*i.e.*, he is a family member, a neighbor, or someone at school). The average age of girls who are abused is 10 years old and the average age of boys is 7 years old.

When a child reports being abused, this is not only a cry for help, but also an act of courage. Children do not fabricate stories about detailed sexual activities. Thus, sexual accusations by a preadolescent child should be believed. It happens only rarely that a disturbed adolescent lies about being sexually abused. Children describing sexual encounters will use language appropriate to their developmental stage. Visual aids such as special coloring books or anatomically correct dolls will help a child in telling his story. Above all, children should be given the benefit of the doubt about sexual abuse even if their account contradicts an adult's statements.

In all cases of suspected child sexual abuse, as in other types of abuse, the pediatrician should have a high index of suspicion. If a child does not report an incident directly, there are indirect ways of detecting that sexual abuse has occurred. Any genital injuries, irritations, or discharge may indicate sexual abuse, and all venereal disease should be considered *prima facie* evidence of such abuse. The venereal diseases include *Neisseria gonorrhoeae*, syphilis, *Trichomonas vaginalis*, condyloma acuminatum, *Chlamydia trachomatis*, herpes simplex type II, *Mycoplasma hominis*, and ureoplasm urealyticum.

Common childhood problems, although nonspecific, could indicate sexual abuse at home. These problems include difficulty with friends, failure at school, isolation from peers, enuresis, or encopresis. Certain changes in behavior have been associated with sexual abuse. Examples are the sudden appearance of symptoms such as night terrors, fear states, clinging behavior, sudden school phobias, anxiety, depression, and insomnia. In adolescents, one may see acting-out behavior, teenage pregnancy, running away from home, drug abuse, suicide attempts, sexual acting out, or fear of any sexual activity.

If there is a suspicion of sexual abuse, a complete physical examination should be done. An examination of the genital area should be performed last. The skin should be examined closely for the presence of injuries such as abrasions, excoriations, bruises, or suction petechiae on the breasts or the neck. Edema or laceration of the frenulum of the lips may be identified so as to corroborate the child's story of not being able to scream because his mouth was covered by a hand. The abdomen should be examined for tenderness or the presence of masses. In the male, signs of genital or anal trauma should be noted, and the presence or absence of urethral discharge should be determined. For prepubescent girls, a careful inspection should be done of the labia, vagina, hymen, anus, and adjacent skin. In pubescent girls, special attention should be given to signs of pregnancy such as increased uterine size or bluish discoloration of the cervix. A relatively elastic hymen may allow penile penetration without injury. On the other hand, a normal hymen may be innocently traumatized or absent as a result of accidents unrelated to sex. Therefore, the presence or absence of the hymen is not a diagnostic criterion.

In many cases, the findings on physical examination will be normal even though there is a history of sexual abuse. Younger pediatric patients usually show few physical signs, because they are often victims of fondling only. Furthermore, the sexual assault often happens days, weeks, or months before being mentioned by the child. The longer the time between the sexual assault and its revelation, the less likely it is that pertinent positive physical signs of sexual abuse will be discovered. The child should be believed, however, even if there are no abnormal findings on physical examination.

Emotional Abuse

Emotional abuse is the parental act of chronic denigration of a child. Continual verbal attacks deprive a child of love, security, and the feeling of being wanted. Emotional abuse whittles away at a child's spirit and self-esteem. This is probably the most common form of child abuse, the least often reported, and the most difficult to document.

NEGLECT

Child neglect is the type of maltreatment reported most frequently to state agencies, and it causes the greatest morbidity in children.

Medical

Medical neglect includes refusing or denying treatment for serious acute illnesses such as meningitis. It also includes not treating life-threatening, chronic disorders such as diabetes mellitus or asthma when appropriate treatment is known and available. Withholding treatment such as bracing, physical therapy, occupational therapy, and speech therapy for disabling or handicapping chronic diseases, such as cerebral palsy, or for potentially fatal illnesses, such as cancer, for which there is an accepted medical treatment, is also considered medical neglect.

One cannot hold all parents responsible for meeting the optimal standards recommended by the American Academy of Pediatrics for well-baby care. However, at a minimum, the child should have received immunizations (unless contrary to religious beliefs) and should have seen a physician within the first 5 years of life.

Supervisional

Supervisional neglect is expressed in morbidity and mortality of children as a result of accidents. For the first 3 to 4 years of a child's life, his environment needs to be controlled. Leaving a child at home alone without supervision can result in serious injuries and poisonings, many of which could have been prevented if the child were better supervised by an adult.

Emotional

Emotional neglect is the lack of a loving relationship between the parents and the child. Children who are emotionally deprived are usually withdrawn and listless, and many have developmental delays. It is difficult to define the minimum responsibilities of a parent with regard to love. There are cases of parents who are mentally ill or mentally limited and who are thus incapable of assuming the role of parents. Whatever the reason for this deficient relationship, when the child's growth and development are adversely affected, the case is one of emotional neglect.

Educational

Educational neglect of school-aged children is defined as more than 25 days of school absenteeism in the year. The child or adolescent is often made to stay at home to babysit younger siblings. All children should attend school by 6 years of age. Children with special needs, such as disabilities, should be in school by 3 years of age, as provided by federal law.

Physical

Physical neglect is the lack of provision of adequate food, clothing, and shelter. Abandonment, when a parent cannot or will not take care of a child, is the ultimate form of physical neglect. Typically, the child is left with a member of the family or a baby-sitter, and the parent does not return.

In all forms of neglect, the pediatrician's role is to intervene and to be an advocate for the child. The physician, in his best judgment, must decide whether the neglect is hindering the growth and development of the child. Intervention may initially take the form of social service involvement but may at times require the state's child protective services.

Failure to Thrive

Failure to thrive (FTT) is the failure of an infant to grow and develop. Every child needs both adequate nutrition and "love" in order to grow and develop normally. Children who do not thrive are usually less than 2 years old. The first evidence of failure to thrive is usually a subnormal weight gain. The absence of physical clues is often indicative of "non-organic" FTT (see Chap. 184).

OTHER FORMS OF MALTREATMENT

Fetal neglect is considered a form of maltreatment in some states. This occurs when a baby is born showing signs of alcohol or drug withdrawal from maternal substance abuse. In all states, the suspicion of denial of reasonable medical care to a defective newborn may be reported to the Child Protection Agency. Another form of maltreatment is exploitation of a child, which includes forced exposure to drugs, alcohol, and pornography, as well as child labor.

EVALUATION AND TREATMENT

When the physician suspects child abuse or neglect, he must report this suspicion to the state Child Protective Agency and may also refer the child to a local hospital that has a child abuse team. Most victims of suspected child abuse or neglect should initially be admitted to the hospital. The hospital assumes the responsibility for protecting the child, following up on the reported problem, and providing social service support for the child and his family. A hospital admission also allows time for a medical and social evaluation and affords an opportunity for in-depth planning for the future welfare of the child. If a parent refuses admission or threatens to remove his child from the hospital, the physician may need to take protective custody.

During hospitalization, the staff should record the child's history and the results of a physical examination, with specific attention to description of all lesions on the child's body, including their color, type, location, and shape. Clinical photographs should be taken if the child is injured or malnourished. Parental consent is not required for these photographs. Clotting studies should be performed if bruises are present. A skeletal survey should be done on children who have signs of trauma, particularly on children who are less than 3 years old. Exact documentation of growth and development is necessary, particularly if a child appears malnourished or deprived.

If there is suspicion that a child has been sexually abused, a Gram stain of any discharge from the vagina, urethra, or anus for detection of gram-negative diplococci should be done. Specimens from the cervix (in adolescents), vagina (introitus), urethra, anus, and throat should be cultured for *Neisseria gonorrhoeae* and *Chlamydia trachomatis*. Other tests that are indicated include a serologic test for syphilis, a pregnancy test in postmenarcheal females, a wet preparation to test for trichomonads, and testing for the presence of semen. The state's forensic collecting kit should be used if a sexual assault has occurred within the previous 72 hours. Potentially evidential specimens should be obtained, including samples of clothing, diapers, pubic hair, scrapings of blood, and so forth, as indicated.

CHILD PROTECTION AND LEGAL SYSTEMS

In all 50 states, if a physician *suspects* that a child has been abused or neglected, the physician is required to notify the state's Child Protective Agency. After making the report, the physician is protected by law from being sued by the alleged abusive parents. In some states, if a physician fails to report a possible case of child abuse or neglect, he could be jailed, lose his medical license, or become liable to a malpractice suit.

Once the report has been made, the Child Protective Agency has the responsibility for investigating the case. The state case worker will talk with the physician and other medical personnel and with the family, neighbors, and the child. The case worker decides whether the allegation of abuse or neglect has credence and whether to take the case to juvenile court.

In juvenile court (or family court, in some jurisdictions), the judge rules on child abuse on the basis of "preponderance of evidence," and makes decisions concerning custody issues. If the child abuse has consisted of homicide, extreme battery, or sexual abuse, the case may also be adjudicated in criminal court. In criminal court, the judgment is based on evidence "beyond a reasonable doubt" against the alleged perpetrator.

If the physician must go to court to testify, he should be subpoenaed. Preparation for the court appearance includes gathering of medical evidence, including a copy of medical records, laboratory reports, radiographs, and photographs. The physician can make notes from the records and may refer to these while on the witness stand. The physician will usually be questioned by three attorneys: the prosecutor (Assistant State's Attorney), the defense attorney for the parents, and the guardian *ad litem* (for the child). The judge ultimately makes a decision in the best interest of the child. The decision is based on the testimony at the court hearing, especially the important input by the physician.

The physician's responsibility for the patient continues past reporting and possibly testifying in court. The physician should have concern about placement of that child (*i.e.*, whether the placement should be with the natural parents or in a foster home). The overall goal is a permanent and supportive environment for the child. Continued followup with the pediatrician is essential to ensure the optimal growth and development of the child.

ANNOTATED BIBLIOGRAPHY

Day DW: Child abuse: The development of suspicion. Pediatric Digest 13–19, 1976 (Review of history and signs of abuse.)

Ellerstein NS (ed): Child Abuse and Neglect, A Medical Reference. New York, John Wiley & Sons, 1981 (Excellent medical reference.)

Kempe CH, Silverman FN, Steele BN et al: The battered child syndrome. JAMA 181:17, 1962 (The original article describing the syndrome.)

Kerns DL: Child abuse and neglect: The pediatrician's role. JCE Pediatrics 21(7):11–27, 1979 (Review of types of abuse.)

Leake HC, Smith DJ: Preparing for and testifying in a child abuse hearing. Clin Pediatr (Phila.) 16(11):1057–1063, 1977 (Guidelines for the pediatrician in preparing for court.)

Sarles RM: Sexual abuse and rape. Pediatrics in Review 93–98, 1982 (Review of the diagnosis and management of sexual abuse.)

Schmitt BD: Current pediatric roles in child abuse and neglect. Am J Dis Child 133:691–696, 1979 (Discussion of the child abuse team and its role.)

Wilson EF: Estimation of the age of cutaneous contusions in child abuse. Pediatrics 60:750, 1977 (Article on describing the color changes over time of a bruise.)

4

Behavioral Pediatrics

21
Patient Education in Primary Care
EDWARD R. CHRISTOPHERSEN

Historically, primary health care providers have had the major responsibility for educating patients about risks to their health and well-being. Although many providers have been motivated for such a mission, the optimal way for teaching health education has not been developed. Numerous studies have already shown that health education requires more than the simple provision of information. The time factor is an important practical constraint since the average pediatrician spends only a short time on anticipatory guidance. Thus, the fact that the pediatrician does not have much time to include a process (health education) that he knows little about and that has not been effective in the past, underscores the difficulty of achieving success.

Primary care providers have several places where they are responsible for patient education and where the effectiveness of that education can substantially affect the outcome with the patient. A discussion follows on the primary educational opportunities for the primary provider with recommendations on how to maximize the effectiveness of each.

PRENATAL COUNSELING

Most hospitals with obstetric services offer prenatal classes. Information that needs to be conveyed to all expectant couples can be included in these classes with little additional effort. At the University of Kansas Medical Center, for example, the prenatal classes include one 1-hour lecture (out of a total of six 2-hour classes) on parenting. This lecture includes a discussion about normal infant behavior and development and also information on automobile and home safety practices. Using this group format, much more information can be covered during a 1-hour class than a pediatrician could cover during a one-on-one prenatal visit. The pediatric staff should also be able to work with the nursing staff who teach the prenatal classes to include certain information without involving the pediatrician in giving lectures.

Office-based prenatal counseling, although recommended by many individuals over the years, cannot replace group prenatal classes, because the pediatrician does not have the time to cover all of the material necessary during each prenatal visit. Rather, an individual prenatal visit, after a couple has attended the group prenatal class, can be used to answer the couple's personal questions, to discuss concerns on breast-feeding, working mothers, and so forth.

ANTICIPATORY GUIDANCE

After numerous investigators demonstrated that brief "educational" encounters are of little practical value, several models were proposed for the delivery of well-child care that hold more promise. One innovative approach is group well-child care. The delivery of lectures on well-child care in groups has several advantages. The groups allow the pediatrician to spend significantly more time with each family, averaging 45 minutes per visit compared to about 15 minutes with traditional one-on-

one care. The mothers in the groups learn from the other mothers in the groups and they are comforted to learn that other mothers also have similar questions regarding their children. Pediatricians who run the groups commonly report that they learn from the groups because they have the opportunity to observe the mothers interacting with their children over a longer time, and they are able to observe the mothers in a larger social situation where it is possible to make objective comparisons between the mother–child dyads. When the effect on home safety practices (*e.g.*, safe hot water heater settings and smoke detector installations) was evaluated, the well-child groups demonstrated the effectiveness of their counseling. Success was attributed to more time for interaction between the health care provider and the family, as well as more time for the provider to observe and comment on the practices that the families were already engaging in.

Well-child visits provide the most "natural" opportunity to conduct well-child groups. The physical examination portion of the appointment is usually conducted at the beginning or end of the group appointment, so that the examinations do not interrupt or interfere with the groups. Lastly, convening "special" groups such as providing parents with information about parenting may be highly successful.

Several points should be considered by the pediatrician who prefers one-on-one well-child care or who is unable to offer group well-child care. A necessary, though insufficient, point is that a provider needs adequate time if he is to be an effective communicator. Recipients of health care recommendations need to be made aware of the seriousness or importance of an issue; to believe that they can follow their pediatrician's recommendations successfully; and to have time to consider the issue and to make up their minds. In addition, families should be given realistic appraisals of how both compliance and noncompliance with the provider's recommendations will affect them. As a practical application for child passenger safety, the combination of addressing both the positive and negative aspects of accident prevention is superior to either approach by itself.

At least an equally important consideration is the amount of effort that a health education strategy takes for parents to implement. The less amount of effort required by the parent, the more likely the parent is to follow the pediatrician's suggestions. Parents, for example, are more likely to insert plastic outlet covers than to install child safety latches on kitchen cabinet doors.

Another important factor in health education efforts is the distinction between active and passive approaches. Active approaches require varying amounts of effort on the part of the parent. Passive approaches, in contrast, require little or no effort. For example, traditionally, seat belts have involved an active approach: They have required that the driver exert effort every time that he entered the vehicle. With a passive approach to seat belts, the seat belt is drawn around the driver when the driver shuts his door; no effort is required from the driver. The air bag is another example of a passive restraint. The air bag is completely automatic or passive in that the driver does not even know it is there, nor does he have to do anything in order to render it effective. An additional variation on the active/passive theme is legislation (which may require manufacturers to install devices that will automatically protect a person). Substantial gains have been realized through legislative efforts in several areas of health education.

ACUTE CARE REGIMENS

Before researchers began actually measuring compliance with health care instructions, many providers assumed that their patients were dutifully following their physicians' recommendations. Now it has become well known that large numbers of patients/families do not follow their physicians' recommendations. In one study in a pediatric outpatient clinic over 50% of patients stopped taking penicillin by the third day of a 10-day regimen, 71% stopped by the sixth day, and by the ninth day 82% of patients were not taking their medication.

Several areas need to be addressed by the physician in order to maximize patient compliance.

Parent/Patient Education

In order for a patient to follow a physician's recommendations, he must understand and remember them. Patient or parental understanding and recall can be increased by more efficient presentation of medical information. Whenever possible, patients should be provided with instructions and advice at the start of the information to be presented. The provider should stress how important it is that the patient follow the regimen exactly. He should use short, easily understood sentences and should provide concrete examples whenever possible. In one recent study (Finney et al, 1985) compliance on a regimen for acute otitis media was investigated. While the control group received their instructions in the standard way, with the physician telling the patient what to do, the experimental group received a written copy of the physician's recommendations and had a monitoring sheet on which they were to keep track of the medications and when they were given. The control group had 49% compliance compared with 82% compliance by the experimental group.

Increased Follow-Up

To reduce the possibility of poor compliance over time, the pediatrician can have nurses or office personnel telephone parents after the first few days of therapy and encourage them to continue the prescribed course of medications. This telephone contact should be handled carefully so as not to put parents on the defensive. During the phone call, parents can be asked about how their child is feeling and if they have any questions. Within this context of inquiring about the child's progress, the parents can then be encouraged to continue therapy even though their child is asymptomatic. Explain to parents that most people have a tendency to stop therapy when they or their children are feeling better. Parents should then be given a brief rationale about why it is important to continue therapy. The total time for this follow-up call can usually be limited to 2 or 3 minutes unless the parent has additional questions.

Physician–Patient Interaction

Some correlative data show that patient satisfaction and compliance may be related to patterns of physician–patient interaction. For example, noncompliance has been found to be related to unmet expectations of mothers who brought their children to pediatricians. Generally, the pediatrician should make sure that he finds out what the parents' concerns and expectations are, and then he should provide information both about the diagnosis and the cause of the illness. A friendly, conversational attitude, coupled with a lack of medical jargon, may also improve compliance.

CHRONIC DISEASE REGIMENS

Two important characteristics that distinguish chronic care regimens from acute care regimens are that the chronic care regimens are typically much more complex and they must be carried on for a longer time. Compliance may be facilitated by the following steps.

Regimen Checklist

A written list of the recommendations that the physician usually makes, with a space to check off those that apply in a particular instance, may make it easier for the parents to follow the physician's recommendation. The parents then have a written product that they can take with them when they leave the office which will serve as a reminder of what they are supposed to be doing. Interestingly, many physicians will report that they have always had some "compulsive mothers" who insisted on writing down everything that the physician said; yet, it is difficult for parents to follow a complex regimen without some kind of written reminder. Similarly, there are some regimen components that parents have little knowledge of and that require more guidance from the physician. When parents are advised to increase the fiber in their child's diet because of constipation, a list of dietary suggestions should be provided. Many parents do not know which foods are high in natural fibers. In these instances, the use of a written list of suggested foods and food preparation suggestions may greatly facilitate the parents' attempts to comply with the physician's recommendations.

Behavioral Rehearsal

When the physician recommends a complex set of procedures for the parents to follow, those elements that can easily be rehearsed in the office should be. Whether a parent is instructed to give a diabetic child an insulin injection, provide postural drainage exercises for a child with cystic fibrosis, or monitor exercises for a child with rheumatoid arthritis, asking the parent to practice the procedures in the office, and rehearsing with them while in the presence of the office nurse can help substantially with complex regimens.

Gradual Implementation

The physician should be aware of "information overload." Each parent can only assimilate so much information at any one time. The regimen components can be introduced in a step-by-step fashion as the parent masters prior steps in a sequence of components ordered in terms of difficulty and necessity. Although there is a temptation to tell the parent everything during one visit, this is the hardest style for parents to accommodate. For example, the parents of a newly diagnosed diabetic can be instructed and given the opportunity to rehearse giving the insulin injections. The next day, for an inpatient, the parents can be instructed in and allowed to rehearse the procedures for measuring their child's blood glucose levels.

Tailoring of Regimens

Tailoring refers to the practice of adapting the regimen to the personal habits and routines of a patient and his family. If possible, medications can be prescribed at times when well-established habits occur, such as when the patient eats, takes vitamins, or brushes his teeth. For example, parents of children with cystic fibrosis may do their postural drainage exercises while their child is watching one of his favorite television shows. Pediatricians can decide how to tailor regimens by inquiring about the daily routines of a particular patient and discussing with parents convenient times to conduct regimen components. The time that a physician spends tailoring a regimen may have long-range benefits since the patient may continue to comply with the treatment regimen without further effort by the physician.

Increased Supervision

Increased supervision in the form of more frequent follow-up appointments may also improve compliance. By giving more frequent, shorter appointments, the physician can better monitor the patient's progress and attend to compliance problems. For example, selected diabetic patients may be asked to return to the endocrine clinic to have their Hgb A_1c checked at monthly intervals. When the results of the assay are available, a nurse calls the patient/parents to give them feedback about the patient's current degree of metabolic control. The visits may be brief but the cumulative effect of visits may further convince patients and their parents that the physician is concerned and ready to help. A telephone call may be substituted for a clinic visit to decrease the cost to parents and to take up less of the physician's time.

WHY IMPROVE HEALTH EDUCATION EFFORTS?

Compliance failures are costly from a therapeutic and an economic standpoint. An obvious consequence of noncompliance with medical regimens is that patients fail to receive the benefits of effec-
tive therapies and thereby may adversely affect their health. Incomplete antibiotic therapy, for example, may result in a greater probability of recurrent infections. Abrupt discontinuation of medications such as prednisone can result in life-threatening side effects. The accumulation of unused medications in the home can increase the probability of accidental poisoning of young children. Physicians may also inadvertently conclude that a particular treatment is ineffective when in fact an adequate trial of that treatment was not possible because the patient did not adhere to the treatment regimen. The cost-effectiveness of medical care is also affected by patient compliance. Money is spent on unused medications and parents may incur the expense of additional diagnostic and treatment procedures that may not have been necessary with optimal patient compliance. Poor compliance can also lead to more frequent hospitalization that results in increased costs to parents. The cost of hospitalization is indirectly passed onto other families in the form of increased insurance premiums and the cost of health maintenance organization services.

Obviously, with preventive health care recommendations such as accident prevention strategies, no benefits can be realized if the patient does not implement the strategies or if the physician fails to adequately inform the parents about the importance of implementing the strategies. The combination of the use of existing groups, like hospital prenatal classes and provider health education efforts, represents the most effective and least costly alternatives available.

Most physicians also report increased satisfaction with their practices when they are not constantly confronted with the frustration of patient noncompliance. The routine use of strategies to improve patient compliance may well result in increased satisfaction for both the physician and the patient.

ANNOTATED BIBLIOGRAPHY

Christophersen ER: The Baby Owner's Manual: What to Expect and How to Survive the First 30 Days. Shawnee Mission, KS, Overland Press, 1984 (Written as a text to accompany prenatal classes, the manual includes a discussion and examples about normal infant behavior [vision, hearing, self-quieting], home and automobile safety practices, and a self-assessment quiz for parents on newborns.)

Finney JW, Friman PC, Rapoff MA, Christophersen ER: Improving compliance with antibiotic regimens for otitis media: Randomized clinical trial in a pediatric clinic. Am J Dis Child 139:89–95, 1985 (Results of a carefully controlled study of medical compliance with pediatric patients. The methodology and the results may be useful to primary providers interested in medical compliance.)

Osborn LM: Group well-child care. Clin Perinatol 12(2):355–365, 1985 (Concise discussion of some of the features of group well-child care that makes it so appealing to some pediatricians. Dr. Osborn, a practicing pediatrician, was one of the first advocates of group well-child care.)

22
Divorce and Single Parents
LINDA V. ROSS

By 1990, it is estimated that 33% of the children under the age of 18 (1 million per year) in the United States will experience their parents' divorce. The divorce rate in the United States is the highest in the world with approximately 40% of current marriages of young adults ending in divorce. Children will live an average of 6 years in a single-parent home created by marital disruption. Although there are differences of opinion, there is strong evidence that divorce can have negative effects on a child's cognitive, emotional, and social development.

Mechanisms by which the negative effects on child development can occur include a lowered socioeconomic status, the loss of a father or mother in the home, conflict in parent–child relationships, loss of external social support systems, stress- and crisis-related problems, and disruption in the nuclear family including possible separation from siblings. Some of the negative effects of divorce on children include a lowered self-esteem, increased aggression or delinquency, particularly in boys, depression, feelings of guilt and responsibility for the divorce, fear of abandonment by the custodial parent, fantasies of reuniting the divorced parents, regression in toilet training and other developmental tasks, academic difficulties, and social withdrawal. Factors related to a child's adjustment to parental divorce include age, sex, predivorce cognitive and emotional functioning, parental adjustment, parental communication about child-rearing, extent of environmental changes required, cultural and family beliefs, and social support available within and outside the family. In general, a young male child whose parents do not adjust well to the divorce and remain in conflict over child rearing and who is required to move away from his home or social support has the poorest prognosis for a healthy adjustment to his parents' divorce. On the other hand, the most important variable related to

satisfactory adjustment to divorce among children seems to be a positive relationship with the custodial parent. Individual differences including the child's cognitive and behavioral abilities mediated by family variables are important in describing why children react differently to the stress of parental divorce.

PRESENTATION

Parents may present to the primary health care provider with specific questions or problems regarding a pending divorce. More often, however, the provider will become aware of a pending or recent divorce when the custodial parent comes with nonspecific questions or recurrent problems and does not tell the physician of the divorce. Billing problems are often the reason the family health care provider learns that there has been a change in marital status. Other presenting problems often encountered include regression in the accomplishment of toilet training, bedtime problems, temper tantrums, or frequent minor illnesses. Occasionally, the noncustodial parent will call the physician for information regarding the physical or mental health of his child.

DIFFERENTIAL DIAGNOSIS

In determining the effects of divorce on children, the primary health care provider needs to rule out preexisting conditions that might impede a healthy adjustment. Children who have been exposed to a long-term marital conflict may have already developed behavior patterns that require professional intervention. Temper tantrums, bedtime problems, and noncompliance with parental instructions can become exaggerated at the time of divorce when the level of stress is elevated. In general, the child who has a history of maladjustment preceding the divorce is more likely to respond with long-lasting emotional disturbance following the divorce. These problems need to be anticipated because early and timely counseling will minimize long-term problems.

WORK-UP

Plotting the child's weight and height on a standard growth chart allows the pediatrician to reassure the mother that the child's growth is normal. Several scales and screening tests that have been developed to help the primary care physician assess the effects of divorce on the child are summarized in Table 22-1. Most physicians, however, perform only the Denver Developmental Screening Test (DDST) in their offices, choosing to refer to psychologists for further testing. Problems detected in the screening procedures should alert the provider to the need for referral.

The primary health care provider should determine what stresses the children of the divorcing couple will be or have been exposed to. Questions regarding economic changes, living arrangements, who will be the custodial parent, noncustodial parent visitation, school and day care arrangements, disciplinary decisions, extended family support, and other forms of social support need to be addressed at the first opportunity. The answers to these questions will help the provider identify areas in which the family is in need of counseling. The provider should have available resources such as written handouts, books written for lay people, local mental health professionals well-versed in divorce counseling, and community workshops for divorced families to which families can be referred. The physician can attempt to keep the noncustodial parent involved in the child's health maintenance by suggesting conferences in the office and periodic telephone calls regarding the child's health status (see Chap. 23 for a discussion of the effects on children of mothers working outside the home).

PRINCIPLES OF MANAGEMENT

Management of the effects of divorce on children requires the primary health care provider to focus on the needs of the children rather than to become involved in parental disputes. Knowledge of normal child development and skill in educating and counseling parents and children are prerequisites for the provider who intends to assist families adjust to divorce. Management will be determined by the stresses experienced and the predivorce status of the child and his parents. In general, if the custodial parent is able to make a satisfactory pre- and post-divorce adjustment and maintain a positive relationship with the child, the prognosis for the child is good.

The physician can convey directly to the child a compassionate recognition of his feelings, fears, and concerns. Such acknowledgement may diminish the child's sense of loneliness and the lack of adult support. Parental and child adjustment can be improved when both parents and children are in-

Table 22-1. Screening Tests to Assess the Effects of Divorce on Children

NAME	KIND	TIME	AGE	REFERENCE
Achenbach Child Behavior Checklist	Behavioral	30–45 min	4–5 yr 6–11 yr 12–16 yr	Achenbach and Edelbrock (1981)
ANSER	Developmental Health	Varies	School-age	Levine (1983)
Denver Developmental Screening Test	Developmental	15–25 min	Birth–6 yr	Frankenburg (1983)
Eyberg Child Behavior Inventory	Behavioral	10–20 min	2–12 yr	Robinson, Eyberg, and Ross (1980)
Home Screening Questionnaire	Home environment	15 min	Birth–3 yr 3–6 yr	Frankenburg (1983)
Denver Prescreening Developmental Questionnaire	Developmental	5 min	3 mo–6 yr	Frankenburg (1983)

volved in support groups aimed at developing problem-solving skills.

The primary health care provider may sometimes be involved in child custody decisions. Several studies have investigated variables affecting decisions about child custody. Laws vary from state to state and have been summarized by Howell and Toepke (1985). Important issues include joint, shared, or one-parent custody; the best interests of the child; and the acceptance of psychological or physician investigations. Some considerations in the custody decisions are which parent is most likely to foster visitation and respect for the other parent; to maintain continuity of child contact with friends, relatives, neighbors, and school; to provide productive support, guidance, and discipline; to maintain emotional and environmental security; to be aware of resources available for parent support; and to demonstrate flexibility and adaptability with regard to the current situation and the future. The provider is encouraged to maintain the role of the advocate for the child rather than to take sides with either parent. In this role, the professional will be able to provide care and advice to either parent and to the child without being biased by considerations concerning fault in the divorce proceedings.

INDICATIONS FOR REFERRAL

Most acute responses to a divorce, such as anger, fear, depression, and guilt, are considered normal and usually begin to resolve after the first year following a divorce. However, continued exposure to adversity with multiple stresses may lead to developmental disruptions requiring special intervention. Some indications for referral include persistent antisocial behavior; academic failure; symptoms of depression such as insomnia, appetite disturbance, or weight loss; and coercive parent–child interactions. Results of the aforementioned screening procedures will alert the provider to the need for referral.

MANAGEMENT

Management of children and their families following a divorce will depend on the age of the child, the custodial arrangements, and the adjustments of the parents and children. The following discussion centers on common issues relating to divorce and children.

Telling the Children about Divorce

What and how to tell the children is a question often asked by parents contemplating divorce. Some authorities suggest that each child in the family be told separately with both parents present to answer questions, whereas others recommend that siblings be told together. The children should be told that the parents will be living apart and will no longer be married. They should be told what the living arrangements will be and how often they will see the absent parent. Children should not be asked their opinions about where they are going to live nor whether their parents should get a divorce. In the case of older adolescents, their opinions on living arrangements may be taken into consideration in legal decisions, but the parents should not expect their children to make the decisions. Questions of loyalty and abandonment are problematic for children of all ages.

Financial arrangements often result in environmental changes such as a new residence, a mother returning to work, the necessity for day-care or after-school programs, and depleted resources for extra activities such as club memberships and dance lessons. Parents need to be aware of the effects of such environmental changes on their children and reassure them that they will continue to be cared and provided for despite the changes in economic resources.

Visitation

It is important that the child visit as often as possible with the noncustodial parent unless that parent has been abusive or is a substance abuser. Details of visitation such as scheduling, picking-up and delivering children, vacations, grandparent visits, a child's refusal to visit, and debriefing following the visitation should be worked out by the parents with professional assistance, if necessary. The absence of the noncustodial parent (most often the father, although recently more fathers are receiving custody of their children) will have various effects such as fears that he has abandoned the child or has had some mishap. The father–child interaction is often very different postseparation. In some cases, the relationship between absent fathers and their children improves after divorce. This relationship can be fostered by including the fathers in decisions about their children's health, education, discipline, and general child-rearing. The frequent availability of the father is associated with positive adjustment, especially in boys. "Bribes" in the form of excessive gifts, trips, or weekend outings should be discouraged as they introduce unrealistic expectations and place additional stress on the other parent.

Discipline

Discipline of children following divorce may be difficult for various reasons. A mother who has returned to work may have added household responsibilities as well as job responsibilities with less time to devote to her children. Thus, children may experience the loss of both mother and father immediately following a divorce. Disruption of the parenting routine is one factor leading to adjustment problems in children of divorcing parents. It is important to the child's adjustment that stability and organization of the home accompanied by nurturance be restored as quickly as possible. Concrete types of discipline such as a brief time-out period are recommended because the use of lectures and frequent reprimands may lower the self-esteem of a child already at risk. Older children may benefit from the need for greater self-sufficiency in a single-parent family if the mother does not make excessive or inappropriate demands for emotional sustenance. It is important to monitor children frequently and praise appropriate behaviors. Physical touch is one of the best ways of communicating love, acceptance, and understanding to children of all ages.

One common practice that should be discouraged is that of having the child sleep with the custodial parent after the separation or divorce. Since it is unpleasant to remedy this situation once it has occurred, the professional can provide anticipatory guidance to the parent to prevent the habit from developing. Related to sleeping with the parent is the tendency to have the same sex child replace the absent parent symbolically. Forewarning the parent of this possibility may avert the problem. The same advice may prevent the parent from identifying the same sex child with the absent parent.

Feelings

Children may have feelings of guilt about having caused the divorce. They may also feel that they can cause their parents to reunite if they behave in certain ways. It is important that parents be aware of their children's tendencies to feel responsible and not contribute to such fantasies. Parents should not involve the children in their own disputes nor should they use the children as their confidants.

Children will have feelings of anger, fear, sadness, hurt, and loneliness. It is important that parents recognize these feelings as normal reactions to the loss of the family unit and the noncustodial parent. Such feelings are not indicative of parental incompetency. However, if ignored, such feelings may persist and lead to maladaptive responses such as antisocial behavior or depression or academic failure. In the case of maladaptive responses, the parent should be encouraged to seek professional help for the entire family.

Step-Families

The number of children living in step-families is growing. Over 70% of divorced men and women remarry, creating a step-family when children are involved. Much has been written recently regarding the problems involved in joining children of previous marriages into a step-family. Some problems that step-parents may face include hostile step-child behaviors; complications with the spouse's ex-husband or wife; who makes decisions regarding discipline and other child-rearing questions; visitation; and attachment or lack thereof. Some characteristics of step-sibling relationships are that they are instantaneous; they lack a shared family history; they bring into the new family a common experience of loss in their original families; there are conflicting loyalties; there may be shifts in sibling position roles and functions; and there is an abrupt change in family size. The primary care provider may provide anticipatory guidance to parents who are about to become step-parents and direct them to books and community resources to help the family adjustment process.

ANNOTATED BIBLIOGRAPHY

Achenbach TM, Edelbrock CS: Behavioral problems and competencies reported by parents of normal and disturbed children aged four through sixteen. Monogr Soc Res Child Dev 46 (1, Serial No 188), 1981 (Complete discussion of the Achenbach Child Behavior Checklist is presented with data from studies using the scale.)

Einstein E: The Stepfamily: Living, Loving, and Learning. Boston, Shambhala Publications, 1982 (Excellent book to recommend to parents contemplating remarriage or who have already created a stepfamily. Discusses topics such as dating, remarriage, family traditions, noncustodial parents, step-sibling relationships, and signs of trouble.)

Frankenburg WK: Developmental assessment. In Levine MD, Carey WB, Crocker AC, Gross RT (eds): Developmental-behavioral Pediatrics, pp 927–937. Philadelphia, WB Saunders, 1983 (Presents a two-stage developmental screening procedure that may be useful to the pediatrician assessing the effects of divorce on preschool children.)

Howell RJ, Toepke KE: Summary of the child custody laws for the fifty states. Am J Family Therapy 12(2):56–60, 1984 (Summarizes state custody laws and discusses problems often encountered.)

Levine MD: The developmental assessment of the school age child. In Levine MD, Carey WB, Crocker AC, Gross RT (eds): Developmental-behavioral Pediatrics, pp 938–947. Philadelphia, WB Saunders, 1983 (Pre-sents the ANSER screening instrument that may be useful to the pediatrician assessing the effects of divorce on school-aged children.)

Robinson EA, Eyberg SM, Ross AW: The standardization of an inventory of child conduct problems. J Clin Child Psych 2:22–29, 1980 (Discusses the Eyberg Child Behavior Inventory that may be useful to the pediatrician assessing behavioral effects of divorce on children.)

Teyber E: Helping your Children with Divorce: A Compassionate Guide for Parents. New York, Pocket Books, 1985 (Written for parents who are preparing their children for divorce. Discusses topics such as common fears, symptoms of depression, custody and visitation, and common childhood fantasies about reconciliation.)

23

The Working Mother

LINDA V. ROSS AND
EDWARD R. CHRISTOPHERSEN

An increasing number of women are joining the work force in the 1980s and a large percentage of these women are combining careers with motherhood. Among mothers of children less than age 18, 35% work outside the home and 45% of those working mothers have children of preschool age. Of the many reasons why women have chosen to combine careers with motherhood, the most important one is economic necessity. Because it is becoming increasingly more difficult for a family to sustain a comfortable life-style on the earnings of one family member, women are continuing to work after their children are born. The combination of a career with motherhood poses several problems for families as well as society. The problems include the provision of adequate child care for children of all ages from infancy through adolescence; possible detrimental effects of the mother working on the health and development of children; and possible detrimental effects of the mother working on the wife, the husband, and the marital relationship. Solutions to these problems could have substantial economic and emotional impact on the family and society.

The primary health care provider is in a unique position to assess, evaluate, and intervene with the family in which the single mother or father works or both parents work. Ideally, the question of child care should be raised with expectant parents during the prenatal period. Many parents, however, will not have reached a decision about the mother working outside the home until after their infant is born. If the provider has known the family prior to the time the mother goes to work, he may know of preexisting problems that might complicate the child's adjustment to the mother's employment. For example, if the mother is seeking employment to avoid dealing with her child's behavioral problems, the provider should provide consultation or referral in order to ameliorate the behavioral problems and counsel the mother to choose employment for more valid reasons such as economic need or personal satisfaction.

Providers can help parents select the type of child care that will be best suited to the child and the family. The provider can give anticipatory guidance that may prevent or diminish any possible deleterious effects of the mother working outside the home. Having children in day care can affect their development both positively and negatively. Most studies have indicated that no differences were found in intellectual or social development between day-care-reared children and home-reared children. Hopefully, as more infants and preschoolers experience day care, further research will be done to determine the positive and negative effects on child development. Pediatricians must, of course, be sensitive to when they are counseling parents from a data base versus a personal bias.

The provider must make a distinction between the deleterious effects of maternal employment and preexisting problems that are unrelated to the mother's working status. The primary health care provider who has had an ongoing contact with families has an advantage in making this decision. Families who have made good adjustments to previous changes are more likely to adjust well to the mother working outside the home. On the other hand, those families who have had difficulty coping with crises are more likely to manifest behavioral or emotional problems that underscore the importance of obtaining a good family history.

Divorce is one of the possible problems complicating the family's adjustment to the mother working outside the home. Divorce and parental separation may be the cause of the mother seeking employment and may contribute to the presenting problems (see Chap. 22). Other problems that may complicate the family's adjustment to maternal employment include parental conflict over the mother's decision to pursue a career outside the home and parental feelings of anxiety and guilt when both parents decide to work. Such problems can create behavioral or emotional disturbances in the children.

ASSESSING THE IMPACT OF EMPLOYMENT

The American Academy of Pediatrics (AAP) published a statement on the mother working outside the home that included a discussion of questions that may be asked by the mother (American Academy of Pediatrics, 1984). The questions and the AAP's answers follow:

1. Is working harmful to the child? Answers will depend on whether a safe, caring environment is provided for the child and whether the mother is satisfied with her work, her family support, and her ability to nurture her children at the end of each work day.
2. How does a mother evaluate a substitute caregiving situation? Answers should include information about the care-giver, safety, sanitation, and nutrition.
3. What are some of the possible negative effects on children of mothers working outside the home? Answers to this question must include an evaluation of the quality of the child care and care-givers and the mother's energy available for optimal parenting.
4. When is it acceptable to return to work after the birth of a child? Answers will be determined on the basis of the mother's physical health, the infant's physical health, practical and financial considerations, the development of a satisfactory mother-infant relationship, family support, and adequate child-care arrangements.
5. What kinds of reactions can be expected in the mother and other family members if the mother works outside the home? Answers will be most helpful if the provider is aware of the frequent feelings of loss, inadequacy, and guilt experienced by mothers who work. Pointing out positive effects of quality day care and suggesting ways for the mother to spend quality time with her children may decrease the intensity of such negative feelings.
6. Are there special factors that the mother should keep in mind before going to work? The provider can provide answers to this question by recommending that the mother have a frank discussion with other family members about the change in her status and about the necessity of sharing child-care and housework responsibilities.

The pediatrician can use the AAP (1984) leaflet, *The Mother Working Outside the Home*, in several ways. For example, the mother who is considering returning to work might be given the leaflet to review. For the mother who is already working, the leaflet could be given and the questions covered in the AAP handout could be discussed during a subsequent well-child visit. When potential problems are identified during the discussion, an appointment could be scheduled to allow more time for consultation and testing that might not be possible during a well-child visit, or a referral could be made.

After a mother has been working for some time, the health care provider can assess the effects of maternal employment on the child's development by taking a complete family history, plotting physical growth, administering developmental tests, and making behavioral observations (see Chap. 22 for a detailed discussion of a two-stage screening procedure). Problems detected during the assessment should help alert the provider to the possible need for referral.

FINDING QUALITY CHILD CARE

Good child care can be identified in many ways such as through community referral services, referrals from friends or other health care professionals, university child development departments, or local parenting centers or classes. The mother needs to decide whether she wants family day care, live-in help, a babysitter in the home, a day-care center, or a nursery school program. The advantages and disadvantages of each of these types of child care are summarized in Table 23-1. Once the parents have decided on the type of care they prefer, they should screen the facility or person by telephone for obvious positive or negative features and then visit or interview several facilities or persons. Adequate time should be allotted and the child should accompany the mother to the final choices so that she can see her child's reaction to the environment and the care-giver's response to her child. The environment should be clean, cheerful, and safe, and the care-giver should be caring, patient, and responsive to the children in her care.

Other concerns should be staff turnover, individualized attention, stimulating activities and equipment, and an appropriate adult:child ratio for the age level (*e.g.*, 1:3 for infants and 1:4 or 5 for older children). Once the child is being cared for in a day-care facility or by a care-giver in the home, the mother should telephone regularly and drop in unannounced occasionally. If the facility or care-giver objects to unannounced drop-ins, the mother should reconsider her choice. Proximity to the work place may allow the mother to spend occasional lunch hours with her child. Periodic conferences should be scheduled between the care-givers and the mother to monitor the child's adjustment and

Table 23-1. Advantages and Disadvantages of Different Types of Day Care

TYPE OF CARE	ADVANTAGES	DISADVANTAGES
Family day care	Some licensed Most have children of their own One caring adult Least costly: on sliding scale May have flexible hours	Licensing focuses on environment, not social, psychological factors Illness of family child; day care child Taking child out in bad weather Less convenient if more than one child
Live-in help	No early morning hassles Child's illness less problem Often does housekeeping too More flexible hours Good for more than one child More control as employer	Costly Family gives up some privacy Hidden expenses (food, utilities) Often deal with personal problems of employee Difficult to find good help Turnover Fewer children for stimulation
Babysitter in home	Often also does housekeeping Child illness less problem Good for more than one child More control as employer	Transportation difficulties Difficult to find good help Hidden expenses (food, utilities) Fewer children for stimulation
Day-care center	Child has experience with other children; socialization Planned activities spread through day Long hours, seldom closed Continuity of program Sometimes offer special services	No provision for illness Taking young child out of home in bad weather Long day in non-home environment
Nursery school programs	Geared toward cognitive development Child has experience with other children Sometimes offer special services	No provision for illness More costly than day care Taking young child out of home in bad weather May not have summer or vacation arrangements

(Adapted from Ashery RS, Basen MM: The Parents with Careers Workbook. Washington, DC, Acropolis Books Ltd,1983)

progress. The mother should listen attentively to her child during quiet times when he is likely to express feelings and concerns about the child-care situation.

PRINCIPLES OF MANAGEMENT

The focus of family management by the primary health care provider should be on the prevention of possible deleterious effects of the mother working outside the home on the entire family. If the provider possesses optimal skills in counseling and developmental and behavioral assessment, he will be able to advise families more effectively about the possible results of maternal employment. Familiarity with children prior to maternal employment can alert the provider to factors that may interfere with a satisfactory adjustment to changes for the child such as child care outside the home, maternal absence, or increased household responsibilities. Preexisting problems may complicate the management of the family and dictate referral to specialists.

INDICATIONS FOR REFERRAL

The primary health care provider should refer families in which there are significant psychological, behavioral, or developmental problems to appropriate specialists. Indicators of the need for referral include evidence that a child is consistently failing to reach developmental milestones; repeated reports by child-care providers that the child has a behavioral problem; multiple complaints from the parents about their child's behavior at home; or symptoms of serious childhood adjustment problems such as depression or delinquency.

If a child is repeatedly treated for infectious diseases, the provider should investigate the health practices and sanitation of the child-care facility. It may be necessary to notify public health authorities if many cases of infectious disease are encountered from one particular day-care center.

Primary health care providers must be familiar with available community resources to which families can be referred such as government agencies, community support groups, and child advocacy committees. In many metropolitan areas, organizations such as the United Way publish directories such as *Where to Turn* that list most of the service agencies with specific information on the types of referrals and the ways to refer.

MANAGEMENT

The health care professional should provide specific guidance to mothers in order to facilitate the best adjustment for the working mother and her children. The type of guidance varies with the ages of the children involved.

Infant

Mothers should be allowed and encouraged to take paid maternity leave of 4 to 6 months and paternity leave should be granted to fathers to establish their role in caring for their infants. The United States is the only developed nation that does not have a statutory maternity leave policy. Current recommendations from many health care providers include a minimum of 6 months maternity leave for mothers of both natural and adopted infants.

Working mothers should establish daily quality time with their infants to maintain a good mother-infant relationship. High quality time is defined as time when the mother and child are engaged in promoting the child's intellectual, social, or emotional development and in encouraging a warm, accepting maternal attitude toward the child's feelings and behaviors. Working mothers should be encouraged to set priorities for how they will spend their time at home. It is essential that the mother establish the relationships with her infant and her husband as higher priorities than household tasks such as cleaning and laundry. Dividing household tasks with the father, finding outside help, or decreasing expectations for neatness may allow the mother to have more time with her infant.

Preschool Child

The mother of the preschool child may be concerned about such tasks as language development, toilet training, and peer associations. Language may be stimulated in a high quality child-care environment, but mothers should still be encouraged to talk to and listen to their children during the time they have together. Toilet training can be accomplished easily by looking for readiness characteristics such as following two- or three-step directions, finger and hand coordination in removing and replacing clothing, and ability to stay dry several hours. Peer associations may be enhanced in child care settings but the mother may also invite her child's friends to the home so that she can monitor her child's social skills.

Quality time continues to be important at this age. The Child's Game is one method of increasing the quality of the time a mother spends with her child (Forehand and McMahon, 1981). During the Child's Game the parent is taught to engage in any activity the child chooses and to allow the child to determine the nature and rules of the interaction for a short time (*e.g.*, 5 to 10 minutes daily). During that time the parent is asked to describe and praise the child's play, to provide physical contact, and to avoid asking the child questions or giving the child commands. Mothers should also be advised to encourage their children to engage in play by themselves by rewarding brief periods of appropriate play.

School-Aged Child

Although the school-aged child may be in school most of the time the mother is working, she should be encouraged to find child care before and after school. The health care provider should discourage "latch-key" arrangements that expose the child to many risks during unsupervised times. The provider can recommend various community programs that may be available such as the public school system, church facilities, YMCAs, and so forth. For older children who must be unsupervised at times, the mother can be advised to teach her child about fire safety, emergency numbers, stranger avoidance, neighborhood contacts, simple first aid, and routine telephone check-ins with the mother.

Adolescent

The adolescent usually does not require day care unless he has a handicap; however, the adolescent continues to need the mother's quality time. Quality time can include setting aside a designated time each evening during which the adolescent does his homework and the parents work on budgets, correspondence, or other paperwork. Telephone calls, television, and visitors should be discouraged or prohibited during the designated time. In this way, the parents can serve as role models for the adolescent who is developing work habits for adulthood. Delegation and sharing of appropriate household tasks can also encourage increased responsibility in the adolescent.

ANNOTATED BIBLIOGRAPHY

American Academy of Pediatrics: The mother working outside the home. Pediatrics 73: 874–875, 1984 (Official statement of the AAP that may be used as a handout for working mothers.)

Ashery RS, Basen MM: The Parents with Careers Workbook. Washington, DC, Acropolis Books Ltd, 1983 (Excellent practical workbook for parents; covers child care, home management, and parent and career issues.)

Forehand RL, McMahon RJ: Helping the Noncompliant Child: A Clinician's Guide to Parent Training. New York, Guilford Press, 1981 (A book for professionals that describes strategies for training parents in child management.)

Lerner JV: When both parents work: Effects on the development of children. Children Are Different: Behavioral Development Monograph Series (No 12). Columbus, OH, Ross Laboratories, 1985 (Many useful suggestions for parents and professionals when both parents work.)

Wong DL: Guiding parents in selecting child day care. Child Care Newsletter 4:4–6, 1985 (Practical suggestions for the professional to use in advising parents selecting day care.)

Zigler E, Muenchow S: Infant day care and infant-care leaves. Am Psychol 38:91–94, 1983 (Reviews the current status of infant day care.)

24

Working With Difficult Parents
KENNETH H. TELLERMAN

Pediatric practitioners continuously deal with parents who appear angry, anxious, or depressed. Stressed parents may also present themselves through noncompliance with appointments and medications, or alternatively they may repeatedly express seemingly trivial concerns (the "hidden agenda"). Stress may surface from a child's acute or chronic illness or from ongoing psychosocial problems within the family.

Several components of intervention are required for the primary care physician to deal effectively with these "difficult" parents.

1. Acknowledge that you are sensitive to parental concerns.
2. Explore parental concerns.
3. Help resolve parental concerns.

All of these approaches may be integrated into one session for acute problems. For more complex problems, however, these approaches may need to be adapted over a longer time frame.

ACKNOWLEDGING PARENTAL CONCERNS

When dealing with parents experiencing emotional turmoil, it is important for the physician to convey to parents the message that their feelings and concerns have been recognized. Several effective communication techniques can be used to convey this message.

Pacing

The physician may wish to "pace" body language and statements to that of the parent in order to establish rapport. If the parent is anxious and frenetic, the physician may wish to respond in an animated fashion. If the parent is weepy and depressed, the physician may wish to approach the parent in a soft, gentle manner.

Reflective Statements

Reflective statements reflect back feelings that parents have verbally or nonverbally expressed and convey to parents the message that the physician is aware of their emotional state.

Examples

"You seem really upset."
"It sounds like you are pretty angry."
"I noticed tears in your eyes while you were speaking."

Empathic Statements

Empathic statements are supportive statements that convey to parents the message that the physician is aware that the situation is difficult for them.

Examples

"It must be frightening to you when your daughter's fever gets that high."
"You must be exhausted after staying up all night."
"This must be very difficult for you."

Active Listening

Active listening is the technique of identifying and reiterating the feelings and concerns inherent in seemingly neutral statements made by the parent ("listening between the lines").

Examples

Parent: "This is the third ear infection he has had in 3 months."
Practitioner: "You are upset because he has had so many ear infections in a short amount of time."
Parent: "Every doctor I see tells me something different."
Practitioner: "You are frustrated because you have been given so much different advice."

Using the Parent's Sensory Representational System

People often communicate in a sensory (*i.e.*, visual, tactile, or auditory) modality. Rapport with the parent may be potentiated by using the same sensory modality.

Examples

Parent: "I just can't *picture* going through another night like last night."
Practitioner: "I can *see* that last night's experience with your child was quite distressing for you."
Parent: "Sometimes I *feel* like I am being *pulled* in a hundred directions."
Practitioner: "I have a *feeling* that you are right."

All of these approaches convey to parents the message that the physician is sensitive to their duress. Once the physician has established this ground work, the next step is to explore the nature of their difficulty.

EXPLORING PARENTAL CONCERNS

Direct Approach

The direct approach is best for many parents for getting to the root of the problem. Examples of direct questions include: "Can you tell me what you are concerned about?"; "Why did you bring your daughter to the office today?"; "What worried you about her?"; "Why did that worry you?" It is also prudent to ask what the parent hopes will be accomplished as a result of the visit. The parent's expectations may influence the intervention. If the parent's expectations are unrealistic, it is important to explain why his expectations cannot be met.

Indirect ("Third-Person") Approach

When dealing with reserved or less articulate parents, one may use the "third-person" approach, whereby the suspected concerns of the parents are verbalized by the practitioner. This approach allows issues to become apparent that parents might not themselves raise.

Examples

"Some parents are concerned that high fevers can seriously harm their infant. Do you have such concerns?"

"When some parents have experienced a death or illness in their family, they are concerned that their child may die. I wonder if you have such concerns about your child?"

Additional techniques can be used to further delineate parental concerns as the interaction proceeds.

Clarification

When clarification techniques are used, the parent is required to elaborate on unclear points.

Examples

"I am not sure I understand what you mean by that."

"You seem upset. I wonder what is bothering you?"

"You have become quiet. I wonder what you are thinking about?"

"I saw a tear in your eye. Can you tell me what upset you?"

Summarizing Techniques

Summarizing techniques allow the physician to recapitulate what the parent has said in order to validate the accuracy of the assessment.

Example

"Let me see if I understand what you are saying . . . you had a niece who died of meningitis, so whenever your baby gets a high fever, you become worried that she has meningitis as well."

Once parental concerns have been acknowledged and delineated, the final aspect of the interaction should direct the parents toward a resolution of their concerns.

RESOLVING PARENTAL CONCERNS

An effective intervention has occurred when the parent leaves with the hope of a productive change and feeling in better control of the problem. This objective can be achieved in several ways.

Viewing the Problem from a New Perspective

Implicit in the concerns of most parents experiencing duress is the fear of a "bad outcome" to the problem. A key point of intervention is to accept with the parent that although the situation is bad, *the problem is not as bad as it seems* (providing, of course, that this is the case) and to help the parent to view the problem from a new perspective. A classic example is related by the psychotherapist, Milton Erikson. He allayed his 3-year-old son's anxiety following a laceration by getting the child to defocus on how many sutures he would require and to reflect instead on whether he would require "as many sutures" as his older siblings had received for their lacerations.

For the parent distressed by infantile colic, one might accept with the parent that the infant appears to be in discomfort (the situation is bad), but that colic *will not* harm the infant (the situation is not as bad as it seems) and that indeed crying for some infants is a developmentally healthy mode of tension release (new perspective on an old problem.)

For the parent overwhelmed by a hyperactive child, one might accept with the parent that raising a hyperactive child is a difficult endeavor (the problem is bad). One might proceed to help the parent identify his child's strengths and positive features (the problem is not as bad as it seems). In addition, one might help the overwrought parent view the problem from the child's perspective and gain an empathic view of how hyperactivity places the child in a position of poor school achievement and peer rejection.

Conveying an Expectation of Improvement

In addition to helping parents gain a new perspective on a problem, it is helpful to convey to the parent (if the prognosis is not dismal) that the situation is capable of improving. The suggestion that the situation is promising for positive change can be a powerful intervention. The implicit message to convey is that "things will get better." If, for example, the parent is overwhelmed by a child with colic, the physician can convey to the parent that colic is a self-limited phenomenon and that an improvement can soon be expected. For an acutely ill child, it is helpful to give the parent a time range over which to expect improvement. For the child with an ongoing behavioral disorder, one might review the child's strengths and assure the parent that with work, the child is capable of improving his behavior.

Helping Parents to Regain Control

Problems and concerns can often become magnified to the point of overwhelming a parent. The physician can help parents regain a sense of control over their problems by the following methods.

Setting a Realistic Plan of Action. The most important aspect of this intervention is to convey to parents that they have choices. The physician may actively engage parents in problem-solving strategies by having them review all of their options, review the advantages and disadvantages of each option, and select a realistic plan of action. This plan should be as specific as possible regardless of whether it is a treatment regimen for acute gastroenteritis or a "time-out" strategy for a child with behavioral problems. It is helpful to anticipate what problems may occur despite the plan and how the parent will deal with such problems. For some parents, it is helpful to have them recount the plan to ascertain whether they understand it. If the physician lets a parent leave with "something to do" about the problem, the parent's stress can be markedly alleviated.

Ongoing Availability of the Practitioner. A parent's sense of control can be enhanced when he is assured of ongoing physician availability and that resolution of the problem is viewed as a cooperative venture. It is important to the parent that the physician can be reached if a concern arises.

Positive Feedback. Parental sense of control can be enhanced by bolstering their confidence. It is helpful to convey to parents that their physician feels that they are competent and capable of handling the problem, for example by saying: "I know that this has been difficult, but you are doing an excellent job." or "I know that you are a caring parent."

WHEN TO MAKE A REFERRAL

If a parent's or child's problem seems extreme, or if the problem is refractory to the aforementioned primary intervention, it is prudent to refer the family to a mental health consultant (see Chap. 28 for further discussion on making a mental health referral).

ANNOTATED BIBLIOGRAPHY

Green M: The pediatric interview. In Green M, Haggerty RJ(eds): Ambulatory Pediatrics III. Philadelphia, WB Saunders, 1984 (Nice overview of methods of conducting a pediatric psychosocial interview.)

King M, Novik L, Citrenbaum C: Irresistible Communication. Philadelphia, WB Saunders, 1983 (Excellent and unique book on psychosocial communication techniques for medical professionals.)

Korsch B, Freeman B, Negrete VF: Practical implications of doctor-patient interaction analysis for pediatric practice. Am J Dis Child 121:110, 1971 (Summary of practical guidelines for effective communication with parents based on Korsch's classic work on communication with parents.)

Poole SR: The "overanxious" patient. Clin Pediatr 19:557, 1980 (Helpful guidelines for working with anxious parents.)

Schulman J: The management of the irate parent. J Ped 77:338, 1970 (Good practical guidelines for working with difficult parents.)

Wender E: Interviewing. In Levine M et al (eds): Developmental-Behavioral Pediatrics. Philadelphia, WB Saunders, 1983 (Nice overview of methods of conducting a pediatric psychosocial interview.)

25

Chronic Illness

PAULA KIENBERGER JAUDES

A chronic illness may be defined as a physical disorder that continues for 3 months or more, requires hospitalization for more than 1 month, or is expected at the time of diagnosis to last for more than 3 months.

Approximately 10% of all individuals under 21 years of age in the United States have a chronic illness or disability. For more than two million children, chronic conditions cause some degree of limitation of their daily activities. These conditions include arthritis, asthma, autism, central nervous system injury, cerebral palsy, chronic renal failure, cleft lip and palate, congenital heart disease, cystic fibrosis, diabetes mellitus, Down's syndrome, hearing impairment, hemophilia, leukemia, mental retardation, muscular dystrophy, neural tube defects, phenylketonuria, sickle cell disease, seizure disorders, and visual impairment. Asthma is the most common of these conditions.

A pediatrician in private practice will examine between 200 and 300 chronically ill children per year. Because of measures such as vaccinations and effective antibiotic treatment, which have resulted in decreased morbidity from acute illnesses and an increase in the survival rate of children with chronic illness, chronic disease has both increased and become more evident than formerly in medical practice. Parents, physicians, educators, and society are also more aware of chronic disease.

The Vanderbilt Institute for Public Policy Studies has examined the issues concerning the care of chronically ill children and has identified three principles related to public policy concerning such children. These principles are also applicable to the care of these children: "(1) Children with chronic illnesses and their families have special needs which merit attention, beyond that provided to the health needs of able-bodied children. (2) Families have the central role in caring for their own members, and the goal of policy [care] should be to enable families to carry out their responsibilities to nurture their children and encourage their most effective development. (3) Policy (care) should encourage professional services of a highly ethical nature. Key elements include truth-telling, confidentiality, maintenance of dignity and respect for family preference, professionals' recognition of their own effectiveness, and emphasis on collaboration." (Hutchins, 1985)

There are issues in the care of chronic disease that can be faced in common by the child and his family, by society, and by the pediatrician. Any chronic illness may cause severe psychologic disruption of the child and may profoundly alter the life of the family. It has also been shown that the impact of chronic illness on children and their families is similar regardless of the specific type of illness. Issues that need to be faced in all cases of chronic disease include the effects on the child's growth and development; the parents' emotional reactions to the child's illness; the impact of the illness on siblings, parents, and the life of the family; worry about the future; and the choice and comprehension of the appropriate treatment.

The effect on the child and family in relation to the issues mentioned and the role of the pediatrician in the care of these children now follow.

THE CHILD

The goals in all therapeutic intervention on behalf of a child with a chronic illness should be to minimize the biologic manifestations, complications, and progression of the illness and to enable the child to function as independently as possible. The care of the chronically ill child is directed not at a cure, which may be unattainable, but at optimal function. Children with chronic illnesses should be regarded as children with special needs and not as special children.

The effect of a specific chronic disease on the development of the child is determined by the nature of the illness, its severity, the limitations that it imposes, the experience of pain, the treatment modalities, isolation and separation from others, and the visibility of the illness. The developmental problems faced by a 1-year-old are different from those of a school-aged child or an adolescent. A visible deformity (cerebral palsy) may have a different impact than an invisible illness (asthma). Children with an invisible chronic illness may have stress and adaptive problems because although they appear as normal they have limits and restrictions caused by illness. Thus, the children cannot always behave like their peers. At each stage of development, a child must accomplish certain tasks of cognition, social and emotional development in order to advance to the next stage. Chronic illness can interfere with the child's development by delaying or interrupting these sequences.

The main purpose in any therapeutic plan is to regard the child as a whole person, not only considering medical care, but also devoting attention to psychosocial function. Psychosocial adjustment is adequate for most chronically ill children and adolescents. Adjustment not only refers to the ability to adapt to the medical problem but also indicates that an individual is free from disabling psychiatric or social abnormalities. Treatment strategies should be aimed at promoting adjustment.

Maladjustment to a chronic illness was previously considered to be caused by the nature and severity of that disability. It is now apparent from population surveys that, compared to their healthy peers, children with chronic illnesses are generally at increased risk of experiencing significant psychological or social problems. Children who have a poor functional status have more difficulty in making a good psychological adjustment. The degree of psychological adjustment also seems to bear little relationship to traditional measures of morbidity, such as the number of days in the hospital. Among children within a medical diagnostic category, there is a great variability in adjustment; therefore, the medical diagnosis may provide little information, or may even be misleading, regarding the psychological and social status of the patient. Personality attributes that can be regarded as assets, such as intelligence, diminish the likelihood of psychosocial problems, whereas liabilities such as low intelligence or unattractiveness serve to increase the probability of maladjustment. The most important factor in adjustment involves how the family functions with the child and how together they can adapt to the child's illness and its demands.

THE FAMILY

A common characteristic of children with chronic illnesses is their potential to disrupt the life of the family. Research on families with a chronically ill child has focused on the psychopathology of the family members, with little awareness of the positive aspects of the way in which the families adapt. Research has also been done on how families function within specific diagnostic categories as opposed to generic problems faced by families who have a child with a chronic disease.

Both mothers and fathers experience successive or simultaneous reactions after learning of the diagnosis of a chronic illness in their child. These reactions may include shock, anger, resentment, self-blame, denial, sadness, and acceptance. During this process of grieving and reattachment, parents may stop at any one of these stages and may need help to complete this process.

Mothers, who are usually the primary caretakers, vary greatly in their response to their child's illness. Most research has focused on maternal response. Their response is likely to depend on the mother's own developmental history and on her relationship with her own parents. The relationship to her chronically ill child may range from rejection to overprotectiveness to adapting well. The reactions of fathers have been less well studied. Fathers are usually not the primary caretakers but they are usually psychologically involved with the chronically ill child.

Studies on the incidence of divorce in families of chronically ill children have failed to show a consistent increase in the divorce rate. This topic is controversial and has only minimally been studied; the divorce rate may be elevated in families of children with certain diseases. However, parents of chronically ill children seem to have more marital stress than that experienced by families without chronically ill children.

The effects on growth and development of siblings of chronically ill children are varied. Problems for siblings can include fear of catching the disease, guilt, resentment of the burden inflicted, jealousy at attention to the affected child, a real or imagined fear of stigmatization, and problems at school. Factors that may affect the adjustment of siblings include the severity of the illness and the sex, birth order, and age of the affected sibling.

SERVICES NEEDED

Children with chronic illnesses and their families need medical, educational, financial, and advocacy services.

Medical

The child with a chronic illness needs general pediatric care and, in many cases, subspecialty care. The pediatrician provides ongoing health care to the child and family, whereas the subspecialist provides technological expertise in the treatment of the particular disease or deformity. The generalist and the subspecialist complement each other's role in meeting the medical needs of the child and family.

Educational

The patient and the family need to understand the medical aspects of the chronic illness, because they must live with the illness. It is important for them to be educated and to educate themselves, so that they can make appropriate choices concerning schooling, housing, financial matters, equipment, and medical care. The parents may also need this information for the purpose of advocacy.

In 1975, the Educational Act (PL 94–142) for All Handicapped Children was signed; it became fully effective in 1978. The major assumptions from which the law was developed are that all children have the right to education, and that all children, no matter how profoundly handicapped they may be, are able to learn. The law mandates that the states provide appropriate free education for all handicapped children in minimally restrictive environments, with the concurrence of the parents.

All states are mandated to implement educational programs for handicapped children 3 years of age and older. In some states, education is available for these children starting at birth.

Specifically, the law states that a public school must make a multidisciplinary assessment of each child, on the basis of which an individual educational plan (IEP) will be formulated. According to the IEP, the child is then placed in an environment that will enhance his development. The child's educational progress is monitored according to the IEP. The parents participate in all major decisions, and they have the right to appeal placement decisions. The IEP is based on information about the child's illness, developmental status, capacity for daily functioning, and perceived academic potential.

The physician, who is usually the first person to identify children with chronic diseases, will refer a child needing services to the local school district. For physicians, becoming involved in the education of their patients may be a new role. The school forms must be filled out, with information provided about the specific services that will be needed for the child. The physician may, in some cases, have to be the child's advocate to obtain these services from the school system. The physician may also have to educate the school professionals about the illness and he should be prepared to be active in helping to plan the best educational program for the child.

Finally, the community must be educated to the needs of the chronically ill child. The community needs to understand the nature of chronic illness and should respond by removing barriers, both by providing access for handicapped persons and by breaking down stereotyped views of the chronically ill.

Financial

Chronic disease can place major financial stress on a family. Expenses arise not only for direct health care, but also for home care, transportation, extra telephone bills, loss of time from work, special diets, counseling, and so forth.

The extent to which these items are reimbursable—and some never are—depends on the parents' insurance coverage, income, state of residence, and the child's specific medical condition. Private insurance frequently does not cover primary health care, counseling, or home health care.

The pediatrician can advise a family that needs financial help to investigate the availability of funding from Medicaid (Title XIX funds), crippled children's services (Title V), supplemental social security income programs, disease-oriented voluntary associations, or special state programs. The possible public funding sources differ among states and have different eligibility requirements. A resource for the pediatrician could be a nurse/social worker who works for the state agency that handles funding for children with chronic diseases, or a pediatric social worker at a medical center.

Advocacy

Parents and physicians may need to join in being advocates for the chronically ill child to assure that the child's medical, psychosocial, behavioral, and educational needs are being met. In many cases, the community, government, and society have to be educated and motivated to action to meet these needs. Examples of advocacy include the provision of handicapped accessible sidewalks, making sure that the child is in the appropriate classroom, or petitioning the state for funding of in-home care of a child rather than having the child in a hospital.

Specific Services

The child or family may have other specific needs that depend on the type of chronic illness. For example, a child or family under stress may have psychological difficulties and may need counseling. This counseling may be provided by a physician, psychologist, or social worker.

The child may require treatment by one or more health care professionals such as a speech therapist, physical therapist, occupational therapist, vocational therapist, or infant development specialist. Equipment may be needed which could range from simple bracing to an electric wheelchair or a computerized communication board. The home may have to be modified so that the activities of daily living are optimized and so that space can be allocated for equipment. The child and family may need help with transportation to and from therapy and medical facilities. The necessary service can sometimes consist of the provision of a bus fare or access to specialized vans.

Social service assistance may help the family in coping with medical, educational, financial, and psychological problems. Legal assistance may be needed in advocacy for the child. Examples include ensuring that a child is not denied medical benefits because he is poor or in poor housing facilities.

Home care rather than hospitalization may be the best answer for some children whose chronic illness has high technology needs. With home care, the chronically ill child may have as normal a life as possible with his family so as to maximize growth and development. High technology may include a ventilator, phrenic nerve pacer, hyperalimentation, or respiratory treatment. Several requirements should be met for home care to be successful. These requirements include a family willing to care for the child, a flexible, well-thought-out plan of care with a designated coordinator, a backup plan for emergencies, a mechanism for providing social and emotional support for the child and family, and appropriate alternative respite care.

ROLE OF THE PEDIATRICIAN

The general pediatrician assumes the primary care for the chronically ill child. The often complex medical problems are dealt with by the generalist in collaboration with subspecialists. This teamwork prevents fragmentation of medical care. However, the chronically ill child and the family have needs beyond purely medical ones. The pediatrician, as the primary care provider, is in a position to also recognize problems of adjustment and development.

The pediatrician, together with the family, helps with the case management of the health care of the whole child. Case management includes the management of medical care, the continuity of care, the coordination of comprehensive services, and the support of the family. The parents have the primary responsibility for the care of their child. The pediatrician can lend his knowledge, support, medical expertise, coordination of services, and advocacy to the parents in their efforts to meet the various needs in support of their chronically ill child.

ANNOTATED BIBLIOGRAPHY

Blum RW (ed): Chronic Illness and Disabilities in Childhood and Adolescence. Orlando, Grune & Stratton, 1984 (Many medical disease chapters; emphasizes particularly the adolescent.)

Haggerty RJ (ed): Chronic Disease in Children. Pediatr Clin North Am Philadelphia, WB Saunders, 1984 (Excellent overall review of problems; points by Pless, Sabbeth, Stein, and Jessop are echoed in this chapter.)

Hobbs N, Perrin JM (eds): Issues in the Care of Children with Chronic Illness. San Francisco, Jossey–Bass, 1985 (Defines and examines the opportunities available to families who have a child with a chronic illness.)

Hobbs N, Perrin JM, Ireys HT: Chronically Ill Children and Their Families. San Francisco, Jossey–Bass, 1985 (Findings from a study of public policies affecting chronically ill children and their families.)

Hutchins V: Chronic Illness: Old and New Perspectives. Presented at New Directions in Care of Children with Chronic Illness, sponsored by United Hospital Fund of New York, New York, May 1985 (Keynote address.)

Pless IB, Pinkerton P: Chronic Childhood Disorders—Promoting Patterns of Adjustment. London, Henry Kimpton, 1975 (General discussion on the adjustment to chronic illness.)

Sabbeth BF, Leventhal JM: Marital adjustment to chronic childhood illness: A critique of the literature. Pediatrics 73:762, 1984 (Controversial topic, good review.)

Stein REK, Jessop DJ: Relationship between health status and psychological adjustment among children with chronic conditions. Pediatrics 73:169, 1984 (Excellent research on this topic.)

26
Death in the Family*

EDWARD R. CHRISTOPHERSEN

From the beginning of mankind and long before Kubler–Ross chronicled the stages of grieving, families lost loved ones and continued with their lives. Although the stages of grief have been extensively described, there is little discussion of the major differences between "normal" bereavement and the less well-adapted adjustments of some families. Much of the literature on grieving has been characterized by a lack of scientific rigor, an absence of data, and a dependence on clinical examples. This chapter provides a discussion of normal grieving or "uncomplicated bereavement," major depressive episodes, and also a discussion of several suggestions for helping parents and children cope with grief.

The *Diagnostic and Statistical Manual of Mental Disorders* published by the American Psychi-

* This chapter is dedicated to Peg and my Dad, whom I loved and who died while I was preparing this chapter.

atric Association, begins its discussion of "uncomplicated bereavement" with the following statement:

This category can be used when a focus of attention or treatment is a normal reaction to the death of a loved one. A full depressive syndrome frequently is a normal reaction to such a loss, with feelings of depression and such associated symptoms as poor appetite, weight loss, and insomnia. However, morbid preoccupation with worthlessness, prolonged and marked functional impairment, and marked psychomotor retardation are uncommon and suggest that the bereavement is complicated by the development of a Major Depression.

In Uncomplicated Bereavement, guilt, if present, is chiefly about things done or not done at the time of the death by the survivor; thoughts of death are usually limited to the individual's thinking that he or she would be better off dead or that he or she should have died with the person who died. The individual with Uncomplicated Bereavement generally regards the feeling of depressed mood as "normal," although he or she may seek professional help for relief of such associated symptoms as insomnia and anorexia.[1]

The task for the primary health care provider is to discriminate between families who are experiencing a normal grief process and those in which there is significant pathology requiring a referral to an appropriate mental health practitioner. Unfortunately, in much of the published literature on grieving, the authors never state whether they are dealing with normal grief reactions or the reactions of individuals who present with significant psychopathology.

PRESENTATION

In those instances in which a family member, perhaps a child, has been hospitalized, up to the time of his death, the close family members seldom maintain a normal life-style. Parents who sleep in chairs in their children's hospital rooms, or on sofas in the waiting room outside of a pediatric intensive care unit cannot be expected to look, act, or feel normal. The use of hospital restrooms, showers, and bathtubs, and changing clothes much less frequently than usual exacerbates the acute stress. A parent, under these circumstances, will not get as much quality sleep. He may also exhibit less affect and may have a decreased appetite. Thus, some of the reactions that are interpreted solely as grieving may very well have been a result of the combined effect of the loss and a reaction to the severe disruption in life-style.

It is important to know about any pre-existing pathology in a family who is grieving, because families with significant psychopathology cannot be ex-

pected to behave or adjust in the same manner as families who have not experienced this condition. Primary health care providers have a major advantage in that most of the families whom they follow have been known to them for years, and they usually know which families have had adjustment problems. If a family is known to have had serious emotional problems prior to a death in the family, the provider should consider referring the family to a mental health practitioner for management immediately after a death or, in some cases, during the critical illness period. The pre-existing condition, coupled with the death in the family, may create a condition that is simply beyond the time constraints and the training of a primary provider. The urgency or eventual need for counseling is much reduced in a well-adjusted family. In the absence of prior experience with the family, the decision becomes much more difficult, because the provider must then draw judgments from a history obtained while a family is under significant stress. It is highly desirable to spend time with the family, to listen, to provide emotional support, to help them cope, and to discover emerging or pre-existing problems. Unfortunately, many primary providers are not able to find the requisite time.

DIFFERENTIAL DIAGNOSIS

Probably the most frequently encountered differential diagnosis for the provider to make is between uncomplicated bereavement and a major depressive episode. The *Diagnostic and Statistical Manual of Mental Disorders* states that:

The essential feature (of a major depressive episode) is either a dysphoric mood, usually depression, or loss of interest or pleasure in all or almost all usual activities and pastimes. This disturbance is prominent, relatively persistent, and associated with other symptoms of a depressive syndrome. These symptoms include appetite disturbance, change in weight, sleep disturbance, psychomotor agitation or retardation, decreased energy, feelings of worthlessness or guilt, difficulty concentrating or thinking, and thoughts of death or suicide or suicide attempts. (p. 210)

Uncomplicated Bereavement is distinguished from a major depressive episode and is not considered a mental disorder even when associated with the full depressive syndrome. However, if bereavement is unduly severe or prolonged, the diagnosis may be changed to Major Depression. (p. 213)

WORK-UP

History

Primary health care providers are usually the first resource that families turn to when they experience a death. To emphasize this point, it should be restated that the major advantage that the primary provider has is prior experience with the family. If the provider has seen how a family reacted to a prior serious illness, or hospitalization, or to another kind of stress like a job layoff, then he has a good baseline with which to compare the family's functioning shortly after a death in the family and to anticipate problems. A brief office interview, or a phone conversation, may be sufficient to decide if the family needs a referral. If the family members are very sad, with their lives temporarily disrupted, but there is no reason to suspect any prior history of emotional problems, then the practitioner may assume, for the present time, that the family will eventually be able to adjust. Some practitioners may want to administer a depression inventory (*e.g.*, Beck) to one or both of the parents in order to assist in making a judgment regarding the need for a referral. However, the administration of any such inventory would be best left until at least several weeks after the death, in order to give the family members time to deal with their grief. If, after several weeks, they are not functioning better, then a referral may be indicated.

INDICATIONS FOR REFERRAL

In most cases, the primary provider is in the best position to offer advice and support to parents and children who have experienced a loss. Unfortunately, relatively few mental health professionals seem to have much experience with medical disorders.

If there has been a history of significant adjustment problems, if the family either requests a referral for "counseling" or presents with enough symptoms, then the family probably should be referred to a mental health practitioner for assessment and treatment. The provider should not hesitate to inquire about the training and expertise of a professional prior to referring a family to them, because mental health professionals (even those who practice at tertiary care centers) are not always adept at dealing with grief reactions.

TREATMENT AND MANAGEMENT

Treatment Considerations with Parents. In most families, there will be no presenting pathology beyond normal grief. Few people are competent at grieving. The provider may want to make several suggestions to families who either have a child in critical condition or who have already lost a child due to an accident or illness.

Maintenance of Routines. Many people become accustomed to a routine, and when these individuals have a family member in the hospital, or there is a death in their family, their routine is drastically changed. It is also difficult to ascertain whether changes in the family members' habits are due directly to the emotional trauma of the illness or death or to the fact that the individuals' routines have been so drastically altered. In many instances, I have recommended that parents try to return to their normal schedule, and, although doing so may be difficult, they will usually report that they feel much better after doing so.

When a family member dies, the surviving family members usually gather to discuss the departed member, relive old times, and so forth. While these discussions probably do contribute to an individual's ability to deal with the grief process, the disruption in scheduled activities after a short time may become as big a problem as the death. Survivors should resume their daily schedules as soon as it is practical, with no more than 2 weeks' time lapsing between the death and returning to work. The primary provider may have to deal with support people who think that the individual is going back to work too soon.

Physical Conditioning. Several studies suggest that physical exercise can help substantially in preventing or reducing clinical depression. This is particularly true in individuals who were on active exercise programs up until the time of a disease or trauma. We have frequently recommended that parents go for long walks around the Medical Center in order to get some exercise. Parents who have a lot of trouble sleeping during a child's hospitalization will often be able to cope better if they exercise and if they sleep in their own beds. The combination of exercise and a good night's sleep may also improve their appetite. Hence, the parent who exercises, eats, and sleeps well will begin to feel better.

Emotional Support for the Grieving. Most of the comments that people make to someone who is grieving are of little help and may be tasteless. Physical contact of a gentle, supporting nature is superior to anything that can be said. Holding a parent's hand without saying a word can often be more comforting than nervously babbling on. Encourage family members to express their support with physical contact—physical contact often says what we want to say and can't find the words to express.

Support Groups. Some families appreciate going to a support group and sharing their feelings with others who are in a similar situation. Groups like Compassionate Friends can offer emotional support for families who can gain from group discussions. Other families will never attend a support group for any reason. Support groups are an individual type of experience. The provider has to know a family before making decisions about emotional support. This knowledge of a family usually comes about prior to a crisis. If this knowledge is not available, regardless of the reason, then the provider will need to spend some time with the family prior to deciding whether to refer the family to such a group.

Treatment Considerations with Children. Children usually need much less time than adults to discuss a death: they do much better if they resume a routine as soon as possible. Rather than one or two lengthy discussions about death, children may want to discuss it briefly, and episodically, over a period of months or longer. How the child wants the format of the discussions should be respected. Naturally occurring discussion, rather than programmed marathons, will be much better received by the child and will be easier for the parent to cope with. Parents should be discouraged from lying to their children. Grandma is not asleep, nor is her state anything like sleeping. Children can only learn the meaning of words like "death" by having them used in a correct and meaningful context. Death should neither be glorified nor made worse than it really is. A death should certainly not be used as a warning to a surviving sibling to improve his behavior.

Egocentricity of Children. Children may appear to act inappropriately in asking for some of the toys from a deceased sibling, but they do not understand or appreciate that their parents cannot deal with the death, much less face the task of deciding what to do with a deceased child's belongings. They may also make inappropriate remarks about a sibling, saying that they are "glad he's gone," or that he "sure won't miss him!" The parents need to decide as soon as possible if they want to tolerate such behavior: If they do not, then they will have to resume limit setting.

Discipline and Limit-Setting. Families typically get very lax in their discipline and limit-setting following a death in the family. The enforcement of house rules, as soon as possible after a death, will help toward restoring normality in a household. Results are often dramatic. There are few, if any, situations that warrant the suspension of usual and customary family rules.

Some parents allow their children to sleep with them after a death in the family. Typically, this practice stems from the fact that the parents do not feel like arguing with the children. However, once the parents allow this kind of a habit to be well established, it takes a good deal of effort to break it. It is usually better not to allow the bad habit to start. Some well-intentioned professionals will actually recommend that families begin bad habits (like encouraging the children to sleep with the surviving parent), with the implication that doing so will somehow make a death easier to cope with. There is no support for such a recommendation in the literature.

No matter who is responsible for the children's caregiving during the time around a death, children need to continue with their lives. They may want to, and should be allowed to, engage in normal recreational activities. The need to do so, in children, represents a very good coping mechanism that should not be circumvented by a well-intentioned adult. A few "hot laps" around a go-kart track may do more for a child than hours of verbal discussion. Such recreational activities are also excellent therapy for the adults who accompany the children.

Obnoxious Child. Typically a child who is obnoxious during a wake or a funeral, was obnoxious before the death. The fact that his parents are preoccupied with a death exacerbates a pre-existing condition. A child whose behavior was unremarkable before a death in the family and who suddenly develops a behavior problem is easy to manage. The child can be placed with a babysitter who is unrelated to the family and who is unaffected by the death. The behavior will usually show a dramatic improvement if the babysitter engages in regular activities and places limits on the child. If the child's behavior shows such an improvement, then the main reason for the acting-out behavior was probably that the family acted in a very different manner with him during their grieving. Since the child has the rest of his life to learn to deal with the loss, there is no hurry. Acquaintances who do not know the family well will often offer to "help in any way they can." These are excellent people to use as babysitters. They will feel as though they are doing something to help the family and the child is removed from a setting that is obviously not beneficial to him. Just because a child knew someone before he died does not mean that the child is going to experience a profound sense of loss. If a child honestly acts as though the death did not have a real impact, it is probably better to leave him alone than to assume that he needs to "learn to cope with his grief." Consider that the adults may be projecting their sense of loss, rather than evaluating the child's feelings correctly.

Dealing with a Child's Guilt. When parents are concerned about their child feeling guilty about a death, they need to ask themselves whether they said anything to encourage that guilt. It is not unusual for a parent to say things under stress that have an entirely different meaning to a child. The fact that thousands of families lose loved ones every day and continue without significant disturbances in their children is sufficient evidence that children will ordinarily do very well in time. Most children who are verbally fluent (beyond about 4 or 5 years of age) are entitled to a brief, accurate explanation of how the family member died and to have their questions answered at that time. During this discussion, the parents (or other relative) can state specifically what was the cause of the family member's death and that there was probably nothing more that anyone in the family could have done. If the same question (about guilt) arises continuously, it means either that the child really does feel guilty or that he is getting a lot of attention from bringing up guilt. Many parents will deny that a child would use guilt just to get attention. If the physician suspects that the behavior is meant to attract attention, it is better to mention this possibility and then drop the subject, having planted a seed that the parents will probably think about and may very well admit to later. One method for separating attention-getting behavior from honest questions about a death is to provide many opportunities for such discus-sions when no apparent secondary gain can be made. For example, a discussion at bedtime about a death may be used by a child as a reason to stay up later, whereas the same discussion at lunch the next day would not.

The Funeral. Most experts agree that children should attend funerals for members of their families. They should be involved in the funeral activities; however, as mentioned above, if the immediate family members are really emotional, it is a good idea to identify a more distant individual to chaperone the child(ren). A child should be allowed to choose whether or not he wants to spend time with a deceased family member. Some children can carry on a perfectly lucid conversation with a deceased sibling, much to the amazement of the adults in the family.

ANNOTATED BIBLIOGRAPHY

American Psychiatric Association: Diagnostic and Statistical Manual of Mental Disorders, 3rd ed. New York, American Psychiatric Association, 1980 (Definitive source on psychiatric diagnoses: there is no other source that is more highly recognized.)

Beck AT, Rush AJ, Shaw BF, Emery G: Cognitive Therapy of Depression. New York, Guilford Press, 1979 (Good review of the literature on depression. Includes a depression inventory that can be administered conveniently in the office.)

Miles MS: The Grief of Parents when a Child Dies. Oak Brook, IL, Compassionate Friends, 1978 (This brief booklet, available for less than $2.00 per copy, is appropriate for distribution to parents and family members. It nicely deals with topics that will be faced by grieving parents and is short enough that parents will probably read it.)

27

Children in Foster Care
EDWARD L. SCHOR

Most children who enter foster care do so because their parents are unwilling or unable to provide for their physical and emotional needs. They come most often from single-parent households, where poverty, lack of formal education, and absence of social support lead to inadequate and inappropriate child care. Over 80% of the children have experienced physical or sexual abuse or neglect. Previous health care is likely to have been frag-mented. As a consequence foster children are likely to have unrecognized or untreated chronic disorders, a high rate of emotional problems, and impaired school performance.

The foster care system is managed by child welfare agencies. These agencies are usually branches of larger public or private social service departments which, in general, operate with severely limited resources. As the first step in the process of placing a child in foster care, social workers determine a family's need for social services such as counseling, public housing, and so forth. Should the application of these resources fail to, or appear unlikely to improve a home situation deemed detrimental to a child's well-being, the social worker may recommend the removal of the child from his home. The purpose of this removal is to assist the family to remediate the circumstances that prevent adequate child rearing so that the child may be returned to the care of his family. Court-imposed separation of children from parents is a decision intended to be based on the best needs of the child. The burden of responsibility for reconstitution of the family is placed on the parents. A child so removed may be placed in a home with a foster family or in an institution (*i.e.*, group home, under the supervision of a staff of child care workers). Most children are placed in foster home care. The child's case worker is then responsible for assisting the biologic family prepare for the return of their child, for supervising the care of the child provided by the foster parent, and for assuring that the child's health and educational needs are being met. An individual social worker may have several dozen or more children in her case load, and therefore, may be unable to meet all of her responsibilities.

Good foster homes, able to provide the appropriate mix of structure and nurturance to distressed children, are in short supply. Despite this shortage agencies do their best to exclude prospective foster parents who are emotionally unsuited for the demands to be placed on them. Foster parents ordinarily receive limited training prior to receiving children and scanty continuing education. They receive an allowance from the state for each child in their care; the rate of support barely covers the cost of providing shelter, food, and clothes for the child, and it does not presume to be a salary for professional child care. Medical care is paid for by Medicaid programs. Foster parenting, therefore, is essentially a voluntary program heavily dependent on the good intentions and intuitive abilities of altruistic lay people.

PRESENTATION

Foster children may present for medical care at several points during the chronology of their foster care placement. Since most children in foster care come to public attention through reports of abuse or neglect, pediatricians may first become involved in the emergency assessment of these children. The subject of child abuse is discussed in detail in Chapter 20. This encounter may present the only opportunity for a physician to obtain a detailed and accurate history of the child.

Because the care of children in foster care is time consuming and reimbursement is poor, agencies have difficulty identifying physicians willing to provide ongoing care for these children. The absence of an organized system of medical care for children in foster care makes the pediatrician's role more difficult. The lack of a documented intake pediatric history, the turnover of caseworkers, the movement of the child from one foster home to another, and the exclusion of biologic parents from child care decisions once a child has been placed in a foster home may cause the continuing care of a child to rest on an insubstantial data base. These same constraints interfere with the completion of referrals for specialized care and with effective communication among all of those individuals involved in the ongoing care of the child.

The health problems of foster children do not differ substantially from those of other children from similar socioeconomic backgrounds. However, their previous lack of comprehensive health care, the family disorganization and abuse they experienced, and, ironically, the separation from their families inherent in foster care placement lead to a considerably increased rate of chronic medical conditions, educational problems, and, most notably, emotional disturbances. In addition, because most of the children who enter foster care are adolescents, health problems of this age group are seen with greater frequency than in the usual pediatric practice.

Short stature is twice as common in foster children as in the general population. They also have a higher rate of auditory and uncorrected visual acuity deficits. Dermatologic, allergic, and orthodontic problems, dental caries, and musculoskeletal deformities are also common chronic disorders. Foster children appear to have a higher rate of developmental disabilities and consequent educational failures. Comprehensive investigation and management of these disorders is time-consuming and requires an organized system of follow-up and consultation. Whether due to their disorganized lives or to superimposed physical and emotional problems, children in foster care are also likely to be behind the expected grade level in school. No data are available on the incidence of specific learning disabilities in these children although it seems to be increased.

The most significant factor in the health care of foster children, which some investigators have found to be almost universal, is emotional disorders. Over one third of foster children have moderate to severe emotional problems, and another third have evident, although less severe, disabilities.

The spectrum of emotional disorders is wide and is related to the age and personality of the child. For a brief interval after their initial placement or subsequent replacement, evidence of emotional disturbance may subside and the foster parents may then experience a "honeymoon" of good behavior by the foster child. This phase passes rapidly and existing mental health problems reemerge. Infants and young children will often fail to thrive or they will have sleeping and eating disorders. Preschool and early school-aged children will have problems of discipline, toileting, and "hyperactivity." Older children and adolescents often present with exaggerations of usual adolescent behaviors, testing the limits of acceptable social behavior through truancy, delinquency, substance abuse, destructive and violent activities, and sexual experimentation. Psychosomatic symptoms such as headache and recurrent abdominal pain are common. The pediatrician, however, should not be lulled into a false sense of security by the absence of these more overt signs. Depression is common among foster children and withdrawal and social isolation strongly suggest emotional disability. These signs are accentuated during times of uncertainty and stress.

The underlying insecurity of foster children is often aggravated when foster parents, having been pushed to the limit of their tolerance or parental abilities and not receiving sufficient professional support, threaten the child with their single greatest fear—removal from their home—in an effort to control the child's behavior. This tactic is usually ineffective and may precipitate behavior requiring removal. Occasionally, physical or sexual abuse of foster children occurs in foster homes, and this possibility should be considered by the pediatrician when a child's behavior deteriorates.

The frequency and severity of emotional problems is strongly related to the child's sense of security and permanence in his life. Foster children commonly have exacerbations of psychobehavioral disturbances when they have contact with their natural parents. These visitations are usually isolated, unnatural contacts in unfamiliar settings under the watchful eye of a caseworker. This surreal experience, connected as it is to decisions of reuniting the family, compounds the stress on both the child and the parent.

WORK-UP

History

The health evaluation of children in foster care extends beyond the physical, emotional, and educational problems that may be present; it must also allow for cognizance of the child's legal status and communication with the multiple people responsible for the child. Previous health care records should be requested, and the child, caseworker, foster parent, and natural parent should all be sources of information. Others, such as relatives and school teachers, can help in developing a complete picture of the child's life and problems. Much can be learned by interviewing these individuals separately, although having the opportunity to watch their interactions can be helpful in understanding the stresses in the child's life and the nature of the supports available to him.

Central to the health and well-being of a foster child is his placement status. The pediatrician should learn the details of the child's foster care history (*e.g.*, the age and circumstances under which the child came into foster care). Since many foster children have had a succession of caseworkers and have lived in several foster homes, the number of these replacements and the circumstances that led to them should be determined. Foster children often feel unjustifiably responsible for their being in foster care and for whatever alterations in their placement that subsequently befall them. In the process of developing relationships with foster children, it is helpful to understand their feelings and perceptions about being in foster care. The pediatrician should ascertain whether there are plans for a child to return home and, if so, when and under what circumstances, or whether the child is free to be adopted and what progress is being made in this regard. Long-term foster care should be avoided if possible because of its inherent insecurity.

Natural parents, although absent, are central to the lives of foster children. The pediatrician should learn the frequency and nature of children's contact with their parents. In their absence, natural parents become fantasy figures imbued with various attributes. A complete understanding of the foster child's sense of self requires that information about their parents be obtained. One should also obtain information about the child's natural siblings. Siblings are often separated and little effort is made by agencies to assure meaningful contact between them.

A description of the child's life within the foster

home should be obtained. This inquiry takes the form of the usual family social history, with the following modifications: physical accommodations and sleeping arrangements should be noted, as should other issues such as chores and allowance that relate to the integration of the child into the home. The foster parents' previous experience in that role, as well as with children of their own, should be explored. The composition of the foster family and the child's perceptions of the entrance or exit of other foster children from the home should be elicited. The types of rewards and punishments being provided by foster parents is important information, because behavior that often appears to foster parents and caseworkers as intolerable, can be understood and remediated by altering the approach to discipline.

A complete school history is essential because school problems are frequent among foster children. Unfortunately, caseworkers and foster parents often have less communication with the child's school than would be optimal, thus early signs of learning problems and school failure may not be noticed. Careful inquiry may provide clues to difficulties in the school setting and prompt the pediatrician to contact school personnel directly. Disparate reports between classroom and home behavior warrant further investigation.

Physical Examination

The physical examination should be comprehensive. Areas in which positive findings are likely should receive particularly careful evaluation. These include growth parameters, vision and hearing, dental examination, and musculoskeletal and neurologic assessment. Young children should be screened with a standardized developmental assessment. Additionally, adolescents should have assessments of maturation, of fitness for sports, and breast, gynecologic, and genital examinations.

PRINCIPLES OF TREATMENT

If the child's emotional, physical, or educational problems are treated as though they are separable from the foster child's life circumstances, the results will be unsuccessful. By being a sympathetic, objective advocate for the child, the physician can be a source of support, advice, and stability in the child's otherwise precarious world. His knowledge and skills offer the opportunity to recognize and address problems, both emotional and physical, which would otherwise handicap the child's future

development. He can also educate and influence the other adults who share responsibility for the child's welfare so that their decisions are consistently in the child's best interest.

Medical care of foster children cannot occur in isolation from the other professional services directed toward the child and his natural and foster families. Unlike serving as a primary care provider for the average child, pediatricians caring for foster children can expect to routinely invest much time acting as an advocate for the child and as a coordinator of an array of services involving the child's health, education, and welfare. The pediatrician must be cautious to avoid a situation in which the child and those responsible for his day-to-day care are lost in an unintegrated mixture of specialists' opinions that do not take account of the child's unique circumstances. The pediatrician may also find himself in conflict with social service agencies, schools, or the judiciary and he should not hesitate to lobby for his patient in these arenas. It is unfortunately not unusual that the best interests of the child are subverted by conflicting interests and bureaucratic obstacles.

INDICATIONS FOR REFERRAL

The nature and frequency of the health problems of foster children identified by pediatricians make referral or consultation a customary part of their care. The frequency of referral to other medical specialists depends partly on the constraints and capabilities of the primary physician. Many of the chronic medical problems will require the input of a subspecialist. Educational problems demand the coordinated services of psychologists and educators. At least 20% of foster children have emotional problems serious enough to warrant referral for ongoing psychotherapy. On occasion, the input of lawyers will be helpful in buttressing the advocacy role of the primary care pediatrician.

TREATMENT AND MANAGEMENT

The practice in which foster children are seen should be organized to accommodate their special needs. Appointment systems should allow sufficient time for the comprehensive care these children require. Counseling services and family planning should ideally be integrated into the primary care setting. Because of the nature of the health problems of foster children and the transient nature of their living situation a great deal of patient education is necessary; this is particularly important with regard to the self-management of chronic illnesses and in the area of sex education. Problems identified by the primary care pediatrician that require subspecialty consultation should be promptly referred and should then be integrated into the child's ongoing health care plan. The anticipation of a return to his natural parents should not delay appropriate medical assessment and care because, as a rule, these plans are rarely implemented in a timely fashion.

The system of record keeping employed by social service agencies will vary. Pediatricians should keep careful office records of foster children, because it is likely that the child's care will be transferred at some point to another physician, or that information will be requested by the agencies or the courts. It is also recommended that foster children, through their foster parents, retain an abbreviated medical record that travels with them through their various placements and their return home. The American Academy of Pediatrics has available such a record.

In his role as a child advocate the pediatrician caring for foster children may wish to participate in the broader, community-based aspects of foster care. Within his office he may identify and recruit families whom he believes would be effective foster parents. He may participate as a member of a citizens' review board that monitors the planning done by agencies on behalf of children in their care. Finally, he may work, independently or through his professional organizations, with local social services agencies. In this capacity he may participate in continuing education programs for agency staff and foster parents, or help develop standards and procedures for health care for foster children in his community.

The final arena in which pediatricians may deal with foster children occurs when these children leave foster care. Children may return to their natural home, in which case an organized transfer of medical responsibility should be initiated. They may also leave foster care at their legal age of majority to enter the adult world. Alternatively, they may be freed for adoption. This latter course is often a complicated process requiring the termination of parental rights by the courts. In general, well-formulated plans should provide children in foster care with a sense of permanency. When children in care are eligible for adoption, the pediatrician may be asked to support the adoption appli-

cation of the child's foster parents. This consultation should be based on knowledge of the foster parent–foster child relationship and on established principles of parent–child attachment.

Many children remain in foster care though they are legally eligible for adoption. These are the "hard to place" children who are older and who have emotional, cognitive, or physical handicaps. Prospective adoptive parents are often reluctant to assume the additional burden these children may present over what they anticipate are the needs of young, healthy infants. In order to facilitate adoption of children with special needs, Congress has enacted legislation allowing their medical care to continue to be financed by the federal Medicaid program after they leave foster care. The philosophy of adoption agencies is that prospective adoptive families exist for each of these children. Pediatricians should encourage families to consider adopting foster children in those situations in which such a process would be in the best interest of the child and the family.

ANNOTATED BIBLIOGRAPHY

Fanshel D, Shinn EB: Children in Foster Care: A Longitudinal Investigation. New York, Columbia University Press, 1978 (The major prospective study of children in foster care which is concerned with issues of placement and how children fare developmentally during long-term separation from their parents.)

Goldstein J, Freud A, Solnit AJ: Beyond the Best Interests of the Child. New York, Free Press, 1973 (Application of principles of child psychology to legal decisions regarding child placement in adoption, foster care, and divorce; required reading.)

Goldstein J, Freud A, Solnit AJ: Before the Best Interests of the Child. New York, Free Press, 1979 (Considers the legal and psychological aspects of the child–parent relationships and the intrusion of the State into what should be a vigilantly protected area.)

Kavaler F, Swire MR: Foster Child Health Care. Lexington, MA, DC Heath Co, 1982 (Much cited cross-sectional study, the largest of its type, of the health of foster children in New York City.)

Knitzer J, Allen ML: Children Without Homes. Washington, DC, Children's Defense Fund, 1978 (Compilation of valuable data on foster children and the foster care system; not specifically focusing on health issues.)

Schor EL: The foster care system and health status of foster children. Pediatrics 69:521–528, 1982 (Review of the history of foster care and of data describing the health problems of foster children.)

28
The Constant Complainer
KENNETH H. TELLERMAN

The pediatrician frequently encounters children who experience recurrent pain. Abdominal pain, headaches, and limb pains are the most common recurrent pains in childhood, occurring in 10%, 15% to 20%, and 7% to 15% of children respectively. Latency aged children are typically affected. An identifiable organic etiology is discovered in less than 7% of children (see Chaps. 104, 105, 136, and 145 for the evaluation of abdominal pain, headaches, and muscoloskeletal pain).

The evaluation and treatment of pain are dealt with in Chapter 182. In this chapter an approach is given to the "constant complainer" (*i.e.*, the child whose pain does not have a discernible etiology [functional pain]) and to the child whose pain is of organic etiology with a psychogenic component.

ASSESSMENT

When a child presents with recurrent pain, the practitioner must perform a thorough history and physical examination to assess for organic etiology. Such an approach also conveys the message to the child's family that their concerns have been taken seriously, thus establishing the basis for potential psychosocial intervention.

Several indicators of organically induced pain include pain that is constant or well localized or pain that awakens the child from sleep. The presence of constitutional signs or symptoms such as fever, arthritis, vomiting, bloody stools, jaundice, rash, growth arrest, or weight loss are serious indications for organic illnesses. The approach to the child with pain *and* constitutional or organic signs has a markedly different orientation (*i.e.*, sense of time urgency and aggressive laboratory investigations) than the child with pain alone.

During the assessment, the practitioner should explore the following factors:

- When do the pains occur? Pains that occur on mornings prior to school may be psychogenic. Do the pains occur during weekends or during pleasurable activities?
- Are there precipitating stressors? Do the pains occur after disagreements with family members

or peers? Do the pains occur prior to anxiety-provoking events such as school examinations or athletic activities? The parents or child may be instructed to maintain a daily diary for a short time, documenting the nature of the pain, the times of occurrence, and the events or thoughts that are associated with the onset of pain.
- Does the child miss school frequently? School absenteeism is frequently an indication of underlying psychosocial issues (see Chap. 40).
- What is the child's personality like? Recurrent pains may occur in a child who is anxious or depressed. Is the child high-strung, uptight, overly dramatic, or an over-achiever? Is the child withdrawn or displaying a sleep or appetite disturbance consistent with depression?
- What is the family "climate"? Is the family experiencing potent stressors such as financial difficulties, marital discord, death, or chronic illness? How do parents respond to the child's pain? Are family members preoccupied with pain? Are there other family members ("models") experiencing recurrent pain?
- Is there evidence of secondary gain? Recurrent pain symptoms may be reinforced by a secondary gain that the child receives. Parents may also attain a secondary gain from the child's symptoms. Such parents may inadvertently reinforce their child's recurrent complaints.
- *Nurturance issues*: Do the child's symptoms elicit caring and nurturant responses from family members? Do the parents inadvertently reinforce the child's symptoms in order to maintain a "caregiving" role?
- *Separation issues*: Are the child's symptoms a component of separation anxiety and do they serve to maintain proximity with parents? Do the parents inadvertently reinforce the symptoms in order to prevent separation? In the "vulnerable child" syndrome, there is parental difficulty with separation, overprotectiveness, and bodily over-concerns. Children at risk include those who experienced a serious illness in which the parent believed the child would die, those who represent for the parent a significant person from the

past who died prematurely, and those whose mothers have had a threatened miscarriage, a spontaneous abortion, or a stillbirth.

• *Control issues*: Does the child use the symptom as a means of gaining control over parents (*e.g.*, "Give me what I want or I will get ill.")? Do the parents inadvertently reinforce the child's symptoms as a means of maintaining control over the child (*e.g.*, "You are too sick to go out and play.")? For some children, high parental expectations of achievement (*e.g.*, academic or athletic) may lead to recurrent pain symptoms as a means of reacting to or thwarting parental control.

• *Attention seeking*: Does the child use the symptom to gain attention or does the child use the symptom to avoid negative attentions (*e.g.*, missing school in order to avoid embarrassment due to scholastic underachievement)? Do the parents inadvertently reinforce the child's symptom in order to gain attention from peers or medical personnel? For some parents, repeated interaction with a physician or social interaction in an office or hospital setting may meet specific needs or a hidden agenda for the parent.

• *Marital discord*: Parents in conflict may inadvertently reinforce their child's pain symptoms. This frequently occurs, by either becoming overly preoccupied with their child's symptoms in order to avoid dealing with their own conflict or by utilizing their child's symptoms as a means of extending their own conflict. Such parents may take conflicting attitudes about their child's symptoms and use the child as a fulcrum, rather than confronting the more relevant sources of their marital conflict.

MANAGEMENT

If the assessment suggests that the recurrent pains are of psychogenic etiology, several effective primary care approaches are available.

First, it is important to acknowledge with the family that the child's pain is real (whether it be organically or psychogenically induced). The pediatrician should be careful not to convey the message that the child is "making it up" or that the pain is simply "in the child's head." By asking both parents and child what they think is causing the pain, an opportunity is provided to dispel any anxiety-provoking fears and fantasies. With less articulate families, the pediatrician may wish to use the "third person" technique to raise hidden concerns. For example, the pediatrician might state: "It

sounds like you are quite concerned about your son's chest pains. Many families fear that chest pain is a sign of a serious heart condition. I wonder if you are concerned that your son has heart disease?"

When the family's concerns have been addressed, the pediatrician can often reassure the parents that although the problem seems bad, it is not as bad as they thought. The pediatrician might address the family by saying: "I have listened to your son's medical complaints and I have examined him thoroughly, and I do not believe that your son is displaying signs of a serious illness." He might proceed to say: "It seems like your son has been under a lot of stress. You have talked about problems at home and at school. Sometimes pains such as your son is experiencing can be worsened by stress."

It is helpful to leave open the possibility of a physical disorder should the signs and symptoms change. The pediatrician might add: "I would like to continue to monitor these pain episodes and if they change, we may need to consider a further evaluation. For now, I think it would be helpful to examine the stress-related issues going on in your son's life."

The practitioner can be helpful in delineating precipitating stressors and developing a problem-solving strategy with the family to reduce stress. He might help the family to evaluate their options, review the advantages and disadvantages of each option, and select a plan of action. Strategies might be as simple as finding an after-school tutor for a child with an academic difficulty or planning constructive time with busy parents of a child who is seeking attention.

Recurrent pain symptoms are frequently seen among children of overprotective parents. In addition, such parents are often overly involved with the child's symptoms, overly anxious, and over-indulgent. Unresolved fears of separation often exist and many of these children meet the criteria for the "vulnerable child syndrome." Overinvolvement between family members and overprotectiveness are characteristic features of "psychosomatogenic families." Recurrent pain symptoms are often an outgrowth of psychosocial dynamics in such families. In families with overprotective and overly indulgent parents, some of the goals of intervention are to diminish the overextended parent's preoccupation with the child's symptoms and to encourage the family to foster age-appropriate behaviors. This will often lead to improvement in the child's pain symptoms.

Means of improving an inappropriate relationship between overprotective parents and the symptomatic child include (1) encourage the family to allow the child to engage in age-appropriate activities outside of the home such as scouts, church groups, and athletic activities; (2) return the child to school if absenteeism is an issue. Strict criteria should be set for when a child can remain home or be sent home from school (*e.g.*, fever, vomiting); (3) encourage the parents and child to spend "positive time" together, engaged in activities that are enjoyable and not focused on pain. Parents should be counseled to defocus on the child's pain symptoms and they should be advised not to inquire about the child's pain or remind the child of his symptoms. Parents need to become aware of how they respond to their child's symptoms and how their response may foster the child's symptoms; (4) in situations where one caretaker is overly involved with the child, it is often helpful to encourage the less involved parent to spend more time with the child and free up the overly involved parent to pursue alternate interests; (5) encourage parents to diminish overly indulgent behaviors. The child's recurrent symptoms will frequently improve when the parents learn to develop appropriate parent–child boundaries.

Some parents may need specific advice on limit setting and may be helped by using such behavioral approaches as "time out." Overly indulgent parents may need to be advised to relegate age-appropriate responsibilities to the child such as participation in household chores.

If the parent–child relationship can be redirected towards a more appropriate interaction, frequently the practitioner will witness regression of the child's symptoms. It is important to remember that many families may require several sessions of counseling before a productive change is noted. Many of the aforementioned approaches can be individually introduced over the course of several counseling sessions.

MENTAL HEALTH REFERRAL

Mental health referral should be considered when the patient's symptoms are refractory to primary care intervention; if the parents are experiencing significant marital discord; or if the parent(s) or child is displaying severely disturbed behavior.

If the family has been introduced early on to the possibility that there is a psychogenic overlay to the pain, the recommendation for referral may be greatly facilitated. It is often more palatable to the family to convey the message that the child's symptoms may be stress-related rather than caused by an emotional problem. For example, the pediatrician might state: "It appears that your child is experiencing a number of stressful occurrences in his life. Pain can sometimes be influenced by stress factors. There is no clear indication of a serious physical illness causing the pain, but we should stay alert for changes in the nature of your son's symptoms. At this point, I believe that counseling will help your family to examine and deal with some of the factors that are contributing to your son's recurrent pain."

Referrals should be made to a specific consultant with a message clearly conveyed that the practitioner will remain available. Recommendations for referral to a mental health consultant should be stated firmly and the practitioner should avoid being apologetic about making such a referral. Some families may require time to process the recommendation, and the practitioner should be sensitive to this need.

ANNOTATED BIBLIOGRAPHY

Allmond B, Buckman W, Gofman H: Psychosomatic conditions. In Allmond B et al: The Family is the Patient: An Approach to Behavioral Pediatrics for the Clinician. St. Louis, CV Mosby, 1979 (Excellent chapter with practical guidelines for the pediatric practitioner on working with psychosomatic families.)

Apley J: The Child with Abdominal Pains. London, Blackwell Scientific Publications Ltd, 1975 ("Classic" on the child with recurrent abdominal pain.)

Green M: Sources of pain. In Levin M et al (eds): Developmental-Behavioral Pediatrics. Philadelphia, WB Saunders, 1983 (Nice review of the evaluation of children with recurrent pain, with a focus on psychosocial issues.)

Green M: Vulnerable child syndrome and its variants. Pediatrics in Review 8:75, 1986 (Excellent review and update on the identification of "the vulnerable child" syndrome.)

Green M, Solnit AJ: Reactions to the threatened loss of a child: A vulnerable child syndrome. Pediatrics 34:58, 1964 ("Classic" article defining "the vulnerable child" syndrome.)

Minuchin S: Families and Family Therapy. Cambridge, Harvard University Press, 1974 (Presents a family therapy model of psychosomatic illness.)

Schecter N: Recurrent pains in children: An overview and an approach. Pediatr Clin N Am 31:949, 1984 (Comprehensive review.)

29
Sleep Disturbances
MARC WEISSBLUTH

Falling asleep, staying sleeping at night, and napping should best be considered as active processes that develop when there is a harmonious synchronization between parental behaviors and the young child's developing sleep/wake rhythms. Disturbances in this process interfere with the evolution of healthy sleep patterns in the older child. Sleeping patterns change as the child grows and many sleep problems in older children originate in early-onset sleep disturbances. This chapter will therefore focus on infancy and early childhood in order to help prevent, recognize, and manage sleep disorders from the perspective of an office-based pediatrician. Child psychiatrists, psychologists, and neurologists often have different views of sleep disturbances.

PRESENTATION

The major complaint of parents whose child does not sleep well is that the child has difficulty in falling asleep or staying asleep. For children under 12 to 16 weeks of age, the complaint may simply reflect parents' misperceptions. They do not appreciate the natural irregularity of sleep/wake cycles at this early age. Night sleep becomes organized after 6 weeks of age and day sleep becomes regularized after 12 to 16 weeks. After the first few months, parents of children who do not sleep well may continue to complain of abnormal sleep schedules, frequent or prolonged awakenings at night, brief durations of night or day sleep, increased resistance to falling asleep, and an apparent failure to fall asleep except in their arms or in the parent's bed; of note is the infrequent complaint of the harmful effects of sleep deprivation. They may or may not perceive that the trend of mood changes towards increasing reflex irritability, fussiness, peevishness, or crying is the direct result of disturbed sleep. Other parents will notice and complain of the increased fretfulness, excitability, and wakefulness but they do not attribute this behavior to sleep deprivation. Such parents may incorrectly assume that both the disturbed sleep and daytime restlessness are caused by teething pain or that they have a "hyper" baby.

During the remainder of the first year of life, parents may further complain that their child cannot sleep without a pacifier, which is always dropping out, that their child rolls over away from his preferred sleeping position and cannot roll back, that their child pulls himself to standing but cannot get down by himself to sleep, or that he awakens too early in the morning.

After the first birthday, the parents might complain that their child is climbing out of his crib or bed and wanting to stay up to play with them or get into their bed to sleep with them. Another issue that parents often worry about after 1 year is whether the child should take only one nap instead of two. Parents of 2- to 4-year-old children often wonder how these behaviors might be related to fears of darkness, death, or abandonment or that they might be associated with other stresses such as toilet training or the arrival of a new baby in the family.

Parents of young children in preschool and school might describe their child's disturbed sleep in terms of his being an "owl" or a "night" person because he likes to stay up late watching television, reading, or listening to music. Decreasing school performance, low self-esteem, or depression may be associated with longstanding impaired sleep quality in these older children.

DIFFERENTIAL DIAGNOSIS

The diagnosis of disturbed sleep rests on the determination whether the child's sleep pattern is age-appropriate and sufficient for the particular child. Norms are available for all age groups; however, the range of normal sleep patterns for any age is wide.

Is there impairment of mood or performance? These changes may represent a combination of chronic fatigue plus the accumulation of "nervous energy" due to the expected physiologic response to the chronic sleep loss. Thus, the adolescent might have features of depression whereas the much younger child may have features of hyperactivity. Extreme temper tantrums or noncompliant behavior might be the sign of an overly-tired toddler. Therefore, the differential diagnosis of common behavioral or emotional problems at any age should include a consideration of whether disturbed sleep is an associated feature. Often, in the younger child but less so in the adolescent, a determination based on which came first, the disturbed sleep or the disturbed behavior, allows the pediatrician to decide which is the primary problem and which is a complication.

The need for this distinction is most clearly made in children with allergies, large adenoids or tonsils, or birth defects causing partial or complete airway obstruction during sleep. These children present with snoring, mouth breathing when asleep, sweating when asleep, restlessness during sleep, frequent awakenings, and in longstanding or severe cases, bedwetting and signs of hyperactivity.

It is important to distinguish between persistent or chronic snoring from transient mouth breathing caused by a seasonal allergy or a sequence of overlapping viral upper respiratory infections during the winter. Airway obstruction during sleep causes poor quality sleep and results in excessive daytime sleepiness that interferes with development or academic performance. When the nocturnal breathing problem is corrected, these children sleep better and dramatically improve their mood and performance.

In many other children it is unclear whether the sleep disturbance reflects a problem within the child or represents problems between the parents. An example of a common sleep problem within the child is the postcolic baby who has learned to expect parents' soothing attention to help him fall asleep. Examples of problems between parents or within the family presenting as a childhood sleep disturbance include marital discord, maternal ambivalence about breast-feeding, maternal guilt about working outside the home, life-styles that view sleep schedules as too inconvenient or artificially restrictive, or parental difficulties in allowing their baby to develop independence. For example, when there is marital discord, the non-sleeping child who clings to the mother at night provides solice to the unloved or unappreciated wife. The family bed may be associated with too much commotion contributing to the sleep disturbance, while at the same time helping parents avoid issues of sexuality, intimacy, or further children. Although a parent may complain that the child is not sleeping, it may serve as a secondary gain or some useful function or reflect a longstanding problem within the family.

Thus, the three major areas to consider when a child does not sleep well are (1) innocent parental errors involving inconsistency, irregularity, or oversolicitousness, (2) a child's difficulty in breathing during sleep, and (3) family problems creating and maintaining a sleep disturbance for the child. These three types of problems may coexist. Less common medical problems such as severe anemia, acquired hypothyroidism causing excessive daytime sleepiness, or impaired mood and school performance associated with psychiatric or neurologic problems should also be considered.

WORK-UP

It is essential to have a detailed written report that includes night sleep durations, night sleep schedule, and the frequency and duration of night wakings. The schedule and duration of naps, the time required to put a child to sleep at naps and at night, the parents' behaviors when the child does not fall asleep at naptime and bedtime, and the parents' behaviors when the child awakens at night are also important.

Specific questions should be directed towards snoring, mouth breathing when asleep or mouth breathing when awake, and cessation of breathing while sleeping. Parents can tape breathing sounds during sleep.

Questions should also be directed to what agreements or disagreements exist between both parents regarding the sleep problem. Questions should be asked about the parents work schedules, child-care routines, their marriage, and time away from their children. Two issues often confuse parents: (1) distinguishing between the child's need to sleep at night and day versus the child's wanting to enjoy more of his parents' company, and (2) encouraging the development of the healthy capacity to experience being alone versus thwarting independence out of fear that the child will feel abandoned. These areas should be explicitly discussed because they might not spontaneously surface. Other issues to consider are: Is one parent an insomniac searching for night-time company?; Does the mother view naps as a waste of time, depriving the child of time from being in mom-and-tot groups or does she view nap time as restricting her social activities?

The history of disturbed sleep often begins with naturally occurring disruptive events such as vacation trips, moves, or frequent common illnesses. Hospitalizations, severe illnesses, death of a family member, or changes in school may also be important precipitating events. Thus, a detailed history is often important.

The work-up for a child with suspected respiratory deficits during sleep might include an endolateral radiograph to determine airway patency, a formal sleep study to evaluate the quality of breathing during sleep, an allergy work-up, or referral to an otolaryngologist.

PRINCIPLES OF MANAGEMENT

The major principle of management is to educate parents that sleep patterns are a health habit that they can encourage or discourage. Just as with other health habits such as tooth brushing and hand washing, there may occur times when the child does not want to cooperate. It is hard not to give into the demands of the child when everyone is tired. However, when the parents understand that sleeping well directly helps the child in terms of being more relaxed, calmer, more attentive, and better able to learn, then they are more motivated to establish healthy sleep habits.

Several hours may be required for counseling. If the physician or family cannot accept this time commitment, the child's sleep problem will likely continue. Counseling is so time-consuming because it must address issues of parental mismanagement, parental guilt, and strong contradictory feelings surface when the child cries at night. The crying always confuses the issues because it bothers parents so much. They have to be repeatedly told: "We are letting the child learn to sleep better; we are letting him cry but we are not making him cry in the sense of hurting him." This attitude of tough love is hard for many parents to accept. The written sleep diary may be invaluable in helping the parents cope; parents can see that compared to the baseline, improvement has occurred. The observed improvement also helps support them to be firm without fear of creating a resentful or angry child.

The behavioral approach to helping the child sleep better should be delayed if there is a suspicion that the child has an abnormal breathing pattern during sleep. When there is a partial or complete airway obstruction during sleep, the night wakings or light sleep states represent protective arousals that prevent asphyxiation. After the airway obstruction is reversed, it is possible that longstanding unhealthy sleep patterns persist because they have become habitual or a part of the family's life-style. When the child is no longer having nocturnal respiratory problems, his sleep habits can be changed by reducing parental reinforcing behaviors.

INDICATIONS FOR REFERRAL

A fatigued family may readily accept only those suggestions that do not add further stresses to their frayed relationships. If it is thought that the chron-icity or severity of the sleeping problem has seriously disturbed all family members, or if the parents are in substantial disagreement about how the problem evolved or how to solve it, then a referral should be made to an expert in pediatric sleep disorders. Alternatively, neurologists, psychologists, psychiatrists, and pediatricians who have developed skills in dealing with pediatric sleep problems may be consulted; they are usually affiliated with academic hospitals for children.

TREATMENT AND MANAGEMENT

Much has been written about young children who do not sleep well because of prenatal factors, mild obstetric problems in the newborn period, constitutional features such as low sensory threshold, colic during the first few months, and food allergies. However, the most common cause of disturbed sleep in infants and toddlers is parental mismanagement. There is unanimity in published reports that when parents change their behaviors and ignore protest crying from their child, the child's sleep habits do change. It has been amply documented, and bears restatement, that there is no psychological or emotional harm to the child when the parents do not respond at those times when the child needs to sleep.

The focus of treatment is not to impose a rigid arbitrary sleep schedule, but rather to develop an orderly routine that reasonably synchronizes caretaking activities with the child's circadian sleep/wake rhythms and, most importantly, that ensures that the child's sleep habits meets his needs. The question that should be answered as treatment proceeds is not how many hours the child should sleep, but rather whether or not the child's behavior indicates that he is well-rested.

Between 4 to 15 months of age, parents should expect their child to begin sleep between 7 PM and 9 PM and to awaken between 5 AM and 7 AM. Many children awaken once around midnight for a brief feeding, and they and their parents immediately return to sleep. A midmorning nap and an early afternoon nap are typically at least an hour. Parents usually spend about 20 minutes soothing their child to sleep at naps and at bedtimes.

If parents stop attending to all but one night waking, put the child down awake or asleep after the predetermined soothing period, and maintain this schedule, protest crying will rapidly disappear. Parents usually prefer a fade procedure whereby they gradually reduce their soothing efforts but they often begin to observe that they are somewhat inconsistent. The inconsistency reflects the fact that their exhaustion overrides their patience in maintaining a planned withdrawal of parental attentiveness. Nevertheless, some improvement is usually observed and many parents now have the courage to try an extinguishing procedure.

After 15 months, children usually take only one nap but now parents may observe an increasing resistance to napping or going to bed at night. The child may soon start to climb out of his crib as he becomes more independent and curious.

Parents who firmly and calmly maintain healthy sleep habits and gently place the child back in the crib silently whenever he gets out teach the child that certain behaviors are unacceptable. Silence and an emotionless attitude help reduce the social rewards that reinforce night waking. Consistency in doing the same behaviors or rituals at sleep times and reasonable regularity when the child is tired helps establish structured sleep habits. It is important to remind parents that they can establish a programmed routine regarding sleep but that they cannot force the child to sleep. Once established, however, the child will usually then sleep.

After about 2 years of age, parents should add positive reinforcing efforts to reward cooperation in maintaining a healthy sleep pattern. Rewards might include keeping the door open wider, a brighter night light, extra time playing with a parent, extra amounts of favorite foods, toys, stars on a chart, or snacks.

The exact management strategy should be tailored to each family. For all families, it is essential that parents keep a sleep log or diary before and during the treatment process. The diary should be examined not only in terms of the duration of sleep but also in terms of sleep schedules and specific parent behaviors. Parents often fail to note that intervals of wakefulness are too long and the result is overstimulation leading to a failure to easily fall asleep or stay asleep. The diary helps improve and adjust the treatment plan to meet the specific sleep needs and family's routines. The parents are rewarded with a better behaved, rested child.

ANNOTATED BIBLIOGRAPHY

Guilleminault C, Winkle R, Korobkin R, Simmons B: Children and nocturnal snoring. Evaluation of the effects of sleep related respiratory resistive load and daytime functioning. Eur J Pediatr 139:165–171, 1982 (Respiratory deficits cause *reversible* sleep disturbances, excessive daytime sleepiness, and impaired school functioning.)

Richman N, Douglas J, Hunt H et al: Behavioral methods in the treatment of sleep disorders—a pilot study. J Child Psychol Psychiatry 26:581–590, 1985 (Parents do not cause more anxiety in their children when they give them less attention at night.)

Weissbluth M: Crybabies. New York, Arbor House, 1984 (Second half of the book discusses fade procedures and extinguishing procedures to promote healthy sleep.)

Weissbluth M: Healthy Sleep Habits, Happy Child. New York, Fawcett Columbine, 1987 (Age-specific guidelines to prevent and correct sleep disturbances.)

Weissbluth M: Modification of sleep schedule with reduction of night waking. A case report. Sleep 5:262–266, 1982 (Presents age-specific normal data for sleep schedules.)

Weissbluth M: Sleep duration and infant temperament. J Pediatr 99:817–819, 1981 (Sleep patterns and personality are associated at age 4 months.)

Weissbluth M, Davis AT, Poncher J: Night waking in 4 to 8 month old infants. J Pediatr 104:477–480, 1984 (Most night waking is due to postcolic sleep problems or partial airway obstruction.)

Weissbluth M, David AT, Poncher J, Reiff J: Signs of airway obstruction during sleep and behavioral, developmental, and academic problems. J Dev Behav Pediatr 4:119–124, 1983 (How sleep deficits harm the child.)

30
Common Feeding Problems in Young Children
DAVID I. BROMBERG

Few areas cause as much parental concern and consternation as those involving feeding and nutrition in infancy and childhood. All parents enter the feeding relationship with their children with a set of experiences and expectations. Based on these, they make decisions about nutrition and feeding practices for their families. Many parents, for example, have grown up hearing about the starving children in Europe (Asia, Africa, or Appalachia may be substituted) or they may be members of the "Clean Plate Club." These parents, therefore, feel it is important for their children to finish a serving presented to them. Similarly, parents have been presented with nutritional "truths" about the role of milk or red meat in a diet and they plan their children's diets based on these "truths." Infants and children bring to the dinner table a set of nutritional and caloric needs as well as certain emotional and developmental requirements. These needs may be in direct conflict with parental expectations with resulting family conflict and behavioral difficulties. The pediatrician is in an important position to educate and counsel about these differing viewpoints and to resolve many common feeding problems.

Chamberlain reviewed problem behaviors that middle-class parents experienced in their preschoolers. Between one quarter and two thirds of all parents of 2-, 3-, and 4-year-olds reported concerns over eating behaviors. These parents ranked eating problems fifth as a major cause of frequent parent–child conflict and ranked it ninth as a problem that worried or concerned them. Eppwright reviewed eating behaviors in preschool children. Over one third of the mothers interviewed expressed concerns about their children eating a limited variety of food and dawdling over their meals. Over 20% of the mothers voiced concern that their children ate too little fruits, vegetables, and meat and too many sweets.

DEVELOPMENTAL ISSUES

Three major developmental areas: (1) temperamental factors, (2) neuromaturational factors, and (3) psychosocial/emotional factors impact on eating behavior and feeding problems. Infants clearly differ from one another in their ability to adjust to new situations and with the intensity that this adjustment occurs. This may reflect on the ease of introduction of new foods and textures. Differences in biologic regularity impact on the ease of meal scheduling and the ability to deviate from schedule. Once some infants start a task, (e.g., eating breakfast) they stay on the task easily, whereas others are distractable and have a short attention span varying from eating to playing to crying.

New feeding behaviors often require increasing neurologic skills or the disappearance of primitive reflexes. The ability of self-feeding necessitates increasing eye–hand coordination and a fine pincer grasp. Until the infant develops these abilities at 9 to 12 months, he will be unable to feed himself. Should these milestones be delayed, the ability to self-feed will correspondingly be altered. The extrusion reflex, present from birth until about 4 months, causes an infant to expel solids placed in his mouth. This expulsion may be viewed by parents as a refusal to feed if solids and the spoon are introduced before this primitive reflex has disappeared.

Psychosocial factors also play a significant role. As the infant approaches his first birthday, he has increasing autonomy needs. This is often reflected in his "need" to feed himself and his desire to not allow his mother anywhere near him with a spoon. At this same time, the infant begins to develop the concept of object permanence, which is partly learned by repetitive games (e.g., peek-a-boo). The game is fun for parents when played with toys or faces, but it may become less fun when played with food thrown from the high chair. When the child is almost 2 years of age and his autonomy needs increase, he often becomes selective in his choice of food. The child often decides at each meal what he chooses to like or reject at that time. Children develop increasing social awareness and social skills around the preschool age. Increasing chattiness at the dinner table about the day's events may result in a decreased food intake. The child's desire to use a knife and fork may well cause increased frustration at meal time.

COMMON PROBLEMS

The most frequently voiced concern about eating behavior is that children do not eat enough or that they eat too limited a variety of foods. In early infancy, nursing mothers may fear that they are not providing enough milk for their babies. They may misinterpret infant cues and misread crying after eating as hunger or lack of satisfaction with a meal. In preschoolers, aged 3 to 5, the growth velocity dramatically decreases, with a concomitant decrease in caloric needs and appetite. Parents will report that their 3-year-old does not eat enough to sustain his activity level. Parents may resort to harsh threats or ineffective cajoling in an attempt to encourage intake. The result may be tense conflicted mealtimes with deteriorating behavior on the part of the child.

Parents also express concern about their children's nutritional balance. This may be reported as a youngster's refusal to eat green vegetables or what a mother might consider inadequate milk intake. Many of these concerns stem from nutritional myths or misinformation. For example, parents, not recognizing the protein content of peanut butter, may have concerns about protein intake when their child eats peanut butter but little meat, Occasionally, the concerns center on a lack of variation in the diet or difficulty in getting a child to try new foods. Concerns about nutritional balance may be warranted and should be investigated by the practitioner. Serious nutritional deficiencies may result, especially when families are committed to faddish or unusual diets.

Mealtime behaviors and table manners are frequently a source of conflict in families. Typical complaints at mealtime include dawdling over meals, messiness, gulping down food, sitting with poor posture, playing with food, or an unhappy mood. Parental expectations and the family's mealtime routine play a large role in the genesis of these problems. For example, large portions and the need to finish everything on the plate may encourage dawdling and playing with food.

Spitting or vomiting are common problems in infancy and often cause parents grave concern. The spitting commonly presents as "wet burps" of 5 ml to 10 ml of regurgitated stomach contents shortly after a feeding. Inadequate weight gain, hematemesis or hematochezia, aspiration pneumonitis, or marked irritability with regurgitation indicates a more significant form of gastroesophageal reflux. Spitting in infancy is usually self-limited and largely disappears by 9 months. Intermittent vomiting may continue in some children throughout childhood. These children often present with a history of vomiting unaccompanied by nausea. They may vomit daily or several times a month. The vomiting does not appear to be under voluntary control. A careful history looking for a relationship to dietary, emotional, or environmental factors should be undertaken although frequently no relationship is found. This process, too, is self-limited and in the presence of adequate growth, reassurance may be the only necessary intervention.

The entities of *rumination* and *cyclic vomiting* are more uncommon and represent a more serious pathology. Rumination is a voluntary self-induced vomiting usually occurring in infancy. The reverse peristaltic wave is encouraged with oral movements and occasionally self-gagging. Rumination is thought to represent a self-stimulating behavior and can seriously interfere with adequate nutrition and normal growth. Serious disturbance of the mother–infant relationship is thought to exist. Treatment involves addressing the underlying social and emotional causes and the use of behavioral techniques

to gain control of the vomiting. Cyclic vomiting is a disorder characterized by recurrent bouts of vomiting not caused by biologic causes. Each of these episodes may be sustained and can result in acute dehydration. Psychopathology is thought to play a significant role and psychiatric treatment is indicated. Colic, overeating and overweight, and failure to thrive are discussed in separate chapters.

DIFFERENTIAL DIAGNOSIS AND WORK-UP

Feeding problems are frequently uncovered during routine health screenings. Open-ended questions about mealtime and nutrition can be helpful in eliciting parental concerns. Once parents have expressed worry about feeding or nutrition, a detailed dietary and feeding history should be obtained. The pediatrician should have a clear picture of what mealtime is like. What are the typical portion sizes and what is the expectation that they will be finished? Are there frequent distractions such as television and telephone calls? How long does a typical meal last? Is the youngster required to eat the entire meal? Are there special mealtime rules, such as finishing dinner before dessert? A detailed 3-day food diary recording of what was served at each meal and how much the child ate can be helpful.

In performing a thorough physical examination, the physician should be looking for both underlying physical abnormalities and also for consequences of poor nutrition. In most of the feeding problems discussed, the etiology lies in difficulties in the parent–child interaction. As such, the examination of these youngsters is frequently unremarkable. However, the therapeutic implications of a normal physical examination in reassuring concerned parents cannot be overstated. A careful neurologic examination looking for a central nervous system dysfunction is warranted in infants who experience difficulties in the transition to solid food and who demonstrate persistent or excessive extrusion reflexes past 4 months of age. In the presence of persistent vomiting, careful consideration should be given to the possibility of increased intracranial pressure, intermittent intussuseption, malrotation, and volvulus. These diagnostic possibilities can usually be excluded on the basis of sustained good growth, a negative history, and a normal physical examination.

The most helpful diagnostic study in the evaluation and management of feeding problems is the meticulous use of the growth chart. Repetitive charting of height and weight over time compared to established norms gives us the most sensitive indicator of the significance of a feeding problem. A feeding problem exists (*e.g.*, undereating, too many sweets, not enough vegetables, dawdling at dinner, and so forth) when it is viewed as such by parents. However, a feeding problem in the presence of a consistent weight gain and an appropriate weight for height may be managed very differently from one in which weight has substantially fallen off the curve. Educational and counseling interventions may suffice in the first situation whereas more intensive counseling and behavioral treatments may be necessary in the latter case.

TREATMENT

Children, when allowed to make their own choices regarding food, tend to select a calorically and nutritionally balanced diet. In most families who complain of feeding problems, the children are adequately nourished and are growing well. The difficulties frequently stem from misconceptions about nutrition or family traditions that are in conflict with the developmental needs of the child. The approach to management should be reassurance and education. Reassurance should begin with a confirmation of health and nutritional status and a review of the growth record. The physician can then demonstrate the developmental level of the child and balance it against the parental expectations. A 1-year-old cannot be expected to eat in a carpeted dining room and keep all his food off the floor. A 4-year-old may not be able to sit civilly through a dinner involving several courses. Once this is recognized, the parent and pediatrician can develop alternative eating strategies.

When pickiness or poor intake is the concern, especially if accompanied by inadequate growth or poor nutritional balance, several behavioral interventions can improve and change the diet, such as reinforcement, portion control, shaping, and modeling techniques. Behavior modification strategies can also be helpful in improving mealtime behavior. The physician can help the parent identify desired behaviors that are positively reinforced and undesirable behaviors that are punished (*e.g.*, with a time-out period). A discussion of specific mealtime routines with parents can also be useful. This discussion might include setting appropriate time limits for eating, determining appropriate portion sizes, creating calm atmosphere, and including children in the dinner conversation.

Nutritional interventions can be helpful in alleviating feeding difficulties. Nutritionally equivalent substitutes can be found for nonpreferred foods. Preferred foods can be embellished with supplemental calories if inadequate calories are the problem. Vitamin supplements can be used when specific inadequacies are suspected. Although often requested by parents, no tonics are available to increase appetite.

INDICATIONS FOR REFERRAL

Most feeding problems are appropriately handled by the pediatrician in the primary care office. Through the use of pediatric diagnostic and counseling skills, most common problems (especially in infants and children with normal growth) can be resolved to the parent's satisfaction and the youngster's benefit. However, assistance from other professionals in developing a comprehensive management plan may occasionally be valuable. This is especially true in the presence of growth retardation or a nutritional deficiency. Dietitians can be especially helpful in assessing nutritional adequacy and in planning nutritional interventions. The pediatrician and dietitian can work together as an effective team in treating common feeding problems.

Attitudes about eating are often deeply ingrained and even with excellent education and counseling parents may be resistant to change. When the physician is faced with a lack of progress concerning a significant feeding problem or if a parent is dissatisfied with the outcome of treatment, referral to a mental health resource is indicated. Child psychiatrists, child psychologists, and feeding disorder teams (often including psychiatrists, psychologists, developmentalists, and dietitians) would all be appropriate referral sources. Psychiatric referral is also indicated for most cases of rumination and cyclic vomiting. Consultation with a gastroenterologist may be indicated when significant vomiting is a component of the problem.

ANNOTATED BIBLIOGRAPHY

Chamberlain RW: Management of preschool behavior problems. Pediatr Clin North Am 21:33, 1974 (Overview of behavioral concerns in the preschool age group and a pediatric approach to counseling.)

Davis CM: Self-selection of diet experiment; its significance for feeding in the home. Ohio State Med J 34:862, 1938 (Often-quoted reference suggesting children's self-selection of a balanced diet given the opportunity.)

Dunn J: Feeding and sleeping. In Rutter M (ed): Scientific Foundations of Developmental Psychiatry, pp 119–128. Baltimore, MD, University Park Press, 1981 (Interesting review of the biologic and psychological factors influencing feeding patterns and their relationship to the development of feeding problems.)

Eppwright ES: Eating behavior of preschool children. J Nutr Educ 1:16, 1969 (Reviews food amounts, food types, and eating behavior in preschoolers.)

Finney JW: Preventing common feeding problems in infants and young children. Pediatr Clin North Am 33:775. 1986 (Review of the behavior modification techniques available for use in the amelioration of feeding problems. Good examples of parent education material about issues of feeding and mealtime behavior are included.)

Fraiberg SH: The Magic Years, pp 72–76. New York, NY, Charles Scribner's, 1959 (Delightful review of child development from an analytic perspective. Feeding issues are presented as they would be perceived by a toddler.)

Ilg FL, Ames LB: Child Behavior, pp 69–83. New York, NY, Harper & Row, 1955 (Thoughtful review of eating behavior from a developmental perspective. Discusses several specific problems and makes management recommendations.)

31
Speech Disorders
JONATHAN SCHWARTZ

The development of speech is considered by parents and physicians to be a sensitive measure of a child's intellectual potential. Parents eagerly anticipate their child's first word and often remember for many years a particular string of words that their child created early in life. Because of the central role of speech in social, intellectual, and emotional development, pediatricians should be familiar with the components of speech so that they are comfortable assessing speech development, especially when a problem is suspected.

Speech refers to the transcription of language into sounds. Speech disorders may result either from a problem in the acquisition or comprehension of language or from a problem in producing sounds. The presence of intact hearing is also crucial to the development of normal speech.

The distinction between psychological and neurologic causes of speech disorders may be difficult to make. Several psychosocial factors may adversely affect the quantity or quality of a child's speech. In most cases, the pediatrician can narrow the differential diagnosis considerably by taking a careful history, by conducting a thorough physical examination, and by assessing the child's speech.

DEFINITIONS

Disorders of speech can be divided into those of sound and of language production. Disorders of sound production include articulation disorders (dysarthria), voice disorders (dysphonia), and fluency disorders (dysrhythmia). Dysarthria refers to the incorrect enunciation of distinct syllables and words; dysphonia implies a loss of voice, usually due to hoarseness; and dysrhythmias are disorders in the rhythm or fluency of speech. Stuttering is the most common form of dysrhythmia that requires treatment.

Disorders of language production include both delays in the onset of speech and abnormalities in the understanding and production of formal spoken language.

CLINICAL PRESENTATION AND DIFFERENTIAL DIAGNOSIS

Significant *delay* in the development of speech may be caused by intellectual retardation, hearing loss, psychosocial deprivation, autism, or developmental aphasia. *Intellectual retardation* is the most common cause of delayed speech acquisition. The more severe the retardation, the slower is the acquisition of communicative speech. A high proportion of intellectually retarded children also have other problems that may contribute to delayed speech development. Psychosocial deprivation and hearing loss are both more common among intellectually retarded children than among children of normal intelligence. Therefore, it should not be assumed that intellectual retardation is the sole cause for delayed speech development.

Hearing loss is also a common cause of delayed speech acquisition. Although screening tests to detect early hearing loss have been increasingly utilized, many children who are referred to speech clinics at 3 or 4 years of age are found for the first time to have impaired hearing. Many children with retarded speech development have a history of recurrent or chronic otitis media, or a perforated eardrum.

Psychosocial deprivation may contribute to speech that is immature with respect to articulation, vocabulary, sentence length, and grammar, as well as to a delay in the onset of speech. Children generally begin to speak more slowly in families that place little emphasis on verbal stimulation.

Infantile autism is a rare cause of failure to develop speech. Babbling is often delayed, echolalia (repeating of the last few words said) is prolonged, and 50% of these children may not acquire communicative speech if they are left untreated. In addition to the delay in onset, the speech of an autistic child tends to be formal and is delivered in monotonous flat tones. These children also misuse pronouns; for example, using "he" or "it" instead of "I." The autistic child may occasionally appear to develop speech normally at first, only to regress before 3 years of age. The cause of autism is unknown.

Developmental aphasia has been increasingly appreciated as a cause for speech delay. There is a delay in the maturation of the central neurologic process required to produce speech. This term is generally reserved for those children who have no words by the age of 18 months or no phrases by 30 months despite normal intelligence, good emotional relationships, adequate hearing, and normal articulation skills. There is usually no difficulty in the comprehension of spoken language. Speech development may not only be deviant but also delayed, and the severity of the delay may vary widely. A family history of late speech acquisition without sequelae is often found. Consultation with a speech pathologist should be sought when difficulty in speech comprehension (developmental receptive aphasia) is present or there is no evidence of word sound acquisition by the expected age.

Dysarthria should be suspected when a child's speech is difficult to understand, although the quantity and loudness is normal. Children normally may omit consonants or substitute incorrect consonants up to 5 years of age. When dysarthria persists beyond this age, the pediatrician should suspect the presence of a diagnosable cause for dysarthria. The most common causes are either neurologic abnormalities or local structural abnormalities affecting the mechanics of speech production. Neurologic abnormalities, such as upper motor neuron lesions, may be suggested by an early history of difficulty with sucking or swallowing.

The child may be observed to have abnormal muscle tone, especially of the palatal and pharyngeal muscles, and poor coordination of muscle groups used during speech. These difficulties are accentuated when the child is asked to increase the speed of his speech. Local abnormalities include cleft palate, malocclusion resulting from abnormalities of the upper or lower jaw, or an excessively large jaw. Dysarthria may also result from hearing loss.

Stuttering is a frequent concern of parents who notice that their child begins to repeat words or hesitate before starting a word. Between the ages 2 to 4, when children are rapidly acquiring new vocabulary and grammar, a certain amount of dysrhythmia (including hesitations, repetitions, and prolongations) is normal. This dysrhythmia is symptomatically similar to stuttering. The diagnosis of stuttering should be made only if the dysrhythmia persists into the school years. When a child continues to struggle with the rhythm of his speech, secondary symptoms may begin to develop, especially when negative attention is focused on his speech efforts. These symptoms, which are attempts to avoid the embarrassment of stuttering, include various facial movements, such as grimacing and blinking, and actual avoidance of situations that require the child to speak.

Dysphonia usually presents as hoarseness and affects girls more often than boys. The quality and loudness of the child's voice often fluctuates in pitch and volume from hour to hour. There is frequently a history of recurrent laryngitis, and an examination of the pharynx often reveals signs of inflamed nodules on the vocal cords.

Elective mutism is apparently the only disorder of speech with a strictly functional cause. These children usually speak freely and normally at home, but do not speak at all in certain other settings, such as at school. This disorder can persist for months or years. Such children usually manifest other symptoms of poor adjustment such as poor peer relations or overdependence on their parents. The child's developmental milestones and intelligence are usually normal. No neurologic abnormality is apparent.

WORK-UP

History

It is important to take a careful medical history, including a history of the pregnancy and prenatal course, as well as a psychosocial history. The medical history should be sufficiently thorough to reduce the likelihood that a neurologic insult may have resulted in a delay or defect in speech development. Prematurity and significant illness during the neonatal period may increase the likelihood of abnormal milestones and suggest that a speech disorder is only a part of the clinical picture. A history of middle ear disease should always be noted.

The psychosocial history should include a fam-

Table 31-1. Milestones of Speech Acquisition

AGE	SPEECH ACQUISITION
Birth–1 mo	Mainly involuntary distress responses (*e.g.*, crying)
2–3 mo	Produces consonants; voluntary nondistress responses
7–10 mo	Reduplicated monosyllables (*e.g.*, ma-ma); babbling
11–18 mo	Two-word combinations
36 mo	Simple sentences with subject, verb, and object

ily history, especially a history of speech development and speech disorders among family members. Stuttering is more common among family members of stutterers than it is in the general population. The child's emotional and social development should be evaluated. Children who are delayed in their speech development are usually anxious and shy in social settings, whereas an autistic child shows little emotional response. An intellectually retarded child will usually be immature in his social and emotional responses. The child who has an elective mutism may be anxious and shy or unreactive in social situations.

The child's home life and relationships with family members should be reviewed and an evaluation should be made of the extent to which the child is stimulated and encouraged to develop speech and language skills.

Examination

The presence of intact hearing bilaterally should always be determined. The development of the child's speech should be assessed with respect to both the timing and the normality of the speech itself. It is useful to access three aspects of speech: the child's understanding of languages, the development of the child's own language, and his capacity to articulate properly with the correct rhythm. The pediatrician can usually access each of these in the office, by listening carefully and by noting the child's responses to particular questions or commands (Table 31–1).

PRINCIPLES OF MANAGEMENT

Management of speech disorders is aimed at correcting any underlying anatomic defects, such as a cleft palate, or at creating an environment that will promote the development of normal speech.

Parents may benefit from instruction in techniques for stimulating their child's speech by certain sound or word games. Some parents should be encouraged to place their child in day programs that will provide increased stimulation for the child's speech. A professional program of speech therapy should be undertaken when a child's speech is deviant or delayed for reasons other than inadequate stimulation. The earlier this step is taken, the more likely it is that the child will develop normal or communicative speech. The age at which a child should be referred for evaluation depends on the clinical finding; for example, a child who has acquired no spoken language by 20 months should be referred to a speech pathologist once all the medical and surgically treatable conditions have been ruled out. "Stuttering" speech, however, is a normal finding in the preschool child and the parents of preschool children who are dysrhythmic should be gently reassured that such errors are within the range of normal and may well become a more serious problem if the child is made to feel ashamed of his mistakes. It is best either to ignore the mistakes or to be gently encouraging.

INDICATIONS FOR REFERRAL

A child should be referred for a surgical consultation when a structural abnormality may be impairing speech. A neurologic consultation may be helpful if a neurologic cause for delayed or defective speech is suspected. Psychological testing should be requested when intellectual retardation is suspected, regardless of the patient's age. The patient should be referred for psychotherapy when elective mutism is diagnosed or when a child's speech disorder is accompanied by anxiety or depression, which may often be the case for patients who stutter. Psychotherapy may also be helpful for parents of these children, particularly when parental distress is upsetting to the child or complicates his treatment.

The pediatrician should have a low threshold for referring patients with delayed or deviant speech for a specialized evaluation by a speech pathologist. Speech pathologists are best able to distinguish between normal variations in speech and problems that warrant treatment. The advantages of earlier intervention have been increasingly appreciated in the past decade.

ANNOTATED BIBLIOGRAPHY

Bax M, Hart H: Assessment of speech and language development in the young child. Pediatrics 66 (3): 350–354, 1980 (Guide to the evaluation of speech in preschool children.)

Hubatch L, Johnson C: Early language abilities of high-risk infants. J Speech and Hearing Disorders 50: 195–207, 1985 (Discussion of language delay in children with a history of prematurity and respiratory distress in children.)

Morley ME: Development and Disorders of Speech in Childhood. Baltimore, Williams and Wilkins, 1972 (Thorough and authoritative text.)

Rutter M, Martin EJ: The Child with Delayed Speech. Philadelphia, JB Lippincott, 1972 (Nontechnical and readable chapters on the causes, evaluation, and management of speech disorders.)

32
Enuresis

DAVID I. BROMBERG

Enuresis is a common, complex problem of childhood. The clinician treating enuresis is faced with a confusing array of etiologic considerations and an abundance of treatment possibilities. Because it is an essentially benign, self-limited disorder, there is a tendency to downplay or ignore this condition. There may, however, be significant psychosocial morbidity associated with enuresis that the primary care physician may be able to prevent.

Enuresis is usually defined as the involuntary passage of urine, more frequently than once a month, in children over the age of 5. It is *primary* if it had always existed without periods of dryness, or *secondary*, if a youngster had been consistently dry for a period of from 6 to 12 months before beginning to wet. Enuresis is termed *nocturnal* when the wetting occurs at night (bedwetting), or *diurnal* when wetting occurs during the day. Most enuretics are primary (70% to 75%) and nocturnal.

The prevalence of enuresis varies widely. Estimates range from 9% to 22% of 6-year-old males, and 5% to 18% of 6-year-old females. The male to female ratio ranges from 1.5:1 to 2:1. At 11 years old, 13% of white and 22% of black males and 9% of white and 12% of black females are enuretic. The trend in enuresis is clearly for the prevalence to decrease with increasing age. Estimates of 10% to 15% spontaneous "cure" rate per year have been made, and by age 18, the prevalence of enuresis is less than 3%.

The prevalence of enuresis increases with lower socioeconomic class and is higher among black youngsters, both male and female, even when controlling for socioeconomic level. Many other etiologic factors must be considered to understand the clinical entity of enuresis. These can be divided into developmental, biologic, and psychologic factors.

DEVELOPMENTAL FACTORS

The ability to control urinary flow involves several component tasks that are generally mastered at different ages. Between 1 and 2 years of age children become aware of micturition. It is generally not until age 3, however, that most children can consistently postpone micturition. Children are closer to age 4 before they can voluntarily urinate on command and are often 5 to 6 years old before they can withhold urination with any degree of bladder distention.

BIOLOGIC FACTORS

Over three quarters of children of both parents with a history of enuresis will be enuretic. The specific mode of inheritance remains elusive. Further support for biologic factors comes from the association of other biologic variables in children with enuresis. These variables include a lower mean bone age, a later sexual maturation, and a lower average height.

Children with enuresis have a reduced functional bladder capacity; as a result, they void more frequently during the day and can only hold a reduced bladder volume at night. Bladder volume appears to be functionally, but not anatomically, reduced.

Enuresis has also been conceptualized as representing a disorder of arousal from sleep or as a sleep disorder. Parents frequently describe their enuretic children as being extremely sound sleepers. Several studies, including some that used extensive sleep polygraphy, have failed to demonstrate this relationship. Thus, the role of sleep abnormalities in enuresis remains unproven.

PSYCHOLOGICAL AND PSYCHOSOCIAL FACTORS

The relationship of enuresis with psychological antecedents and sequelae has received a great deal of attention and remains largely unresolved. Enuresis is not primarily a psychiatric disease. Large population studies, most notably those of Rutter on the Isle of Wight, demonstrate that although the incidence of psychiatric illness is higher in populations of enuretic children, most children with enuresis do not have a significant psychiatric disease. The relationship of enuresis and emotional disturbance is higher in girls than in boys; it is higher in youngsters with secondary enuresis; and it is higher in youngsters with diurnal enuresis. Emotional stress can precipitate secondary enuresis and early stress factors (family disruption, separations from mother, and multiple hospitalizations) may be important in the development of primary enuresis.

Enuresis often engenders feelings of shame and low self-esteem in affected children. Enuresis may cause emotional disturbance. An enuretic child is stressful to many families.

PRESENTATION

The clinician may become aware of a patient's enuresis under several different circumstances. The complaint of enuresis may accompany several other physical or behavioral complaints, or it may be the chief complaint of a visit. Enuretic children are generally anxious about the possibility of wetting while at camp and may want to discuss their problem at a precamp physical examination. Enuresis will often be discovered as part of health screening at routine well-child visits.

Each of these different presentations dictates a slightly different evaluation and treatment approach. Gearing the evaluation and treatment to the degree of the family's concern and to associated findings is important. The child who presents with secondary enuresis in addition to social withdrawal and school refusal should have a thorough psychosocial and psychological evaluation. Similarly, the youngster who has secondary enuresis, polyphagia, and polydipsia should be carefully evaluated for diabetes mellitus. The 5-year-old who has primary enuresis may only require educational counseling, reassurance, and a follow-up plan.

DIFFERENTIAL DIAGNOSIS

The most important differential feature in evaluating enuresis is its primary or secondary nature. For the child with secondary enuresis, greater emphasis should be placed on evaluating recent psychosocial and emotional factors.

Most children with enuresis, both primary and secondary, have a functional problem in the absence of organic pathology. It has been estimated that only 1% to 3% of all enuretic children have organic disease. Urinary tract infection is the most significant of these organic problems, and should be considered especially in the girl with secondary enuresis. Other urinary tract abnormalities are unlikely to present as enuresis. Disorders that greatly increase urinary output may result in enuresis, and especially in the child with secondary enuresis, consideration should be given to the diagnosis of diabetes insipidus, diabetes mellitus, and sickle cell disease. Drugs that have a diuretic effect, either as a primary action or as a side effect, may cause enuresis. Consideration should also be given to any neurologic condition that may alter the innervation to the bladder, such as meningomyelocele.

WORK-UP

History

The management of enuresis begins with a careful history obtained in a supportive fashion. The history should begin by defining the problem as primary or secondary and noting nocturnal and diurnal features. Careful documentation of the degree and frequency of wetting is essential in establishing a baseline from which to gauge the results of treatment. Frequently, the family has tried several interventions before presenting the problem to the physician. These methods should be discussed and their effectiveness should be determined.

In view of the multifactorial etiologies of enuresis, the data base should include developmental, biologic, and psychosocial information. Any associated developmental delays should be documented. The family history will frequently reveal a close relative with a history of enuresis. Knowledge of this is supportive to the youngster who often feels isolated with this problem. In secondary enuresis, the history of recent psychosocial stresses may help the family understand the child's symptom. A history of toilet training including the family's perception of the ease with which it was accomplished may be useful.

In order to develop an appropriate treatment strategy, it is essential for the clinician to understand the impact of enuresis on the child and on the family. Has being enuretic kept the child from participating in peer or family activities (*e.g.*, sleepovers, camp experiences, or family visits)? Has extra laundry from an enuretic child been a stress on the family? Are the parents angry or frustrated with the child and the problem? Do the parents agree regarding their approach to wetting?

Physical Examination

The physical examination should focus on possible urinary tract abnormalities and neurologic dysfunction. Subtle neurologic differences may be associated with developmental delays. More definitive neurologic findings may suggest a pervasive neurologic problem that causes a neurogenic bladder. Abnormalities of the external genitalia can be associated with other urinary tract abnormalities. The physical examination will usually be entirely normal. It must be remembered, however, that patients consider their physicians to be experts in physical problems. A careful, thorough examination is an essential part of an evaluation of enuresis and provides the necessary reassurance to the child and the family that the child appears to be anatomically and medically healthy.

Laboratory Tests

A complete urinalysis and a clean-caught urine culture are a necessary part of the evaluation. A urinary tract infection may result in enuresis and may not be suggested either by the history or physical examination. Other laboratory studies should be obtained only if indicated by the history or physical examination. There is no indication for routine radiographic studies unless the history suggests an abnormality of the urinary tract.

PRINCIPLES OF MANAGEMENT

The mortality of functional enuresis is zero. There is, however, a significant psychosocial morbidity associated with enuresis. Bedwetters frequently are ashamed of their wetting and have feelings of low self-esteem and poor self-worth. They may exhibit withdrawn and acquiescent behaviors. The presence of enuresis may significantly interfere with age-appropriate peer activities. Thus, evaluation and treatment strategies for enuresis should have as a primary goal the prevention or alleviation of psychosocial morbidity. Educational interventions should teach the multifactorial nature of enuresis. Parents often blame themselves or the child for the bedwetting. Children may fear that they wet because they are bad or lazy. The understanding

that bedwetting is a problem that runs in their family and that it represents a difference in nervous system development can be useful. Optimism should be maintained throughout because of both the spontaneous resolution in enuresis and the successful treatment interventions available. Helping a youngster get control of his bedwetting and succeed at mastering it can provide him with an important boost in self-esteem.

INDICATIONS FOR REFERRAL

Functional enuresis is an entity that should be managed by the primary care provider in an ambulatory setting. Historical or physical findings that suggest an abnormality of the urinary tract may require further diagnostic studies. A urinary tract abnormality (*e.g.*, obstructive uropathy, reflux, or congenital abnormalities) warrants a referral to a urologist. A urology referral in the absence of strong supportive evidence of an abnormality may be harmful in both subjecting the child to possible unnecessary procedures and in suggesting the likelihood of organic problems. There is a similar danger in psychiatric referral in otherwise uncomplicated enuresis. Psychiatric referral is warranted when enuresis is accompanied by a serious secondary individual or family pathology or when there are serious accompanying pathologic behaviors. The combination of symptoms of enuresis, firesetting, and cruelty to animals is of particular concern and suggests significant psychopathology.

TREATMENT

General Considerations

In describing their enuretic youngsters, parents will often talk of the child's easy acceptance of the symptom and his nonchalance about wetting the bed. In actuality, most enuretic children are ashamed that they wet and are anxious to stop bedwetting. Rather than asking children if they are sad or embarrassed about wetting, we should assume that they are, and we should then begin to educate them about the problem. One method of informing a 7-year-old child of how common a problem enuresis is, is to tell him that three or four of his classmates also wet their beds. An explanation should then follow as to why we think children wet their beds. The goal is to explain bedwetting in a nonjudgmental way that removes blame both from the child and the parents.

Latency aged children (6- to 12-year-olds) are

confronted with the developmental challenge of being industrious (*i.e.*, being faced with a job and accomplishing it). Overcoming bedwetting may be presented as a challenge to the child, thereby giving him responsibility for the symptom as well as the satisfaction of mastering it once it is overcome. Parental participation is needed in most of the treatment protocols; however, the choice of whether or not to begin treatment and the responsibility for following through with the program can be the youngster's.

"Home" remedies that are often tried to control enuresis include limiting fluids after dinnertime, taking the child to the bathroom when the parents go to bed (lifting), limiting carbonated beverage or milk in the diet, and rewarding a period of dry nights. The success rate with most of these interventions is low. If these methods are working, they need not be discouraged; however, there is little reason to promote them as a primary treatment.

Behavior Modification

Many children can consciously control their enuresis. This is evidenced by their ability to achieve a limited period of dryness in order to obtain a desired reward (*e.g.*, bicycle, doll). In the absence of a systematic program to alter their wetting behavior, however, there is a high recitivism with this approach. Helping parents structure a standard behavior modification program may yield somewhat better results. The program should be discussed with the child before it is started and emphasis should be placed on the desired goal of dry nights. This heightened awareness of trying to stay dry may increase the child's rate of success. Positive reinforcement of a dry bed in the morning should include social praise and perhaps a visual reinforcer (a sticker on a calender). The youngster may then be challenged to increase his run of dry nights and may be further rewarded for specified goals (*e.g.*, 4 nights of staying dry in a week). Negative reinforcement, both social disapproval and punishment, should be eliminated. The success rate with this type of system has been estimated at about 25%, although no firm figures are available. This method is particularly appropriate for the younger child (between the ages of 5 and 7) in the family who wants to try some intervention.

Urine alarms offer a more formalized behavioral intervention that yield a much higher success rate. The alarms involve an apparatus that is either worn by the child or is located in the bed. When the child wets, an electrical circuit is completed and either a buzzer sounds or a bell rings. When the alarm sounds, the child goes to the bathroom and finishes urinating. He then returns to bed, changes into dry nightclothes, and resets the alarm. This method can be explained to the child and his family as an attempt to teach the child to respond to the stimulus of a full bladder. Motivation on the part of the child and at least one parent is essential. It should be emphasized that the alarm is not a punishment for wetting. Dry nights are recorded and socially reinforced. The newer alarms (*e.g.*, Wet-Stop from Palco Laboratories, Scotts Valley, CA) are miniaturized, more reliable, and more sensitive to small amounts of urine. Success rates of up to 70% with the newer alarms have been documented. Relapse rates range from 10% to 15%. The alarms provide an excellent intervention for the motivated youngster over the age of 7.

A third behavioral approach described as dry bed training has been reported by Azrin and associates. This technique involves a practice phase whereby the youngster practices going to the bathroom. During the following night, intensive training occurs whereby the child is awakened every hour and is encouraged to urinate. On awakening, dryness is reinforced; wetness elicits cleanliness training whereby the child changes his bed and his clothes and practices going to the bathroom. Subsequent training involves other protocols using nighttime awakening, positive reinforcement, cleanliness training, and practice sessions. The program is complex and demanding, especially in the initial phases. Success rates up to 85% have been reported. Some of the techniques of dry bed training (*e.g.*, positive practice, cleanliness training) can be used in combination with urine alarms.

Bladder Stretching Exercises

Decreased functional bladder capacity has been demonstrated in enuretic children. Based on this finding, exercises to increase bladder capacity have been recommended for the treatment of enuresis. Children are instructed to try to avoid urinating for as long as possible during the day. Their progress is monitored by recording voiding volumes on a daily basis. They are encouraged to increase the average volume of their voidings. A 35% cure rate using bladder exercise techniques has been demonstrated.

Pharmacotherapy

Imipramine (Tofranil) has a definite antienuretic effect. In doses of 25 mg to 75 mg ½ to 1 hour before bedtime, 40% to 70% of enuretic children will be dry. The mechanism of action is unclear and has variously been postulated as an anticholinergic effect, an antidepressant effect, or an alteration in sleep cycle. The response to imipramine is rapid and occurs usually in the first week of treatment. The drug is usually continued for 3 months and then its use is gradually tapered. The remission rate is high; up to 50% of responders will again wet once the drug is discontinued. An extensive list of toxic effects of imipramine paired with a low therapeutic index in children discourages the use of this drug for treatment of enuresis. Imipramine may play a limited role in the short-term management of bed-wetting on special occasions for older children.

The antidiuretic effects of vasopressin analogues have been considered in the treatment of enuresis. Studies using intranasal desmopressin have demonstrated a reduction in the frequency of wetting. Remission on stopping the drug has been high. Oxybutynin (Ditropan), a bladder antispasmodic, has also been partially successful in controlling enuresis. The implications for the use of these agents in the management of enuresis is not presently clear.

ANNOTATED BIBLIOGRAPHY

Azrin NH, Sneed TJ, Foxx RM: Dry-bed training: Rapid elimination of childhood enuresis. Behav Res Ther 12:147, 1974 (Complete review of the behavioral dry-bed training techique.)

Brazelton TB: Is enuresis preventable? Clin Dev Med 48/49:281, 1973 (Explores the possible connection between enuresis and toilet training.)

Cohen M: Enuresis. Pediatr Clin North Am 22:545, 1975 (Good overview of enuresis from a pediatric perspective.)

Gross RT, Dornbusch SM: Enuresis. In Levine MD, Carey WB, Crocker AC, Gross RT (eds): Developmental-Behavioral Pediatrics, pp 573–586. Philadelphia, WB Saunders, 1983 (Clear overview of enuresis with an in-depth look at the clinical associations of enuresis demonstrated by the National Health Examination Survey.)

Rutter M, Yule W, Graham P: Enuresis and behavioral defiance: Some epidemiological consideration. Clin Dev Med 48/49:137, 1973 (Interesting epidemiologic analysis of data from the Isle of Wight which examines the connection between enuresis and psychopathology.)

Schmidt BD: Nocturnal enuresis: An update on treatment. Pediatr Clin North Am 29:21, 1983 (Excellent analysis of treatment options presenting a rational approach to the age-appropriate treatment of enuresis. The parent handouts that the author uses in his practice are included.)

Shaffer D: The association between enuresis and emotional disorder: A review of the literature. Clin Dev Med 48/49:118, 1973 (Insightful and well-organized review of a complicated subject.)

Shaffer D: The development of bladder control. In Rutter M (ed): Scientific Foundations of Developmental Psychiatry, pp 129–137. Baltimore, MD, University Park Press, 1981 (Careful look at the developmental issues in the etiology of enuresis. Epidemiologic factors and other etiologic theories are also reviewed.)

Starfield B, Mellitis EE: Increase in functional bladder capacity and improvements in enuresis. J Pediatr 72:483, 1968 (Presents an intervention for increasing functional bladder capacity and the implications for a group of enuretic children.)

33

Encopresis

PAUL K. BRUCHEZ

Encopresis in a pediatric outpatient setting is a common problem and may be resistant to standard pediatric or mental health intervention. The incidence of all encopresis has, at times, been estimated to be as much as 3% of a pediatric clinic population. It is a presentation that requires a sensitivity both to the stigma of the symptom and to the apparent inertia toward its resolution.

Encopresis is defined as "repeated voluntary or involuntary passage of stool into places not appropriate for that purpose in the individual's own sociocultural setting."[1] It is classified as a primary type when a child has never achieved bowel control and as a secondary type when a child has previously achieved regular control but has discontinued that behavior.

PSYCHOLOGICAL MECHANISMS

Encopresis has been viewed as a classic conversion symptom with the child attempting to maintain infantile pleasure of withholding and then rebelling. It often presents as a symptom of childhood stress. Studies indicate that in as many as one half of the cases, the onset of secondary encopresis is often associated with beginning school, adjustment difficulties in school, separation from the mother, or birth of a sibling. School transitions (from grade to grade or from primary to secondary), and the onset of a marital separation or divorce are also frequent precedents and contributory factors. The stress-induced presentation of encopresis, when addressed early by parental education, support, and guidance, responds well and quickly. It is the more stable family system with the more engrained control struggle or possible covertly expressed rebellion that is more difficult to treat and requires a more prolonged and close interdisciplinary approach.

DIFFERENTIAL DIAGNOSIS

In establishing the diagnosis of functional encopresis, the following organic causes of encopresis, which may manifest as fecal soiling without retention, must be considered: diarrheal disorders causing accidental incontinence, diseases of the central nervous system, and sensory or motor defects in the anorectum or pelvic floor muscles. The following causes of chronic retention with or without soiling should also be ruled out: Hirschsprung's disease, intestinal pseudo-obstruction syndrome, hypothyroidism, hypercalcemia, chronic codeine or phenothiazine use, disease of the intestinal smooth muscle, and anal/rectal stenosis or fissure.

WORK-UP

The work-up must include a complete developmental and social history. A thorough physical examination including a careful inspection of the anus, a rectal examination, and a neurologic examination should be performed. A urinalysis and urine culture should be ordered for all girls because a urinary tract infection is a frequent concomitant condition in encopretic girls. When palpitation cannot establish the presence of retained stool, a plain view roentgenogram of the abdomen can help to rule out the presence of retained stool. A rectal biopsy should be considered *only* if there are signs that truly suggest an aganglionic megacolon. Some experts recommend that a rectal biopsy not be performed unless the symptoms have not improved after long-term optimal medical management. The yield from biopsy is low even in such instances.

TREATMENT

The initial education of the family and the patient can go far to promote the resolution of the problem of encopresis. If, as is frequently the case,

the encopresis is the result of chronic constipation, a complete bowel clean-out is recommended to try and return to the patient the lost physical sensations to muscle tone that allow for normal, routine defecation. Thus, it is important to first establish a nonimpacted colon. Levine's widely accepted regime for the initial outpatient treatment of moderate to severe stool retention recommends three to four cycles of the following: 1 to 2 Fleet's enemas on the first day; Dulcolax suppositories BID on the second day; and one Dulcolax suppository on the third day. Mild retention may be treated by a stool softener daily for up to 14 days. If the stool retention is severe, or if the above regimen fails, hospitalization with saline enemas may be necessary to achieve initial catharsis. (For an expanded discussion on the management of chronic constipation, see Chapter 108.)

The physician must be seen as the patient's ally. This can be achieved in several ways, such as Levine's idea of the physician acting as coach to aid the child in strengthening his colonic muscles. The physician can also be supportive and can maintain clearly that the soiling problem is common and that many children have been helped through this approach to the problem. In addition, by the judicious use of stool softening agents, the physician can eliminate painful stools as a precipitant of the interruption of normal defecation.

The physician *must* be seen as the patient's ally: This can be achieved in several ways, such as by the physician acting as a coach to aid the child in strengthening his colonic muscles. The physician can also be supportive and maintain clearly that the soiling problem is common. Many children have been helped through this approach to the problem of soiling. Since the interruption of normal defecation can be caused by painful stools, a stool softening agent will be given to assure that defecation will not be painful.

After adequate catharsis has been achieved, light mineral oil for several months (several tablespoons daily are usually necessary to assure that stools are soft) along with multivitamins to prevent a fat-soluble vitamin deficiency are recommended. A daily routine of sitting on the toilet for 10 minutes two times a day should then be established. If a previous bowel pattern existed, it would be best to have this coincide with the child's pre-encopretic pattern. A good time to try to establish a pattern if one did not exist before, is 1 hour after a meal. Other recommendations include increasing high fiber in the diet, increasing clear fluids, and decreasing diuretic fluids such as cola and cocoa. Copious praise should be given for the appropriate behavior. Parents should be encouraged to give the child a small tangible reward (*e.g.*, stickers or stars) for success of bowel movement in the toilet and another reward if he successfully keeps his pants clean for a day.

Sondheimer's most common causes of treatment failure are worth noting: (1) treatment of the patient with stool softeners without adequately cleaning the bowel; (2) adequate bowel clean out, but without follow-up maintenance of stool softeners; and (3) poor or inadequate patient education, guidance, and follow-up.

These interventions are often successful in the more situational disturbance/adjustment disorder types of problem. A psychiatric interview is recommended if these interventions fail and physiologic causes have been ruled out. A developmental history with milestones should be reviewed with an emphasis on control struggles and aggressive expression (*e.g.*, terrible 2-year-old autonomy struggle, toilet training, temper tantrums, and meal- and sleep-time behavior.) Any situational alterations should also be pursued: These might include but might not be limited to parental disruption, job loss, separation, divorce, family illness, death of a close family member or friend, a family move, school changes, sibling births, and hospitalizations.

There is a strong interface between psychology and medicine in the contributory factors of encopresis. A psychologically proactive stance by the pediatric practitioner will often combine all the elements necessary for a bimodal attack of psychology and medicine on this problem which is difficult to resolve.

INDICATIONS FOR REFERRAL

Psychiatric referral should be considered in children who present with a concomitant learning disability or hyperactivity, children with marked fearless, risk-taking, and disobedient behavior, and children with frequent incontinence in school. Children who have fecal incontinence without impaction or adolescent encopresis should also be considered for prompt psychiatric consultation.

REFERENCES

1. American Psychiatric Association: Diagnostic and Statistical Manual of Mental Disorders, 3rd ed. Washington, DC, American Psychiatric Association, 1980

ANNOTATED BIBLIOGRAPHY

Bemporard JR, Kresch RA, Asnes R, Wilson A: Chronic neurotic encopresis as a paradigm of a multifactorial psychiatric disorder. Nervous and Mental Disease 166: 472–479, 1978 (Useful review of psychological perspectives on encopresis.)

Bornstein PH, Balleweg BJ, McLellarn RW et al: The "bathroom game": A systemic program for the elimination of encopretic behavior. Behav Ther Exp Psychiatry 14 (1): 67–71, 1983 (Behavioral intervention using intermittent positive rewards for bowel movements in toilet, and clean pants.)

Levine MD: Encopresis: Its potentiation, evaluation, and alleviation. Pediatr Clin North Am 29(2), April 1982 (Thorough, excellent review; comprehensive presentation of inpatient and outpatient medical management of all ranges of problems.)

Sondheimer JM: Helping the child with chronic constipation. Contemp Pediatr pp 12–28, March 1985 (Succinct treatment approach; strong on patient education.)

34
Attention Deficit Disorder
MICHAEL S. JELLINEK

Pediatricians have diagnosed many thousands of children as having attention deficit disorder (ADD), hyperactivity, or minimal brain dysfunction (or disorder). In the early part of the century, the terms were applied to children with neurologic damage after encephalitis or trauma ("organic drivenness"). In the 1940s through the 1960s the diagnosis of hyperactivity broadened to include children with various difficult behaviors manifested at home or in school. Over the last 15 to 20 years, extensive research efforts to validate disorders have led to a narrowing of the diagnostic criteria and an emphasis on the cognitive component of the children's difficulties. Despite the many years of research and experience with the cluster of symptoms that include inattention, impulsivity, motor hyperactivity, and learning difficulties, the diagnosis remains imprecise and the treatment largely remedial rather than curative.

The cause of ADD remains unknown. The diagnosis, as currently applied, probably includes several distinct disorders with multiple neurologic, genetic, temperamental, environmental, and behavioral factors variously contributing to the etiology of the yet-to-be-defined subgroups. There has been much speculation that sugar or food additives contribute or even cause ADD. Although case report data suggest that a small group of children may respond to an elimination diet, formal studies on groups of children with ADD have shown little or no effect of limiting sugar or food additives. ADD symptoms are rarely caused by medical disorders but are occasionally manifested as a part of temporal lobe epilepsy, postconcussion syndrome, thyrotoxicosis, and hypoglycemia. Among common environmental factors, lead exposure may contribute or possibly cause ADD.

Using the current criteria for ADD, there is strong suggestive evidence of a genetic pattern for at least some children. The pattern of inheritance is not defined and has not been differentiated from other defined genetic influences in depression, alcoholism, and conduct disorder. The male:female ratio for ADD is approximately 10:1, and the estimated prevalence ranges from 1% to 10% of children, depending on diagnostic criteria.

PRESENTATION

The preschool child is usually brought to the pediatrician by exhausted parents who complain that their child acts as if "driven by a motor." A shortened attention span and impulsivity will be manifested as disobedience, excessive need for supervision, and accidental rather than intentional destructiveness. Some parents will try to adapt to the child's disorder by lowering expectations for activities that require the child to sit still (e.g., at dinner or at religious services) or by providing additional child-proofing in the home. The parents may also have a greater tolerance for the child's need for supervision, structure, and outlets for physical activity. Other parents are less accepting of a young child's ADD and will interpret the child's behavior as inconsiderate and intentional misbehavior. These parents, because of their beliefs or because they are exhausted, may maintain unreasonable expectations and thus become trapped in cycles of repeated disappointment and punishment.

The school-aged child usually presents in first grade when higher expectations stress their cognitive and behavioral abilities. The child with ADD will have a shorter attention span than his peers and will require frequent teacher intervention to keep him "on task." Despite the teacher's efforts, the child will withdraw from work that requires sustained attention or that challenges his learning disability. He may daydream, walk around the room, talk out of turn, engage others to join him in play, or (possibly in a manner similar to children with conduct disorder) he may begin to misbehave and disrupt the class. The short attention span, impulsivity, and occasional destructive behavior will also be disturbing at home by preventing the family from relaxing during the "prime time" of 5 PM to 8 PM and setting up daily arguments about homework or chores. School-aged children with ADD will also often have motor hyperactivity with fidgetiness and an impressive need "to get the energy out."

Adolescent onset ADD in the absence of obvious neurologic insult is not a primary diagnosis. It usually represents continuing symptoms from childhood, ADD-like symptoms secondary to a learning disability elicited by academic demands for abstract/organizational thinking, or one symptom of a primary psychiatric diagnosis (e.g., anxiety, agitated depression, mania, and so forth).

DIFFERENTIAL DIAGNOSIS

The current *Diagnostic and Statistical Manual of Mental Disorders*, published by The American Psychiatric Association, lists criteria for ADD. Several possible modifications in these criteria have been suggested by recent research. The current list of behaviors tends to overlap with criteria for conduct disorder and thus there is either a subgroup with ADD/conduct disorder or the boundaries of the two disorders are not sufficiently clear. Since the number of children with ADD without hyperactivity is relatively few, a more useful distinction may be drawn between *situational* and *pervasive* ADD. The diagnosis of *situational* ADD would apply to those children who meet ADD criteria in one setting but not in another and reflects (1) the clinical finding that ADD symptoms may be reported in school but not with a tutor or at home, and (2) there can be a low correlation between a teacher's and parent's ratings of ADD symptoms for groups of children. There is a small group of children with symptoms of ADD present in every setting (e.g., home, school, and clinic) or at an earlier age of onset (preschool). These children have greater impulsivity, minor neurologic abnormalities, and possibly derive more benefit from psychopharmacologic treatment.

The differentiation of learning disabilities and ADD can present a complex problem. A child with an undiagnosed specific learning disability can, secondary to the frustration of not meeting classroom expectations, begin to manifest ADD symptoms, especially fidgetiness, short attention span, and "calling out in class" impulsively. An appropriate education plan for such a child will relieve the stress and the ADD symptoms will ease or disappear. In addition, up to 80% of children with ADD have associated learning disabilities and therefore all children presenting with ADD symptoms require intelligence and achievement testing.

WORK-UP

ADD is a clinical diagnosis based primarily on a history and secondarily on observation and psychological testing. After excluding the rarer neurologic, physiologic, and environmental etiologies, the most valid diagnoses of ADD depends on a consistent pattern of short attention span, impulsivity, and motor hyperactivity that is present both at home and at school. It is not unusual for the child to be able to override ADD symptoms for short periods of time or under highly structured circumstances such as individual tutoring, although the same set of symptoms are present on other days. The age of onset can be as late as 7 or 8 years of age but earlier onset is more confirmatory.

Although observation in the office and a neurologic examination may be contributory factors, these procedures are insufficient to confirm or rule out the diagnosis. Many children will have ADD-like symptoms in a physician's office or even in several settings for a short duration secondary to stress or anxiety. Neurologic "soft" signs, although more common in the postulated "pervasive" ADD subtype, are not pathognomonic.

Intelligence and achievement testing is an essential part of the treatment planning, and projective psychological tests can help define the impact of the disorder on the child's defenses and self-esteem. Neuropsychological testing can help confirm the diagnosis by carefully assessing the child's cognitive style and is helpful for children with complex learning disabilities.

PRINCIPLES OF MANAGEMENT

ADD is a 24-hour-a-day disorder and its management includes psychological/family issues, an educational plan, and frequently psychopharmacologic intervention. Given the complexity, chronic nature, and the changing impact of the child's development, the management of ADD requires a substantial initial time commitment and follow-up at regular intervals.

Children with ADD are at serious risk for an ongoing sense of failure, rejection, and damaged self-esteem. The child is difficult to manage in the home and requires special planning for physical activity, and increased parental presence for supervision, daily support for academic work, and often a conscientious effort at setting limits for disruptive behavior. In school, the child is constantly being reminded to pay attention, complete assignments, sit still, and stop disrupting the class. Given the likelihood of associated learning disabilities, the child may also be under major stress trying to keep up with the rest of the class, having to work especially hard to understand assignments, and being identified as "a poor student" or as "not trying" either by the teacher or because of having to leave the room for special help.

The pediatrician must look at the child's entire day and carefully assess the parent's and teacher's level of expectations. Using the severity of ADD, the key trouble points at home as identified by the history, and the insights available from the psychological testing, the pediatrician should help to establish a specific, reasonable set of expectations. The pediatrician should ascertain what the parents' expectations are regarding the time allowed for dinner, homework, music or religious lessons, the orderliness of the child's room, or how long a friend can visit. Children with ADD will do best with increased parental structure and support that is titrated so as not to be overbearing or inhibit potential autonomy. Usually a period of "mindless" relaxation such as sports and television is essential after a school day with homework organized into manageable 10- to 30-minute subunits. Rules are best divided into "squirrels and elephants"—squirrels being the minor infractions that are allowed to go by and the elephants being the small number of major rules that require very clear enforcement. It is essential that both parents agree on all of the "squirrels" and "elephants" so that manipulation and discord are minimized. The more detailed implementation of these guidelines requires an understanding of any associated learning disabilities, the range of variability in the child's daily performance, the child's developmental level, the parent's personality, and the family background.

Developing the child's educational plan requires careful diagnostic testing that hopefully will be part of the school's evaluation. If the local school system does not seem to have the necessary expertise or the educational plan does not seem to be effective, then it is often helpful to get a second opinion from an experienced educational consultant or neuropsychologist who can then work with the school to set reasonable expectations for the child's academic program. With changes in teachers, courses, and the child's development, the educational plan should be reviewed on a yearly basis. If stimulant medication is part of the overall plan, it is important to discuss the reasons and minimal risks with the school administration to assure that the medication will be given and with the teacher so that the child is not subtly criticized for needing drugs.

Although the use of stimulants to treat ADD is considered the first and most successful psychopharmacologic approach, the treatment is not curative or specific. The first step in prescribing a psychotropic drug for ADD is to clarify the target symptoms that are the goal of the treatment. Psychotropic drugs have several behavioral effects that are helpful for many children, including a decrease in motor hyperactivity, a better control of impulsivity, and an increased attention span. Therefore, for many children, the use of medication will improve daily school performance, limit disruptive behavior, and if used in the evening will make the child more "livable" during valuable family time. A secondary benefit of medication may be to improve self-esteem (with the decrease in criticism). There is no strong evidence that psychotropic drugs improve long-term educational achievement nor remedy specific learning disabilities. Research using neuropsychological testing indicates that the effects of medication on learning are more complex than originally thought. If this evidence is substantiated in classroom studies, future decision-making on which drug and what dosage may depend more on testing and less on observation.

Stimulants are the first line of pharmacologic treatment. Dextroamphetamine and methylphenidate have a therapeutic effect for 2 to 4 hours (a slow-release preparation of methylphenidate may last longer). For some children, the short length of action is a problem because of re-emerging behavior, mood swings, and because up to three doses, including one in school midday, may be necessary. Pemoline is a longer-acting stimulant but may be less effective. It has a delayed therapeutic onset of several weeks. Dosage should be titrated starting at a low dose (dextroamphetamine and methylphenidate 0.3 to 1 mg/kg/day in divided doses; pemoline 0.5 to 2 mg/kg/day as single dose) with objective tracking of target symptoms on a weekly basis to assess for optimum therapeutic effect. Adverse effects from stimulant medication are usually mild and tolerable (e.g., decreased appetite, sleep disturbances, questionable minor effect on growth). Reports suggest that the use of stimulants may be associated with onset of Tourette's syndrome and thus may be contraindicated in families with a history of tics. If discontinued, stimulants such as other psychotropic drugs should be tapered to assess for behavioral change.

For some children, stimulants may not be well tolerated and the length of action may be too short. Antidepressants, especially imipramine and desipramine, have been tested for the treatment of ADD. These antidepressants seem to have the same behavioral benefits as the stimulants, require only one dose a day because of a 10- to 17-hour half-life, which also permits blood level measurement to assess for toxicity and compliance. This treatment approach, however, is not approved by the FDA, and should only be undertaken within a specialized treatment center or under research protocol.

Antipsychotic agents, especially thioridazine, have been used in the treatment of ADD most commonly for young children and sometimes in combination with stimulants. As with antidepressants, the use of antipsychotics or mixed drug regimens should be limited to a specialized setting.

Even with the best efforts at interventions in the home, school, and using medications, the child with ADD will have and must be aware of his shortcomings (which will also be pointed out by peers or siblings). As the child gets older and certainly in grade school, the pediatrician should try to develop a relationship with the child and include the child's perspective in assessing the efficacy of the treatment plan. Most children with ADD will identify what is helpful and, for example, despite their inclination not to take medication, will readily affirm the need for stimulants if they are helpful. In addition, it would be useful to find areas of special interest (e.g., sport, mechanical ability, hobby, and so forth) that the child can gradually develop into real areas of skill that will foster self-esteem or become positive shared experiences with parents or peers.

INDICATIONS FOR REFERRAL

Caring for a child with ADD requires time and expertise, and some pediatricians may refer to a child psychiatrist, psychologist, or behaviorist for the comprehensive treatment of the child and family. If the pediatrician has the expertise and is able to devote the time necessary for interviewing, reviewing psychological test results, contacting the school, assessing the medication, and providing follow-up, then the care of the child with ADD can be among the most interesting and gratifying aspects of pediatric practice. Recent follow-up studies have showed that providing comprehensive care does combine to make a real impact on the child with ADD. Self-esteem can be preserved, an appropriate level of educational achievement is possible, and outcome in adult life after graduating from the special demands of a school setting can be successful.

If the pediatrician is the primary caregiver, referral should be selective to meet special needs or if an aspect of the treatment plan is not effective. Specific criteria for referral include help in addressing a stubborn behavioral problem, family counseling, or the trial of alternative medication.

ANNOTATED BIBLIOGRAPHY

American Psychiatric Association: Diagnostic and Statistical Manual of Mental Disorders, 3rd ed. Washington, DC, American Psychiatric Association, 1980 (Official diagnostic manual that sets criteria for all psychiatric disorders for adults and children. Supporting sections give current perspectives on diagnostic methodology.)

Barkley RA: A review of stimulant drug research with hyperactive children. J Child Psychol and Psychiatr 18:135–165, 1977 (Although written 8 years ago, this review is an excellent critical summary of over 100 drug trials.)

Biederman J, Jellinek M: Psychopharmacology in children. N Engl J Med 310:968–972, 1984 (Well referenced review of psychiatric medications in children that covers the practical use of stimulants and antidepressants in the treatment of children with ADD.)

Silver L: The relationship between learning disabilities, hyperactivity, distractibility, and behavioral problems. J Am Acad Child Psychiatry 20:385–390, 1981 (Excellent study demonstrating the frequency of learning disabilities in children with ADD.)

Taylor E: Syndromes of overactivity and attention deficit. Rutter M, Hersov L (eds): Child and Adolescent Psychiatry, Modern Approaches, 2nd ed., pp 424–441. London, Blackwell Scientific Publications, 1985 (Outstanding review of ADD emphasizing a sophisticated, critical review of the literature. Helpful start for an in-depth review of any aspect of ADD with an extensive bibliography.)

Weiss G: Long-term outcome: Findings, concepts, and practical implications. In Rutter M (ed): Developmental Neuropsychiatry, pp 422–436. New York, Guilford Press, 1983 (Thoughtful review of what is known about the long-term outcome of children with ADD.)

35

Depression and Suicide

RICHARD M. SARLES

Depression during the childhood and adolescent years is not uncommon and represents between 10% and 20% of patients seen in child psychiatric outpatient settings. In "normal" school samples, approximately 1.5% to 4% of children and adolescents meet the diagnostic criteria for depression.

Depression may be defined broadly as a condition in which painful feelings of loss are accompanied by a lowered sense of self-esteem with feelings of helplessness and hopelessness and a sense that the world has lost its meaning. Depression may also be defined from a biologic perspective as a genetically vulnerable central nervous system that is depleted of biogenic amines (dopamine and norepinephrine).

The *Diagnostic and Statistical Manual*, 3rd edition (DSM-III) of the American Psychiatric Association, defines depression as a dysphoric mood or pervasive loss of interest or pleasure accompanied by at least four of the following symptoms: change of appetite, difficulty in sleeping, psychomotor agitation or retardation, loss of interest in usual activities, loss of energy, feelings of self-reproach or guilt, complaints or evidence of diminished ability to concentrate, and recurrent thoughts of death or suicide. Associated features, such as separation anxiety and fears in the prepubertal age group, and restlessness, sulkiness, withdrawal from social activities, reluctance to cooperate with family activities, lack of attention to schoolwork, and lack of attention to personal appearance in the adolescent age group are also listed.

The concept of "masked" depression popular in the 1970s listed symptoms, such as an increase in psychosomatic complaints that are unsubstantiated by a careful physical examination and laboratory data (*e.g.*, recurrent headaches or recurrent abdominal pain), reversal of affect in which the child or adolescent takes an uncharacteristic, foolish, provocative, or clowning behavior, a sense of feeling rejected by peers, teachers, or family, low frustration tolerance, self-punitive behaviors, aggression, a decrease in school performance and grades, listlessness, and a loss of interest in friends, hobbies, and school. Adolescents may also manifest symptoms that may "mask" the underlying depression, such as delinquency, runaway behavior, substance abuse, and dangerous (abusive) sexual behavior. Many normal adolescents may also demonstrate "normal" depression as part of their developmental struggle. Seldom do children and adolescents recognize the dysphoria, but reveal their depression in these other forms.

"Normal" depression of adolescents may be the reaction of the adolescent to the process of the dependence–independence struggle in which they vacillate between feelings that their independence is not being achieved fast enough and feelings that it is approaching too fast. The normal adolescent is also confronted with the struggle for self-identity and self-image in which he often cannot meet his own (and often his parents') goals and expectations professionally, scholastically, and sexually, thus leading in many cases to normal feelings of depression. As the adolescent moves toward young adulthood and the adult world, the adolescent may experience anger toward the adult world, which is often directed at the "mess the world is in," inflation, war, famine, and pollution. Depression, anger, and guilt may also result from the values and restrictions their own parents place on them. The adolescent, in the consolidation of the developmental concept of death, begins to understand the finiteness of life, which is often reinforced by the deaths of peers in automobile accidents.

MAJOR DEPRESSION

The average duration for a major depression is approximately 32 weeks, usually preceded by good premorbid functioning. Most patients recover fully within 18 months; however, 70% of these patients will have another episode of major depression within 5 years.

In contrast, a dysthymic disorder manifests only mild to moderate impairment, generally has an earlier age of onset than major depression, and usually demonstrates a long history of emotional problems and family discord. The average duration of a dysthymic episode is approximately 36 months, and 70% of these patients will have an episode of major depression within 5 years.

Both major depression and dysthymic disorder have a high correlation with other childhood disorders, especially anxiety disorders and conduct disorders, the interaction of which is not fully understood. The differential diagnosis, therefore, is often complex and unclear and may include overlapping symptoms of attention deficit disorder, anxiety disorders, and conduct disorders. Unfortunately, even child psychiatrists are hampered in the differential diagnostic work-up because of these overlapping conditions and by the lack of reliable laboratory tests for children and adolescents. For example, tests such as the EEG Sleep Study, the dexamethasone suppression test (DST), urinary methoxyhydroxyphenylglycol (MHPG), and growth hormone assay, which are often helpful in the diagnosis of adult depression, have led to unreliable and unreproducible results with children and adolescents. Certain psychological tests including projective tests may, however, provide additional diagnostic help as may the semistructured diagnostic interviews, such as the Beck's Depression Inventory (BDI), and the Depression Inventory Schedule for Children (DISC).

SUICIDE

Suicidal behavior in children and adolescents covers a spectrum of behaviors and may be defined broadly as thoughts and actions that, if carried out, may lead to serious self-injury or death.

The spectrum of behaviors begins with the benign, almost universal, *nonsuicidal thought about death* coinciding with the developmental understanding of death and dying as the child matures. The *wish to be dead* is also probably a normal occurrence in many children and adolescents when, on occasion, feeling so bad, upset, humiliated, or angry they wish to be dead. Suicidal ideation, however, represents a quantum leap from normal thoughts of death to the actual thinking of killing oneself. *Suicidal threats* are usually well beyond the scope of normality and usually indicate serious signs of danger that may lead to overt or covert suicidal gestures and attempts. Lastly, and most tragically, in the spectrum of behaviors is *completed suicides*.

RISK FACTORS

No single factor can dictate the appropriate treatment or predict the outcome for the suicidal patient. The practitioner is faced with the difficult clinical decision based on a weighing of various factors in the clinical equation.

How then can the busy primary care physician identify the child or adolescent who is at risk for suicidal behavior and how does the practitioner deal with the patient who expresses suicidal thoughts, actions, and behaviors?

If the primary care physician suspects signs of depression as previously outlined, it is important to determine if the patient experiencing suicidal thoughts is contemplating suicide, or if he has previously attempted suicide. A series of empathetic questions can often elicit important information that the patient is often eager to share in his quest for help, because the suicidal patient often feels that no one is willing to listen and no one wants to help or understand.

The physician can begin by asking or commenting that the patient really appears "blue," "down in the dumps," or depressed. The patient can be asked if he ever felt so depressed that he wished that he were dead. Then the patient can be asked if he had ever thought of killing himself. If the patient denies such thoughts, it is helpful to ask why the patient has not been depressed or has not thought of killing himself. The answer may indicate coping skills and ego defense mechanisms providing strengths to the patient in times of stress. Should the patient admit to suicidal thoughts, it is important to ask how far the thoughts have been taken; for example, is there a plan or a method and date? It is also critical to learn if the patient has made previous attempts, in what fashion, who knew, and what response was elicited. Verbalizations by the patient, such as "nothing matters anymore, it's too late," "I won't be a problem much longer," or "I'd be better off dead" should signal the need for mental health intervention. If the patient gives away favorite possessions stating "I won't need these anymore," considerable alarm should be given as this may indicate a serious suicidal potential. Each of these questions and statements provides important data for the practitioner to determine an appropriate treatment plan and recommendation.

Thirty percent of people who have attempted suicide have made previous attempts, and the risk of a successful suicide increases with each attempt. Fifty percent of adolescents who attempt suicide abuse drugs or alcohol, 50% are "in trouble with the law," and 66% not only abuse substances but are also in legal difficulties. In addition, 30% of suicidal patients demonstrate signs of depression during the 3 months preceding the suicidal behavior.

For those patients contemplating suicide or who have attempted suicide, the method of the attempt gives some indicators of the intent and lethality; therefore, the more lethal the method, the greater the risk factor. Wrist cutting, house gas, and nonprescription pills are of relatively low lethality compared to carbon monoxide, hanging, and firearms that are highly lethal. The patient who has a well-thought-out plan, method, date, place, clothes, and so forth, and who has the means to carry out the attempt (*e.g.*, a gun, a noose, a long bayonet knife, or has picked a high building or a bridge) is at a high risk for lethality.

INDICATIONS FOR REFERRAL AND TREATMENT

In general, the treatment of the depressed or suicidal child and adolescent is usually beyond the expertise or interest of most pediatricians. Even those practitioners who have had significant behavioral pediatric training or elective training in child psychiatry and have a particular interest in psychosocial aspects of pediatrics find that the time demands involved in intensive psychotherapeutic intervention exclude them from this type of work in a busy pediatric practice.

The pediatrician who has a strong clinical impression or who has diagnostic criteria to indicate a major depression, a dysthymic disorder, or suicidal behavior of the child or adolescent should present his honest appraisal of the situation. Appropriate recommendations for mental health consultation and intervention should be made without trying to please or appease the patient or parents by avoiding a discussion of the true assessment of the clinical situation. The physician should explain to the patient and the parents that the patient's behavior signals a marked departure from the norm. Nonargumentative firmness on the part of the physician concerning the need for consultation is essential. Although the primary care physician may acknowledge the patient's anger or dismay about needing to see a "shrink" or other mental health professional, the practitioner needs to assert his professional responsibility to render the best medical opinion, even if it is not to the liking of the patient. It is often seemingly paradoxical that a sturdy posture in this regard is reassuring to the patient for it conveys the idea that someone (the practitioner) is listening and hearing the patient's trouble and is concerned about the behavior.

The patient and the parent often question the primary care physician regarding what type of treatment should be offered to the depressed or suicidal patient. Should the patient be given an antidepressant, is the preferred treatment hospitalization, family therapy, individual or group therapy, cognitive or behavioral therapy, or a combination of these treatment modalities? Is a special day school for the emotionally disturbed indicated or is a brief or long-term intensive hospital treatment necessary? What should be the professional background of the consultant, physician, psychologist, or social worker? All of these important questions must be addressed and vary widely, depending on the nature and severity of the problem, the family support systems, financial considerations, and the availability of mental health resources within the community.

It is beyond the scope of this chapter to discuss treatment modalities. However, the referring physician should be familiar with the mental health resources that exist in his community. This knowledge should include the therapeutic approach that is used, the level of professional competency, and the fee structure. It is highly desirable for the physician to have an ongoing personal relationship and contact with a specific mental health facility or professional. The selection and ongoing relationship with a mental health professional is critical to optimal patient care and may represent the most important role that the primary physician can assume in caring for a child or adolescent with emotional difficulties.

ANNOTATED BIBLIOGRAPHY

American Psychiatric Association: Facts About Teen Suicide. Washington, DC, American Psychiatric Association, (This fact sheet, provided free by the American Psychiatric Association, is a concise, readable overview of signs and symptoms that should alert peers, parents, teachers, and professionals to the troubled adolescent at risk for depression and suicide.)

Curran BE: Suicide. Pediatr Clin North Am 26(4):737–746, 1979 (Directed specifically to the practicing pediatrician and provides a nice overview of the problem with important diagnostic issues and treatment strategies.)

Kashani JH, Husain A, Shekim WO et al: Current perspectives in childhood depression: An overview. Am J Psychiatry 138(2):143–153, 1981 (Excellent overview and summary of the issues of diagnosing childhood depression. The article discusses the historical background leading up to current thinking.)

Poznanski E, Mokros HB, Grossman J, Freeman LN: Diagnostic criteria in childhood depression. Am J Psychiatry 142(10):1168–1173, 1985 (Current state-of-the-art paper on the diagnostic aspects of childhood depression.)

Sarles RM, Friedman SB: The process of consultation and referral. In Gellert E(ed): Psychosocial Aspects of Pediatric Care, pp 145–154. New York, Grune & Stratton, 1978 (Discusses broad indications for consultation and referral and gives specific suggestions to facilitate the selection of a consultant.)

5

Developmental Pediatrics and School Health

36
Detection and Assessment of Developmental Disabilities

BRUCE K. SHAPIRO

Developmental disorders are a group of disorders whose common factor is a dysfunction resulting from a "static" central nervous system disorder that manifests in childhood and that has a chronic course with a high likelihood of functional limitations. There is no universally accepted classification of developmental disorders; most are based on the disorder's most obvious manifestations. Classification is difficult because central nervous system (CNS) lesions are likely to be diffuse in children (*e.g.*, from asphyxic, genetic, or metabolic disorders) and multiple disorders may coexist. Diagnoses may also be accompanied by lesser degrees of dysfunction that do not result in additional diagnoses but are important for management. Classification is further limited by CNS maturation. Children may "grow into" disorders. For example, the neurologic substrate for a specific learning disability exists before school but the diagnosis cannot be established until academics commence. Children may also "outgrow" disorders; however, residual dysfunction is common. Early delays in motor or language areas may not prove handicapping but may be "markers" for other dysfunctions in learning and behavior. Early diagnosis is important in order to group children with similar disorders and thereby further delineate the natural history of the disorder, identify etiologic factors, design treatment programs, and prognosticate. A clinically applicable classification is presented in Table 36-1.

PRESENTATIONS

Efforts to detect developmental disability as early as possible have been an integral part of treatment programs, schools, and legislation (*e.g.*, P.L. 94–142—The Education for All Handicapped Children Act). As part of this effort, screening of asymptomatic populations during well-child visits has been advocated. However, it is unclear that this action substantively improves the detection of a developmental disability or that remediable secondary problems occur in presymptomatic children.

The age at which developmental disabilities can be detected is decreasing despite a lack of routine screening. Postulated reasons for this include the better visibility of handicap, an increased awareness of pediatricians, greater availability of services, preschool experiences, and more stringent parents who are unwilling "not to worry" in the expectation that their child will "outgrow it."

Formal screening tests are limited by applicability to only certain ages or poor test qualities. Most initial screenings are done by the parent. The results of these screenings will be shared if the pediatrician inquires whether there are concerns about the baby or if he asks the mother to estimate how old the baby/child is acting (divide this age by the chronologic age to obtain a reliable overall rate of development).

Developmental disabilities usually present as a

Table 36-1. Classification of Developmental Disorders (Prevalence/1000)

A. Disorders primarily manifesting a motor handicap
  1. Cerebral palsy (2)
B. Disorders primarily manifesting a cognitive handicap
  1. Mental retardation (30)
C. Disorders having globally normal cognition but showing specific deficits in processing
  1. Peripheral disorders of processing
    a. Deafness (1)
    b. Blindness (0.4)
  2. Central processing disorders
    a. Motor
      1. Minimal cerebral palsy
      2. Central hypotonia
      3. Apraxia
      4. Clumsy child syndrome
      5. Complex tic disorders
    b. Language
      1. Autism (0.4)
      2. Preschool communication disorders (40)
      3. Articulation disorders (?)
      4. Developmental dysphasias (?)
        a. Expressive
        b. Receptive
        c. Mixed
      5. Specific learning disability
    c. Minor perceptual dysfunction (visual motor dysfunction) (?)
    d. Behavioral
      1. Strauss syndrome (100)
      2. Hyperkinetic syndrome (100)
      3. Attentional deficit disorders (100)
      4. Oppositional disorders (?)
D. Seizures (10)

result of the failure of the child to meet age-related expectations. The earliest presentations are those related to a dysfunction in major organ systems (*e.g.*, coarctation of the aorta in Turner's syndrome), physical anomalies (*e.g.*, Down syndrome), or physiologic imbalance (*e.g.*, maple syrup urine disease). Slightly later presentations are failure to establish proper feeding, periodicity, and colic. Poor interaction with caretakers or the environment may indicate vision and hearing deficits. Gross motor failures, such as an inability to sit, predominate after 9 months with most children referred by 15 months. Although a motor dysfunction is the presenting symptom, these children commonly have additional abnormalities in thought and language. At this age, however, moderate degrees of dysfunction in nonmotor areas are usually not evident to the caretakers. However, language delay becomes the major reason for referral between 21 and 30 months. These children may also show behavioral disorders, which are usually dismissed as

"terrible twos." Behavioral and preacademic areas are the major concern with 3- to 5-year-old children, and often result when a child is unable to match the performance of his peers in preschool. Underachievement is a major reason for evaluating young school-aged children for developmental disabilities. Behavioral dysfunction may accompany academic underachievement and may be severe enough to mask a learning dysfunction.

DIFFERENTIAL DIAGNOSES

Developmental Disability Syndromes

Cerebral Palsy. Cerebral palsy is the most common movement disorder of childhood. It is a disorder of movement or posture and results from a static lesion to the immature central nervous system. In addition to physiologic and topographical categories, cerebral palsy is also classed by further (additional) neurologic defects. In cerebral palsy, the motor disability may not be the greatest handicap.

Mental Retardation. There is a significant subaverage intellectual functioning manifested during the developmental period and associated with deficits in social/adaptive function. Most retarded people are mildly affected. Behavioral dysfunction is usually the major impediment to successful adaptation.

Blindness and Deafness. These categories do not refer to total end organ failure. Thus, the definitions for these disorders (vision less than 20/200 corrected or visual fielded less than 20°; and hearing loss to a level of 100 dB) can be viewed as arbitrary. Although these disorders affect peripheral organs, the etiology may also cause a central dysfunction.

Central Processing Disorders. Central processing disorders preclude function at a level predicted by intelligence (IQ) alone. Thus, a bright child with an IQ of 125 may not learn to read. The central processing disorders form a spectrum across age of presentation and severity: autism to preschool communication disorder to developmental dysphasia to specific learning disability. Some disorders change category with time (*e.g.*, preschool communication disorders to specific learning disability). More precise definition of the neural mechanism of these dysfunctions awaits a better understanding of how humans learn. Most of these disorders (except the most severe) are compatible with independent life function. Aberrant behavior, however, may be more of a problem than the neurologic dysfunction. Attentional peculiarities (ranging from short attention to perseveration), hyperactivity, impulsivity, and emotional lability may be part of abnormal neurologic development and not secondary reactions to disability.

WORK-UP

If there are concerns about a child's development, an assessment is the appropriate action. An assessment entails the quantification of the child's abilities for the purpose of a diagnosis and, if indicated, a comprehensive management (habilitation) program. A proper assessment will yield clues regarding the etiology of the child's condition, provide a diagnosis, and delineate areas of strength and weakness. An assessment of areas other than those of primary concern is required because, in children, neurologic dysfunction is diffuse. An incomplete assessment leads to incomplete counseling, incorrect treatment goals, unsuccessful programs, and frustration.

In developmental disorders, the history usually gives the diagnosis. A diagnosis, however, reveals little about the etiology and degree of impairment. Thus, the history should also review family prenatal and perinatal histories, past medical history, current functioning, and assess behavioral disturbances. In addition, attempts should be made to exclude progressive neurologic processes, metabolic disorders, and chronic underlying illnesses. Physical examinations should be comprehensive with particular attention to dysmorphisms, pigmentary abnormalities, and an expanded neurologic examination. Laboratory screening is unlikely to yield

Table 36-2. Usual Ages of Attainment of Developmental Milestones

1 mo	GM	Head up in prone	9 mo	GM	
	FM			FM	Object constancy
	LAN	Social smile (6 wks)			Bang cubes together
2 mo	GM	Chest up in prone			Rings bell for fun
	FM	Follows across midline		LAN	Gesture games
	LAN	Coos	10 mo	LAN	Dada (discriminately)
3 mo	GM	On elbows in prone	11 mo	FM	Plucks pellet
	FM	Follows in a circle		LAN	First word (other than ma/da)
		Blinks to visual threat	12 mo	GM	Walks independently
	LAN	Up on wrists in prone		FM	Places pellet in bottle
4 mo	GM	Rolls prone to supine			Voluntary release
		Orients to voice (E)			Marks with a crayon
	LAN	Laughs out loud (4½)			Immature jargon
5 mo	GM	Rolls supine to prone		LAN	Imitates squeezing a doll (E)
	FM	Transfers		P.S.	Drinks from a cup
		Pulls down ring			Assists with dressing
	LAN	Orients to sound (E)	15 mo	GM	Runs
6 mo	GM	Sits (unsupported)		FM	Dumps pellet from bottle
	FM	Unilateral reach		LAN	Directed pointing
	LAN	Babbles			4–6 words
7 mo	GM	Comes to sit (7.5)	18 mo	FM	Scribbles spontaneously
	FM	Attempts pellet			Uses tools
	LAN				3-cube tower
8 mo	GM	Crawls; pulls to stand		LAN	3 body parts
	FM	Attains pellet			Parallel play
		Inspects bell			Domestic imagery
		Understands "no"			7–20 word vocabulary
	LAN	Dada (indiscriminate)			Mature jargon (16 mo)
				P.S.	Uses spoon
			21 mo	LAN	2-word phrases
					50-word vocabulary
					Points to pictures (E)
			24 mo	FM	3-cube train
				LAN	2-word sentences

FM = fine motor/problem solving; GM = gross motor; LAN = language; P.S. = personal/social. Gross motor and personal/social milestones are historical. Fine motor/problem solving are elicited. Language milestones are historical save where noted by examiner (E).

positive findings in the absence of historical clues. Therefore, no "routine" laboratory battery can be employed for developmental disorders.

An assessment is usually based on the child's "best" performance on standard tests. An alternative means of obtaining data is through parental recall of the child's developmental milestone attainment (Table 36-2). Historical milestones are not widely used for several reasons: (1) they may not be recorded accurately; (2) practitioners are not taught how to use them; and (3) their variability in the normal population obscures their consistency in delayed children. This technique depends on parental recall but requires less time and obviates the need to secure the child's cooperation. Old records and baby books may supplement poor memory.

Milestones can be grouped into four major categories: gross motor, language, fine motor/problem solving, and personal/social. *Gross motor milestones* are directed towards independent locomotion. Gross motor delay is necessary for the diagnosis of cerebral palsy, but the age of motor milestone attainment is not predictive of later cognition. *Language milestones* relate to the development of symbolic thought. They can be further subdivided into expression (that which is said), reception (that which is understood), speech (the manner in which things are said), and visual language (nonverbal communication, *e.g.*, play). Language is the best predictor of later cognition. *Fine motor/problem solving milestones* interweave visual maturation, hand function, problem solving, and visual motor abilities. These milestones are not easily obtained by a history, but do have a good relationship to cognition. They form the basis for most of the infant intelligence scales. *Personal social abilities* are the end result of problem solving, motor and language. These milestones reflect an increasing mastery of the child over his environment and relate to feeding, dressing, and hygiene: These depend on environmental factors but are associated with cognitive thresholds.

Pediatricians should record milestone attainment data at each well-child examination. Usually four or five questions need to be asked about language, motor, and personal social development. If concerns arise from the questions then fine motor/problem solving skills can be elicited. Ascertaining milestone achievement in the various categories of development permits a rate to be assigned to each category. Rates can be calculated by dividing the expected age of achievement by the actual age of achievement. Viewing developmental rates across time allows the detection of degeneration or acceleration.

Quantification of milestone achievement can lead to 3 types of abnormalities: delay, dissociation and deviance. Delay is the most common reason for referral and indicates a significantly subaverage (usually less than 75%) rate of development. Delay is a symptom and requires further evaluation. The delay can be global or may affect only one stream of development. Dissociation is that state which exists when one phase of development is out of synchrony with the others. Table 36-3 demonstrates the use of dissociation to achieve early diagnosis. Deviance refers to nonsequential development, as in the case of the child who walks without crawling, and is most commonly seen in processing disorders.

Limitations

Diagnoses are not fixed until the CNS matures. Variability of diagnosis is particularly true of children with normal or near-normal rates (greater than 65%). (A change in diagnoses is possible in children with slower rates but is less likely.) Prognostication in young infants is difficult because conclusions are based on small amounts of behavior. Repeated measures over time are indicated if prognosis is the goal of assessment.

Prematurity affects developmental assessment in inconsistent fashions. As a result there can be no single formula to correct for "premie catch up."

Table 36-3. Dissociation: An Aid to Early Diagnosis

| | STREAMS OF DEVELOPMENT | | | |
DISORDERS	Gross Motor	Language	Problem Solving	Personal Social
Cerebral palsy	D	N	N	N to D
Mental retardation	N	D	D	D
Communication disorder	N	D	D	N to D

The table demonstrates the use of rates of development to achieve early diagnoses. N = normal, D = decreased. *Normal* and *decreased* are relative terms because developmental disabilities that occur multiply and therefore the number of combinations is greater than shown on the table.

Correcting for most prematures (over 32 weeks' gestation) is not critical after 12 months of age because there will be little effect on clinical decisions. Children with unstable baselines (*e.g.*, those who fail to thrive, who are oxygen dependent, and who are in compensated heart failure) may also demonstrate developmental delays. Although an assessment is important to document their current level of function and decide if developmental interventions are required, prognostication is poor if the child is not physiologically stable.

Some children will not perform when asked. Shy children are another source of noncompliance. Studies have shown that excessively shy children may be unable rather than unwilling to perform. Both of these scenarios point to the value of historically derived data. Having the parent participate in the assessment may also be helpful.

Although gifted children generally attain milestones at a faster rate, it is not clear that developmental assessments in the first 2 years can detect gifted children. No harm is done to the gifted child if detection is delayed until giftedness is obvious; whereas problems are likely to ensue in the child who is incorrectly identified as "gifted." Thus, an assessment for giftedness is unwarranted in the first few years.

INDICATIONS FOR REFERRAL

Children with a *motor dysfunction* require delineation of the motor deficit by a developmental pediatrician, neurologist, or a motor therapist. They also require an evaluation of cognitive processes by a psychologist, with or without a speech pathologist. Audiologic, ophthalmologic, and orthopedic referrals may be required. The child with *language delay* requires an audiologic evaluation to exclude significant hearing loss and psychologic testing to rule out mental retardation. A pediatric speech pathologist may assist defining the nature of a language disorder and developing a treatment program. Professionals trained in neurobehavioral problems can teach parents techniques for dealing with behavioral disorders. Children with *academic underachievement* require an expanded neurologic examination to assess subtle abnormalities, and an evaluation of their cognitive potential (IQ) and achievement (academic performance) if a specific learning disability is suspected. Psychiatric intervention may be indicated if secondary behavior disturbances are significantly interfering with the child's function.

TREATMENT AND MANAGEMENT

There is no cure for developmental disorders, therefore treatment should be viewed as palliative. The broad goals of treatment are to allow a person to function to the maximum level permitted by his impairment and to prevent secondary dysfunctions (social or biologic). These goals, however, must be further refined based on a knowledge of the diagnosis and the constellation of problems with which the patient presents. Short-term objectives must be clearly defined and be consistent with long-term goals.

The pediatrician's role in management/treatment is not limited to prevention, diagnosis, evaluation, and treatment of medical conditions (including pharmacotherapy). Comprehensive management (habilitation) plans transcend traditional health issues and interaction with educational and social agencies is frequently required. As a result, competing management goals underscore the need to prioritize these plans. The pediatrician is in an ideal position to coordinate services and act as an advocate for his patient because of his knowledge of the family and ability to view the "total" child.

Chronic disorders require ongoing monitoring. Treatment programs need to be reviewed to ensure that they are still relevant. Goals may need to be readjusted. Periodic reviews afford the opportunity to assess health status, family function, school performance, and behavior. New information, reflecting therapeutic advances or age appropriate concerns, may be provided during these visits. Reviews should be undertaken by pediatricians whenever a child is not meeting expectations or at least semiannually in infants, annually in preschoolers, and biannually in school-aged children.

ANNOTATED BIBLIOGRAPHY

Accardo PJ, Capute AJ: The Pediatric and the Developmentally Delayed Child: A Clinical Text Book on Mental Retardation. Baltimore, University Park Press, 1979 (Presents an approach to developmental disabilities and questions for language assessment [see also Clin Pediatr 17:847, 1978])

Capute AJ, Shapiro BK, Palmer FB et al: Normal Gross Motor Development I: The influence of race, sex and socioeconomic status. Dev Med Child Neurol 27:635–643, 1985 (Contains questions for assessment of motor development and current motor milestones.)

Drillien CM, Drummond MB: Neurodevelopmental Problems in Early Childhood. London, Blackwell, 1977

(Basic text describes a neurodevelopmental examination, specific entities, and therapies.)

Illingworth RS: The Development of the Infant and Young Child, 7th ed. Edinburgh, Churchill Livingstone, 1980 (Comprehensive review of development and assessment focusing on children under 5 years of age.)

Shapiro BK, Batshaw ML: Mental retardation. In Gellis S, Kagan B: Current Pediatric Therapy, 12. Philadelphia, WB Saunders, 1986 (Illustrates principles of management of developmental disabilities using mental retardation as an example.)

Shapiro BK, Palmer FB, Wachtel RC, Capute AJ: Issues in the early identification of specific learning disability. J Dev Behav Pediatr 5:15–20, 1983 (Reviews temporal components of development.)

Thompson G, Rubin IL, Bilenker RM: Comprehensive Management of Cerebral Palsy. New York, Grune & Stratton, 1983 ("Total child" approach to cerebral palsy and its manifestations.)

Wing L (ed): Early Childhood Autism: Clinical Education and Social Aspects, 2nd ed. New York, Pelham Press, 1976 (Best single source on the topic.)

37

School Readiness

BRUCE K. SHAPIRO

Failure to develop school readiness at the appropriate time frequently portends serious academic and behavioral dysfunctions in the primary grades and has been associated with difficulties extending through adolescence into adulthood. Despite this, school readiness has not been a major pediatric issue. Two excuses given for the traditional lack of involvement are that most children perform adequately in school and that the pediatric role in school problems is not clear. School readiness has become an area of concern because parents are more aware of deviant development: unready children can be identified and alternatives to traditional school may be implemented earlier.

School readiness indicates that the child has the necessary psychoneurologic processes for academic learning to proceed. Psychologic abilities are developing rapidly during this period. Language abilities expand from limited communication (750 words, 3-word sentences) to nearly mature usage. Visual skills show marked maturation, particularly in visual motor areas. Abstract reasoning appears. Expectations are not specific to the individual but a group; performance is measured against peers. The determination of school readiness uses psychoneurologic processes to predict educational progress. This approach to school readiness is based on two hypotheses: (1) deviations can be detected; and (2) these processes relate to school performance. Further delineation of predictive processes and charting of their natural history in preschool children represents a major research direction.

PRESENTATIONS

Unreadiness for school may be associated with delays in motor or language areas. These delays are usually not handicapping and are modest in degree (associated with developmental rates above 75%). Delays may occur in only one aspect of development (e.g., expressive language).

Gross motor dysfunction is usually associated with abnormalities of tone. Hypotonia is most common and is reflected in clumsiness. Awkward running or reticence in engaging in motor activities may result from minimal spasticity or asymmetric tone. Preschool children who "trip over the cracks in the sidewalk" or experience multiple episodes requiring sutures may have motor dysfunction, hyperactivity, or attentional problems.

Fine motor/visual motor dysfunction may be seen in children who experience difficulty with buttoning, delayed shoe tying (over age 5 years), or poor cutting or pencil grasp. An inability to copy figures or solve puzzles may reflect a motor dysfunction or a lack of the brain's ability to interpret visual information accurately (visual motor dysfunction). In preschool children reversing letters occasionally is not unusual, although excessive reversals should be investigated.

Language and behavior are the major areas of developmental concern in preschool children. By this time most mild to moderate motor disorders have resolved, although central hypotonia may persist. Clumsiness is difficult to define and other motor dysfunctions (e.g., tic disorders) present at a latter age. Visual perceptual delays may coexist with language and behavioral problems, but go unnoticed unless the child has had a school experience.

Delayed language abilities are common in preschool children, with an estimated 3% prevalence. Disorders may affect articulation (clarity of speech), expression (that which is said), or reception (understanding). Most articulatory and expressive disorders resolve, but receptive disorders are usually associated with deficits in expression and articulation. Defining articulatory disorders is best done by speech pathologists. Subtle manifestations of receptive disorders may be reflected in a difficulty in following instructions or a poor memory.

Although language disturbances are common, disordered behavior is the most common presenting symptom of school unreadiness. Behavioral manifestations may be poor play skills, unwillingness to share or take turns, or inability to play by the rules. Attentional peculiarities consisting of a short attention span, "tuning out," or perseveration may begin to be noted. Components of behavior contributing to poor peer interaction include degrees of emotional lability, "negativeness," impulsivity, or activity that are excessive for age. These behavioral aberrations may also lead to suboptimal responses to discipline and create major parental stress.

"Late bloomers" cause transitory concern to their parents and physicians. These are children whose development has been delayed sufficiently to raise concerns, but who prove not to have handicaps (*e.g.*, 20-month-old walkers or 30-month-old talkers). They achieve a functional level (threshold) and concern may diminish incorrectly because they have "closed the gap." In some children, if abilities are measured carefully, the gap persists. Many "late bloomers" are evidencing abnormal central nervous system (CNS) maturation and not simply individual variation. Late bloomers commonly evidence difficulties in academic areas.

Perhaps the most dramatic presentation of school unreadiness is the child who is expelled from nursery school because he "isn't ready" because of "immaturity." Immaturity is not well defined but is generally applied to the child who evidences sufficient delay to prevent effective competition with age peers but not enough to be called "delayed." Immaturity is most commonly used to describe behavior but may be applied to other aspects of development.

DIFFERENTIAL DIAGNOSIS OF SCHOOL UNREADINESS

School readiness is not a single entity. It is a concept that is not easily measured because it is the end result of multiple processes that mature at different rates. Although many etiologies are responsible for failure to achieve school readiness, school unreadiness is usually expressed as dysfunctions in processing or intellectual limitation.

A hearing loss should also be considered among the causes of school unreadiness, although this is not common. Preschool children constitute a "high-risk" group for mild intermittent hearing loss because of the large number of children with fluid in the middle ear. Whether an intermittent hearing loss can result in lasting dysfunction in language processing is unclear. The child with a sensorineural hearing loss is less controversial. These children may have a communicatively significant hearing loss that interferes with language processing. Even minimal losses of this type should be monitored since their hearing loss may progress.

Eye problems are usually *not* a primary cause of school unreadiness. Major visual deficits are usually manifested in infancy. Although the preschool period is important for detecting preventable/treatable conditions, such conditions are not causes of, but are associated with, school unreadiness. Most of the problems with visually presented material result from a neurologic rather than an ophthalmologic dysfunction.

In the past, mental retardation was a major cause of school unreadiness. Although mentally retarded children are still delayed in their attainment of school readiness, they are being identified earlier and therefore infrequently present *de novo*. The intellectual limitation now associated with school unreadiness is usually in the borderline range (IQ equivalent 70–80).

Minimal brain dysfunctions (MBD) or processing disorders are the most common causes of school unreadiness. These disorders represent deficits in CNS function that express themselves in a more limited fashion than the more global disorders (*e.g.*, cerebral palsy, mental retardation). The classification of these disorders is descriptive. However, symptomatology is not specific and it is likely that each cerebral dysfunction represents a family of disorders. Classification is further clouded by the coexistence of disorders (*e.g.*, hyperactivity and communication disorder). Further definition of the neural mechanisms of these disorders may lead to a more useful classification.

Insufficient experience is commonly invoked as an etiology of school unreadiness; however, this is an unproven cause. In the absence of extremes, it is unclear that experience exerts a major influence on the development of school readiness. The argument (*e.g.*, Head Start) is more compelling in the marginal cases such as those children who border on intellectual limitation or processing disorders or those from socially unstable situations. However, the type and amount of experiences needed to ensure school readiness remain to be defined.

Intellectual limitation, minimal brain dysfunctions, and hearing loss may each result from many etiologies. Although usually associated with static encephalopathies arising in early life, these conditions may be acquired later (*e.g.*, brain infection or automotive trauma) or result from progressive processes. Central nervous system degeneration, infection, ischemia, metabolic and nutritional disorders, neoplasia, physical agents and toxins, and immunologic processes have all been implicated in the failure to achieve school readiness.

WORK-UP

The basic work-up for the child whose school readiness is questioned is a comprehensive history and physical examination. Modifications of usual techniques may be necessary because of the age of the child and because the history may reflect varying views (*e.g.*, parents and teachers, mother and father) of the child. Further evaluations and tests will depend on the clinical findings.

Although some clinicians attempt to develop a history of the present illness, this may prove difficult if there is no clear onset to the child's problem. Others find that reviewing the child's development from the earliest beginnings to the present is the most useful technique. Regardless of the approach, the history of the clinician should be able to detail the nature of the problem, know when the parents became concerned, establish a course (worsening/improving), and delineate associated problems.

The family history should focus on the academic progress of first- and second-degree relatives. Parents should be queried about their academic attainment, grades repeated, early school performance, and whether they are recreational readers. Early school performance of siblings, uncles, aunts, and cousins should also be reviewed. Late walkers (over 18 months) and later talkers (over 30 months) should be noted, as should "late bloomers." Cer-

ebral palsy, mental retardation, learning disorders, and early childhood deaths should be noted.

Pregnancy, birth, and neonatal histories may be of limited value although conditions arising during this time have been related to adverse developmental outcomes. Questions should review maternal factors (*e.g.*, age, infertility, chronic diseases), pregnancy factors (*e.g.*, glycosuria, abnormalities of placentation), potentially toxic agents (*e.g.*, infections, alcohol), labor and delivery complications, gestational age, birth weight, and neonatal disorders. Special attention should be paid to early feeding difficulties.

The past medical history is usually unremarkable; however, a pattern of repeated episodes of minor trauma, sutures, or ingestions occasionally emerges. The past history should also identify factors (significant illnesses or hospitalizations) that might be responsible for altering a child's developmental rate (*e.g.*, head trauma or seizures).

A developmental history documents the child's pattern of development. Early delays are noted in the acquisition of motor, language, and self-help skills, as is the presence of deviant (nonsequential) development. Some children who lack school readiness show a pattern of plateaus and spurts. A history of a loss of skills suggests a degenerative disease.

The behavioral history attempts to detect abnormalities in the development of behavior and assess components of current behavior. Unusual fetal activity, prolonged colic, and difficulty in establishing periodicity may be noted. Excessive or prolonged stranger and separation anxiety is not uncommon. Delays in interactive play and socialization are common. Qualitative aspects of behavior (*e.g.*, lability, hyperactivity, and distractibility) may be difficult to quantitate because these criteria are age dependent and parents show wide variations in their judgments. Parents and teachers may have discordant views of the child that reflect the differences in home versus group behaviors.

A complete review of systems and previous evaluations is indicated to more completely delineate the scope of the problem and identify other disorders that may contribute to the lack of school readiness.

The goals of the physical examination of the child who exhibits school unreadiness are to detect possible etiologies for the clinical picture, identify curable conditions, and assess brain function. Growth parameters (including head circumference) may indicate chronic disease, fetal alcohol syndrome, or Soto's syndrome. Mild dysmorphisms (*e.g.*, high palate or posteriorly tipped ears) are more frequent in children with cerebral dysfunction. A comprehensive physical examination is indicated.

An assessment of brain function includes examination of the cranial nerves, motor function, sensation, and other aspects of processing. A cranial nerve examination may reveal strabismus, facial asymmetry, or decreased tongue movements. Vision and hearing assessments are indicated. Motor assessment may show abnormality of tone, focality of findings, or difficulty in modulating movement. The sensory examination in the preschool child is visually limited to the primary modalities. Higher cortical functions such as laterality, stereognosis, extinction, and finger identification are not reliably assessed in preschool children. Processing may be addressed by various pencil and paper tasks, block constructions, and memory tasks.

The Sprigle School Readiness Screening Test (Sprigle and Lanier, 1967) and the Pediatric Examination of Educational Readiness (Meltzer LJ et al, 1981) were developed to identify children who lack school readiness. Both tests show good relationships with selected aspects of kindergarten function. However, the ability of these tests to predict school performance has not been demonstrated. Studies of the Denver Developmental Screening Test also show a relationship with school performance; however, there is disagreement over how well it predicts later school problems. None of these tests permits a diagnosis to be made, nor do they define a specific course of treatment.

INDICATIONS FOR REFERRAL

The major differential diagnoses of school unreadiness are cognitive limitation and MBD. A pediatric psychologist can provide an estimate of the child's cognitive potential and make qualitative statements about processing. Although a large number of instruments may be used, the minimum should include either the Wechsler Preschool and Primary Scale of Intelligence (WPPSI) or the Stanford Binet, a measure of social-adaptive behavior (*e.g.*, Vineland), quantitation of the child's behavior and a screening of family function. Supplemental tests are frequently used to assess language and visual processing abilities.

Although the differential diagnoses are few, the manifestations are many. Consequently, consults must be brokered carefully to prevent the "gang" approach to management. Audiologic and ophthalmologic referrals may be indicated if office screening tests were failed. Speech pathologists may help if articulation problems are significant and they may help to further define language disorders detected by psychological testing. Psychiatrists, behavioral pediatricians, psychologists, and social workers may assist with associated behavioral problems. Motor therapists are available to try to diminish the clumsiness and improve the quality of movement.

PRINCIPLES OF MANAGEMENT

Children who fail to successfully make the transition into school are likely to experience lasting difficulty. Unfortunately, there is no method to instill readiness. Treatment is aimed primarily at the prevention of secondary problems while ensuring that the child is in a situation that will allow his potential to be achieved.

Children who lack school readiness commonly exhibit dysfunctions in several areas. A comprehensive treatment program is needed to deal with the varied manifestations of an abnormal CNS. Attempting to treat each manifestation as a separate problem fails to prioritize treatment goals and mandates that even trivial (in terms of long-range function) problems be treated. This may lead to delays in parental acceptance of the developmental dysfunction because focusing on transitory phenomena may obscure the true nature of the deficit. Unless a comprehensive plan is instituted, parents are frequently overwhelmed by the number of "problems," confused when new problems appear (*e.g.*, reading difficulty), and frustrated by the therapist's inability to cure their child.

Although each program must be individualized, certain general principles of treatment can be delineated: (1) Parents must have a clear understanding of the child's dysfunction and the causes. (2) They must be reassured that the child's problems are not primarily the result of inept parenting. (3) Questions of etiology, inheritability, and prognosis need to be answered. (4) Alternate strategies for dealing with the child's behavior and techniques for saying "yes" should be established. (5) The child's strengths must not be lost in his dysfunctions.

Children who lack school readiness may be eligible for special educational services through the Education for All Handicapped Children ACT (PL 94–142). This law provides for special services to children over age 3 in most jurisdictions (several states have lowered the age to the time of identification of a handicap). The eligibility criteria and type of service are determined by the local educational agency.

The role of pharmacotherapy in preschool children is controversial. Stimulant medication may assist distractability, attentional problems, and hyperactivity, although most parents initially prefer to try a behavioral approach. Dextroamphetamine sulfate may be used in children older than 3 years of age and is available as an elixir. Methylphenidate is not approved by the FDA for children younger than 6 years. Major tranquilizers may have adverse effects on learning. If used, medications should be an adjunct to a comprehensive program.

Unless the child's progress is monitored, the program is likely to fail. Parents will need to have questions answered about their child's progress. Aspects of the treatment program will need modification. For example, the diagnosis of a specific learning disability may be made. Special programming in school is likely to be needed. The latest "fad" cures will require discussion.

The management of the preschooler who lacks readiness is not the end of the process; the unready preschooler is likely to need management as a school-aged child with learning disorders. However, properly identifying and managing preschool issues is likely to make the transition into school easier.

ANNOTATED BIBLIOGRAPHY

Drillien C, Drummond M: Development Screening and The Child with Special Needs. Clinics in Developmental Medicine 86. Philadelphia, JB Lippincott, 1983 (Population study of over 5000 children. Follow a cohort into school. The bibliography is selective, fairly current, and useful in determining the outcome of preschoolers who lack readiness.)

Meltzer LJ, Levine MD, Palfrey JS et al: Evaluation of a multidimensional assessment procedure for preschool children. J Dev Behav Pediatr 3:67–73, 1981 (Outlines development of this test.)

Shapiro BK, Palmer FB, Wachtel RC, Capute AJ: 1981 Issues in the early identification of specific learning disability. J Dev Behav Pediatr 5:15–20, 1984 (Suggests that neurologic substrate for learning disability is detectable before school age and reviews studies suggesting relationships between early development and learning problems. Extensive bibliography.)

Sprigle HA, Lanier J: Validation and standardization of a school readiness test. J Pediatr 70:602–607, 1967 (Outlines development of this test.)

Sturner RA, Green JA, Funk SG: Preschool Denver Developmental Screening Test as a predictor of later school problems. J Pediatr 107:615–621, 1985 (Bibliography contains articles for and against the use of DDST to detect school problems.)

38

Consulting to Day Care Centers and Schools

MURRAY M. KAPPELMAN

The primary care physician shares a common goal with educators at each stage of the child's development, that is, the successful passage of the youngster through that psychosocial/educational time frame. The training and skills of the physician differ from those of the educator so that each brings a different component to the overall support of the child during the school years. Recognizing that the child's physician possesses professional information not only about the specific child but also about children in general, the educational community frequently seeks out the physician's advice on various issues related to the youngster.

The questions asked of the physician and the action/reaction of the medical primary care professional differ significantly relative to the age of the particular young person. Thus, the typical school consultation regarding a preschool child will possibly differ from that concerning a high-school junior. The format of this discussion varies from the standard in this text because of the general nature of the topic and the need not only to use age-related categories but also divergent types of services and problems.

PRESCHOOL CHILD

Physical Problems

In this first school contact age period, the physician not uncommonly is required to assist the school in delineating the potentials and limitations possessed by children with chronic physical problems. Consultations on the exercise levels for children suffering from congenital cardiac problems, asthma, early onset diabetes, and sequelae of central nervous system (CNS) problems such as cerebral palsy are common and important areas of cross-communication so that the preschool child can be permitted the maximum physical activity within reason considering the organic problem.

Sensory Problems

This preschool encounter may be the first indication that the child has an intrinsic sensory deficit such as diminished or dysfunctional vision or hearing. Once discovered, the physician must alert the parent and school to continually observe and be aware of problems related to these deficits. The primary care physician should also be prepared to screen and refer appropriately all children sent to him by the preschool teacher with the concern that the youngster has a sensory deficit.

Social Problems

Separation of the parent and child may occur first at this preschool period. Helping the school differentiate between the normal developmental separation anxiety concordant with this age period versus an excessive and, therefore, socially alarming separation problem may form the focus of the social consultation at this age.

Behavioral Problems

Social settings tend to be somewhat more restrictive than the home environment; therefore, the child's behavior may be accentuated or may actually change within the preschool setting. The normally active child at home may seem like the "hyperactive" child within the school room. The child who controls at home may find that his inability to act in the same way is intolerable within the school setting. The personality of the authority figures within the two settings may differ significantly and confuse and alarm the child into either acting-out or closing-inward behaviors. The preschool may request that the parent consult the primary care physician (or may communicate directly with the physician) to elicit help in understanding the child's maladaptive behavior in the specific preschool setting.

Learning Problems

Certain children can be directly compared to peers for the first time within the initial school environment. Developmental delays, usually of a subtle nature, that are manifested by the lack of ability to keep pace with peers, surface and often become

the basis of a worried and hurried phone call to the physician for a consultation regarding the youngster's developmental progress and learning abilities. The problem is often behavioral, situational, or environmental rather than developmental; however, the physician must be prepared not only to study the child using his own knowledge of development, but also to elicit advice from professionals trained in other aspects of child development. These include a psychologist, a speech therapist, and an educational specialist, among others, who may be intrinsic to a school system or referred to as external consultants.

ELEMENTARY SCHOOL CHILD

Physical Problems

For those children who have not had a preschool experience, the kindergarten or first-grade entry level may introduce the same issues of dealing with a chronic illness within the elementary school setting both to parents and teachers/school administration. The pediatrician finds that the first exposure to a cohort of other children, whether preschool or early elementary school, increases the number of minor respiratory and gastrointestinal illnesses for the average young child and causes missed days of school with resulting loss of learning time and increasing parental concern about the child who suddenly appears "sickly." Reassurance of parents about the normality of this situation and assistance at the school level in the management of "epidemics" of illness of a minor nature from both the medical and educational standpoint will become an important part of the daily practice of the primary care pediatrician.

More serious issues will also arise regarding the communicability and preventability of major illnesses within the preschool and, particularly, the elementary school population. An outbreak of a communicable disease such as chickenpox will require the pediatrician to keep the parents and school informed regarding future expectations relative to prevention, occurrence, school return, and communicability. The importance of previous immunization will become the focus of telephone calls from the school and parent with the break-through case of rubeola, rubella, mumps, or polio-like symptoms in a classmate. When one of the children develops *Hemophilus influenzae* type B meningitis, the issue of rifampin prophylaxis, and "other parent" reassurance through information puts the pediatrician "front and center" in consulting with the school. The concerns about children who have had contact with or carry the antibodies to hepatitis surface antigen or HIV (with or without autoimmune deficiency syndrome (AIDS)-related symptoms) bring the pediatrician in contact with the school and the parents for consultation. The risks to the other children and reasonable precautions within the school setting are major issues and incite much concern.

Safety within the schools should be a key focus of the pediatrician who consults with a school or school system. Assisting the school personnel in creating a physically safe environment for the children permits the primary care physician to practice the key element of good medicine—preventive pediatrics. The pediatrician should also be prepared to help the elementary school set up appropriate responses to injury, physical illness, and emotional crises in the school child.

Sensory Problems

Again, if this is the first contact the child has had with the school environment, the detection and complications of major congenital or acquired vision or hearing losses become the pediatric consultants' concern. Intermittent diminution of hearing secondary to repeated or persistent otitis media may create problems between the school child and the learning environment that are not immediately linked to decreased auditory acuity. The pediatric consultant to the family and school must be alert to diagnose each child whose learning or behavioral problems in school have a hearing deficit as the etiology.

Social Problems

School phobias may begin with the entry into elementary school if there has been no preceding school or child-group experience for the youngster. Alerting the parent and school about the necessity of a quick return of the school-avoiding child into the classroom will allow appropriate therapy both for the child and the parent suffering from the acute separation problem. Helping the school distinguish between the child who works well and happily alone for part of the interactive school time versus the shy or withdrawn child will enable the teacher and other school personnel to identify the child who needs social encouragement or psychological investigation and possibly treatment.

The school will often ask for the pediatrician's advice on the maladaptive child. Primary versus secondary socially maladaptive behavior alerts the pediatrician to long-standing child/family issues in the former in contrast to acute situational issues in the latter. Examples of the issues causing secondary social maladaptation are parental separation or divorce, illness or death of a family member, or emergence of learning disabilities within the child with recurrent poor school performance. These acute situational crises are also the cornerstones for the school avoidance syndromes that manifest later in the school child who had previously gone willingly to elementary school. The pediatrician consulting with the school on these problems not only assists in diagnosing the specific child but also, by example and information transfer, performs in-service education with the teachers and school administration that will assist them in discovering and referring future cases.

Behavioral Problems

Once more, if this is the first large-group restrictive situation for the child, the level of the youngster's activity may become an issue for the pediatrician called by the school as a consultant. Whether or not the child suffers from the attention deficit disorder (ADD) is often the primary concern of school and is transmitted to the parent. The "overactive" child in the lower elementary grades may have many reasons (only one of which is ADD) for activity above the mean for the peer classmates. The pediatrician consulting with the school on the specific child will analyze not only the child's relationship with the school environment but also the opposite; thus, the school is offered insight relative to the totality of child/teacher interaction in this situation (which may have an important bearing on other similar child/teacher interactions within the same classroom and same school.)

As noted above, acute situational crises can activate aberrant or unacceptable behaviors in the previously well-adjusted and integrated school child. The results can be school avoidance, daytime wetting, peer withdrawal, encopresis, acting-out behavior in the classroom or playground, developmental regression, or learning problems. The pediatrician is often viewed as the front-line consultant in these situations.

Learning Problems

Elementary school children have many varied reasons why they have difficulty in learning. It often becomes too convenient for the educators or parents to label the child as having developmental or neurologic bases for the youngster's failures to keep pace with peer achievement. Working together with the school, the parent, and the child, the pediatrician can become the focal point around which a thorough analysis is made for specific etiologies of the child's learning problems. The pediatric consultant must be cautious in forming conclusions based on previous performance (*e.g.*, in the case of the fourth-grade child who has done well previously and seems to begin to have real learning problems: These problems need not be situational but could be caused by a specific perceptual learning disability that has surfaced because of the increasing complexity of the learning tasks). Knowing all of the possibilities enables the pediatrician to be the ideal consultant to an educational system that does not always train the teachers in the causes of learning failure to the degree that they can make these differentiations by themselves within the classroom.

JUNIOR HIGH-SCHOOL CHILD

Physical Problems

The pediatrician has the distinction of working with children in an age group that passes from infancy into adulthood. One of the aspects of this passage is the development of sexual characteristics. The school often requests the pediatrician to consult with the system as a sex educator in an effort to provide a back-up to the parents' expected sex education within the home and prevent the expression of the complications of careless early adolescent sexual experimentation (*i.e.*, pregnancy, abortion, and sexually transmitted diseases). In addition, the pediatrician as sex educator assists the developing adults to recognize, understand, and accept the physical and emotional changes taking place within their bodies and minds.

Physical activities escalate at this age with the introduction of competitive and noncompetitive sports. The prevention of injury to the young participants by consulting with the school as well as talking with the coaches and the young players to create a safe sports atmosphere becomes a high priority for the pediatrician acting as consultant to schools.

Unfortunately, too many young people begin experimenting with drugs and alcohol at this age. The pediatrician, with the school, should begin addressing the high risks associated with substance abuse. The junior high-school youngster often feels both invulnerable and invincible. The school personnel with the parents and the pediatric consultant must introduce reality into their thinking so that they develop the beginnings of responsibility and an understanding of the consequences of their actions.

Sensory Problems

During this age period, most progressive school systems begin to attempt the mainstreaming of sensory impaired youngsters who were probably in special school environments previously. The pediatrician is the most appropriate consultant to prepare the other children, the teachers, and the school administration for the integration of these special children. Helping the sensorily handicapped child in his adaptation process also requires the assistance of the physician consultant to the school system. Too few pediatricians and primary care-givers fully understand the child with sensory handicaps. This is often not sufficiently addressed in their training, and yet they will be asked for expert advice. It will often be necessary for the pediatric consultant to seek outside educational help relative to these areas as part of a self-learning experience to be competent in the consultant role.

Social Problems

The school consultant faces different issues when consulting with schools dealing with early adolescents rather than with younger children. The issues of drugs, alcohol, and sexuality have been mentioned. The other three issues that confront and often confound the pediatric consultant are aggression and acting-out behavior, adolescent depression and suicide, and dropping out of school. The schools often request that the pediatric consultant act as the triage officer who seeks and finds appropriate referral pathways for the children presenting with these disturbing early adult problems. It becomes the responsibility of the community pediatrician to find and establish networks of professionals in the other disciplines necessary to assist in the diagnosis and the treatment of these serious behavioral/social problems.

Behavioral Problems

Within the adolescent age period, the social and behavioral issues become so intertwined that it becomes not only confusing but also unnecessary to attempt to make the differentiation. One feeds clearly into the other. Thus, the social issues of parental divorce or other social disruption impacts on responsive behavior resulting in aberrations seen within the school environment. Some issues may be endogenous rather than situational such as certain adolescent depressions; however, most behavioral abnormalities in young adults are related directly to situational issues whether obvious or complex and subtle. Extremes such as anorexia or obesity form the framework of the often hyperbolic adolescent reaction to situational stress. School failure is often merely a signal of more serious concerns to which the young adolescent desperately wants attention to be paid. The pediatrician who acts as a consultant in these cases is often asked by the school system to be the individual who leads the young person toward the appropriate means of assistance and remediation. As noted above, that becomes the pediatrician's role for which preparation must be made.

Learning Problems

Because the young person has passed through the elementary school age does not mean that the potential for specific learning problems is no longer an issue. Many youngsters are diagnosed in the elementary schools and carry their learning disabilities like heavy baggage dragging them downward within the junior high school environment. Some young adolescents begin their educational decompensation with the rising complexity of the junior high school educational demands (and often multiple teacher environments). The learning problems, however, are often expressed differently in this age period with social and behavioral acting out or withdrawal as primary manifestations. Misdiagnosis of these behaviors as complete unto themselves without consideration of the possibility of learning disorders as the basis will cause many young people to "give up" and leave the system, with often disastrous personal and social consequences. The pediatric school consultant may thus offer the school advice on "working-up" these behaviors.

HIGH-SCHOOL CHILD

Physical Problems

As with the junior high school student, the pediatric consultant no longer deals only with the young person's response to congenital or chronic illness but must assist the school in coping with or-

ganic issues related to emotional crises, drug and alcohol issues, truancy, sexually related problems, eating disorders, sports and vehicular injuries. The consultant physician must deal first with education as a form of prevention and ultimately with the school's response system and referral network.

Sensory Problems

Mainstreaming the sensory impaired young adult still remains a primary school issue needing pediatric consultation and assistance.

Social Problems

Those social problems outlined for the junior high school student are not only present as issues but are also increased significantly in number. Some of the serious problems no longer remain because the system has failed the child rather than the reverse; the youngster is no longer in school but in the community and all too often he is inadequately prepared for life or survival.

Behavioral Problems

The issues are the same as for the junior high school cohort. The pediatric consultant works simultaneously as an educator and a crisis intervener, both for the high school student and the faculty/administration.

Learning Problems

The previously diagnosed (or undiagnosed in a few cases) young adults with specific learning disabilities may remain within the school system if the system has adapted to their specific needs. All too many are out on the streets feeling inferior as students and as human beings. Commonly, they feel that they have little worth saving; that is, the "nothing-to-lose" syndrome that leads to delinquency and self-abuse. Assisting the schools in coping with the need of these young people for an appropriate vocational education that prepares them to live as contributing members of our society versus closing the door to the learning disabled drop-out problem becomes one of the most important goals of the physician consultant to the high-school administration.

Dealing with the gifted as well as the average student falls within the combined interdisciplinary responsibility of the school administration and the physician consultant. All too often the physician, as well as the school personnel, view the role of the physician consultant to the senior high school as one that deals with the physical aspects of the young adult. The true pediatric consultant to the senior high school (as well as to all levels of the school system) deals with the whole child/young adult encompassing their physical, emotional, and social health; all aspects fit within one consultancy role.

It becomes obvious that consulting with day-care centers and school systems requires the pediatrician to offer not only medical information, diagnosis, and referral but also involvement in the educational, social, and career aspects of the child's life. These elements become interdigitated, and the complete pediatrician acting as consultant to the school assumes many different roles such as the role of the diagnostician combined with that of the educator. Prevention mixes with treatment. Child–physician interaction blends with interdisciplinary teaming. The physician realizes that he is working in a different system, one unlike the structure within which his original training took place, so that adaptability and flexibility and acceptance of alternative rules and standards may be necessary to reach the desired end-product—the healthy school child who is able to reach a maximum level of educational achievement commensurate with that child's potential. That ideal must be the goal of the pediatric consultant to the day-care center and the school system. To reach that goal requires integration into the school environment, understanding the issues facing the professionals working within the system, knowing the rules and standards of the other profession, learning to work intimately with trust and appreciation of the other professionals, and never lowering the quality or expectations of primary care provided for the children within the schools.

The pediatrician must take on this responsibility within the community. Clearly no other professional can perform the tasks outlined above as well or can advocate across such broad areas of concern as the pediatric consultant within the school system. What becomes the challenge to the pediatrician is to be appropriately trained, prepared, and available to perform the job well. The child of the present and the citizen of tomorrow will be the physician's beneficiaries.

ANNOTATED BIBLIOGRAPHY

Brent DA, Howell M: Data based program evaluation in a project involving mental health consultation to schools. J Am Acad Child Psychiatry 22:447, 1983 (Review of school health from a mental health perspective.)

Committee on School Health. American Academy of Pediatrics Guidelines for Urgent Care in School. Pediatrics 74:148, 1984 (Essential guidelines for the physician consultant relative to crisis intervention.)

Kappelman M et al: The school health team and the school health physician. Am J Dis Child 129:191, 1975 (Perspective on the definition of "school health.")

Low MB: The Education for all Handicapped Act of 1975: A pediatrician's viewpoint. Pediatrics 65:271, 1978 (Assists the pediatrician in the interpretation of the handicapped child legislation.)

Nader P: A pediatrician's primer for school health activities. Pediatr Rev 4:82–92, 1982 ("State-of-the-art" article on school health.)

Senn M: The role and prerequisites and training of the school physician. Pediatr Clin North Am 12:1039, 1965 (Early "ground-breaking" article on school health.)

Walker DK: Care of Chronically Ill Children in Schools. Pediatr Clin North Am 31:221, 1984 (Addresses the important issue of the chronically ill child in an appropriate manner.)

Weitzman M et al: School absence: A problem for the pediatrician. Pediatrics 69:739, 1982 (Deals with truancy.)

39
Learning Disabilities
CHARLES N. SWISHER

Learning disability represents a large area of morbidity in the pediatric population, estimated from 3% to 7% of the general population. Its presentation is multifaceted. School failure, behavioral disorders, and clumsiness are common presenting features.

The focus in this chapter is on "cognitive" learning disability as opposed to the learning disabilities resulting from attention deficit disorders (ADD) or hyperactivity and the learning disabilities resulting from global developmental delay or retardation. However, it should be clearly understood that there is a considerable overlap between these various etiologies, and the "final common pathway" of a learning disability has several possible precursors in addition to the cognitive problems discussed in this chapter.

PATHOPHYSIOLOGY

From the neurologic perspective, the most concrete data have come from the work of Geschwind and Galaburda (Duffy and Geschwind, 1985). "Disconnection syndromes" in the brain have been demonstrated in adults following stroke, and "disconnections" in the form of heterotopias have been found in the brains of learning disabled individuals following accidental death. This anatomic variability demonstrated neuropathologically may relate to the behavioral characteristics delineated by the neuropsychologist, including such specific areas of difficulty as attention, memory, reasoning, communication, reading, writing, spelling, calculation, social competence, and emotional maturation. Learning disabilities are not due primarily to visual, hearing, or motor handicaps, mental retardation, emotional disturbance, or environmental disadvantage, although they may occur concurrently. A strong familial pattern has been noted in the expression of learning disability and, as with infantile autism and ADD, males are predominantly affected. However, it is obvious that environmental factors have a considerable influence on the phenotypic expression of various learning disabilities, and parental attitudes and behaviors as well as parental genes influence the success or failure of a child with learning disabilities.

CLINICAL PRESENTATION

Recognition of the child with a cognitive learning disability, in contrast to the child with ADD, occurs when the parent or educator assesses skills at the preschool or early school level. Approximately one third of children with cognitive learning disabilities have motor problems characterized by clumsiness, left–right confusion, and eye–hand coordination problems so that they may be slightly delayed in walking and may develop expected motor skills (such as throwing or catching a ball or riding a bicycle) poorly or late. They are frequently the last chosen in intramural athletics and their problems with motor performance add to the low self-esteem that they develop quickly when confronted with their learning problems in the school setting.

In view of the paucity of data on the intrinsic nature of learning disabilities, various classifications are available. Perhaps the most widely used, if not the most sophisticated from an etiologic standpoint, is the current classification in the *Diagnostic and Statistical Manual of Mental Disorders* (DSM-III):

1. Attention deficit disorder (see Chap. 34)
2. Developmental reading disorder
3. Developmental arithmetic disorder
4. Developmental language disorder
   a. Expressive type
   b. Receptive type
5. Developmental articulation disorder
6. Mixed specific developmental disorder
7. Atypical specific developmental disorder

This classification equates developmental reading disorder with dyslexia and considers there to be a significant reading impairment in children between 8 to 13 years if there is a 1- to 2-year discrepancy in reading skill to chronological or mental age. As the time of acquisition of basic reading skills varies widely, it is preferable to avoid a clear designation of dyslexia or reading disability prior to the age of 7 or 8. Although not a component of learning disability *per se*, emotional problems such as low self-esteem, depression, and withdrawn and apathetic behavior are frequently present. There may also be aggressive or acting-out behavior as a result of frustration with the education process or parental expectations.

DIFFERENTIAL DIAGNOSIS

By definition, cognitive learning disabilities exclude specific causes that make the acquisition of reading, arithmetic, language, or articulation skills difficult or impossible such as vision, hearing or motor handicaps as well as psychiatric disturbance, global mental retardation, and environmental disadvantage.

The most controversial differential diagnosis is that of an underlying neurologic disorder. In the 1960s, the term *brain damage* was frequently used interchangeably with learning disability, because certain patterns of functioning ("scatter" or variable performance) on psychological subtests were considered similar to the patterns of performance demonstrated in patients who had recovered from acquired traumatic injury to the brain. Subsequent study has more strongly suggested a pattern of developmental delay in the development of certain cognitive skills such as reading and arithmetic, although some inconsistent performance is seen occasionally in both the injured brain and the learning-disabled child. However, the correlation between prior brain injury, such as perinatal asphyxia, postnatal meningitis, or head trauma with cognitive learning disability is not high.

Psychiatric disturbance is another controversial differential diagnosis. All too frequently the child with poor cognitive performance in the classroom is considered to have a motivational or discipline problem suggesting an underlying psychiatric disturbance. Determining the primary condition is often a chicken-or-egg problem because school failure quickly leads to low self-esteem, depression, frustration, and acting-out behavior.

Global mental retardation is distinguished from learning disabilities by a uniform delay in all areas of cognitive development, in contrast to the scattered areas of strength and weakness illustrated by the learning disabled child. The mentally retarded child acts more or less like a younger child, whereas the learning-disabled child has striking inconsistencies in performance.

WORK-UP

The evaluation and treatment of learning disabilities is best managed with an interdisciplinary team approach ideally including teachers, psychologists, pediatricians and pediatric neurologists, as well as speech and language pathologists, psychiatrists, occupational therapists, and social workers. This interdisciplinary activity may be informal or formal depending on the location of one's practice. Informally, one should utilize past evaluations and recognize that medical evaluation and management is only one part of a multifaceted approach to the learning-disabled child. Formally, there exists in many communities the opportunity for comprehensive interdisciplinary evaluation of learning-disabled children through specialized programs based in school districts, hospital outpatient clinics, or private settings. Although the primary care pediatrician cannot expect to master the intricacies of the psychological testing, the pediatrician can prove valuable or detrimental in the proper management of the child. Insofar as the pediatrician explores community resources and selects competent services for referral, together with maintaining an ac-

tive interest as the child's advocate, the child will benefit; if the pediatrician abdicates this role and fosters a pessimistic approach, the child will either remain incompletely evaluated or improperly managed. Alternatively, the parents may gravitate to the practitioners of unproven therapies and expensive, fad-oriented approaches that prey on parents anxious for remediation.

History

A careful family history often reveals learning disabilities and should be carefully explored. The history of development of motor and language milestones is also important as language and motor delays are frequently present. Additionally, one should inquire into current patterns of behavior, peer relations, school strengths and weaknesses, and home activities and hobbies.

Physical Examination

A physical examination may show some mild dysmorphic features, such as abnormal dermatoglyphics. Particular attention is paid to the visual, auditory, and tactile sensory examination, as specific sensory deficits can mask as learning disabilities. Subtle motor signs suggestive of delayed maturation (such as clumsiness), choreoathetoid movements of the upper extremities (particularly when the arms are held outstretched or when the patient is asked to run), difficulty with rapid alternating motions and other tests of fine motor coordination, errors in cortical sensory tests (such as stereognosis and graphaesthesia), are often present. The basic pediatric hearing and vision screening evaluations are, of course, essential parts of the examination.

Laboratory Tests

Even though psychological testing is expensive and time-consuming, any child in whom there is a strong suspicion of learning disabilities should be evaluated by a qualified clinical psychologist. The tests selected by the psychologist depend on the age of the patient and the presenting learning difficulties, but frequently include the Stanford–Binet or Wechsler intelligence tests or the Peabody Picture Vocabulary Test. These tests, however, may be inappropriate for a child with language deficit, and thus more specialized tests may be administered. An aid to referral is a screening evaluation by the pediatrician. Such a screening evaluation could include a test of reading, such as the Gilmore Oral Reading Test (reading and answering questions regarding short, grade-appropriate paragraphs), a test of perceptual-motor skills, such as the Berry–Buitanika Test of Visual Motor Integration (copying figures of increasing complexity such as a circle for 3-year-olds, a triangle for 5-year-olds, a diamond for 8-year-olds) and the Denver Developmental Screening Test for children under the age of 6. Any interpretation of test results should be tentative and should take into account the child's past history of educational progress and environmental stress.

At present, electrophysiologic evaluation of children with learning disabilities has limited diagnostic usefulness. An electroencephalograph (EEG) may be useful to distinguish between those children who are inattentive from seizure activity, either abortive focal seizure activity or generalized (petit mal) and those who are unresponsive related to anxiety, auditory processing problems, or distractibility. A number of EEGs in normal children may be read as "borderline" and unless convincing paroxysmal unresponsiveness or inappropriate behavior is noted, anticonvulsant medication is not indicated. Evoked potential testing, primarily of utility in the testing of vision and hearing in very young or retarded children, has research interest but little clinical use at this time. Likewise, the Brain Electrical Activity Mapping (BEAM) has considerable research interest, but presently has unproven clinical use.

PRINCIPLES OF MANAGEMENT

Allocation of the pediatrician's time in the office setting is an important initial consideration in the management of the learning-disabled child. Because learning disabilities are complex, controversial, and present a chronic pattern of school difficulties interspersed with crisis periods relating to new school settings, parent–teacher controversies, and secondary emotional distress, these issues are difficult to resolve in the usual length of time for general pediatric visits. Depending on the interests and practice patterns of the pediatrician, special time may be set aside for a 1-hour initial session, and subsequent visits may be ½ hour or more. Regardless of where the evaluation is performed, the pediatrician should have a good knowledge of the community resources available for the evaluation and subsequent management of the child. By law (PL 94-142), school districts are required to

evaluate and provide an adequate program of remediation for all children with prominent learning disabilities. Private programs have a distinct advantage as mediators when controversy exists (as is not infrequently the case) between parental expectation and school assessment of a child's appropriate educational placement.

Considerable controversy exists regarding the "correction" of motor deficits as an aid to enhancing educational progress. Eye movement exercises and vestibular stimulation are two therapies where efficacy is currently questioned.

Unlike the use of medication in the treatment of many children with ADD disorders, the role of medication in children with cognitive learning disabilities is much more limited. If attention deficits coexist and do not appear to be secondary to anxiety or problems with language or memory difficulties, medications may be used (see Chap. 34). Medication may again be indicated if emotional lability or depression is a feature. In the former case, methylphenidate, pemoline, or imipramine may be used. In the latter, imipramine or amitriptyline may be useful.

INDICATIONS FOR REFERRAL

As discussed, the evaluation and management of the learning-disabled child is an interdisciplinary process and depends on the local facilities and the nature and the degree of the learning disability. Children over 2 years of age with language delays and normal hearing should be referred for a speech and language evaluation. Children with gross and fine motor delays and apparent difficulty with following directions and socialization may benefit from a "zero-to-three" infant stimulation program. After the age of 3, if speech and language or learning problems are present, a preschool program including a psychological assessment and input from special educators, speech and language pathologists, as well as physical and occupational therapists, may be indicated. Subsequent school programs for learning-disabled children include both self-contained classrooms for children with prominent learning disabilities who require a full-time program of remediation, or resource room placement for one or several hours each day where the learning-disabled child receives assistance in reading or other cognitive tasks. Ongoing assistance is also usually available in the school from clinical psychologists, social workers, and counselors who periodically evaluate or offer supportive psychotherapy for the child.

PATIENT EDUCATION

After psychological testing has been reviewed, it is important to emphasize the child's areas of strengths to the parents and to encourage successful experiences for the child in those areas in which they do well. For example, a child with poor co-ordination and good cognitive but poor reading skills may not enjoy competitive team sports. However, this child may enjoy individual sports such as swimming or hiking and activities such as Boy Scouts and museum visiting. The parent frequently assumes the role of the tutor for the learning-disabled child. Although this has some limited value, it often leads to frustration and recrimination on both sides when things do not go well. The parent should be advised to limit, if possible, extra academic work at home and if special homework projects are required, to engage a tutor (who could be an interested high-school student) as a more objective enhancer of the child's progress.

ANNOTATED BIBLIOGRAPHY

Accardo P: A Neurodevelopmental Perspective on Specific Learning Disabilities. Baltimore, University Park Press, 1980 (Excellent critical review of the neurodevelopmental perspective in learning disabilities.)

Brutten M, Richardson SO, Mangel C: Something's Wrong with My Child. New York, Harcourt Brace, 1973 (Excellent guide for the parent and other interested laypeople regarding learning disabilities.)

Duffy H, Geschwind N: Dyslexia, A Neuroscientific Approach to Clinical Evaluation. Boston, Little Brown, 1985 (Presentation of recent research and new diagnostic aids as well as an historical perspective of learning disabilities.)

Frederiks JAM (ed.): Handbook of Clinical Neurology, vol 2 (46): Neurobehavioral Disorders. Chaps 4, 5, and 7. New York, Elsevier, 1985 (Comprehensive discussions of clinical presentation and evaluation of aspects of learning disabilities.)

Gabel S, Erickson M: Child Development and Developmental Disabilities. Boston, Little Brown, 1979 (Comprehensive textbook written from the interdisciplinary standpoint with various specialists contributing to an overview of normal and pathologic development, including learning disabilities.)

Gaddes WH: Learning Disabilities and Brain Function, 2nd ed. New York, Springer, 1985 (Learning disabilities viewed from the neuropsychological perspective with much information on the appropriateness and effectiveness of test results.)

Kinsbourne M, Kaplan P: Children's Learning and Attention Problems. Boston, Little Brown, 1979 (Sensitive and practical guide to evaluation and management.)

Rapin I: Children with Brain Dysfunction. New York, Raven, 1982 (Well-written perspective on some of the more complex areas of language and cognition from the standpoint of etiology and evaluation; written for the practicing pediatrician.)

40
School Phobia and School Refusal

DAVID VAN BUSKIRK

When a physically healthy child fails to attend school, the primary care physician may be puzzled by the inconsistent attitudes brought to him. For example, the pediatrician may find the child unconcerned, the parents greatly frustrated, and the school ready to take action. The pediatrician must determine the origins and nature of the reaction in order to assess such a complicated situation. Despite the various manifestations, the same issues relating to separation underlie both school phobia and school refusal. The peak incidences occur when children leave a familiar situation to begin elementary or junior high schools.

PSYCHOLOGICAL MECHANISMS

Separation anxiety is normal in the infant and toddler. A child cries, clings, refuses to get out of the car, and may develop somatic symptoms such as a stomach ache in response to the anxiety over separation. The very young child links survival to the availability of mothering and the loss of mother is as terrifying as the prospect of death. The first encounter of the child with the extended and regular separations demanded by nursery school or kindergarten tests the thoroughness of mastery derived from early, briefer separations.

The child who is vulnerable to separation is so overwhelmed by the stress of such separation that he activates an intertwined series of defense mechanisms, particularly regression, displacement, and avoidance. Regressed as he is, he feels immersed in the psychic state of being 2 years old, an age when feelings and thoughts have magical powers. His anger is so intense that he fears it may destroy the mother who sent him away to school. Displacement diverts the strong feeling of upset and rage from his mother to his school. This defensive step amounts to converting the school into the cause of separation, perceiving the school as a hostile and dangerous place. Thus, the school is the incidental recipient of this displacement of the child's intolerable feelings. On other occasions the hostile or dangerous object might be strange dogs or dark rooms. No logic can dislodge such phobic conviction. Once the vulnerable child has created a phobia incorporating all the power derived from his belief that loss of his mother is equivalent to death, a most formidable pattern of avoidance has entered the life of the child, his family, and his school.

The young child who becomes school phobic has a pre-existing characterological and possibly biologic vulnerability antedating symptoms connected to school. Current symptoms may have their roots in life experiences occurring during the second year of life, which is a crucial time for the mastery of strong affect in connection with separation and individuation. Severe stresses during that developmental period such as the birth of a sibling, the departure of a father, a life-threatening illness, or the death of a grandparent leave an indelible imprint on the psychological development of the toddler. Such interruptions in the usual flow of preschool life thwart the mastery of fluid separations and reunions.

The older child who fails to attend school presents a different picture. While progressing through primary school, he has outgrown much of his parent's influence on his behavior. By puberty, the child's own control over school attendance is far greater. For preteens and high-school students, the preferred diagnostic label is now *school refusal* to emphasize the conscious motivation of such children not to attend school. In the younger children, one presupposes a predominantly unconscious mechanism with anxiety and fear usually evident.

Older children demonstrate a *dislike* of school, disavowing those same feelings that are so overwhelming to the young phobic.

There are two dissimilar groups among older school refusers. One group of the older *refusers* are antisocial young teenagers who may already be substance abusers or involved with the juvenile courts. Their school refusal is often referred to as truancy, because they appear to show minimal anxiety or fear related to school avoidance. A second group persists in manifesting early separation problems and as these children enter adolescence, they become generally more anxious, constricted, and avoidant.

Immediate Precipitating Stresses

Since separation is so important to the syndrome of school phobia and refusal, it is not surprising that the current loss of a parent (by disease, death, marital disruption, or geographic distance) is the most common immediate precipitant or stressor. Those children who were overwhelmed by earlier losses will be more vulnerable to regression when such trauma occurs subsequently.

In other children, a phobic reaction may develop subsequent to a somatic illness as minor as an upper respiratory infection or as major as neoplasms or multiple fractures. Symptoms, in some cases, seem to be far out of proportion to the minimal stress.

Mediating the development of the symptom of school phobia or school refusal requires the participation of the school itself. A susceptible child's anxiety can be raised by starting school (phobias are most common in the first months of the school year), transferring to a new school, or changing teachers. The capacity of a school to react with support but firm expectations that the child is to once again behave appropriately for his age may lessen symptomatic phobic behavior.

PRESENTATION

The initial complaint to the primary care physician is frequently of a somatic nature. The sore throat, stomach ache, anorexia, or vomiting that may be symptoms of acute separation anxiety may distract the physician temporarily from the underlying situation. A careful history unmasks the crucial timing: the stomach hurts before breakfast and disappears when the child returns home at the end of the school day, or the headache never occurs on a weekend. It is important for the physician to reconstruct the essential family and life events behind these symptoms. He should inquire about the loss of a parent by death or family disruption, about the arrival of new siblings, about illnesses in any of the family, about moves to new dwellings, and about changes in school.

DIFFERENTIAL DIAGNOSIS AND WORK-UP

Somatic Illnesses

Since the child who presents as phobic most frequently will have somatic complaints, laboratory tests such as complete blood counts and throat cultures are commonly the first step both in ruling out organic illness and in assisting the physician in communicating the degree of his own concern to parents whose fears of organic disease are sometimes concrete. School-initiated behavioral programs commence with the premise that the physical springs from the emotional, that sending a child to school will not neglect the treatment of a physical illness in that child. Nonmedical care-givers responsible for subsequent management need reassurance that there is no evidence for somatic illness.

Childhood Depression

Child psychiatrists have become sensitized to the occurrence of depression in children. Failure to attend school may occasionally be observed as a manifestation of this complex disorder even when the more common signs of depression are not apparent. The presence of withdrawal, isolation from peers, sleep disturbances (difficulty falling asleep, awakening in the midst of sleep, as well as difficulty arising), tearfulness, vulnerability to rejection, low energy, and low self-esteem are strongly suggestive of this syndrome not only in children but also in adults. In a childhood depressive reaction, persistent sad facial expressions, erratic moods with periods of great activity, and aggressive behavior may also be present.

Psychotic Children

Bizarre behavior indicating self-absorption is the most common presenting symptom of the autistic or schizophrenic child. Observant adults notice twirling, echolalia, or public masturbation at school, in the street, or at home.

Anxiety Disorders

Psychiatric nosology classifies many different symptom clusters under adult anxiety disorders, but there is no consensus as to whether it is useful to distinguish the more generally anxious and inhibited children from the phobic ones. Follow-up of these groups of children into adult life has revealed that a significant number of phobic or refusing children will later become agoraphobic or substantially impaired by psychiatric disorders. The nervous systems of phobic children are apparently unable to handle extreme anxiety. Whatever the combination of nature (central nervous system proclivity) and nurture (prior stresses), these children are vulnerable to stresses that involve separation.

Sexual or Physical Abuse

The avoidance of school may stem from a persistently traumatic interaction at home. The intimidation of the child by an abusive parent or other adult can become a way of life. Inhibition may spread to any area of the child's existence in which incest or alcohol or domestic violence might be revealed, and the child stays home to keep secrets hidden.

PRINCIPLES OF MANAGEMENT

Recent onset school phobia is an emergency. Various studies of this condition have demonstrated that the younger child with recent onset of failure to attend responds to immediate interventions while any delay in intervention leads to greater resistance. In his first telephone contact the pediatrician can discuss with the parents steps toward identifying any possible physical illness and support immediate school collaboration to effect a rapid return of the child to class.

After further evaluation and familiarity with the situation, he may suggest tolerance for such symptomatic behavior as vomiting after breakfast. Permission to have pain (or perhaps to throw up) will give the child support in his mastery of the fear of separating. The pediatrician's message is that strong feelings as well as physical discomfort can be lived with as part of growing up. Precipitating events (e.g., a recent marital quarrel, a fight at school, or viral illness) need not be pursued in depth until after the avoidant behavior is being corrected.

Parental Involvement

The parents of a child with a school attendance problem should be involved immediately and urgently in the attempt to return the child to school. When the primary care pediatrician encounters a child who has been out of school, he must include both parents in helping to develop a more comprehensive plan. For example, the pediatrician might suggest a shift of the responsibility for delivering the phobic child to the school from the mother to the father. It is important to support the parent's participation in whatever team approach the school may initiate. The unconscious fostering of avoidance by the anxious parent can be counterbalanced when parents join with other adults who share the objective of returning the child to school at the earliest possible time.

School Intervention

In many communities, public schools are sensitized to the need for rapid intervention and may only rely on the pediatrician to assess the physical state of the child. Once that assessment demonstrates no organic disease, the school system, through an integrated team including parents, teacher, school psychologist, nurse, and administrator, may develop a series of increasing expectations of attendance using a behavioral protocol. An experienced school system is ready to go to court for legal support if the parents fail in their efforts to get a child back into school.

INDICATIONS FOR REFERRAL

Two weeks is an adequate trial of unassisted school-based intervention in situations where there is no immediate physical illness or emotional trauma. If progress has not occurred during that time, the pediatrician should consider a referral to a mental health specialist.

Other indications for referral would be related more to the nature of the child or family than with the failure of an initial concerted effort to correct behavior. The suspicion of either childhood depression or psychosis as well as the possibility of abuse or other substantial family issues are reasons for referral to a child psychiatrist. Comprehensive psychiatric care progresses from treating the acute phobic symptoms to dynamic therapy with the aim of lessening the impairment of emotional and cognitive development. The pediatrician has a key role in supporting the commitment of the family during the process of transition from crisis to long-term care.

A child psychiatrist might use one of the tricyclic medications (*e.g.*, Imipramine, up to 2.5 mg/ kg daily) for a school-aged child whose anxiety does not respond to other interventions. This is the preferred psychopharmacologic approach since the benzodiazepams do not treat underlying depression, frequently require larger and larger doses, and do not produce longstanding substantial improvement. Current opinion holds that it is the antianxiety or antipanic rather than the antidepressant property of a tricyclic agent that is effective in phobic disorders.

Psychotherapy, as family or as individual play therapy, is indicated for many of the phobic or school-refusing children. The phobic child may turn out to be the expressor of an overwhelming family discord, and the focus of care may move from the child's fear of school to the mother and father's troubled relationship.

The longest follow-up study of school phobia indicates that school phobic children may follow a deteriorating spiral from primary school phobia to high school refusal to adult behavioral constriction including agoraphobia. An early working through of the dynamics of separation and loss can prevent such future disability.

ANNOTATED BIBLIOGRAPHY

Blagg NR, Yule W: The Behavioral Treatment of School Refusal—A Comparative Study. Behav Res Ther 22 (2): 119, 1984 (Carefully designed protocol for school refusal with rapid and successful results.)

Coolidge J et al: A Ten-Year Follow-Up Study of Sixty-six School Phobic Children. Am J Orthopsychiatry 34:674–684, 1964 (This group was followed through acute and long-term difficulties. The study demonstrates the need for a guarded prognosis where phobia or refusal persists.)

Hersov L, Berg I (eds): Out of School. New York, John Wiley & Sons, 1980 (Most comprehensive overview of the subject with excellent chapters on several aspects. See particularly Waller D, Eisenberg L: School Refusal in Childhood—a Psychiatric–Pediatric Perspective; Lewis M: Psychotherapeutic Treatment in School Refusal; Gittleman–Klein R, Klein D: Separation Anxiety in School Refusal and its Treatment with Drugs. (An overview of the psychopharmacologic management.)

Kolvin I, Berney TP, Bhate SR: Classification and Diagnosis of Depression in School Phobia. Br J Psychiatry 145:347, 1984 (Older children with school phobic symptoms reveal a disproportionate number of symptoms consistent with childhood depression.)

Waldron S Jr et al: School Phobia and Other Childhood Neuroses: A Systematic Study of the Children and Their Families. Am J Psychiatry 132:8, 1975 (Twice as many school phobic children compared with other neurotic children show excessive separation anxiety, dependency and depression.)

41
School Failure
MURRAY M. KAPPELMAN

In addition to the child's physical and emotional health, parents correctly expect that the primary health care-giver will also advocate for the child's educational health with equal expertise and enthusiasm. If one considers the community within which the child and family live and interact, who better should take the objective role as an investigator and source finder in cases of school failure than the child's personal physician? It, therefore, becomes imperative that the pediatrician become aware and knowledgeable regarding the potential "failure factors" possible in the children whose grades plummet and whose achievement is inadequate.

Zuckerman has designed an outline created to provide a framework on which the physician can insert information gleaned from appropriate and relevant questions and begin the process of diagnosis, referral, and remediation in the case of an individual child's school failure. Modifications and additions to the original proposed outline have been made to expand and clarify the etiologies of poor school performance in the school-aged child.

LEVEL OF MATURITY

Could the child have entered school at too early an age (see Chap. 37)? This is a fairly common problem in the early grades. The child whose birthday is in November or December, but who is registered for school with other children born potentially 11 months earlier, may be less prepared for the pace or the social and educational demands of a system geared for children at a more advanced level of age and maturity. Each child develops educational skills at his own pace; some move quickly, others more slowly. The ultimate result is usually the same—each reaching a satisfactory range of assimilating and adapting information at some point during the first few years of school. If a youngster has entered school at an early age and has normal but relatively sluggish learning skills or emotional adaptability, the child may find the peer group advancing at a more rapid pace. This child could easily fail despite serious and earnest efforts to succeed. This child wants to be like the peer group, to do well in school, and not to be the slowest in the class; but he cannot "put it all together" at quite the same rate as the slightly older peers. The result may be anger, frustration, withdrawal, and, ultimately, failure which may adversely influence the child's later education.

As the child's pediatrician, what do you recommend in this situation? One must balance the potential impact on the child of "holding him back" one year versus the continuing frustration of the youngster trying to race with a peer crowd faster and more mature. If social and learning maturity are the key factors in the child's early grade failure, then suggesting that the child be retained to repeat the early grade successfully could have several positive features. Having experienced the material before, the child will likely experience success and esteem the second year. In addition, the child's age will be more in keeping with that of the older youngsters in the new cohort in terms of social maturity, peer acceptance, and coordination in games and sports. When appropriate, the immature child could benefit clearly from repeating the year in a very early grade. The key issue for the pediatrician is to be sure that this recommended approach is not viewed as a failure on the part of the teachers, parents, or child. Everyone must be convinced, after careful analysis, that the suggestion is merely for a delay and reassignment to a more appropriate group according to the age and level of learning maturity. A vital rule of communication between parent and the failing child in this situation is optimism. The pediatrician's role after suggesting the potential school response is to protect the child's self-esteem.

NEUROLOGICALLY BASED SENSORY AND MOTOR DISTURBANCES

Hearing Impairment

Many professionals and parents are unaware what an isolating handicap severe hearing impairment can be to the growing child. This is particularly true with congenital deafness or severe hearing loss with associated impaired language formation. Communication with the outside world has been cut off through two of the most sensitive modalities; hearing and speech.

The child with congenital deafness and poor speech formation is usually diagnosed long before entry into a school situation requiring pass/fail criteria. These youngsters are often sent to separate classes or schools within which attention is paid to the child's need for alternative teaching techniques, speech development, and socialization skills enhancement.

The youngster who presents the challenge to the pediatrician is the child who is failing because of diminished hearing acuity due to congenital or acquired reasons that are not serious enough to identify the child during preschool play. Acquired diminished hearing may result from trauma, sequelae to bacterial meningitis, persistent or recurrent otitis media, or foreign material in the outer ear canal. The post-rubeola hearing loss is now rarely seen due to rubeola prevention programs. It is the pediatrician's responsibility to attempt to diagnose these losses BEFORE the school failure and clearly not to overlook the possibility after the child receives poor grades.

Visual Impairment

Serious visual impairment or blindness will be diagnosed long before school in most cases; however, more subtle but significant visual abnormalities such as myopia, hyperopia, astigmatism, and significant strabismus can be missed and form the basis of a child's failure within the school situation. Appropriate office screening at 4 years of age and attention to eye muscle movement and coordination with each physician/child contact will alert the pediatrician that trouble exists that could lead to reduced acuity with resultant poor school performance. A thorough assessment of potential visual impairments using a history and an examination and visual screening should clearly be a part of every pediatrician's work-up of the failing child.

Motor Impairment

The child with cerebral palsy or hypotonic syndromes is rarely missed until school time. The pediatrician faces the task of working with the parents and the school system to find the educationally and motorically ideal school setting for the child with motor handicaps. So much has been accomplished by children growing into productive adulthood with severe motor problems that anything less than a herculean effort by parent, child, pediatrician, and school system to help the child reach maximum potential is unacceptable at this time.

COGNITIVE DISORDERS

Mental Retardation

The pediatrician will find the differentiation between the child with mild mental retardation from the peer with learning disabilities or emotional/situational problems to be difficult. Generally, the youngster whose development has been sufficiently slow to warrant the label of moderate to severe and profound retardation has come to the attention of the parents and the pediatrician during regular office visits when history, observation, and such tests as the Denver Developmental Screening Test are employed as part of the child's assessment. Moderate to severe brain dysfunction resulting in childhood autism must also be distinguished from mental retardation because of the somewhat different prognosis in some cases and the educational approach in most. Mental retardation is static but deserves the correct educational approach; autism (usually neurologic rather than emotional) can be dynamic, and correct approaches may make a considerable difference in the ultimate educational and social level of performance.

The pediatrician should be alerted to the potential of mild mental retardation when there is a lag or dysfunction in the growing youngster's levels of fine-motor coordination and more complex speech development (use of pronouns, syntax development, association of words and shapes). School failure may be the first sign of slow development at the level of mild mental retardation. The work-up of the failing child will include the referral to the clinical psychologist. The pediatrician becomes the child's advocate for maximal mainstreaming with appropriate resource in areas needing special assistance in learning. Vocational training that begins early to create independent citizens may also require encouragement from the pediatrician working closely with the school system.

Minimal Brain Dysfunction

Specific Learning Disabilities. It is estimated that between 5% and 10% of school children suffer from specific learning disabilities sufficiently serious to affect their learning. Specific learning disabilities are dealt with in Chapter 39; however, in this section, consideration must be given to prevention and diagnosis because it relates so clearly to school failure. The learning-disabled child awakens every morning painfully aware that he will be going to class to "fail" often despite an innate sense that better work could be done but is being blocked and detoured outside of the child's control.

Prevention of failure from specific learning disabilities is based definitively on early suspicion and diagnosis. Recent work suggests that language development not only plays a key role in the expressive language area but also in the area of reading. Dyslexia is more often a result of abnormalities in the auditory-verbal perceptual axis than related to visual-motor difficulties as previously believed. Delayed speech development, early signs of poor coordination, clumsiness beyond the norm, impaired use of writing instruments and toys, delayed fine-motor development (tying shoes, buttoning buttons)—these are but a small list of clues that alert the pediatrician to watch this child for subsequent school problems and then take specific action. Overt developmental signs pointing to future learning disability can be referred earlier than the preschool years; however, most youngsters can wait until peer group interaction and expectations suggest the diagnosis. This means early action so that proper educational assistance can be programmed for the learning-disabled child.

Currently, there are two nonstandardized but useful screening tests that measure the neuromaturational development of children at various ages which have been designed for pediatricians to administer and score. These tests are Levine's Pediatric Early Educational Readiness (PEER: ages 5 to 7) Test and the later Pediatric Early Elementary Examination (PEEX: ages 7 to 9) plus Shaywitz's Yale Neuromaturational Screening Test. These instruments do not provide valid "numbers": They are designed to make the pediatrician more aware that a specific child may have learning disabilities and that further investigation may be required using standardized instruments. They are screening instruments for the pediatric office. These tests do not, in any way, replace the psychologist's standardized tests, the educator's instruments, or the speech pathologist's important screening.

The longer the pediatrician waits to make this diagnosis and begin remediation, the more often the child will see "Failure" on his report card, and the more educational and emotional hurdles will be constructed to prevent satisfactory educational and emotional outcome for the child.

Attention Deficit Disorder. Clearly, too many overly active youngsters who are doing poorly in school are labeled as attention deficit disorder (ADD) children. The challenge to the pediatrician is to analyze carefully each case and, if appropriate, refer to other professionals expert in learning and behavior problems in children. The diagnosis of ADD is best made after considerable thought and after working with a team of experts. Poor attention span, impulsivity, inability to finish tasks, and easy distractibility are components of this "syndrome" that may be present without excessive or misdirected activity. Any one or combination of these behaviors can obviously lead to poor performance in the school setting and eventual failure (see Chap. 34).

Psychoactive drugs (Ritalin, Dexedrine, Cylert) have demonstrated satisfactory results at controlling the activity and attention issues in most children if monitored carefully; however, unless the other elements often associated with this problem (specific perceptual weaknesses, peer and family rejection, emotional overlay, speech problems, medical issues, sense of low self-worth) are addressed simultaneously with the medication, the pediatrician may merely be slowing the child down to better recognize his failures.

ENVIRONMENTAL INTERFERENCE

Poor School Environment

Several issues may play a role in creating a school environment that is conducive to failure in a specific child, and these possibilities should be investigated. Clearly, poor instruction looms large as a potential for inadequate information transfer; however, this is too often the first accusation made by the parent without a school visit and first-hand observation. In actuality, poor teaching ranks low on the list of frequent causes of school failure among children in the educational system. The adequate child often learns despite the teacher in some cases. A poorly-controlled, noisy classroom could be another cause. Personality conflicts, real or imagined, between teacher and child can form the basis of diminishing motivation to perform and they can result in a poor report card. If a child is bullied or shunned, this may create emotional barriers to learning in an environment perceived to be hostile by the child. The pediatrician, by talking to parent, teacher, and child (alone) may uncover one of these as possible reasons for the school failure.

Education Not in the Dominant Language

This has become a serious problem in our current school system, particularly in the lower grades. The young child is confronted with English as the dominant language of communication after preschool years of another language being the primary or exclusive form of verbal interchange. Quick answers cannot be given to this problem. The parents' English is often poor to nonexistent. The school must start with these youngsters as bilingual, with English clearly the weaker of the two languages. The pediatrician can alert those parents of the impending problem and encourage them to teach their children to speak English. If no progress is being made in the bilingual equilibrium of the child, the pediatrician needs to alert the school of the child's special language needs. Schools often make accommodations; occasionally, the family is isolated in an English-speaking world.

School Absence

This problem has three basic causalities requiring investigation by the pediatrician. The first reason for persistent significant school absence is chronic illness in the child. At times, these absences are unavoidable (*e.g.*, severe asthmatics), but too frequently the parents keep the chronically ill child away from school too long after an illness and too often when he only has minor symptoms. In the former, home teaching can be suggested by the pediatrician; in the latter, the pediatrician needs to educate the parents and lower their level of anxiety. Parents must realize that their child is subject to the serious potential problem of educational deprivation.

The second school absence occurs when the parent, due to personal or social crises, is unable or unwilling to ensure that the child attends school. The depressed parent, the recently separated single parent, the rural farming parent needing extra hands are examples of parents who inappropriately and willingly encourage or suggest school absence. The pediatrician will need assistance from the social work professional to deal with these parents. Poverty and lack of school clothing is another social reason why children stay away from school, re-

creating the cycle of lack of education, poor job potential, and low incomes.

Truancy is the third reason for frequent school absences. This increases with the increase in age and grade. If the child stays away from school in this manner, it need not be sociopathic behavior; it may indicate trouble within the school environment. This trouble could be learning disabilities with persistent failure, serious emotional or physical taunting or teasing, sexual harassment or panic, drugs or alcohol, unannounced pregnancy, or merely a serious problem with self-esteem realistically or unrealistically based on intellect, appearance, or sociability. It is essential to regard truancy as a signal and work with the parents and the school to discover the basic reasons behind the willing withdrawal from the learning environment. Returning the young person to the same environment without working on remediating the underlying concerns only leads to truancy, recidivism, and early school dropout. This is the ultimate school failure.

Family Dysfunction

The child who has family issues on his mind and cannot concentrate on schoolwork will most likely have problems with his school performance. Poor school performance commonly accompanies parental separation and divorce, illness of a close family member, the death of a loved one, physical violence within the household, the involvement of a family member with police with or without incarceration, family incapacity due to drugs or alcohol, and disruption due to a family member moving away (*e.g.*, father in service). These family issues are examples of common child concerns that crowd out the information to be learned from the child's thought processes. These problems often only require quick medical and educational assessment of the family situation; but, on occasion, a one-on-one interview with the child (sometimes several to build trust) will be necessary to uncover the basic anxiety that is preventing learning and precipitating school failure.

As noted above, the very dysfunctional family often cannot see school as a priority; therefore, the child misses school so often that failure ensues. Another serious issue in this type of family is the poor role modeling toward educational achievement and often the low priority given to educational achievement. This is a "no-win" situation as long as the child remains in such a household.

The pediatrician often makes the diagnosis and may be able to assist in the resolution of some family issues; more often, however, he needs the assistance of other professionals (*e.g.*, social worker, protective services, psychiatry, lawyers, and so forth) to deliver the comprehensive family remediation needed to relieve the child's anxiety and permit the youngster's attention to be redirected toward learning in school.

EMOTIONAL DISORDER

Lack of Motivation

Motivation often stems from family enthusiasm over learning and solid home role models. Even with these in place, however, some children appear to lack the motivation to learn. More careful investigation will often reveal that the lack of motivation shields the child from his own poor self-concept as a learner, his fear of failure in a family with high standards, competition from siblings, underlying undiagnosed learning disabilities, or interest in areas far removed from those taught within the school environment. "He just doesn't care about getting good grades" may be one of the most dangerous statements that can be made about a failing child. Of course, he cares; why he is doing poorly in school is the issue that must be discovered by the team of parent, teacher, and pediatrician.

"Bad Crowd" Syndrome

A frequent complaint by parents and teachers is that a young person has begun to do poorly in school because he associates with a group of peers who are also doing poorly in school, who are truant, or who are school dropouts. This argument does have solid bases in the school performance slide of some youngsters; however, the pediatrician must remember that the young person may have selected his friends because of his perception of their similarity to himself. He is living a self-fulfilling prophecy of his own learning inadequacy. The reasons for this may need the pediatrician's attention rather than the "bad crowd."

Depression

Poor school performance is a cardinal sign in the depressed youngster and adolescent. It may be one of the first and only signs before the child takes major self-destructive action. The unexpected decline in school grades in the older child clearly points toward an investigation of the young person's state of emotional well-being. Whether the depression is endogenous or acutely situational in origin, the sudden falling school grades must cause the team of parent, teacher, and pediatrician to investigate the young person's status and refer for treatment expediently if depression is the apparent cause of the poor school performance (see also Chap. 35).

Psychosis/Thought Disorder

Again, one of the early signs of serious emotional illness may be withdrawal from learning within the school environment and school failure. Careful questioning by teacher and pediatrician should uncover a child with disordered thinking and a dysfunctional mental status requiring intensive therapy often within residential settings where the young person's educational needs are addressed simultaneously with the emotional rehabilitation. The pediatrician has the responsibility to make the diagnosis and initiate the expedient referral. School failure in this youngster is just an indication of many problems.

The challenge of school failure in the pediatric patient is a large one; in many ways it turns the pediatrician into a detective teaming with other professionals and the parents and often the child to discover the clues that will lead to the diagnosis or multiple diagnoses regarding the causes behind the poor grades on the child's report card. This requires considerable time, but it gives the pediatrician his distinctive role.

ANNOTATED BIBLIOGRAPHY

Feagans L: A current view of learning disabilities. J Pediatr 102(4):487–493, 1983 (Provocative and controversial article by a psychologist.)

Hartzell H, Compton C: Learning disability: 10 year follow-up. Pediatrics 74(6):1058, 1984 (Long-term effect of learning disabilities addressed in a sensible manner.)

Levine M et al: The pediatric early elementary examination: Studies of a neurodevelopmental examination for seven- to nine-year-old children. Pediatrics 71(6):894, 1983 (Dr. Levine's neurodevelopmental testing instrument for early detection of learning disabilities offers help to the pediatrician.)

Levine M et al: The dimension of inattention among children with school problems. Pediatrics 70(3):387, 1982 (Interesting perspective on the issue of attention deficit disorder.)

O'Quinn AN: Management of Chronic Disorders of Childhood. Chicago, GK Hall, 1985 (Several valuable and well-written chapters, especially on diabetes and closed head injury.)

Learning Disabilities. Pediatr Clin North Am 31:2, 1984 (Excellent compendium of articles on the subject.)

Shaywitz S et al: Current status of the neuromaturational examination as an index of learning disability. J Pediatr 104(6):819, 1984 (Another pediatric screening instrument of some value for learning disabilities.)

Zuckerman B, Chase C: Specific Learning disability and dyslexia: A language-based model. Advances in Pediatrics. Chicago, Year Book Medical Pub, 1984 ("Ground-breaking" article that predicts subsequent findings.)

6

Adolescent Medicine

42
Contraception
ARTHUR ELSTER

The dramatic changes in sexual behavior of American youth since the 1960s have been well documented. More adolescents are unquestionably having sexual intercourse and at earlier ages. With the downward trend in the age of puberty and the upward trend in the age of marriage, the "culturally-based" sexual abstinence and infertility period imposed by society has lengthened. It has been difficult (and unusual) for adolescents to pass through the interval from menarche to marriage without engaging in sexual intercourse. In fact, around 22% of girls have had sexual intercourse by 15 years of age and 57% by the age of 18. Rates for males are even greater, with 66% having had intercourse by the age of 18. Major racial differences exist for both sexes, with black youths sexually active at earlier ages than white youths.

Because of the high rate of sexual behavior and the low rate of contraceptive usage, the United States has one of the highest adolescent pregnancy rates of all Western countries. Approximately one million teenagers, representing about one female in 10 aged 15 to 19, become pregnant each year in the United States. Half of these pregnancies occur within 6 months of the first sexual encounter (see Chap. 44). The role of the pediatrician, and the health care field in general, must clearly be expanded in order to address the delivery of contraceptive services.

ETHICAL ISSUES

A major issue confronting practitioners is the practical and ethical question of whether to involve parents when providing birth control to uneman-

cipated minors. Legally, U.S. Supreme Court decisions during the 1970s, which ensured the right of unemancipated minors to receive an abortion, also had the effect of establishing that women could receive reproductive health services regardless of age and without parental consent. Although these decisions have been challenged, the basic principle still stands. Although the adolescents' sexual activity is often known by their parents, many adolescents who need birth control are in living situations estranged from parents or are victims of physical or sexual abuse. In these situations, the involvement of parents may be impossible, unrealistic, or unwarranted. Practitioners should take a flexible approach and they should appraise and respond to the various social circumstances that arise with individual patients.

ISSUES OF NONUSE AND NONCOMPLIANCE WITH CONTRACEPTION

Most adolescent pregnancies are unplanned. Only half of sexually active teenagers use contraception at first intercourse and only 34% use birth control on a regular basis. Once a contraceptive method is prescribed, the compliance rate tends to be low. Teenagers who have a stable relationship with their partner and are self-motivated are more compliant than others. When questioned about their nonuse of birth control, adolescents often state that they did expect to have sex, they did not think they could get pregnant, or they felt that birth control was wrong or dangerous. Few teenagers claim they did not know about contraception or where it could be obtained, or that their partner objected. It appears that a combination of impulsive behavior along with misinformation separates teenagers who successfully use contraceptives from those who have become pregnant.

Males present a somewhat different picture. Most know about the efficacy of birth control, including condoms, but maintain the attitude that contraception is the female's responsibility.

Adolescents, both males and females, often have false ideas regarding contraception and pregnancy. Some of this may be developmental in that teenagers may lack the cognitive ability to comprehend complex information about reproductive physiology. Risk-taking behavior, in which adolescents think that adverse consequences happen only to others and not to themselves, is also related to the self-centeredness of adolescent development. Sporadic intercourse, which did not result initially in conception, only serves to reinforce the false belief that they are safe from becoming pregnant and need not use a contraceptive. Misinformation also results, however, because most learning about sex comes from friends and not from parents or health professionals.

CHOICE OF CONTRACEPTIVE METHOD

A thorough understanding of a teenager's social adaptation and sexual history is essential prior to counseling about contraception. This can be learned by questioning about school performance and vocational goals, interaction with peer group and parents, and involvement with drugs and alcohol. The number of partners and frequency of sexual intercourse can provide information regarding the stability of social relationships and the risk of sexually transmitted diseases. With this type of information, the pediatrician can assess the teenager within a more comprehensive social and developmental structure, thus allowing counseling to be more appropriately directed.

The major types of birth control methods currently in use are described in Table 42-1. Each method has advantages and disadvantages for adolescents. The following discussion describes these methods and highlight aspects that pertain to use by adolescents. The difference between the effectiveness when the method is used optimally and what actually occurs with the typical person is important to note. The greater the difference, the more problem the teenager will have with compliance.

Rhythm and Abstinence

The rhythm method (also referred to as fertility awareness) requires the monitoring of changes in cervical mucous and body temperature as markers of ovulation. This method is used reasonably successfully by adult women who are highly motivated and is attempted by only a small percentage of teenagers. Rhythm is not well suited for adolescents because it requires a high degree of motivation and planning. As reported previously, total abstinence is practiced by many school-aged females. A discussion of abstinence should be included when counseling about contraception because some adolescents may respond well to knowing they are not alone if they refrain from sexual intercourse and may, as a result, alter their sexual practices.

Withdrawal

Withdrawing prior to orgasm is a contraceptive method practiced by a substantial percentage of adolescents. Its advantage is that it is safe and does not need physician intervention. The disadvantages are that it requires self-control based on a strong desire to prevent pregnancy and that sperm are emitted with the pre-ejaculation fluid.

Barrier Methods

Diaphragms, condoms, and vaginal sponges are all reasonably effective methods especially if used in combination with contraceptive foam or jelly. These methods tend to be well tolerated by older adolescents and young adults who are comfortable manipulating their external genitalia, but are not as well accepted by more embarrassed, younger adolescents.

There are many advantages of these methods, especially pertaining to the control of sexually transmitted diseases and minimal to no physician involvement. Since the frequency of sexual intercourse among adolescents is sporadic, these methods are ideal in that they do not require continuous usage (as with birth control pills or an intrauterine device [IUD]). Unfortunately, the poor acceptance of barrier methods and the inability of adolescents to use these methods effectively eliminates their use except by the most motivated teenager.

Intrauterine Device

Considerable research data document that the IUD leads to increased risk of pelvic inflammatory disease among adolescents. Some teenagers, how-

Table 42-1. Major Birth Control Methods

DESCRIPTION	RHYTHM	WITHDRAWAL	BARRIER METHODS	IUD	INJECTABLE STEROIDS	PILLS
Effectiveness Use*	76%	77%	Diaphragm—81% Condom—90% Sponge—80%–90%	95%	99.5%	98%
Theoretical†	80%–98%	84%	Diaphragm—98% Condom—98% Sponge—90%	98.5%	99.5%	99.5%
Major Advantages	Safe No cost	Safe No cost	Prevents STD Use related Low cost Few side effects Involves partner Minimal/no involvement with a physician	Compliance Convenient	Compliance Allows menstrual regulation	Highly effective Noncontraceptive benefits
Major Disadvantages	Requires comfort manipulating genitals Requires discipline Requires monitoring of body changes Requires regular ovulation	Requires self-control Sperm in pre-ejaculate fluid	Interrupts sex	Expulsion PID Cramps	Risk of malformations High rates of menstrual irregularity Needs prescription	Expensive Many side effects Daily administration Guilt Needs prescription
Percent Who Use The Method	5%	36%	Diaphragm—1% Condom—34% Sponge—unknown	1%	Unknown	19%
Comments	Not realistic for teenagers	Gives teenagers a false sense of security	Very safe, but undesirable to most teenagers	Not recommended for teenagers	Not approved by FDA	Socially the most acceptable method to teenagers

* The actual (observed) rate of preventing pregnancies.
† The rate of preventing pregnancies if used appropriately.
The effectiveness rates used in this table are based on a summary of contraceptive failure rates reported by Hatcher et al, 1986.

ever, such as those who have been unsuccessful with previous methods of contraception, will want an IUD because of the convenience of not having to worry about daily medication or barrier methods. Adolescents should generally be counseled away from using the IUD.

Injectable Steroids

Depo–Provera (150 mg IM every 3 months) is an effective method of regulating menstrual flow. Because it has not been approved by the FDA for use as a contraceptive agent, the primary use of Depo–Provera in the United States is with mentally handicapped adolescents who have difficulty with menstrual hygiene. It has also been used in patients who have abnormal platelet function to prevent bleeding from menses.

Birth Control Pills

Realistically, the choice of contraception for the sexually active adolescent comes down to birth control pills. The newer low dose combination pills (containing 30μg to 35μg of estrogen with progesterone) are highly effective and have relatively few major side effects. Compliance with taking a pill at the same time each day is often difficult for the adolescent who may be ambivalent about contraception. It is important to remember that what may appear to be a minor medical side effect to a physician may, in fact, be perceived by an anxious adolescent as a major problem. Thus, weight gain, yeast vaginitis, intermenstrual bleeding, and nausea may excessively frighten a teenager because of "all the bad things I had heard" and cause her to stop taking the pill without first checking with her physician for advice. In addition to medical concerns, the adolescent may feel that since sex should be spontaneous, taking the pill connotes the unacceptable impression that she is "looking for sex." Because of the medical risks and risks of noncompliance, adolescents on birth control pills should initially be seen every 1 to 3 months and once a compliance pattern is established, every 6 months. It is important for the physician to emphasize to the teenager that during the first several months of using birth control pills, physically minor side effects are common and should be anticipated.

Because of the manner in which the packages are designed, and not necessarily for physiologic reasons, birth control pills should be started on the Sunday after menses has begun. Using 28 pills per packet rather than 21 pills assists the teenager to establish the habit of taking a pill each day of the cycle. It is essential that the pill be taken at the same time each day; this is usually better accomplished at bedtime. If the teenager notices she missed taking a pill, then she should take it at that time; if it is not noticed until time for the next pill, then two should be taken simultaneously. In no circumstance should more than two pills be taken at the same time. In the event that she goes more than 24 hours without a pill, a back-up method of contraception should be used.

A low-dose triphasic preparation (which has a fixed amount of estrogen and varying amounts of progestin) will generally be the preferred pill for most teenagers. Absolute contraindications for birth control pills include active or chronic hepatitis, unexplained uterine bleeding, and a history of thromboembolism. Relative contraindications include a history of migraine headaches, hypertension, diabetes mellitus, seizure disorders, or teenagers who have not yet had their growth spurt. In each of these situations, the potential benefits of hormonal therapy—such as pregnancy prevention and reduction in risk of iron deficiency anemia, menstrual difficulties, endometrial and ovarian cancer, ovarian cyst, breast disorders such as fibrocystic disease and fibroadenoma, rheumatoid arthritis, and pelvic inflammatory disease—should be weighed against the potential deleterious effects, such as thromboembolism, elevation of blood pressure, elevation of lipid profiles, and altered carbohydrate metabolism.

The use of birth control pills in the lactating adolescent presents a special problem. Although exogenous hormones can reduce breast milk production, birth control pills can be used safely if begun after lactation is well established (*i.e.*, 2 to 4 weeks postpartum). The irregularity with which many adolescents breast-feed and their frequent resumption of sexual activity prior to the routine 6-week postpartum examination places responsibility on the pediatric provider to initiate contraception at the 2-week well-child visit.

Steroidal hormones adversely affect the metabolism of various minerals and vitamins in the body. Due to their frequent poor dietary habits, adolescents on birth control pills should be observed closely for nutritional disorders such as megaloblastic anemia.

Unfortunately, the costs of birth control pills are many, including financial costs, the inconvenience of having to see a physician, uncomfortable side effects, and guilt. Compliance may be especially difficult for teenagers who are concrete in their cognitive thought processes and are not able to perceive future consequences or for those teenagers who lack self-esteem and view pregnancy as an attractive alternative to school. Physicians should ensure, as much as possible, that obstacles interfering with effective contraceptive use are reduced.

ANNOTATED BIBLIOGRAPHY

Chilman CS: Some psychological aspects of adolescent sexual and contraceptive behavior in a changing American society. In Lancaster JB, Hamburg BA (eds): School-Age Pregnancy And Parenthood: A Biosocial Perspective. New York, Aldine de Gruyter, 1986 (Comprehensive review of sexual attitudes, behavior, and contraceptive use and how these have changed over the years.)

Ch'iu Lyle K, Segal SJ: Contraceptive use-effectiveness and the American adolescent. J Reprod Med 22:225, 1979 (Discussion of the effectiveness of the various contraceptive methods with special reference to use by adolescents.)

Greydanus DE: Alternatives to adolescent pregnancy: A discussion of the contraceptive literature from 1960 to 1980. Semin Perinatol 5:53, 1981 (Complete review of the current state of contraceptive technology.)

Hatcher RA, Guest F, Stewart F et al: Contraceptive Technology: 1986–1987. Irvington, New York, 1986 (Excellent "cookbook" for how to use each method of contraception.)

Kastner LS: Ecological factors predicting adolescent contraceptive use: Implications for intervention. J Adolesc Health Care 5:79, 1984 (Study reporting on factors that influence contraceptive decision making.)

Morrison DM: Adolescent contraceptive behavior: A review. Psychol Bull 98:538, 1985 (Thorough review of the psychological literature regarding adolescent contraception.)

Zelnik M, Kantner JF: Sexual activity, contraceptive use, and pregnancy among metropolitan-area teenagers: 1971–1979. Fam Plann Perspect 12:230, 1980 (Report on the sexual behaviors of a national sample of American youth and how these changed over the course of several years.)

43

Pelvic Examination of the Adolescent

ARTHUR ELSTER

The performance of pelvic examinations and the provision of gynecologic care to adolescents are issues which, until recently, have been largely ignored by pediatricians. With a re-emphasis on comprehensive, holistic patient care, the acceptance that adolescents are an integral aspect of pediatric practice, and the understanding that many adolescent problems are gynecologic, pediatricians are changing their practice patterns and office settings so that they can perform pelvic examinations.

The indications for performing a pelvic examination and the preparation of both the pediatrician and the adolescent for this procedure are the topics addressed in this chapter. Specific gynecologic disorders are discussed in Chapters 120 through 122.

INDICATIONS FOR PERFORMING A PELVIC EXAMINATION

Any teenager who is sexually active should have a yearly pelvic examination, including a Pap smear and cervical culture for gonorrhea (GC). Even though the rate of cervical cancer among adolescents is low, the pediatrician should be aware of the possibility of gynecologic cancer and he should include a Pap smear as part of routine screening. Because of increased risk of cancer, more frequent examinations, as often as every 6 months, should be performed on teenagers who have had a genital herpes infection, venereal warts, or multiple types of sexually transmitted diseases (STD). Epidemiologic studies show that genital chlamydia infections are more common than GC. In high-risk populations, such as teenagers who have had multiple sexual partners or past histories of STD, testing for chlamydia should be routinely included.

Pelvic examinations should be done on nonsexually active teenagers if there is a need to screen for cervical cancer. One recommended approach is to perform a teenager's first pelvic examination at the time she separates from the pediatrician, usually at graduation from high school. This ensures that the procedure is done by the person who knows her best and, therefore, that it will be performed in the most sensitive and reassuring manner. Routine examinations should be performed on teenagers who have been exposed to intrauterine diethylstilbestrol (DES). Although such cases are now relatively rare, the history of maternal DES use during the first trimester should still be questioned. Because of the risk of cervical changes that are not well detected by a Pap smear, these females should be referred to a gynecologist for special detection procedures, usually after menstruation begins.

Pelvic examinations are necessary to evaluate the causes of abnormal sexual development. Examples include the adolescent who has delayed breast development (no breast development by age 13 years), pubic hair development (no pubic hair by 13.5 years), or menarche (menstruation has not begun by age 15 years).

Lower abdominal pain is a relatively frequent complaint in the adolescent. Ovarian cyst, endometriosis, ectopic pregnancy, pelvic inflammatory disease (PID), pain of ovulation, and psychogenic pain secondary to sexual abuse must be considered in the differential diagnosis.

Vaginal discharge with or without itching is also common among adolescents and younger children. It is important to differentiate an infectious cause of vaginal discharge, such as monilia, trichomonas, GC, chlamydia, nonspecific (Gardnerella-associated) vaginitis, or foreign body from physiologic leukorrhea, which is seen in early puberty. Vaginal secretions increase secondary to estrogen stimulation of the cervical mucosa, usually about 6 to 12 months prior to menarche, producing a clear and nonirritating discharge. The diagnosis of leukorrhea is made from taking the patient's history (normal progression of pubertal events) and from a microscopic examination of the discharge that reveals no white blood cells or bacteria.

Menstrual problems requiring a pelvic examination include irregular menses, primary or secondary amenorrhea, or dysmenorrhea. Irregular menstrual periods, usually not associated with cramps, are common among young adolescents and are the result of anovulatory cycles. As many as 50% of females do not ovulate by 2 years postmenarche. An evaluation for irregular menses should include a pelvic examination in adolescents who are greater than 2 years postmenarchal or in those females who previously had been regular. Once ovulation is established, menstruation becomes regular and cramping usually worsens.

Dysmenorrhea is reported by around 60% of adolescents and appears to present as a major disability in as many as 14%. Cramping and associated symptoms, such as diarrhea, fatigue, and irritability, may occur at the time of, or preceding, menstruation. Primary dysmenorrhea is caused by increased levels of endometrial prostaglandin, whereas secondary dysmenorrhea is related to pelvic pathology, such as endometriosis, PID, or uterine tumor. In teenagers who are not sexually active, a bimanual examination can suffice to eliminate mass lesions or infection as the cause of the menstrual pain.

A pelvic examination needs to be performed on any child or adolescent who has been sexually abused. Pediatricians should be suspicious of abuse whenever a teenager presents with chronic, unexplained abdominal pain or is excessively anxious about having a pelvic examination. Physicians must be especially sensitive to the emotional needs of the teenager who usually has feelings of guilt, depression, confusion, and distrust. There may be few signs of abuse noticeable on a pelvic examination, especially if it is an ongoing situation. If the abuse has occurred recently, attention should be given to obtaining proper laboratory specimens for the detection of semen or sperm, either through microscopic evaluation of vaginal fluid or by fluorescense of ultraviolet light.

The last indication listed in the box, Indications for Performing a Pelvic Examination, is to confirm pregnancy and ascertain the length of gestation. Around 10% of adolescents aged 15 to 19 become pregnant each year, and a much larger number have "false alarms." A teenager concerned with the possibility of pregnancy who has not yet told her parents often presents with vague abdominal or menstrual concerns. Physicians should routinely ask about sexual behavior and the regularity of menstruation, preferably without the parent in the room. Associated signs of pregnancy include an increased frequency of urination, nausea, and breast tenderness. An enlarged uterus and cervical changes can usually be appreciated by 8 to 10 weeks' gestation.

Indications for Performing a Pelvic Examination

Health surveillance and education

Exposure to sexually transmitted diseases (STD)

Contraception

Maternal exposure to diethylstilbestrol (DES)

Abnormal pubertal development

Unexplained lower abdominal pain

Vaginal discharge

Menstrual problems

Sexual abuse

Diagnosis of pregnancy

PREPARATION

The Practitioner

In order for a pediatrician to perform an adequate pelvic examination, he needs a knowledge base and technical skills that are not always taught in residency programs. He should have a thorough understanding of gynecologic problems, normal adolescent growth and development, and the more commonly used medications, such as hormones, antiprostaglandins, and antibiotics for STD. He needs to be able to use a vaginal speculum, perform a bimanual examination, and perform a microscopic examination of wet mounts of vaginal discharge. He then needs to be able to synthesize the data and develop a treatment plan. Superceding all this, a pediatrician must have the communication skills and the confidence to interact with adolescents concerning gynecologic and sexual issues. Because of the sensitive nature of pelvic examinations, teenagers often prefer a female provider; thus, in particular, female pediatricians should develop their gynecologic skills. Practicing pediatricians can acquire the knowledge and technical skills to perform pelvic examinations in various ways, including working at a family planning clinic, doing a mini-fellowship at an adolescent medicine training program, or attending conferences on office gynecology. Various drug companies have also excellent teaching material and films.

The Patient

Adolescents, especially those having their first pelvic examination, are anxious due to self-consciousness (including concerns about undressing, personal cleanliness, and embarrassment), feelings of vulnerability, and potential aversive consequences (including pain and discovery of pathology). The level of anxiety, however, is often related to other issues in the adolescent's life, such as feelings of anger, depression, and negative self-esteem unrelated to the examination itself. Pelvic examinations are also difficult for adolescents because they are struggling with issues of sexuality, body image, and identity. In addition, information about pelvic examinations comes predominantly from friends and tends to emphasize the negative, technical aspects, especially pain. Interacting with these patient-related obstacles is the personal feelings of the provider, who himself may also be uncomfortable performing an examination.

The most effective way to perform an adequate pelvic examination is to take time before the examination—while the teenager is still dressed—and discuss both the technical and emotional issues. The openmindedness and willingness of the physician to discuss emotional concerns creates within the adolescent a feeling that the physician has a personal interest in her that leads to increased satisfaction and reduced anxiety. The use of drawings or visual aid devices such as a plastic model of the pelvis also helps the teenager to better understand the procedure as well as her body. Although a teenager may generally prefer to have a female provider, the quality of the physician—patient interaction can overcome much of this concern.

To provide teenagers with some degree of control, it is best to allow them the option of whether or not to have a chaperone in the room during the examination. Younger patients tend to want a family member present; older teenagers—who are being examined by a male—would rather have a nonparent chaperone than be alone. In general, teenagers do not want a friend in the room.

Before the examination, it is best to inquire what the adolescent knows about pelvic examinations and the female reproductive anatomy. If she has had a previous examination, that experience should be reviewed. The patient should be told exactly what will be done and she should be shown the speculum.

Pelvic examinations can be performed legally without parental consent in all states in order to diagnose STD and pregnancy. It is still best, however, to obtain parental consent whenever possible. This alleviates the possibly awkward situation of having to explain to parents that their daughter may have a serious gynecologic disease when they did not even know that she had been examined.

WORK-UP

Examination of the External Genitalia

Inspection of the external genitalia should proceed in the following order:

- Note the distribution of pubic hair and assess the level of physical development (Tanner staging).
- Inspect the skin of the perineum and perianal region for rashes, warts, or sores.
- Note the size of the clitoris as a sign of virilization.
- Observe and palpate for lumps or masses around the urethra (Skene's gland) and around the labia minora (Bartholin's gland).
- Spread the labia and note the presence of discharge or erythema.

Speculum Examination

A good light source and an appropriate examination table is necessary to perform an adequate speculum examination.

Almost all examinations on adolescents can be accomplished using a Pederson speculum, rather than a larger, spoon-shaped Graves' speculum. The Graves' speculum is only necessary with fairly large or parous adolescents. The speculum should be warm, but not hot to the touch. For preadolescents, a regular pediatric otoscope is well tolerated for performing examinations of the vagina. Whatever speculum is used, it should be inserted without a lubricant because the jelly can interfere with obtaining appropriate vaginal cultures, especially GC.

Most examinations are performed in the traditional supine position. With some adolescents, however, using the semi-sitting position may help to alleviate anxiety, especially with a male provider. In preadolescents, some experts recommend having patients in the knee–chest position because it allows better visualization of the vagina.

Insert one finger into the introitus and apply gentle pressure to the posterior vagina to help the teenager relax. Ask the patient to tighten and then relax those muscles on which she feels the pressure. Repeating this procedure several times is usually all that is needed to obtain proper relaxation. While the finger is in the introitus, feel for the depth and direction of the cervix. This provides the "map" for inserting the speculum and locating the cervix, which for the pediatrician is usually the most difficult technical part of the examination.

Insert the Pederson speculum horizontally and observe the vaginal mucosa for lesions. The mucosa on the posterior wall is ruggated, whereas that of the anterior wall is smooth. This can be useful if there is difficulty in visualizing the cervix. Observe the color and consistency of any discharge found in the vaginal vault. Observe the cervix for erosions (areas that are red and inflamed), ectropion (an extension of the endocervical cells to the external os, which can also appear red), the presence and color of any discharge or blood from the os, and the color of the cervix (a bluish color of the cervix, Chadwick's sign, can be an early sign of pregnancy).

Cells from the endocervical canal should be obtained for a Pap smear using procedures recommended by the local pathology laboratory. If indicated, samples of vaginal discharge to test for GC and chlamydia should be obtained. Any vaginal discharge should be plated on a glass slide and examined microscopically with both KOH (for yeast) and saline (for trichomonads, clue cells, and white blood cells).

Bimanual Examination

Insert two fingers of one hand into the vagina and note the position and size of the uterus and the presence of pain with movement of the cervix. Also determine the firmness of the cervix—a soft, boggy cervix can be an early sign of pregnancy. A normal size uterus is about the size of a small fist; a 12-week gravid uterus is palpated at the pelvic brim; a 16-week uterus is midway between the symphysis pubis and the umbilicus; a 20-week uterus is at the level of the umbilicus.

Using both the internal and external examining hands, palpate the adnexae for masses and pain. Having the teenager take slow, deep breaths may relax the pelvic and abdominal muscles, allowing the provider a more adequate bimanual examination. An attempt should be made to palpate the ovaries; in adolescents, especially those who are anxious, this may not be successful.

A rectovaginal examination does not need to be done routinely. It should be performed, however, if endometriosis is suspected in order to palpate the uterosacral ligaments for nodularity.

INDICATIONS FOR REFERRAL

Referral to a gynecologist is necessary when there is doubt regarding the presence of abnormal findings on the pelvic examination, a history of maternal ingestion of DES, no clinical improvement in patients with treated PID, an abnormal Pap smear, or a pelvic mass. As with any area of medicine, the physician's level of comfort managing gynecologic problems will determine how frequently and under what circumstances a referral will be made.

ANNOTATED BIBLIOGRAPHY

Emans SJ, Goldstein DP: The gynecologic examination of the prepubertal child with vulvovaginitis: Use of the knee–chest position. Pediatrics 65:758, 1980 (Description of how to examine the prepubertal child.)

Emans J: Pelvic examination of the adolescent patient. Pediatr Rev 4:307, 1983 (Good review of the technical aspects and the normal and abnormal findings associated with pelvic examinations.)

Hein K, Schrieber K, Cohen M, Koss LG: Cervical cytology: The need for routine screening in the sexually active adolescent. J Pediatr 91:123, 1977 (Reports on the frequency of abnormal findings from Pap smears, thus justifying the need for routine screening.)

Phillips S, Friedman SB, Seidenberg M, Heald FP: Teenagers' preference regarding the presence of family members, peers, and chaperones during examination of the genitalia. Pediatrics 68:665, 1981 (Reports on how the preference for the type of chaperone differs with factors such as the age of the teenager and the sex of provider.)

Sarrel PM: Indications for a first pelvic examination. J Adolesc Health Care (editorial) 2:145, 1981 (Brief discussion on reasons for performing a teenager's first pelvic examination.)

Seymore C, DuRant RH, Jay S et al: Influence of position during examination, and sex of examiner on patient anxiety during pelvic examination. J Pediatr 108:312, 1986 (Reports on factors influencing a teenager's anxiety during a pelvic examination.)

44

Teenage Pregnancy

JEAN BRODNAX

Teenage pregnancy has been a focus of national attention since the early 1970s. The United States has the highest teenage pregnancy rate of six industrialized nations studied by the Alan Guttmacher Institute. This epidemic of children bearing children has medical, socioeconomic, educational, and vocational ramifications that ultimately affect all of American society. Health professionals caring for children and adolescents must attempt to prevent or identify teenage pregnancy issues and approach them in a helpful and supportive manner.

MAGNITUDE OF THE PROBLEM

Teenage pregnancy is pervasive in this country, affecting all races and socioeconomic classes. Currently, over 1 million pregnancies occur in teenage girls each year in the United States; 80% are unintended and 80% are out of wedlock. Although the teenage pregnancy rate increases with age, the problem is not limited to older teenagers. Approximately 30,000 pregnancies/year occur in girls under age 15.

It is predicted that if current trends continue, four in ten young girls who are now 14 years of age will get pregnant as teenagers and two in ten will give birth. Nearly one half of all black females will get pregnant by the age of 20. By age 18, 22% of all black teenage girls have given birth compared to 8% of white teenagers.

One half of teenage pregnancies occur in the first 6 months after initial intercourse and one fifth occur within the first month. The younger the adolescent, the more likely she will become pregnant soon after her first intercourse (largely due to poor use of contraceptives), and the greater will her risk be for having repeat pregnancies during the teenage years (see also Chap. 42).

Over one half of all teenage pregnancies in the United States result in abortions. When compared to other industrialized nations, the teenage abortion rate in the United States is exceedingly high, and the youngest teenagers have the highest abortion rates. Adolescents account for one third of all legal abortions performed in the United States. Forty-five percent of teenage pregnancies conclude as live births. Birth rates increase with increasing age and are highest among blacks who are less likely than whites to abort. Some teenage pregnancies end in miscarriage.

Prenatal care among teenagers is generally poor. Most receive no prenatal care in the first trimester and one fifth have none before the third. This is due mainly to denial of the pregnancy or a delay in diagnosis.

Most teenagers who give birth keep their babies and this trend continues to increase. In 1971, 13% chose adoption compared to 4% in 1978. Blacks are much less likely than whites to opt for adoption.

CAUSES

One major contributing factor to the rise in adolescent pregnancy is the increase in sexual activity over the last two decades. The incidence of sexual intercourse among unmarried teenage women increased by two thirds during the 1970s. In 1982, one half of teenage women aged 15 to 19 were sexually active. The mean age of first intercourse for teenage women is just over 16 years and is even younger for blacks. Only 20% of young women report planning their first intercourse, and for most it "just happens." One half of all sexually active teenage women report having more than one partner and one sixth report having four or more partners. Most teenagers engage in sexual intercourse less than once a month, but one fifth have sex more than once a week.

In spite of the increase in sexual activity and the availability of contraception, birth control use among teenagers in this country remains poor. Only 40% of teenagers use any contraceptive method at first intercourse. Some reasons that adolescents give for non-use of contraception include a lack of expectation that they will have intercourse, their youth, infrequent sex, difficulty in obtaining contraceptives, and disbelief that they will get pregnant.

The situation of high sexual activity rates and poor contraceptive use among teenagers is unique to this country when compared to other industrialized nations. For example, in Sweden, greater proportions of teenagers are sexually active at every age but abortion, birth, and pregnancy rates are much lower. Birth control is much more available and sex is dealt with in an open and realistic manner, in contrast to the ambivalent messages that teenagers receive in this country. In addition, most teenagers are not knowledgeable about basic reproductive biology and contraception.

Thus, it is imperative that the health care providers do not wait for an adolescent to seek contraception before addressing issues of sexuality, but rather that they reach adolescents early, ideally before they have initiated sexual activity. Since the youngest sexually active adolescents are at greatest risk for premature pregnancy, maximal effort must be aimed at this group.

CONSEQUENCES

Many studies have addressed the possible medical, social, and economic consequences of teenage pregnancy. Unfortunately, most fail to adequately control for important variables such as age and socioeconomic status. Thus, the adverse consequences of teenage pregnancy tend to be overstated in the literature.

Obstetric

The pregnant adolescent is at increased risk for obstetric morbidity and mortality. These risks are more pronounced in pregnant girls less than 15 years of age. For this group, the risk of maternal death is 60% higher than it is for women in their early 20s. The most common medical complications of teenage pregnancy are pregnancy induced hypertension (PIH), iron deficiency anemia, and delivery of low-birth-weight (LBW) (<2500 g) babies.

PIH, seen in 15% to 40% of teenage pregnancies, is the most common medical complication and may manifest in one of two forms. Pre-eclampsia is seen most frequently in primigravidas and is common among adolescents of low socioeconomic status. A diagnosis of PIH is made typically when the blood pressure exceeds 140/90 and there is concomitant 2+ proteinuria. Eclampsia is diagnosed when convulsions appear with hypertension and proteinuria. The treatment of PIH includes hospitalization for bed rest and observation and treatment with anticonvulsant medication ($MgSO_4$), if indicated, to prevent seizures. The termination of pregnancy leads to a resolution of symptoms.

The iron deficiency anemia is largely a result of nutritional deficiency. Iron supplementation and a frequent assessment of the patient's hemoglobin identifies and corrects this condition.

Low-birth-weight infants from prematurity are more common than small-for-gestational-age babies. Fourteen percent of infants born to mothers less than 15 years old are LBW compared to 9.9% of infants born to mothers 15 to 19 years of age and 6.5% of infants born to women 20 to 29 years of age. Maternal factors associated with LBW babies in teenagers include inadequate prenatal care, low prepregnancy weight, placental growth retardation, amniotic fluid infection, anemia, narcotic use, smoking, and being a primigravida. Demographic factors include ethnic origin (nonwhite teenagers have a higher incidence) and unmarried status.

Many investigators have shown that the aforementioned medical complications are not due to any unique biologic disadvantage of young age, but rather are due to factors mainly related to low socioeconomic status (e.g., inadequate prenatal care, poor nutrition, low prepregnancy weight, and poor pregnancy weight gain). When controlled for these factors, many studies demonstrate that teenagers are at no more increased risk for complications of pregnancy than older women. Even for the youngest teenagers, early prenatal care and good nutrition significantly improve the outcome of teenage pregnancy.

Medical

Perinatal, neonatal, and infant mortality rates are higher for offspring of teenage mothers than for those of older mothers. This is greatest in the 15 years and younger age group. Again, this cannot be attributed to age alone, but is largely influenced by socioeconomic factors. Perinatal mortality rate rises sharply with subsequent teenage births. For the first birth in the teenage years, it is 6:1000, for the second-born during the teens it rises to 71:1000 and for the third-born it is 143:1000. This increase is mainly attributable to worsening socioeconomic conditions with subsequent births.

Infant mortality (death between 1 month and 1 year of age) is twice as high for infants of teenage mothers as for mothers in their 20s. Deaths are most commonly due to sudden infant death syndrome (SIDS) [infants of teenage mothers are five times more likely to have SIDS than children of older mothers], infections, and accidents.

Infant morbidity is somewhat higher among infants of teenage mothers. This is largely attributed to factors such as adolescent immaturity and unwillingness to accept responsibility for the care of the infant or lack of knowledge and experience concerning infant care.

Physical growth of children born to adolescent mothers is the same as that of older mothers by the time children reach 7 years of age.

Some studies have shown that teenage mothers have suboptimal maternal behavior if observed for touching, vocalization, and closeness to the infant. Most studies show that cognitive development of the child is adversely effected by young maternal age. This is true even after controlling for socioeconomic variables. It is important to note that studies do not substantiate any increase in child abuse among adolescent mothers.

Social and Economic

Early childbearing is associated with curtailing education, low paying jobs or unemployment, marital instability, and subsequent repeat births at a young age. After delivery, many girls cannot return to school because of a lack of child care assistance. Teenage fathers are also less likely than other male teenagers to graduate from high school. Poor education leads to poor vocational skills and lower paying jobs or unemployment for teenage parents, approximately two thirds of whom live below the poverty level. On average, the income of teenage mothers is half that of women in their 20s, and many remain below the poverty level throughout their adult lives. Many maintain a single parent household, restricting income even more.

Teenage marriages are adversely effected by early parenthood. Nearly one half of women who give birth as teenagers are separated or divorced within 15 years, which is threefold higher than women who delay their childbearing until after the age of 20. Young, separated, or divorced mothers

are less likely to receive child support from the father than older mothers who are separated or divorced.

Repeat pregnancy is another negative social outcome of teenage pregnancy. Fifteen percent of pregnant teenagers become pregnant again within 1 year and 30% within 2 years. If the pregnancies conclude as live births, a downward socioeconomic spiral is reinforced.

The aforementioned social and economic consequences of teenage pregnancy are eased somewhat if the young family lives with or gets financial, psychological, and child care assistance from extended family members. The children of teenage parents also do better physically, cognitively, psychologically, and socially in an extended family setting.

PREVENTIVE APPROACHES

Clearly there is no single or simple solution to the problem of teenage pregnancy. Prevention may be approached on three levels: primary, secondary, and tertiary. The goal of primary prevention is to prevent a teenage pregnancy. Once a pregnancy has occurred, one may intervene with options for resolution of the pregnancy in an atmosphere that promotes good decision making (secondary prevention). Once a teenager makes the decision to carry to term and keep a baby, tertiary prevention may be exercised by offering interventions with the goal of preventing the adverse outcomes of teenage pregnancy.

Primary prevention is the optimal solution to the teenage pregnancy issue. Education is the most important component of primary prevention. This includes instruction on feelings, anatomy, sexuality, sexually transmitted diseases, and birth control. Such instruction may come from several sources such as schools, churches, community organizations, and importantly, primary health care providers. Information should be offered in a nonjudgmental manner, so that the teenager does not feel threatened or disapproved of. This education should be directed at both sexes and should start ideally at a young age before sexual activity has begun. The availability of contraception is the second important component of primary prevention. If discussions of issues of sexuality are routinely included in adolescent well-child visits, the pediatrician may determine when contraception is necessary, again preferably before the teenager has initiated sexual activity. In recent years, some cities have offered contraception to teenagers through school-based programs. This is obviously an efficient way to reach a large number of adolescents. In these geographic areas, teenage pregnancies have declined dramatically, by as much as 40%. School-based contraceptive programs have unfortunately met with some opposition from parents, churches, and local officials.

DIAGNOSIS OF PREGNANCY

A primary care pediatrician should know how to diagnose a pregnancy. Some teenagers will schedule a medical visit because of a concern of possible pregnancy. Many adolescents, however, exercise denial about a possible pregnancy, thus a pediatrician should be alert to possible signs and symptoms of pregnancy during other types of medical visits. During a routine history, an adolescent female should be questioned about her sexual activity, her last menstrual period (LMP), the duration and character of its flow, and the presence of symptoms of pregnancy including nausea, vomiting, dizziness, fatigue, breast soreness, expanding waistline, and urinary frequency. A missed menstrual period is an indication for further investigation of a possible pregnancy, even if the teenager denies sexual activity (as some do for fear of parental discovery or disapproval). Pregnancy is by far the most common cause of secondary amenorrhea. Signs of pregnancy on a routine physical examination include tender enlarged breasts, darkened areolae, enlargement of the nipples, galatorrhea, and enlarged fundus on abdominal examination. If pregnancy is at all suspected and a fundus is not felt on abdominal examination, it is important first to perform a pelvic examination. The patient should be instructed to empty her bladder. Signs of pregnancy on the pelvic examination include thick cervical mucus, bluish hue to cervix (Chadwick's sign), softening of the cervix, and enlargement of the uterus.

Even if the physical examination is nonconfirmatory, a pregnancy test should be performed if there is *any* suspicion of a pregnancy.

PREGNANCY TESTING

Most standard laboratory tests for the determination of pregnancy are based on measurement of the beta subunit of human chorionic gonadotropin (HCG) in serum or urine. HCG is produced by the placenta and appears in maternal serum and urine about 9 days after conception. Most of the recently developed pregnancy tests that use radio-immunoassays (RIA) or enzyme immunoassays (EIA) of HCG will be positive at, or soon after, this time. Urine tests for HCG are qualitative whereas serum measurements are quantitative. HCG increases in the serum until about 12 weeks of gestation, at which time it declines sharply. Thus, a positive but low serum measurement indicates either an early first trimester or a second or third trimester pregnancy. Home test kits have become available in the last several years. Older home tests are agglutination-inhibition type assays and do not detect pregnancy before the sixth week of gestation (*i.e.*, 6 weeks after the LMP). More recently, home test kits based on EIA have become available: These have the advantage of a color endpoint and they become positive at an earlier gestational age. HCG levels are low in ectopic pregnancies and home test kits may give a false negative result.

ECTOPIC PREGNANCY

Ectopic pregnancy should be suspected if there is abdominal pain, irregular vaginal bleeding, or a tender adnexal mass in the presence of a missed period. A diagnosis is made by serum or urine beta subunit measurement in combination with pelvic ultrasound. The treatment is by laparotomy with surgical excision of the pregnancy.

SPONTANEOUS ABORTION

Spontaneous abortion should be suspected in any pregnant adolescent with bleeding and crampy pelvic pain. Quantitative measurement of the β subunit of HCG and ultrasound may help to establish the diagnosis. Treatment consists of dilatation and curettage to remove any remaining contents of the uterus.

DETERMINATION OF GESTATIONAL AGE

Gestational age can be determined in several ways. One method is to count backwards by weeks to the first day of the LMP. This method, however, is imprecise. A more reliable method is sizing by abdominal or pelvic examination. Given an inverted or midposition uterus, this is accurate within 2 weeks. A retroverted uterus is more difficult to size. The uterus is just perceptibly enlarged at 6 to 8 weeks, grapefruit size at 10 weeks, felt just above the symphysis pubis at 13 weeks, midway between the symphysis pubis and umbilicus at 16 weeks, and at the level of the umbilicus at 20 weeks. Ultrasound is the most accurate way to determine gestational age. Several fetal parameters may be used to reflect menstrual weeks of pregnancy including crown–rump length, biparietal diameter, and femur length.

OPTIONS

After a pregnancy is diagnosed and the gestational age is determined, three options should be presented to the patient: induced abortion (if gestational age permits), continuation of the pregnancy with adoption after birth, or continuation of the pregnancy with the prospect that the teenage mother will keep and raise the child. The pediatrician should discuss the advantages and disadvantages of each option carefully and objectively with the adolescent. In most instances she may have input from the father of the baby, grandparents, and any extended family that may be involved. The final decision, however, should be made by the teenager herself and she should be advised of the same by the pediatrician.

After discussion of the procedure, if abortion is chosen the pediatrician should refer the adolescent to an appropriate clinic or office.

Induced Abortion

Induced abortion was legalized in the United States in 1973. Since then, the number of abortions performed has increased yearly, though at a decelerating pace. Induced abortions may be divided into four types: menstrual regulation, standard first-trimester vacuum curettage, mid-trimester curettage, and mid-trimester abortion by amnioinfusion.

Menstrual regulation (also known as menstrual extraction, menstrual induction, and menstrual aspiration) is an early abortion performed within 6 to 7 weeks of the LMP. The procedure is performed with minimal cervical dilatation and minivacuum aspiration using a plastic syringe and cannula. This procedure is more likely to result in failed or incomplete abortion than other types of abortions, but is less likely than later abortions to produce a life-threatening complication.

A first-trimester standard vacuum curettage can be performed up to 13 weeks of gestational age. Frequently, laminaria tents (stems of seaweed) are placed in the cervix the day before the procedure to induce some dilatation. Anesthesia used for the abortion may be local (e.g., paracervical block), general, or by varying degrees of sedation. The cervix is progressively dilated prior to the insertion of a vacuum cannula that evacuates the contents of the uterus. A metal curette is then passed into the uterus to ensure that the cavity is empty. A second suctioning is then done. The most common complications of first-trimester abortions include retained tissue, infection, perforation, vasovagal reaction, heavy bleeding, and uterine hypotonia (postabortal syndrome).

Mid-trimester curettage (performed at 13 to 15 weeks) differs from first-trimester curettage in that greater cervical dilatation is necessary and some fetal and placental parts must be removed by forceps. A risk of perforation of the uterus is greater because of a larger, softer uterus.

Amnioinfusion (gestational age 16 to 22 weeks) is done by instilling hypertonic saline or prostaglandins directly into the amniotic sac. This induces fetal wastage with subsequent passing of the fetus and placenta. The complications of this method are mostly related to retained placenta and toxic actions of the drugs used. This procedure occasionally results in the birth of a live fetus.

Second-trimester abortions of either type account for less than 10% of all induced abortions in this country, but unfortunately they are more common among teenagers due to a delay in diagnosis.

The mortality rate from legal abortions ranges from 0.4 per 100,000 at 8 weeks or less to 16 per 100,000 at 21 weeks or more. Deaths associated with complications of childbirth are significantly higher than those associated with first- or early second-trimester abortions.

Most of the literature in the field documents that legal abortion induced in the first trimester does not carry a significant risk of psychological trauma. Feelings of guilt and depression are usually mild and transitory and are often accompanied by a sense of relief.

Tertiary Prevention

When a teenage pregnancy is diagnosed and the adolescent elects to carry to term, she should be referred expediently for prenatal care. Adolescents generally require more frequent prenatal visits than older women to monitor nutritional status, possible anemia, infection, and toxemia. Social service consultation is often useful to help the teenager with school, work, or day-care plans. Parenting education should also be part of the prenatal care program. A teenager should ideally be referred to a clinic or hospital that offers a teenage prenatal program with comprehensive obstetric, psychosocial, and outreach services.

ANNOTATED BIBLIOGRAPHY

Alan Guttmacher Institute: Teenage Pregnancy: The problem that hasn't gone away. New York, 1981 (Compilation of statistics on teenage pregnancy with brief interpretations of data. Good overview.)

Fursteberg F, Lincoln R, Menken J: Teenage Sexuality and Childbearing. Philadelphia, The University of Pennsylvania Press, 1981 (Excellent collection of articles on teenage pregnancy.)

McAnarney E: Premature Adolescent Pregnancy and Parenthood. New York, Grune & Stratton, 1983 (In-depth analysis of several aspects of teenage pregnancy.)

45
Eating Disorders of Adolescents
RICHARD M. SARLES

Eating disorders of adolescents are usually more prevalent in women who are preoccupied with weight and food and who develop abnormal eating patterns. The two most prevalent eating disorders, anorexia nervosa and bulimia, are the primary disorders within this category, and although somewhat related and overlapping, they appear to be distinct and different entities.

ANOREXIA NERVOSA

The term *anorexia nervosa* is actually a misnomer. Anorexia means loss of appetite, yet most of these young women do not experience loss of appetite but a profound disorder of body image and eating patterns. The German word *pubertätmagersucht* better defines this condition as a relentless pursuit of thinness or a seeking or passion for the leanness of puberty.

Case Presentation

Laura M, a 15½-year-old high school sophomore, was examined by her pediatrician because of a marked weight loss over a 3-month period. Laura insisted that she felt well and that she had no physical complaints.

Laura was a tenth grade student, a class officer who generally achieved an A to B average. She was an avid tennis player, she competed on the school swimming team, and she had a part-time job at a fast-food chain. She was described by her parents as a happy teenager who never gave them any trouble and who seemed like the "perfect child." Laura seemed to be liked by her peers and often received phone calls from them each evening. She helped in the house and often prepared meals for the family. Laura's early childhood growth and development were completely normal.

During the summer vacation, Laura felt that her thighs were too large and decided to "cut back" on sweets and junk food. Her routine, preschool sports physical examination revealed that her weight had dropped from 118 lb to 112 lb and that her menstrual periods had stopped for the prior 2 months, but she appeared in good physical health and still fell easily within normal limits on the growth chart.

In early November, Laura's mother accidentally saw her undressing and was shocked by Laura's marked thinness. Laura could not understand her mother's great concern, insisting instead that she still had fat thighs and a pot belly, and, in fact, admitted to running 5 to 7 miles each day and doing calisthenics each evening prior to bed. When Laura stood on the bathroom scales she weighed only 82 lb. She had lost approximately 36 lb.

Mr M, her father, was a 41-year-old insurance executive who owned his own agency and had gained professional recognition and marked financial success through real-estate dealings. He was president of his fraternity and captain of the tennis team in college. His interest in sports continued as an avid spectator at the professional baseball and football games and as an active participant in tennis.

Mrs M was a 39-year-old successful member of a large advertising agency. She had graduated *cum laude*, Phi Beta Kappa, and had won two journalism awards. She entered graduate school to pursue her Master's and Doctorate work in journalism but completed only 1 year before getting married. She became pregnant soon after being married.

Mr and Mrs M were an attractive couple; Mrs M always dressed stylishly, expensively, and impeccably; Mr. M dressed conservatively and neatly. Both admitted that appearances were important to them and achievement was the mark of success. They admitted to being "wed to their work," managing to go out to dinner together or spending time alone only "once in a great while." Family vacations had denied them time to vacation alone as a couple for the past 7 years.

When Laura was examined by her pediatrician, the following physical findings were noted. Laura appeared as a very thin and wasted, but well-groomed adolescent with absent normal female body contours. Her axillary and pubic hair patterns were normal and a thin, silky body hair was present. Her skin was cold, dry, and cracked. Her temperature was 96.2°F; her blood pressure was $^{68}/_{48}$; her pulse was 52. Laboratory studies including hemoglobin, hematocrit, WBC and differential, urinanalysis, stool specimen for blood, ova, and parasites, and liver studies were all within normal limits.

Laura represents a typical example of the adolescent girl with anorexia nervosa. A well-behaved girl in a high achieving family, she developed an overwhelming need for thinness of delusional proportions resulting in profound weight loss.

The American Psychiatric Association Diagnostic and Statistical Manual (DSM-III) Criteria for Anorexia Nervosa include an intense fear of becoming obese with an age of onset prior to age 25, which does not diminish as weight loss progresses, a disturbance of body image, a refusal to maintain body weight over a minimal normal weight for age and height, a weight loss of at least 25% of original body weight, and no known illness that would account for the weight loss. Amenorrhea is usually present, although 25% of these girls cease their menstrual periods prior to the onset of weight loss. Bradycardia, hypotension, hypothermia, dry cracked red skin, thinning of scalp hair with an increase in fine body hair, and loss of female body contours are other physical signs. Laboratory data usually show no major abnormalities until severe starvation and physical deterioration result.

Other signs and symptoms include excessive ritualistic exercising that may be in addition to organized school sports and an excessive preoccupation with food such as preparing the family dinner, working in food establishments, and gourmet cooking. The adolescent has often a marked disturbance of body image and body concept of delusional proportions claiming absolute denial of pathologic weight loss or thinness. Anorectic adolescents often see themselves as fat even with a marked weight loss and often misjudge their own waist size as overly large by at least 50%. Curiously, these adolescents can correctly observe other persons' body size and the size of inanimate objects. Anorectic adolescents often have an inaccurate or confused perception of body stimuli in

that they often believe that food, once in the stomach, will multiply. The adolescent, for example, may think that four Cheerios for breakfast is ample and filling.

The marked and progressive weight loss despite parental or physician intervention is often so striking that the diagnosis of anorexia nervosa is usually made without difficulty.

BULIMIA

Bulimia is defined as episodic binge eating followed by vomiting (usually self-induced), abdominal pain, use of laxatives, and deep sleep. Like anorexia nervosa, the age of onset is usually prior to age 25 and is found predominantly in women. However, unlike the anorectic patient whose weight loss is most profound and noticeable, weight loss is not obvious with bulimic patients and marked overt physical symptomatology is usually absent. The binge-eating bulimic often consumes large amounts of high-caloric, usually sweet, soft, and easily digested food in rapid fashion with little chewing. Their eating is usually secretive and inconspicuous and is often unknown to their families or friends. Their excessive binging is terminated by intense abdominal pain, social interruption, or sleep. Self-induced vomiting often occurs which helps relieve the abdominal pain. Bulimia is often associated with substance abuse, particularly barbiturates, amphetamines, and alcohol use. There is a high correlation with depression, and self-deprecating thoughts and a depressed mood often precede and follow the binge period. In contrast to the anorectic, the bulimic has a clear awareness that his eating habits are abnormal and has an ingrained fear of not being able to stop and control his eating.

On physical examination, the primary care physician is often able to discern side effects of the bulimic behavior, such as parotid enlargement, hypokalemia, rectal bleeding, destruction of dental enamel, and alopecia.

Although anorexia nervosa and bulimia share broad, general characteristics and often co-exist, personality features have been described that distinguish the two groups. Anorectic patients tend to be more perfectionistic, compliant, conforming, academically successful, and generally well liked by their teachers, yet they often have difficulty in forming relationships outside of the family, and social isolation is a common occurrence. Anorectic patients are also more introverted, display little overt psychiatric symptomatology, and deny hunger more often than their bulimic counterparts.

Bulimics, on the other hand, are more extroverted, tend to vomit more frequently, and exhibit more somatic complaints. The bulimics also manifest greater anxiety, depression, and guilt. Of special importance, an impulse control disorder, kleptomania, is a common problem among bulimic patients and seldom if ever is seen with anorectic patients.

ETIOLOGY OF EATING DISORDERS

Although many etiologic factors have been offered for the explanation of the various eating disorders, no single theory is applicable or universally accepted. The concept of biopsychosocial etiology can best be applied to the eating disorders. Biologic factors have been demonstrated in case reports of anorexia nervosa occurring in twins, siblings, and parent–child pairs. Further evidence of biologic factors points to the temporal relationship of the pubertal endocrine changes with clear findings of hypothalamic dysfunction in anorectic patients. Whether any of these hypothalamic alterations is primary and precedes the anorexia, or secondary to starvation effects, is not completely understood. Further evidence for biologic factors contributing to eating disorders includes the high preponderance of affective disorders in patients with eating disorders and their families. Bulimic patients, in particular, appear to be at significant risk for primary affective disorder, and in one study, more than 40% of bulimic patients had previously sought therapy for depression.

SOCIOCULTURAL FACTORS

Sociocultural factors have also been implicated in the etiology of eating disorders. Although surveys indicate that the average American adult woman is 5'4" in height; wears a size 14 dress; and weighs 144 lb, the media continue to extol and emphasize the concept that a woman's value depends on her having a young, thin, alluring body. Women's magazines constantly allude to successful diets, and the centerfold photographs of women in *Playboy* have become thinner during the last 10 to 15 years. Thus, young women are bombarded with the message to remain thin and "perfect." A recent United States National Health survey of 17-year-old girls revealed that 50% would like to be thinner. A survey of friends and relatives of anorectic patients demonstrated envy in 50% of those questioned for the self-control and discipline the anorectic exerts toward food. In addition, the mass media is bombarded with advertisements for diet sodas, diet foods, and diet drugs. One seldom sees an overweight model, an overweight actress, or an overweight Miss America.

PSYCHODYNAMIC ETIOLOGIES

Psychodynamic theory points out that the anorectic patient's behavior and starvation can be viewed as a mechanism to deny the assumption of the female sexual role and mature adult role. The loss of the normal hourglass feminine curve, the diminution of apparent breast fullness, and the amenorrhea all contribute to the "negative" feminine image. Additionally, the normal biologic urges of puberty may be defended against by the intense obsessive-compulsive control that the anorectic directs towards dieting and food intake.

TREATMENT

Eating disorders represent a biopsychosocial disorder and therefore demand both medical and psychiatric treatment.

The first priority of treatment, however, is a complete and thorough medical evaluation that may be accomplished on an outpatient basis, or if weight loss is severe, on an inpatient basis. Medical personnel must inform the patient and the parents that the eating disorder is not of organic etiology but that serious physical consequences can and do occur. In addition, the medical team should emphasize the biopsychosocial nature of this disorder and the importance of cooperative work between the medical and psychiatric personnel. The decision to hospitalize a patient must take into account the patient's physical condition and if there is profound weight loss with physical symptoms, such as marked hypotension or bradycardia. Hospitalization should also be considered if the patient or family refuse to comply with the medical and psychiatric treatment and a significant and serious weight loss continues. Depending on the severity and the nature of the presenting symptoms, the decision to use family therapy, group therapy, individual therapy, antidepressant medication, behavior modification, or cognitive therapy may be employed. Because there is no single precise etiology for the eating disorders, there is no single clear-cut effective therapy.

The type of psychotherapy and the possible use of antidepressant medication should be left to the expertise of a professional involved in the mental health aspects of eating disorders. Although many patients can be successfully treated by the primary care physician, the very nature of this biopsychosocial disorder suggests that a cooperative venture between physical health care specialists and mental health care specialists would lead to an optimal treatment program and a greater potential for a successful outcome.

ANNOTATED BIBLIOGRAPHY

Bruch H: The Golden Cage. Howard University Press, 1978 (Easily read book by one of the leading authorities in the field of eating disorders. Vignettes of almost biographical flavor are balanced by keen clinical insights into the illness of anorexia nervosa. A book applicable to both the professional and lay public.)

Dickstein LJ: Anorexia nervosa and bulimia: A review of clinical issues. Hosp Community Psychiatry 36(10):1086–1092, 1985 (Summary of theoretical and clinical issues concerning eating disorders with an excellent bibliography.)

Lucas RL: Toward the understanding of anorexia nervosa as a disease entity. Mayo Clinic Proc 56:254–264, 1981 (Provides an interesting historical review of anorexia nervosa and presents the clinical material from a broad and varied point of view.)

Minuchin S, Baker L, Rossman B et al: A conceptual model of psychosomatic illness in children. Arch Gen Psychiatry 32:1031–1038, 1975 (Classic paper in the psychosomatic literature; gives an interesting family dynamic perspective to eating disorders.)

46
Rebelliousness and Out-Of-Control Behavior
JOSEPH J. JANKOWSKI

Rebelliousness may be defined as an externally directed behavior against parents or their surrogates, including the establishment, society, authority in general, teachers, or a therapist. It can be difficult to evaluate clinically because within a behavioral spectrum, it could be considered both normal and abnormal. At points along this spectrum, rebelliousness behavior changes almost imperceptably from being acceptable to that of increasing concern. As this occurs, parents, teachers, and other human service providers tend to refer the child initially for a medical examination. As a result, the pediatrician is often the first clinician to examine such children and he is expected to make clinical judgments regarding the seriousness of the behavior and the need for intervention. This chapter is intended to help the pediatrician make these clinical decisions.

PRESENTATION

Rebellious behavior usually first occurs at the developmental stage of identity formation, around the age of 13, when the adolescent is struggling to become a separate individual from his parents. Rebelliousness often begins insidiously and escalates slowly until it either reaches a resolution with psychological integration or progresses to a more serious problem manifested by out-of-control behavior.

The course of clinically significant rebellious behavior is not predictable. In some, it occurs intermittently and does not become serious; in others, it smoulders for several years before either slowly burning out or progressively leading to a more serious problem.

Adolescents separate from their parents and develop their own identities at variable rates. Both intrapsychic and interpersonal factors greatly influence this process. Reality issues such as acute and chronic medical problems, sexual or physical abuse, disfigurement, physical and emotional handicaps, and the loss of a parent through separation, divorce, illness, or death often play critical roles.

Rebelliousness is less serious when this behavior includes the selection of clothing, music, and grooming styles that are at variance with parental expectations. A progression towards more serious behavior includes experimentation with drugs and alcohol, irritability, and unprovoked fighting with the parents or taking a totally different life-style from that of the parents. If left unchecked, this latter behavior might escalate to lying, cheating, stealing, truancy, and running away. If it becomes out of control, the patient might run away, overdose on substances, talk about suicide, or become assaultive. At the extremes, the patient can demonstrate overt homicidal or suicidal behavior and can lose contact with reality. Such patients are unable to care for themselves and are at high risk of being injured, arrested, hospitalized, or incarcerated. Thus, at times what appears on the surface as rebellious behavior might actually represent symptoms of a more serious underlying psychiatric disturbance, such as anxiety, panic, depression, mania, or psychosis.

DIFFERENTIAL DIAGNOSIS

The differential diagnosis of rebellious and out-of-control behavior is as follows:

*   *Developmental disorders* are usually first present in the early grades. If reading, arithmetic, and language deficits are still prominent in adolescence, the patient will invariably have problems in relating to parents, peers, and teachers. These adolescents tend to develop a poor self-esteem and become rebellious because they are frustrated by not being able to function adequately in a learning environment and by not being understood by others.
*   *Personality disorders* occur in adolescents suffering from personality deficits that result in an impairment of social relationships with parents, peers, teachers, and others with subsequent oppositional, rebellious, or withdrawn behavior. Stress superimposed on such disorders usually exaggerates the symptoms and can mimic more serious psychiatric illnesses.
*   *Oppositional disorder* includes a pattern of disobedience, negativism, and oppositional reactions; for example, temper tantrums, argumentativeness, and stubbornness.
*   *Identity disorder* encompasses the impairment of social or academic functioning as a result of difficulty in identity formation such as definition of goals, career, moral, value, and friendship choices, sexual orientation, and group loyalties.
*   *Attention deficit disorder* includes attentional deficits with or without hyperactivity in acute or residual states. Such children display problems with impulse control as manifested by acting before thinking, quick shifts from one activity to another, difficulty organizing one's work because of competing external stimuli, and difficulty in postponing gratification.
*   *Adjustment disorder* is the result of a poor adaptation to psychosocial stressors. Symptoms often include a depressed mood, anxiety, anger, disregard for rules or societal norms, work inhibition, or withdrawal.
*   *Substance abuse disorder* includes patients abusing drugs or alcohol either socially or continuously. They are often secretive, untruthful, and committed to continuing their pattern of abuse with physiologic or psychological dependency. Personality changes and deterioration in school attendance, grades, work, and interpersonal relationships are usually observed.
*   *Conduct disorder* is characterized by a repetitive aggressive pattern of violating another's rights such as the destruction of property, vandalism, rape, assault, breaking and entering, or by a repetitive nonaggressive pattern of violating societal norms or rules; for example, lying, stealing, persistently running away, truancy, substance abuse, and the disregard for rules at home and school. Rebelliousness is often confused with conduct disorder.
*   *Anxiety disorders* are usually noted as the adolescent separates from the parent. Symptoms of anxiety can be manifested as fighting with parents, siblings, peers, school avoidance, phobias, or increased fear during separation experiences such as changing schools, graduation, moving or parental separation, and divorce.
*   *Post-traumatic stress disorder* is manifested by symbolic behavioral events that represent the re-experience of psychological trauma, which was severe enough initially to evoke significant prior reactions of distress. This may occur after being sexually abused. Post-traumatic symptoms often include promiscuity, hypersexualized behavior, or perpetrating sexual abuse on others. Those who have been physically abused often express post-traumatic symptoms of overaggressiveness, self-destructiveness, and injurious or violent behavior directed at others.
*   *Affective disorder* indicates an abnormal variation of two moods, manic and depressive. During manic phases the patient is unusually active, demonstrating a physical restlessness, a flight of ideas, grandiosity, a decreased need to sleep, and easy distractibility. Depressive patients report a decreased appetite, insomnia, loss of energy, loss of libido, unusual fatigue, feelings of poor self-esteem, and an inability to concentrate. In a bipolar disorder, manic and depressive phases are alternatingly present.
*   *Schizophrenic disorders* present as social isolation, bizarre ideation, blunted affect, peculiar behavior and impairment in personal hygiene progressing to the point of bizarre, controlling, somatic, grandiose, or persecutory delusions. Auditory or visual hallucinations may also be present. Such patients frequently cannot achieve or maintain prior levels of functioning in school

or work and become embattled with parents, peers, and teachers.

- *Other psychotic disorders* include such entities as schizophreniform disorder and brief reactive psychosis, both presenting as schizophrenic-like disorders. Schizophreniform patients have no prior recognizable psychosocial stressors. The illness lasts for more than 2 weeks but less than 6 months. Brief reactive psychosis appears immediately following a stressor with symptoms lasting from days to weeks with a general return to premorbid levels of functioning. Included in this category are schizoaffective disorders that combine schizophrenic-like and affective symptoms.

WORK-UP AND DIAGNOSTIC EVALUATION

Before an evaluation can proceed, the clinician must develop a trusting relationship and an alliance with the adolescent and an assurance of confidentially. Once these prerequisites are in place, essential components of the work-up include the following:

- *Chief complaint* defines the adolescent's problem by establishing the level of rebelliousness or out-of-control behavior. Information can be obtained by meeting both with the adolescent alone and together with the parent(s) as well as relatives, school personnel, or other human service providers.
- *Past history of patient* includes a past medical, developmental, educational, and psychiatric history obtained from the patient, parents, and records of other human services providers.
- *Past family history* includes the development of a genetic history of medical and psychiatric illnesses to help better establish a differential diagnosis. This history should include data on parents, aunts, uncles, cousins, and grandparents and can be provided by both the patient and the parent.
- *Current family functioning* is determined through interviews with the patient and parents. An assessment is made of the family's capability to allow the patient to separate gradually. Is the family so enmeshed that it cannot allow a member to separate without a severe disruption or is separation perceived as an abandonment? Are there current problems within the family that might negatively affect separation experiences (*e.g.*, medical or psychiatric illness, death, marital separation, or divorce)?

- *Psychosocial environmental influences* include the type of activities experienced in the peer group and the patient's personal interests (*e.g.*, sports, music, acting, and photography). The type of community in which the patient lives and the social factors inherent in such a locale (*e.g.*, poverty, affluence, and expectations) can be important forces in shaping behavior. It is also helpful to know whether adequate supervision is provided in the environment.
- *Medical examination* should include observation for birth defects, physical deformities, and highly visible problems (*e.g.*, acne that has a high psychological impact). It is also important to determine the usage of prescription and over-the-counter medications. Screening for venereal disease is mandatory if the examiner suspects sexual abuse or promiscuity.
- *Mental status examination* is used to evaluate the patient's pattern of thinking, including the presence of delusions, hallucinations, and suicidal or homicidal behavior. A determination should also be made regarding whether the adolescent is oriented to time, place, and date. Abnormalities in the patient's mood (*e.g.*, depressed, agitated, hypomanic or manic states) should be described.

PRINCIPLES OF MANAGEMENT

- *Mild rebellion* includes behavior at variance from parental expectations such as choice of music, hair-style, dress, and clothing. An increased amount of time is also spent with peers. This behavior is within the range of normal and parents are cautioned not to overreact or interfere with it. In most cases, the parents can benefit from support to help them tolerate these variances, and not reject the adolescent or overinterpret the behavior as negative.
- *Moderate rebellion* includes behavior that might have an adverse effect on the adolescent such as experimentation with alcohol, smoking, staying out excessively late, provocativeness, and fighting with parents. In this stage, it is necessary to set firm limits to help prevent the adolescent's behavior from becoming self-destructive. The parents often require guidance to understand that their child is not psychiatrically disturbed and support not to worsen the existing problem. Parents usually have difficulty in dealing with their child at this stage of rebellion and require professional consultation. They must be cautioned

against fighting with their child as if he were a peer.

- *Severe rebellion* includes behavior that definitely has an adverse effect on the adolescent such as truancy, substance abuse, stealing, promiscuity, and lying. Parents will need professional help to deal with these symptoms before their child becomes alienated or driven out of the home. Such adolescents can be treated as outpatients if the parents are understanding and stable. The child must, however, be capable of responding to limits and of utilizing the anxiety generated in outpatient psychotherapy to progress developmentally without severe regression. If severe regressive behavior occurs, the child may need to live away from the family or be hospitalized in order for psychiatric treatment to proceed. Parental rejection is often a reaction to this phase of adolescent rebellion.

- *Out-of-control behavior* has a self-destructive effect on the adolescent. Examples include suicidal, assaultive, or running away behavior, school dropout, pregnancy, or living on the streets. During this stage, the child will likely require placement in an alternative living arrangement because he often cannot live at home. Such adolescents often require inpatient hospitalization, and afterwards, placement in a residential treatment facility. Their needs for intensive psychiatric treatment usually necessitate a special clinical setting where a therapeutic milieu, psychotherapy and psychopharmacologic agents are available. Treatment often avoids criminalization and placement in a correctional facility.

INDICATIONS FOR REFERRAL

- *Mild rebellion*—The pediatrician can discuss the adolescent's behavior with the parents and help them to understand and better tolerate these normal developmental changes. It must be pointed out to parents that with this behavior, their child is slowly separating from them in an orderly and nondestructive fashion. These children do not require a referral elsewhere.

- *Moderate rebellion*—The pediatrician can meet either with the child and parent together or separately to discuss the rebellious behavior and attempt to help the parent set appropriate limits. Follow-up meetings with the child and parent on a weekly basis for several months is important. A child psychiatrist can be consulted if needed. Early intervention is important because procrastination often leads to more severe problems.

- *Severe rebellion*—The child and parents should be referred to a child psychiatrist for diagnosis and development of a treatment plan. Severely rebellious adolescents require a complete psychiatric evaluation including assessments of the individual child, child–family interaction, and current family functioning. In most cases, the child will require individual and family psychotherapy that can be provided on an outpatient basis.

- *Out-of-control behavior*—In this extreme clinical condition, the child should be referred immediately to a child psychiatrist or to a child psychiatry emergency service or inpatient facility. In this stage, the child will require a comprehensive diagnostic assessment followed by intensive psychiatric treatment including psychotherapy and psychopharmacologic agents. This treatment is best provided initially within an inpatient child psychiatry setting that has the capacity to contain the child and prevent him from running away. Children in this stage of rebellion often do not accept psychiatric services of their own volition. They might, in fact, need to be court ordered into a treatment facility with the help of a child psychiatrist and attorney.

Children at any stage of rebellion can be referred to a clinical psychologist for cognitive assessments and projective testing.

- *Cognitive assessments*—A battery of psychological tests are used. The results of the Wechsler Intelligence Scale for Children—Revised (WISC-R) allows the clinician to determine a patient's current cognitive and potential intellectual functioning. Learning disabilities can be assessed by the Diagnostic Reading Scales (also referred to as Spache), Halstead Neuropsychological Test, and the Gates–MacGinitie Reading Test. Achievement tests such as the Gray Oral Reading Test, Wide-Range Achievement Test (WRAT), and Key-Math Diagnostic Arithmetic Test can also be helpful.

- *Projective tests*—Tests such as the Rorschach Test help to determine either the existence of, or to establish the parameters of, psychopathological thinking.

ANNOTATED BIBLIOGRAPHY

Baittle B, Offer D: On the nature of male adolescent rebellion. Adolesc Psychiatry 1:139–160, 1971 (Contemporary paper on adolescent rebellion.)

Blos P: The function of the ego ideal in adolescence. Psychoanal Study Child 27:93–97, 1972 (Important developmental paper on understanding adolescent behavior including rebelliousness.)

Freud A: Adolescence. Psychoanal Study Child 13:255–278, 1958 (Treatise on general adolescent development with a section on rebellious behavior.)

Freud S: Three essays on the theory of sexuality. Standard Edition 7:132–243, 1905; London, Hogarth, 1953 (Earliest reference to adolescent rebellion.)

Johnson A, Szurek SA: The genesis of antisocial acting out in children and adults. Psychoanal Q 21:323–343, 1952 (Landmark paper concerning etiology of antisocial and rebellious behavior as related to unconscious parental influences.)

Offer D: The Psychological World of the Teenager. New York, Basic Books, 1969 (Important work dealing with normal adolescent behavior.)

Offer D, Offer JB: From Teenage to Young Manhood: A Psychological Study. New York, Basic Books, 1975 (More advanced study of normal adolescent behavior including a section on rebelliousness.)

7

Allergy, Immunology, and Drug Reactions

47
Allergic Rhinitis
IRVING W. BAILIT

Of the estimated 17 million people in the United States with allergic rhinitis, 10% to 20% are children. Symptoms usually begin in the pediatric age group and often in the preschool period. Early recognition and treatment will provide necessary control measures. Only 5% to 10% of children with allergic rhinitis "outgrow" their sensitivity. Allergic rhinitis may be seasonal, perennial, or both. Genetically predisposed children in the temperate climates may develop seasonal hypersensitivity to trees (in April through May), grass (in May through July), ragweed (in August through October), or to the molds (in Spring through Fall). Perennial causes include animal danders, feathers, house dust, and indoor molds. The dust mite is probably the most antigenic factor in house dust. Sensitivity may be to a single allergen but more often multiple allergens are involved. Foods are seldom causes of nasal allergy.

Associated nasal hyperreactivity predisposes the allergic child to several nonallergic stimuli such as sudden temperature changes, positional changes, smoke, aerosols, odors, and airborne particulate matter. Food allergy, atopic dermatitis, and bronchial asthma are also often present.

PATHOPHYSIOLOGY

Sensitization to inhalant antigens produce specific IgE antibodies that attach to the abundant mast cells found in conjunctival and nasal tissues and to the circulating basophils. On re-exposure to the antigen, a series of enzymatic reactions occurs causing the disintegration of the mast cells and the release of chemical mediators (histamine, kinin, prostaglandin D_2, leukotriene C, and TAME esterase). The effects are increased nasal edema, vasodilation, mucorrhea, and infiltration of eosinophils. Reactions may be both immediate and late phase responses occurring 3 to 12 hours after provocation. Added parasympathetic responses increase nasal obstruction and rhinorrhea.

CLINICAL PRESENTATION

Rhinorrhea is clear and bilateral. Because of the congestion, nasal speech and mouth breathing are common, as are manifestations of postnasal drip such as throat clearing, and nocturnal and early morning coughing. Paroxysmal sneezing and nasal itching are characteristic of the allergic nose.

DIFFERENTIAL DIAGNOSES

Acute and chronic respiratory infections are the most common causes of upper airway symptoms. In the presence of purulent secretions, look for foci of infection in the ears, nose, throat, and sinuses. Nasal smears and cultures may indicate infection.

Sinusitis is a complication and a differential diagnosis of chronic allergic rhinitis. Approximately half of allergic children with chronic nasal symptoms were found to have abnormal sinus films. Chronic purulent nasal discharge, fever, and cough

211

are suggestive of sinusitis. A Water's view of the sinuses may be necessary for diagnosis.

Nasal obstruction from choanal atresia, foreign body, septal deviation, or hypertrophied adenoids must be considered. A lateral x-ray view of the nasopharynx may be necessary to exclude adenoidal hypertrophy.

Eosinophilic nonallergic rhinitis may present with classical symptoms of allergy and with nasal eosinophilia. An allergy work-up is completely negative. This condition is seen less frequently in children than in adults. *Vasomotor rhinitis* is a nonallergic rhinitis associated with profuse rhinorrhea and nasal obstruction caused by an autonomic nerve imbalance. It is also only rarely seen in the pediatric population.

Nasal polyps are uncommon in childhood but do occur in 10% to 20% of children with cystic fibrosis. A sweat test should be performed when polyps are identified. The triad of nasal polyps, aspirin hypersensitivity, and asthma appears occasionally in the adolescent.

The overuse of topical nasal decongestants may produce rebound swelling (rhinitis medicamentosa). Local vasoconstrictor drops should not be used for more than 3 to 5 days.

WORK-UP

History

A comprehensive history should indicate the relationship of symptoms to season, place, time of day, activity, and exposure to both specific allergens and nonspecific irritants. The onset, duration, and progression of symptoms, and the complications and the response to previous management are important details. The family history and past history of allergy will help confirm the presence of atopy. An environmental history should disclose potential allergens in the home, school, and outdoor environments.

Physical Examination

Although somewhat variable, findings associated with acute seasonal allergic rhinitis are pallor and edema of the nasal turbinates, clear nasal secretions containing eosinophils, conjunctival injection, tearing, and lid swelling. An examination with chronic allergic rhinitis may reveal frequent swiping of the nose (the "allergic salute"), a transverse nasal crease (the "allergic crease") and facial elongation, gaping mouth and malocclusion from chronic nasal obstruction ("allergic facies"). Darkening beneath the eyes (allergic shiners) may result from venous engorgement.

Laboratory Tests

Children with suspected allergy should be skin tested. The prick method of testing to the inhalants is safe, accurate, and noninvasive and is more sensitive and cost-effective than in vitro radioimmunoassays (RAST). With a strong clinical history, follow-up selected intracutaneous testing may be necessary. Food tests are less reliable and should be performed by prick test only. Positive skin test reactions are only meaningful if there is a clinical correlation. There is no age limitation to skin testing for allergies. However, in the preschool child, testing should be limited to those allergens that relate to the history of exposure or symptoms. Prick skin testing should be considered to identify the atopic child, to determine the presence of specific allergens for avoidance, and to measure the intensity of skin reactions prior to immunotherapy.

The presence of eosinophilia and elevated IgE may be helpful but not necessarily diagnostic or necessary to perform as part of a routine work-up. Serum IgE levels over 20 IU/ml at 1 year of age and over 100 IU ml at 3 years of age suggest atopy. Nasal eosinophilia may help distinguish an allergy from an infection.

TREATMENT AND MANAGEMENT

The control of allergic symptoms should be directed towards the avoidance of exposure and the use of symptomatic medication and immunotherapy when indicated.

The avoidance of indoor allergens such as animals, feathers, and house dust will often be sufficient to alleviate symptoms. Parents should be provided with detailed instructions for environmental control, especially of the child's bedroom. Nonspecific irritants such as aerosol sprays, tobacco smoke, and wood-burning stoves should be avoided. Humidification in the winter and air conditioning in the summer may be helpful. Electronic air cleaners are seldom necessary.

Antihistamines that competitively inhibit the effects of mediator release by binding to the H1 receptors are the primary sources of symptomatic relief. The effects of these drugs are unpredictable, and trials with representatives of the six classes of antihistamines may be necessary. The addition of an oral nasal decongestant (pseudoephedrine, phenylpropanolamine, or phenylephrine) may be beneficial. Tachyphylaxis and excessive sedation may limit the use of oral antihistaminics. Several newer agents, such as terfenadine (Seldane) 60 mg bid, do not cross the blood–brain barrier and do not cause sedation.

Allergic conjunctivitis may require flushing with artificial liquid tears or require topical ophthalmic antihistamine-decongestants to supplement the antihistamines. Ophthalmic corticosteroids are not usually necessary or recommended.

Cromolyn sodium 4% (Nasalcrom) is available in a pump spray and should be used locally in each nostril 4 to 6 times a day for the prevention of nasal symptoms. There are no significant side effects, but supplementary antihistamines may be needed for optimum effect.

The topical nasal corticosteroids have proven to be effective when other measures fail. Hypothalamus-pituitary-adrenal axis suppression, mucosal atrophy, or candidiasis rarely occurs. A therapeutic trial should extend at least 2 weeks. The usual dose is two sprays to each nostril twice daily. (Beclomethasone [Vancenase]; Beconase—400 μg/day; or flunisolide [Nasalide] 200 μg/day). Alternatively, beclomethasone may be administered as one spray in each nostril two to four times a day. The dose should be reduced to the lowest effective amount. Short-term side effects of capillary bleeding and local irritation may occur but tachyphylaxis has not been reported. Dexamethasone nasal spray (Decadron Turbinaire) may be used short-term but only because one third of this drug is absorbed systemically.

Many double-blind placebo-controlled studies have shown that immunotherapy is over 80% effective in children with seasonal allergic rhinitis. Perennial nasal allergy often responds to immunotherapy with house dust and house dust mites but is less responsive to animal dander injections. Monthly maintenance injections should continue for 3 to 5 years. Newer formaldehyde modified antigens and polymerized antigens hold promise for less injections and less reactions. These modified antigens await FDA approval. Immunotherapy should be restricted to those children who have a proven sensitivity, intense and prolonged symp-

toms, and who are unresponsive to other forms of treatment.

Otitis media and serous otitis occur more frequently in the allergic child secondary to eustachian tube obstruction and dysfunction. Hearing, speech, and learning may be affected and should therefore be monitored carefully.

Approximately 3% to 10% of children with allergic rhinitis will develop allergic asthma. In addition, up to 40% of children will note exercise-induced wheezing.

INDICATIONS FOR REFERRAL

A referral to an allergist should be considered for children with symptoms of sufficient intensity and duration and who are unresponsive to treatment. Consider referral of children with chronic or recurrent infections for possible underlying allergic hypersensitivity, especially in the presence of a past or family history of allergy. Although some pediatricians do skin testing, allergy diagnosis must not be solely based on positive skin tests. Follow-up intracutaneous testing (usually best performed by an allergist) is often necessary to uncover suspected allergens.

ANNOTATED BIBLIOGRAPHY

Bailit IW: Pediatric Aspects of Allergic Rhinitis Allergy Proceedings 3:468–471, 1982 (Review of the incidence, causes, complications, and treatment of allergic rhinitis in the child.)

Kawabori I, Pierson W, Conquest L et al: Incidence of exercise-induced asthma in childhood. J Allergy Clin Immunol 58:447, 1976 (Study of the high incidence of exercise-induced asthma in childhood allergic rhinitis.)

Rachelefsky G, Goldberg M, Katz R et al: Sinus disease in children with respiratory allergies. J Allergy Clin Immunol 61:310–314. 1978 (Study on the high incidence of sinus disease in the allergic child.)

Norman P: Review of nasal therapy: Update J Allergy Clin Immunol 72:421–432, 1983 (Excellent review of the recent therapy for allergic rhinitis.)

Siebohm P: Allergic and nonallergic rhinitis. In Middleton E, Reed CE, Ellis EF (eds): Allergy Principles and Practice, pp 868–876. St. Louis, CV Mosby, 1978 (Lucid classification and description of allergic, nonallergic, and vasomotor rhinitis.)

48
Asthma
ALLEN LAPEY

Asthma is the most common chronic lung disorder of children and the most frequent cause of medical hospital admission for children in the United States. Prevalence studies show that 5% to 10% of all children are affected. The incidence peaks from ages 10 to 12 and then gradually subsides during adolescence and young adulthood. Recent epidemiologic data suggest an increasing prevalence over the past 10 years, especially in black children and in urban areas. Correspondingly, increasing numbers of children have been hospitalized with asthma. Risk factors include a history of atopy, bronchiolitis, parental smoking, and recurrent croup. Over 50% of asthmatic children have their first attack of wheezing before 2 years of age. The common perception that most children grow out of their asthma is unfortunately a misconception. Although over 50% of intermittent childhood wheezers are asymptomatic by the age of 21, most retain their bronchial hyperresponsiveness on methacholine challenge and are apt to become symptomatic with viral, exercise, or antigen provocation in later years. The natural history is discouraging for those children who are persistent wheezers or highly atopic. Less than 5% have any likelihood of a long-term remission.

PATHOPHYSIOLOGY

The fundamental abnormality shared by asthmatic patients of all ages is airway reactivity, resulting in varying degrees of smooth muscle spasm, increased mucous secretion, and inflammation. Normal subjects may demonstrate a similar response following an appropriate infectious or inflammatory insult. Hyperresponsiveness, however, always returns to normal in time. This does not occur with the asthmatic airway; it always demonstrates an abnormal response to a cholinergic, cold air, or immunologic challenge. This clear distinction between normal and asthmatic is the rationale for methacholine challenge, the infrequently used but highly specific test of bronchial hyperreactivity.

The theories of β-adrenergic unresponsiveness and increased cholinergic airway responsiveness have been proposed as alternative explanations for a basic underlying genetic defect common to all asthmatic patients. Neither fits well with known data.

Viral infections, especially respiratory syncytial, parainfluenza, and rhinoviruses, are the most important triggers of asthma in children. Bacterial infections, on the other hand, have not been implicated as triggers of acute bronchospasm. It is important to differentiate between the mechanism of airway obstruction induced by viral insults and that from cold air or methacholine challenge. The latter is characterized by the pure spasm of a large airway smooth muscle. The former is an inflammatory insult with mucous membrane disruption and a tremendous mucous hypersecretion.

The hyperpnea of exercise is another common trigger of asthma and is most bothersome in adolescents. The bronchospasm is associated with heat loss from the airway surface and is, therefore, more pronounced in cold, dry air.

Airborne antigens, notably ubiquitous perennial indoor agents, begin to play a more important role in school-aged and adolescent children. Animal danders, dust, and house dust mites are frequently implicated, whereas seasonal pollens have yet to be conclusively implicated in pure childhood asthma without rhinitis.

Many nonspecific, poorly defined environmental irritants are also involved. Cigarette smoking, strong fumes or odors, smoke from defective wood stoves, and outdoor air pollution are frequently mentioned. A sudden change in the weather appears to be another factor and may be the explanation, along with viruses, for the epidemic of childhood asthma that peaks every year in October and November. Emotional factors must also be considered; for example, joy and sorrow can both precipitate bronchospasm.

Characteristically, the asthmatic response to an antigenic challenge is immediate, occurring within 5 to 10 minutes, mediated by IgE, and associated with the release of preformed and membrane-bound mediators that bring about smooth muscle spasm and recruitment of eosinophils. This is often followed by a late asthmatic response, more likely to occur in patients with frequent or chronic asthma. The late response peaks 8 to 10 hours after challenge, long after the subject has recovered from the immediate phase.

In clinical practice, early and late responses most likely coexist and blend into one another. Late responses involve an inflammatory and cellular mechanism. They are more persistent and difficult to treat, and they respond poorly both to theophylline and β-agonist drugs.

Several physiologic and anatomic considerations can help differentiate the small child's asthmatic reaction from that of the adult. First, there is the application of Poiseuille's law: the resistance to airflow through a tube varies inversely with the fourth power of the radius. Small airways are more easily obstructed. Second, collateral ventilation through pores of Kohn and channels of Lambert are poorly developed in early childhood. This may help explain why the child's lung is more susceptible to atelectasis. Third, anatomic studies have shown that there is an increased percentage of mucous glands in the bronchial mucosa of children compared to adults. The increased secretions are another factor predisposing to obstruction.

CLINICAL PRESENTATION

A typical presentation of acute asthma is the rapid onset of wheezing, cough, tachypnea, and retractions in a previously well child, 2 days after the first signs of an upper respiratory infection (URI). Other common scenarios include the athlete who runs without stopping up and down the field and who cannot catch his breath 15 minutes into the game and the allergic child who has recently been exposed to an animal and has both an early and late response. The child develops itchy eyes and sneezing associated with a constant irritative cough within an hour. The cough responds to a β-adrenergic inhalant and the prompt return home of the child. That night, however, 8 to 10 hours later, the patient develops progressive chest tightness and wheezing, but has little relief from the inhaler.

Many children with asthma respond with cough or perhaps mucous hypersecretion rather than wheezing. Such patients typically cough at night; they seem better during the day, but they cough again with hard play or excitement. The diagnosis is established when the cough responds to maintenance bronchodilator therapy. Other asthmatic children are apt to be mislabeled as having recurrent pneumonia because every viral URI results in a cough, patchy segmental infiltrates on a chest roentograph, and perhaps a fever. Infiltrates are frequently in the right middle lobe or lingula. In reality, these infiltrates represent atelectasis from retained secretions, characteristically in those lobes that drain the least efficiently. Most of these patients have a history of wheezing, though not necessarily with each illness.

DIFFERENTIAL DIAGNOSIS

Just as not all asthmatic children wheeze, all children who wheeze are not asthmatics. The differential diagnosis between bronchiolitis and asthma in the young child is difficult, even when a documented respiratory syncytial viral infection exists. On the other hand, if clinical bronchiolitis recurs, the infant more than likely has asthma. Cystic fibrosis is an important cause of wheezing and cough and is often brought on by respiratory viral infections. Such patients can be recognized because they generally respond slowly and incompletely to bronchodilators. The diagnosis of cystic fibrosis is confirmed by a positive sweat test.

The wheeze and cough of foreign body aspiration begin abruptly. The chest examination generally yields asymmetric findings. Non-radiopaque objects are suspected when supine films or fluoroscopy show asymmetric emptying due to trapped air on the involved side. Bronchoscopy with a rigid scope is indicated if suspicion exists.

Gastroesophageal reflux has been incriminated as a cause of chronic or recurrent pulmonary disease, but its role in otherwise healthy children remains unsettled. The pediatrician should remember that gastroesophageal reflux is a normal age-related phenomenon; the various tests for pathologic reflux are inconclusive; and the medical management of reflux is generally safe, allowing the physician to "buy time." Surgical intervention, with potentially serious sequelae and no proven pulmonary benefits, should be avoided if possible.

Several anatomic lesions can sometimes be confused with asthma. Although many congenital and acquired airway lesions can cause wheezing, they are not common. Tracheomalacia is caused by hypercompliant respiratory tract cartilage that vibrates during expiration and sometimes during inspiration. The patients are chronically noisy breathers, accentuated by excitement, but without retractions or distress. They are frequently labeled "happy wheezers" and outgrow their problem. Extrinsic airway compression can be caused by vascular anomalies impinging on the airway, hilar nodes, or mediastinal masses. The wheezing is characteristically fixed. In the case of vascular rings, it is both inspiratory and expiratory. Chest fluoroscopy with barium and possibly a CT scan will confirm the diagnosis.

Finally, mention should be made of pseudoasthma, a functional problem usually in older children and adolescents. Wheezing is simulated by laryngospasm and is usually more noticeable when the patient is under stress. The obstruction can usually be overcome by asking the patient to *pant* rapidly, at which time the noise will clear. The clue in these patients is the unusually noisy and occasionally stridorous nature of their breathing, and total unresponsiveness to standard aggressive bronchodilator therapy. An evaluation should involve laryngoscopy to confirm normal glottic structure and function followed by a referral for behavior modification.

WORK-UP

History

The history is the most important aspect of the asthma work-up. Past wheezing episodes are carefully reviewed for age of onset, time of year, associated illnesses or allergic exposures, response to and side effects from therapy, and patient status between attacks. Are there other features to suggest atopy, such as eczema or rhinitis? Is there a past history of bronchiolitis or recurrent croup? Is there asthma or atopy in the family? Do the parents smoke? Is the child in day care? The answers to these questions should give the pediatrician a good idea of the mechanism triggering the child's asthma. The frequency and severity of past episodes, as well as the status between attacks, will guide the decision of whether to use maintenance drugs or medication as needed.

Physical Examination

Between episodes, the child with asthma may appear entirely normal. Airway lability can often be brought out, however, by insisting that the patient expire forcefully, which frequently uncovers end-expiratory wheezing. Chest deformities may develop when asthma becomes chronic. Pectus carinatum, increased A-P diameter of the thorax, elevated shoulders, and slouching habitus are not uncommon. Despite chronic hypoxemia, digital clubbing is rare and should suggest cystic fibrosis.

The allergic child with asthma generally has fa-

cial clues: allergic shiners (bluish discoloration beneath the lower eyelids), a transverse nasal crease (secondary to chronic upward rubbing because of an itch), and gaping facies due to nasal obstruction and chronic mouth breathing. The nasal mucosa may be pale and swollen with a clear discharge. If the nasal mucosa is red with purulent discharge, sinusitis is a consideration. The presence of nasal polyps in a young child who is wheezing should suggest cystic fibrosis.

An examination of the acutely ill asthmatic reveals a marked prolongation of the expiratory phase and air hunger. A pulsus paradoxus of over 20 mm Hg indicates severe airway obstruction. The pediatrician should remember to check for neck crepitus caused by subcutaneous emphysema and precordial crunch caused by pneumopericardium. Asymmetry of breath sounds between the right and left lung is not unusual in uncomplicated asthma, but unless it resolves promptly with treatment, this should suggest pneumothorax or a foreign body.

Laboratory Tests

The complete blood count may reveal eosinophilia, but is otherwise usually normal. Total IgE is helpful in clarifying the allergic component of the patient's disease. Pulmonary function testing to determine the degree of airflow obstruction and its reversibility is the single most important test in evaluating the asthmatic patient. Pulmonary function, including at least FVC, FEV-1, and reversibility with inhaled bronchodilator are repeated annually and more frequently if necessary. (For a further discussion on pulmonary function tests, see Chap. 167.) In complicated or refractory cases, a sweat test to rule out cystic fibrosis and sinus films to rule out sinusitis should be obtained.

TREATMENT AND MANAGEMENT

Acute Asthma

For the therapy of acute bronchospasm, repeated inhalations of nebulized β2-adrenergic agents has become the preferred initial therapy. Isoetharine 0.5 ml, albuterol 0.5 ml, or metaproterenol 0.2 to 0.3 ml in 2 ml saline have consistently been shown to be as effective as subcutaneous epinephrine, but with considerably less tachycardia, pallor, excitement, and nausea. Aerosol therapy is effective even in severe bronchospasm with little air movement and in patients who have become unresponsive to inhaled β2-agonists on the outside. In uncooperative subjects, many now prefer terbutaline 0.01 mg/kg subcutaneously to epinephrine because of fewer side effects and a longer duration of action. Tremor may be a problem, however.

Inhalation treatments are repeated every 20 minutes as necessary. If there has not been a sufficient improvement following the second treatment, theophylline is added. Children likely to tolerate oral medications can be given 5 mg/kg of a short-acting preparation po and watched for the next 2 to 3 hours. Sicker patients should be given IV aminophylline, 7 mg/kg over 20 minutes remembering that every 1 mg/kg in the loading dose will raise the serum theophylline level by 2 μg/ml. Patients who have received po theophylline over the past 24 hours should first have a stat theophylline level and the loading dose adjusted to achieve a final serum concentration of 14 μg/ml. Any patient ill enough to receive IV aminophylline should at the same time begin corticosteroid therapy. Methylprednisolone 1 mg/kg or hydrocortisone 5 mg/kg IV are both effective. Aminophylline can then be continued as a constant infusion of 1.1 mg/kg/hr for ages 1 to 6, and 0.9 mg/kg/hr at ages 7 to 12. Treatment with aerosol β2-agonist should be continued, as the steroid bolus should begin to restore β-receptor responsiveness after 1 hour. If, after 4 hours of observation, there is not a satisfactory improvement, hospitalization for continued IV therapy is indicated. All aspects of the above described acute management scheme can be carried out in an office setting, with the possible exception of stat theophylline level determinations.

Once satisfactory acute control is achieved, the patient can be sent home receiving one drug more than he had previously been using at the time of the attack, that is: β-agonist if on nothing, β-agonist plus maintenance theophylline if previously on β-agonist, and both of the above plus prednisone if previously on β-agonist and theophylline. Any patient requiring steroids in the past for acute asthma can generally be assumed to need steroids again for subsequent acute attacks. Finally, patients using aerosolized beclomethasone who break through with asthma must be considered steroid dependent and they should be treated with systemic prednisone until the airway obstruction has subsided and aerosolized medications can again be reintroduced.

Many preschool patients are seen with recurrent episodes of cough, some fever, diffuse wheezing and, at times, rales. Segmental infiltrates on chest roentographs are common, more likely the result of atelectasis than pneumonia. Although acute bronchospasm is not usually associated, this nonetheless represents asthma. Therapy should involve an aggressive use of bronchodilators with consideration of corticosteroids acutely and anti-inflammatory prophylaxis with nebulized cromolyn chronically. It appears that most of these episodes are triggered by viral illnesses. Despite the radiographic abnormalities, there is little to justify the use of antibiotics.

Chronic Asthma

The goals of long-term asthma management are to prevent hospitalization and emergency room visits, minimize school absenteeism, encourage full physical activity and sports participation, discourage secondary gain from chronic illness, and to do all this with the least amount of medication and minimal side effects. The mainstay of asthma therapy is pharmacologic. There are four classes of drugs: β-adrenergic agents, theophylline, cromolyn sodium, and corticosteroids.

β-Agonists. For mild asthma with intermittent wheezing less than half the time, oral or inhaled β-agonist is the preferred drug. Either albuterol or terbutaline is preferred, given their enhanced β2 selectivity and longer duration of action. Children over the age of 8 years are encouraged to use metered dose inhalers rather than oral drugs, as systemic side effects are less and bronchodilation is prompt, at one tenth the oral dose. Most children with mild asthma can be effectively controlled on two inhalations every 6 to 8 hours. Optimal airway deposition of the inhaled agent, which at best is no more than 15% of that expelled from the device, is dependent on a proper inhaler technique; this must be demonstrated and patiently reinforced by the physician and his staff. The correct method involves a single slow inhalation from end expiration (FRC) rather than from residual volume, with the mouth piece held 1 inch from the open mouth. The lips should not touch the inhaler. Inhalation is followed by a 10-second breath hold and the entire procedure repeated 3 minutes later. In younger patients or those that find inhaler coordination difficult, various useful spacer devices have been developed. For the preschool aged child, many parents much prefer the improved control they can enjoy using a home compressor and nebulizer to administer β-agonist aerosol by mask or mouthpiece. With this equipment, β-agonist inhaler solution such as isotharine 0.5 ml, albuterol 0.5 ml, or metaproterenol 0.2 to 0.3 ml is diluted in 2 ml saline and the medication is nebulized for a 5- to

10-minute treatment of quiet breathing. This procedure requires essentially no cooperation from the child other than sitting reasonably still.

β2-adrenergic aerosols are also the preferred drug for prevention of exercise-induced asthma. Two inhalations from a metered dose inhaler immediately before anticipated activity frequently permits the athlete to participate successfully in strenuous physical exercise that he would otherwise have to avoid. Inhalers have the potential for abuse, especially when used by adolescents. The danger with the newer selective β2-agonists is not as much the direct toxicity of the drug, as it is the failure of the patient to recognize that an inadequate short-lived response to therapy is an immediate indication to seek medical attention, not to continue taking more of the drug. This problem can be avoided with proper education and reinforcement.

Theophylline. The development of sustained release theophylline preparations with essentially total bioavailability has greatly simplified the management of childhood asthma. Most physicians consider theophylline the preferred bronchodilator for maintenance therapy of moderate (*i.e.*, persistent or frequently intermittent) asthma. However, the drug has a low therapeutic index (*i.e.*, a narrow range between therapeutic and toxic serum concentrations). Furthermore, many patients, not infrequently younger children, experience side effects of hyperactivity, gastrointestinal upset, and insomnia at therapeutic or even subtherapeutic serum levels.

It is prudent to begin therapy with two thirds of the recommended dose. The dose can be increased in incremental steps every 3 to 4 days until a satisfactory clinical response is achieved or a peak recommended dose is attained. Children aged 1 to 9, with relatively shorter theophylline half-lives, usually require TID administration of a sustained release preparation with maximal dose of 24 mg/kg/day. Older children and adolescents can usually be managed with BID administration at a dose of 18 to 20 mg/kg/day up to 800 mg/day. Theophylline levels should be checked when the conventional dose causes signs of toxicity or it fails to produce a good response. Standard anhydrous theophylline liquid or tablet preparations are rarely indicated in asthma management. There are many reliable sustained-release products now available, including bead-filled capsules that can be opened and sprinkled on food for younger children. Both Slo-BID and Theodur are particularly reliable in their absorption characteristics and can provide continuous

Increased and Decreased Theophylline Clearance

INCREASE THEOPHYLLINE CLEARANCE

Phenobarbital
Phenytoin
Intravenous isoproterenol
Low carbohydrate, high protein diet
Cigarette and marijuana smoking

DECREASE THEOPHYLLINE CLEARANCE

Erythromycin
Troleandomycin
Cimetadine, not ranitidine
High fever
Liver disease
Heart failure
High carbohydrate, low protein diet

therapeutic levels with BID administration in older children and TID administration in children ages 1 to 9. Although the therapeutic range of serum levels is stated as 10 μg/ml to 20 μg/ml, it is preferable to aim for levels in the lower end of the range. Otherwise, a temporary reduction in clearance could result in toxicity. Drugs and other factors that commonly affect theophylline clearance are listed in the box, Increased and Decreased Theophylline Clearance. Remember that there is nothing magical about a therapeutic level. Many mildly involved patients have complete control of their asthma with no side effects on low doses and "subtherapeutic" levels. When to stop the drug is usually not completely clear; it is wise to have the patient symptom-free for at least 1 week before maintenance therapy is discontinued.

Cromolyn. Cromolyn has become popular again as an alternative to theophylline for first-line maintenance therapy of asthma. Much of the interest has grown from the realization that theophylline is not tolerated by many patients. In contrast, cromolyn is essentially nontoxic. Furthermore, it has become increasingly clear that cromolyn is effective in controlling nonspecific airway hyper-reactivity. Formerly available only as an aerosol powder that was often irritating when inhaled, cromolyn is now also available as a 20% aerosol solution for use with a power-driven nebulizer and as a metered dose inhaler. The aerosol solution, when administered TID or QID with or without an added β-agonist, is often effective in controlling asthma in smaller children who are unable to use inhalers. Many comparative studies have consistently shown that cromolyn is as effective as maintenance theophylline and that it has no side effects. As a first-line drug roughly equivalent to theophylline in efficiency, cromolyn is unlikely to benefit the poorly controlled asthmatic who is already receiving full doses of adrenergic agents and theophylline. Such a patient will probably need corticosteroids. Cromolyn is not indicated for acute asthma; its use is strictly prophylactic, and as such has been shown to prevent both the early and late bronchial response to inhaled antigen challenge.

Corticosteroids. Oral corticosteroids are the last drugs to be started and the first to be stopped in asthma management. Unfortunately, they are often not started soon enough. Steroid therapy is *indicated*: (1) for patients in relapse despite full doses of theophylline and β-agonist, (2) for patients with a history of steroid therapy for past episodes, (3) for patients in trouble despite inhaled steroids, (4) for chronic low-grade asthma that simply persists despite optimal therapy. One regimen is prednisone 2 mg/kg/day, up to 60 mg/day, for 3 to 5 days until the asthma resolves, then tapering over 3 to 4 more days. The tapering process prevents the psychological withdrawal and musculoskeletal aching that patients experience occasionally, even following 7-day courses of therapy. A brief steroid course is remarkably effective in clearing asthma and restoring responsiveness to β-agonist agents and the risks are minimal. For the occasional severely involved chronic asthmatic, low-dose alternative day prednisone or daily inhaled beclomethasone can free him to lead a relatively normal life without leaving the crippling side effects of daily steroid therapy. The patient is cleared generally with a 7-day course of prednisone, following which he remains on 15 mg to 20 mg given at or about 8AM every 48 hours. The dose can then be slowly withdrawn in increments of 2.5 mg every 1 to 2 weeks, depending on the patient's response. Alternatively, beclomethasone by aerosol, in a dose of four inhalations twice a day or two inhalations four times a day has been shown to have significant steroid-sparing effects on previously steroid-dependent asthmatics. The drug is extremely surface-active in small doses, and although absorbed, it is rapidly metabolized by the liver. Hypothalamic-pituitary-adrenal suppression is absent or insignificant at doses up to eight inhalations a day. Many patients, especially children, are controlled on only four inhalations a day.

Side effects include oral candidiasis, which is preventable by rinsing the mouth after use. Hoarseness is also occasionally seen and disappears when the drug is discontinued.

The effectiveness and relative safety of steroid therapy in the treatment of asthma, whether in alternate day, topical, or short course high doses, cannot be emphasized enough. The most tragic outcomes in childhood asthmatics come from a lack of treatment, not from the therapy itself.

INDICATIONS FOR REFERRAL

Asthma is often a chronic disease requiring a comprehensive and long-term therapeutic approach. Episodic intervention must be replaced by anticipatory care. For physicians willing to devote the time, long-term asthma management can be one of the most gratifying experiences in pediatrics. In this respect, referrals are generally unnecessary and may actually interfere with physician–patient communication. This is certainly true of mild and moderate asthma. Referral is more likely necessary for management of severe chronic, steroid-dependent asthma, and for diagnostic clarification of suspected allergic factors in asthma.

It should be remembered that there is no evidence that therapy of any sort, even by the most sophisticated subspecialist, influences the natural history of the disease. Nonetheless, proper patient and family education, stressing anticipatory care and self-management, has been effective in improving patient self-esteem and the overall quality of life.

ANNOTATED BIBLIOGRAPHY

Cropp GJA: Special features of asthma in children. Chest 87:555, 1985 (Particularly strong discussion of epidemiology, risk factors, and prognosis.)

Ellis EF: Asthma in childhood. J Allergy Clin Immunol 72:526, 1983 (Lucid, concise discussion by one of the acknowledged leaders in the field.)

Rachelefsky GS, Siegel SC: Asthma in infants and children, Parts I and II. J Allergy Clin Immunol 76:1–14, 409–425, 1985 (This two-part review presents the allergist-immunologist point of view. The section on therapy is comprehensive and well referenced.)

Weinberger M: The pharmacology and therapeutic use of theophylline. J Allergy Clin Immunol 73:525, 1984 (Honest overview, emphasizing not only pharmacokinetics but also practical aspects of theophylline dosing.)

49

Anaphylaxis—Outside the Emergency Room

IRVING W. BAILIT

Anaphylaxis is the most frightening unanticipated and potentially fatal hypersensitivity reaction. Reaction time may occur within minutes after provocation. The rapidity of the reaction is related directly to the intensity. Because of the imminent danger of such reactions, the physician must be knowledgeable of the causes and the means of prevention, and he must be prepared to offer emergency treatment.

PATHOPHYSIOLOGY

A massive release of the chemical mediators of anaphylaxis may be the result of specific antigen–antibody (IgE) interaction from prior sensitization or may occur from a number of non-IgE mediated mechanisms. In either type of reaction there is a basophil and mast cell disintegration and a release of histamine, leukotrienes, prostaglandins, and platelet activating factors. Nonallergic responses may involve immune complexes and the activation of complement (anti-IgA reactions), the direct basophil and mast cell release of mediators (radiocontrast reactions), or arachidonic acid metabolism (aspirin hypersensitivity). The major pathologic findings are edema of the larynx and upper airway (the primary cause of death in children), acute pulmonary hyperinflation, and cardiovascular collapse secondary to hypovolemia and shock. The site of the reaction is more dependent on the host than on the provoking source.

CLINICAL PRESENTATION

Initial symptoms begin with flushing, increased warmth, generalized pruritus followed by urticaria and angioedema. Reactions may lead to stridor and hoarseness, dyspnea and wheezing, dysphagia, vomiting, cramps and diarrhea, lightheadedness, and loss of consciousness.

WORK-UP

History

The following is a list of the most common causes of anaphylaxis and the history should explore recent exposure to these offending agents:

- Drugs—Penicillin and its synthetic derivatives are the most common causes of anaphylaxis followed by aspirin and the nonsteroidal anti-inflammatory agents. The cephalosporins may cross-react with penicillin. Other drugs include insulin, ACTH, codeine, morphine, and the non-β lactam antibiotics (see Chap. 50).
- Biologicals—Antiserum, toxoids, egg-based vaccines, gammaglobulin, and chymotrypsin
- Diagnostic agents—Radiocontrast materials
- Foods—Especially milk, egg, nuts, legumes, fish, shellfish, and berries (see Chap. 51)
- Hymenoptera venoms—Honey bee, yellow jacket, hornet, wasp, and fire ant (see Chap. 70)
- Allergy extracts—Diagnostic and therapeutic allergens given by injection
- Physical agents—Cold-induced and exercise-induced anaphylaxis
- Injectables—Dextran and nitrofurantoin. Blood transfusion in sensitized IgA-deficient patients
- Idiopathic—Despite extensive studies, the cause of many anaphylactic reactions is unknown.

Physical Examination

Depending on the severity and duration of an episode, an examination will reveal flushing and regional or generalized urticaria with or without associated angioedema. Edema of the tongue, uvula, or larynx may cause stridor, retraction, or cyanosis. Lower airway obstruction will be manifested by a cough and wheezing. Cardiovascular effects are hypotension, a thready or irregular pulse, and signs of shock.

The presence of these clinical manifestations combined with the history of a compatible temporal association to a likely etiological agent is diagnostic of an anaphylactic reaction. However, remember that many such episodes are idiopathic in origin. The diagnosis of the cause is based on a history and studies to determine allergic antibody. Laboratory studies are not usually necessary for diagnosis of the acute episode but may be helpful in monitoring the reaction.

TREATMENT

The possibility of an anaphylactic reaction must be anticipated in all patients receiving drugs or diagnostic or therapeutic materials. The atopic patient is more susceptible to anaphylaxis. Early identification and treatment is important. Necessary medications and equipment should be readily available for monitoring and treatment. Necessary office equipment should include tourniquets, needles and syringes, arm board, intravenous tubing, parenteral fluids, oxygen, ambu bag, oral airways, and a cricothyrotomy tube or No 12 needle.

The most important drug is epinephrine (Adrenalin) 1:1000 0.1 to 0.5 ml max (0.01 ml/kg) given subcutaneously or intramuscularly. Dose may be repeated at 15- to 20-minute intervals three times. In the presence of cardiovascular collapse, epinephrine is diluted in 10 ml saline and 1 ml to 2 ml is given slowly over several minutes intravenously. If the antigen is introduced by injection or venom sting on an extremity, then epinephrine may be given subcutaneously (0.1 ml to 0.2 ml) at the site. A tourniquet should be applied proximally to reduce antigen absorption.

In the presence of urticaria and angioedema, follow epinephrine with diphenhydramine (Benadryl). This drug may be administered orally or intramuscularly 10 mg to 25 mg in younger children and 25 mg to 50 mg in older children. With severe reactions, treat intravenously (2 mg/kg) up to 50 mg/dose over several minutes. Benadryl should be continued orally for the next 48 hours (5 mg/kg/day).

In the presence of wheezing unresponsive to epinephrine, isoetharine (Bronkosol) or a β-2 agonist such as metaproterenol (Alupent) may be given by nebulization. Continued wheezing would warrant the use of aminophyllin intravenously (5 mg/kg to 7 mg/kg) in IV solution over 20 minutes and followed if necessary with an infusion of 0.6 to 1.0 ml/kg/hr. Theophylline levels should be monitored.

Treatment of hypotension is by rapid infusion of intravenous saline or volume expanders. Vasopressor agents such as metaraminol (Aramine) 0.4 mg/kg given slowly in 500 ml of 5% D/W or levarterenol bitartrate (Levophed) 1 mg (1 ml) in 250 ml of 5% D/W at 0.5 ml/min in children or 4 mg (4 ml) to 1000 ml 5% D/W at a rate of 1 to 2 ml/min in adults may be necessary to control hypotension. Blood pressure and cardiac rate should be closely checked.

Corticosteroids are not useful as initial treatment of anaphylaxis but may be indicated for secondary or delayed symptoms. Either hydrocortisone (Solu–Cortef) 7 mg/kg followed by 7 mg/kg/ 24hr at 4- to 6-hour intervals or methyl prednisolone (Solu-Medrol) 2 mg/kg followed by 2 mg/kg/24 hr may be used.

It is important that vital signs be monitored frequently. Oxygen should be available and used when needed. Acute upper airway obstruction may require a cricothyrotomy tube or a No 12 needle to establish a temporary airway. Initial treatment of anaphylaxis should be started in the office. Unresponsive patients should be transferred to hospital intensive care units for continued care.

PREVENTION

Most anaphylactic reactions are preventable. A complete history should uncover previous history of anaphylaxis, adverse drug reactions, allergic reactions to foods, venoms, vaccines, and diagnostic agents.

Drugs

Although only 10% to 25% of drug reactions are allergic, any history of adverse drug reactions must be considered as a possible cause of anaphylaxis. A review of previous medical records or skin testing may rule out drug allergy. Use alternative drugs whenever possible. Oral medications are less likely to cause systemic reactions. In serious clinical situations where penicillin is mandatory, testing to both the major and minor antigenic determinants of penicillin is both safe and accurate. Children with negative reactions may be safely treated with penicillin. Positive skin reactors should avoid penicillin and its derivatives or undergo oral desensitization. Unfortunately, testing to most drugs is not possible.

Vaccines

Routine childhood immunizations should be maintained so that heterologous antiserum does not become necessary. Children with known egg hypersensitivity may react to viral vaccines grown on chick embryo. Skin testing with diluted and undiluted vaccine should precede administration.

Foods

Foods should be introduced cautiously to atopic children. Known food reactions should be avoided. Questionable reactions may be proven by prick skin testing or by radioimmunoassay testing (RAST), although delayed reactions may require dietary elimination and challenge for diagnoses. Although most food sensitivity clears with increasing age, certain food allergies such as to nuts and fish may persist for a lifetime.

Radiocontrast Material

Previous reactors should avoid reexposure. However, when repeated studies become necessary, pretreat with prednisone 50 mg orally every 6 hours for 3 doses before the study and diphenhydramine (Benadryl) 50 mg IM 1 hour before the procedure.

Hymenoptera

Children with urticarial responses only to venom stings are not felt to be at risk for increasing anaphylaxis and immunotherapy is not recommended. Children with upper or lower airway obstruction or with cardiovascular symptoms and reactive to venom testing should be immunized to the specific venoms.

IMMUNOTHERAPY

Physicians who administer inhalant antigens and venoms by injection must be prepared to treat systemic reactions. Such reactions may be reduced by observing the size of local reactions as a guideline to antigen tolerance, reducing antigen dose during high pollen seasons and with new extracts, and observing the patient for 20 minutes after injection.

EXERCISE-INDUCED ANAPHYLAXIS

This physical condition is now being recognized with increasing frequency. Incidence is greater when exercise occurs after meals and sometimes after specific foods (*e.g.*, celery, shrimp). Treatment is by limitation of exercise duration, avoidance of foods for 4 hours prior to exercise, and the availability of an epinephrine syringe.

Children with a history of anaphylaxis should wear an identifying bracelet. This may be obtained from the Medic-Alert Foundation in Turlock, California. These children should also have an epinephrine kit available (Epi-pen, Epi-pen Jr from Center Laboratory or an AnaKit from Hollister–Steir Laboratory) for emergency use. The parent and child should be instructed regarding the technique of administration and indications for use.

ANNOTATED BIBLIOGRAPHY

Bailit IW: Anaphylaxis. In Gellis SS, Kagan BM (eds): Current Pediatric Therapy, Vol 11, pp 641–643. Philadelphia, WB Saunders, 1984 (Concise review of measures of prevention and treatment.)

Sale SR, Greenberger PA, Patterson R: Idiopathic anaphylactoid reactions. JAMA 246:2336, 1984 (Excellent treatise on idiopathic anaphylaxis—the scope of the problem, work-up, and management.)

Sheffer AL: Anaphylaxis. J Allergy Clin Immunol 75:227–233, 1985 (Current knowledge of immunologic mechanisms of anaphylaxis.)

Yaffe SJ et al: Anaphylaxis. Committee on Drugs Am Acad Pediatrics 51:137–140, 1973 (Review of causes and treatment by the Committee on Drugs of the American Academy of Pediatrics.)

50
Drug Allergy
STEVEN M. MATLOFF

Adverse drug reactions are an important clinical problem. This chapter focuses on the small subset of adverse drug reactions that can be demonstrated to have an immunologic mechanism, and the term *drug allergy* is used to refer to these reactions. Allergic drug reactions account for the minority (5% to 10%) of all adverse reactions to drugs, whereas the majority (90%) of all drug reactions are not immunologically mediated. Most of these latter reactions are due to either excessive dosage (leading to toxicity), side effects, intolerance, idiosyncracy, or drug interactions.

An exact incidence of adverse drug reactions is not known, but estimates in hospitalized patients indicate a prevalence of as high as 6% to 15% and drug-induced reactions may account for as many as 3% of hospital admissions. Thus, these reactions cause significant morbidity and mortality.

The epidemiology of drug allergy is made difficult for several reasons. First, it is not always possible to determine if a symptom or sign could be caused by the drug or by the disease being treated. Second, many patients are often treated with more than one medication simultaneously and it is difficult to determine which medication is responsible for the reaction. Third, ambulatory patients who have drug reactions are seldom reported and therefore accurate statistics are difficult to obtain.

Certain factors may be important in determining whether an individual will have a greater chance of developing an allergic drug reaction, although in most instances it is not entirely clear why a drug allergy occurs in a particular patient. Those individuals who have had a history of an allergic reaction to one drug seem to be at increased risk for developing repeated allergic reactions to the same drug and also to other drugs. The drug itself is important because some drugs (*e.g.*, penicillin) appear to be more allergenic than others. Genetic factors may play a role, but this is still not clear. Atopic patients do not appear to have a higher incidence compared to nonatopic patients. Multiple courses of a drug increase the chances of developing an allergic reaction to that drug. Certain disease states may increase the risk of reactions to certain drugs.

PATHOPHYSIOLOGY

Allergic drug reactions are characterized by the generation of an immunologic response to a drug or drug metabolite. This, in turn, produces a clinically significant adverse reaction that is manifested by the appearance of various signs or symptoms that do not resemble the known pharmacologic effects of the drug. Most immunologic reactions can be categorized according to the well known Gell's and Coombs' classification. Type 1 reactions, manifested as anaphylaxis, are those mediated by the presence of an IgE antibody directed against specific drug-related antigens. IgE is bound to the surface of mast cells and basophils, and when the drug antigens attach to specific antidrug IgE, vasoactive mediators (*e.g.*, histamine, leukotrienes, and so forth) are released from these cells, leading to anaphylaxis that can vary in severity from trivial to life-threatening and fatal. The manifestation and treatment of anaphylaxis are discussed in Chapter 49. These reactions occur within minutes to several hours after initiation of drug treatment, but reactions may also appear days after the drug is started. There is usually a history of prior exposure to the drug, but often this history cannot be elicited. The most common medication to cause severe and fatal anaphylaxis is penicillin.

Anaphylactoid reactions have similar symptoms compared to IgE-mediated anaphylactic reactions. In these cases, the drug is capable of directly or indirectly causing non-IgE dependent vasoactive mediator release. The spectrum of symptoms are the same as those seen with true anaphylaxis. Examples of diagnostic agents and medications that may cause these types of reactions include radiographic contrast material, codeine and other narcotic analgesics, aspirin and the nonsteroidal antiinflammatory drugs.

Type 2 immunologic reactions are those mediated by the production of cytotoxic antibody (IgG, IgM) which is able to cause damage by binding to cell membranes and causing complement activation or by inducing mononuclear cell activation. Penicillin-induced hemolytic anemia is an example of this type of reaction.

Type 3 reactions are caused by an immune complex formation (drug antigen–antibody complexes) that subsequently activates the complement cascade, leading to the generation of anaphylotoxins C3a and C5a, with subsequent mediator release and inflammation. Serum sickness is the classical clinical presentation and can be caused by several medications, but most commonly with penicillin and other antibiotics. Manifestations include lymphadenopathy, fever, urticaria, exanthem, arthralgia or arthritis, and general malaise.

Type 4 reactions are classical delayed hypersensitivity reactions and include T-cell mediated immunity. Delayed skin reactions or contact dermatitis from topical medication exposure are examples of this type of drug-induced immunologic reaction.

WORK-UP

The history and physical examination are the most important tools in diagnosing a drug allergy. A clear history of the symptoms and their temporal relationship to drug administration, prior drug use, and prior history of drug reaction are all important. The drug dosage, the duration of therapy, the disease being treated, and concomitant medication use should be determined. Other underlying medical disorders (*e.g.*, hepatic or renal dysfunction) should be known.

Symptoms or signs of drug allergy may be present while an individual is taking a drug and the diagnosis of a drug allergy is a clinical one in most instances, because there are usually no immediate diagnostic tests that can help confirm the diagnosis.

The patient will often have a history of drug allergy. It is best to avoid the drug, unless it is considered essential for treatment and no acceptable alternatives are available, or if the alternative medications themselves have caused unacceptable adverse reactions.

If no acceptable alternative therapy is available that is well tolerated and equally effective, the patient should then be referred for further evaluation for diagnostic testing (if available) or desensitization or test dosing (if appropriate). The following discussion reviews selected aspects of the most common allergic drug reactions. (For an exhaustive review, see any of the three references listed in the bibliography.)

PENICILLIN

Although penicillin and other β-lactam antibiotics may cause various adverse reactions, their propensity to cause immediate anaphylactic reactions is a major concern. Anaphylactic reactions may occur when the drug is administered for the first time, implying that the patient was sensitized by way of an occult source (foods, or by intrauterine exposure). Patients will often give vague histories of penicillin allergy but are unable to recall the details. These patients should often be assumed to be allergic and penicillins should be avoided in these patients as well as in those with more convincing histories.

If a patient with a positive history requires penicillin, penicillin skin testing should be performed with both the major and minor metabolites of penicillin. The three reagents currently in use for skin testing include benzyl penicilloyl–polylysine, penicillin G, and a minor determinant mixture (MDM) containing benzylpenicilloate and benzylpenicilloylan–propylamine. (MDM is not commercially available at this time).

A positive skin test to any reagent, but especially the minor determinant, indicates that the patient is at high risk (50% to 70%) for developing an anaphylactic reaction if penicillin is administered. Patients with positive skin tests can be desensitized by administering small amounts of penicillin and cautiously increasing the dose until full therapeutic doses are achieved. This procedure involves considerable risk and should only be performed in an ICU setting with an open IV line in place, resuscitation equipment, and personnel in attendance. It must be made clear in the medical record that no acceptable alternative therapy is available to the patient, and it is best if this is stated by an Infectious Disease Consultant. Most patients can be successfully desensitized but it must be emphasized that the desensitization applies only to the present course of antibiotic therapy, and the patient would

need to be re-evaluated at a later time if it became necessary to administer penicillin again. There are few clinical situations in which penicillin would be the only acceptable alternative medication, and these situations occur generally in hospitalized patients with serious life-threatening systemic infections.

If the skin tests are negative, patients are at a low risk of developing immediate IgE-mediated reactions within the first 72 hours of penicillin administration. However, false negatives occur rarely and for this reason patients with negative test results should also be given penicillin cautiously by giving small test doses and gradually increasing to full therapeutic doses. Skin test results cannot predict the likelihood of developing delayed adverse reactions, which may occur more than 72 hours after the initiation of penicillin treatment and this should be made clear to patients before beginning a course of treatment.

Penicillin skin testing should not be done if alternative non-β lactam antibiotics can be used in a patient. Penicillin testing should only be considered if alternative therapy has failed or is not well tolerated. An urticarial reaction will often occur while a patient is taking both penicillin and another drug, and in this situation, penicillin testing may be useful to help determine if penicillin is the likely offending agent.

Caution should be exercised in administering cephalosporins and semisynthetic penicillins to patients with documented penicillin allergy. These antibiotics should be avoided in such patients if an alternative therapy is available, but could be cautiously administered if essential, by using similar test dosing or desensitization schedules. The exact incidence of cross-reactivity between cephalosporins and penicillin is not known.

AMPICILLIN

Ampicillin can cross-react with penicillin and cause anaphylactic reactions. A major cause of concern is its frequent cause of delayed skin rashes, usually maculopapular, that may occur after several days of therapy. These are usually not IgE mediated and may not reappear on subsequent administration. They occur more frequently in patients with infectious mononucleosis, hyperuricemia, or if taken concomitantly with allopurinol. Alternative therapy would be recommended. Skin testing can help in assessing the risk of developing immediate IgE-mediated reactions.

ASPIRIN AND NONSTEROIDAL ANTI-INFLAMMATORY DRUGS

These medications can cause severe life-threatening anaphylactoid reactions, bronchospasm, and generalized urticaria. There is a significant degree of cross-reactivity between aspirin and the nonsteroidal anti-inflammatory drugs (NSAID). It is therefore advisable for an individual who is sensitive to aspirin to avoid NSAID unless the drugs are considered absolutely necessary because of their anti-inflammatory effects and because no acceptable alternative agents are available.

If there is doubt about the clinical diagnosis of aspirin hypersensitivity, and it becomes essential to use this medication, the patient can be tested by cautious oral challenge, beginning with small doses (1 mg or less) and gradually increasing the dosage every 30 minutes. It must be emphasized that this is a high-risk procedure and should only be performed by individuals skilled in its administration and should be done in a hospital intensive care setting. Informed consent is necessary, and unequivocal indications for performing the challenge must be clearly recorded in the medical record.

SULFONAMIDES

This group of antibiotics is a common cause of immunologic reactions, manifested primarily by generalized skin eruptions ranging from minor urticaria to life-threatening exfoliative dermatitis or Stevens Johnson syndrome. Other manifestations, such as serum sickness, blood dyscrasias, and anaphylaxis, are also observed.

The treatment involves withdrawal of the medication and strict avoidance of these medications in the future. Test dosing can be performed, but it involves considerable risk and should only be done if there are no acceptable alternative medications. Cross-reactivity may occur with the thiazide diuretics, some oral hypoglycemic agents, and acetazolamide, and should be avoided in sulfa-allergic patients.

LOCAL ANESTHETICS

Patients with a history of an adverse reaction to a local anesthetic will often be referred by dentists or other health care providers. In most instances, the reactions that have occurred have been non-immunologic. Many of these reactions are due to vasovagal reactions, hyperventilation, central nervous system stimulation or depression, cardiovascular side effects, or side effects from other components of the local anesthetic such as epinephrine. IgE-mediated hypersensitivity occurs rarely and it is almost always possible to find an alternative local anesthetic that the patient will be able to tolerate by performing appropriate subcutaneous challenges. It is important to perform challenges with this group of drugs, if appropriate, so that they will not unnecessarily be avoided because of a history of a nonallergic adverse reaction. When true immediate (IgE-mediated) hypersensitivity can be demonstrated, other agents may at times need to be substituted, such as a local injection of benadryl or general anesthesia.

IMMUNIZING AGENTS

Various adverse reactions to both passive and active immunizing agents have been reported. These can be either immunologic or nonimmunologic, and fortunately they are seen rarely. One major concern is the use of egg protein containing vaccines in the patient with known or suspected egg allergy manifested by anaphylactic symptoms after eating eggs. These vaccines include measles, mumps, influenza, and yellow fever. Patients who can eat eggs without allergic symptoms can be immunized with these vaccines without prior testing. Those with definite adverse reactions to egg ingestion or suspected reactions should be evaluated on an individual basis, weighing the risks of vaccination and the risks of not being immunized against the benefits of immunization.

Skin testing can be performed with measles vaccine and a desensitization protocol has been reported to be successful at administering measles vaccine to children with a history of egg allergy and positive skin tests to measles vaccine.

Some vaccines such as MMR and OPV contain trace amounts of neomycin. A history of anaphylactic reaction to neomycin would contraindicate the use of these vaccines. DPT may rarely induce urticarial or anaphylactic reactions.

Immune globulin can be rarely associated with adverse reactions of the anaphylactoid type. Patients with IgA deficiency are at increased risk for adverse reactions with immune globulin.

RADIOGRAPHIC CONTRAST MATERIAL

Radiographic contrast material (RCM) may cause anaphylactoid reactions in a small percentage of patients. Patients with a prior history of anaphylactoid reaction to RCM should avoid future use if possible, since they are at increased risk of developing repeat reactions. If a diagnostic study is considered absolutely necessary, and no acceptable alternative diagnostic procedure can be performed, patients can be pretreated with diphenhydramine, ephedrine, and corticosteroids before RCM administration. This will significantly reduce but not eliminate their risk of anaphylactoid reactions. If emergency RCM administration is necessary in patients with prior reactions to RCM, pretreatment is also recommended, but its effectiveness is still uncertain. Informed consent and documentation of the absolute need for the procedure needs to be clearly recorded in the chart.

PREVENTION

The best treatment of drug allergy is prevention. Patients should be questioned carefully before drugs with a propensity to cause allergic reactions are prescribed. It is important to establish a definite need for a drug before it is prescribed so that unnecessary drug administration can be avoided. On the other hand, it is important not to unnecessarily withhold appropriate drug therapy if indicated, for fear of a possible drug reaction.

Acute reactions are best managed by the withdrawal of the suspected drug and symptomatic control with antihistamines, epinephrine, and corticosteroids as appropriate. Patients should be made aware of their history of drug allergy and advised of the importance of future avoidance. Medical records should have drug allergies prominently displayed. Patients should be encouraged to obtain a medic-alert bracelet to identify drug allergy in the event of emergency treatment.

ANNOTATED BIBLIOGRAPHY

DeSwarte RD: Drug allergy. In Patterson R (ed): Allergic Diseases: Diagnosis and Management, 3rd ed, pp 505–661. Philadelphia, JB Lippincott, 1985 (State-of-the art review; well referenced.)

Goldstein RA, Patterson R (eds): Supplement symposium proceedings on drug allergy: Prevention, diagnosis, treatment. J Allerg Clin Immunol 74(4), 1984 (Excellent coverage of various clinically relevant topics.)

Vanarsdel PP Jr: Adverse drug reactions. In Middleton E Jr, Reed CE, Ellis EF (eds): Allergy: Principles and Practice, Vol 2, 2nd ed, pp 1389–1414. St. Louis, CV Mosby, 1983 (Excellent overall review of drug reactions.)

51

Adverse Reactions to Foods

STEVEN M. MATLOFF

A great deal of misinformation and confusion exists on the subject of food allergy, which often compounds the difficulty in affirming or refuting the diagnosis. Patients may come to the primary care physician or allergist convinced that a particular symptom or group of symptoms is caused by food ingestion. The physician's task is to determine if the presenting symptoms or signs are attributed to ingestion of foods, or if other causes explain the symptom complex. If the adverse reaction is found to be food related, the physician must then also determine if the etiology is immunologic or nonimmunologic. The term *food allergy* should be reserved for those reactions due to an immunologic mechanism. *Food intolerance* is the term applied to nonimmunologic mechanisms.

Although an accurate prevalence of allergic and nonallergic adverse food reactions is not known, these reactions are relatively uncommon. In general, this problem seems to be more common in children, but the onset of allergic and nonallergic food

reactions can occur at any age. The difficulty in accurately identifying prevalence figures is due largely to the heterogeneity of presenting clinical features; the range of these include minor nuisances to lethal events, types of adverse food reactions, and lack of unequivocal means for diagnosis.

PATHOPHYSIOLOGY

The most common immunologic reaction that leads to classical food allergy is the type I immediate hypersensitivity reaction, mediated by food allergen specific IgE. An IgE antibody directed toward a specific food allergen is produced in a patient probably as a result of a poorly defined genetic or acquired susceptibility. There may be an alteration of the normal gastrointestinal immunologic or nonimmunologic processing of food antigens in these individuals. It is not clear what predisposes an individual to develop an allergic response to food. The food specific IgE will, by itself, cause no direct symptoms, but will strongly adhere to specific receptors on the cell surface of mast cells and basophils. When the patient is reexposed to the same or a similar cross-reactive food allergen, these allergens will bind to cell-bound IgE, initiating a cascade of biochemical events that results in the local and systemic release of histamine and other vasoactive mediators. These chemical mediators, in turn, exert their effects on the blood vessels, respiratory tract, myocardium, and gastrointestinal tract, accounting for the range of symptoms of anaphylaxis.

Nonallergic reactions may produce symptoms by leading to the direct, non-IgE-mediated release of mast cell mediators or may produce symptoms by other non-mast cell dependent mechanisms. A detailed discussion of these nonallergic mechanisms is beyond the scope of this discussion.

CLINICAL PRESENTATION

The symptoms may be localized to one site or one organ system or may include the full constellation of anaphylactic symptoms, that is cutaneous symptoms (angioedema, urticaria, pruritus) and respiratory symptoms (laryngeal edema, oropharyngeal pruritus or swelling, wheezing, chest tightness, or cough).

Anaphylactic food reactions are the easiest to recognize, because the symptoms and signs are generally well defined and often striking, and the presence of allergen-specific IgE can almost always be confirmed. The most common foods that produce this type of allergic reaction include (but are not limited to) milk, eggs, fish, nuts and peanuts, soy, and certain fresh fruits. The clinician will typically see the patient either during the acute episode when clinical symptoms are manifest or after their resolution. It is important to establish the temporal relationship between the time of food ingestion and the onset of symptoms, as the shorter this time interval is, the more likely that the food can be confirmed to be the trigger of the adverse reaction (allergic or nonallergic).

DIFFERENTIAL DIAGNOSIS

Adverse reactions to foods can be produced by many medical conditions (see the box, Differential Diagnosis of Adverse Food Reactions). Various gastrointestinal disorders such as reflux esophagitis, gastric or duodenal ulcer, celiac sprue, lactose intolerance, cholelithiasis, and achalasia will be

Differential Diagnosis of Adverse Food Reactions

1. Food allergy
   a. IgE mediated
   b. Other immunologic mechanisms
2. Pseudo-allergic conditions
   a. Foods containing vasoactive mediators
   b. Foods causing direct histamine release
3. Additive reactions
4. Gastrointestinal disorders
5. Infectious diseases
6. Metabolic conditions
7. Toxins
8. Psychogenic conditions

manifested by food-induced symptoms. Many infectious diseases produce prominent gastrointestinal symptoms such as infection with salmonella, shigella, vibrio parahemolyticus, giardia, trichinella, hepatitis, and botulism. Various food toxins, both endogenous and exogenous, may be implicated. Examples are scombroid poisoning, mushroom poisoning, and paralytic shellfish poisoning. Many foods contain endogenous pharmacologically active ingredients, such as histamine, dopamine, and serotonin, that may produce symptoms similar to classical IgE-mediated anaphylactic symptoms.

Psychological reactions to foods are not uncommon. Further studies are needed to determine the relationship of diet to the development of attention deficit disorder (hyperactive child syndrome), tension fatigue syndrome, enuresis, and neuropsychiatric disorders.

There is no evidence to attribute food allergy as a cause of cardiac arrhythmias, disorders of the musculoskeletal system, obesity, and sudden infant death syndrome.

Migraine headaches are often triggered by various foods, usually induced by the pharmacologic amines or stimulants that they contain, or due to their intrinsic ability to release histamine. IgE-mediated reactions have not been demonstrated to be a chronic cause of vascular headaches.

WORK-UP

History

The history is the most important diagnostic aid in the work-up of food-induced reactions. Meticulous attention should be given to the presenting signs and symptoms, their severity, their temporal relationship to the intake of concomitant foods, beverages or drugs ingested, and the state of the food (*e.g.*, processed, cooked, fresh, or uncooked). The relationship of exercise to eating, the presence of atopic disease, and the potential contamination of the food by toxins, additives, or antibiotics are important historical features. A thorough analysis, if possible, of a food or meal may be necessary to elucidate the source of a food reaction. A determination should be made if the child has had consistent or similar serious reactions to the same food. This will identify the patient who is predisposed to food allergy and also allows for review of a nonallergic reaction to a preservative, food coloring, or additive, rather than to a specific food. A patient, therefore, may be having adverse reactions to various apparently unrelated foods, but in fact the reaction may be to an unifying preservative or additive that is contained in and common to different foods. The physician can only make an accurate diagnosis by examining the list of offending foods and by attempting to link them by knowing that they may contain the same preservative.

Patients with immediate IgE-mediated reactions to foods will often describe an immediate awareness of something being seriously wrong after a bite or slight taste of the food. Exquisitely sensitive patients may develop symptoms by merely inhaling the odors from the food, such as fish or peanut butter (see page 232 for a list of foods that commonly cause allergic reactions).

Physical Examination

During an acute allergic episode, the following may be observed: urticaria, angioedema, oropharyngeal or laryngeal edema, hyperactive bowel sounds, increased abdominal girth, distension, bronchospasm, rhinoconjunctivitis, hypotension, and symptoms of generalized systemic anaphylaxis with shock. The physical examination is usually normal when the patient presents for a diagnostic evaluation.

Laboratory Tests

Immediate hypersensitivity skin testing detects the presence of a food allergen specific IgE antibody. Skin test results should not solely be relied on to make a diagnosis of food allergy. A negative skin test will usually exclude a severe IgE-mediated food allergy, but coupled with a strikingly positive history, the latter should be assumed to be the more reliable diagnostic indicator. False-positive and false-negative results occur, but if correlated with the history, will generally provide sufficient information to recommend a trial of elimination from the

diet, with anticipated improvement. If the patient is able to tolerate a food that gives a positive skin test reaction, the skin test result should be disregarded.

The patient with a history of anaphylaxis to a specific food should not be skin tested unless the specific cause of the reaction is unclear (*e.g.*, when the patient ate several foods at the same time, each being a potential offending agent, and other safer methods of diagnosis [*i.e.*, radioallergosorbent test or RAST] have failed to reveal a likely cause).

RAST, which detects allergen-specific IgE in the patient's serum, should be performed as the initial diagnostic procedure in a patient with a history of severe anaphylaxis, or in individuals who are unable to be skin tested because of severe eczema or dermatographism. These tests, however, are not as sensitive as skin tests; they are more expensive; and the results take longer to obtain. They are also only as good as the quality of the allergen used in the assay, and since they measure allergen-specific IgE in the serum, patients with significant concentrations of cell-bound IgE, but small amounts in the serum, may be missed.

ORAL CHALLENGE

If the history and results of skin or RAST tests are still equivocal, oral challenges with the food or additive in question may be necessary. The challenge is usually performed in either an open (physician and patient aware of the food), single blind (patient not aware), or double blind fashion (patient and physician not aware). The latter approach is the most objective because the patient and physician bias is eliminated. Oral challenges should never be done if the history reveals anaphylaxis. Freeze-dried food inserted into opaque dye-free capsules is generally used for the testing.

It is beyond the scope of this chapter to describe these methods in detail. In office practice, the physician seldom needs to proceed to oral challenge, although in many cases, particularly where psychogenic factors are felt to be causative, this is a useful method to refute the diagnosis of an adverse food reaction.

ELIMINATION DIETS

Various types of elimination diets, ranging from the elimination of a single food to instituting an elemental diet, may be used both as a diagnostic and as a therapeutic trial. The patient needs to be reliable and compliant in order for an accurate assessment to be made. Foods can be added back gradually and removed a second time if the symptoms reappear. This approach can be time consuming but is often worth the temporary inconvenience.

CONTROVERSIAL TECHNIQUES

Presently, cytotoxic testing and provocative subcutaneous and sublingual testing are unproven diagnostic techniques and they should not be performed.

TREATMENT AND MANAGEMENT

When a particular food has been confirmed to be the cause of an adverse food reaction, avoidance is obviously the preferred treatment. It is important for the patient to be aware of potentially cross-reacting foods (see the box, Partial List of Cross-Reacting Food Groups). If a suspected food cannot be confirmed as causing the adverse reaction, it is best to eliminate that food for a limited time. The food should be eliminated if the symptoms improve or return when the food is reintroduced.

Partial List of Cross-Reacting Food Groups

1. Dairy Products
   Milk
   Butter
   Cheeses
   Yogurt
   Ice cream
2. Legumes
   Peanuts
   Peas
   Soybean
   Lentil
   Licorice
   Beans
3. Cashew Family
   Cashew
   Mango
   Pistachio
4. Plum Family
   Plum
   Prune
   Almond
   Apricot
   Cherry
   Peach
   Nectarine
5. Nightshade Family
   Pepper
   Eggplant
   Tomato
   Potato
6. Parsley Family
   Caraway
   Carrot
   Celery
   Dill
7. Walnut Family
   Walnuts
   Pecan
   Hickory nut
   Butternut

Patients should be given a list of all foods that are in the same food group, since they can all potentially cross-react, producing allergic symptoms of greater or lesser severity. The degree of cross-reactivity in a particular patient is variable. (Adapted from *Adverse Reactions to Foods*, AAAI and NIAID Report US Department of Health and Human Services, NIH Publication No. 84-2442, July 1984, pp 21–25.)

Particular vigilance must be emphasized when the patient is eating away from the home (*e.g.*, at restaurants, friend's or relative's homes, office or school parties). In these settings, patients may not be aware of all the ingredients used in cooking (*e.g.*, walnuts contained in a stuffed mushroom or coffee cake) and severe anaphylactic reactions will most commonly occur in individuals already known to be allergic to a particular food. The patient should be clearly warned and advised that when in doubt, they should avoid that particular food. Health education must emphasize that future reactions could be potentially lethal. This warning is generally well accepted by patients who have had a severe anaphylactic reaction, and these patients usually become appropriately cautious. Thus, the elimination of the specific food(s) is central to effective treatment.

In the case of adverse reactions to additives, preservatives, and so forth, it is important to become aware of those foods that contain them. This information will often not be on the label of a food or indicated on menus in the restaurant setting (*e.g.*, salad bars treated with the sulfiting agent preservatives); thus, awareness is necessary to avoid potentially severe reactions. Consultation with a nutritionist is helpful in learning which foods to avoid.

It is important for the physician not to induce a state of unnecessary caution and elimination, unless specifically indicated, particularly in the adolescent and young adult who might be at risk for, or is presently suffering from, an eating disorder. Some of these patients may rationalize their eating disorders because of confirmed or unconfirmed food allergies, and they begin to feel, without foundation, that they are allergic to virtually all foods. Psychiatric referral, to avoid exacerbation of an underlying eating disorder, is necessary in these atypical cases. A food allergy, however, has not been demonstrated as a primary cause of an eating disorder.

All patients with documented food-induced anaphylaxis should be given an H1 antihistamine (diphenhydramine or chlorpheniramine) and self-injectable epinephrine (ANA-Kit or Epi-Pen) to use in the event of accidental ingestions. The treatment of acute anaphylaxis is reviewed in Chapter 49. Gastric lavage is rarely necessary because most patients will spontaneously vomit the residual gastric food contents. An osmotic cathartic, such as magnesium citrate, may sometimes be used. Observation for 24 hours or longer for delayed symptoms may be necessary, depending on GI transit time and the severity of the symptoms.

The young child with a food allergy should be re-evaluated every 6 to 12 months by the allergist, because a food allergy presenting at a young age is more likely to spontaneously remit with time than a food allergy that has its onset in late childhood or adulthood. However, a food allergy in some individuals may remain present for life.

A medic-alert bracelet should be worn by the patient so that the recognition and treatment of a reaction will be immediate.

Immunotherapy using food extracts has not been demonstrated to be effective and should not be used. Preventative pharmacologic treatment may need to be tried in rare refractory cases, but this cannot be recommended as a standard treatment and it is often not effective.

Reassurance and psychological support for the patient and family are important aspects of the overall treatment plan.

INDICATIONS FOR REFERRAL

The patient with confusing symptoms, an unclear association of symptoms with food, and a lack of response to treatment should be referred for an appropriate work-up. The allergist should be consulted in all cases where the diagnosis of a food allergy is seriously entertained but not easily confirmed, or in the patient who has had a severe anaphylactic reaction to a food. If an allergy evaluation fails to reveal an immunologic etiology, other nonimmunologic cases of adverse food reactions

need to be considered, particularly if the symptoms recur.

A multidisciplinary team approach with consultation by a gastroenterologist, infectious disease specialist, food technologist, nutritionist, and psychiatrist may occasionally be necessary.

With all of the new food additives, flavorings, colorings, and sweeteners continuously being introduced, the clinician should be aware of their possible roles in the production of food-related symptoms. An understanding of the heterogeneity of adverse food reactions will help the clinician focus the work-up in an appropriate direction without performing numerous expensive and unnecessary tests.

ANNOTATED BIBLIOGRAPHY

Adverse Reactions to Foods, AAAI and NIAID Report, NIH publication No. 84-2442, July 1984 (Excellent, state-of-the-art reference source, reviewing all aspects of adverse food reactions, including pathophysiology, diagnosis, and treatment; excellent appendix of diseases transmitted by foods that is well referenced and indexed.)

Bock SA: Prospective appraisal of complaints of adverse reactions to foods in children during the first 3 years of life. Pediatrics 79:683–688, 1987 (Two important findings: (1) most reactions were nonimmunoglobulin-E-mediated and (2) most reactions occur during the first year of life and with rechallenge, by the third year they don't usually recur.)

Symposium Proceedings on Adverse Reactions to Foods and Food Additives. J Allergy Clin Immunol 78 (1), July 1986 (Excellent overview of the subject.)

52
Urticaria, Angioedema, and Serum Sickness

RAOUL L. WOLF

Urticaria and angioedema are common occurrences in pediatrics; as many as one quarter of the general population will experience an episode. The two conditions are examples of an acute allergic reaction, initiated by several allergenic substances. The response manifests itself by an accumulation of fluid in the epidermal or dermoepidermal regions.

By contrast, serum sickness is an unusual problem, predominantly occurring in response to drug administration. It is important to recognize the con-

dition when it occurs and to remove the offending agent when possible.

PATHOPHYSIOLOGY

The development of urticaria and angioedema is similar in both conditions. The response is mediated by IgE and depends on prior sensitization. These molecules of IgE are fixed to mast cells. With cross-linking by a specific antigen, they initiate the release of potent vasodilator substances, such as histamine and slow-reacting substances (now known as leukotrienes). The result of this is local edema and swelling; in urticaria, this lies within the epidermis and in angioedema, at the dermoepidermal junction and subcutaneous tissue. The stimulation of nerve endings gives rise to pruritus.

Serum sickness arises because of a completely different mechanism. This is an IgG-mediated reaction that occurs mostly to injected antigens (such as penicillin) or occasionally to ingested substances. Antigens and antibodies normally form complexes in the presence of excess antibody, giving rise to an insoluble lattice that is removed by the action of phagocytic cells. When antigen is present in excess, however, or there is deficient or delayed antibody production, the complexes remain soluble. This phenomenon is an example of a circulating immune complex disease. The complexes deposit in blood vessels and tissues, primarily skin, joint tissues, and lung. This activates the serum complement cascade, releasing substances that are chemotactic for polymorphonuclear cells. With the resultant release of enzymes and prostaglandins, an inflammatory response occurs. This gives rise to the characteristic fever, rash, and joint pain. This type of reaction was a common result of injections of vaccines prepared in horse serum, but now the penicillin group is probably the most common cause.

CLINICAL PRESENTATION

The patient with urticaria usually has an abrupt onset of symptoms, often within 10 to 15 minutes of exposure to antigen. Pruritus is the first sign and may be intense. This is followed by the appearance of macular or elevated multiform lesions, ranging from 2 mm to several cm in size, with a wide surrounding erythema. Even apparently uninvolved areas of skin may be pruritic. Fever is not a usual accompaniment to the condition and, if present, should raise suspicion about an underlying disease process.

Chronic urticaria is present when the condition has persisted for longer than 6 weeks. This problem is more common in adults than in children. The cause is usually elusive and difficult to determine, and the condition is often refractory to therapy.

Angioedema may have a more gradual onset and is often associated with drug reactions. Pruritus is not as prominent; rather, a burning or painful sensation is noted. Swelling often begins about the lips

or hands and is diffuse. The swelling may spread to involve the tongue and, in extreme cases, may cause laryngeal edema and acute respiratory distress. The time from exposure to emergence of the lesions can vary, and it is often more difficult for the patient to pinpoint the offending agent than in urticaria. The patient, however, will sometimes note lip and tongue swelling that occur almost immediately on tasting a food that causes an allergic reaction. Angioedema on an allergic basis is usually associated with urticarial reactions at the same or at distant sites, making identification easier.

The clinical pattern of serum sickness is distinct from urticaria and angioedema. Fever is the initial event, and the temperature may be high (103° to 105°), often spiking in nature, returning to the baseline or below between spikes. A headache is usual. A rash accompanies the fever. This is usually red, diffuse, and punctate, but is often urticarial. The lesions may involve the palms and soles. Lymphadenopathy is seen and may involve any nodes, including the supraclavicular and epitrochlear nodes. Arthritis involves large joints, especially knees and hips. This feature may be prominent, causing significant pain and discomfort. Encephalitis and peripheral neuropathy are rare manifestations. Renal involvement presenting with hematuria occurs rarely and is seldom a major feature (in contrast to the features of experimental models for serum sickness).

DIFFERENTIAL DIAGNOSIS

The lesions of urticaria are characteristic and easy to distinguish. The difficulty is in determining the cause. Examples of the more common causes are listed on page 232. The distribution and pattern of the lesions may be helpful. Lesions that start around the lips and tongue may indicate sensitivity to a food. The usual foods involved are nuts and dairy products, fish and shellfish. In considering the possible foods that might be causative, one should keep in mind that cross-reactivity occurs within families of foods, for example peanuts belong in the legume family. Insect stings are a relatively common cause for urticaria and angioedema, but the patient is usually aware that this is the cause of the problem. Physical urticaria, such as cholinergic or solar, often forms a characteristic pattern with fine punctate wheals in clusters. There is usually a history of exposure to heat or cold.

The swelling seen in angioedema is less typical of an atopic reaction than it is in urticaria. Other

Common Causes of Urticaria and Angioedema

Foods
  Nuts
  Dairy products
  Shellfish
  Berries

Drugs
  Penicillins
  Sulfa drugs
  Iodides

Insect stings

Physical stress
  Heat
  Cold

Infestations

causes of diffuse swelling, such as hypoproteinemia, must be excluded. The intermittent nature of angioedema is a clue, as is the uneven distribution of the lesions.

Many diseases, especially those with an immunologic basis, such as rheumatoid arthritis, can present with urticaria. Since this is a relatively uncommon subgroup, it is difficult to decide when to investigate for these disorders. The presence of fever, especially with high spikes, should indicate the possibility of an autoimmune disorder. Chronic or recurrent episodes of urticaria should suggest infectious hepatitis or infectious mononucleosis or a parasitic infestation. The latter is usually accompained by eosinophilia. Repeated ingestion or exposure to a drug should be looked for where the lesions are recurrent.

Recurrent angioedema, especially on cold exposure, raises suspicion of hereditary angioedema. In this autosomal dominant condition, there is a deficiency of an inhibitor of activation of the complement pathway. As a result, there is spontaneous complement activation with formation of active vasodilator substances. This condition can be life-threatening because of laryngeal edema. The measurement of serum complement levels will confirm the diagnosis.

Serum sickness is less typical in appearance than urticaria and angioedema, making positive diagnosis difficult. Systemic inflammatory diseases such as juvenile rheumatoid arthritis (JRA) may also present with joint swelling and fever. This onset is generally slower and a migratory pattern of joint involvement is noted. There are often nodules associated with rheumatoid diseases. The ultimate differential usually is made only by long-term observation; signs and symptoms persist in JRA. Systemic lupus erythematosus (SLE) presents with fever and arteritis, but multiple organ systems are involved. Renal involvement is frequent, whereas it is rare in serum sickness. The rapid onset and history of drug or infectious exposure indicates serum sickness. The absence of positive rheumatoid serologic tests does not exclude JRA, as these tests are often negative in this form of the disease. On the other hand, negative serology does exclude SLE. In distinguishing the various causes of serum sickness, drug reactions are the most common, especially to penicillin and phenytoin (Dilantin). Vaccines and various sera are also causes.

WORK-UP

History

A careful history is the key to diagnosing urticaria and angioedema. Most identifiable causes can be traced to within 30 minutes of onset of the lesions. For example, the patient may describe a shrimp dinner that ended abruptly when his lips and tongue became swollen and urticarial lesions appeared. Other examples would include exposure to a drug or contact agent, such as a cat, with rapid emergence of the lesions. A history that is helpful in determining a diagnosis is a reaction to iodides in soap or contrast media. This is predictive of a severe reaction with use of injected radiocontrast media and must be sought in all patients who will undergo these procedures. Where the history is not so helpful, and a reaction to a food is suspected, the patient may be asked to keep a food diary, recording everything eaten and annotating the log with the times and dates of allergic reactions. Theoretically, this is a helpful procedure; in practice, it often fails because patients do not keep the record or attempt to fill it in from memory a week later. This technique is thus useful if the patient is diligent.

A history of drug reactions should be sought. Other atopic diseases such as allergic rhinitis, eczema, contact reactions, and asthma should be elicited. Although not diagnostic, such a history increases the possibility that a suspicious reaction is urticarial.

In evaluating serum sickness, the onset of symptoms from 10 days to 2 weeks after drug exposure or an infectious episode is suggestive of the condition. There is often a history of previous episodes with spontaneous resolution or in response to therapy. Family history or a history of atopic disease does not correlate with serum sickness.

Physical Examination

The clinical appearance of urticaria has already been noted. Some aspects of the physical presentation may be helpful. The distribution of the lesions may indicate the source. Lesions beginning around the mouth or tongue imply that an ingested agent, such as nuts or berries, may be responsible. The location on the skin, such as in the underwear area, suggests a reaction to a laundry detergent. Hand, mouth, and tongue involvement, especially an exposure to cold or physical stress, should raise suspicion of hereditary angioedema. Pruritus is the most helpful sign associated with urticaria.

Physical causes for urticaria can be excluded by hot or cold contact tests or to pressure. Signs of systemic disease, such as splenomegaly, lymphadenopathy, and hepatomegaly, are unusual in urticaria and should be taken as indicators of an underlying disorder such as rheumatoid disease. These features are not uncommon in serum sickness, however, and do not indicate a need for extensive investigation.

Laboratory Tests

Laboratory investigations are generally of limited value in these conditions and tests should be reserved for specific indications. Allergy skin testing is unlikely to be helpful, other than to confirm a suspected IgE-mediated response to a food. It will not be of any value in detecting food or other allergens unsuspected from a careful history. The skin test assay is a sensitive measurement of specific IgE bound to mast cells in the skin. In urticaria, however, the reaction may not correlate well with actual causes for the condition. Specific IgE can also be measured from serum by means of a radioallergosorbent (RAST) test. This test is sensitive. It too, may not be helpful in delineating the cause and it is a more expensive assay than skin testing. A complete blood count (CBC) with differential may reveal a high eosinophil count, suggesting a parasitic infestation or underlying atopic state. Where a suspicion of systemic disease is entertained, an erythrocyte sedimentation rate (ESR) is a good screening test. More specific assays, such as rheumatoid factor and antinuclear antibody, should be done if there is an elevated ESR with a prolonged course for the disease.

Low serum complement levels, namely total hemolytic complement, C4 level and C3 (BIC) levels indicate hereditary angioedema. All will be reduced during an acute attack, but between episodes only C4 will be low.

The investigation of serum sickness should include CBC and ESR. The CBC may show eosinophilia or neutropenia or thrombocytopenia in response to the etiologic agent. A positive Coombs' test and anemia should arouse suspicion of SLE. A urinalysis is essential to differentiate from conditions which more frequently involve the kidney such as SLE, though mild proteinuria is seen in serum sickness. Other investigations should be conducted either to confirm or disprove clinical suspicion, such as rheumatoid serology, if rheumatoid disease seems likely. Serum complement values may be transiently low in serum sickness, but it is not usually necessary to perform this test.

TREATMENT AND MANAGEMENT

The initial therapy for urticaria and angioedema consists of removing the patient from the cause, if possible, and preventing a progression of the condition. If an insect stinger is present, it should be removed with a scalpel blade, not tweezers or fingers, to avoid breaking it off and thereby injecting more venom.

Where there is a significant swelling or a threat that swelling may spread, epinephrine 0.01 ml/kg of a 1/1,000 dilution to a maximum of 0.3 ml is given subcutaneously. This can be followed by diphenhydramine (Benadryl) at 5 mg/kg/24 hours for 3 to 5 days. In cases where pruritus is a major symptom, this is better controlled by hydroxyzine (Atarax, Vistaril) at 2 to 5 mg/kg/24 hr. This should also be continued for 3 to 5 days or longer if resolution of the lesions is delayed.

Chronic urticaria is much more difficult to treat and is often refractory to antihistaminics. Some authors have indicated that histamine H_2 receptors are present in skin blood vessels. (H_1 receptors are found on smooth muscle and H_2 receptors are part of the regulation of gastric acid secretion and are found on mast cells). Cimetidine, an H_2 blocker, has been used in conjunction with an H_1 blocker with some success in refractory cases of urticaria.

Steroid therapy does not have a place in acute urticaria, although it may be helpful in refractory cases. In angioedema, the presence of laryngeal edema or severe swelling of face and lips is an indication for using Prednisone 1 mg/kg/day or dexamethasone (Decadron) 0.1 mg/kg/day in a short course of 4 to 5 days. The drug can be discontinued without tapering if such a short course is used.

Serum sickness is usually self-limited and requires supportive therapy. Salicylates at 80 mg/kg/day are effective in controlling joint symptoms and fever and may be used for about 1 week beyond the resolution of symptoms. Diphenhydramine is useful to treat an urticarial component. In the presence of severe symptoms, neurologic involvement or significant renal involvement, Prednisone at 2 mg/kg/day should be used. Following the resolution of symptoms, the Prednisone dose can be tapered over 2 to 3 weeks.

INDICATIONS FOR REFERRAL OR ADMISSION

Most patients with urticaria will recover spontaneously and will not have another episode. In recurrent or refractory episodes, a consultation and an extensive work-up and history may be beneficial.

Admission is indicated in the patient with angioedema or serum sickness, accompanied by a low or unstable blood pressure. Severe reactions, even with a stable circulatory system, are an indication for admission and observation for 24 hours. The patient who does not respond or who has further episodes will benefit from a work-up for an underlying disease. At times, this may be accomplished best in a hospital.

ANNOTATED BIBLIOGRAPHY

Bock SA: The natural history of food sensitivity. J Allergy Clin Immunol 69:173–177, 1982 (Important review of the natural history of food sensitivity.)

Fauci AS: Serum sickness. In Parker CW (ed): Clinical Immunology, pp 486–490. Philadelphia, WB Saunders, 1980 (Overall review.)

Goldstein RA, Patterson RJ (eds): Drug allergy: Prevention, diagnosis treatment. Symposium. J Allergy Clin Immunol (Oct suppl), Vol 74, 1984 (Wide coverage of the topic.)

Kaplan AP: Urticaria and angioedema. In Middleton E Jr, Reed CE, Ellis EF (eds): Allergy, Principles and Practice, pp 486–490. Philadelphia, WB Saunders, 1980 (Broad-based discussion of the problem.)

Lewis J, Lieberman P, Treadwell G, Erffmeyer J: Exercise induced urticaria, angioedema and anaphylactic episodes. J Allergy Clin Immunol 68:432–437, 1981 (Interesting look at a rarer problem.)

Metcalfe DD: Food hypersensitivity. J Allergy Clin Immunol 73:749–766, 1984 (Sober look at a topic fraught with myth and misunderstanding.)

Sheffer AL: Anaphylaxis. J Allergy Clin Immunol 75:227–236, 1985 (Recommended as a post-graduate review.)

8

Cardiovascular Problems

53
Heart Murmurs
HERBERT E. COHN

The incidence of congenital heart disease is approximately 6 to 8: 1,000 live births or less than 1 in 100 children. Cardiac murmurs are noted in 50% to 70% of children who are active, healthy, and asymptomatic. Most of the latter have insignificant or "functional" cardiac murmurs that represent vibrations of normal structures within the heart. It is essential to differentiate these from the significant cardiac murmurs that reflect underlying congenital heart lesions and that warrant referral to a pediatric cardiologist for further evaluation. One should be able to do this by means of a history, cardiovascular examination, and basic laboratory information consisting of an electrocardiogram, chest roentgenogram, and hemoglobin determination.

PATHOPHYSIOLOGY
AND CLINICAL PRESENTATION

The vibratory murmur is produced at the aortic valve as blood ejected in systole passes over the free margins of the open aortic valve leaflets. An open aortic valve is not circular, but rather has a triangular configuration when open. It is the valve leaflets that form the sides of the triangle that vibrate in systole. The pulmonary systolic ejection murmur takes its name from its chest wall location at the upper left sternal edge over the pulmonic valve. Some phonocardiographic studies have suggested that this murmur's origin is actually in the left ventricular outflow tract and that its mechanism is similar to that of the vibratory murmur. In both cases, the cardiac murmurs reflect vibrations of normal structures. There are no pressure or volume

overloads. No compensatory mechanisms operate, thus no additional physical or laboratory findings should be present.

The murmurs of valvar, aortic, and pulmonic stenosis stem from significant turbulence as blood is ejected from a ventricle in systole across thickened stenotic valve leaflets. When sufficient vibration occurs, it causes the anterior chest wall to vibrate; this palpable sensation is called a *thrill*. The area of greatest turbulence is distal to the stenotic valve, and dilatation of the arterial wall occurs there. As the thickened valve *domes* or pops open in systole causing a jet of ejected blood to strike the dilated, tensed arterial wall distal to the valve, a high frequency sound called an *ejection click* is produced.

Atrial septal defects produce systolic ejection murmurs at the pulmonic valve. Blood flows from left to right through the defect at the atrial level and produces a right ventricular volume overload. As right ventricular volume increases, there is a relative stenosis at the pulmonic valve. Thus, more blood is presented to the pulmonic valve orifice than can readily pass, which accentuates the physiologically occurring vibrations at the pulmonic valve. Since right ventricular volume is increased on an absolute basis, right ventricular ejection time and pulmonic valve closure are delayed and there is wide splitting of the pulmonic component of the second sound. If the degree of left to right shunting is significantly large (a pulmonary to systemic flow ratio above 2 to 1), a relative tricuspid stenosis also occurs and an early diastolic flow murmur is audible at the tricuspid area (lower left sternal edge). This

235

Differential Diagnosis of Systolic Ejection Murmurs in Childhood

1. Vibratory, musical murmur (innocent, functional)
2. Basal pulmonic ejection murmur
3. Valvar aortic stenosis
4. Valvar pulmonic stenosis
5. Atrial septal defect
6. Ventricular septal defect
7. Hypertrophic subaortic stenosis

diastolic murmur is commonly referred to as a *flow rumble*.

The murmur of a ventricular septal defect reflects the turbulence of blood flow through the defect itself, commonly located in the membranous ventricular septum. The vibrations are harsh and pansystolic (*i.e.*, has almost the same pitch and intensity throughout systole as opposed to peaking in intensity in midsystole as do ejection murmurs). Blood flow produces a right ventricular pressure and volume overload, increased pulmonary arterial pressure and flow, and a left ventricular volume overload as it flows from left to right through the defect. If the blood flow is sufficiently large (a pulmonary to systemic flow ratio above 2 to 1), a relative mitral stenosis occurs and a mid-diastolic murmur or flow rumble is audible at the apex.

The murmur of hypertrophic subaortic stenosis is associated with a diamond-shaped systolic ejection murmur heard along the lower left sternal edge. The hypertrophied muscular portion of the ventricular septum obstructs the left ventricular outflow tract in systole. Events such as the Valsalva maneuver that transiently decrease left ventricular filling intensify the obstruction and accentuate the murmur. A bifid pulse wave is palpable at the radial pulse and reflects the pattern of left ventricular emptying during systole. (See the box, Differential Diagnosis of Systolic Ejection Murmurs in Childhood.)

WORK-UP

History

The detection of a cardiac murmur frequently leads the pediatrician to conduct a more thorough evaluation of the cardiovascular system. One needs to obtain a careful history and cardiovascular system review, including a review of the pre- and perinatal history. Inquire into the child's level of activity and endurance, which often reflect cardiovascular performance. A history of recurrent pneu-

monitis or lower respiratory infections may be found, especially in patients with left to right shunt lesions. The rate of linear growth and weight gain can be reduced in the presence of increased caloric expenditure associated with increased cardiovascular workload or congestive heart failure. Linear growth is not usually affected, but slower than normal weight gain is common. Cardiovascular signs and symptoms such as syncope or chest pain may indicate significant left or right ventricular outflow tract obstruction. Cyanosis associated with exposure to cold or prolonged bathing, chest pain which is "sticking" in quality and brought on by deep inspiration, and palpitations associated with anxiety may appear to reflect cardiac pathology, but are rarely of cardiac origin in childhood.

Previous cardiologic evaluations, previous hospitalizations, or studies such as electrocardiograms and chest films may provide baseline data for comparison with current findings. A review of the family history is important. A parent or sibling with known congenital heart disease significantly increases the probability of a patient having a congenital heart lesion.

Physical Examination

Clinical findings that reflect structural cardiac lesions are often present, but may be subtle. Neither the intensity nor the quality of sound of most cardiac murmurs provide reliable criteria by which the significance of the murmur can be determined. Furthermore, lesions such as mitral valve prolapse or bicuspid aortic valve may not produce a cardiac murmur. A significant congenital heart lesion requiring surgery may be asymptomatic. Therefore, an approach that includes a search for other physical findings such as abnormal precordial impulses or chest deformities, an assessment of the second heart sound components in terms of intensity and movement with respirations, and the presence of ejection clicks or diastolic flow murmurs is necessary to yield an accurate assessment of the child's cardiovascular status.

An inspection of the child's chest for an asymmetric precordial bulge may reflect underlying ventricular hypertrophy. A palpable ventricular impulse reinforces the high index of suspicion for ventricular hypertrophy. Abnormalities of the second heart sound, both in terms of intensity and movement with respirations, are valuable means of assessing right ventricular hemodynamics. A widened split of the second heart sound generally indicates a right ventricular volume overload. An increased intensity of the second heart sound indicates an elevated pulmonary arterial pressure. When the pulmonary arterial pressure is sufficiently elevated, an increased intensity often results in a palpable second heart sound along the upper left sternal edge. The presence of an ejection click generally reflects a dilated aorta or pulmonary artery in the vicinity of the click. This is commonly found with obstructive valvular lesions such as aortic or pulmonic stenosis. Clicks are found in other conditions causing dilatation of a great vessel such as truncus arteriosus where the aortic root is dilated.

The assessment of a cardiac murmur should include at least six characteristics: (1) timing; (2) quality; (3) intensity; (4) duration; (5) location; and (6) radiation of sound. Timing may be described as systolic, diastolic, or continuous, the latter referring to a murmur being present in systole and continuing beyond the second heart sound into diastole, even if it is not present throughout all of diastole. Quality refers to the characteristics of the sound such as harsh, soft, vibratory, or musical. The intensity of systolic murmurs is graded on a scale of 1 to 6 whereas the intensity of diastolic murmurs is graded on a scale of 1 to 4. The duration refers to the amount of systole or diastole in which the murmur is heard, such as holosystolic or midsystolic. The location refers to the area where the murmur is loudest. The radiation of sound is usually in the direction of flow. Murmurs of pulmonic stenosis, for example, are heard in the pulmonary area and over both lung fields posteriorly and murmurs of mitral insufficiency are heard in the left axilla.

The most common innocent or functional murmur is a vibratory systolic ejection murmur. It is of low to medium pitch with a musical quality and is best heard along the lower left sternal edge, third to fourth left interspace, and toward the apex. It is short, midsystolic, and ends well before the second heart sound. It is heard best in the supine position and diminishes in the upright position; it is intensified by fever or excitement. There are no precordial impulses or deformities, normal first and second heart sounds are present, and no clicks or extra sounds are noted.

The basal or pulmonary systolic ejection murmur is higher in pitch and less uniform in quality than the vibratory murmur. It is best heard in the supine position and is intensified by fever or excitement. These systolic murmurs are usually less than grade 3/6 in intensity and are usually not transmitted to the back. They are associated with a normal second heart sound whose two components

widen in inspiration and narrow with expiration. As noted, there are no associated cardiovascular findings on physical examination. The electrocardiogram and chest films are normal.

The continuous murmur known as a venous hum is also considered a functional murmur. It extends through systole into diastole. It is best heard in the upright position at the upper left or right sternal edge and can be obliterated by placement of a thumb over the external jugular vein just above the clavicle or by having the patient turn his head laterally. This murmur disappears in the supine position and there are no other associated physical findings.

Diastolic flow murmurs are noted with large left to right shunt lesions associated with a pulmonary to systemic flow ratio of greater than 2 to 1. Similar phenomena occur if there is a left to right ventricular volume overload associated with mitral or tricuspid valve regurgitation and relative stenosis at either valve.

The murmurs reflecting atrial septal defects and mild valvar pulmonic stenosis may closely resemble the pulmonary systolic ejection murmur. The associated findings, however, differentiate these lesions. Atrial septal defects have wide splitting of the second heart sound components that do not narrow to a single sound on expiration. The tapping impulse of the right ventricular volume overload is felt over the left precordium along the left sternal edge. There may be a slight left precordial bulge evident. The electrocardiogram shows a minor right ventricular conduction defect or incomplete right bundle branch block pattern and evidence for a right ventricular hypertrophy. Chest roentgenograms show increased pulmonary vascular markings and a fullness to the pulmonary arterial segment. The heart size is generally normal, but may be slightly increased. Valvar pulmonic stenosis is associated with an ejection click along the left sternal edge from the fourth left intercostal space to the pulmonic area. The click precedes the systolic ejection murmur which is harsh and diamond-shaped, and which is best heard along the upper left sternal edge at the second to third left interspace. A palpable impulse reflects right ventricular hypertrophy. A thrill reflects turbulence at the pulmonic valve but does not convey reliable information about severity. The electrocardiogram shows evidence of right ventricular hypertrophy. The chest P-A and lateral roentgenograms may show decreased or normal pulmonary vascular markings and the overall heart size is generally normal.

The ventricular septal defect, uncomplicated by

pulmonary arterial hypertension, may have a harsh pansystolic murmur beginning with the first heart sound and lasting throughout the aortic component of the second heart sound. This murmur is often associated with a thrill and is best heard at the lower left sternal edge, radiating to the xiphoid region. The pulmonary component of the second heart sound is neither accentuated nor obscured and is best heard at the lower left sternal edge. If the magnitude of left to right shunting is sufficiently large, a diastolic flow rumble may be audible at the apex. There is no ejection click unless the ventricular septal defect is closing by aneurysm formation in the ventricular septum. Electrocardiographic findings may show left ventricular hypertrophy or combined ventricular hypertrophy. The chest P-A and lateral films show increased pulmonary vascular markings and ventricular enlargement.

Laboratory Tests

The electrocardiogram provides several different kinds of information. The heart rate and rhythm can be determined by inspection. The intervals of the P, QRS, and T waves and characteristics of the electrical conduction system can be measured. The presence and severity of ventricular hypertrophy can be interpreted by voltage criteria and pattern recognition. The type of physiologic adaptations, such as pressure of volume overload made by each ventricle can be distinguished. The electrical axis in a three dimensional plane can be determined, which is valuable in understanding both the conduction system and the adaptations of ventricular hypertrophy.

The chest roentgenogram provides information on cardiac size and silhouette, the pulmonary vasculature, and the location and configuration of the aortic arch. The boot-shaped upturned apex of right ventricular enlargement, and the figure 8 or *snowman* configuration of supracardiac total anomalous pulmonary venous return are two examples.

The hemoglobin determination provides information on anemia or polycythemia and is a sensitive indicator for chronic hypoxemia.

These laboratory studies are readily available in the primary care setting and provide independent sources of information that may support information derived from the history and physical examination. For example, the presence of a right ventricular impulse, evidence for right ventricular hypertrophy on the electrocardiogram and an upturned apex on the cardiac silhouette all support the impression of a real abnormality in cardiovascular function and help to distinguish the patient with a structural congenital heart lesion from a patient with an insignificant cardiac murmur.

Noninvasive Studies

The various forms of echocardiography provide much detailed physiologic data on cardiovascular anatomy and function that can be obtained noninvasively. The M-mode echocardiogram gives information on chamber dimensions and wall motion as well as the pericardial space and the presence of an effusion. The information is printed on paper and measurements of myocardial contractility can be made.

The two dimensional echocardiogram provides a picture, usually on videotape, of intracardiac anatomy such as the septal and valvular structures, chamber walls, and chamber dimensions. Septal defects, thickened valve leaflets, or membranous structures can be visualized directly.

Doppler echocardiography can detect specific sites of turbulence within the heart or circulation. It can measure the velocity of blood flow at an obstructive site. From these data, one can estimate the pressure difference across the obstructive site which produced an increased flow velocity. This technique provides a graphic picture, on screen or on paper, of the turbulence associated with increased blood flow.

Echocardiographic studies are not generally available in the primary care setting and are costly. The application of these techniques is best reserved for the pediatric cardiologist when the patient's clinical findings require these studies.

INDICATIONS FOR REFERRAL

The primary care provider can generally differentiate those patients with insignificant murmurs from those with structural congenital heart lesions. Children identified as having structural congenital or acquired heart disease should be referred to a pediatric cardiologist for further evaluation and therapy as necessary. Children with borderline findings in which a more definitive evaluation is necessary in order to distinguish whether they have a significant congenital heart problem should also be referred. Children with known congenital heart disease whose disease severity and course need to be monitored with respect to medical management, the timing of surgery, or changes in the patient's clinical course also warrant referral to a pediatric cardiologist.

PATIENT EDUCATION

If the cardiovascular evaluation detects structural congenital heart disease, the child should receive appropriate bacterial endocarditis prophylaxis. If the child is found to have a cardiac murmur that is insignificant and no real structural congenital heart lesion is noted, it is important to emphasize that the child has no cardiac disease. The emphasis should be on health and fitness rather than on a finding that carries undertones of morbidity and negative psychosocial values.

ANNOTATED BIBLIOGRAPHY

Caceres CA, Perry LW (eds): The Innocent Murmur, A Problem in Clinical Practice. Boston, Little, Brown, 1967 (Interesting book that relates diverse views on the characteristics and causes of an innocent murmur.)

Gooch AS, Maranhao V, Goldberg H: Clues to Diagnosis in Congenital Heart Disease. Philadelphia, FA Davis, 1969 (150 diagnostic puzzles based on clinical findings in patients with congenital heart disease.)

Moss AJ, Adams FH, Emmanouilides GC: Heart Disease in Infants, Children and Adolescents, 2nd ed. Baltimore, Williams and Wilkins, 1977 (Exhaustive, multiauthored reference for pediatric cardiologists.)

Nadas AS, Fyler DC: Pediatric Cardiology, 3rd ed. Philadelphia, WB Saunders, 1972 (Concise, thorough discussion of cyanotic and acyanotic congenital heart disease and a useful reference.)

Perloff JK: The Clinical Recognition of Congenital Heart Disease. Philadelphia, WB Saunders, 1970 (Emphasis on physical examination findings and relationship to physical measurements such as carotid pulse tracings, phonocardiography, and cardiac catheterization data.)

Stein PD: A Physical and Physiological Basis for the Interpretation of Cardiac Auscultation: Evaluations Based Primarily on the Second Sound and Ejection Murmurs. Mount Kisco, New York, Futura Publishing Company, 1981 (Detailed discussion on turbulence and cardiac murmurs that reflect it.)

54
Cardiac Disease in the Neonate
VICTOR C. BAUM

Congenital heart disease is relatively common, affecting approximately 0.8% of all newborns. This excludes lesions presenting in later life (mitral valve prolapse, nonstenotic bicuspid aortic valve), and patent ductus arteriosus in premature infants. Congenital heart disease can present in the infant as congestive heart failure, cyanosis, dysrhythmia, airway obstruction, or as an asymptomatic murmur. An evaluation of infants is particularly difficult for various reasons. Up to 60% of all newborns will have a murmur on the first day of life, about 1% of all infants will have a dysrhythmia noted on a 10-sec ECG rhythm strip, and up to 13% will have ectopic beats. Most of these murmurs and dysrhythmias are asymptomatic and resolve spontaneously. Signs of congenital heart disease may be mimicked by various noncardiac disease processes. The degree of findings (*e.g.*, loudness of murmurs) may bear no relation to the severity (present or future) of the underlying cardiac defect, and murmurs themselves may be due to normal transitional physiologic processes. Almost all electrocardiographic variables have age-related normal values that change rapidly in the first few weeks of life. A stable physiologic state may change drastically with spontaneous closure of a patent ductus arteriosus if certain congenital defects are present. The normally rapid neonatal heart rate makes auscultation difficult for the inexperienced, and finally some are intimidated by the complex anatomy and physiology of the neonatal cardiovascular system and the complex congenital cardiac lesions.

This chapter is not intended to cover all of the possible congenital cardiac diseases; rather, it will be an overview of lesions presenting in the neonatal period and those problems that can masquerade as cardiac disease in the newborn.

PATHOPHYSIOLOGY AND DIFFERENTIAL DIAGNOSIS

Since heart disease in the neonate involves several distinct entities, the pathophysiologies must be considered separately.

Structural Abnormalities

A direct etiologic agent or disease can only be ascribed in about 10% of cases of congenital heart disease. These are due to chromosomal (*e.g.*, Down, Turner, trisomy 13 and 18 syndromes) and single gene (*e.g.*, Holt–Oram and Ellis–van Creveld syndromes) abnormalities, in utero infection (*e.g.*, rubella), and maternal teratogens (*e.g.*, ethanol, lithium). Rare families have been described in which a ventricular septal defect (VSD), atrial septal defect (ASD), patent ductus arteriosus (PDA), or primary pulmonary hypertension are transmitted as autosomal dominant characteristics. Cardiac abnormalities may also be included as components of a recognizable and named dysmorphic syndrome. In most of the congenital cardiac malformations, the etiology is ascribed to multifactorial inheritance. The fetal pulmonary arteries normally see only a small fraction of the cardiac output due to shunting by way of the foramen ovale and the ductus arteriosus. When these close, the branch pulmonary arteries must remodel to accommodate the increased blood flow. Until this is completed after the first few months of life, a murmur may be generated by a turbulent flow across these vessels (peripheral pulmonic stenosis).

Cyanosis

Visible cyanosis is present when greater than 3 to 5 g/dl of desaturated hemoglobin is present. Cyanosis, given a constant hemoglobin oxygen saturation, is more readily apparent with polycythemia and less readily apparent with anemia or the presence of fetal hemoglobin, which shifts the oxygen–hemoglobin saturation curve. A neonate may not be visibly cyanotic until the arterial Po_2 falls below 35 mm Hg. Cyanosis in the infant with congenital heart disease is almost always caused by right to left shunting of blood so that systemic venous blood returning to the heart bypasses the lungs before returning to the systemic circulation. This shunting may be at the atrial (ASD or patent foramen ovale), ventricular, or great vessel (PDA) level. The shunting is accompanied usually by decreased pulmonary blood flow. However, some specific lesions such as the transposition of the great arteries (TGA) and total anomalous pulmonary venous return (TAPVR) may have normal or increased pulmonary blood flow because of their specific physiology. Uncommonly, a congenital heart defect may result in pulmonary edema that may itself contribute to cyanosis in an otherwise acyanotic lesion. Cyanosis may also be caused by increased pulmonary arterial pressure, for example from pulmonary disease or polycythemia, resulting in right to left shunting through a normally patent ductus arteriosus or foramen ovale. When pulmonary arterial hypertension results in cyanosis from right to left shunting in an otherwise normal heart, it is known as persistent

fetal circulation (PFC), or more accurately, as persistent pulmonary hypertension. Pulmonary disease is always in the differential, and usually results in respiratory distress, an abnormal chest roentgenogram, and hypercapnea. Increased venous pressure may result in decreased local blood flow with venous suffusion and cyanosis. (See Chap. 189 for a detailed discussion of noncardiac causes of cyanosis.)

Heart Failure

Congestive heart failure in the older neonate is most often caused by lesions producing a large left to right shunt through a VSD or PDA. However, in the newborn, shunting through these defects is severely restricted by the normally elevated pulmonary vascular resistance and these lesions do not produce signs of heart disease until shunting is increased coincident with the fall in pulmonary vascular resistance, typically at 1 to 2 months of age. Heart failure on the first day of life is commonly due to metabolic abnormalities (*e.g.*, anemia, polycythemia, neonatal thyrotoxicosis, hypothyroidism, hypocalcemia, hypomagnesemia, and hypoglycemia), or in utero dysrhythmias (usually paroxysmal supraventricular tachycardia or complete heart block). Structural defects that result in heart failure on the first day of life are those of severe left-sided outflow obstruction (critical aortic stenosis, hypoplastic left heart), and large arteriovenous malformations (cerebral or hepatic). Various disease processes may result in a cardiomyopathy with resultant heart failure in the neonatal period. A peripartum asphyxial insult may result in myocardial damage with resultant heart failure, predominantly of the right ventricle with transient tricuspid insufficiency. Myocarditis can affect individuals at any age, including neonates. Endocardial fibroelastosis (EFE) is a disease of unknown etiology that is noted for a marked thickening of the endocardium. Although uncommon, it may produce heart failure from birth. If the left coronary artery arises anomalously from the pulmonary artery rather than from the aorta, it will result in inadequate myocardial perfusion and myocardial ischemia as the pulmonary arterial pressure falls at 1 to 2 months of age. Hypertrophic cardiomyopathy (idiopathic hypertrophic subaortic stenosis or IHSS) is typically a disease of the ventricular septum and left ventricle in older children and adults. Occasionally, however, it may be present in the neonate. Pompe's disease, one of the glycogen storage diseases (α-1, 4-glucosidase deficiency) is the only glycogen storage disease that has a major cardiac as well as voluntary muscle involvement. Finally, infants of poorly controlled diabetic mothers may have massive cardiomegaly and decreased myocardial function at the time of birth.

Dysrhythmias

Dysrhythmias may not have a recognizable etiology. Paroxysmal supraventricular tachycardia (PSVT) is most common during the first month of life. The involved bypass tract is manifest as the Wolff–Parkinson–White syndrome only about one half of the time. Congenital heart block may be associated with maternal connective tissue disease, most commonly systemic lupus erythematosus.

CLINICAL PRESENTATION

The signs of heart failure in infants are somewhat different than in older children and adults. Tachypnea is a common early sign. Other common signs are tachycardia, diaphoresis (especially with feeding), hepatomegaly, poor feeding and easy tiring with feeding, and failure to thrive. When heart failure is advanced, pulmonary crackles and a gallop may be noted and the infant will be oliguric. Unlike adult patients, peripheral edema is rare and the distinction between right-sided and left-sided heart failure is not clear. Since the liver is normally easily palpable in the infant about 2 cm below the right costal margin at the mid-clavicular line, palpation of liver size tends to be a good indicator of the degree of heart failure.

Cyanosis may not be present until low arterial Po_2s are reached. A differentiation should be made between central cyanosis and peripheral or acrocyanosis. Central cyanosis may be normal until 2 to 3 hours of life but persistence beyond that time should raise concerns that the infant may have cyanotic congenital heart disease. Infants with cyanotic lesions are often tachypneic and hyperpneic but without respiratory distress. Their arterial pCO_2 is typically normal or even low.

Although not all of the congenital cardiac lesions can be discussed, salient points for lesions representing most patients encountered are presented below.

Acyanotic Lesions

Ventricular Septal Defect (VSD). Although the most frequent congenital cardiac defect seen in childhood, an isolated VSD is usually asympto-

matic in the nursery and may cause only a trivial or even no murmur. Only as pulmonary vascular resistance falls in the first 1 to 2 months does increasing shunting through the defect and increasing pulmonary blood flow result in a murmur and, if the shunt is great enough, signs of increasing congestive heart failure. These are often noted for the first time on a routine well-baby examination.

Atrial Septal Defect (ASD). Simple, uncomplicated (secundum) atrial septal defects are not symptomatic in the newborn period and do not generate a murmur. They are not detected on a routine physical examination, electrocardiogram, or chest roentgenogram in the neonatal period.

Patent Ductus Arteriosus (PDA). In the term newborn, these are usually asymptomatic due to the normally elevated pulmonary vascular resistance, similar to ventricular septal defects. At 1 to 2 months of age a murmur, which was previously very soft or absent, becomes the typical PDA murmur in the left infraclavicular fossa. If there is major shunting through the PDA, congestive heart failure develops. In the newborn, the murmur, if present, tends to be softer, systolic only, and heard lower down along the left sternal border than in older infants and children. It may be impossible to differentiate the murmur of a PDA in the newborn from that of a VSD at this age. Because much of the pulmonary arterial musculature develops at the end of gestation, pulmonary vascular resistance in the premature infant falls more rapidly than in term infants. This explains the development of congestive heart failure in premature infants with a PDA as they recover from respiratory distress syndrome in the first week or two of life. It must always be remembered that a PDA in a premature infant does not exclude the presence of other congenital cardiac defects that may be masked by the PDA and that may even be "ductal dependent," that is pulmonary or aortic blood flow depends on patency of the PDA.

Coarctation of the Aorta. Infants with coarctation typically present at 7 to 14 days of age, coincident with obstruction to descending aortic blood flow with closure of the ductus arteriosus. The hallmark of coarctation is the disparity of arterial pulses and blood pressure between the arms and the legs, although the left subclavian artery, supplying the left arm, may be variably involved by the narrowed area. Occasionally, the difference in pulses may not be apparent by palpation, and blood pressures must always be obtained in both arms and one leg to exclude the presence of a coarctation.

Aortic Stenosis. Only the most severe degrees of stenosis ("critical aortic stenosis") result in problems in the neonatal period, and this is a rapidly life-threatening defect when it becomes manifest so early in life. These infants have poor cardiac output with poor peripheral pulses throughout. There may be a systolic ejection click. A murmur will not be generated if cardiac output is low.

Peripheral Pulmonic Stenosis. This asymptomatic condition has a murmur similar to a soft neonatal VSD or PDA murmur, but it is heard particularly well at the periphery of the lungs.

Endocardial Cushion Defect. This lesion, or more precisely, group of lesions (primum ASD ± basal VSD ± cleft mitral valve ± cleft tricuspid valve) has a variable presentation depending on its specific components. If a major atrioventricular valve insufficiency is present, the infant may present with early heart failure. Endocardial cushion defects are common in infants with Down syndrome and are present in approximately 25% of these cases (approximately one half of Down syndrome infants who have congenital defects).

Arteriovenous Malformations (AVM). Though not strictly cardiac defects, large AVMs present with severe congestive heart failure in the first few days of life. These infants have a very hyperdynamic precordium, bounding pulses with a wide pulse pressure, and a bruit is often, but not always, heard over the affected organ, typically the brain or liver.

Hypoplastic Left Heart. This lesion, due to atresia of the mitral or aortic valve, results in heart failure in the first few days of life. These infants have poor pulses throughout, poor peripheral perfusion, metabolic acidosis, and do poorly with early mortality.

Anomalous Origin of the Left Coronary Artery. In this lesion, the left coronary artery originates from the main pulmonary artery. The low oxygen content in this blood supplying the myocardium is surprisingly well-tolerated. However, inadequate myocardial perfusion occurs at the time of the normal fall in pulmonary arterial pressure at 1 to 2 months of age. The increased exercise and energy expenditure associated with feeding may cause angina in these young infants, which may manifest as crying, pallor, and diaphoresis.

Vascular Rings, Pulmonary Arterial Sling. These defects cause difficulty by encircling the trachea, alone or in combination with the ductus arteriosus or ligamentum arteriosum. These infants may have evidence of upper airway obstruction with inspiratory stridor in the nursery, or they may develop it in the first few months.

Pompe's Disease. These infants present with hypotonia and cardiomyopathy. They usually present at a few months of age.

Infant of a Diabetic Mother. Infants of poorly controlled diabetic mothers may have a murmur and major cardiomegaly. It is uncommon for them to be symptomatic from cardiac involvement and the cardiomegaly resolves spontaneously over several weeks.

Myocarditis. These infants present with profound, rapidly progressive heart failure. There are poor peripheral pulses, a quiet precordium, and cardiomegaly. There may be a murmur of mitral insufficiency.

Transient Myocardial Ischemia. Occasionally, infants who have undergone a peripartum anoxic insult will develop ischemic injury to the myocardium. Unlike older patients with ischemic insults, these infants have predominantly right ventricular involvement and present with cardiomegaly and tricuspid insufficiency. As in other cases of myocardial injury, CPK-MB isoenzyme levels in the blood are elevated.

Hypertrophic Cardiomyopathy (IHSS). Uncommonly, this disease may present with heart failure in the neonate.

Cyanotic Lesions

Transposition of the Great Arteries (TGA). These typically large infants with a male predominance present with cyanosis from the time of delivery without the normal resolution over the first few hours. They are surprisingly without distress despite their profound cyanosis. Their physical examination, electrocardiogram, and chest roentgenogram can be close to normal. If there are associated lesions that allow for increased shunting between the pulmonary and systemic circulation, they may be less cyanotic.

Tetralogy of Fallot. The age at presentation depends on the severity of the pulmonary stenosis. Most often, pulmonary stenosis is not well-developed at birth and these infants do not become cyanotic until several months of age, or they may present only with the murmur of a VSD. If pulmonary stenosis is severe, they will present with cyanosis from birth. Hypercyanotic "Tet. spells" are distinctly unusual in the first few months of life.

Total Anomalous Pulmonary Venous Return. If associated with obstruction to pulmonary venous return, typically with TAPVR below the diaphragm, infants present in the first week of life with cyanosis and tachypnea. The chest roentgenogram looks much like pulmonary edema, but the cardiac silhouette is normal or small in size. The arterial Po_2 of these infants can increase significantly in response to increases in the inspired oxygen.

Persistent Fetal Circulation. These infants have already had another insult such as peripartum asphyxia or aspiration. A cardiac examination is essentially normal, although there may be a differential cyanosis of the upper and lower body with a large right to left ductal shunt. This differential cyanosis may not be discernible, particularly if there is also a significant atrial right to left shunt.

Tricuspid or Pulmonary Atresia. These infants present with cyanosis. There may be adequate pulmonary blood flow by way of the patent ductus arteriosus to allow them to remain stable, but these newborns can deteriorate rapidly on ductal closure at about 7 to 10 days of age.

Ebstein's Anomaly. This defect of tricuspid valve formation presents with signs related to tricuspid insufficiency and right to left atrial shunting. They have cyanosis, massive cardiomegaly, and may have atrial dysrhythmias related to atrial distention. The dysrhythmias and often the cyanosis resolve with the fall in pulmonary vascular resistance and decreasing tricuspid insufficiency. Ebstein's anomaly is often associated with the Wolff–Parkinson–White syndrome.

Dysrhythmias

Protracted in utero tachycardia or bradycardia can result in nonimmune hydrops fetalis. The specific cardiac rhythm can be determined by fetal echocardiography. Perhaps the most common "dysrhythmias" detected in the nursery are sinus arrhythmia and sinus bradycardia. Sinus arrhythmia is a normal finding that is more pronounced in children than in adults. There is sinus slowing during inspiration. Sinus slowing can be so pronounced

that junctional or even ventricular escape beats are noted on the ECG. Although newborns are typically considered as having relatively high resting heart rates, healthy term newborns can have sleeping heart rates descend into the 70s. Sinus bradycardia can also accompany yawning, defecation, or apnea. If the heart rate responds appropriately to stimulation of the infant, and is not associated with apnea, it is of no concern. As mentioned above, over 10% of newborns will have atrial or ventricular premature beats. Some of these will be noted on routine auscultation of the chest or palpation of the pulses. Almost all ectopy will resolve spontaneously by 1 month of age.

The most common "pathologic" dysrhythmia in the neonate is paroxysmal supraventricular tachycardia (PSVT). The heart rate in infants with PSVT is higher than that in older children and adults and is in the range of 210 to 300. These infants may present *in utero* with hydrops fetalis or may present at any time with heart failure and tachycardia. Since these infants cannot complain of tachycardia, they often do not come to medical attention until the tachycardia has been present for one or more days and they have developed congestive failure. Although it may be difficult to differentiate the rhythm at this time from an appropriate sinus tachycardia, the heart rate in PSVT tends to be higher, and there is little if any beat to beat and second to second variability in the heart rate.

Exact diagnosis of the structural cardiac malformations depends on rigorous physical, x-ray, electrocardiographic, and echocardiographic examinations as well as cardiac catheterization in difficult cases. However, a simplified approach using the presence of a murmur, cyanosis or heart failure, the age at presentation, the pulmonary blood flow on chest roentgenogram, and the electrocardiogram is offered in the box, Diagnostic Clues in Neonatal Heart Disease. These are guidelines; a significant individual variation may exist.

WORK-UP

Although the temptation is to immediately call for a pediatric cardiologist and order an echocardiogram whenever heart disease is suspected in a newborn, much progress can be made in determining the presence or absence of heart disease and making a specific diagnosis using the basics of the history, physical examination, ECG, and chest roentgenogram. In addition to being intellectually

Diagnostic Clues in Neonatal Heart Disease

Cyanosis (severe), pulmonary blood flow normal or increased ± narrow mediastinum:
TGA

Mild cyanosis, increased pulmonary blood flow:
TAPVR, truncus arteriosus, TGA with large VSD, doble outlet right ventricle, common ventricle

Cyanosis, pulmonary venous congestion, small heart:
TAPVR

Cyanosis, decreased pulmonary blood flow:
Massive cardiomegaly: Ebstein's anomaly, pulmonary atresia with tricuspid insufficiency
Left ventricular hypertrophy: pulmonary atresia
Superior QRS axis [0 − (−90)]: tricuspid atresia
QRS axis 30–90, no murmur: pulmonary atresia with intact ventricular septum
Right ventricular hypertrophy, QRS axis 30–90, murmur: pulmonary stenosis
Right ventricular hypertrophy, QRS axis >90, systolic murmur: VSD with pulmonary stenosis (tetralogy of Fallot)
Right ventricular hypertrophy, QRS axis >90, continuous or no murmur: pulmonary atresia with VSD

Cyanosis, normal cardiac exam, upper to lower body pO₂ difference:
PFC

Cyanosis, abnormal abdominal situs:
heterotaxy, usually asplenia

Heart failure, first week:
Metabolic
In utero dysrhythmia
Tricuspid insufficiency murmur, elevated CPK-MB: transient myocardial ischemia
Bounding pulses, hyperactive precordium ± bruit: arteriovenous malformation
Upper to lower pulse disparity: coarctation
Decreased pulses, left ventricular hypertrophy ± ejection click: critical aortic stenosis
Decreased pulses, right ventricular hypertrophy, active precordium: hypoplastic left heart

Heart failure, 2–4 weeks:
Acyanotic, murmur: VSD, PDA, endocardial cushion defect
Acyanotic, no murmur:
Left ventricular hypertrophy: EFE
Low voltage QRS: myocarditis
Q wave or T wave inversion leads I, avL, and V5–V6: anomalous origin of left coronary artery
Left ventricular hypertrophy, short PR, hypotonia: Pompe's disease
Desaturated or cyanotic:
No murmur or soft murmur: TAPVR
VSD murmur, right ventricular hypertrophy: double outlet right ventricle, TGA with VSD
Biventricular hypertrophy: truncus arteriosus

satisfying, this allows appropriate therapeutic measures to be begun at an earlier stage.

History

The history may provide clues to various lesions even in neonates. Specific points include a history of maternal drug usage (licit and illicit), connective tissue disease, rashes or other infectious diseases during pregnancy, diabetes, thyroid disease, and a family history of heart disease (structural or EFE). The presence of in-utero tachycardia or bradycardia should be investigated, and the chart should be reviewed for evidence of peripartum asphyxia (*e.g.*, low Apgar). The age at onset of heart disease provides an important clue to the specific lesion present.

Physical Examination

A complete physical examination is crucial. Is there gross evidence of a dysmorphic syndrome? Are the vital signs normal for age? The blood pressure must be taken in both arms and a leg. With the ready availability of Doppler and oscillometric blood pressure devices, the flush technique of estimating the blood pressure in infants is obsolete. If cyanosis is present, is it acrocyanosis or central cyanosis? If central, is it generalized or does it affect primarily just the upper or the lower body? Is the skin warm and well perfused or is it cold and mottled, suggesting the presence of heart failure? Are there cutaneous hemangiomas that might be accompanied by internal arteriovenous malformations? Are the peripheral pulses symmetric in the arms and the legs? Are the pulses weak and thready, or are they bounding, suggesting an aortic runoff lesion? Although an examination of the jugular veins is often not productive in infants due to their short, fat necks, the scalp veins may become distended with severe congestive heart failure. Are the lungs clear, or is there evidence of pulmonary disease or pulmonary edema? Is the precordial activity increased? Are there bruits heard over the skull or liver? Despite the normally rapid heart rate in neonates, cardiac auscultation is made easier by the routinely loud cardiac sounds transmitted by the thin chest wall. The first heart sound is normally narrowly split, and this should be differentiated from a systolic ejection click. The second sound should be easily detectable. It is normally more narrowly split and the pulmonic component louder than in older children due to the elevated pulmonary vascular resistance and pulmonary arterial pressure in neonates. Murmurs should be listened for and characterized as in older patients. If the infant is on a ventilator, disconnecting the ventilator tubing from the endotracheal tube for a few seconds will markedly increase the quality of the auscultatory examination at no risk to the infant. The abdomen should be examined for hepatosplenomegaly. The liver is normally palpable approximately 2 cm below the right costal margin in the midclavicular line. It is best palpated by gentle pressure of the fingers on the abdomen and moving the hand cephalad and caudad. The fingers will fall off the edge of the liver, which will be felt better than by direct, deep palpation.

Laboratory Tests

Chest Roentgenogram. A single frontal view of the chest will suffice. Very little useful information regarding heart disease is obtained from the lateral chest roentgenogram in young infants. The film should be examined for cardiac size and position, evidence of abdominal situs (manifested by stomach and liver position), a narrow mediastinum, pulmonary blood flow, and the side of the aortic arch (right sided arches are associated with tetralogy and double outlet right ventricle). In addition, the pulmonary vascular pattern can be examined to see if it looks like the cascading pattern of normal pulmonary arteries, or the more horizontal pattern of bronchial collateral vessels. It must be remembered that films taken in exhalation and the normally large neonatal thymus may both give the appearance of cardiomegaly. The pulmonary blood flow in an expiratory film will also appear to be increased.

Electrocardiogram. All patients with congenital heart disease should have an electrocardiogram

(ECG). It must be remembered that all ECG variables have age (and sometimes rate) related normal values. Some of the more important values are listed in Table 54-1. The change in R wave predominance with age reflects the gradual resolution of the normal fetal right ventricular predominance. The T wave is normally upright in lead V1 until the fourth day, and then again after about 10 years of age. Persistence or resumption of its upright position is a sign of right ventricular hypertrophy. The QT_c interval (<0.4 sec) is the same in infants as in older children. The electrocardiogram of the premature infant shows a shorter PR interval (0.10) and QRS duration (0.05) with lower QRS amplitude and a more rapid shift to left ventricular predominance. The P wave axis should be the same as in older patients. An upright or rightward P wave axis may be seen with the heterotaxy syndromes.

Arterial Blood Gases. Arterial blood gases are critical, particularly to confirm a clinical diagnosis of cyanosis and to monitor response to therapy. Severe heart failure will result in metabolic acidosis. Cyanosis and a normal arterial Po_2 suggest methemoglobinemia or an abnormal hemoglobin. If congenital heart disease is suspected, samples should be obtained from preductal (right radial or right temporal arteries) and postductal (umbilical artery) sites to assess right to left ductal shunting. The arterial Po_2 is normally 45 mm Hg by 1 hour of age and 60 mm Hg by 1 day of age. If the sample is obtained with the infant crying, the Po_2 may be much lower than a resting sample even in normal infants. If this is a problem, a small amount of subcutaneous local anesthetic can be infiltrated near the artery and the infant will not cry during blood sampling.

Echocardiography. Echocardiography, often combined with Doppler evaluation of blood flow,

Table 54-1. Selected Age-Related Normal ECG Values

	1 DAY	1–30 DAYS	1–3 MONTHS
QRS axis	110–170	70–120	30–110
PR interval (sec)	0.11	0.11	rate 91–110:0.14 rate 111–130:0.13 rate 131–150:0.12 rate >150:0.11
QRS duration (sec)	0.08	0.08	0.09
R V$_4$R (mm)	5–13	4–8	2–9
R V$_1$ (mm)	6–19	5–17	6–17
R V$_5$ (mm)	5–15	4–22	12–25
R V$_6$ (mm)	2–10	3–15	7–19

has made major contributions to the early, non-invasive diagnosis of even the most complex congenital cardiac defects. The availability of echocardiography and a skilled pediatric echocardiographer does not make the preliminary evaluation any less necessary.

MANAGEMENT

The specific surgical approach to structural heart disease depends on the specific lesion, as well as the current practices of the cardiac surgeon. However, some general approaches to medical management can be made.

Ductal Dependent Lesions. Any time there is a concern that a congenital cardiac lesion is present which requires ductal patency for supply of either systemic or pulmonary blood flow, ductal patency should be maintained pharmacologically with prostaglandin E_1 (PGE_1, Prostin-VR) until a definitive diagnosis and surgical palliation or correction is undertaken. This can be life saving. Even if a later examination (echocardiography, catheterization) shows that a ductal-dependent lesion is not present, PGE_1 can be discontinued with little if any detriment. Ductal-dependent cyanotic lesions include TGA, pulmonary atresia or severe pulmonary stenosis, and tricuspid atresia. The acyanotic lesions include coarctation of the aorta, hypoplastic left heart, and critical aortic stenosis. The beginning dose of PGE_1 is 0.1 µg/kg/min. After a therapeutic response is achieved (as determined by increased Po_2 or increased peripheral pulses), the dose can be decreased to 0.05 µg/kg/min, and some infants may even be controlled with lower doses. The most common complications of PGE_1 are apnea, fever, and cutaneous flushing.

Heart Failure. The general approach to the neonate with heart failure is the same as for any patient. In the nursery, specific additional measures include the use of supplemental oxygen, an infant seat, assuring a neutral thermal environment, correcting acidosis, hypoglycemia or infections if present, and normalizing hematocrit. Critically ill neonates will occasionally require intubation, mechanical ventilation, and rarely even sedation and paralysis to control severe heart failure with metabolic acidosis. Other measures applicable to all young children include a salt-limited diet, diuretics, and digoxin. Fluid restriction should not be used if it results in a diminished intake of calories. Caloric supplementation, either by use of 24 cal/oz formula or by supplementing regular formula with medium

Table 54-2. Digoxin Doses (mg/kg)

AGE	DIGITALIZING PARENTERAL	DIGITALIZING ORAL
Premature	0.02	0.03
Term–2 weeks	0.03	0.05
2 weeks–6 months	0.05	0.06

chain triglycerides will provide much needed extra calories. Several commerically available infant formulas have a lower salt content than others (7 vs 11 meq/l). The most widely used diuretic is furosemide (Lasix) at a dose of 1 mg/kg 2 to 3 times per day intravenously or orally, although some infants will require more, particularly if given orally. Potassium depletion is a concern as in older patients. The schedule for digitalization depends on the age of the infant and the mode of administration. One half the total digitalizing dose is given followed by one fourth in 8 hours, and one fourth 8 hours after that. It may also be given in three equal doses 8 hours apart. After the total digitalizing dose has been given, the maintenance dose is begun. The normal maintenance dose is one fourth the digitalizing dose, if both are administered by the same route (oral or parenteral). If the infant was digitalized intravenously and the maintenance dose was given orally, the daily maintenance dose is one third the digitalizing dose. The daily dose is usually given in two divided doses, every 12 hours (Table 54-2). Digoxin levels are usually not useful in neonates. The usual therapeutic levels are higher than in adults.

Infants who have a lesion that could result in congestive heart failure in the first few months (VSD, PDA) should be seen at least monthly for the first 3 months.

Indomethacin (Indocin), useful for ductal closure in the preterm infant, is not useful in term and post-term infants.

Congenital Heart Block. If a congenital heart block is diagnosed prenatally, a pediatric cardiologist or a pediatric surgeon should be notified in case emergent transvenous pacemaker placement is required. If the heart rate is >60, no therapy is usually required. An isoproterenol (Isuprel) infusion may be used as a temporizing measure, but results are usually minimal.

PSVT. The therapy is the same as for older children, using vagal maneuvers, digoxin, propranolol and, in critically ill children, electrical cardioversion. Verapamil, though very effective, is contraindicated in neonates due to the high incidence of profound hypotension. The diving seal reflex (application of ice water to the face) tends to be more effective in neonates than in older children. The dose of digoxin is the same as for treating heart failure. The dose of intravenous propranolol is 0.1 mg/kg. Conversion by overdrive pacing, either transvenous or transesophageal, should be reserved for specialized centers. Once the rhythm is successfully terminated, these infants are usually maintained on digoxin for 6 to 12 months. It is then discontinued if the infant has no further episodes.

PFC. This is treated by hyperventilation to produce a significant respiratory alkalosis. Occasionally these infants also require treatment with tolazoline (Priscoline), a vasodilator. The dose is 1 mg/kg intravenously into a vein draining to the superior vena cava (arm or scalp) followed by an infusion of 1 to 2 mg/kg/hr. Most infants are controlled successfully with hyperventilation alone.

PATIENT EDUCATION

Parents of infants who are at risk of developing heart failure should be given a list of the signs of congestive heart failure with instructions to contact the physician should any of these signs develop. Parents should also be reassured that if heart failure develops, it will be over a period of days to weeks and not as an acute emergency. It might also be worthwhile to explain that the term heart *failure* is not as ominous as it may sound. The families of all infants with congenital heart disease should receive appropriate counseling regarding the risk of recurrence in future pregnancies.

ANNOTATED BIBLIOGRAPHY

Braudo M, Rowe RD: Auscultation of the heart—early neonatal period. Am J Dis Child 101:67–78, 1961 (Describes the common occurrence of murmurs in normal newborns.)

Davignon A, Rautaharju P, Boisselle E et al: ECG standards for children. Percentile charts. Pediatr Cardiol 1:133–152, 1979–1980 (Lists age-related normal values for a wide range of ECG variables.)

Fyler DC: Report of the New England Regional Infant Cardiac Program. Pediatrics (suppl) 65:375–461, 1980 (Epidemiologic report from a large multicenter data base.)

Lees MH: Cyanosis of the newborn infant. Recognition and clinical evaluation. J Pediatr 77:484–498, 1970 (Discusses the pathophysiology of cyanosis, particularly in the neonate.)

Moller JH, Neal WA: Heart Disease in Infancy. New York, Appleton–Century–Crofts, 1981 (Text devoted to cardiac diseases in the infant.)

Southall DP, Johnson AM, Shinebourne EA et al: Frequency and outcome of disorders of cardiac rhythm and conduction in a population of newborn infants. Pediatrics 68:58–66, 1981 (Discusses the incidence, distribution, and prognosis of abnormal rhythms noted in the nursery.)

55
Chest Pain
HERBERT E. COHN

Chest pain in children is a common complaint in primary care settings and creates anxiety in patients, their parents, and pediatricians. Although a physician evaluating a child with chest pain may think first of angina pectoris or myocardial infarction, these are unlikely as chest pain in childhood infrequently stems from heart disease. In assessing chest pain, one must be careful not to increase the child's anxiety level. This can best be done by a careful history with an emphasis on letting the patient express the symptoms in his own words. The physical examination may yield a full explanation, but is usually normal.

PATHOPHYSIOLOGY, CLINICAL PRESENTATION, AND DIFFERENTIAL DIAGNOSIS

Musculoskeletal causes of chest pain can occur through muscle strain, as in an overuse injury producing chest wall pain. Direct trauma to the chest (*e.g.*, from diving, swimming, gymnastics, or soccer) has often been forgotten by the patient when the bruising becomes symptomatic.

Costochondritis may arise through exercise, coughing, or sneezing, and causes a tenderness or inflammation over the junction between the anterior ribs and the sternum. It is associated with sharp, anterior chest pain at the costochondral junctions. In Tietze's syndrome, there is a local swelling of a particular costochondral junction. Rib fracture is often associated with severe chest pain and follows a known episode of chest trauma or a period of severe or protracted coughing. Slipping rib syndrome is thought to be a sprain disorder produced by trauma to the costal cartilages of the eighth, ninth, or tenth ribs. The patient describes a slipping movement of the ribs and can sense a clicking and popping when bending or flexing the trunk. One can reproduce the pain by performing a "hooking" maneuver in which the affected rib margin is grasped and then pulled anteriorly.

Pleural causes of chest pain usually manifest as a pain worsened by deep inspiration and coughing, and include such entities as the "precordial catch" syndrome, pleurisy, and pneumothorax. The "precordial catch" syndrome refers to a pattern of left anterior chest pain in young, healthy individuals. The pain is sharp, severe, sudden in onset, and localized to the left precordium near the apex. It occurs at rest, especially with bending, and is worsened by attempting to take a deep breath, as if something "catches" or sticks. The pain most likely arises from the parietal pleura although there is no apparent correlation with previous illnesses, physical abnormalities, or evidence of a cardiac origin. In pleurisy, there is inflammation of the parietal pleura innervated by intercostal nerves carrying pain fibers. The pain is made more intense by deep and rapid breathing that causes greater excursions of the lung against the inflamed parietal pleura. In pleural effusion, the pain usually arises from pressure on the diaphragm. Pain is felt posteriorly in the shoulder when the central part of the diaphragm is involved, and in the side or back when the anterior part of the diaphragm is involved. Marked inflammation of the lung parenchyma produces no chest pain unless the parietal pleura is involved. The pain of pneumonitis is the pain of pleurisy.

Inflammation of the bronchi may manifest in several different forms. Tracheobronchitis may be associated with a burning pain on coughing. "Asthmatic bronchitis" may be associated with a sensation of pain or tightness in the chest during inspiration.

Intercostal nerve pain is most commonly seen in a child with herpes zoster infection, and follows a specific dermatome distribution. It may be sensed as an ache over a portion of the chest wall. Its distribution can be mapped by touch or pinprick. In herpes zoster, the pain may precede the appearance of skin lesions by several days.

Cardiovascular causes of chest pain, although the least common, are among the most serious. Structural congenital heart lesions that can cause chest pain include the left ventricular outflow tract obstructive lesions such as valvar and subvalvar aortic stenosis, and cardiomyopathies including idiopathic hypertrophic subaortic stenosis (IHSS). To a lesser extent, pulmonic stenosis can also be associated with chest pain. These lesions are not generally associated with chest pain at mild or even moderate degrees of severity, and one is not likely to find symptomatic left ventricular outflow tract obstruction if cardiac signs have not been noted previously on physical examination. Children who have a known aortic or pulmonic stenosis whose congenital heart disease is increasing in severity may begin to complain of chest pain on a cardiogenic basis and need surgical relief of their severe obstructive lesions. The pain is caused by myocardial oxygen deprivation leading to myocardial insufficiency and ischemia. Coronary arterial anomalies, such as an anomalous left coronary artery arising from the pulmonary artery, are rare. Although they may be difficult to diagnose, the usual signs and symptoms are those of myocardial ischemia and congestive heart failure. Thus, the patient is often acutely and severely ill and needs urgent care. Pallor, irritability, chest pain, and signs of acute congestive heart failure, together with the characteristic ECG pattern (deep Q waves in lead I and aVL) usually assist in making the diagnosis in an infant under 1 year old. Of all infants born with this type of anomaly, 15% to 20% reach adulthood.

Mitral valve prolapse is often associated with chest pain in the adult population but is much less frequently associated with chest pain before adolescence. The pain occurs with or without exertion. Its etiology is not clear; it may result from papillary muscle dysfunction or through noncoronary causes such as autonomic dysfunction and instability.

Pericarditis and myocarditis can occur in any child. In pericarditis, the chest pain is due to a large effusion causing great tension on the pericardial sac. It is associated with a dull ache over the heart, especially the mid to left precordium. Acute pericarditis is also associated with severe, sharp midsternal pain and can be referred to the left infraclavicular or subscapular areas of the chest. These children often appear sick and uncomfortable and have other findings of cardiovascular involvement.

Supraventricular tachycardia, at rates above

200/min, may cause chest pain and hypotension through inadequate myocardial oxygen delivery, leading to myocardial insufficiency and ischemia. At rates from 140 to 200/min, supraventricular tachycardia is unlikely to cause chest pain. Extrasystoles do not usually cause chest pain unless they are occurring successively or in runs of ventricular tachycardia. Palpitations may be felt by the child if the cardiac rhythm is irregular.

Esophageal reflux of gastric contents may be associated with a retrosternal burning sensation referred to in lay terms as *heartburn*. This sensation is usually in the xiphoid region of the upper abdomen. In adults, this area is a frequent source of confusion in differentiating between gastrointestinal and cardiogenic causes of pain. In childhood, this area is an infrequent source of pain.

Psychogenic causes of chest pain are common in childhood. The pain can mimic angina pectoris in its characterization, and the distribution may be similar to that described by an adult in the child's family.

Miscellaneous causes of chest pain include sickle cell crises with anginal pain secondary to vascular occlusion, tumors involving the lung and chest wall such as Hodgkin's disease, or bony infiltration of ribs and sternum by sarcomas or leukemic involvement. Inflammatory myopathies such as trichinosis can also produce intercostal myalgia.

Idiopathic causes of chest pain make up a large percentage of pediatric complaints of chest pain (45% in one prospective study). This group includes the complaints of chest pain not associated with exercise or syncope and present in a child with an otherwise normal history, physical examination, and laboratory studies such as an electrocardiogram, a chest roentgenogram, and a hemogram. In most cases, symptoms appear to be self-limited and tend to diminish or resolve within 1 year.

Differential Diagnosis of Chest Pain in Childhood

1. Musculoskeletal causes
    a. Muscle strain
    b. Direct trauma
    c. Costochondritis
    d. Rib fracture
    e. Slipping rib syndrome
2. Pleural causes
    a. Precordial catch syndrome
    b. Pleurisy
    c. Pleural effusion
3. Pulmonary parenchymal causes
    a. Referred pain from pneumonitis
    b. Tracheobronchitis
    c. "Asthmatic bronchitis"
4. Intercostal nerve causes
    a. Herpes zoster infection
    b. Radiculitis
5. Cardiac causes
    a. Left ventricular outflow tract obstructive lesions
        1. Aortic stenosis, valvular and subvalvular
        2. Hypertrophic cardiomyopathy
    b. Right ventricular outflow tract obstructive lesions
        1. Pulmonic stenosis, valvular and subvalvular
    c. Coronary artery anomalies
        1. Anomalous left coronary artery arising from the pulmonary artery
    d. Mitral valve prolapse
    e. Pericarditis
    f. Myocarditis and other inflammatory disorders
    g. Kawasaki disease, including coronary arteritis
    h. Dysrhythmias
        1. Supraventricular tachycardia
        2. Extrasystoles, ventricular and AV junctional in origin
6. Esophageal causes
    a. Esophageal reflux
    b. Esophagitis
7. Psychogenic causes
8. Miscellaneous causes
    a. Sickle cell crisis
    b. Thoracic tumors, including lung parenchyma and chest wall
    c. Inflammatory myopathies
9. Idiopathic

WORK-UP

History

A careful history is necessary in differentiating the causes of chest pain in childhood. One should have a description of the chest pain: what it feels like and its precipitating factors, as well as its location and duration. Is it exercise-induced and is it associated with other symptoms such as lightheadedness? Has the chest pain been associated with syncope? Chest pain associated with exercise or syncope is likely to reflect an underlying structural cardiac lesion, such as a left ventricular outflow tract obstruction. Has there been prior drug use? Has there been recent illness, a heart attack or death in a relative or friend? Is there an underlying source of anxiety in the child's daily life? Family, friends, and school-related stresses should be asked about. It is especially important to observe and listen as much as to ask. Anxiety may be reflected in a worried expression, a quiet child, a tachycardia, hyperventilation, or a lack of congruence between the child's appearance and behavior. An active child, who is talkative and eager to play, is probably well. Have you noted differences from prior interactions during the visit (child–parent, child–physician, and parent–physician)? Who is most stressed? Is the atmosphere tense and emotional, or relaxed and more rational? Have you considered your own feelings and openness to any diagnosis? Have you prejudged that there is nothing wrong?

Physical Examination

Clinical findings that reflect the etiology of chest pain are not usually evident. The child's appearance is important and can be assessed as the physician measures the pulse, respiratory rate, and blood pressure. The respiratory rate and effort may reflect the degree of illness and discomfort. A dyspneic child has driven, hard respirations and is likely to have an underlying respiratory or cardiovascular problem. The clinical picture of hyperventilation, sweaty palms, and a dry mouth is likely to reflect anxiety (which could also be caused by the patient's concern about his chest pain). Asthma, with its prolonged expiratory phase and greater use of the accessory muscles in breathing, can often be easily diagnosed. An inspection of the patient's chest may yield signs of recent trauma. A prominent costochondral junction may reflect costochondritis. Chest wall assymetry due to an underlying cardiac lesion is easily missed unless the physician looks at the supine patient from the feet toward the head.

Palpation of the midsternal area may elicit tenderness over the costochrondral junctions. Palpation over the supraclavicular areas may elicit crepitus from subcutaneous air secondary to a pneumomediastinum. Palpation of the precordia for abnormal cardiac heaves, impulses, or thrills, may provide evidence of a structural congenital heart lesion. An examination of the breast tissue and other soft tissue of the chest for tenderness, particularly in the adolescent, may provide an explanation for the chest pain. Anterior–posterior or lateral compression of the chest wall may reproduce the pain of recent rib cage trauma.

Percussion of the chest provides information on the lung parenchyma. Dullness to percussion is often associated with underlying consolidation, atelectasis, or pleural effusion. Tympany may reflect hyperaeration as from asthma most commonly. Resonance to percussion suggests a normal quality of the underlying lung parenchyma.

Auscultation provides evidence of bilateral air exchange. Wheezing reflects bronchospasm. Decreased breath sounds may reflect pneumonitis, atelectasis, or pneumothorax.

The cardiovascular examination should be directed toward evidence of an inflammatory disorder such as pericarditis or myocarditis, a dysrhythmia, and findings of a structural congenital heart lesion. Tachycardia, muffled heart sounds, or the presence of a pericardial friction rib are useful clues for pericarditis. The quality of the heart sounds and the presence of a gallop rhythm might also reflect a myocarditis. The rhythm should be described as regular or irregular, and if the latter, the particular pattern should be noted. Children with supraventricular tachycardia may experience chest pain during a period of rapid heart rate. Patients with ventricular or supraventricular extrasystoles are generally asymptomatic, but may describe palpitations. Insignificant cardiac murmurs are common in childhood. Few congenital heart lesions are likely to produce chest pain and it is more likely that a child with chest pain from any cause could have a cardiac murmur of the insignificant type that is wholly unrelated to the chest pain. On the other hand, the presence of an ejection click, a prominent cardiac impulse, or hepatomegaly related to congestive heart failure would be important clues to an underlying structural congenital heart lesion. Any of the left or right ventricular outflow tract obstructive lesions are likely to be associated with significant cardiac murmurs as well as ejection clicks, ventricular impulses, alterations of the second heart sound, and other positive cardiac findings.

Laboratory Tests

An electrocardiogram should not be considered a routine study as part of an evaluation of chest pain, but is valuable if clinical clues suggest its usefulness. It can document the cardiac rate and rhythm, the electrical conduction pattern, and the presence of chamber hypertrophy. It may also provide clues in the presence of an anomalous coronary artery from the pulmonary artery or other coronary abnormalities such as seen in Kawasaki disease; ST and T-wave changes suggest pericarditis or myocarditis. In perspective, however, the electrocardiogram may be entirely normal in any of these conditions early in the illness; subtle changes may be appreciated only when several studies are obtained sequentially as the illness evolves.

The chest roentgenogram is also valuable in the assessment of chest pain, but should be considered only if the history and physical findings warrant this study. The chest film may corroborate the physical findings of a pulmonary process such as pneumonitis, effusion, or pneumomediastinum. A chest film might also show evidence of chest trauma such as rib fracture, displacement, or bony callus formation.

Noninvasive Studies

Additional noninvasive cardiovascular studies may be useful, particularly in the child whose chest pain is associated with exercise or syncope. Two-dimensional echocardiography is valuable in assessing ventricular function and anatomic abnormalities such as aortic or pulmonic stenosis, other intracardiac abnormalities, and coronary artery anomalies. It is also valuable in documenting the presence and magnitude of a pericardial effusion. A treadmill ECG (stress test) is valuable in assessing cardiac dysrhythmias such as supraventricular tachycardia. The acute stress of the study may provoke and hence document the dysrhythmia. This type of study may also demonstrate the degree to which the child can perform before evoking any chest pain and may provide some degree of reassurance to the child and parents regarding strenuous activity in the face of a recent complaint of chest pain.

MANAGEMENT AND INDICATIONS FOR REFERRAL

Any child in acute distress complaining of chest pain should be evaluated in the Emergency Ward where cardiovascular support can be provided if the patient develops circulatory collapse. The child with recurring chest pain associated with exercise, syncope, lightheadedness, palpitations, easy fatigue, or a history of known congenital heart disease should be referred to a pediatric cardiologist for further evaluation. Children with findings suggestive of an acute inflammatory process such as pericarditis or myocarditis should also be referred. Patients in whom esophagitis is secondary to reflux, caustic ingestion, or a foreign body ingestion leading to retrosternal chest pain, as well as patients with chest wall trauma, pleural effusion, or pneumothorax may be managed by the pediatrician in conjunction with a pediatric surgeon for further

evaluation and treatment of the underlying condition. Children whose chest pain is on a musculoskeletal basis secondary to trauma, but not associated with any bony fracture, can generally be managed with rest, analgesics, and simple supportive measures. Those children whose chest pain is on a psychogenic basis can be helped as they are listened to and allowed to feel that their symptomatology is being taken seriously. Gentle questioning as to what the child sees as the cause of the chest pain often leads to acceptance of the physician's reassurance that the child's pain is not on a cardiogenic basis and that he is not in imminent danger (see Chap. 28).

Despite the descriptions of each of these entities, nearly one half of childhood complaints of chest pain are called "idiopathic" since no specific explanation can be given. A course of watchful observation usually shows that the child remains free of any impairment of cardiovascular function or performance.

ANNOTATED BIBLIOGRAPHY

Coleman WL: Recurrent chest pain in children. Pediatr Clin North Am 31:1007, 1984 (Extensive discussion of the causes and pathophysiology of recurrent chest pain in childhood.)

Driscoll DJ, Glicklich LB, Gallen WJ: Chest pain in children: A prospective study. Pediatrics 57:648, 1976 (The authors conclude from this prospective study that chest pain in children rarely signals serious disease which is not apparent from a thorough history and physical examination.)

Fyfe DA, Moodie DS: Chest pain in pediatric patients presenting to a cardiac clinic. Clin Pediatr 23:321, 1984 (This study shows that in pediatric patients, chest pain is infrequently due to underlying cardiac disease.)

Miller AJ, Texidor TA: Precordial catch, a neglected syndrome of precordial pain. JAMA 159:1364, 1955 (Thorough description of this common source of chest pain in young, healthy individuals.)

Selbst SA: Evaluation of chest pain in children. Pediatr Rev 8:56, 1986 (Clearly written review of the subject with a rational approach to the management of children with chest pain.)

56
Hypertension

JULIE R. INGELFINGER

In 1987, the American Academy of Pediatrics Second Task Force on Blood Pressure Control in Childhood published new normative data for children ranging in age from early infancy to late adolescence. These data are shown in Figure 56-1 and they have been compiled by pooling the blood pressure data from nine different studies involving >70,000 children in order to obtain norms that are meaningful for the entire United States' population. The Task Force recommends measuring blood pressure in all children over the age of 2 as part of a normal physical examination, and for infants whenever they are ill or have an unexplained health problem. Blood pressure should be considered elevated if it is on several occasions clearly 2 standard deviations above the mean for age. Furthermore, blood pressure between the 90th and 95th percentile should be considered suspicious, especially if the child is not heavy or tall for his age. Note that the new blood pressure nomograms depict the 90th percentile for height and weight under each month or year of age: This is so that the child with a blood pressure between the 90th and 95th percentile who is unusually large for age will be spared the label of "hypertensive," because blood pressure is often "high" in those children because of size alone.

Blood pressure should be measured with the child as relaxed as possible with a well-maintained, appropriately sized blood pressure cuff. For each child, the cuff should completely encircle the arm, and the inner bladder should go more than halfway around the arm. Width should cover at least 75% of the upper arm (shoulder to olecranon). Cuffs are available in sizes for newborn, infant, child, adult, and large adult. Blood pressure readings should be taken at least 2 to 3 times prior to calling the measurements at a particular visit elevated. Unless blood pressure is exceedingly high (more than 3 standard deviations above the mean for age) an elevated pressure should be confirmed on three separate occasions before labeling someone as hypertensive. A markedly elevated blood pressure will require immediate diagnostic and therapeutic intervention.

Data linking systolic and diastolic blood pressure levels and cardiovascular risk do not yet exist. The high frequency of hypertension in the adult American population, however, has led the Second Task Force on Blood Pressure Control in Childhood to recommend following blood pressure levels annually in all children over age 2. If this recommendation is followed, it is clear that both youngsters with definite hypertension will be identified and that those with borderline hypertension will also be noted. It is a widely held belief that essential hypertension has its roots in childhood, and an office evaluation of blood pressure should always be an integral part of pediatric health care.

CAUSES OF ELEVATED BLOOD PRESSURE

In the first year of life nearly all hypertension is secondary in origin. As age increases, a larger proportion of children with blood pressure elevation have primary (essential) hypertension. The commonest causes for sustained hypertension vary by age group in pediatric and adolescent populations. In newborns, most common causes are renal artery thromboses, renal artery stenosis, congenital renal abnormalities (including polycystic kidney disease), coarctation of the aorta, and bronchopulmonary dysplasia-associated hypertension. In the infant to 6-year-old patient, renal parenchymal diseases (structural, inflammatory, as well as tumors), coarctation, and renovascular diseases are most common. Among 6- to 10-year-olds, renal parenchymal diseases and renal artery disease, as well as primary hypertension, are most frequent. In adolescence, primary hypertension, followed by renal parenchymal diseases, constitutes the most frequently seen cause for sustained hypertension.

The recommended evaluations for suspected primary or secondary hypertension differ, and thus the astute physician must be aware of the different diagnostic possibilities for sustained hypertension. Acute hypertension, on the other hand, is often due to iatrogenic or factitious (self-induced) causes, as well as to acute renal failure in nephropathies such as hemolytic uremic syndrome, nephritis, or acute tubular necrosis.

WORK-UP

In establishing the etiology of hypertension, a good history and physical examination are among the most effective tools.

History

A family history of hypertension may direct the evaluation. Thus, one should try to establish whether there is a history of essential hypertension in the family or hypertension secondary to a genetically transmitted systemic disease associated with high blood pressure such as neurofibromatosis. One should ask for medical history in several different ways, especially with adolescents, in order to find toxic exposures or drug experimentation that might cause hypertension. Some of the historical findings associated with particular hypertensive diagnoses include family history of primary hypertension or of systemic diseases such as multiple endocrine neoplasia (pheochromocytoma-associated), glomerulonephritis, or toxemia. A family history of hyperlipidemia or early complications of hypertension may suggest added cardiovascular risk. Neonatal history of umbilical artery cathethers or severe postnatal course may alert the physician to consider a renovascular etiology of hypertension. A review of symptoms for edema, abdominal pain, headaches, dizziness, epistaxis, weight loss, flushing, muscle cramps, weakness, or constipation may be helpful.

Physical Examination

On physical examination one must take four extremity blood pressures and search for pulse delay to rule out coarctation. A physical examination should attend to skin lesions and other physical findings that suggest an etiology of elevated blood pressure. A general examination should evaluate for signs of endocrinopathy, edema associated with renal disease, and bruits over vessels. Hypertensive retinal changes, Bell's palsy, and hemiparesis would all suggest marked, chronic hypertension.

Laboratory Tests

When one suspects primary hypertension, the recommended evaluation is to screen for the most common organic causes of hypertension, and then to screen for other cardiovascular risk factors. Thus, the Task Force recommends doing a careful urinalysis and culture; performing a measurement of renal function such as a creatinine; checking electrolytes to be sure there is not hypokalemia or increased tCO_2, which would suggest primary or secondary aldosteronism; and then checking a lipoprotein electrophoresis. Even though there may be a family history of hypertension, a very young child with an elevated blood pressure should have a further evaluation including some anatomic study of the urinary tract. Since primary hypertension is a diagnosis of exclusion, a child might be temporarily classified in this category but worked up later in more detail should the blood pressure elevation continue to be a problem.

An evaluation for secondary hypertension should be phased. The initial evaluation is similar to the one already described, but the higher the blood pressure and the younger the child, the more complete the evaluation should be. If secondary hypertension is suspected, the first series of tests should include a complete blood count (CBC), urinalyses and culture, serum electrolytes, tCO_2, and BUN/creatinine. A uric acid may be helpful, as it may be elevated in renal disease. Echocardiography to assess left ventricular mass should be obtained to determine possible target organ damage. Subsequent to the initial evaluation, radiologic and radioisotope studies need to be considered, as well as hormonal studies. To rule out renal parenchymal disease, some form of urinary tract imaging study—either an ultrasound and radionuclide study or an intravenous pyelogram—should be performed. If renovascular disease is suspected, renal angiography may be necessary; one may choose arteriography or digital subtraction angiography. If not highly knowledgeable about juvenile hypertension, the Task Force recommends that the primary care physician discuss the sensitivity, specificity, and utility of each specialized test with an expert in order to expedite a cost-effective evaluation. Should endocrine causes of hypertension be suspected, measurement of appropriate hormones in plasma and/or urine should be undertaken. If all tests for secondary hypertension were performed in all children, the cost of the work-up would exceed several thousand dollars. Thus, the evaluation should be focused on defining the most likely suspected secondary cause. The types of evaluation available will vary from center to center, and so, for example, the anatomic studies of the urinary system should depend on what tests are best performed. A hypertensive IVP is less sensitive and specific than a radionuclide renal scan for evaluating unilateral renal artery disease, but some centers have little experience in doing the scans in a

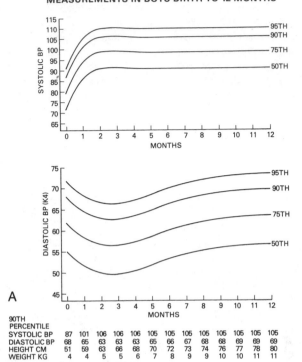

AGE-SPECIFIC PERCENTILES OF BLOOD PRESSURE MEASUREMENTS IN BOYS BIRTH TO 12 MONTHS

90TH PERCENTILE													
SYSTOLIC BP	87	101	106	106	106	105	105	105	105	105	105	105	105
DIASTOLIC BP	68	65	63	63	63	65	66	67	68	68	69	69	69
HEIGHT CM	51	59	63	66	68	70	72	73	74	76	77	78	80
WEIGHT KG	4	4	5	5	6	7	8	9	9	10	10	11	11

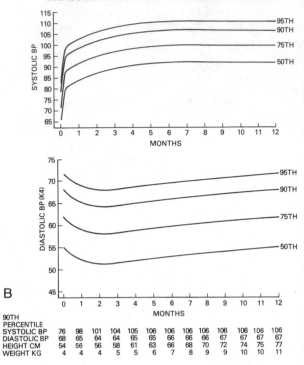

AGE-SPECIFIC PERCENTILES OF BLOOD PRESSURE MEASUREMENTS IN GIRLS BIRTH TO 12 MONTHS

90TH PERCENTILE													
SYSTOLIC BP	76	98	101	104	105	106	106	106	106	106	106	106	106
DIASTOLIC BP	68	65	64	64	65	65	66	66	66	67	67	67	67
HEIGHT CM	54	56	56	58	61	63	66	68	70	72	74	75	77
WEIGHT KG	4	4	4	5	5	6	7	8	9	9	10	10	11

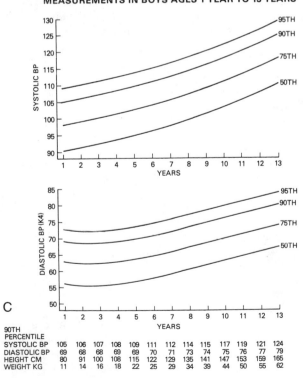

AGE-SPECIFIC PERCENTILES OF BLOOD PRESSURE MEASUREMENTS IN BOYS AGES 1 YEAR TO 13 YEARS

90TH PERCENTILE													
SYSTOLIC BP	105	106	107	108	109	111	112	114	115	117	119	121	124
DIASTOLIC BP	69	68	68	69	69	70	71	73	74	75	76	77	79
HEIGHT CM	80	91	100	108	115	122	129	135	141	147	153	159	165
WEIGHT KG	11	14	16	18	22	25	29	34	39	44	50	55	62

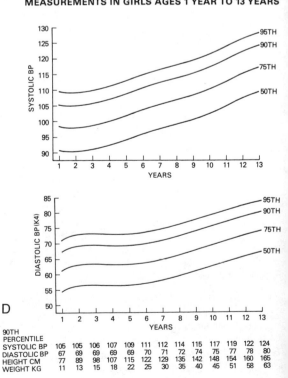

AGE-SPECIFIC PERCENTILES OF BLOOD PRESSURE MEASUREMENTS IN GIRLS AGES 1 YEAR TO 13 YEARS

90TH PERCENTILE													
SYSTOLIC BP	105	105	106	107	109	111	112	114	115	117	119	122	124
DIASTOLIC BP	67	69	69	69	69	70	71	72	74	75	77	78	80
HEIGHT CM	77	89	98	107	115	122	129	135	142	148	154	160	165
WEIGHT KG	11	13	15	18	22	25	30	35	40	45	51	58	63

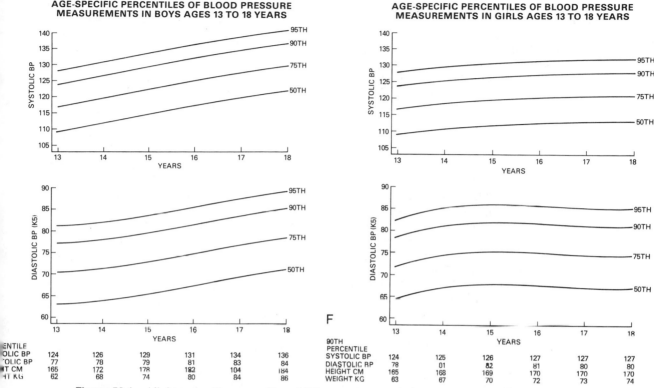

AGE-SPECIFIC PERCENTILES OF BLOOD PRESSURE MEASUREMENTS IN BOYS AGES 13 TO 18 YEARS

AGE-SPECIFIC PERCENTILES OF BLOOD PRESSURE MEASUREMENTS IN GIRLS AGES 13 TO 18 YEARS

ENTILE						
OLIC BP	124	126	129	131	134	136
OLIC BP	77	78	79	81	83	84
T CM	165	172	178	182	184	184
HT KG	62	68	74	80	84	86

90TH PERCENTILE						
SYSTOLIC BP	124	125	126	127	127	127
DIASTOLIC BP	78	01	82	81	80	80
HEIGHT CM	165	168	169	170	170	170
WEIGHT KG	63	67	70	72	73	74

Figure 56-1. (*A*) Age-specific percentiles of BP measurements in boys—birth to 12 months of age; Korotkoff phase IV (K4) used for diastolic BP. (*B*) Age-specific percentiles of BP measurements in girls—birth to 12 months of age; Korotkoff phase IV (K4) used for diastolic BP. (*C*) Age-specific percentiles of BP measurements in boys—1 to 13 years of age; Korotkoff phase IV (K4) used for diastolic BP. (*D*) Age-specific percentiles of BP measurements in girls—1 to 13 years of age; Korotkoff phase IV (K4) used for diastolic BP. (*E*) Age-specific percentiles of BP measurements in boys—13 to 18 years of age; Korotkoff phase V (K5) used for diastolic BP. (*F*) Age-specific percentiles of BP measurements in girls—13 to 18 years of age; Korotkoff phase V (K5) used for diastolic BP. (Report of the Second Task Force on Blood Pressure Control in Children, 1987. Reproduced by permission of Pediatrics 79:1–25, 1987 © 1987)

young child. In that instance, an IVP ought to be performed.

Exercise Testing

Exercise tolerance should be quickly screened in a hypertensive child. If systolic pressure exceeds 200 or diastolic exceeds 100 mm Hg to 110 mm Hg, further study is needed.

A quick evaluation of the effect of exercise may be done in the office. It consists of having a child do jumping jacks for 120 seconds. Many children will not be able to do this in a sustained fashion for the entire time, but an evaluation as close to it as possible ought to be done. Blood pressure and pulse are obtained in a standing and seated position be-fore the exercise and immediately thereafter. While this does not provide electrocardiographic or echocardiographic data, the peak diastolic and systolic pressures and the rapidity of the fall to normal may be obtained.

Office Stress Testing

Several maneuvers may be done in the office and provide a good index of the labile hypertensive child. With a hand grip from an athletic store, have the youngster squeeze it with one hand and take blood pressure serially in the other arm at 3- to 5-min intervals. The youngster with labile hypertension will have a marked and prolonged increase in blood pressure, whereas most children will have a mild increase. One may place the hand of the arm not having blood pressure taken into a little basin of ice water. Serial blood pressures at 2- to 3-min intervals will identify some youngsters with labile hypertension. The rapidity of return to normal will also be helpful. Serial substraction of 7s or 3s from 100 should also be performed while blood pressure is being taken. In our experience, serial substraction from 100 is the most stressful of these in-office tests.

TREATMENT

A child with mild, yet sustained hypertension is best managed with nonpharmacologic intervention. A weight control program, with the entire family involved, is often all that is needed to lower blood pressure in the overweight child with mild blood pressure elevations. Recognizing that weight loss may be difficult, the physician should find ways for frequent follow-up while a child is on such a program and he should plan additional intervention should the weight loss approach not be followed.

Although data are from adult populations, it would seem likely that about half of youngsters with primary hypertension are salt sensitive and respond with decreases in blood pressure to sodium chloride restriction. The mechanism of the salt sensitivity is unknown, though there is evidence that it could be related to a number of physiologic abnormalities including red cell membrane abnormalities, sodium flux channels (either sodium potassium or sodium calcium or sodium sodium), sensitivity to angiotensin II, or adrenergic receptor number or response. Thus, a youngster with blood pressure elevation may be placed on a no-added salt diet with improvement in blood pressure control. Other dietary interventions such as increased potassium and increased calcium in the diet recommended for adults with high blood pressure have not been adequately evaluated in children. Further dietary changes such as a low cholesterol diet are often advocated, because hyperlipidemia would be an additional problem for the at-risk hypertensive child.

Dynamic exercise is felt to be a beneficial adjunct in blood pressure control if used in a training program for the mildly hypertensive youngster. Some studies also show that a training program of isometric exercise results in lower resting blood pressure in youths with mild blood pressure elevation. However, the diastolic pressure during dynamic exercise drops while that in isometric exercise rises, leading some to recommend only dynamic exercise programs for the hypertensive youngster. It is worth mentioning that a youngster with moderate or marked elevation in blood pressure should have some form of exercise testing prior to doing competitive sports (see above for screening). If blood pressure responses (during *peak* exercise) are high (systolic greater than 200, diastolic greater than 100 to 110 during *peak* exercise), antihypertensive pharmacotherapy should be initiated before participation in a sports program is approved.

Relaxation or meditation is an effective means of lowering blood pressure in the motivated patient. Various behavior modifications techniques to induce relaxation ranging from biofeedback to meditation to psychotherapy have been used. The relaxation response, as described by Dr. Herbert Benson, is easily taught to school-aged children and adolescents. A surprising number of children and their families seem interested in this modality and it should be explored as a powerful means of blood pressure control.

Pharmacologic Therapy

The pharmacologic agents now available for the drug therapy of sustained hypertension are numerous (Table 56-1). Many hypotensive agents have *not* been tested in children and adolescents, but the Federal regulations permit their use on a case-to-case basis. Pediatric doses are listed in this table. The approach to therapy has often been step-care in the past decade. This concept means that one drug is used initially and then others are added step by step until blood pressure control is achieved. As compliance with therapy is a major problem in the treatment of hypertension, it is our opinion that the simplest regimen possible should be undertaken in all instances. Thus monotherapy, or therapy with one drug at a time, offers certain advantages over step-care. In general, if a child requires more than two drugs for effective therapy or more than maximal therapy with a single agent, referral to a specialist for further treatment, if not further evaluation, is indicated. Another general principle is that the longer an antihypertensive agent has been used in children, the more is known about it and thus the less likely one is to encounter undescribed side effects of the medication that may, for example, interfere with a child's development or school functioning. Initial treatment is generally begun with a thiazide-type diuretic, especially in black patients, asthmatics, or diabetics, or with an adrenergic

Table 56-1. Antihypertensive Medications*‡

	DOSE	NO. OF TIMES/DAY	ROUTE
Diuretics			
Hydrochlorothiazide (Hydrodiuril, Esidrix)	1–2 mg/kg	2	Oral
Chlorthalidone (Hygroton)	0.5–2 mg/kg	1	Oral
Furosemide (Lasix)	0.5–2 mg/kg	2	Oral, intravenous (IV)
Spironolactone (Aldactone)	1–2 mg/kg	2	Oral
Triameterene (Dyrenium)	1–2 mg/kg	2	Oral
Adrenergic Inhibitors			
β-adrenergic antagonists			
Metoprolol (Lopressor)	1–4 mg/kg	2	Oral
Atenolol (Tenormin)	1–2 mg/kg	1	Oral
Propranolol (Inderal)	1–3 mg/kg	3	Oral, intravenous with caution (max 1 mg)
Central adrenergic inhibitors			
Methyldopa (Aldomet)	5–10 mg/kg	2	Oral
Clonidine (Catapres)	0.05–0.40 mg	2	Oral
Guanabenz (Wytensin)	0.03–0.08 mg	2	Oral
α₁-Adrenergic Antagonist			
Prazosin hydrochloride (Minipress)	0.5–7 mg	3	Oral
Vasodilators			
Hydralazine (Apresoline)	1–5 mg/kg	2 or 3	Oral, intramuscular, IV (drip)
Minoxidil (Loniten)	0.1–1.0 mg/kg	2	Oral
Diazoxide (Hyperstat)†	3–5 mg/kg/ dose		IV (bolus)
Nitroprusside (Nipride)†	1–8 µg/kg/min		IV (drip)
Angiotensin-converting Enzyme Inhibitor			
Captopril			
<6 mo of age	0.05–0.5 mg/kg	3	
>6 mo of age	0.5–2.0 mg/kg	3	Oral

* Not to exceed usual adult dosage with all drugs.
† Primary use is in hypertensive emergencies.
‡ This is a partial list. Additional β-adrenergic antagonists, α plus β blockers, α blockers, calcium channel blockers, and new angiotensin-converting enzyme inhibitors are not listed because these have had limited use in children.

blocker, especially in adolescents with hyperkinetic-type primary hypertension.

Once a child's blood pressure is controlled, it is often possible to use lower doses of medication than were needed initially. Thus, after blood pressure has been controlled for 6 to 12 months, a "stepping down" procedure from the maximal dose is helpful. Several youngsters may have had the cycle of the pathophysiology causing their hypertension interrupted and can be taken off medication entirely.

Treatment of Acute Hypertension

Treatment of acute hypertension should involve therapy of potentially life-threatening blood pressure elevation with concomitant evaluation for the cause. Blood pressure rarely needs to be decreased precipitously. Whenever undertaking parenteral therapy, the physician must remember that too rapid lowering of blood pressure may cause cerebrovascular insults, visual changes, and acute renal failure. If previously normal blood pressure has become acutely and severely elevated, the patient may be at risk to have hypertensive encephalopathy. In that instance parenteral therapy is clearly required. Thus, the current recommendations for parenteral antihypertensive therapy include acute severe hypertension such as may be observed in acute glomerulonephritis, hemolytic-uremic syndrome, or head injuries. A patient who has accelerated hypertension as well as previous hypertension may respond to increasing antihypertensive dose and close monitoring. If a child requires acute parenteral therapy, hospitalization is usually re quired, often in an intensive care unit for the first 24 hours. The doses of diazoxide and nitroprusside are given in Table 56-1. Either agent is often first used. Alternatively, hydralazine (0.15 mg/kg IM or IV) or sublingual nifedipine may be used.

COMPLIANCE

For adults, half those with hypertension drop out of all care within a year of discovering their hypertension; of the remaining half, most do not have adequately controlled blood pressure. The statistics on pediatric patients with hypertension are equally dismal. Various modalities may be helpful in ensuring compliance with blood pressure evaluation and control in those youngsters that need it. Most importantly, education in the form of written materials and teaching sessions may be helpful. An introduction to home blood pressure monitoring may be useful, because it will generate empirical data for the youngster and family to follow. The data obtained may also be invaluable in selecting a treatment plan. Other aids to compliance include making necessary office visits as convenient as possible, and including the patient as a colleague in deciding acceptable therapy. For instance, some patients will have many side effects to one form of therapy and should be able to share any difficulties they have. Such patients should share in the choice of subsequent therapy.

ANNOTATED BIBLIOGRAPHY

Ingelfinger JR: Pediatric Hypertension. Philadelphia, WB Saunders, 1982 (Single author book on hypertension in childhood; detailed discussion on pathophysiology.)

Lieberman E: Clinical assessment of the hypertensive patient. In Kotchen TA, Kotchen JM (eds): High Blood Pressure in the Young, pp 237–248. Boston, John Wright, PSG Inc, 1983 (Review for assessment.)

Loggie JMH: Systemic hypertension. In Adams FH, Emmanoulidies GC (eds): Moss' Heart Disease in Infants, Children, and Adolescents, 3rd ed., pp 692–707. Baltimore, Williams & Wilkins, 1983 (Good review.)

Loggie JMH, Horan MJ, Gruskin AB et al (eds): NHLBI Workshop on Juvenile Hypertension. New York, Biomedical Information Corp, 1984 (Symposium on Childhood Hypertension with general information.)

Report of the Second Task Force on Blood Pressure Control in Children—1987. Pediatrics 79:1–25, 1987 (New blood pressure norms and recommendations for evaluation and intervention in primary and secondary hypertension.)

The 1984 Report of the Joint National Committee on Detection, Evaluation and Treatment of High Blood Pressure. Arch Intern Med 144:1045–1057, 1984

9

Dermatologic Problems

Amy Paller, Section Editor

57

Topical Preparations and Applications: General Principles

AMY PALLER

Dermatologic problems seen by pediatricians are often responsive to topical agents, but the pediatrician must be aware of the most appropriate agent to select. The absorption of topical preparations is increased greatly by occlusion, whether from plastic wraps or natural occlusion of skinfolds (axillae, inguinal), and the strength of the agent must be tailored accordingly. Agents that are well-tolerated on intact skin, such as corticosteroid creams and topical tars, are often irritating to acutely inflamed or denuded skin, and only bland emollients and compresses may be tolerated. The pediatrician should be aware that topical agents may aggravate an underlying condition by irritation or by causing allergic contact dermatitis. The allergic contact dermatitis is often not caused by the active ingredient itself, but by the vehicle, stabilizers, preservatives, or perfumes present in the medication. Among the most common allergens found in medications are ethylenediamine, lanolin, parabens, thimerosal (merthiolate), benadryl, "caines," and neomycin (see Chap 61). If a dermatologic condition appears to be aggravated by an agent that contains one or more of these common sensitizers, the preparation should be changed to one without the allergen.

When choosing a topical preparation, the vehicle and ingredients should be chosen to suit the individual patient. Ointments or emollient creams are most appropriate for patients with dry skin. The less occlusive creams or lotions are preferable if the skin is not very dry, or in summer when excessive occlusion may cause blockage of normal sweating and miliaria (prickly heat). Acute weeping dermatitis is dried and relieved by cool compresses.

In general, preparations of lower concentrations should be used first if appropriate. Although it would be ideal to have the pharmacist compound ingredients to individualize each preparation, the cost is usually prohibitive and the most appropriate available agent is preferable. Generic agents are often just as effective as the more expensive brand names.

One of the most common patient complaints is itching, and various topical agents, in addition to systemic antihistamines, may be helpful. Environmental factors that may cause or exacerbate the pruritus should be identified. Excessive bathing, especially with bubble baths, is often a cause of dryness and irritation and may be easily eliminated. Other frequently implicated irritants include wool (in clothing, blankets, and rugs), cold, sweat, dryness, and retained laundry products. Home remedies may aggravate the condition. The pruritus of dry skin may be relieved by the use of mild soaps (such as Dove), bland emollient creams and lotions, and topical preparations with antipruritics. Topical antihistamines (especially benadryl) and "caine" anesthetics should be avoided, since they often cause contact sensitization, but menthol 0.125% to

259

0.25% may be added to ointments or lotions and pramoxine 1% is a nonsensitizing topical anesthetic. Topical corticosteroids are helpful for patients with moderate to severe pruritus.

AVAILABLE TOPICAL AGENTS

Topical therapeutic agents may be applied as liquids (wet dressings, lotions) or solids (powders, creams, ointments). *Wet dressings* cool and dry oozing and vesicular eruptions, debride crusts, and help relieve itching. Medications applied to the moist skin after compresses are more effectively absorbed. Plain tap water, saline solution (parents may add one teaspoon of salt to a pint of lukewarm water), or Burow's solution (one Domeboro tablet in one pint of water makes a 1:40 solution) are the most frequently used compressing solutions. Potassium permanganate or silver nitrate 0.5% are other antiseptic drying solutions, but they stain. Wet dressings are best applied with strips of clean sheets or handkerchiefs to promote evaporation. The total time of compressing should be 20 minutes, with dressings applied three to four times daily. The cloth should be soaked in the lukewarm solution (cool solutions cause heat loss), wrung out, and applied. After 5 minutes, before the dressing is dry, the cloth should be wetted again and reapplied. After the compresses, the skin should be gently patted dry. The child should be distracted during the sessions to increase compliance. *Baths* are useful for widespread skin eruptions. Baking soda, oatmeal, or Aveeno colloidal oatmeal may be added to bathwater to ease pruritus. Bath oils, such as Alpha–Keri, Lubath, or Domol, are lubricating, but should not be used in young children and must be used with care in older children because they cause the bathtub to become slippery. Tar baths (Zetar, Polytar bath, Balnetar) are useful adjunctive agents for psoriasis.

Lotions are mixtures of powder in liquids and are best used to provide cooling by evaporation for acute dermatitis. Shake lotions, such as calamine, are effective in drying as well as cooling and soothing and are often discontinued when the acute dermatitis has subsided after a few days. *Emulsion lotions* are lotions with oil that are less occlusive and more drying than creams or ointments. Corticosteroids and antifungal agents are available in these forms.

Creams and ointments are the most commonly used bases for topical medications. Creams are mixtures of oil droplets in water and ointments are water in oil or pure preparations of oils (*i.e.*, pe-

trolatum). The oil component is usually lanolin or petrolatum. When the emollient agent is applied to the skin, the water evaporates, leaving the protective or occlusive film of oil. Various bland ointments and creams, such as Aquaphor, Eucerin and Nivea, may be used as lubricants or as bases for adding corticosteroids, antibiotics, keratolytics, and other active ingredients. *Gels* are combinations of propylene glycol, hydrocarbon polymers and water, acetone, or alcohol that are best used for hairy areas. Benzoyl peroxide, corticosteroids, tars, and keratolytics are available in a gel form. *Oils*, such as mineral oil, may be useful as mild keratolytics (removing psoriatic scalp scale) or to clean surfaces (removing zinc oxide paste in the diaper area of patients with irritant dermatitis), but are too occlusive to be recommended as emollients.

Powders are finely divided solids that are absorptive and reduce friction. Cornstarch is useful for diaper dermatitis, but talcum power should be avoided for infants because of the risk of inhalation. Powders, such as Zeasorb, are effective agents for hyperhidrosis. *Pastes* are combinations of powders and oils that are drying (powder) and protective (oil). Pastes are thick, sticky, and difficult to apply and remove, but are useful for irritant diaper dermatitis (zinc oxide paste, Lassar's paste—25% zinc oxide, 25% talc, 50% petrolatum, or a combination of Burow's solution, Aquaphor, and zinc oxide paste in a ratio of 1:2:3). Forty percent salicylic acid *plaster* is incorporated into an occlusive backing for treating warts, calluses, and corns.

Mild *shampoos*, such as Castille soap, DHS, Ionil, Sebulex, Purpose, and Neutrogena, may be preferable for patients with atopic dermatitis and scalp dryness. Tar shampoos are useful for psoriasis and seborrhea. Superfatted *soaps* with lanolin, oils, cold cream, or Aquaphor added are less drying, as are glycerine soaps (Purpose, Neutrogena). Nonsoap bar cleansers, such as Lowila and Cetaphil cleanser, are alternatives. Sulfur or salicylic acid are added to acne soaps to remove oil and peel skin. These soaps alone will not control acne and may cause irritant dermatitis.

ACTIVE INGREDIENTS IN TOPICAL AGENTS

Of all the available topical preparations, *corticosteroids* are most important for their anti-inflammatory, antipruritic and vasoconstrictive properties. Pediatricians should not avoid corticosteroids if they are indicated, but must be careful in choosing their strength, especially in infants, and to stop the corticosteroids as soon as the condition is ade-

Table 57-1. Examples of Topical
Corticosteroid Preparations

POTENCY (%)	GENERIC NAME
Lowest Potency	
1.0	Hydrocortisone
2.5	Hydrocortisone
Low Potency	
0.2	Hydrocortisone 17-valerate (Westcort)
0.1	Hydrocortisone butyrate (Locoid)
0.1	Clocortolone (Cloderm)
0.01	Fluocinolone acetonide (Synalar)
0.025	Fluandrenolide (Cordran)
0.01	Triamcinolone acetonide (Kenalog)
Moderate Potency	
0.025	Fluocinolone acetonide (Synalar)
0.1	Betamethasone valerate (Valisone)
0.05	Desonide (Tridesilon)
0.02	Triamcinolone acetonide (Kenalog)
Potent	
0.05	Fluocinonide (Lidex)
0.25	Desoximetasone (Topicort)
0.1	Amcinonide (Cyclocort)
0.1	Halcinonide (Halog)
0.05	Diflorasone diacetate (Maxiflor)
0.05	Betamethasone diproprionate (Diprosone)

quately treated. Local side effects include atrophy, telangiectasias, folliculitis, striae, hypertrichosis, acneiform eruptions, hypopigmentation, and secondary infections. Topical corticosteroids may mask the erythema of bacterial, fungal, yeast, or mite infections or infestations while encouraging the proliferation of organisms.

Very mild corticosteroids, such as hydrocortisone, should be used on the face and intertriginous areas (Table 57-1). Fluorinated steroids on the face produce atrophy and acneiform eruptions. Mild corticosteroids are usually also effective on the body for dermatitis in infants, but moderate strength or even strong corticosteroid preparations may be required for limited periods of time in older children for more severe eruptions. The vehicle chosen should be appropriate for the underlying condition (*e.g.*, ointment for dry skin and cream for exudative dermatitis). Occlusion may be indicated for recalcitrant plaques in chronic conditions. The corticosteroid (usually in ointment form) should be applied and topped with occlusive plastic film (such as Saran wrap). Gauze wrap, socks, gloves, or stockinettes may be used to maintain occlusion.

Tars and anthralin preparations are useful in older children and adolescents, especially for psoriasis, but should only be prescribed by a dermatologist. Tars may darken skin and stain light-col-

ored hair yellow. Potential side effects include irritation, folliculitis, and photosensitivity.

Most cutaneous infections require systemic antibiotics. *Topical antibiotics* should be used alone for minor infections, but otherwise as adjuctive agents to systemic medications. Topical antibiotics that contain neomycin (*e.g.*, Neosporin) may cause contact allergy. Topical erythromycin, clindamycin, meclocycline, and tetracycline in alcohol, cream, and ointment vehicles are frequently effective for patients with mild inflammatory acne.

Topical antifungal and antiyeast agents are effective, but systemic agents such as griseofulvin or ketoconazole should be used if lesions are widespread or if the scalp or nails are involved. Imidazole (miconazole, clotrimazole, econazole) creams, lotions or solutions are used to treat dermatophyte, candidal, and pityrosporum infections. Nystatin is available as a cream, ointment, or powder for cutaneous candidal infections, but the imidazoles are of equal or greater efficacy. Less expensive agents, such as selenium sulfide lotion, are equally effective for pityrosporum (tinea versicolor) infections (see Chap. 65). *Topical acyclovir* is helpful for treating herpetic infections, but is most useful for primary infections and is expensive. Immunocompromised children should be treated with systemic acyclovir; topical acyclovir has minimal additional value. *Antiparasitic agents* may be used topically for lice and scabies. Lindane (1% gamma benzene hexachloride, Kwell) is the most commonly used scabicide. To avoid CNS toxicity, it should be left on only 4 to 6 hours and should never be used in infants under 1 year of age or by breast-feeding mothers. Six percent precipitated sulfur in petrolatum is a safe alternative for patients unable to use lindane, but must be applied nightly on 3 sequential nights. Ten percent crotamiton lotion (Eurax) may be less irritating and more antipruritic than lindane or sulfur. Pyrethrin (RID) or lindane shampoos are used for head or pubic lice infections (see Chap. 70).

Sunscreens protect the skin from ultraviolet light and are important for use in children, especially with fair skin, to help prevent the later development of cutaneous aging changes, precanceroses, and skin cancers. The most widely used chemical sunscreens contain para-aminobenzoic acid (PABA) or PABA esters and are most effective against ultraviolet B light (290 nm to 320 nm). Among PABA-containing sunscreens are Eclipse, Sundown, and Presun. Water Babies is a hypoallergic (PABA-free) sunscreen. Benzophenones block ultraviolet A light (320 nm to 390 nm) and include Solbar and Uval. Some sunscreens contain both PABA or PABA esters and benzophenones. Physical sunscreens, such as zinc oxide paste, RVPaque, and A-Fil, protect the skin from all wavelengths of ultraviolet light. Sunscreens that offer high sun protection factors (SPF 15 and higher) are most effective.

Masking preparation such as Covermark (Lydia O'Leary) and Dermablend cover disfiguring lesions. They are especially useful for teenagers with port wine stains, areas of hypo- or hyperpigmentation and scars.

58
Atopic Dermatitis
AMY PALLER

Atopic dermatitis is a chronic, severely pruritic disorder characterized by dry skin, eczematous patches, lichenification, and a predisposition to staphylococcal pyodermas. The term *atopic* refers to the fact that affected children frequently have elevated IgE levels and a family or personal history of other atopic disorders, especially allergic rhinitis or asthma. The disorder usually begins in infancy, but occasionally occurs later in childhood or even in adulthood. Atopic dermatitis affects 1% to 3% of the pediatric population. The diagnosis is made by the characteristic distribution and clinical features of the rash.

PATHOPHYSIOLOGY

Despite considerable strides in studying atopic dermatitis, the primary cause remains unknown. Abnormalities of the adrenergic/cholinergic axis, IgE levels, and cell-mediated immunity have been noted. Basophil and mast cell histamine and perhaps other chemical mediators, such as prostaglandins and leukotrienes, are thought to participate. The decreased levels of cyclic adenosine monophosphate (cAMP) have been related to increased levels of leukocyte phosphodiesterase. The elevation of IgE may be due to deficient T lymphocyte suppression of IgE-producing B cells. Whether the T cell anomalies are primary or secondary to increased histamine and decreased cAMP levels is unclear.

CLINICAL PRESENTATION

Atopic dermatitis begins between 2 and 6 months of age in 60% of affected children. Lesions are typically intensely pruritic, dry, scaling, erythematous patches, often characterized by edema and linear excoriations. The lesions are poorly defined; their borders fade gradually into the surrounding normal skin sites. In some children, especially black children, the rash may be papular. Rarely, the dermatitis takes the form of an exfoliative erythroderma. In infants, the rash is frequently exudative, even without a secondary infection. In older children and adolescents, well-circumscribed patches of eczema (nummular eczema) may develop and evidence of chronic changes, such as areas of thickened skin with exaggerated skin markings (lichenification) and hyperpigmentation, may be seen (Fig. 58-1). If the atopic dermatitis becomes secondarily infected with bacteria, yellow exudate and crust overlie the rash.

As the child gets older, the areas of predilection change. In infancy, the eruption may be widespread or limited to areas with maximal irritation, such as the perioral area and cheeks. By the second half of the first year of life, the crawling infant is most severely affected on the extensor surfaces of the arms, wrists, and legs. By childhood and adolescence, the rash localizes to the flexural areas at the antecubital and popliteal folds, the wrist, and around the neck. Not uncommonly, the hands and feet become involved during childhood with extreme dryness, erythema, and hyperkeratosis with fissure formation. "Dyshidrotic eczema" may occasionally develop with tiny vesicles and pustules on the palms, soles, and interdigital areas, probably due to exposure to sweat and other irritants.

The rash of atopic dermatitis is aggravated by several factors. The process of rubbing or scratching leads to more rash and more pruritus. Patients with the disorder have extremely dry skin, due at least in part to increased transepidermal water loss. The dermatitis often becomes aggravated by the low humidity in winter. The skin is easily irritated so that exposure to wool, saliva, and sweat can markedly exacerbate the dermatitis. Some patients have an exacerbation of the eczema in the summer

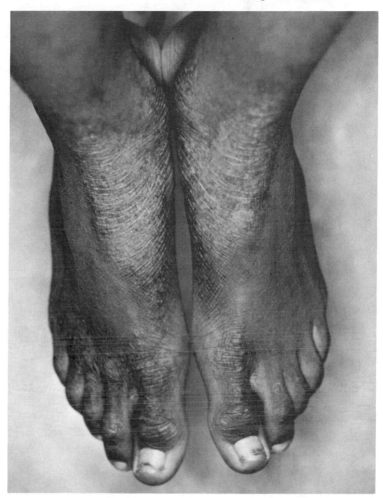

Figure 58-1. Lichenification on the dorsal aspect of the feet of a teenager with atopic dermatitis.

due to the irritant reaction to sweat and sweat retention. Other flare factors include infections and superimposed allergic contact dermatitis.

OTHER FEATURES OF ATOPIC DERMATITIS

Besides the generalized dryness, dermatitis, and excoriations, patients with atopic dermatitis display various other clinical features that are not pathognomonic to the disorder. On the face, an extra line may be found under the eyelid (Dennie's pleat, Morgan's fold), presumably due to lower eyelid edema or chronic dermatitis. The eyelids may also appear hyperpigmented (allergic shiners). In addition, affected children show midfacial pallor, probably because of increased vascular permeability and edema. Pityriasis alba are slightly scaly, hypopigmented circular patches that are most commonly found on the face, trunk, and upper arms due to mild inflammation. Follicular hyperkeratosis with mild to moderate inflammation (keratosis pilaris) is common and usually found on the upper anterior thighs, the upper extensor arms, and on the cheeks in younger children. The palmar creases of affected individuals are accentuated due to dryness and thickening of the skin. Ichthyosis vulgaris with fine white scaling, which is most prominent on the lower legs, and palmoplantar keratoderma have been associated with atopic dermatitis. Children with atopic dermatitis also demonstrate the phenomenon of "white dermographism." When the skin of a dermographic person without atopic dermatitis is stroked firmly, the "triple response of Lewis" occurs, characterized by a red line, a flare, and then a wheal. Children with atopic dermatitis have a paradoxical response with the initial red line replaced by a white line without any wheal within approximately 10 seconds. This phenomenon helps in making the diagnosis of atopic dermatitis, but may also be observed in nonatopic individuals. Finally, there appears to be an increased risk of the development of asymptomatic bilateral, central anterior subcapsular cataracts (<5% and usually in adults) even without corticosteroid use, and keratoconus (elongation of the corneal surface, <1%).

Atopic dermatitis clears by school age in 50% of the patients who develop the disorder in early infancy. In an additional 25% of children, the dermatitis may resolve by puberty, but 25% of patients continue to have difficulty into adulthood.

The most common complication of atopic dermatitis is secondary bacterial infection of affected areas of skin, especially at excoriated sites. The usual organism is *Staphylococcus aureus*, followed by group A β-hemolytic streptococci. Studies have shown that 93% of lesions of atopic dermatitis harbor *S. aureus*, and that 76% of samples of uninvolved skin also yield the organism by culture. Although children may show complicating bullous impetigo (coagulase-positive staphylococcus), the typical lesions of impetigo are erythematous with superficial yellow crusts and sometimes small superficial pustules. Patients with a secondary infection will often not respond to appropriate therapy for the underlying eczema unless the infection is cleared with systemic antibiotics.

Eczema herpeticum (Kaposi's varicelliform eruption) is a severe complication of atopic dermatitis, characterized by the abrupt development and rapid spread of the vesicles of herpes simplex. The lesions are usually multiple groups of intact or umbilicated vesicles and pustules overlying erythematous bases. The diagnosis may be confirmed by the finding of multinucleated giant epithelial cells (and occasionally intranuclear viral inclusion bodies) on a Tzanck test. This rapid test is performed by lifting the roof of the vesiculopustule, by scraping the base, and by applying the material to a slide that is stained with Giemsa. Viral cultures of lesional material will further verify a herpes infection. The high risk of eczema vaccinatum that was associated with having a smallpox vaccination or being exposed to a vaccination recipient has been virtually eliminated since the vaccination is now rarely given.

Children with atopic dermatitis have an increased risk of the development and spread of molluscum contagiosum, dermatophyte infections (tinea), and warts. This propensity appears to relate to T-lymphocyte abnormalities, the abnormal cutaneous barrier, and the tendency towards easy spread because of pruritus and scratching.

DIFFERENTIAL DIAGNOSIS

The diagnosis of atopic dermatitis is facilitated by the intense pruritus and characteristic pattern and appearance of lesions. Other types of cutaneous inflammation in children may resemble that of atopic dermatitis. *Seborrheic dermatitis* is a common eruption of infants that often develops within the first month of life. It tends to be nonpruritic with greasy, yellow scales that are typically found on the scalp (cradle cap) and in intertriginous areas. Seborrheic dermatitis usually clears by the second year of life. *Irritant contact dermatitis*, although it is frequently one of the manifestations of atopic dermatitis, may be noted in normal infants and children after exposure to saliva (cheeks), urine and feces (groin area) or exposure to harsh soaps, detergents and sheets (cheeks, extensor surfaces). Irritant dermatitis without associated atopic dermatitis is less dry and less pruritic. *Allergic contact dermatitis* is rare in young children and often involves well-circumscribed erythematous vesicles and papules that follow the distribution of the contactant. The dry, scaly, fissured eruption of *juvenile plantar dermatosis* may resemble eczema on the feet of children with atopic dermatitis. The eruption occurs symmetrically at pressure sites on the plantar surface of the feet and does not involve other sites.

Psoriasis commonly develops during childhood, but may be distinguished from atopic dermatitis by the minimal pruritus and well-circumscribed brightly erythematous lesions topped with the thick white scale of psoriasis. Areas of predilection include the scalp, elbows, knees, and intertriginous areas. The nails may be pitted and dystrophic. The perioral and acral vesicular lesions of infants with *acrodermatitis enteropathica* may be distinguished by the associated failure to thrive, alopecia, diarrhea, irritability, and lethargy. Patients frequently have secondary candidal and bacterial infections and respond rapidly to zinc administration. Many infants and children with *scabies* develop eczema from rubbing and scratching. The clues for making a diagnosis of scabies are the clinical characteristics and distribution of the lesions and the associated linear burrows. The mite, eggs, or feces may be found in skin scrapings with mineral oil.

The most common cutaneous manifestation of *histiocytosis X* in infants (Letterer–Siwe disease) is a scaly, erythematous eruption on the scalp and intertriginous areas. The rash may be differentiated from atopic (and seborrheic) dermatitis by the hemorrhagic character, vesicles, and ulcerations as well as the simultaneous occurrence of gingival and visceral abnormalities. The *Wiskott–Aldrich syndrome* is an X-linked recessive disorder characterized by severe eczema, thrombocytopenic purpura, an increased susceptibility to recurrent pyogenic infections, and abnormalities of both humoral and cell-mediated immunity. The eczema closely resembles that of atopic dermatitis, but also has petechiae and purpuric areas. Interestingly, the atopic dermatitis-like eruption resolves in patients treated successfully by bone marrow transplantation with T-lymphocyte engraftment. The severe eczematous rash of the *hyperimmunoglobulin E syndrome* tends to be more intertriginous and is associated with cutaneous abscesses. Atopic-like eczema is often seen in patients with *phenylketonuria* and *ataxia–telangiectasia*.

EVALUATION

The history of a child with atopic dermatitis will often include a family (70%) or personal history of allergic rhinitis, asthma, atopic dermatitis, or hives. Questions regarding the time of onset (after the first 2 months), the degree of pruritus, and the sensitivity to irritants and seasonal variations may help to establish the diagnosis. Determining the bathing habits and past experiences with trials and topical corticosteroid preparations and antibiotics will help in management. Attention should be paid to the distribution and character of lesions on physical examination as well as to the coexistence of secondary infection or other abnormalities that may suggest a systemic abnormality (see differential diagnosis). No routine laboratory tests are necessary. Suspected bacterial, herpetic, or fungal infections should be cultured. Tests to eliminate the possibility of other disorders, such as Wiskott–Aldrich syndrome and the hyperimmunoglobulin E syndrome, may be considered.

TREATMENT

Physicians should discuss the exacerbating factors and therapeutic measures with parents and children. Families must understand that the disorder is chronic and that quick cures do not exist. They should be reassured, however, that therapy can result in dramatic improvement and prevent the disfiguring lichenification. Teenagers should avoid choosing occupations that involve frequent handwashing or exposure to irritating chemicals. Personal or family counseling is advisable for people in emotionally stressful home situations.

General Measures

Many patients with atopic dermatitis benefit from a daily bath or shower, which adds water to the outer layer of skin, followed immediately by the application of lubricants. In winter the skin tends to be particularly dry due to the decreased ambient humidity, and heavy emollient creams, such as Eucerin or Nivea, or vaseline may be required. Harsh soaps should be substituted with mild or superfatted soaps. The bath water should be lukewarm, because hot water increases skin dryness. Bubble baths are best avoided, because they irritate the skin. Older children may benefit by the addition of bath oils. Humidifiers are also helpful during dry winter months; however, they must be cleaned regularly to avoid the dissemination of molds.

The treatment of a patient with atopic dermatitis should be tailored to the individual child. Although most patients are more troubled by the dryness and pruritus in winter, some children have more difficulty in summer and find that the irritation of sweat is a major problem. These patients may experience more pruritus with thick lubricants and benefit from lubricating lotions, such as Shepard's lotion, which are less occlusive. Such patients are also helped by the use of air-conditioners in the summer. Similarly, most patients improve with the regimen of daily baths followed immediately by lubrication. Other children, especially with many excoriated sites, cannot tolerate water at all and benefit from avoidance of water and the use of Cetaphil lotion as a cleansing and lubricating agent.

Corticosteroids

Anti-inflammatory topical corticosteroid preparations are usually necessary to clear the inflammatory lesions. The strength and base of topical preparation depend on the location and severity of the rash and also on the age and tolerance of the patient. Fluorinated corticosteroids should never be used for more than a few days on the face or intertriginous areas because of the risk of skin atrophy. Younger children and patients with milder eruptions may clear with the weak, nonfluorinated agents only, whereas patients who are older or who have more severe pruritus and inflammation may require a moderate or high strength corticosteroid (see section on Topical Preparations and Applications in Chap. 57). Most children with dry skin prefer ointment bases or emollient bases, especially during the winter, whereas some prefer to use cream bases covered with lubricating agents. Corticosteroid gels and lotions are usually too drying for patients with atopic dermatitis. Systemic corticosteroids are rarely indicated and should be used only for short periods of time by patients with a severe, generalized, intractable disease. Exacerbations following discontinuation of systemic corticosteroid therapy are a further disadvantage of this therapeutic approach.

Other Topical Agents

Other topic agents that have been helpful for children with atopic dermatitis include ultraviolet light, mild tar preparations, and keratolytics, such as urea or salicylic acid, for lichenified plaques.

Weeping dermatitis is often caused by a secondary infection and requires compresses to dry and cool the areas and to remove crusts and debris. Burow's solution or cool saline compresses should be applied two to three times daily for 20 to 30 minutes using a man's handkerchief or torn bedsheets to allow for evaporative loss. Topical corticosteroid or lubrication may be applied after the compresses. If *bacterial infection* is suspected and involves more than a small area, the patient should be treated with systemic antistaphylococcal antibiotics, such as erythromycin or dicloxacillin. The treatment of *herpetic infections* depends on the extent of involvement. Compresses and topical antibiotics (*e.g.*, Polysporin) should be used in all patients. If patients have rapidly spreading vesicles, fever, or evidence of visceral involvement, such as elevated transaminases, systemic acyclovir should be administered. The use of topical acyclovir five times daily will also decrease the spread and duration of lesions, but it is not needed along with systemic acyclovir. Secondary bacterial infection of herpes simplex lesions should be treated with systemic antistaphylococcal antibiotics.

Antipruritics

Antihistamine preparations, especially hydroxyzine and diphenhydramine, may be valuable, especially for their sedative effects. Many children cannot tolerate antihistamines during the day be-

cause of sedation, but find these agents invaluable at night when scratching is most intense. It is also advisable to keep one's nails short.

Diet Therapy

Dietary therapy is helpful in a small percentage of patients and is best reserved for patients with severe eczema who do not respond to more traditional measures, because compliance with dietary manipulation is difficult. The foods most commonly implicated are milk and eggs. By 3 or 4 years of age, many children no longer require food restriction and the avoided foods may be added gradually. Skin testing and hyposensitization are of minimal value. Experimental therapies, such as topical phosphodiesterase inhibitors, oral evening primrose oil and papaverine, require more study before they can be recommended.

INDICATIONS FOR REFERRAL AND ADMISSION

Patients who are difficult to manage or who require more than moderate strength topical corticosteroid preparations should be referred to a dermatologist for management. Patients with severe atopic dermatitis who cannot be managed effectively as outpatients may respond to the intensive topical or systemic management of brief hospitalization. Patients with eczema herpeticum or severe secondary bacterial infections may also require observation and treatment in the hospital.

ANNOTATED BIBLIOGRAPHY

Buckley RH, Matthews KP: Common "allergic" skin diseases. JAMA 248:2611, 1982 (Includes a good review of the clinical features of atopic dermatitis.)

Dahl MV: Atopic dermatitis: The concept of flare factors. South Med J 70:453, 1977 (Review of the flare factors that patients should be counseled to avoid.)

Hanifin JM: Atopic dermatitis. J Am Acad Dermatol 6:1, 1982 (Excellent review of the histopathologic, immunologic, and pharmacologic features of atopic dermatitis.)

Rassmussen JE: Recent developments in the management of patients with atopic dermatitis. J Allerg Clin Immunol 74:771, 1984 (Review of new ideas for therapy of atopic dermatitis.)

Seborrheic dermatitis is a common disorder, characterized by scaling and erythema in a "seborrheic" distribution, that is, in areas with the highest concentration of sebaceous glands and sebum production, including the face, scalp, upper chest, retroauricular and intertriginous areas. The disorder occurs in infancy and adolescence.

PATHOPHYSIOLOGY

Despite the localization of lesions of seborrheic dermatitis, there is no clear relation between sebum and the dermatitis, and the cause of seborrheic dermatitis remains unknown. Some authors have postulated that sebum or a breakdown product irritates the skin. Recent evidence suggest an association between the inflammatory reaction and *Pityrosporum orbiculare*, a lipophilic yeast that is a normal inhabitant of the skin. The yeast is found in increased numbers and therapy with topical ketoconazole decreases both the yeast and the inflammation. However, many investigators consider that the yeast is a secondary invader without any etiologic role.

CLINICAL PRESENTATION

In infancy, the dermatitis usually begins between the second and tenth week of life. "Cradle cap" and diaper dermatitis with erythema and greasy yellow or dry white scaling of the scalp and inguinal region, respectively, are the most common manifestations. Some infants have more widespread involvement with lesions across the entire face and scalp, and intertriginous and presternal areas. Secondary bacterial or candidal infections are common. Pruritus is minimal and the child is otherwise well. Most infantile cases either clear spontaneously after weeks to months or respond quickly to topical medication. Seborrheic dermatitis is rarely seen in prepubertal children beyond 18 months of age.

In addition to infancy, the disorder may begin in adolescence during or after the onset of puberty. The scalp is the most common site and seborrheic dermatitis is found in the form of fine white scaling or dandruff. In addition, the nasolabial folds, eyebrows, forehead, external ears, and retroauricular areas are frequently inflamed and scaly. Intertriginous sites and the presternal area may become involved. The dermatitis is bilaterally symmetric. Blepharitis and conjunctivitis are occasional complications. Although often asymptomatic, the rash is pruritic for some individuals. Lichenification is unusual and oozing and crusting, especially of intertriginous sites and the ear canals, suggest secondary bacterial infection.

Leiner's disease is a severe, exfoliative form of seborrheic-like dermatitis associated with diarrhea, failure to thrive, and gram-negative bacterial and candidal infections. Most affected infants are breast-fed. Within the first weeks of life, scales and erythema resembling seborrheic dermatitis develop on the scalp, face, and intertriginous areas, followed by a generalized extension of the rash. The disorder appeared to be due to a dysfunction of the fifth component of complement in opsonization. More recently, this disorder has been shown to be a heterogeneous group of immunodeficiency disorders, including severe combined immunodeficiency, hyperimmunoglobulinemia E, and C_3 deficiency in addition to C_5 dysfunction.

DIFFERENTIAL DIAGNOSIS

The differential diagnosis of seborrheic dermatitis and dandruff in infants and teenagers includes tinea capitis and corporis, atopic dermatitis, pediculosis, contact irritant and allergic dermatitis, psoriasis, drug eruptions, and histiocytosis X. In teenagers, tinea versicolor, lupus erythematosus, and other photosensitivity disorders, pityriasis rosea, Darier's disease, and pemphigus foliaceus should be considered. *Tinea capitis* may manifest as fine white scaling of the scalp without erythema or alopecia. *Atopic dermatitis* may mimic scalp seborrhea, but the flexural lichenification and positive family history of atopy help to confirm the diagnosis. *Pediculosis* may be differentiated by the nits and excoriations. *Contact dermatitis* shows sharp borders, conforming to the distribution of the offending agent. Plaques of *psoriasis* tend to be well-demarcated in contrast to the erythema and scaling of seborrheic dermatitis; the clinical course, predilection for sites of trauma, and skin biopsy are helpful in the differential diagnosis. The lesions of *pityriasis rosea* tend to follow skin lines and are not typically found in sites of seborrheic dermatitis, except in the inverse pattern. Plaques and patches of *lupus erythematosus* have telangiectasia, and the superficial crusting of *pemphigus* can be differentiated from infected seborrheic dermatitis by skin biopsy and immunofluorescence microscopy. *Darier's disease* is an autosomal dominant condition characterized in adolescence by greasy, scaly papules in a seborrheic distribution, but with oral and nail changes as well. The hypo- and hyperpigmented circular macules of *tinea versicolor* may be confused with seborrheic dermatitis, but microscopic examination of skin scrapings reveals the spores and hyphae of *Pityrosporum orbiculare*.

The most important disorder to distinguish from seborrheic dermatitis in infants is the Letterer–Siwe form of *histiocytosis X*. The cutaneous eruption usually begins as scaling and erythema on the scalp, retroauricular, axillary and diaper areas. The concomitant petechiae and purpuric papules, pustules, and ulcerations should lead one to suspect the diagnosis. Not infrequently, the palms and soles are affected, in contrast with the typical sparing of palms and soles in seborrheic dermatitis. Other manifestations of histiocytosis X include gingival ulcerations, fever, hepatosplenomegaly, adenopathy, lytic lesions of bone, pulmonary infiltration, and hematologic suppression. Histopathologic examination of cutaneous lesions shows a proliferation of well-differentiated histiocytes with other inflammatory cells, especially neutrophils and eosinophils. By electron microscopy, tennis racket-shaped "Birbeck granules" or "Langerhans' granules" are seen in the cytoplasm of the histiocytic cells. The greatest mortality occurs in infants with widespread visceral involvement and thrombocytopenia.

TREATMENT

The therapy of seborrheic dermatitis depends on the site and extent of involvement. The disorder is self-limited in infants, but chronic and recurrent when it begins in adolescence. If moderate or symptomatic inflammation and scaling are present in infancy, the scalp is best treated with a mild antiseborrheic shampoo, such as those with selenium sulfide or zinc pyrithione. The shampoo should be used three to four times a week and left on the scalp for five minutes before rinsing. If the crusts of "cradle cap" are thick, warm mineral oil or baby oil applied for 10 minutes prior to shampoo may be helpful. Skin lesions are best treated with hydrocortisone 1% cream twice daily. For teenagers, the same general measures are employed, but more vigorous therapy may be necessary, such as tar shampoos or the use of preparations for cutaneous lesions with stronger nonfluorinated topical corticosteroids. Low-dose ketoconazole (*i.e.*, 200 mg twice weekly) has been used in teenagers and adults with good results. Secondary infection with bacterial or candidal organisms should be treated with compresses and antistaphylococcal antibiotics or antifungal agents, respectively.

INDICATIONS FOR REFERRAL AND ADMISSION

Infants or adolescents who do not respond readily to antiseborrheic shampoos and nonfluorinated topical corticosteroids should be referred for dermatologic consultation. Hospitalization is indicated only in patients with severe seborrheic dermatitis with secondary infections, Leiner's disease, or disorders that may resemble seborrheic dermatitis but do not respond to routine therapeutic measures, such as histiocytosis X.

ANNOTATED BIBLIOGRAPHY

Ford GP, Farr RM, Ive FA et al: The response of seborrheic dermatitis to ketoconazole. Br J Dermatol 111:603–607, 1984 (Seborrheic dermatitis responded well to ketoconazole therapy, suggesting that yeast contribute to the disorder.)

Geiser CF: The histiocytosis syndromes. Pediatr Ann 8:54–64, 1979 (Good review of the clinical manifestations of histiocytosis X.)

Lipton JM: The pathogenesis, diagnosis, and treatment of histiocytosis syndromes. Pediatr Dermatol 1:112–120, 1983 (Current review of the manifestations, therapy, and prognosis of histiocytosis X.)

Marks R, Pearse AD, Walker AP: The effects of a shampoo containing zinc pyrithione on the control of dandruff. Br J Dermatol 112:415–422, 1985 (Seborrhea cleared much more readily on the area treated with zinc pyrithione, and clearance correlated with a significant reduction in the number of *Pityrosporum orbiculare*.)

Miller ME, Koblenzer PJ: Leiner's disease and C₅ dysfunction. J Pediatr 80:879–880, 1972 (These authors demonstrate the dysfunction of the fifth component of complement in opsonizing yeast.)

One of the most common problems of infants is diaper dermatitis. Irritant contact dermatitis is the usual underlying cause, but the dermatitis is frequently superinfected with candidal organisms.

PATHOPHYSIOLOGY

Several factors encourage the development of diaper rash. Infants with an atopic or seborrheic background tend to be more susceptible. The diaper area is occluded, especially by plastic pants or plastic-covered diapers, and moisture is trapped with resultant alteration of the stratum corneum layer, maceration, and cutaneous erosion. Irritation is produced by friction in the inguinal area, and further promoted by the wetness of the area. The moist, warm environment encourages the overgrowth of *Candida albicans* and bacteria. In the past, urinary ammonia was thought to be a prime factor in causing irritant diaper dermatitis. Although ammonia does produce more inflammation on wet skin with altered barrier properties than saline solution, it is now known that the concentration of ammonia and the pH of the urine are the same in infants with and without diaper dermatitis.

CLINICAL PRESENTATION

The history and physical examination provide the clue to the underlying cause of a diaper rash. It is often necessary to culture the inguinal area, since secondary candidal or bacterial infections of irritant dermatitis are common.

Primary irritant contact dermatitis appears on convex surfaces with sparing of the folds. It is usually not seen until after 3 months of age and relates to trapped moisture and to friction at sites of contact with the diaper. Ammonia and its irritant products from bacterial enzyme catabolism may contribute to the irritation. Tightly applied diapers, especially with occlusive edges, and rubber or plastic pants that overlie diapers increase the risk of irritant contact dermatitis. The erythema has a shiny appearance and tends to wax and wane. Pustules, nodules, and erosions are frequently found,

and erythematous papules may be present, especially at the periphery of the rash. Infants with frequent diarrheal stool may have intense perianal and even medial buttock inflammation. If the inguinal area folds are affected by a rash as well as convex surfaces, *intertrigo* due to the heat, maceration, and sweat retention of folds must be considered. Intertrigo appears in the folds as erythema with maceration and erosions. The hot humid diaper environment may also cause cause prickly heat with tiny vesicles (*miliaria crystallina*) or erythematous papules and pustules (*miliaria rubra*) due to sweat retention, often in association with intertrigo. *Allergic contact dermatitis* is unusual in infants, but has been reported following the use of contact sensitizers, such as neomycin (in Neosporin) and parabens (preservatives in creams). The diaper rash of allergic contact dermatitis from a topical medication often manifests itself as an exacerbation of the previous rash under treatment despite adequate therapy and involves sharply demarcated areas exposed to the sensitizing agent. Allergic contact dermatitis begins as tiny superficial vesicles that rupture and appear eczematous within a few days after the onset of the eruption.

Candidal infections are the most characteristic of the diaper rashes. The infection may be the primary cause of dermatitis or secondary to other inflammatory processes, especially irritant dermatitis or seborrheic dermatitis. The rash is intensely red, has sharp borders with satellite pustules and papules beyond the borders, and involves the inguinal folds. The infant may have concomitant oral thrush, candida in the gastrointestinal tract, or have been exposed to maternal vaginal candidiasis. Perianal erythema with papules and pustules suggests candidal infection with seeding from the gastrointestinal tract. Many infants with candidal infections have a recent history of antibiotic use, often for recurrent otitis media. Occasionally, scattered plaques or patches of scaly erythema are seen elsewhere in conjunction with a candidal diaper rash. This "id" reaction is a hypersensitivity response to the candidal antigens and no candida can be cultured from the plaques.

Seborrheic dermatitis commonly occurs in the diaper area of infants, beginning at 3 or 4 weeks of age. The rash (usually nonpruritic) starts in the folds and extends to convex surfaces with a poor demarcation from surrounding skin. The scale is yellow and greasy, and other sites, such as the scalp (cradle cap), face, retroauricular areas, axillae, neck folds, and umbilicus may be affected. In infancy, secondary yeast infections are common. Seborrheic dermatitis usually clears by 6 months of age and almost always by 18 months. *Letterer–Siwe disease*, the malignant form of histiocytosis X seen in infants, often involves the diaper area and resembles seborrheic dermatitis. The concurrent erosions and purpuric areas help to distinguish the conditions, in addition to the presence of gingival erosions, hepatosplenomegaly, lymphadenopathy, pulmonary interstitial infiltrates, and hematologic abnormalities. The lesions of histiocytosis X do not respond readily to mild topical corticosteroids, in contrast to the rash of seborrheic dermatitis. A skin biopsy is diagnostic. The severe seborrheic dermatitis of *Leiner's disease* is much more extensive than the diaper area and is associated with diarrhea, failure to thrive, and gram-negative bacterial and candidal infection. Affected infants demonstrate defective opsonization of yeast by the fifth component of complement.

Atopic dermatitis may first become manifest in the diaper area due to the increased susceptibility to irritation. The eruption begins after 2 months of age and is characterized by marked pruritus and secondary bacterial infections with oozing and crusting. Frequently, other sites are affected by the dry, pruritic rash, especially the face and extensor surfaces. *Psoriasis* occasionally begins in infancy, usually in the diaper area since it is the site of greatest trauma (Koebner phenomenon). The typical well-demarcated scaly plaques of psoriasis may not be scaly in the diaper area due to maceration and moisture. Other sites of involvement, including the scalp and nails, as well as characteristic skin biopsy changes may be found, but often the diagnosis only becomes apparent by a recurrence of the rash beyond infancy.

Large vesicles or bullae in the diaper area may be due to infection with *Staphylococcus aureus* (bullous impetigo). The bullae tend to be flaccid and rupture easily, leaving a denuded red base. *Staphylococcal scalded skin syndrome* is most commonly found in infants and is due to a blood-borne toxin produced by the organisms in a localized infected site. Exfoliation typically begins periorificial, including in the perineal and perianal areas. The rash begins as tender patches of erythema. Superficial vesicles and pustules develop and rapidly rupture to form yellow crusts overlying the erythema. Infants with widespread blistering may develop fluid and electrolyte imbalances as well as sepsis (see Chap. 64).

Granuloma gluteale infantum is characterized by large, firm, dusky red nodules in the perineal area, buttocks, and inner thighs. The condition tends to resolve spontaneously after several months. Although the cause of this disorder is not known, in many affected infants topical fluorinated corticosteroids had been used for long periods of time before the appearance of lesions.

Acrodermatitis enteropathica is a rare autosomal recessive disorder due to abnormal absorption and metabolism of zinc. Affected infants have erythema and crusting at acral and periorificial sites, as well as hair loss, diarrhea, and failure to thrive. Secondary candidal infections are common. Infants with zinc deficiency due to inadequate zinc intake (hyperalimentation without trace minerals, hypozincemia in breast milk) exhibit identical manifestations. The response to zinc supplementation is rapid. Finally, infants with *scabies* frequently have papules, burrows and secondary dermatitis in the inguinal area. Usually other sites are affected, especially the trunk and axillae, and the mites, eggs, or feces are found in mineral oil scrapings of affected areas.

TREATMENT

The treatment of diaper dermatitis is most successful if the cause of the rash is determined. Since friction and occlusion are detrimental in all forms of dermatitis, the diaper area should be kept dry and occlusive pants or plastic-covered diapers should be eliminated. Studies comparing cloth versus disposable diapers are contradictory, although a double-blind study found that disposable diapers decreased the incidence of rashes. The diaper area should be dried gently and exposed to air to dry completely following urination. Washing of the diaper area with each urination is excessive and may be irritating. Cleansing after bowel movements is necessary, but only mild soaps should be used. Commercial wipes should not be used if they prove irritating.

Ointments such as zinc oxide paste or A & D ointment may be helpful to reduce friction and prevent the skin from contact with irritants. Petrolatum may be too occlusive and may encourage the trapping of moisture. Cornstarch may be useful for decreasing friction and does not encourage the growth of candida as was once thought. Talcum powder should not be used because it has been associated with aspiration pneumonitis in infants. Baking soda should also be avoided, because its use in diaper rash has led to metabolic alkalosis.

Irritant and allergic contact dermatitis are best treated with avoidance of the offending agent and twice daily application of a mild nonfluorinated topical corticosteroid cream, such as 1% hydrocortisone. The diaper dermatitis of seborrheic dermatitis and psoriasis also responds to 1% hydrocortisone cream. Corticosteroid ointments are best avoided in the diaper area, because they are often too occlusive. Fluorinated corticosteroid preparations should not be used in the groin area because of the high risk of local side effects, especially skin atrophy.

Candidal infections are best treated by keeping the area dry and by application of a topical antifungal preparation, such as clotrimazole, for 3 weeks. If thrush is present or the gastrointestinal tract is suspected to be the source of candidal organisms, oral suspensions of nystatin 200,000 units four times daily for 7 days is helpful. Possible sources of candida should be identified and eliminated (*e.g.*, treatment of maternal mastitis or vaginal infection). The id reactions are best treated by anticandidal therapy to the diaper region and other involved intertriginous sites and 1% hydrocortisone cream to the plaques. Mycolog cream should be avoided because it contains a fluorinated corticosteroid.

INDICATIONS FOR REFERRAL AND ADMISSION

Infants with diaper dermatitis that is not responsive to general measures and selected anti-inflammatory or anticandidal therapy should be referred to a dermatologist for further evaluation and management. Patients with severe generalized dermatitis, staphylococcal scaled skin syndrome, or histiocytosis X may warrant hospital admission.

ANNOTATED BIBLIOGRAPHY

Gonzalez J, Hogg RJ: Metabolic alkalosis secondary to baking soda treatment of a diaper rash. Pediatrics 67:820–822, 1981 (Reminder of the potential development of metabolic alkalosis from the use of baking soda.)

Leyden JJ: Cornstarch, *Candida albicans*, and diaper rash. Pediatr Dermatol 1:322–325, 1984 (Cornstarch did not encourage the growth of *Candida albicans*.)

Leyden JJ, Katz S, Stewart R et al: Urinary ammonia and ammonia-producing microorganisms in infants with and without diaper dermatitis. Arch Dermatol 113:1678–1680, 1977 (These authors found no difference in the amount of ammonia in the diaper area of infants with and without dermatitis.)

Mofenson HC, Greensher J, DiTomasso A et al: Baby powder—a hazard! Pediatrics 68:265–266, 1981 (Good review of the problem of baby powder inhalation.)

Stein H: Incidence of diaper rash when using cloth and disposable diapers. J Pediatr 101:721–723, 1982 (In a blind prospective study comparing cloth and disposable diapers, the author found less diaper rash with the disposable diapers.)

61
Contact Dermatitis
AMY PALLER

Dermatitis caused by exogenous agents may be irritant (nonimmunologic) or allergic (delayed hypersensitivity) in nature. In infants, most contact dermatitis is irritant. In older children and adolescents, it is more likely to be due to a contact allergy.

Irritant contact dermatitis in infants usually involves the diaper area and is due to contact with urine or feces (see diaper rash). Saliva or fruit juices are the most common irritating agents on the face or neck. In older children and adolescents, irritant dermatitis is less common because of thicker, less irritable skin, but may occur after exposure to irritating solvents, deodorants, or medications (*e.g.*, acne preparations). Other agents that may produce primary irritant dermatitis include harsh soaps, detergents, bubble baths, bleaches, fiberglass, acids, and alkalis. Children with atopic dermatitis are most susceptible to irritant dermatitis. The development of irritant dermatitis depends on the concentration, duration, frequency, and site of exposure to the contactant, as well as local factors, such as occlusion and sweating.

Allergic contact dermatitis, in contrast to irritant dermatitis, only requires a brief exposure to a small amount of the causative agent. It is much less common in children than in adults. The incidence clearly increases as the child gets older, but documented contact allergic dermatitis has been described in young infants.

PATHOPHYSIOLOGY OF ALLERGIC CONTACT DERMATITIS

Allergic contact dermatitis is a cell-mediated (type IV) hypersensitivity response. A sensitization period of exposure of the allergen to skin takes a week to months, depending on the strength of the allergen. For many cutaneous allergens, this sensitization phase requires antigen processing by the epidermal Langerhans cells and complexing to a haptenic carrier before proliferation of specific T lymphocytes occurs. Upon second exposure to the antigen, the elicitation phase occurs with activation of the T lymphocytes, release of inflammatory mediators and subsequent erythema, edema with occasional blister formation, and cellular infiltration. Typically, the dermatitis may be seen within 24 hours after exposure to the allergen and persists for approximately 2 weeks.

CLINICAL PRESENTATION

Allergic contact dermatitis may be acute, subacute, or chronic, and the appearance of lesions depends on the phase. Acute dermatitis is characterized by intense erythema, papules, vesicles, and oozing. In subacute dermatitis, the lesions are scaling and crusting with less vesiculation, and in chronic dermatitis, the reaction may include mild erythema, scaling, fissures, pigmentary alteration, and lichenification. The reaction is usually limited to the site of contact with the allergen and the distribution provides a clue to the cause of the dermatitis. For example, reactions to nickel appear on the earlobes, fingers, and neck. Reactions to leather tanning agents or to the rubber of shoes are seen on the dorsa of the feet, and to cosmetics, nail polish, or topical medications on the face and eyelids.

Common Allergens

The most common cause of contact allergy in children is *Rhus plant dermatitis* (poison ivy, poison oak, poison sumac) (Fig. 61-1). The poison ivy plant has three notched leaflets. Poison sumac is a shrub or tree with 7 to 13 leaflets arranged in pairs along a central stem and is found east of the Mississippi in wooded areas. Poison oak is an upright shrub found on the West coast. The eruption follows contact with damaged leaves, roots, or stems, which contain the plant oleoresin and its active compound pentadecylcatechol. The oleoresin is spread on the skin by scratching, and vesicles and erythema often have a linear distribution. The face, hands, and feet are usually affected, although boys will commonly have lesions over the genital and perigenital area. Commonly, the dermatitis becomes secondarily infected with streptococcal or staphylococcal organisms.

Besides allergy to the Rhus family of plants, the frequency of allergy to specific agents is determined by patch testing. In the United States, the most common contact allergens in children are nickel, rubber chemicals, formaldehyde, ethylenediamine, balsam of Peru, benzocaine, mercuric bichloride, paraphenylenediamine (PPD), potassium dichromate, para-aminobenzoic acid (PABA) preservatives and neomycin. The major sources of these agents are jewelry, shoes, cosmetics, and topical medications.

The incidence of contact sensitivity to *nickel* is 2.5% in children aged 5 to 13. Sources of nickel allergy include jewelry, eyeglass frames, metal fasteners, and belt buckles. The patient is often not aware that metal (such as in earrings) contains nickel. The presence of nickel may be ascertained by painting the metal with 10% dimethylglyoxine, which causes a pink color. Although stainless steel is an alloy of nickel and chrome, the two metals are tightly bound and stainless steel does not cause contact allergy. If nickel cannot be eliminated, sensitivity may be diminished by coating the nickel with several layers of clear nail polish.

Shoe dermatitis is usually caused by contact with *rubber chemicals*, including accelerators (mercaptobenzothiazole and thiurams) and antioxidants. The reaction most commonly involves the dorsa of the feet with sparing of the interdigital webs and plantar surface. *Adhesive agents* and *potassium dichromate*, a chemical used to tan leather, may also be responsible for shoe dermatitis. Sweating exacerbates the dermatitis by increasing percutaneous absorption of the allergen or causing superimposed irritant dermatitis. The rubber compounds may also be found in bandages and adhesive tape. In susceptible children, non-rubber acrylate bandages, Dermicel or Micropore tape, and Steri-strips may be used.

Cosmetic dermatitis often affects the eyelids, even when the agents are applied to the hands or scalp, by transfer of the allergen to an area of greater permeability. Allergy to the organic dye

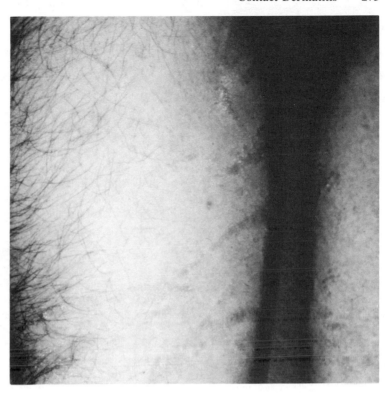

Figure 61-1. Linear pattern of contact dermatitis due to poison ivy.

PPD usually develops in teenaged girls after exposure to hair dyes, with erythema, edema, and vesiculation of the posterior neck, ears, face, and scalp. Occasionally, PPD may be used to dye textiles, stockings, and shoes with resultant contact allergy. *Formaldehydes* are used as preservatives in shampoos, cosmetics, and glues. Topical medications may contain contact allergens, and disorders may appear to be aggravated because of the development of a superimposed contact allergic dermatitis. *Balsam of Peru* is occasionally found in topical medications. It cross reacts with fragrances in cosmetics and can cause hand or facial dermatitis in children. *Parabens* (derivatives of aminobenzoic acid) are antimicrobial preservatives found in cosmetics and topical medications. Although the use of *mercury compounds* has decreased, they are strong sensitizers and are still used as disinfectants in topical preparations, such as Merthiolate. *Benzocaine* is a topical anesthetic that is used for relief of sunburn and pruritus. *Neomycin* is a topical antibiotic, most commonly found in Neosporin. Topical preparations that contain *diphenhydramine*, such as Caladryl, may cause contact reactions when the topical agent is applied or with later use of the oral antihistamine.

Clothing dermatitis is usually irritant, but allergic contact dermatitis occasionally occurs. *Formaldehyde* and *formaldehyde-releasing substances* in permanent press fabrics (polyester-cotton) may cause clothing dermatitis, especially in areas with a tight fit, such as the axillae and the inner thighs. *Rubber compounds* may cause waistband dermatitis from the elastic waistband of underwear following washing with bleach.

DIFFERENTIAL DIAGNOSIS

Conditions that may resemble allergic contact dermatitis include irritant dermatitis, dyshidrotic eczema, bacterial or candidal infections, juvenile plantar dermatosis, and phytophotodermatitis. The distribution, history of exposure, and later results of patch testing aid in confirming the diagnosis. Bacterial and candidal infections may be ruled out by culture of lesions. Juvenile plantar dermatosis is usually found in school-aged, prepubertal children and is characterized by symmetric erythema, scaling, and fissuring of the weight-bearing areas of the feet with sparing of the insteps and interdigital spaces. Most affected children are athletic, have hyperhidrosis, and wear occlusive socks and shoes.

Allergic dermatitis due to shoes, atopic dermatitis, and tinea pedis must be considered in the differential diagnosis. The treatment of juvenile plantar dermatosis includes topical corticosteroid ointments, antibacterial ointment to fissures and agents, such as aluminum chloride, to decrease hyperhidrosis. Phytophotodermatitis is a toxic reaction due to exposure to certain plants and sunlight. The furocoumarins that cause phytophotodermatitis are released on crushing the plant and are found in limes, lemons, figs, celery, and parsnip plants. Lesions are typically well-circumscribed patches of erythema and hyperpigmentation in a sun-exposed site.

EVALUATION

The history of exposure to the allergen is critical in suspecting the diagnosis. The distribution and appearance of lesions by physical examination further confirms the diagnosis of contact allergy and suggests the contactant. Patch testing by the dermatologist provides corroborative evidence that a suspected allergen is responsible. Patch testing should be deferred until the acute reaction has cleared to prevent exacerbation from absorption of the test material. Aluminum-backed strips with disks containing the individual allergens are applied to the back for 48 hours and read 30 minutes after removal. Reactions are graded on the basis of erythema and edema. For patients with nickel allergy, applying dimethylglyoxine to a suspected metal will determine nickel content.

TREATMENT

Management of contact allergy, whether irritant or allergic, involves treatment of the dermatitis and elimination of the offending agent. Topical corticosteroid creams of moderate potency (unless the lesions are on the face or intertriginous sites) should be applied two to three times daily until the rash has cleared. If extensive areas are involved, such as in widespread Rhus dermatitis, prednisone 1 mg/kg/day for 10 to 14 days is the most effective treatment. Weeping lesions should be compressed with saline solutions or Burow's solution 1:20 to 1:40 (one Domeboro tablet to one pint of lukewarm water is a 1:40 solution). Shake lotions, such as Calamine, are also helpful to dry lesions and decrease oozing. Systemic antihistamines may decrease pruritus. Secondary bacterial infection should be treated with systemic antistaphylococcal antibiotics.

To minimize exposure to the Rhus family of plants, affected children should be taught to recognize the plant and to remove clothes and wash rapidly and thoroughly after exposure to remove the oleoresin from fingers and other body parts. The fluid within vesicles does not contain any allergen. Nickel should be avoided or coated with nail polish. Hypoallergenic shoes are available for patients with allergic contact dermatitis to shoe components. These include vinyl and canvas tennis shoes without rubber, moccasins, wooden clogs, and polyvinyl shoes. Special shoes may be ordered from the Musebeck Shoe Company, Foot-So-Port Shoe Division, Forest and Westover, Oconomowoc, Wisc, 53066. Rubber-free insoles or agents used to diminish sweating of the feet, such as tea baths or aluminum chloride solutions, may also help.

INDICATIONS FOR REFERRAL

Any patient suspected of having allergic contact dermatitis that requires patch testing or patients with widespread or recalcitrant dermatitis should be referred to a dermatologist.

ANNOTATED BIBLIOGRAPHY

Coffman K, Boyce T, Hansen RC: Phytophotodermatitis simulating child abuse. Am J Dis Child 139:239–240, 1985 (Two cases of phytophotodermatitis in children.)

Fisher AA: Contact Dermatitis, 2nd ed. Philadelphia, Lea & Febiger, 1973 (Extremely complete text of contact allergens, their manifestations, and cross-reactivity.)

Heskel NS: Contact dermatitis in children. Dermatol Clin 2:579–584, 1984 (Review of allergic contact dermatitis in children, citing the overdiagnosis of the condition.)

Mackie RM: Juvenile plantar dermatosis. Semin Dermatol 1:67–71, 1982 (Review of juvenile plantar dermatosis.)

Weston WL, Weston JA: Allergic contact dermatitis. Am J Dis Child 138:932–936, 1984 (Review of contact dermatitis, suggesting that allergic contact dermatitis is more common than suspected.)

62
Papulosquamous Eruptions
AMY PALLER

Papulosquamous eruptions include various childhood dermatologic problems that are all characterized by small, elevated lesions with scaling. Among the more common papulosquamous disorders of children are psoriasis, pityriasis rosea, Mucha–Habermann disease, lichen nitidus, and lichen striatus.

PSORIASIS

Psoriasis is one of the most common dermatologic abnormalities (1% to 3% of the population) and 37% of patients first develop the disorder during childhood, especially during the second decade of life. The diagnosis, nevertheless, is often missed by pediatricians. The disorder is chronic with periods of spontaneous remissions and recurrences. Although there is a familial predisposition, the inheritance pattern of psoriasis appears to be multifactorial.

The underlying cause of psoriasis is unknown. Both epidermal alterations with accelerated epidermal proliferation and dermal vascular abnormalities are thought to be contributory. Recent research has focused on the role of leukotrienes in causing the inflammation. It is clear that environmental factors may improve or exacerbate psoriasis. Cutaneous trauma may induce lesions after a lag time of 1 to 3 weeks, a phenomenon called the *isomorphic response* or *Koebner phenomenon*. The sudden appearance of small widespread psoriatic plaques (acute guttate psoriasis) can follow streptococcal infections, especially in adolescent patients (Fig. 62-1). Although sunlight in moderate amounts may help to clear psoriatic lesions, sunburn is another environmental response that is associated with the Koebner phenomenon. Certain drugs may also aggravate the condition, such as systemic corticosteroids (especially on withdrawal), lithium, and some of the nonsteroidal antiinflammatory agents.

Psoriasis may manifest in various cutaneous alterations, some of which are found only in children. The most common variant is typical plaque-type psoriasis (psoriasis vulgaris) with well-circumscribed erythematous papules and plaques with loosely adherent shiny white scale concentrated at the center of lesions. The plaques of children are usually less scaly and thinner than those of adults. When the scale is removed, pinpoint sites of bleeding are uncovered (Auspitz sign). The lesions are symmetric and are found at sites of trauma, especially the elbows, knees, buttocks, umbilical, intergluteal and presacral areas, and palms and soles. The scalp is another common site and may be the only site of initial involvement. Lesions frequently encircle the hairline and are found on the retroauricular area and external ears. Well-demarcated, thick adherent crusts are found occasionally on the scalp (tinea amiantacea). Seborrhea and fungal infections of the scalp must be differentiated from the well-defined plaques and thick scaling as well as by KOH examination and cultures. In contrast to its rarity in adults, the face is commonly involved in children. Many patients with psoriasis have dystrophic nails with discoloration, thickening, distal fractures, ridging, and pitting (Fig. 62-2). In patients with nail alterations but no cutaneous psoriatic plaques, fungal or bacterial infections, trauma to the nail, lichen planus, alopecia areata, atopic dermatitis and 20 nail dystrophy of childhood must be considered.

Psoriasis in the diaper area of infants (napkin psoriasis) usually appears eczematous and is often mistaken for seborrheic dermatitis, irritant dermatitis, or candidal infection. Just as psoriasis vulgaris is seen at the sites of trauma in children and adolescents, psoriasis in infants is most commonly manifest in the diaper area, a site of considerable trauma. Napkin psoriasis is more recalcitrant to mild topical corticosteroids than contact dermatitis and seborrheic dermatitis. The rash usually affects the inguinal and intergluteal folds. Psoriatic plaques are also often found on the scalp and trunk. They must be differentiated from seborrheic dermatitis and the id reaction of candidal diaper dermatitis. All lesions should be cultured for *Candida albicans*, because the yeast is a common cause of secondary infection in infants with psoriasis.

The acute guttate (teardrop) form of psoriasis is the first sign of psoriasis in 15% of patients, al-

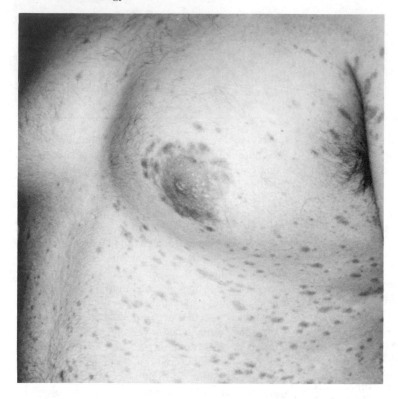

Figure 62-1. Acute guttate psoriasis in a teenager following streptococcal pharyngitis.

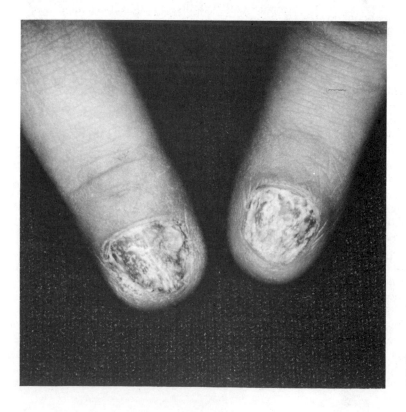

Figure 62-2. Psoriatic nails of a child with a single psoriatic plaque in the periungual area.

though it occurs more frequently in patients with known psoriasis. Teenagers and young adults are commonly affected. The lesions are round to oval erythematous scaling papules that range in size from 2 mm to 10 mm. The papules are widespread and symmetric. Lesions may be present on the face and are more common on the trunk and proximal extremities, but the palms and soles are usually spared. Two thirds of patients report pharyngitis 2 to 3 weeks before the eruption develops, and streptococcal organisms are often found by pharyngeal cultures. Guttate psoriasis should be differentiated from psoriasiform drug reactions, pityriasis rosea, and secondary syphilis.

Pustular psoriasis is an unusual form in childhood and may be generalized or localized. Although pustular psoriasis in adults usually follows years of plaque-type psoriasis, pustular psoriasis in children is often the initial manifestation of psoriasis. Some children have a history of psoriasiform seborrheic dermatitis. Episodes of generalized pustular psoriasis are frequently accompanied by malaise, fever, and leukocytosis. Sheets of 1 mm to 2 mm pustules appear suddenly and overlie erythema and scaling. Cultures of the pustules yield no organisms. The localized form of pustular psoriasis involves the palms and soles, often in association with more typical plaques elsewhere on the body. Staphylococcal pustulosis, dyshidrotic eczema, contact dermatitis, infantile acropustulosis, and fungal infections should be considered.

Exfoliative erythroderma is a rare form of psoriasis that is characterized by generalized desquamation and erythema. Children who are most affected have a past history of psoriasis. Drug reactions, severe seborrheic or atopic dermatitis, contact dermatitis, and pityriasis rubra pilaris must be considered.

Psoriatic arthritis in children is unusual, but has been recognized with increasing frequency. It is defined as an inflammatory arthritis beginning before the age of 16 years associated with psoriasis, either preceding the onset of psoriasis or occurring within the subsequent 15 years, usually with the absence of rheumatoid factor in the serum. The peak age of onset is 9 to 12 years, and the arthritis is more prevalent in girls. Nearly one half of the patients have a positive family history of psoriasis. Cutaneous psoriasis may be absent or mild, and patients are frequently given the erroneous diagnosis of juvenile rheumatoid arthritis. Joint disease is usually asymmetric and monoarticular or oligoarticular, although polyarticular arthritis often develops later.

Sausage digits, tendon sheath involvement, and distal interphalangeal joint changes are typical. Some patients have sacroiliitis or spondylitis (especially with HLA–B27). Iridocyclitis is the most common extra-articular feature (9%), but other systemic manifestations, such as fever, hepatosplenomegaly, lymphadenopathy, and cardiopulmonary alterations, are rare. The long-term prognosis is good, with minimal permanent joint destruction for most patients. Most children who have psoriatic arthritis respond to aspirin and nonsteroidal anti-inflammatory agents in addition to physical and occupational therapy.

A histopathologic examination of lesional skin supports the clinical diagnosis of psoriasis, although many biopsies, especially of treated lesions, may not show classic features. The typical microscopic features of psoriatic plaques include a thickened stratum corneum with layers of retained keratinocyte nuclei (parakeratosis), hyperplastic epidermis, dilated capillaries, and intracorneal and subcorneal collections of polymorphonuclear leukocytes (Munro abscesses).

Psoriasis tends to be a chronic disorder and onset in childhood often suggests a more complicated, recalcitrant course in adulthood. Many patients tend to have a mild form of the disease, however, and spontaneous remissions occur for variable periods of time in almost one half of patients.

Management

One of the most important aspects of management is the education of parents and patients that psoriasis is a chronic disorder with remissions and recurrences. Injury to the skin should be avoided (Koebner phenomenon) by protective guards when participating in traumatic sports and by choosing occupations that minimize cutaneous injury. Tight elastic undergarments, clothing, and shoes should also be avoided. Patients must be careful to avoid excessive exposure to the sun so that sunburn does not occur.

Since psoriasis is a chronic disease, therapy should be conservative, especially in children. Topical therapy is usually successful, especially corticosteroids, tars, and anthralin. Fluorinated corticosteroids are usually required (except on the face and intertriginous areas) and should be applied three times daily. Arthralin or coal-tar preparations are also useful as adjunctive agents, but may cause irritation, folliculitis, and staining of the skin and clothes. These preparations are available as ointments, pastes, body oils, bath oils, and gels. Thick plaques may require keratolytic agents, such as 3% sulfur or 6% salicylic acid preparations, or intralesional injections of triamcinolone. Scalp psoriasis is best treated with shampoos containing tars and keratolytics used at least every other day. Thick plaques may be softened with mineral oil covered by a warm towel or phenol and saline solutions. Corticosteroids in solutions or ointments may also be useful for scalp psoriasis.

More complicated therapy for psoriasis is rarely needed for children. Patients with lesions that are recalcitrant to topical medications may improve with a combination of tar and ultraviolet B light (Goeckerman regimen). Methotrexate and systemic retinoids may be valuable for children with resistant generalized pustular psoriasis or erythroderma. Systemic corticosteroids are almost never indicated, except in rare cases of erythroderma for acute therapy. Any patient who does not respond to regimens of topical corticosteroids should be managed by a dermatologist. Hospitalization may be required for Goeckerman regimens and initiation of systemic medications.

PITYRIASIS RUBRA PILARIS

Pityriasis rubra pilaris (PRP) is a rare skin disorder in children characterized by salmon-colored scaly plaques surrounding islands of normal skin, pointed follicular papules, and palmoplantar keratoderma. Some juvenile cases are hereditary with an autosomal dominant mode of inheritance. Three forms are described in children and account for 45% of cases. Juvenile forms often relapse, but may remit completely after 3 years. PRP is most commonly mistaken for psoriasis, and there is an intrafamilial (or even personal) occurrence of both disorders. The clinical and histologic appearance of lesions are very similar. Occasionally other disorders, including seborrheic dermatitis, lichen planus, vitamin A deficiency, follicular eczema, atypical keratosis pilaris, and drug eruptions, must be considered in the differential diagnosis.

PRP is often recalcitrant to topical steroids and keratolytic agents, including topical vitamin A derivatives. Oral vitamin A in doses of 50,000 to 150,000 units daily may be effective in children with PRP but its use is limited by potential side effects. Success has also been reported with systemic retinoids (13-cis retinoic acid and etretinate) and methotrexate, but these agents can only be administered intermittently and cautiously in children.

PITYRIASIS ROSEA

Pityriasis rosea (PR) is a common papulosquamous eruption that occurs frequently in children and adolescents. Although a virus is suspected to be causative, no agent has yet been isolated and the risk of contagion is minimal. The eruption often begins with a 1-cm to 5-cm scaly erythematous patch ("herald lesion") that is often mistaken for tinea. A few days to a few weeks later, generalized lesions typically develop, especially on the neck, upper arms and legs, and trunk. The lesions are oval with a collarette of scale at the periphery and follow a typical distribution along skin lines to produce a *Christmas tree* pattern on the back. Lesions are occasionally papular (especially in black children), vesicular, hemorrhagic, or urticarial. The rash may be limited to the extremities and intertriginous areas (inverse PR) or may be localized. Palms and soles are rarely affected, but facial involvement is more common in children. Most patients are asymptomatic or complain of mild pruritus. Pruritus is occasionally intensive and patients have mild constitutional symptoms, such as malaise, pharyngitis, fever, or headache. The eruption is self-limited and tends to clear after 6 to 8 weeks, although transient pigmentary changes may remain.

When PR is atypical in distribution, especially with lesions on the palms and soles, the diagnosis of secondary syphilis must be considered. Other disorders that may resemble PR include drug eruptions, parapsoriasis, seborrheic dermatitis, widespread tinea infections, psoriasis, lichen planus, and scabies with eczematization. Therapy is symptomatic, because the disorder is self-limited and includes antihistamines, emollients, and mild topical corticosteroids.

MUCHA–HABERMANN DISEASE

Mucha–Habermann disease (acute parapsoriasis, *pityriasis lichenoides et varioliformis acuta*, PLEVA) is a self-limited disorder that occurs frequently in children and especially in adolescents. The disorder is characterized by crops of papules and vesicles with central necrosis and crusts. The papulovesicles are usually on the trunk and extremities. Lesions may heal with scars or pigmentary alterations. Each episode lasts for weeks to months, with resolution and recurrences for a few years.

Mucha–Habermann disease must be differentiated from chickenpox, pityriasis rosea, scabies, and impetigo. A histopathologic examination of skin shows a heavy infiltrate of lymphocytes and histiocytes, erythrocyte extravasation into the dermis, and epidermal edema with necrosis and vesicle formation. Pruritus may be decreased by lubricants, mild topical corticosteroids, antihistamines, and lubricants. Tetracycline or erythromycin administered for 3 to 6 months and ultraviolet B light have been helpful in many cases.

Pityriasis lichenoides chronica may evolve from the acute form or *de novo* and usually lasts for 6 months to years. The firm, hyperpigmented papules are more scaly than those of the acute form and resolve without scar formation. Pityriasis rosea, psoriasis, and secondary syphilis should be considered. Many patients improve during the summer and with ultraviolet B light.

LICHEN PLANUS

Lichen planus is a relatively common pruritic dermatosis that occurs occasionally in children. The typical lesion is a small flat violaceous papule covered with a shiny white scale. Fine white lines (Wickham's striae) cross the surface of the papules. Several variants with atrophic, hypertrophic, vesiculobullous, annular, and ulcerated lesions have been reported. Lesions are most commonly found on the flexural surfaces of the extremities, anterior lower legs, dorsum of the hands, and on the genitalia. Mucous membranes, especially the buccal mucosae, are covered by lacy patterns of white papules in most patients and may be the only site of involvement. Up to 10% of patients have nail dystrophy with thinning of the nail plate, longitudinal ridging, and distal splitting. Pterygium formation with fusion of the proximal nail fold with the nail bed is the most typical nail change.

The histopathologic changes of lesional skin are fairly specific. They include hyperkeratosis, focal increase of the granular layer, degeneration of the basal cell layer, a "saw-toothed" appearance of the epidermis, and a linear band of lymphocytes and histiocytes in the upper dermis and lower epidermis. Direct immunofluorescence of skin sections shows ovoid globular deposits of immunoglobulins and complement and a linear band of fibrinogen at the dermal–epidermal junction that suggests an immunologic etiology. Several drugs have caused lichenoid reactions, but none are commonly used in childhood.

Lichen planus tends to resolve spontaneously after months to years. Systemic antihistamines, lubrication, and topical corticosteroids may help to diminish the intense pruritus experienced by most patients. Severely affected children may require a short course of systemic corticosteroids. Griseofulvin has occasionally been reported to have helped a patient.

LICHEN NITIDUS

Lichen nitidus is a benign, asymptomatic dermatosis that is seen usually in children. The papules of lichen nitidus are tiny, sharply demarcated, and skin-colored. The papules are usually hypopigmented in black children. Papules may have a central depression and are often linear in distribution. The forearms, trunk, genitalia, and abdomen are the most common sites of involvement. The histopathology of lichen nitidus is distinct, with compressed epidermis encircling discrete dermal nests of lymphocytes, histiocytes, and giant cells. In children, the differential diagnosis includes flat warts, keratosis pilaris, and the lichen spinulosus pattern of papular eczema. No known therapy is effective, but the disorder clears spontaneously within a few years.

LICHEN STRIATUS

Lichen striatus is a rare dermatosis that is seen usually in school-aged children. A unilateral linear band of violaceous papules develops suddenly, especially on an extremity, and may extend for a few weeks. The eruption is often asymptomatic, but may be pruritic, and regresses spontaneously after 6 months to 1 year. The histopathologic changes are not specific and biopsy is only helpful to eliminate the possibility of other disorders that may resemble lichen striatus, such as inflammatory linear epidermal nevus, flat warts, linear lichen planus, tinea, and psoriasis. Treatment is not necessary, but topical steroids may decrease the inflammation and encourage clearance of the lesions.

ANNOTATED BIBLIOGRAPHY

Farber EM, Jacobs AH: Infantile psoriasis. Am J Dis Child 131:1266–1269, 1977 (Report of psoriasis in 14 infants)

Fox BJ, Odom RB: Papulosquamous diseases: A review. J Am Acad Dermatol 12:597–624, 1985 (Well-written review of the various papulosquamous disorders.)

Griffiths WAD: Pityriasis rubra pilaris. Clin Exp Dermatol 5:105–112, 1980 (Review of pityriasis rubra pilaris with subclassification into three juvenile forms.)

Perlman HH, Lubowe II: Pityriasis rosea in children. J Pediatr 40:109–129, 1952 (Study of pityriasis rosea in a large population.)

Shore A, Ansell BM: Juvenile psoriatic arthritis—an analysis of 60 cases. J Pediatr 100:529–535, 1982 (Review of psoriatic arthritis in children with the suggestion that it is more common than we think.)

Watson W, Farber EM: Psoriasis in children. Pediatr Clin North Am 18:875–895, 1971 (Complete review of psoriasis in children.)

63
Vesicular, Bullous, and Pustular Eruptions
AMY PALLER

The cutaneous disorders with vesicles, bullae, and pustules that occur in infancy and childhood may be benign and self-limited, as transient neonatal pustular melanosis, or chronic and potentially severe, as epidermolysis bullosa. By definition, a vesicle is an elevated lesion filled with clear fluid that measures less than 1 cm in diameter, whereas a bulla is larger than 1 cm in diameter. A pustule is a vesicle or bulla that is filled with purulent material.

TRANSIENT NEONATAL BLISTERING DISORDERS

The most common transient cutaneous abnormality in the neonate is *erythema toxicum neonatorum*, a disorder of unknown cause characterized by erythematous macules and papules, vesicles, and pustules. The lesions usually appear at 2 to 3 days of age and clear spontaneously at the end of the first week of life. The face, trunk, and extremities are usually affected, and the palms and soles are almost always spared. The diagnosis may be confirmed by performing a smear of a vesicle or pustule that will show eosinophils without polymorphonuclear leukocytes, multinucleated giant cells, or bacteria by Wright's, Giemsa, or Gram stains. A histopathologic examination of a skin biopsy shows that the pustule filled with eosinophils is follicular and beneath the horny layer of skin. *Transient neonatal pustular melanosis* is noted usually at birth or within the first 24 hours of life in 5% of all black infants, but in less than 1% of white infants. The neck, chin, palms, soles, and groin area are most commonly affected. The typical lesions are pustules and vesicles with a collarette of scale that resolve as hyperpigmented macules. The vesicles and papules clear spontaneously by 3 days of age and the hyperpigmented macules by 3 months. Scrapings from the vesicles or pustules show neutrophils without multinucleated giant cells or bacteria. A histopathologic examination of a skin biopsy demonstrates that the neutrophils are in and beneath the horny layer of skin.

Miliaria rubra and miliaria crystallina result from obstruction of the immature eccrine sweat ducts and occur in neonates during the first few weeks of life. *Miliaria crystallina* is an asymptomatic eruption characterized by tiny clear vesicles, especially in intertriginous areas, that rupture easily. The duct obstruction in miliaria crystallina is superficial and the vesicle forms beneath the horny layer. There is minimal inflammation and special stains show no organisms. *Miliaria rubra* is a pruritic eruption that is often found on areas of skin covered by clothing and is characterized by erythematous papulovesicles and rarely pustules. The sweat duct obstruction is deeper and histopathologic examination of a skin biopsy shows inflammation surrounding the epidermal eccrine ducts. Special stains for organisms are negative. Miliaria also occurs in older children at areas with excessive sweating that are occluded by clothing. Miliaria may be prevented by regulation of environmental temperature. In neonates, avoidance of overheating and application of lukewarm compresses facilitate the clearing of lesions and decrease discomfort. Older children benefit from the application of cool compresses, calamine lotion, and preparations of ¼% menthol in lotion.

Acropustulosis of infancy is a rare disorder, most commonly seen in black male infants. The disorder usually begins by 10 months of age and may be manifest at birth. The dorsal and plantar aspects of the hands and feet develop pruritic erythematous papules that evolve rapidly into vesicles and pustules. Smears of vesiculopustular contents show neutrophils and occasionally eosinophils, but no organisms by special stains. A histopathologic examination of skin biopsies shows that the pustules are located beneath the horny layer. The lesions tend to remit and recur every few weeks for 2 to 3 years, and the associated pruritus may be severe. Topical corticosteroids are often not effective. Oral antihistamines and dapsone may help, but hematologic tests must be monitored if dapsone is used.

Several infectious processes may develop in the newborn period that are associated with vesicles, bullae, and pustules and must be distinguished from the more benign transient disorders. These are reviewed in detail elsewhere in the text. *Impetigo neonatorum* is staphylococcal bullous impetigo in the neonatal period and is characterized by vesicles, bullae, or pustules on an erythematous base (see also Chaps. 64 and 191). The lesions erode, leaving a moist lesional base with crusting. The intertriginous areas are most commonly affected. Smears of the lesions show polymorphonuclear leukocytes and cultures grow *S. aureus*. Impetigo neonatorum must be treated with systemic antistaphylococcal antibiotics. The vesicles and pustules of *congenital cutaneous candidiasis* must also be considered (see also Chap. 65). The lesions are generalized without accentuation of the diaper and oral areas and are present at birth or appear within a day after birth. The palms and soles are usually involved. The yeast may be found on KOH examination of smears from the lesions and in culture. Congenital cutaneous candidiasis should be treated by the application of topical anticandidal creams and oral nystatin for 10 days. *Herpes simplex* infection in the newborn infant is the most devastating of the vesiculopustular eruptions and must be considered (see also Chaps. 67 and 191). Lesions may be single, but some grouped vesiculopustules should be noted. Tzanck smears of lesional contents show multinucleated epidermal cells and occasionally intracytoplasmic inclusion bodies. Viral cultures are confirmatory. Administration of intravenous acyclovir should be initiated if the diagnosis of Herpes simplex is suspected. *Congenital varicella* infections may also manifest as vesiculopustules in the neonatal period and demonstrate multinucleated giant epidermal cells, but cultures yield the varicella-zoster virus (see also Chaps. 191 and 197). Finally, vesiculobullous hemorrhagic lesions, especially on the palms and soles, are rare but diagnostic of *congenital syphilis* in the neonate or young infant (see also Chap. 191).

MASTOCYTOSIS

The group of disorders characterized by mast cell infiltration of skin is called *mastocytosis*. In children, *urticaria pigmentosa* is the most common form. Urticaria pigmentosa is characterized by solitary or multiple red-brown macules, papules, and nodules that become urticarial or frankly bullous after the lesions are stroked firmly (Darier's sign). The lesions are usually 1 cm to 3 cm in diameter and are located on the trunk. The lesions may resemble bruises and affected children are occasionally mistakenly considered to be victims of child abuse. The reaction is thought to relate to the release of mast cell contents, especially histamine. A histopathologic examination of skin biopsies shows large numbers of mast cells in the dermis and subcutaneous tissues. The mast cell granules stain well with toluidine blue or Giemsa stains.

Most patients develop the lesions of urticaria pigmentosa by school age and the lesions usually clear spontaneously by puberty. With advancing age, there is less of a tendency for blistering of lesions to occur. Systemic involvement, including flushing, gastrointestinal symptoms, headaches, tachycardia, hypotension, and coagulation abnormalities, is rare in children who develop the disorder before 10 years of age. Ten to 30% of older children have systemic symptoms, although they are usually mild. Systemic mastocytosis is rare in children, but 95% of children with systemic mastocytosis have cutaneous lesions. In the systemic form, mast cells may infiltrate almost any organ, although the bone, gastrointestinal tract, liver, and spleen are most frequently affected. Patients may have bone pain with lytic lesions, gastrointestinal ulcers, hepatosplenomegaly, anemia, and eosinophilia.

Most patients with urticaria pigmentosa are asymptomatic and require no therapy. Patients with pruritus, urticaria, flushing, or more severe symptoms are best managed by antihistamine administration and the avoidance of exacerbating factors. Affected infants and children should avoid hot baths and vigorous exercise. Medications that may stimulate mast cell histamine release include salicylates (except in low doses), codeine, morphine, procaine, polymyxin B, and atropine. Cheeses and alcoholic beverages (including cough syrups with alcohol) may also exacerbate the disorder. H1-blocking antihistamines and combinations of H1 and H2 blockers (*e.g.*, cimetidine) may help in preventing or ameliorating systemic symptoms. Topical corticosteroids have been shown to decrease pruritus and clear lesions in adults with urticaria pigmentosa. Oral disodium cromoglycate, a drug that blocks histamine release, has been used successfully in patients with gastrointestinal reactions. Psoralens and ultraviolet A (PUVA) light therapy decreases the number of mast cells in cutaneous lesions, but is not recommended for children. The administration of aspirin in low doses has been suggested, but trials must be attempted with great care because aspirin also stimulates mast cell release of histamine.

In the neonate and young infant, collections of

mast cells usually manifest as *mastocytomas*, nodules that increase in size for months and disappear spontaneously within the first few years of life. The lesions are usually solitary, slightly elevated red-brown nodules that are most frequently located on the trunk or arms. Not uncommonly, the nodules have a pebbly, thickened appearance, and the Darier's sign is positive. Mastocytomas must be distinguished from juvenile xanthogranulomas and, if on the head or neck, from nevus sebaceus. Systemic symptoms are rarely associated. Some cases have been reported to have progressed to generalized urticaria pigmentosa.

ERYTHEMA MULTIFORME AND TOXIC EPIDERMAL NECROLYSIS

Erythema multiforme (EM) minor, EM major (Stevens–Johnson syndrome), and toxic epidermal necrolysis (TEN) are now considered to be related hypersensitivity reactions that are immunologically mediated. *TEN* is unusual in children, almost always occurs after 10 years of age and is usually a complication of drug use. The most common etiologic agents in children are sulfonamides, penicillins, barbiturates, phenytoin, and salicylates. TEN is a rapidly progressive, potentially life-threatening disorder characterized by the development of large flaccid bullae that rupture to reveal denuded tissue. Occasionally, patients initially have the rash and mucosal changes of erythema multiforme, with a rapid evolution into the bullae of TEN. The mucosal surfaces are also usually covered by blisters and crusting. The cleavage of TEN is at the dermal-epidermal junction (in contrast with the intraepidermal level of blistering in the staphylococcal scalded skin syndrome, which was formerly considered to be a form of TEN). This level of cleavage can be easily suspected clinically in black patients by the loss of pigmented skin, consistent with a loss of the entire melanin-containing epidermis.

Erythema multiforme is more common than TEN, and 20% of cases of EM occur in children and adolescents. The lesions of EM begin as erythematous macules that enlarge and develop circumferential pallor. The central portion develops epidermal necrosis and turns a dusky purple, leading to the characteristic "target" lesions or "iris" lesions of EM, with concentric zones of color surrounding zones of pallor. Occasionally, central vesicles or bullae develop. The lesions are symmetrically distributed and begin acrally over the extensor surfaces of the extremities and the dorsum of the hands. The palms, soles, and later the flexural areas, trunk, and ears often become involved. The skin lesions evolve during a 3 to 5 day period. Mild involvement of mucous membranes, especially the lips and oral mucosa, may be seen with the minor form of EM. The cutaneous lesions heal in 2 to 4 weeks with desquamation, crusting, and transient pigmentary alterations, but without scar formation. Symptoms of an upper respiratory infection are described in the week preceding the skin eruption in one third of children.

EM major (*Stevens–Johnson syndrome*) is characterized by more severe mucosal lesions and considerable morbidity. Inflammatory lesions develop suddenly after a prodromal period of up to 2 weeks that includes malaise, fever, sore throat, cough, chest pain, headache, vomiting, diarrhea, myalgias, and arthralgias. The mucosal vesicles and crusts are most commonly found on the lips, oral mucosa, and bulbar conjunctivae. The ocular involvement may be severe and may progress from purulent conjunctivitis to corneal ulceration, anterior uveitis, panophthalmitis, synechiae, and blindness. The nasopharynx, esophagus, respiratory mucosa, and genitourinary tract may also be involved, resulting in refusal to eat, trouble with breathing, and urinary retention due to pain on urination. Pneumonitis and renal disease with hematuria and tubular necrosis have also been reported. High fever and weakness are commonly associated.

The skin lesions of EM major are variable in appearance and include the typical "target" lesions of EM minor, confluent areas of erythema, and the large bullae with desquamation of TEN. A histopathologic examination of skin from lesions of EM major or minor shows epidermal necrosis and perivascular infiltrates of mononuclear inflammatory cells in the upper dermis, but no vasculitis. The lesions of EM major continue to erupt for 10 days to a month and heal after approximately 4 to 6 weeks.

EM may be associated with infections or drugs. The drugs that cause EM reactions in children include sulfonamides (including thiazides), barbiturates, phenytoin, and penicillins. The two infectious diseases that have clearly been associated with EM are *Herpes simplex* and *Mycoplasma pneumoniae*. The EM usually follows the infectious processes by about 10 days. As a drug reaction, EM also occurs 10 days after initiation of a drug for the first time, but may appear within hours after beginning a drug that has been previously administered.

The management of EM and TEN in children is controversial. The most critical therapy is the removal of an offending drug, if one is discovered. In general, EM minor is self-limited and should be treated conservatively with cool compresses and oral antihistamines. Topical corticosteroids are usually not helpful, even for associated pruritus. Children with EM major and TEN should be hospitalized because of the extensive associated tissue necrosis and debilitation. Lukewarm compresses or whirlpool baths are helpful and should be followed by the application of antibacterial ointments to promote re-epithelialization and prevent secondary bacterial infection. If secondary infection occurs, antistaphylococcal antibiotics should be administered, but otherwise any unnecessary systemic drugs should be withheld. An ophthalmologist should be consulted to manage ocular involvement. The use of systemic corticosteroids for severe EM major and TEN in children is controversial and no good prospective studies have been described. Since the disorders can lead to extensive fluid and electrolyte imbalances and secondary bacterial infections with a mortality of up to 50%, many dermatologists recommend high-dose corticosteroid therapy (1 to 2 mg/kg/day), especially if the corticosteroids can be started early in the course, and infection as a cause of the EM is eliminated or adequately treated. The corticosteroids should be tapered during the following weeks as healing occurs. Other investigators have suggested that corticosteroids have no beneficial effect and only lead to complications, especially infection.

CHRONIC BULLOUS DISEASE OF CHILDHOOD

Immunologically-mediated blistering disorders in children are rare, although pemphigus, bullous and cicatricial pemphigoid, dermatitis herpetiforme, and epidermolysis bullosa acquisita have all been described in children. The most common blistering disorder in childhood is *chronic bullous disease of childhood*. This disorder usually occurs before the age of 6 and is characterized by blisters with variable pruritus in the perioral area, lower trunk, upper thighs, and perineum. The blisters are often hemorrhagic and may be large or small and clustered in annular or sausage-shaped patterns. A histopathologic examination of skin sections shows a subepidermal blister with a variable amount of mixed inflammatory cell infiltration. By immunofluorescence microscopy, linear deposits of IgA are seen at the basement membrane zone.

In contrast to other blistering disorders, chronic bullous disease of childhood is self-limited and

clears spontaneously after months to a few years. The preferred management is administration of sulfapyridine or dapsone with or without supplemental prednisone. These drugs should be tapered to a maintenance dose as soon as possible and discontinued when the patient tolerates withdrawal without a recurrence of blisters.

EPIDERMOLYSIS BULLOSA

Epidermolysis bullosa (EB) is a group of inherited disorders in which blistering occurs at sites of mechanical trauma. Subgroups are distinguished by the clinical manifestations, the mode of inheritance, and the level of blistering. The pathophysiology of most forms of EB is poorly understood. The most common forms of EB are the autosomal dominant *simplex* and *Weber–Cockayne* forms. In both of these disorders, the blistering occurs within the epidermis and no scarring results. Blisters in patients with the Weber–Cockayne form are localized to the hands and feet, whereas blisters of the simplex form are usually more generalized. Blisters tend to occur readily after trauma and are increased with hyperhidrosis during the summer. Patients with the simplex form of EB may have blisters at birth or in early infancy, whereas patients with the Weber–Cockayne form often do not develop blisters until later childhood or adolescence.

Junctional epidermolysis bullosa (JEB) is a group of autosomal recessive disorders with cleavage through the lamina lucida region of the epidermal-dermal junction. The most common and most severe type is *EB letalis*. Neonates almost always have blisters at birth, especially of the extremities, as well as intraoral blisters and a loss of nails. The lesions resolve with atrophy, but without scarring or milia formation. These infants are at a great risk of fluid loss and sepsis. Subsequent blisters may develop spontaneously or after minimal trauma. Not uncommonly, the gastrointestinal, upper respiratory, and genitourinary tracts develop blisters that may resolve with tissue stenosis.

The diagnosis of JEB may be made by demonstration with electron microscopy or immunofluorescence mapping of blister formation through the lamina lucida zone of the cutaneous basement membrane. Most affected infants die because of the complications of extensive blistering. The few reported infants with the letalis form of JEB who have survived into later childhood have growth retardation, anemia, and extensive granulation tissue, especially in the perioral area.

The scarring or dystrophic forms of EB may be

autosomal dominant or autosomal recessive in inheritance. The *dominant dystrophic types of EB* may manifest at birth or in early childhood. Lesions resolve with scar formation and milia. The mucous membranes and nails are rarely affected. The *recessive dystrophic form of EB* is severe and mutilating. The blisters are almost always present at birth as large tense, deep blisters that heal slowly, leaving scars and milia. Repeated blistering and scar formation leads to syndactyly (mitten deformity) of the hands and feet by early childhood. Dysphagia due to esophageal involvement is common, and blisters of the pharynx, larynx, and trachea have resulted in hoarseness and upper airway obstruction. Eating may be impaired due to intraoral involvement. Squamous cell carcinomas of the scarred skin or mucosae may develop and are the most common cause of death in patients who survive early childhood. Ultrastructural examination and immunofluorescence mapping of skin biopsies from patients with the dystrophic forms show that the cleavage is below the dermal-epidermal junction.

Patients with forms of EB except the mildest of the epidermal forms should be managed by a dermatologist, as well as by other specialists in the care of patients with epidermolysis bullosa, including pedodontists, pediatric and plastic surgeons, and dietitians. Therapy is primarily supportive and includes wound dressings, the prevention of secondary infection, the management of complications, and the assurance of optimal nutrition. Compresses should be applied to open wounds two to four times a day, followed by the application of topical antibiotics, such as bacitracin–polymyxin B or silver sulfadiazine. Artificial skin barriers, such as Vigilon or Opsite dressings, may be helpful for some patients. Staphylococcal colonization of skin may be diminished by adding chlorhexidine to the bath water. In all patients, trauma must be avoided by using nontraumatic nipples, shoes that fit well, and padding over extensor surfaces and other sites of trauma.

Systemic antibiotics are crucial in patients with secondary infections. Brief courses of topical corticosteroid preparations may decrease inflammation. For patients with the recessive form of dystrophic EB, phenytoin, a drug that decreases collagenase production by fibroblasts, may be useful. Multicenter trials of phenytoin for these patients are now in progress. In addition, surgical repair of the syndactyly should be performed in early childhood and repeated as necessary to restore hand function. Finally, referral of families to the Dystrophic Epidermolysis Bullosa Research Association of America (DEBRA), 2936 Avenue W, Brooklyn, NY 11229, is invaluable.

ANNOTATED BIBLIOGRAPHY

Cooper TW, Bauer EA: Epidermolysis bullosa: A review. Pediatr Dermatol 1:181–188, 1984 (Practical, comprehensive review of the subgroups of epidermolysis bullosa and their management)

Huff JC, Weston WL, Tonnesen MG: Erythema multiforme: A critical review of characteristics, diagnostic criteria, and causes. J Am Acad Dermatol 8:763–775, 1983 (Good review of erythema multiforme)

Rasmussen JE: Erythema multiforme in children: Response to treatment with systemic corticosteroids. Br J Dermatol 95:181–186, 1976 (Retrospective study of the effect of systemic corticosteroids in the Stevens–Johnson syndrome)

Schachner L, Press S: Vesicular, bullous and pustular disorders in infancy and childhood. Pediatr Clin North Am 30:609–629, 1983 (Comprehensive review of the various vesicular, bullous, and pustular disorders in children)

Surbrugg Sk, Weston WL: The course of chronic bullous disease of childhood. Pediatr Dermatol 2:213–215, 1985 (Recent review of chronic bullous disease of childhood)

64

Bacterial Skin Infections

AMY PALLER

The normal skin of infants and children provides an effective barrier against bacterial invasion. When the skin is damaged, pathogenic bacteria can easily invade and proliferate. Spontaneous blistering, as in epidermolysis bullosa, or localized alteration of host defenses due to trauma, as in insect bite reactions and scalp trauma due to traction, are often associated with secondary bacterial infections. The most common organisms are staphylococcal and streptococcal. Children with underlying inflammatory dermatoses, especially seborrheic dermatitis and atopic dermatitis, are also prone to secondary infections. Maceration and abnormally moist skin permit bacterial infections, both gram-positive and gram-negative. Children with alterations in physiologic defenses risk recurrent bacterial infections. Children with alterations in lymphatic drainage, as in chronic familial lymphedema, have chronic infections of the feet and lower legs. Patients with immunologic disorders, especially agammaglobulinemias, chronic granulomatous disease, and deficiencies of the alternate complement pathway or terminal sequence, have severe bacterial infections of viscera and skin. Children who are immunocompromised by a neoplastic disease or drug, especially corticosteroids, have an increased susceptibility to bacterial infections due both to mon and unusual organisms. Finally, infants are more subject to bacterial infections because of an immature immunologic system and also an immature visceral function. The higher frequency of the staphylococcal scalded skin syndrome in infants is thought to be due to inadequate renal clearance and metabolism of the staphylococcal toxin.

GRAM-POSITIVE BACTERIAL INFECTIONS

Most bacterial skin infections of infants and children are due to *Staphylococcus aureus* and group A *Streptococcus pyogenes* infections. *Impetigo* is the most common manifestation and accounts for 10% of all skin problems in pediatric clinics. Impetigo may be bullous, due to phage group II staphylococcus, or vesiculopustular, due to streptococcus or staphylococcus. The bullae of bullous impetigo are tense and filled with purulent material. They rupture, leaving a moist, erythematous base (Fig. 64-1). The superficial vesiculopustules of impetigo rupture easily to form thick yellow crusts and are found most commonly on the lower extremities during the summer. Either form of impetigo may be associated with fever and lymphadenopathy.

Staphylococcal organisms produce the exotoxin exfoliatin, which is responsible for the bullae of bullous impetigo. Staphylococcal organisms also cause furuncles and carbuncles, invade the hair follicles to produce folliculitis, and disrupt the epidermis in the staphylococcal scalded skin syndrome. In neonates, staphylococcus is also responsible for omphalitis, dacrocystitis, mammary abscesses, and paronychia, probably because these are sites of

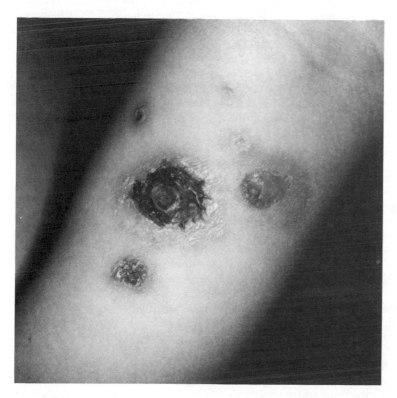

Figure 64-1. The bullae of staphylococcal impetigo rupture leaving a moist, denuded base.

trauma. Streptococcus is responsible for the generalized rash of scarlet fever and local infections, including erysipelas and ecthyma.

Folliculitis in children usually affects the superficial portion of the hair follicle and is characterized by a tiny pustule and erythema centered in a hair follicle. Folliculitis occurs usually on the face, scalp, extremities, and buttocks. Lesions frequently appear in crops and are nontender, but may be pruritic. Most folliculitis is due to Staphylococcus aureus, but streptococcus may occasionally be responsible. *Gram-negative folliculitis* due to Klebsiella, Proteus, or Enterobacter may occur on the periorificial region of the face of teenagers who use broad-spectrum systemic antibiotics for acne. *Hot tub dermatitis* due to pseudomonas may be follicular and has been reported in children who are exposed to infected hot tubs or pools. Superficial folliculitis may also be noninfectious from the occlusion of follicles by oils (as in hair pomades), tars, and occlusive dressings.

Folliculitis barbae is a deep folliculitis caused by staphylococcus of the beard area that occasionally affects adolescent boys. Pruritic follicular papules and pustules with erythema may progress to form crusts and boggy edema (sycosis barbae). Scratching and shaving spread the infection. Warm compresses, topical or systemic antibiotics, and the use of an electric razor or avoidance of shaving are helpful. *Pseudofolliculitis barbae* is an inflammatory process of the hair follicle due to curly hair (especially in black patients) with repenetration of the skin by hair. Pathogenic bacteria are not responsible. Pseudofolliculitis barbae may respond to changing the manner of shaving, use of the chemical depilatories, shaving less closely, or keratolytic agents, such as topical vitamin A acid (Retin-A).

Acne keloidalis or folliculitis keloidalis nuchae is a chronic perifollicular infection that is common in black adolescents and young adults. Collections of pruritic, firm skin-colored or hyperpigmented papules are found at the nape of the neck. Many patients harbor pathogenic staphylococcus, but it is not clear that there is any relation between the organisms and the folliculitis. Patients respond to systemic antibiotics, as in the treatment of acne, and intralesional or strong topical corticosteroids to diminish keloid formation.

Furuncles are painful circumscribed perifollicular staphylococcal abscesses that extend from folliculitis. They occur most commonly in older children on hairy areas subject to trauma, especially on the thighs, buttocks, perineum, face, scalp, nape of the neck, and axillae. They may reach a diameter of 5 cm, become fluctuant, and eventually rupture to release a purulent, sanguineous discharge. *Carbuncles* are deeper staphylococcal abscesses formed by interconnecting furuncles that drain from many sites at the skin surface. The lesions are larger than furuncles and are often associated with extreme tenderness, fever, chills, and malaise. Patients with chronic granulomatous disease have recurrent staphylococcal abscesses that often require repeated incision and drainage procedures as well as systemic antibiotics. Children with the hyperimmunoglobulin E syndrome (and Job's syndrome) also have recurrent abscesses, but are not able to mount a normal inflammatory response, so that the abscesses are only mildly tender and inflamed.

Paronychia or inflammation around the nails is often due to *S. aureus*. Streptococcus or pseudomonas is occasionally causative. Pseudomonas paronychia is characterized by a green discoloration of the nails. Patients who have paronychia and nail dystrophy and whose hands are frequently in contact with water may have candidal paronychia.

The *staphylococcal scalded skin syndrome* (SSSS) is an exfoliative condition most common in infants because of the diminished ability to excrete the responsible toxin produced by phage group II *Staphylococcus aureus*. Three phases occur: erythematous, exfoliative, and desquamative. Many parents report cutaneous tenderness and restlessness before any erythroderma is seen. Cutaneous erythema and tenderness develop initially periorificially and spread rapidly to involve the trunk and limbs. One to two days later exfoliation develops, with yellow crusts around the mouth, eyes, umbilicus, perineum, and perianal area. Two to 3 days later, the skin begins to shed spontaneously or with light stroking (Nikolsky sign). The palms and soles shed last. Affected children are uncomfortable and experience malaise, but are often without fever or other complaints.

The diagnosis of SSSS is made by the typical clinical course and appearance of affected infants and the superficial blistering at the granular level of the epidermis, in contrast to the dermal-epidermal separation of toxic epidermal necrosis. Staphylococcus is usually recovered from the nasopharynx and occasionally the conjunctivae and impetiginous areas of skin, but rarely from the blood or erythematous areas of skin. Many cases are aborted at the erythematous or exfoliative stage by the prompt institution of systemic antistaphylococcal antibiotics. Although the mortality is low, infants may have considerable loss of fluid and electrolytes. Systemic corticosteroids are contraindicated.

The *toxic shock syndrome* is another disorder

with cutaneous manifestations due to a staphylococcal toxin that may be seen by the pediatrician, especially in adolescent girls who use tampons. Patients have fever, hypotension, or postural dizziness and there is evidence of multiple visceral involvement, especially diarrhea, vomiting, myalgia, and renal failure. The mucocutaneous abnormalities include a diffuse scarlatiniform (rough texture with red-brown fine papules) or macular erythematous eruption and subsequent desquamation, edema of the hands and feet, and conjunctival hyperemia. The conditions that are most commonly mistakenly diagnosed are scarlet fever and Kawasaki's disease.

Scarlet fever is a diffuse erythematous eruption due to a toxin produced by β-hemolytic streptococcus, usually in association with streptococcal pharyngitis. Other features are lymphadenopathy, nausea and vomiting, headache, abdominal discomfort, and occasionally splenomegaly. The disease occurs most commonly in children and begins with fever and pharyngitis. One to two days later the rash appears, first on the neck and then on the trunk and extremities. The eruption is characterized by dusky red, blanching tiny papules that have a rough texture. Papules are usually absent from the face, palms, and soles, but the face characteristically shows flushing with circumoral pallor. On the body, the rash is intensified in skin folds and at sites of pressure. In the antecubital and axillary fossae, linear petechiae are seen with accentuation of the erythema (Pastia's lines). The exanthem usually lasts 4 to 5 days and then begins to desquamate, first on the face and last on the palms and soles. *S. aureus* and viral infections may also be associated with scarlatiniform rashes.

Ecthyma, a condition that is usually streptococcal in origin, is characterized by superficial vesicles that rapidly become ulcers with necrotic central crusts. The ulcer spreads centrifugally if it is left untreated. The lesions heal slowly and usually leave scars. The lower extremities are usually affected and associated lymphadenopathy is common. Insect bites and varicella lesions may be precursors of ecthyma.

Cellulitis is an acute inflammation of the dermis and subcutaneous tissues characterized by tenderness, warmth, and erythema with a poorly-defined border. Usually *S. aureus* or group A hemolytic streptococcus is the causative agent. Periorbital cellulitis is often due to *S. aureus* or pneumococcus. Buccal (facial) cellulitis in infants has often a violaceous hue and may be due to *H. influenza*. Violaceous cellulitis has also been described with pneumococcal infections. Tender regional adenopathy is commonly associated with cellulitis and patients may have malaise, fever, and chills. Cellulitis with superficial blisters is usually caused by streptococcus. *Blistering distal dactylitis* is an uncommon form of cellulitis in children due to *S. pyogenes* with purulent blisters and a rim of erythema localized to the volar fat pad of the distal phalanx of the finger. The differential diagnosis includes blisters from friction and burns, herpetic whitlows, staphylococcal bullous impetigo, and epidermolysis bullosa. *Erysipelas* is a distinctive type of cellulitis caused by streptococcus with a sharply demarcated, elevated advancing edge. Affected sites in young children and infants include the face, abdomen, legs, and intertriginous areas.

Erythrasma is a superficial infection due to the gram-positive bacterium *Corynebacterium minutissimum* characterized by well-circumscribed dusky red scaly patches in axillae, groin, and interdigital spaces. Fifteen percent of cases occur in prepubertal children, and the disorder is more common in adolescents. Erythrasma may coexist with candidal infections. The treatment of choice is Erythromycin for 10 days. *Trichomycosis axillaris* is a benign infection of the axillary and pubic hairs due to *Corynebacterium tenuis*. Only postpubertal adolescents are affected. Concretions that are usually white or yellow are found on the hair shaft and patients may complain of hyperhidrosis with an unpleasant odor or red-stained perspiration. Management includes shaving the affected hairs and the use of antibacterial soaps and deodorants.

THERAPY OF STAPHYLOCOCCAL AND STREPTOCOCCAL INFECTIONS

Most cutaneous infections require treatment with systemic antibiotics. Although topical antibiotic ointments may be used as adjunctive agents, they are only appropriate as single agents for very localized impetigo. Usually oral antibiotics suffice for impetigo, folliculitis, and paronychia (except in young infants), but parenteral antistaphylococcal antibiotics must be administered in neonates with any bacterial infection and for more serious infections, such as buccal and periorbital cellulitis, the staphylococcal scalded skin syndrome, and the toxic shock syndrome. Furuncles and carbuncles often respond to incision and drainage procedures in addition to systemic antibiotics. In the acute phase of impetigo, saline or Burow's compresses help to decrease oozing and debride the crusts. Emollient lotions are useful during the desquamation phase of infections, such as the staphylococcal scalded skin syndrome and scarlet fever.

GRAM-NEGATIVE BACTERIAL INFECTIONS

The major gram-negative bacteria that cause infections with cutaneous manifestations are meningococcus, gonococcus, and the gram-negative rods that cause gram-negative folliculitis and hot tub dermatitis. *Gram-negative folliculitis* is an infection with gram-negative rods, especially Enterobacter, Klebsiella, Escherichia, Serratia, and Proteus, that usually occurs as a complication of acne vulgaris. Affected patients have taken oral antibiotics for prolonged periods. Most patients have superficial pustules without comedones on the cheeks, chin, and philtrum. Deep nodulocystic lesions are occasionally seen. Patients respond within weeks to ampicillin or trimethoprim-sulfamethoxazole treatment, which eliminates the causative bacteria. Isotretinoin (Accutane) has also been effective.

Hot tub dermatitis is a rash due to pseudomonas that appears within 2 days after exposure to infected hot tubs, whirlpool baths, and swimming pools. The eruption may be follicular, maculopapular, vesicular, pustular, or polymorphous and is distributed primarily on the lateral aspects of the trunk, the proximal extremities, buttocks, and in the axillae. Patients often have malaise, pruritus, discomfort of the eyes and throat, axillary adenopathy, and occasionally fever, external otitis, mastitis, nausea, vomiting, and abdominal cramps. The disorder is self-limited and lasts 7 to 10 days. Other cutaneous lesions caused by pseudomonas include otitis externa, toe web infections, cellulitis of the foot, and ecthyma gangrenosum. *Ecthyma gangrenosum* is a painless ulceration with a necrotic black eschar and surrounding erythema due to pseudomonas. The lesion is frequently located in the anogenital or axillary region and may be associated with pseudomonas septicemia. Debridement and systemic antibiotics are required.

Skin lesions develop in approximately two thirds of patients with meningococcemia or meningococcal meningitis. The cutaneous lesions may be macular erythema, morbilliform, urticarial, purpuric, or petechial. The petechiae are pinpoint lesions that may have a raised vesicular or pustular center. Lesions are most common on the trunk and extremities, but may also occur on the palms, soles, and mucosae. More fulminant meningococcal infections are often associated with extensive purpuric lesions and with large, well-circumscribed ecchymotic patches covering large areas of the body. Necrotic bullae may develop within the ecchymotic patches with resultant sloughing. Other features of acute meningococcemia include fever, irritability, myalgia, arthralgia, and hypotension. The cutaneous and visceral lesions are due to vasculitis of capillaries and venules. On histopathologic examination of lesional skin, the meningococcal organisms may be seen in blood vessel lumina, thrombi, neutrophils, and the endothelial cells.

Cutaneous lesions occur in more than 90% of patients with chronic meningococcemia, although this disorder is uncommon in children. Crops of erythematous macules and papules often appear with fever and develop purpuric, ulcerated centers. Myalgia and arthralgia are commonly present. The differential diagnosis of the cutaneous lesions includes Henoch–Schönlein purpura, Rocky Mountain spotted fever, gonococcemia, purpura fulminans, erythema multiforme, and typhoid fever. Intravenous penicillin (alternatively, chloramphenicol) is the preferred antibiotic, and patients with shock must be supported with fluids to increase circulating blood volume and vasopressor agents.

The skin lesions of gonococcemia resemble those of meningococcemia. They are small erythematous, hemorrhagic papules or vesiculopustules or petechiae, found primarily overlying the joints of the distal extremities. Lesions are also associated with fever, arthralgia, and myalgia and resolve spontaneously within a week. *Neisseria gonorrhoeae* may be found by a smear or culture of early cutaneous lesions. The preferred treatment is parenteral penicillin (alternatively, tetracycline).

ANNOTATED BIBLIOGRAPHY

Bach MC: Dermatologic signs in toxic shock syndrome—clues to diagnosis. J Am Acad Dermatol 8:343–347, 1983 (Review of the skin changes in the toxic shock syndrome)

Blankenship ML: Gram-negative folliculitis: Follow-up observations in 20 patients. Arch Dermatol 120:1301–1303, 1984 (Discussion of the complication of gram-negative folliculitis in patients with acne)

Chandrasekarm PH, Rolston KVI, Kannangara DW et al: Hot-tub associated dermatitis due to *Pseudomonas aeruginosa*: Case report and review of the literature. Arch Dermatol 120:1337–1340, 1984 (Review of the skin and systemic changes of hot tub dermatitis)

McCray MK, Esterly NB: Blistering distal dactylitis. J Am Acad Dermatol 5:592–594, 1981 (Discussion of the streptococcal infection of children, blistering distal dactylitis)

Tunnessen WW: Practical aspects of bacterial skin infections in children. Pediatr Dermatol 2:255–265, 1985 (Review of cutaneous bacterial infections and their management)

65

Superficial Dermatophyte and Yeast Infections

AMY PALLER

Superficial fungal and yeast infections are limited to the epidermis, hair, nails, and mucous membranes. The three common causes of these infections are dermatophytes (especially Trichophyton tonsurans), *Pityrosporum orbiculare* (tinea versicolor), and *Candida albicans*.

DERMATOPHYTOSES

The dermatophytoses can be subdivided, based on the location of the fungal infection into tinea capitis (scalp), tinea corporis (face and body), tinea cruris (groin), tinea pedis (feet), and tinea unguium (nails). Of these, tinea capitis and corporis are commonly seen in prepubertal children. Tinea cruris, tinea pedis, and tinea unguium almost always occur beyond the onset of puberty or in immunocompromised children.

Tinea Capitis

Tinea capitis is the most common dermatophytosis of childhood and usually affects prepubertal children from 2 to 10 years of age. Fewer than 5% of cases of tinea capitis occur in adults. More than 90% of cases are due to *Trichophyton tonsurans*, passed from human to human (anthropophilic), whereas the remaining less than 10% are mostly due to the zoophilic *Microsporum canis*. *T. tonsurans* affects black much more commonly than white children.

Pathophysiology. Fungal hyphae are transmitted from fallen hairs, scale, and shared fomites, such as combs, towels, and hats. The hyphae spread radially and penetrate the hair follicles from the site of initial infection. *T. tonsurans* spores are formed within the hair shaft (endothrix infection), whereas *M. canis* spores form on the surface of the hair shaft (ectothrix infection). Endothrix infections cause significant weakening of the hair shaft with fracture of the hair near the scalp, resulting in the "black dots" on the scalp. The hair bulb is usually preserved.

Clinical Presentation. The manifestations of tinea capitis due to *T. tonsurans* differ considerably from those of *M. canis* infections. Children with *M. canis* infections have well-demarcated areas of alopecia that fluoresce by Wood's lamp examination. *T. tonsurans* is more variable and often subtle in its appearance. It does not fluoresce. Approximately 20% of children with noninflammatory tinea capitis have the seborrheic type of *T. tonsurans* tinea capitis with fine white scaling and associated pruritus. Alopecia may only occur after years of scaling and infection and is then slowly progressive (Fig. 65-1). The scaling may be localized or generalized and is commonly mistaken for seborrheic dermatitis or atopic dermatitis. The black dots that are characteristic of *T. tonsurans* tinea capitis are seen in 40% of patients and are the best material for diagnosis. The black dots may be hidden under scale or may be almost imperceptible so that alopecia areata is mistakenly diagnosed. Kerions are boggy, erythematous, tender nodules with perifollicular pustules that develop on the scalp in 5% to 30% of patients as a hypersensitivity reaction to the fungus. They may be associated with lymphadenopathy, a generalized papular rash ("id" reaction), fever, and leukocytosis. They are often incorrectly thought to be bacterial cellulitis or folliculitis and are treated with antibacterial antibiotics. Cultures may grow *S. aureus*, but only antifungal agents eliminate the kerions. Many patients with tinea capitis have concurrent tinea corporis.

Differential Diagnosis. The scaling and pruritus of *T. tonsurans* infections may be confused with seborrheic dermatitis, atopic dermatitis, or even with psoriasis. In alopecia areata, the scalp is usually totally normal with a well-demarcated area of alopecia and no scaling, inflammation, or black dots. The black dots may be mistaken for the broken hair shafts of trichotillomania, but perifollicular hemorrhage is not present in tinea capitis. The kerions must be distinguished from bacterial folliculitis and cellulitis, and the appearance of a healing kerion may resemble morphea or the alopecia of discoid lupus erythematosus.

289

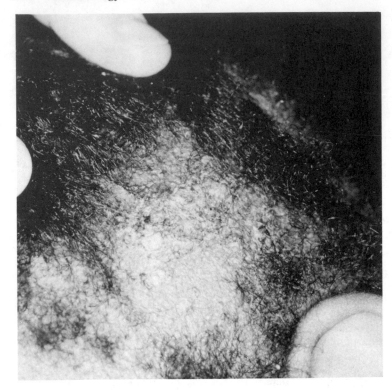

Figure 65-1. Alopecia and scaling of tinea capitis due to *Trichophyton tonsurans*.

Evaluation. The Wood's lamp has been used for years for making a diagnosis of tinea capitis, based on the fluorescence of hairs infected with *Microsporum*. With the marked preponderance of infections due to the nonfluorescent *T. tonsurans*, Wood's lamp examination is of minimal value. The diagnosis depends on the results of a potassium hydroxide (KOH) examination of infected hairs and fungal cultures. The most reliable source of infected hairs is the black dot, which may be found with a magnifying glass and extracted by forceps or gentle scraping with a scalpel or sterile toothbrush. Other hairs that are long enough to be pulled are rarely infected, but may have spores and hyphae at the base. KOH preparations are made by placing the specimens on a glass slide, adding a drop or two of 10% to 20% KOH, heating gently, and examining them under the microscope. The KOH dissolves the cellular material and enables hyphae and spores to be seen. The hyphae and spores are aligned within the hair shaft in parallel orientation in T. tonsurans endothrix infections. The fungi surround the hair shafts in *M. canis* infections.

Despite the result of KOH examination, a fungal culture should be performed. Specimens should be inoculated onto Sabouraud's agar with cyclohexi-

mide and chloramphenicol (Mycosel). Fungal growth is usually seen within 2 weeks. Dermatophyte test medium (DTM) contains a phenol red indicator that changes from yellow to red and allows a rapid diagnosis, but has a high rate of false-positive reactions from saprophytic fungi or bacteria.

When a diagnosis of tinea capitis is made, the entire body should be examined for evidence of tinea corporis. In addition, all family members should be examined for tinea, because untreated family members provide a continuing source of reinfection following adequate therapy. Dermatophytes are isolated from the scalps of 25% of family members.

Treatment. Tinea capitis infections must be treated with systemic griseofulvin. Ketoconazole appears to be equally effective, but may cause liver abnormalities and has not been fully tested in children. Topical antifungal agents are not curative and have no additive value. The microsize form of griseofulvin is available in a suspension of 125 mg/5 ml. The medication should be administered with fatty meals or milk at a single or twice daily dose of 15 mg/kg/day for 6 to 8 weeks. Patients should be followed at 3 to 4-week intervals to evaluate progress.

Children with tinea capitis may transmit the disorder until all spores are cleared. Spores may be cultured for 8 weeks after the initiation of griseofulvin alone. The use of sporicidal shampoos decreases the time that the child must be kept home from school or wear protective head covering. Sporicidal shampoos with selenium sulfide 2.5% (Selsun) clear spores after approximately 2 weeks. These shampoos should be left in contact with the scalp for 5 to 10 minutes after lathering and used 2 to 3 times weekly. Oiling of the hair after shampooing prolongs the carriage of infectious spores.

The use of systemic or intralesional steroids for children with kerions is controversial. Most dermatologists find that the incidence of scarring is negligible and hair regrowth is excellent after kerion resolution with griseofulvin alone. Secondary infection should be treated with erythromycin 30 to 50 mg/kg/day in four divided doses and Burow's compresses to the site to decrease oozing and crust formation.

Tinea Corporis

Tinea corporis is a superficial tinea infection of non-hair-bearing areas that is now usually caused by *T. tonsurans*, often in association with tinea capitis. Tinea corporis is characterized by one or more well-circumscribed scaly patches with a papular, vesicular, or pustular border ("ringworm") and central clearing. Lesions must be differentiated from the papulosquamous plaques of pityriasis rosea, nummular eczema, psoriasis, seborrheic dermatitis, contact dermatitis, tinea versicolor, and granuloma annulare. Any lesion suspected of being fungal should be scraped at the border and examined with KOH and culture. Limited tinea corporis is treated effectively with topical antifungal agents, such as clotrimazole, miconazole, and econazole, for 3 to 4 weeks or until 2 weeks after the clinical manifestations have cleared. For more extensive lesions, a course of griseofulvin should be administered (see tinea capitis).

Tinea Cruris

Tinea cruris (jock itch) is common in adolescent boys and affects the groin, intertriginous folds, and upper thighs. It is often pruritic, especially during hot, humid weather or physical exercise, or when wearing tight clothing. *Epidermophyton floccosum* and occasionally *Trichophyton rubrum* or *T. men-*tagrophytes are the responsible dermatophytes. Tinea pedis is commonly associated. The rash of tinea cruris is usually bilaterally symmetric, well-circumscribed, erythematous, and scaly with a raised border. Tinea cruris must be differentiated from seborrheic dermatitis, intertrigo, irritant or allergic contact dermatitis, psoriasis and erythrasma. The diagnosis is confirmed by KOH examination and culture of scales from the periphery. The fungal infection responds rapidly to topical antifungal agents, applied two to three times daily for 4 weeks. Adjunctive measures include the use of absorbent powders and loose-fitting clothing.

Tinea Pedis

Tinea pedis or athlete's foot is the most common tinea infection of adolescents and adults, but is rarely found in prepubertal children. *T. rubrum* and occasionally *E. floccosum* and *T. mentagrophytes* are the usual causative dermatophytes. Tinea pedis may manifest as a chronic scaling disorder with or without an increased horny layer, intertriginous inflammation, or vesiculopustules. The interdigital area is almost always involved with peeling and maceration of surrounding skin. The dorsum of the foot usually remains clear in contrast to the eruptions of contact and atopic dermatitis. Occasionally, erythema, scaling, and vesicles occur as an "id" reaction on the palms and sides of the fingers and less commonly on the trunk and extremities. Atopic dermatitis, dyshidrotic eczema, juvenile plantar dermatosis, and contact dermatitis must be distinguished by KOH examination and fungal culture. Tinea pedis may be treated with topical antimycotic agents. The warm, moist environment of the feet, however, predisposes patients to recurrent infections. Absorbent powders, such as Zeasorb or powders with undecylenic acid (Desenex) or tolnaftate (Tinactin), are helpful in decreasing moisture. Acute vesicular lesions should be dried and cooled with compresses (*e.g.*, Burow's) three times daily for 3 to 5 days. Severe tinea pedis infections may require systemic griseofulvin. "Id" reactions are best treated with compresses and topical corticosteroids.

Tinea Unguium

Tinea unguium is a chronic infection of the nails caused by *T. rubrum*, *T. mentagrophytes*, or *E. floccosum*. Tinea unguium is rarely seen in prepubertal children unless they are immunocompromised. The infection usually begins distally as a white or yellow patch of the nail. The nail becomes thickened and with subungual debris and friable. The most commonly confused entity is onychomycosis due to *Candida albicans* which is usually associated with paronychia. Fungal infections in children must also be distinguished from nail dystrophy associated with atopic dermatitis, psoriasis, trauma, lichen planus, twenty nail dystrophy of childhood, and ectodermal dysplasias, such as paronychia congenita and the nail-patella syndrome. Scrapings for KOH and culture should be taken from underside of the nail. Tinea unguium is difficult to eradicate and has a high recurrence rate. Topical agents are rarely curative, but help to control spread of the infection. Griseofulvin must be administered for 6 to 9 months for infections of the fingernails and 12 to 18 months for toenail infections. Patients taking griseofulvin for longer than 2 to 3 months should be monitored every 3 months for the rare development of hematologic and hepatic abnormalities.

Tinea Versicolor

Tinea versicolor (pityriasis versicolor) is a common infection caused by *Pityrosporon orbiculare*, a lipophilic yeast that is a normal inhabitant of the epidermis. The infection is most prevalent in adolescents, but may also occur in prepubertal children. Lesions appear during warm, humid weather due to overgrowth of the yeast and are characterized by multiple, coalescent round scaly erythematous macules (Fig. 65-2). The macules usually occur on the anterior and posterior trunk and on the proximal arms. The lesions become more pronounced because of pigmentary changes that result from postinflammatory hyperpigmentation or hypopigmentation due to the production by yeast of azelaic acid, an inhibitor of tyrosinase, an important enzyme for melanin synthesis. The eruption is occasionally pruritic, but is otherwise benign.

The differential diagnosis of tinea versicolor includes postinflammatory hypo- or hyperpigmentation, pityriasis alba, vitiligo, pityriasis rosea, and secondary syphilis. The diagnosis of tinea versicolor can usually be made clinically because of the characteristic appearance of the eruption. A KOH examination should be performed to confirm the diagnosis. Fungal hyphae and spores overlie epidermal cells in a typical, tightly-clustered "spaghetti and meat balls" pattern. Fungal cultures should not be performed, because the yeast is difficult to grow. Lesions fluoresce by Wood's lamp examination.

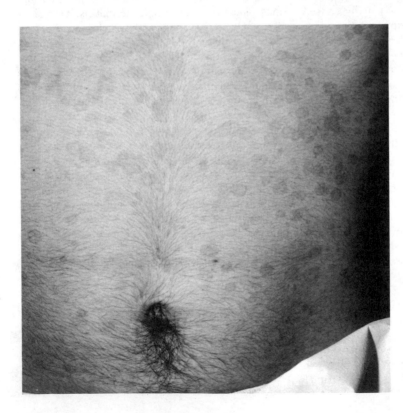

Figure 65-2. Round, scaling erythematous macules of tinea versicolor.

Tinea versicolor responds well to many topical agents. Selenium sulfide lotion 2.5% (Selsun lotion) is the most commonly used preparation. A thin layer may be applied to all affected areas, left on for ½ hour and washed. The lotion should be applied daily for 1 week, weekly for the next month and then monthly for 3 months. Since the infection is due to overgrowth of normal inhabitants of the skin, the lotion should also be applied once monthly during warm months (April through October in northern climates). Alternate therapies include twice daily application for 4 weeks of 25% sodium thiosulfate with 1% salicylic acid (Tinver lotion) or topical antifungal agents, such miconazole, econazole, and clotrimazole, and the monthly administration of a single oral dose of 200 mg to 400 mg ketoconazole.

CANDIDAL INFECTIONS

Candidiasis (moniliasis) is an infection of the skin, mucous membranes, and occasionally the viscera caused by *Candida albicans*. Although not normally found on the skin, candidal organisms may be normal inhabitants of the mucosal surfaces. Candidal infections are more common in neonates, and children with endocrinologic disorders (especially diabetes mellitus), trisomy 21, immunologic deficiencies, acrodermatitis enteropathica, leukemia, or lymphoma or children who are administered corticosteroids or other immunosuppressive agents and long-term systemic antibiotics. Candidal mucocutaneous infections may manifest in various forms (see also Chap. 89).

Oral candidiasis or thrush is especially common in infancy and is noted at the end of the first week of life in 5% of infants, presumably acquired from an infected maternal vaginal area. The lesions are white, curdlike adherent plaques that overlie inflammation of the tongue, buccal and gingival mucosae, and hard and soft palates. KOH preparations demonstrate egg-shaped budding yeast and hyphae or pseudohyphae (nonseptate). Nystatin oral suspension used four times daily for 1 to 2 weeks is effective therapy.

Cutaneous candidiasis usually affects warm, moist intertriginous areas. In the newborn, cutaneous candidiasis usually takes the form of diaper dermatitis (see Chap. 60), especially after the first week of life, with fiery erythema, scaling, and satellite papulovesicles in the diaper area. Occasionally, a congenital form occurs in which the lesions appear within a few days of birth, presumably from intrauterine exposure to candidal organisms. The

lesions of congenital candidiasis are scattered diffusely over the trunk, extremities, scalp, palms, and soles without aggregation in the diaper area. The oral mucosa is usually not involved. The lesions begin as erythematous macules that become papular, then pustular. Constitutional symptoms or signs of visceral involvement are rare, and the papulopustules tend to clear spontaneously with residual desquamation after approximately 1 week.

Erythema toxicum, staphylococcal pustulosis, transient neonatal pustulosis, neonatal herpes simplex, congenital syphilis, and Letterer–Siwe disease are included in the differential diagnosis and may be distinguished by smears and cultures of pustules and scales, as well as by lack of other clinical features. Although the eruption clears spontaneously, oral nystatin and topical anticandidal agents (nystatin, miconazole, clotrimazole) should be applied to decrease the number of cutaneous and gastrointestinal organisms.

Candidal vulvovaginitis is not an uncommon infection of adolescent girls who take contraceptives, systemic antibiotics or have diabetes mellitus. The labia are pruritic and brightly erythematous with white patches on the mucosae. There is often a thick white vaginal discharge. The infection may spread to the perineal and perianal areas and upper thighs. Miconazole cream inserted into the vagina nightly or vaginal tablets inserted twice daily are effective therapies.

Perleche or angular cheilitis is an irritant dermatitis of the corners of the mouth due to saliva. The dermatitis most commonly affects teenagers with braces and is best treated with vaseline and hydrocortisone ointment. Secondary infection by candida occasionally occurs and should be assessed by KOH examination and culture.

Candida paronychia develops most commonly in patients who immerse their hands frequently in warm water. It may also occur in newborns and infants in association with thrush and thumb sucking. The paronychial area is red and swollen, but is often painless. The nail is thickened and discolored. Secondary bacterial infection due to *S. aureus* or pseudomonas may occur. *Erosio interdigitalis blastomycetica* is also encouraged by moisture and is frequently associated with candida paronychia. The eruption affects the interdigital space, and is pruritic, erythematous, macerated, and fissured. Treatment includes the avoidance of moisture and the application of topical antibiotics and anticandidal preparations.

Chronic mucocutaneous candidiasis is a rare disorder due to a dysfunction of the immunologic response to candidal organisms. The disorder is occasionally associated with other immunologic deficiencies or with endocrinopathies, especially hypoparathyroidism and Addison's disease. Widespread candidal infections of the skin, mucous membranes, and nails begin in infancy or childhood. In addition to oral thrush and vaginitis, cutaneous lesions develop that are red and markedly scaly with serpiginous borders, especially on the extremities. The nail folds are chronically red and swollen with dystrophy of the nails. Associated visceral candidiasis is uncommon. In the past, anticandidal agents were either ineffective or dangerous. Ketoconazole clears the infections effectively and rarely causes side effects. Oral clotrimazole may also be efficacious.

INDICATIONS FOR REFERRAL

KOH examinations and cultures should be performed on all patients with suspected fungal and yeast infections. Unless a pediatrician feels competent in performing these examinations, both di-

agnosis and treatment should be managed by a dermatologist.

ANNOTATED BIBLIOGRAPHY

Chapel TA, Gagliardi C, Nichols W: Congenital cutaneous candidiasis. J Am Acad Dermatol 6:926–928, 1982 (Report of a case of congenital candidiasis and review of the clinical features)

DeVillez RL, Lewis CW: Candidiasis seminar. Cutis 19:69–83, 1977 (Review of the various clinical manifestations of candidal infections)

Krowchuk DP, Lucky AW, Primmer SI et al: Current status of the identification and management of tinea capitis. Pediatrics 72:625–631, 1983 (Well-written review of the evaluation and management of tinea capitis)

Solomon LM, Rippon JW, Lucky AW et al: Tinea capitis: Current concepts. Pediatr Dermatol 2:224–237, 1985 (Discussion by several dermatologists of how each treats tinea capitis)

Wyre HW, Johnson WT: Neonatal pityriasis versicolor. Arch Dermatol 117:752–753, 1981 (Tinea versicolor occurred in a 2-week-old infant)

66
Warts and Molluscum Contagiosum
AMY PALLER

Warts and molluscum are among the most common skin lesions found in children. Both are caused by DNA viruses that remain restricted to the epidermis and are transmitted by skin to skin contact. Both may be autoinoculated from one area of skin to another.

WARTS

Warts affect up to 10% of the school-aged children, with a peak incidence during adolescence. The virus that causes warts is a papillomavirus and has an incubation period of 1 to 6 months. The wart viruses have now been classified into more than 40 subgroups based on DNA homology, each one associated with a particular clinical type of wart.

Clinical Types

There are four common clinical types of warts: verruca vulgaris, verruca plantaris, verruca plana, and condyloma acuminatum. Verrucae vulgaris or

common warts are found usually on the hands of children and adolescents, although they may be found anywhere on the body, especially at sites of local trauma and autoinoculation. Verrucae vulgaris are most commonly round with finger-like projections initially (papillomatous) and become markedly rough and hyperkeratotic (verrucous) with time. Within the warts are multiple, tiny black dots that represent thrombosed capillaries. Filiform verrucae vulgaris are long, thin, filamentous warts that are found usually on the face, neck, nasolabial region, and eyelids. Periungual and subungual verrucae vulgaris occur around and under the nails, especially on the hands. Because of the location of periungual and subungual warts at sites of trauma, these warts grow easily and become irritated. They may become secondarily infected and are difficult to eradicate.

Verrucae plantaris or plantar warts occur on the weight-bearing areas of the heels, soles, and metatarsal heads. Because of the location of weight-bearing areas, they extend deeply into the epidermis and develop a smooth horny surface, rather than becoming raised and verrucous. They may become extremely uncomfortable as they enlarge. Plantar warts may be single, but more commonly are mother–daughter warts (primary central warts with satellite warts) or mosaic warts (thick plaques of coalescent small warts, usually found on the heels and soles). Plantar warts must be differentiated from calluses, corns, and scars. Calluses and corns are localized areas of hyperkeratosis that form at points of pressure, especially at the metatarsophalangeal joints. The distinction may be made by paring the lesions. Calluses and corns have a central hard core but no thrombosed capillaries, which appear as tiny black dots. In addition, calluses and corns tend to be most tender to direct pressure, in contrast to maximal tenderness with lateral pressure to warts. Scars result from thickening of the dermis and are thus not hyperkeratotic and easily pared. They have neither a central core nor thrombosed capillaries. Talon noir or black heel must also be distinguished from plantar warts. This condition is most common in teenaged athletic boys, due to capillary rupture. Clusters of brown or black pinpoint hemorrhages are found on the heel or lateral aspects of the feet. The hemorrhages are localized to the horny layer and when the skin is pared, the hemorrhages disappear.

Verrucae plana or flat warts are flat, smooth, slightly elevated warts that range in size from 2 mm to 5 mm (Fig. 66-1). They are most commonly found on the face, arms, and legs. Flat warts are usually multiple and hundreds may be present. Flat warts often coalesce to form small plaques or spread in a linear array by autoinoculation.

Condyloma acuminatum or genital warts are moist, cauliflower-like warts that are found on the mucous membranes and mucocutaneous junctions of the anogenital and inguinal areas (Fig. 66-2). Less commonly, these warts are seen in the mouth, at the urethral meatus, and on the conjunctivae. Genital warts become white and macerated rather than scaly due to their location in moist occluded areas. Before 20 years of age, condyloma acuminatum are found usually on sexually active adolescents, but may also be noted on younger children. Although infants may develop the warts after an incubation period of 1 to 20 months from contact with maternal genital warts during delivery, any child with condyloma acuminatum must be suspected for child abuse and medical and social investigations for abuse must be performed. Laryngeal papillomatosis in infants is contracted during passage of the infant through a maternal genital area that is infected with condyloma virus. The laryngeal papillomas occur on the vocal cords and laryngeal mucosa and may extend into the trachea and bronchi, leading to hoarseness and airway obstruction. Condyloma acuminatum must be distinguished from condyloma lata of secondary syphilis. Condyloma lata are more broad-based, flattened, and smooth than condyloma acuminatum.

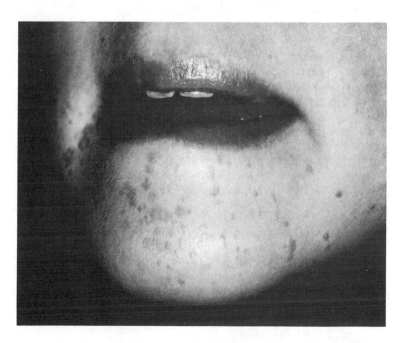

Figure 66-1. Flat warts on the chin of a teenager.

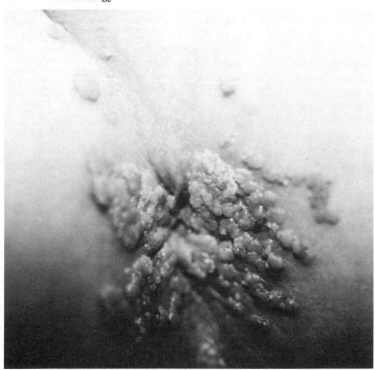

Figure 66-2. Perianal condyloma acuminatum in a 2-year-old boy who was sexually abused.

Treatment

Warts in children have a high spontaneous rate of involution. Twenty-five percent of warts clear by 6 months and 65% of warts clear without therapy by 2 years. Warts that are painful, subject to trauma, enlarging, or cosmetically objectionable should be treated.

No single therapy is effective for warts. Regardless of the form of management selected, warts have up to a 10% recurrence risk. Plantar, periungual, and subungual warts are the most recalcitrant to therapy. Treatment must be adjusted to the maturity and tolerance of the child, since therapies such as liquid nitrogen and electrodessication are painful, but treatment modalities such as cantharidin, salicylic acid, and podophyllin are painless on application.

The most commonly used agents for treating warts are *keratolytic preparations* with salicylic and lactic acids. These preparations (such as Duofilm, which is a combination of 16.7% salicylic acid and 16.7% lactic acid in flexible collodion) are best applied nightly, or twice daily for thick warts, after soaking the affected area to increase permeability.

High concentrations of salicylic and lactic acids are most useful for verrucae vulgaris and plantar warts and are often used alone or in conjunction with cryotherapy. Preparations with lower concentrations of acids (5%) are useful for flat warts. The acids should be applied with a toothpick or wooden applicator directly to the wart with avoidance of surrounding normal skin. If irritation develops, the medication should be stopped for a few days and subsequently applied less frequently. Results are usually noticeable within 3 to 4 weeks. *Forty percent salicylic acid plasters* are useful for plantar warts. The plasters should be cut to the size of the wart and left on for 5 days. Between applications of the plaster, the foot should be soaked in water and pared or rubbed with a pumice stone to remove the excessive horny layer. *Tretinoin (Retin-A)* may be effective for flat warts, probably because it is irritating and causes peeling. The cream of gel may be applied twice daily in increasing concentrations until mild irritation develops.

All other therapy must be applied at the physician's office, preferably by a dermatologist. *Cryotherapy with liquid nitrogen* (-197°C) is highly effective for all forms of warts, although it is painful. Liquid nitrogen is applied to the lesion until the warts and the area surrounding the warts are white. The freezing induces intraepidermal blistering within a week, which removes the wart but leaves the junctional zone of skin intact. Pigmentary changes may result, especially in dark-skinned children, but scarring does not occur.

Cantharidin is a potent blistering agent that derives from beetles and is available as a 0.7% solution in acetone and flexible collodion (Cantharone). Cantharidin is particularly effective for plantar warts and periungual warts, but may induce a ring of satellite warts at the periphery of the primary lesion. Cantharidin is applied with a toothpick or wooden applicator and is allowed to dry, covered with adhesive tape. For thick warts, the adhesive may be removed after 24 to 48 hours. An intraepidermal blister is formed which eliminates the wart and causes no scarring. The adhesive should be removed and the lesion washed before 24 hours if irritation develops, to decrease the risk of excessive blistering.

Bleomycin injected directly into warts is a highly effective therapy, but should be used only for warts that are resistant to more conventional means of treatment. The lesions become necrotic and clear within a few weeks. Scarring rarely occurs. Bleomycin is especially useful for plantar and periungual warts.

Podophyllum resin is a antimitotic cytotoxin that is useful for condyloma acuminatum on mucosal surfaces. A 20% solution in tincture of benzoin is applied to lesions and washed after 4 to 6 hours. Podophyllum is toxic to the kidneys and nervous system and should not be used in large amounts, especially in children. Podophyllum is contraindicated in pregnant women. The therapy may be repeated weekly to monthly, but alternate methods of treatment, such as cryotherapy, electrodessication and curettage, or the application of trichloracetic acid, should be used for condylomas if the lesions do not respond readily. In addition, recurrent or recalcitrant condyloma acuminatum should prompt investigation for condylomas of the anal mucosae by proctoscopy.

The excision of warts is not recommended, but other methods of removing wart tissue, including *electrodessication* and *curettage* and *laser*, are highly effective. Electrodessication and curettage are especially useful for large single warts and require previous injection with lidocaine (Xylocaine). Laser therapy has been highly effective for plantar warts and recalcitrant condyloma acuminatum.

MOLLUSCUM CONTAGIOSUM

The lesions of molluscum are caused by a poxvirus that replicates in the cytoplasm of epidermal cells. The lesions are seen most commonly in children between the ages of 3 and 16, although it has been reported as early as the first week of life. The incubation period is 2 weeks to 6 months. The virus may be contracted in swimming pools as well as by direct skin to skin transmission.

Clinical Presentation

Molluscum are discrete, smooth, pearly, or flesh-colored papules on a mildly erythematous base (Fig. 66-3). The center is often umbilicated, especially in larger lesions, and contains a milky white material with virus and epidermal cells. The papules are usually found on the trunk, axillary, antecubital and crural areas and face. The lesions begin as tiny papules and enlarge up to 3 cm in diameter. Papules may be noted in a linear array due to autoinoculation. Hundreds of papules may be found on patients with atopic dermatitis and in immunologically compromised children. Molluscum are found occasionally on mucosal surfaces, including the oral mucosae and conjunctivae.

Patients may complain of pruritus and excoriations may be seen, especially in children with atopic dermatitis. Dermatitis often surrounds the molluscum. Molluscum may occur near the eyelids and on the conjunctival mucosa, leading to conjunctivitis and superficial keratitis. In addition, lesions may become secondarily infected with staphylococcal or streptococcal organisms.

The differential diagnosis of molluscum includes chickenpox, intradermal nevi, juvenile xanthogranuloma, warts, and milia. Secondarily infected molluscum may be confused with primary pyoderma. Characteristic eosinophilic intracytoplasmic inclusion bodies (molluscum bodies) are found on histopathologic specimens of lesions or smears of the central white material.

Treatment

The treatment of molluscum depends on the age of the patient and the size and distribution of lesions. Although the lesions are self-limited and last from 2 weeks to 1½ years, they spread readily, are a source of secondary bacterial infection, and are cosmetically objectionable. As a result, they should usually be removed.

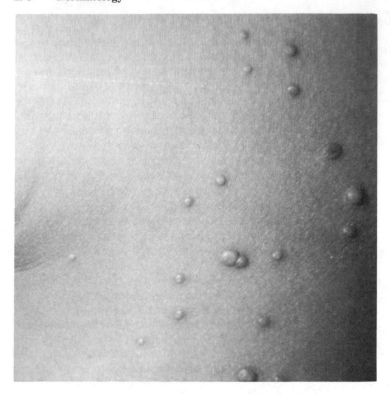

Figure 66-3. Dome-shaped papules of molluscum contagiosum, some with central umbilication.

Most therapeutic regimens for molluscum require destruction of the lesions. Cantharidin is useful for younger children because its application does not cause pain. In contrast to the response of keratotic warts to cantharidin, molluscum lesions blister easily, often within hours after application, and must be washed as soon as blistering begins. Cantharidin should never be used in intertriginous areas or on the face, because the extent of blistering is poorly controllable. As with warts, cryotherapy is helpful and light freezing at intervals of 2 to 3 weeks will eradicate lesions effectively. Individual lesions may be removed by piercing the center of each papule with a needle to remove the viral material or by curettage. Cryotherapy and removal of individual lesions by physical means are both acceptable for facial lesions.

Indications for Referral

Children with warts and molluscum may be referred to a dermatologist if the primary care physician is uncomfortable with the therapy, or if the treatment has been unsuccessful. A gastroenterologist may be consulted to perform proctoscopy in children with condyloma acuminatum in the perianal area. Patients with warts and molluscum should be followed for a period of months for the development of more lesions or recurrent lesions, in view of the viral incubation periods.

ANNOTATED BIBLIOGRAPHY

DeJong AR, Weiss JC, Brent RL: Condyloma acuminatum in children. Am J Dis Child 136:704–706, 1982 (This article reviews 34 cases of condylomas in prepubertal children and stresses the need to consider child abuse.)

Jarratt M: Viral infections of the skin. Pediatr Clin North Am 25:348–355, 1976 (Review of the clinical features and treatment of warts and molluscum.)

Lutzner MA: The human papillomaviruses. Arch Dermatol 119:631–635, 1983 (Discussion of the different subgroups of papillomaviruses.)

Sanders BB, Stretcher GS: Warts: Diagnosis and treatment. JAMA 235:2859–2861, 1976 (Well-written review of the clinical features of warts and their therapy.)

Viral exanthems are generalized or localized cutaneous eruptions that are commonly confused with drug reactions. The rashes may take the form of macules, papules, vesicles, petechiae and purpura, and urticaria. An enanthem and other evidence of viral infection may be associated.

PATHOPHYSIOLOGY

Viral exanthems are often generalized and result from hematogenous dissemination of virus to the skin and cutaneous blood vessels. Alternatively, the rash may represent a hypersensitivity reaction to the virus. Viruses may also reach the skin by nerve fibers, leading to the cutaneous localization of herpes simplex or herpes zoster infections. The reason for the specific distribution of certain viral exanthems, such as the peripheral distribution of Coxsackie virus A16 in the hand, foot, and mouth syndrome or the central localization of echovirus infections, is unknown.

CLINICAL MANIFESTATIONS

Erythematous macular exanthems without papules are unusual and are most commonly related to echovirus infections. Occasionally, the rash of infectious mononucleosis seen in association with ampicillin administration is generalized, macular, and confluent. More commonly, the rash is maculopapular. *Maculopapular eruptions* are the most common form of viral exanthem. The rash may be discrete maculopapules (rubelliform) or confluent maculopapules (morbilliform). The most common cause of maculopapular exanthems is enterovirus, especially echovirus 9. The eruption is usually rubelliform. It starts on the head and upper trunk and spreads peripherally. Fever and aseptic meningitis may be associated. Adenoviruses are a common cause of upper respiratory tract infections in children. Two to 8% of infections are associated with maculopapular rashes that are usually rubelliform. Rhinovirus, influenza viruses, respiratory syncytial virus, and parainfluenza viruses also cause rubelliform eruptions that clear within 2 to 3 days.

Papular eruptions associated with viral infections may manifest as *papular acrodermatitis of childhood* (PAC), a self limited disorder of children characterized by the sudden appearance of nonpruritic flat-topped, flesh-colored to erythematous papules on the extensor extremities, face, and buttocks. PAC was originally described with hepatosplenomegaly, lymphadenopathy, and anicteric hepatitis due to hepatitis B (*Gianotti–Crosti syndrome*). PAC has also been associated with several other viruses, including Epstein–Barr virus, parainfluenza virus, Coxsackie A16, and hepatitis A. The eruption is often preceded by upper respiratory tract symptoms, including fever, cough, and rhinitis. The lesions clear spontaneously after about 2 weeks to 2 months. Children with the eruption of PAC should be questioned about a recent history of an upper respiratory infection and should be evaluated for hepatosplenomegaly and lymphadenopathy. Liver enzyme levels and serologic studies for hepatitis A and B, Epstein–Barr, Coxsackie, and parainfluenza viruses should be performed. No treatment is necessary.

The most common *vesicular exanthem* is chickenpox (see Chap. 197). Generalized vesiculopustular exanthems that heal without crusting have been described with enterovirus infections. Localized vesicles are typical of hand, foot, and mouth disease, and herpes simplex and zoster infections. *Petechiae* and *purpura* may be due to direct damage or immunologic damage by the virus. Alternatively, petechiae may be the manifestation of thrombocytopenia, most common with rubella infections. Petechiae and purpura may be seen with echovirus 9 infections. Bacterial infections, particularly meningococcemia, and rickettsial infections must be considered in the differential diagnosis. *Urticarial eruptions* have been described with infectious mononucleosis, enterovirus infections, mumps, and hepatitis B.

SPECIFIC VIRAL INFECTIONS WITH DISTINCT MORPHOLOGIES

Measles (rubeola) is a disorder of considerable morbidity and mortality that is due to a paramyxovirus. Measles is rarely encountered now because of the vaccination. The incubation period is 10 to 14 days. The prodromal phase, the period of greatest contagion, begins with malaise, headache, cough, coryza, photophobia, conjunctivitis, and a fever that rises during a 4-day period. The classic enanthem (Koplik spots) appears 2 days after the onset of other symptoms and is often gone by the time that the exanthem develops. Koplik spots are tiny white papules, resembling grains of salt, overlying bright red buccal and lower labial mucosae. The vivid red-purple maculopapular rash is discrete at first, but quickly becomes confluent. It begins on the scalp, forehead, and neck and spreads towards the feet over a 3-day period. The rash begins to clear after 4 days, first on the face, and resolves with fine branny desquamation and hyperpigmentation. Generalized lymphadenopathy, especially of the cervical nodes, pharyngitis, otitis media, pneumonia, laryngotracheitis, vomiting, and diarrhea may be seen in association. Subacute sclerosing panencephalitis and encephalitis are rare complications. *Atypical measles* occurs in patients who have been immunized against measles, especially with inactivated virus, and are subsequently exposed to measles. The inactivated virus has not been used since 1967, except in immunocompromised patients. The disorder begins with marked fever for 2 to 3 days, headaches, and myalgia. The exanthem starts peripherally and either does not progress or advances in a cephalad direction, in contrast to the course of typical measles. In addition to erythematous maculopapules, vesicles and petechiae may be seen. Koplik spots do not occur, but edema of the extremities and a typical nodular pneumonia are common. The illness lasts for 1 to 3 weeks.

Rubella (German measles) is also rare due to vaccination. The virus is spread by respiratory droplets with an incubation period of 14 to 21 days. The exanthem is usually the first sign of the illness and lasts between 1 and 5 days. It is characterized by generalized, discrete pink maculopapules that first appear on the face and then spread to the trunk and extremities as the facial rash fades. An enanthem (Forchheimer's sign) is characterized by petechiae on the soft palate and may be seen in up to 20% of patients early in the course. In younger children, slight fever and lymphadenopathy, especially of the suboccipital and postauricular nodes, are associated features. Adolescents and adults often have a prodromal period with fever, headache, coryza, sore throat, mild conjunctivitis, and malaise. Arthritis, particularly of the small joints of the hands and feet, is occasionally a complication of older children and adults. Purpura and encephalitis are also rarely reported.

The most severe complication of rubella is *congenital rubella* by transplacental infection of the fetus during pregnancy. Affected infants are small for gestational age and may have a typical triad of deafness, congenital cataracts, and congenital heart disease. Other features include hyperbilirubinemia, hepatosplenomegaly, thrombocytopenic purpura, pneumonia, bone defects, and meningoencephalitis. "Blueberry muffin" lesions are multiple purple palpable macules or nodules that are noted at birth or within the first 24 hours. Blueberry muffin lesions are located usually on the head, neck, extremities, and trunk and range in size from 2 mm to 8 mm. On histopathologic examination, the lesions show aggregates of non-nucleated and nucleated erythrocytes in the dermis, due to dermal erythropoiesis. Dermal erythropoiesis and blueberry muffin lesions may also be seen in neonates with toxoplasmosis, cytomegalovirus infection, leukemia, and Rh incompatibilities. In rubella, the lesions clear after approximately 1 month. (For a more extensive discussion on these and other congenital infections, see Chapter 191.)

Roseola infantum (exanthem subitum) is the most common exanthem of children under 3 years of age. A single etiologic virus has not been identified, and the response has been related to several viruses, including echoviruses, Coxsackie virus, and adenovirus. The disorder is characterized by high fevers with rapid defervescence when the rash appears on the third or fourth day. The exanthem consists of small pale pink discrete macules or maculopapules that last only 1 to 2 days. The child is otherwise well, but periorbital edema is common. Leukopenia with relative lymphocytosis is common at the time of the rash. Febrile seizures may be associated.

Erythema infectiosum (fifth disease) affects children between the ages of 3 and 12 years. It is characterized by three stages. The first stage develops suddenly as an erythematous blush of the malar area (slapped cheek appearance). The next day the second stage develops, which is a maculopapular rash on the extensor surfaces of the extremities and occasionally on the trunk and buttocks. After about 6 days as this rash fades, the third stage develops and the characteristic lacy pattern of macular erythema is seen. The lacy pattern persists for a few days to a week, but frequently reappears after sun exposure, friction, or temperature change. Constitutional symptoms are mild and no enanthem is associated. Parvoviruses have been implicated as causative.

Hand, foot, and mouth disease is a distinctive disorder caused by Coxsackie A16 and occasionally Coxsackie A5 or A10. The illness is characterized by a fever and a vesicular eruption that follows a 3- to 6-day incubation period, occasionally associated with malaise, low-grade fever, sore throat, and abdominal discomfort. The enanthem begins first with small red macules that rapidly progress to vesicles and then ulcers on an erythematous base. The oral lesions may be seen on the buccal mucosae, tongue, gingivae, soft and hard palates, uvula, and tonsillar pillars. Up to two thirds of affected children have characteristic vesicular lesions on the hands and feet, especially on the dorsal surfaces. The lesions begin as maculopapules and progress to superficial elliptical vesicles surrounded by a red border. Occasionally, high fever, diarrhea, arthralgias, and adenopathy are associated.

Infectious mononucleosis is a common infection in adolescents, but is rare in younger children. It is caused by the Epstein–Barr virus. The illness begins with headache, fever, and malaise followed by pharyngitis. Lymphadenopathy is generalized, although most notable of the cervical nodes. Over one half of patients have splenomegaly, and hepatomegaly is not uncommon. A maculopapular (or occasionally macular) confluent eruption develops in 10% to 15% of patients after approximately 5 days. The trunk and upper arms are most frequently involved, and the eruption tends to persist for a few days. Other cutaneous manifestations of infectious mononucleosis include urticaria, eyelid edema, and the development of a generalized maculopapular rash in almost 90% of patients after ampicillin, and occasionally penicillin, administration. Twenty-five percent of patients develop an enanthem 1 to 2 weeks after the onset of the disorder characterized by discrete petechiae at the junction of the hard and soft palates.

Herpes simplex cutaneous and mucosal infections may be "primary" in patients without previous exposure or circulating antibodies, or "recurrent" when the infection develops again in the area of the primary infection. Primary infections occur most commonly in children between the ages of 1 and 5 years by close contact with infected adults and other children. Primary infections tend to be more painful, extensive, and of longer duration than recurrent infections. The incubation period is 3 to 10 days. Most children and adolescents have primary herpetic gingivostomatitis or recurrent herpes labialis, and the infection is usually due to type 1 herpes simplex. Primary gingivostomatitis begins with fever, sore throat, and irritability followed by the development of painful grouped vesicles overlying erythema on the gingivae, buccal mucosae, tongue, palate, and lips. The vesicles ulcerate and form white plaques overlying marked mucosal erythema. Cervical lymphadenopathy is associated. The fever disappears after approximately 4 days, but the oral lesions of primary herpes persist for up to 2 weeks. Primary herpetic gingivostomatitis must be differentiated from aphthous stomatitis, hand, foot, and mouth disease, erythema multiforme, Vincent's infection, and Behcet's disease (see Chap. 87).

The recurrent infection is due to reactivation of quiescent viruses from regional spinal ganglia and usually manifests as a "cold sore" or "fever blister" with localized grouped vesicles on the lower lip. A few hours to a few days before the eruption appears, patients complain of a burning sensation or itching at the site. Erythema and swelling develop first, followed by vesicles that rapidly become pustular and crusted after 2 to 3 days. Trauma to the lips, sun exposure, menstruation, and stress often precipitate recurrent lesions. Systemic toxicity is not usually associated, and the lesions resolve after 7 to 10 days. Erythema multiforme may be associated with recurrent herpes labialis as a hypersensitivity reaction that follows the herpetic eruption by 7 to 10 days. Painful erosions in the mouth and on the lips and the classic target lesions of the extremities and trunk are the manifestations of erythema multiforme (see Chap. 63).

Herpetic vulvovaginitis and *herpes progenitalis* are rare in children, but are occasionally found in sexually active adolescents. Usually herpes simplex virus type 2 is responsible. The primary forms are characterized by burning pain, edema, grouped vesiculopustules and ulcerations, usually on the vaginal mucosa, labia, or perineum in the girl and on the penile shaft or perineum in the boy. Fever, malaise, and regional lymphadenopathy are usually associated. The lesions form crusts within 7 days and clear in 2 to 4 weeks. Recurrent genital infections in the boy are usually on the prepuce, glans, or sulcus, and in the girl on the labia, vulva, clitoris, or cervix. The lesions tend to be more localized than in the primary forms, and constitutional symptoms or lymphadenopathy are mild. Recurrent lesions usually heal after about 8 days (see Chap. 120).

Primary cutaneous inoculation herpes may appear anywhere on the body, but is most common on the finger (*herpetic whitlow*). The virus is inoculated into traumatized skin of the finger and develops into a painful vesiculopustule or bulla with surrounding erythema. The pain subsides after approximately 1 week, but lesions commonly take up to 3 weeks to resolve.

Eczema herpeticum or Kaposi's varicelliform eruption is a widespread eruption of cutaneous herpes lesions in patients with underlying atopic dermatitis, Darier's disease, or bullous ichthyosiform erythroderma. Clusters of vesicles develop on areas of abnormal skin and spread during a period of about a week (Fig. 67-1). The coalescence of grouped vesicles into sheets of pustules overlying erythema is not uncommon. The lesions often become secondarily infected with bacteria. Lymphadenopathy and fever are usually associated, especially in primary herpetic infections. The lesions heal spontaneously in 2 to 3 weeks. Visceral dissemination is unusual, but occasionally patients demonstrate evidence of hepatic involvement or meningoencephalitis.

Neonatal herpes infections occur in 1 in 3000 to 1 in 15,000 deliveries. The disease is usually caused by type 2 herpes simplex virus, acquired at or immediately before delivery. Infections may be disseminated, with infections involving the viscera with or without involvement of the central nervous system (CNS), or may be localized, involving the CNS, skin, eyes, or mouth. Skin vesicles are seen in 70% to 80% of affected neonates and are often the initial manifestation and the clue to the correct diagnosis. Other features include microcephaly, seizures, respiratory distress with pneumonitis, hepatitis with jaundice, conjunctivitis and petechiae and ecchymoses (see Chap. 191).

DIAGNOSIS OF HERPES SIMPLEX

Rapid diagnosis of herpes simplex can be made by a Tzanck smear. The base of the vesicle is scraped and applied to a slide, which is stained with hematoxylin and eosin, methylene blue, Wright's stain, or Giemsa stain. Multinucleated giant cells and occasionally intranuclear inclusions may be seen. The Tzanck smear is usually not positive once the lesions have become crusted, and cannot differentiate herpes simplex from varicella and herpes zoster. Viral isolation by a culture of scrapings from the base of vesicles is the definitive diagnostic

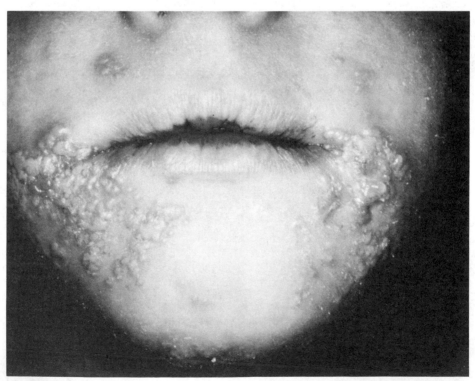

Figure 67-1. Grouped vesiculopustules of herpes simplex in a girl with severe atopic dermatitis and eczema herpeticum.

method and distinguishes herpes simplex from herpes varicella-zoster. A rising serum antibody titer between acute and convalescent sera is necessary to distinguish between primary and recurrent infections.

THERAPY OF HERPES SIMPLEX INFECTIONS

Mucocutaneous herpetic infections are best treated topically by compresses (*e.g.*, Burow's 1:20 to 1:40) three times daily to decrease drainage and relieve discomfort, followed by the application of topical antibiotics, such as Polysporin ointment. If secondary bacterial infection develops, oral antistaphylococcal antibiotics, such as erythromycin or dicloxacillin, must be administered. Oral and topical acyclovir decrease the duration and shedding of primary infections, but have little effect on recurrent oral lesions. Oral acyclovir for preventing recurrent genital herpes may be indicated in particularly severe cases. Topical acyclovir must be applied 5 to 6 times daily, and oral acyclovir has not yet been approved for children less than 12 years of age. The use of acyclovir for primary infections does not prevent recurrences. Oral anesthetics, such as liquid benadryl or 2% xylocaine viscous, decrease the discomfort of oral lesions.

Intravenous acyclovir and vidarabine (Ara-A) decrease the morbidity and dissemination of virus in immunocompromised patients. Trials of the efficacy of oral agents are in progress. At this time, intravenous acyclovir is the preferred drug for immunocompromised patients, including patients receiving immunosuppressants or chemotherapy, patients with eczema herpeticum with evidence of cutaneous or visceral dissemination, and neonates with herpes infections.

Despite the fact that intravenous acyclovir and vidarabine decrease the morbidity and mortality of herpes simplex infections in the neonate, prevention remains the best management. Women with a history of herpes genitalis or with sexual partners with herpes should have weekly cervical and vaginal cultures for herpes beginning no later than 1 month before anticipated delivery. If a woman has clinically apparent lesions or a positive culture within 2 weeks of delivery, the baby should be delivered by cesarean section within 4 hours after rupture of the membranes. If a baby is delivered vaginally from a high-risk mother, fetal scalp monitoring should be avoided to prevent direct inoculation at the site of the monitor. If any suspicion exists that an infant may have been exposed to herpes from an infected mother, serial viral cultures should be obtained from the eyes, mouth, and any skin vesicles, gloves and gowns should be worn and the neonate must be kept from contact with other neonates.

Chickenpox (varicella) is a highly contagious disease of children caused by the herpes varicella-zoster virus. After an incubation period of 10 to 14 days, low-grade fever, malaise, and the characteristic exanthem appear. The exanthem consists of nongrouped erythematous macules that become papular, then vesicular and within 24 hours, ulcerated and crusted. Typically, lesions of various sizes and stages are found in the same vicinity and continue to appear during a 3- to 5-day period. Lesions begin on the trunk, scalp, and face and are pruritic. Involvement of the distal extremities is minimal. Secondarily infected or deeply excoriated lesions may become scars. Ulcers may be present on mucous membranes, especially on the pharynx, palate, and tonsillar pillars. In adults and immunocompromised individuals, chickenpox is usually more severe with hemorrhagic or bullous lesions and disseminated infection, including viral pneumonitis (see Chap. 197).

Herpes zoster (shingles) is the recurrent form of varicella due to reactivation of virus in the dorsal root ganglia through peripheral nerves to the skin. Herpes zoster in children is uncommon and is usually associated with less morbidity than in adults. The risk of developing herpes zoster is greater in children with acute lymphocytic leukemia and children who had chickenpox during the first year of life. Grouped dermatomal erythematous papules rapidly become vesicles and then pustules. New vesicles continue to appear for approximately 7 days and then become crusted. The thoracic and lumbar dermatomes are usually involved. Scattered lesions may be seen outside of the dermatomal borders. In contrast to adults, children with herpes zoster rarely have a prodrome of discomfort or erythema at the dermatomal site. The eruption clears after 2 to 3 weeks. Lymphadenopathy is common, but children rarely develop fever, headache, or postherpetic neuralgia. The lesions of herpes zoster have varicella-zoster virus, so that chickenpox may be transmitted to a susceptible individual. There is no evidence that herpes zoster itself is transmissible. Immunosuppressed individuals may develop dissemination of herpes zoster with widespread lesions, pneumonitis, hepatitis, meningoencephalitis, and purpura fulminans.

The treatment of varicella and herpes zoster is

similar to that of herpes simplex. Shake lotions, such as calamine, or compresses may be useful in drying the lesions of varicella and decreasing pruritus. The dermatomal vesicles of herpes zoster should be managed with compresses and topical antibiotics. Topical corticosteroids creams are useful in diminishing pruritus and inflammation after lesions have crusted. The risk of developing varicella zoster in immunocompromised patients who are exposed to the varicella-zoster virus may be decreased by the administration of zoster-immune globulin. Patients who develop disseminated varicella zoster should be given intravenous acyclovir. A varicella vaccine is currently being tested.

ANNOTATED BIBLIOGRAPHY

Chadwick EG, Shulman ST: Advances in antiviral therapy: Acyclovir. Pediatr Dermatol 2:64–70, 1984 (Review of the status of acyclovir.)

Cherry JD: Viral exanthems. Curr Prob Pediatr XIII:5–44, 1983 (Review of viral exanthems, including skin manifestations.)

Gianotti F: Papular acrodermatitis of childhood and other papulovesicular acrolocated syndromes. Br J Dermatol 100:49–59, 1979 (Discussion of the association of papular acrodermatitis and hepatitis B infections.)

Jarratt M: Herpes simplex infection. Arch Dermatol 119:99–103, 1983 (Review of the clinical and epidemiologic features of herpes infections.)

68
Vascular Nevi

AMY PALLER

Vascular disorders occur in 20% to 40% of newborn infants. These lesions are benign tumors due to faulty communication of angioblastic tissue with surrounding vessels. Telangiectasias are ectatic vessels, and hemangiomas and lymphangiomas are a collection of proliferating endothelium-lined vessels. Although usually confined to the skin, vascular nevi are occasionally associated with systemic complications or as a feature of various syndromes.

STRAWBERRY AND CAVERNOUS HEMANGIOMAS

Hemangiomas vary from small harmless patches to large mutilating and occasionally life-threatening lesions. They are proliferations of immature blood vessels, thought to result from abnormalities at about the 30th day of development. The proliferation of hemangiomas may be due to an angiogenesis factor. In addition, mast cells are thought to participate in hemangioma growth, because they are found in large numbers in biopsies of proliferating but not involuting lesions.

The most common form of hemangioma is the *capillary* ("*strawberry*") *hemangioma* that is characterized as a raised red, firm, well-circumscribed, partially compressible lesion. The face, scalp, and thorax are the usual sites. Most capillary hemangiomas are not present at birth, but appear within the first month or two after birth. The initial lesion may appear as fine telangiectasias surrounded by pallor or as an erythematous patch that resembles nevus flammeus. The surface often develops a lobulated texture as the lesion expands and becomes more elevated during the first 3 months of life. Capillary hemangiomas may be confused with *pyogenic granulomas*, common vascular lesions that are bright red firm, raised, slightly pedunculated papules. Pyogenic granulomas are often associated with focal trauma or infection and are thought to present a reactive process of vascular proliferation. The lesions grow rapidly and bleed easily, but will often clear spontaneously. They usually respond well to electrodessication, cryotherapy, and surgical removal. *Cavernous hemangiomas* are deep, dermal, and subcutaneous collections of large, mature blood vessels lined by thick fibrous walls. The depth of the vascular lesion imparts a blue color. Lesions are commonly present at birth and are characteristically red-blue soft, poorly demarcated compressible lesions. A combination of capillary and cavernous elements often occurs, the *mixed hemangioma*.

Hemangiomas grow rapidly during the first 6 months of life, but usually do not more than double in size. Complications may occur during this period of rapid growth. Larger lesions, especially those that are subject to trauma, may ulcerate. Ulcerated lesions do not tend to bleed significantly, but may become secondarily infected and result in scarring. Good local care of ulcerated hemangiomas, including topical antibiotics such as polysporin ointment or Silvadene cream to prevent secondary infection, should be initiated. A more serious complication that may occur during the period of rapid expansion is the development of thrombocytopenia, microangiopathic anemia, and disseminated intravascular coagulation, thought to be due to platelet trapping within the growing hemangioma (*Kasabach–Merritt syndrome*). Most involved hemangiomas are large and are located on the extremities. Findings that suggest the Kasabach–Merritt syndrome are a rapidly enlarging hemangioma, pallor, ecchymoses and petechiae (especially near the hemangioma), and a bleeding tendency from mucosae and wounds. The hemangioma becomes tense with overlying shiny, discolored skin. An evaluation for the Kasabach–Merritt syndrome should include a complete blood count with blood smear and platelet count, prothrombin and partial prothrombin times, and levels of fibrinogen and fibrin split products. *Disseminated eruptive hemangiomas* develop in crops of up to hundreds of hemangiomas during the first 3 months of life. Visceral hemangiomas, especially of the liver, gastrointestinal tract, spleen, lungs, eyes, and central nervous system, may be associated. Changes on physical examination, especially hepatomegaly, an abdominal bruit or cardiac murmur and rales, are suggestive of visceral involvement. Further diagnostic evaluation should include a complete blood count to check for anemia and thrombocytopenia, and a urinalysis and stool examination for blood. If cardiac failure is suspected, a chest radiograph, electrocardiogram, and echocardiogram should be obtained. Ophthalmologic examination should be performed if lesions are noted to involve the eyes, and computerized tomography should be done if central nervous system lesions are suspected. Abdominal radiographs, ultrasound, liver-spleen scan, and hepatic angiography may help to locate intraabdominal hemangiomas if they seem likely on the basis of an examination.

Most hemangiomas do not enlarge after 12 months of life and subsequently begin to involute spontaneously. In the process of involution, capillary hemangiomas become pale centrally with gray regions within the lesion. Clinical regression is complete in 60% of children by the time that they begin school and in more than 90% of children by 9 years of age. Cavernous and mixed hemangiomas follow a similar course, although cavernous hemangiomas do not tend to grow as dramatically as capillary hemangiomas.

In general, no treatment is indicated for heman-

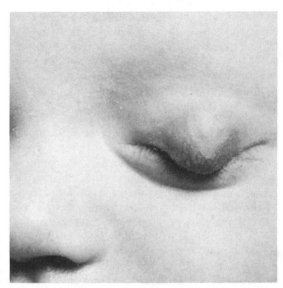

Figure 68-1. Eyelid hemangiomas that obstruct vision or compress the globe require intervention.

giomas. The long-term cosmetic result of a spontaneous involution is usually superior to that of treatment with cryotherapy, sclerosing agents, surgery, or radiation, which often lead to scarring or atrophy. Parents, however, need considerable reassurance, and serial photographs with careful measurements and illustrations of the spontaneous resolution of similar lesions are helpful. Hemangiomas occasionally require intervention because their location or size compromise vital structures, including the eyes, airway, and ear canal. Capillary hemangiomas that are near the orbit and eyelids may cause amblyopia and strabismus. Deeper lesions may cause proptosis, glaucoma, and optic nerve compression (Fig. 68-1). Hemangiomas that obstruct the airway, especially laryngeal hemangiomas, may be associated with cutaneous hemangiomas. The lesions usually cause stridor and other evidence of airway obstruction when they begin to grow towards the end of the first month of life and always by 3 months of age. When therapy is needed, prednisone is usually the most effective agent, in a dose of 2 to 3 mg/kg/day for 1 month followed by every other day doses and gradual withdrawal as tolerated. Involution usually begins by the second or third week. Infants must be followed carefully for the development of complications of corticosteroid use, especially growth retardation, infections, and cataract formation. Intralesional injections of triamcinolone acetonide may also result in involution, but must be administered by an experienced individual, often using general anesthesia for maximal control.

The treatment of the Kasabach–Merritt syndrome must be individualized. Infants with moderate thrombocytopenia may not show signs of active bleeding and may be observed and not vigorously treated. A precipitously dropping platelet count with evidence of bleeding requires intervention. A 2-week trial of prednisone may be attempted if the situation is not emergent. Other treatment modes that have been employed include compressive bandages, surgical debulking of the hemangioma, irradiation, heparin, aspirin and dipyridamole, and the administration of platelets, fresh frozen plasma, and cryoprecipitates. Children with disseminated eruptive hemangiomas without visceral hemangiomas and without signs of cardiac failure do not require therapy. Cardiac failure should be treated with digitalis and diuretics. Corticosteroid therapy should be employed if visceral lesions are present and problematic. Ligation or embolization of hepatic hemangiomas may be necessary.

Several syndromes include hemangiomas. The *blue rubber bleb nevus syndrome* is an autosomal dominant vascular disorder characterized by multiple distinctive hemangiomas of the skin and gastrointestinal tract. The typical hemangiomas of the blue rubber bleb nevus syndrome are elevated, blue or purplish-red thin-walled sacs that contain blood and are easily compressed. Most patients have gastrointestinal tract hemangiomas, especially of the small intestine, resulting in chronic gastrointestinal bleeding and secondary iron deficiency anemia.

Maffucci's syndrome is the association of multiple capillary and cavernous hemangiomas and endochondromas. The hemangiomas often persist. The endochondromas usually affect the small bones of the hands and feet and the long bones, and become apparent in early childhood. Lesions are firm, fixed, easily palpable 1-cm to 2-cm nodules. The endochondromas increase in size throughout childhood and occasionally progress after puberty, causing considerable deformity. From 23% to 30% of patients with Maffucci's syndrome develop an associated malignant disease, especially chondrosarcomas.

The *Bannayan syndrome* is an autosomal dominant disorder characterized by hemangiomas, lipomas, and lymphangiomas in association with macrocephaly, mental retardation, diminished linear growth, and intracranial tumors. *Gorham's syndrome* is a sporadic disorder characterized by multiple cavernous hemangiomas and massive underlying osteolysis with complete or partial replacement of bone by fibrous tissue. *Riley–Smith syndrome* is an autosomal dominant disorder with multiple cavernous hemangiomas, macrocephaly, and pseudopapillomas.

TELANGIECTATIC LESIONS

The *salmon patch*, the most common vascular lesion of infancy, is a transient telangiectatic nevus. It occurs in 40% of infants as a flat pink macule on the nape of the neck ("stork bite"), glabella, or upper eyelids ("angel kisses"). No treatment is needed. Ninety-five percent of salmon patches on the glabella and eyelids disappear within the first years of life, and 50% of the nuchal lesions clear spontaneously.

Nevus araneus (*spider nevus*) is a small telangiectatic lesion with a central arteriole from which blood vessels radiate. Spider nevi are common in school-aged children and often disappear during puberty. Typically, spider angiomas appear on the exposed areas of the face and upper half of the body. Destruction of the central vessel results in the disappearance of the radiating peripheral vessels, so that light dessication of the central punctum will effectively eliminate the lesion.

Cutis marmorata is a normal physiologic response of transient vascular mottling with chilling that occurs during the first weeks of life in neonates, and for longer periods of time in premature babies and patients with Down's syndrome, the Cornelia de Lange syndrome, homocystinuria, and neonatal lupus erythematosus. *Cutis marmorata telangiectatica congenita* (CMTC) is a congenital vascular disorder with prominent venules and capillaries, resulting in a deep red mottling of skin. The telangiectasias often fade with time and may no longer be visible by adulthood. At least 50% of affected patients have associated abnormalities. Most common are limb asymmetry due to hypertrophy or atrophy of an involved extremity, macrocephaly, and mental and psychomotor retardation. In contrast to cutis marmorata, the telangiectasias of CMTC are wider, deeper red, and persistent despite changes in environmental temperature.

Hereditary hemorrhagic telangiectasia (*Rendu–Osler–Weber syndrome*) is an autosomal dominant disorder characterized by the progressive development of mucocutaneous and visceral telangiectasias associated with recurrent episodes of hemorrhage. The skin lesions usually appear after puberty, most commonly on the face, ears, hands, palms, fingers, nailbeds, and forearms. The mucosae of the lips, tongue, buccal mucosa, and nasal septum are virtually always involved. Epistaxis is the most common presenting manifestation, usually during childhood, and is a feature in up to 90% of patients. Forty-four percent of patients have gastrointestinal bleeding, especially of the upper gastrointestinal tract and usually as adults. Twenty percent of patients have pulmonary arteriovenous (AV) fistulas.

Ataxia–telangiectasia (AT) is an autosomal recessive syndrome of progressive oculocutaneous telangiectasias, cerebellar ataxia beginning in early infancy, a tendency towards sinopulmonary infections and selective immunodeficiencies, and chromosomal instability after radiation damage. The initial manifestation is usually cerebellar ataxia, which first becomes apparent when the child begins to walk. Neurologic deterioration is progressive. The characteristic mucocutaneous telangiectasias are usually noted between 3 and 6 years of age, although they have been described at birth. The bulbar conjunctivae are initially affected, and the telangiectasias may appear subsequently on the ears, eyelids, malar prominences, neck, antecubital and popliteal fossae, dorsum of the hands and palate. Progeric changes have been noted in almost 90% of patients, with early loss of subcutaneous fat and premature graying of the hair. Sinopulmonary infections occur in most patients and the most common causes of death are from bronchiectasis and respiratory failure. Patients have a 10% risk of developing neoplasias, especially lymphoreticular and epithelial.

A deficient or absent level of IgA is found in 70% of patients, and many have circulating anti-IgA antibodies. Other immunologic defects include low to absent levels of IgE, defective cell-mediated immunity, and an absent or abnormally developed thymus. Almost all patients with AT have elevated levels of alpha-fetoprotein and carcinoembryonic antigen. The DNA of patients with AT may not be repaired normally after ionizing radiation.

The *port wine stain* (*nevus flammeus*) is a vascular lesion of mature capillaries that is present at birth and grows in proportion to the growth of the child. The lesions are flat and red-purple to blue. They tend to darken in color with advancing age and may develop angiomatous papules. Nevus flammeus does not involute. The vascular lesions may be camouflaged with makeup or treated with laser therapy in adolescence or adulthood for cosmetic purposes.

The *Klippel–Trenaunay–Weber (KTW) syndrome* combines the triad of nevus flammeus, associated hypertrophy of the soft tissue, and bone and venous varicosities. The vascular lesion is unilateral in 85% of patients and usually involves a lower extremity. The bone and soft tissue hypertrophy is probably related to augmented arterial flow associated with the vascular nevus and with venous stasis. Varicose veins develop as collateral channels for obstructed deep veins during the first years of life, when the child spends more time in an upright position. The deep veins may be absent, hypoplastic, or occluded by fibrovascular bands. A few patients with features of KTW syndrome have associated AV shunts. The most common complications of the KTW syndrome are compensatory scoliosis due to hemihypertrophy of a lower extremity and cutaneous ulcerations, edema, stasis changes, and thrombophlebitis due to the venous varicosities. Children with significant varicosities should use elastic support stockings. Varicotomy and vein stripping are not usually indicated in view of the frequently inadequate deep venous supply. These procedures may lead to ankle edema and a rapid recurrence of the varicosity.

The *Sturge–Weber syndrome* (encephalotrigeminal angiomatosis) is a congenital vascular disorder characterized by angiomas of the leptomeninges over the cerebral cortex (usually the posterior parietal and occipital lobes) in association with an ipsilateral nevus flammeus in the distribution of the first trigeminal nerve. Seizures occur in up to 89% of patients, with the majority starting during the first year of life. Typically, the seizures are focal motor seizures or begin with a focus and then generalize. Hemiparesis or hemiplegia contralateral to the nevus are noted in 26% of patients, especially with extension of cerebral atrophy into the major motor portion of the parietal lobe. Intracranial calcifications may be visible by computerized tomography within the first few months of life and by radiographs after 2 years of age. Ocular abnormalities, especially glaucoma, develop more frequently in patients with involvement of both the second and first trigeminal branches. Telangiectatic hypertrophy of oral mucosae is also common.

Coat's disease includes telangiectasias of the face, conjunctivae, nail beds, and breast with retinal telangiectasias and a massive exudation with retinal detachment. *Cobb syndrome* is characterized by nevus flammeus or angiokeratomas in a dermatomal distribution, associated with angiomas of the corresponding segment of spinal cord. *Von Hippel–Lindau syndrome* is an autosomal dominant condition with cerebellar hemangioblastomas, cyst formation, and occasionally port wine stains.

ANGIOKERATOMAS

Angiokeratomas are asymptomatic firm, dark red scaly papules that range from 1 mm to 10 mm in size. Histopathologic examination of lesions shows a thickening of the epidermis overlying vascular ectasia. Solitary or multiple angiokeratomas may occur in childhood after trauma and are usually located on the lower extremities. Disorders involving angiokeratomas are uncommon and include *Fabry's disease, angiokeratoma circumscriptum, angiokeratoma of Mibelli*, and *angiokeratoma of Fordyce*.

LYMPHANGIOMAS

Tumors of the lymphatic vessels may be classified into four types: lymphangioma simplex, lymphangioma circumscriptum, cavernous lymphangioma, and cystic hygroma. Ninety percent are present at birth or appear during infancy. *Lymphangioma simplex* is a solitary, well-demarcated, skin-colored tumor with a smooth surface that is usually located on the head, neck, or proximal extremities. It is often amenable to surgical removal. *Lymphangioma circumscriptum* is the most common form of lymphangioma. The lesions have the appearance of clustered thick-walled vessels and are usually found on the proximal extremities, neck, trunk, and oral mucosae. Hemangiomas are frequently associated, so that lesions may be deep red. Surgical removal often results in recurrence. *Cavernous lymphangiomas* are large, cystic dilations of the deep dermis and subcutaneous tissue that are poorly defined and involve large areas of the extremities, trunk, and face. Surgery must be extensive and often leads to recurrences. *Cystic hygromas* are large, often unilocular lymphangiomas that are commonly located on the neck, axillae, or inguinal regions. Recurrences after surgical removal are uncommon, and cystic hygromas occasionally undergo spontaneous resolution.

ANNOTATED BIBLIOGRAPHY

Esterly NB: Kasabach–Merritt syndrome in infants. J Am Acad Dermatol 8:504–513, 1983 (Review of Kasabach–Merritt syndrome and its treatment.)

Esterly NB, Margileth AM, Kahn G et al: The management of disseminated eruptive hemangiomata in infants. Pediatr Dermatol 1:312–317, 1984 (Discussion of the diagnosis and management of disseminated hemangiomatosis.)

Jacobs AH: Vascular nevi. Pediatr Clin North Am 30:465–482, 1983 (Review of the common vascular nevi.)

Wisnicki JL: Hemangiomas and vascular malformations. Ann Plast Surg 12:41–59, 1984 (Review of the classification, natural history, and treatment of various vascular lesions.)

69

Epidermal Tumors

AMY PALLER

Epidermal tumors include benign lesions of the epidermis, malignant lesions of the epidermis, adnexal tumors (*i.e.*, tumors of eccrine gland, apocrine gland, sebaceous gland, or hair follicle origin), and tumors derived from melanocytes.

MELANOCYTIC LESIONS

Pigmented nevi ("moles") are the most common tumors of childhood. Although congenital melanocytic nevi are present in only 1% of all newborn infants, most people acquire nevi throughout infancy and childhood with a peak average of 20 to 40 nevi per person in later adolescence and young adulthood. Nevi begin to involute later in adulthood. Nevi occur most commonly on sun-exposed areas above the waist and have smooth borders with sharp demarcation from the surrounding skin and usually with homogeneous pigmentation. Pigmented nevi may be classified into three major subgroups: junctional, compound, and intradermal.

Junctional nevi are thought to represent the initial stage of compound nevi and are usually found in children. They are light brown to black macules that are usually devoid of hair but they do not retain normal skin lines. Junctional nevi begin as tiny macules and grow to reach a maximum diameter of 4 mm to 6 mm. Histopathologically, junctional nevi show single melanocytic cells or a nest of nevus cells "dropping off" of the epidermis in an orderly arrangement. *Compound nevi* are usually seen in older children and adolescents, although they are occasionally present at birth. They are more elevated than junctional nevi; they have a warty or smooth surface; and they often contain dark coarse hairs. Compound nevi show nevus cells at the dermal-epidermal border as well as in the dermis. *Intradermal nevi* are seen most frequently in adults, but may develop in childhood. These nevi are dome-shaped with coarse central hairs and a broad or pedunculated base. Clinical differentiation from compound nevi may be difficult. Histopathologically, intradermal nevi show nests of nevus cells in the dermis only. In adulthood with increasing age, intradermal nevi tend to involute and are replaced by fatty or fibrous tissue.

Most pigmented nevi are benign and are of cosmetic concern only. However, congenital pigmented nevi, especially giant congenital nevi, and dysplastic nevi are precursors for malignant melanomas and surgical removal should be performed. *Congenital nevi* are present in 1% of neonates, but most are small or medium-sized nevi. Fewer than 1 in 20,000 neonates have giant congenital pigmented nevi with a diameter of greater than 10 cm to 20 cm. Giant congenital melanocytic nevi are most commonly found on the buttocks, scalp, and paravertebral areas in the distribution of a garment,

especially a bathing trunk. They are usually deeply pigmented and often have scattered satellite lesions. The nevus is usually covered with hair (Fig. 69-1). The histopathologic appearance of congenital melanocytic nevi differs from that of acquired melanocytic nevi. Congenital nevi have nevus cells that extend deep into the lower dermis and often deep into the subcutaneous tissues with an extension between collagen bundles in single rows. In addition, nevus cells are found within hair follicles, blood vessel walls, the perineurium, eccrine ducts and glands, and sebaceous glands.

There is no question that infants with giant congenital nevi have a lifetime risk of developing melanomas by transformation that is at least 6.3%. Seventy percent of these giant nevi transform during the prepubertal years, so that removal as early as possible is encouraged. Because of the depth of congenital nevi, complete excisional removal to the fascia should be performed. Dermabrasion often leads to a better cosmetic result, but does not usually remove the nevus entirely. Although decreasing the number of nevus cells may lower risk the transformation into melanoma, melanomas have developed in dermabraded congenital nevi. Giant nevi must be removed using general anesthesia, so

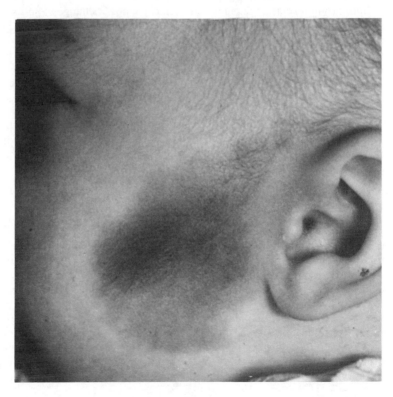

Figure 69-1. Congenital hairy nevus.

that many surgeons prefer to wait until 3 to 6 months of age to decrease the risks of general anesthesia. Atypical areas within the giant nevus during the first 6 months of life should be excised with local anesthesia and examined for possible melanoma. Most giant nevi must be removed with serial grafting of normal skin. Tissue expansion of contiguous areas with the nevus is being employed as a potential source of grafted tissue. Cutaneous lesions that overlie the head and spinal cord may be associated with leptomeningeal melanocytosis that may lead to hydrocephalus, seizures, and melanoma. Computerized axial tomography demonstrates leptomeningeal involvement, but the complete removal of nevus cells from this site is impossible.

The risk of transformation of small and medium-sized nevi into melanoma is controversial. Anecdotal reports suggest that melanomas arise in these congenital nevi, but good prospective studies to study the actual risk and determine the need for removal have yet to be done. Current assessments are based on the history of a congenital nevus at the site of a melanoma and the finding of histopathologic features of congenital nevi at the site of a malignant melanoma. Although there does appear to be an increased risk of transformation into melanoma, the time course of this transformation suggests that it occurs after puberty. The recommendations from dermatologists for management range from removal of all lesions during infancy to removal of all lesions by local anesthesia at or after puberty with annual observation of lesions to removal of selective lesions based on the location and the desires of the patient (*e.g.*, a lesion over a joint is difficult to remove without contracture formation and is easily visible to the patient, but a lesion on the buttocks or scalp is difficult to observe and removal leads to minimal cosmetic defect). Signs of transformation to melanoma include the development of irregular borders, variegate pigmentation, and irregular alteration of topography.

Dysplastic nevi are acquired precursors of malignant melanomas. It has been estimated that approximately 2% of persons in the United States have at least one dysplastic nevus. In addition, 5% to 10% of patients who develop a melanoma have a family history of melanoma. Dysplastic nevi have been found by histopathologic examination in 20% to 35% of all melanomas. Patients with dysplastic nevi have been classified into four subgroups: type A has no family history of dysplastic nevi and no personal or family history of melanoma; type B has other family members with dysplastic nevi but no melanoma; type C has a personal history of both

dysplastic nevi and melanoma, but no family history of either; and type D has other family members with dysplastic nevi and melanomas. The familial types have an autosomal dominant mode of inheritance.

The characteristic clinical features of dysplastic nevi usually appear at puberty, although patients often note large numbers of typical nevi that develop at 5 to 8 years of age. At puberty and subsequently into adulthood, the number of nevi increases further, so that the patient commonly has 25 to 75 nevi (especially in the familial forms) with atypical features, including irregular borders, variegate pigmentation with mixtures of pink, tan, and brown, and indistinct margins. Dysplastic nevi are usually larger than normal nevi and range in size from 6 mm to 15 mm. In contrast to the distribution of normal nevi, dysplastic nevi are most commonly found on the trunk and are also located on feet, scalp, and buttocks. The dysplastic nevi may be macular or may have an irregular rough appearance. Features to suggest that a melanoma has developed are black areas within a lesion and a change in topography developing at the edge of a dysplastic nevus. Any lesion that is suspected of being a melanoma must be removed by excision. Histopathologically, dysplastic nevi show atypical melanocytic hyperplasia with dermal mesenchymal changes and usually nevus cells in the dermis. Patients with suspected dysplastic nevus syndrome should have two or three of the most atypical lesions removed by excisional biopsy to confirm the diagnosis. Subsequently, patients should be followed carefully with serial photographs at least every 6 months, preferably at a pigmented lesion clinic. Scalp lesions should be removed prophylactically, and other lesions should be assessed histologically if clinical changes occur. Patients should avoid exposure to sunlight and oral contraceptives. All family members should also be examined for the possibility of dysplastic nevi.

OTHER MELANOCYTIC LESIONS

Café-au-lait spots are well-circumscribed, homogeneously light brown macules that are present at birth or may appear during the first 5 years of life. Ten percent of all people have one café-au-lait spot, although the presence of greater than two café-au-lait spots is unusual (less than 0.75%). Café-au-lait spots are associated with Albright syndrome (polyostotic fibrous dysplasia) and neurofibromatosis. The café-au-lait spot of Albright syndrome is usually solitary, large, and segmental. The café-au-lait spots of neurofibromatosis are usually multiple (greater than five), scattered, and may be associated with generalized or axillary freckling. Although the café-au-lait spots of Albright syndrome have been distinguished from those of neurofibromatosis by the irregular borders in Albright syndrome, such distinctions are often misleading. A histopathologic examination of café-au-lait spots shows increased epidermal melanin without nevus cells or increased numbers of melanocytes. *Nevus spilus* is a café-au-lait spot with darker macules or papules of pigmentation overlying the light brown patch. Histopathologically, the raised papules usually show nevus cells while the macular areas demonstrate melanocyte proliferation.

Spindle cell nevus (Spitz nevus, benign juvenile melanoma) is a firm, smooth, dome-shaped red-brown lesion that is usually solitary and occurs most frequently in prepubertal children. The lesions are occasionally darker brown and may be confused clinically with malignant melanomas. Spindle cell nevi must also be distinguished clinically from intradermal nevi, pyogenic granulomas, and juvenile xanthogranulomas. Histologically, the spindle cell nevus is a variant of the compound nevus, with nests of nevus cells at the dermal-epidermal junction and in the dermis. Although the lesion is benign, confusion with the histopathologic appearance of melanoma may result from the disordered appearance of nevus cells and the large number of mitotic figures. The presence of spindle and epithelioid cells, sparsity of melanin, dilated dermal blood vessels, and increased maturation of the deeper nevus cells help to differentiate the conditions. Spindle cell nevi may persist into adulthood or become intradermal nevi.

The *halo nevus* (Sutton's nevus) usually occurs late in childhood or during adolescence. A halo of depigmentation appears around a pigmented nevus, probably due to immunologic destruction of melanocytic cells. Halo nevi appear most commonly on the trunk. In most cases, the central pigmented lesion disappears. Rarely, the depigmentation is associated with melanoma.

Mongolian spots are flat, blue-gray, often poorly circumscribed lesions that are usually found on the buttocks, lumbosacral area, and shoulders of infants, especially in black, oriental, and hispanic infants. The lesions are often large and may be single or multiple. A histopathologic examination of mongolian spots shows spindle-shaped melanocytes and melanin deep in the dermis, and the spots are thought to represent melanocytes that have failed to migrate to the epidermis. The blue color results from the depth of the pigmentation and the reflection of blue light (Tyndall effect). Mongolian spots usually disappear within the first 5 years of life, and fewer than 5% of patients have spots that persist into adulthood. Other variants of dermal melanocytosis are the nevi of Ota, nevus of Ito, and blue nevus. The *nevus of Ota* is usually found in black or oriental female patients and is characterized by patchy blue discoloration of the periorbital area, forehead, and upper cheek. The nevus of Ota is usually unilateral. Approximately 50% of patients have the nevus at birth, while most other patients develop the lesion at puberty or pregnancy. The *nevus of Ito* shares the clinical characteristics of the nevus of Ota, but involves the shoulder, upper arms, scapula, and supraclavicular regions. In contrast with the disappearance of mongolian spots, nevus of Ota and nevus and Ito persist and often darken with increasing age. Cosmetic cover-ups are the only indicated treatment. *Blue nevi* are uncommon in children and usually appear during the second or third decades of life, especially in oriental individuals. They are small, round, well-circumscribed nevi that are blue due to the depth of spindle-shaped melanocytes and melanin. Blue nevi are also thought to result from the arrested migration of melanocytes bound for the dermal-epidermal junction. A malignant transformation from blue nevi is rare.

Becker's nevus usually appears at the end of the first decade of life in boys, but has even been reported at birth and may develop in female patients. Brown macular pigmentation develops on the chest, back, or upper arm and spreads irregularly until a size of 10 cm to 15 cm in diameter is reached. Within the next few years, coarse hairs develop in the area of pigmentation. The hyperpigmentation and hypertrichosis are persistent.

Lentigines are small, tan to black oval macules that usually appear in childhood (lentigo simplex). In adults, lentigines are usually sun-induced (solar lentigines, "liver spots"). A histopathologic examination of lentigines shows epidermal melanocytic proliferation. In children, lentigines usually fade or disappear with advancing age. Lentigines are important for their association with syndromes. In the *Peutz–Jeghers syndrome*, characteristic lentigines appear during early childhood on the lips and oral mucosa, nose and periorbital region, on the palms and soles and on the dorsum of the fingers and toes. Associated with the lentigines are polyps, especially of the small intestine. The polyps have a low malignant potential, but may lead to colicky abdominal pain, melena, and intussusception. The

Peutz–Jeghers syndrome has an autosomal dominant mode of inheritance. The *multiple lentigines syndrome* or *LEOPARD syndrome* is another autosomal dominant disorder with variable expressivity characterized by generalized *l*entigines that are usually present at birth or in early infancy, *e*chocardiographic abnormalities, *o*cular hypertelorism, *p*ulmonic stenosis, *a*bnormalities of the genitalia, *r*etardation of growth, and *d*eafness.

EPIDERMAL NEVI

Epidermal nevi usually appear at birth or in early childhood. They may occur anywhere, but are most common on the head and extremities and are often localized to a dermatomal distribution. Lesions tend to be 2 cm to 3 cm or larger; they are usually pigmented to various degrees; and they often appear warty. Epidermal nevi often continue to extend until late adolescence. They do not regress spontaneously and usually become more verrucous in adulthood. Various subgroups of epidermal nevi have been described based on the appearance, distribution, and mixture of epidermal and appendageal components. *Nevus unius lateris* is a linear or curved lesion limited to one side of the body that follows the long axis of the trunk or extremity. The *inflammatory linear verrucous epidermal nevus* (ILVEN) is an erythematous, often pruritic linear epidermal nevus that almost always affects a lower extremity and shows eczematous changes histopathologically. ILVEN must be differentiated from lichen striatus, a benign inflammatory condition that resolves spontaneously after months (see Chap. 62). If a large area of the body is covered with the epidermal nevus, the lesion is a systematized epidermal nevus. *Ichthyosis hystrix* is a form of systematized epidermal nevus that is widespread and usually bilateral with whorls of hyperkeratosis. Epidermal nevi are difficult to remove and often recur, even after full-thickness excision. Malignant transformation of epidermal nevi, usually into basal cell carcinoma, is rare and attempts to remove the lesions are unnecessary except for cosmetic purposes.

The *epidermal nevus syndrome* is a sporadic condition characterized by the association of acquired deformities of the skeletal system, central nervous system, cardiovascular system, and skin. Cutaneous anomalies include epidermal nevi, café-au-lait spots, hypopigmented macules, melanocytic nevi, and hemangiomas. The epidermal nevi may take the form of localized acanthosis nigricans, nevus unius lateris, ichthyosis hystrix, and, when on the face or neck, of linear nevus sebaceus. The most common systemic complications are kyphoscoliosis, mental retardation, seizures, and hemihypertrophy. Patients with the epidermal nevus syndrome must be followed carefully for the development of these systemic abnormalities with careful physical examinations, electroencephalograms, and radiographic studies.

ADNEXAL TUMORS

Adnexal tumors in children are often present at birth or develop in early childhood. Other than the nevus sebaceus, adnexal tumors are usually benign and require removal for cosmetic purposes only. The *nevus sebaceus* (of Jadassohn) is a well-circumscribed, yellow-orange hairless plaque that is usually solitary and located on the scalp, face, or neck. At puberty, the lesion becomes raised and warty. A histopathologic examination of nevus sebaceus shows overgrowth of sebaceous glands and rudimentary hair follicles. Tumors, especially basal cell carcinomas, develop in 10% to 15% of lesions in young adulthood. As a result, it is advisable that all nevus sebaceus be excised by teenage years under local anesthesia. *Trichoepitheliomas* are benign, firm, dome-shaped, skin-colored tumors that are most common on the face. They appear occasionally in childhood, but more commonly develop in adults and can be confused with basal cell carcinoma. Multiple trichoepitheliomas may be inherited in an autosomal dominant manner as epithelioma adenoides cysticum (Brooke's syndrome). *Trichofolliculomas* are solitary skin-colored papules that are also usually on the face, but may be distinguished clinically by a central pore with a woolly tuft of hair. *Syringomas* are benign tumors of the eccrine glands that usually appear during adolescence as skin-colored to yellow tiny papules, usually on the lower eyelids, neck, or upper chest. Syringomas are seen with increased frequency in children with Down's syndrome. *Pilomatrixomas* (calcifying epithelioma of Malherbe) are benign tumors of hair that usually develop during childhood as a hard, skin-colored, or blue nodule on the face, neck, or upper extremities. Pilomatrixomas are usually solitary, but may be multiple, especially in children with myotonic dystrophy.

BASAL CELL CARCINOMA

Basal cell carcinomas are rarely seen in children, except in association with nevus sebaceus, xeroderma pigmentosum, and the basal cell nevus syndrome. The *basal cell nevus syndrome* (Gorlin syndrome) is an autosomal dominant disorder characterized by multiple basal cell carcinomas that develop in childhood in association with musculoskeletal, neurologic, and endocrinologic abnormalities. The basal cell tumors usually appear between puberty and 35 years of age, but may develop as early as the second year of life. The face, neck, and chest are most commonly affected and the basal cell carcinomas appear as skin-colored to brown dome-shaped papules that erupt in crops. Associated tumors include medulloblastomas in infancy and ovarian fibromas.

ANNOTATED BIBLIOGRAPHY

Greene MH, Clark WH, Tucker MA et al: Acquired precursors of cutaneous malignant melanoma. The familial dysplastic nevus syndrome. N Engl J Med 312:91–97, 1985 (Review of the clinical characteristics of dysplastic nevi, including numerous color illustrations.)

Hurwitz S: Epidermal nevi and tumors of epidermal origin. Pediatr Clin North Am 30:483–494, 1983 (Review of the various epidermal tumors.)

Jacobs AH, Hurwitz S, Prose NS et al: The management of congenital nevocytic nevi. Pediatr Dermatol 2:143–156, 1984 (Discussion by several pediatric dermatologists of the management of congenital nevi.)

Rhodes AR: Pigmented birthmarks and precursor melanocytic lesions of cutaneous melanoma identifiable in childhood. Pediatr Clin North Am 30:435–463, 1983 (Review of congenital nevi and their differential diagnosis.)

Solomon LM, Esterly NB: Epidermal and other congenital organoid nevi. Curr Probl Pediatr VI(1):2–56, 1975 (Excellent review of epidermal nevi and other tumors derived from adnexal structures.)

70
Insect Bites and Infestations
AMY PALLER

Bites and infestations are especially common in children and may manifest as papules, nodules, blisters, urticaria, and hemorrhagic lesions. The correct diagnosis is frequently missed. Recognition of these lesions is based on the distribution and grouping of lesions, and history, including exposure to pets and other affected individuals, environmental conditions, childhood habits, seasonal incidence of the lesions, and a recent history of travel. Bites and infestations of dermatologic significance are caused by arthropods, particularly eight-legged arachnids (*e.g.*, mites, ticks, and spiders), six-legged insects (*e.g.*, fleas, mosquitoes, bedbugs, lice, and caterpillars), and helminths.

ARACHNIDS

Mites attack children by burrowing under the skin or by attaching themselves to the skin and causing dermatitis. Mites that most frequently cause dermatologic problems include itch mites (*Sarcoptes scabiei*) and harvest mites (chiggers). The *scabies* mite burrows into the horny layer of skin, especially in areas of skin with a thin horny layer and few hair follicles. The eruption is usually intensely pruritic and manifests as various primary lesions, including burrows, papules, nodules, and vesicles, mixed with secondary excoriations, dermatitis, crusting, and secondary infection (Fig. 70-1). The burrows are the home of the female parasite and the papules represent skin invaded by the scabies larvae. The nodules, vesicles, and pruritus are thought to be hypersensitivity reactions to the mite and do not develop until 3 to 6 weeks after infestation begins. Although adolescents and older children usually have lesions in the interdigital spaces, flexural regions, at the wrists, waistline, buttocks, and around the areolae, infants and young children tend to have more widespread involvement, including lesions on the face, neck, scalp, palms, and soles. The red-brown nodules are especially common in children, particularly on covered parts of the body such as the axillae, groin area, and buttocks. The nodules and their associated pruritus may persist for months, despite adequate antiscabetic therapy. The burrows are found on approximately 10% of adult and adolescent patients, but even less frequently on the skin of young children and infants, due to the elimination of visible burrows by vigorous hygiene and secondary eczematization.

Infants and children frequently develop secondary eczema because of vigorous scratching as well as excessive bathing and application of irritating topical preparations. Atopic children are especially predisposed to develop eczematization and secondary bacterial infections. The administration of topical corticosteroids to unrecognized lesions may diminish the pruritus and erythema, but will encourage the proliferation and transmissibility of the

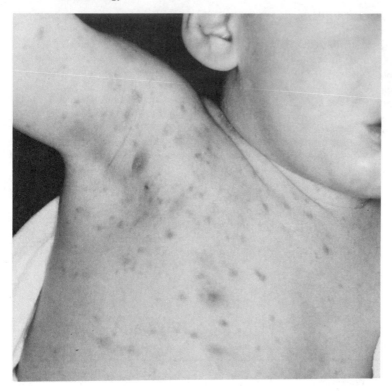

Figure 70-1. Papules, vesicles, and nodules of scabies in an infant.

organism. This phenomenon has been called *scabies incognito*.

Norwegian scabies (crusted scabies) is a form of scabies characterized by lesions covered with thick crusts and scales that are teeming with mites. The buttocks, scalp, palms, soles, elbows, and knees are most extensively involved. Norwegian scabies tends to be less pruritic than classical scabies and occurs with greatest frequency in children with mental or physical handicaps and immunocompromised children (particularly with Down's syndrome). *Canine scabies* is a form of scabies carried by domestic animals, especially the dog. The mite does not reproduce on human skin, but may cause a transient eruption in children on the forearms, thighs, chest, and abdomen. The mite is difficult to identify by skin scrapings, and the diagnosis is often made by a history alone. The infestation clears spontaneously after 4 to 6 weeks.

The differential diagnosis of scabies most frequently includes atopic, contact allergic, and contact irritant dermatitis. Papular urticaria, histiocytosis X, seborrheic dermatitis, and dermatitis herpetiformis may also be considered.

The diagnosis of scabies is often based on the history and the distribution and morphology of le-

sions. A scraping to identify mites, feces, or eggs, however, should always be taken. Fresh papules or burrows are the best sites to scrape after placing a drop of mineral oil on the suspected site. Potassium hydroxide should never be used on scrapings for scabies, since it dissolves the mites, eggs, and feces. Occasionally, a skin biopsy is performed to eliminate the possibility of other diagnoses. A burrow and mite may be found by a histopathologic examination, but this is rare except in Norwegian scabies. Once the diagnosis of scabies is made, all family members must be examined and treated to avoid reinfection.

The most common treatment of scabies is the application of 1% gamma benzene hexachloride (*e.g.*, GBH, lindane, or Kwell). The lotion is applied from the neck down, unless lesions are present on the head, and is washed thoroughly 6 to 8 hours later. The skin should not be soaked before applying the medication so that percutaneous absorption is minimal. A second application may be advisable 1 week later to destroy hatched larvae, but no further applications are necessary unless reinfection occurs. Family members who are in close contact with the patient should also be treated with a second application of GBH. The mite survives up to 48 hours off the body, so that clothing, bedding, and towels that have been used in the 48 hours before treatment should be laundered with hot water. Twenty-four hours after therapy, the patient is no longer capable of transmitting scabies. Evidence of hypersensitivity (*e.g.*, pruritus, nodules, and vesicles) may persist for months. Topical tar preparations, antipruritic lotions such as ¼% menthol in Shepard's lotion, and nonfluorinated topical corticosteroids may ameliorate the pruritus. Because of possible central nervous system and hematologic toxicity of GBH in infants, the medication should not be used in patients under 1 year of age or in pregnant or lactating mothers. Six percent precipitated sulfur in petrolatum is a suitable alternative for these individuals, but it is messy and stains readily. It must be applied nightly for 3 nights. Ten percent crotamiton (Eurax) lotion is an alternate therapeutic agent that is antipruritic, but it is more irritating and probably less efficacious than GBH. Crotamiton should be applied 2 days in succession, each for 24 hours. Systemic antistaphylococcal antibiotics should be administered to patients with secondary bacterial infections.

Harvest mite (chiggers) infestations are usually found in the southern United States and are characterized by intense itching and discrete, bright red tiny papules with hemorrhagic puncta. Purpuric lesions, bullae, urticaria, excoriations, and erythema may be noted. The lesions are most commonly located on the legs and at the waistline, although they may be widespread in children. Mosquito repellants are effective against chiggers. For relief of the pruritus, compresses, topical corticosteroids, antihistamines, and clear nail polish applied directly to the bites have been used.

Ticks may cause local inflammation, systemic symptoms, or may transmit serious systemic disease. The bite is painless, but within days reactions occur due to the introduction of tick saliva. Pruritus and local urticarial reactions are the most common sequelae. A foreign body reaction with nodules may develop if mouth parts are left in the skin. Rarely, patchy hair loss in the area of the tick bite may occur. Serious systemic reactions may result from tick bites, but they subside quickly once the tick is found and removed. These reactions include generalized urticaria, tick bite fever, and tick paralysis. Tick bite fever is characterized by fever, headache, nausea, and abdominal cramping. Tick paralysis is an ascending paralysis that resembles the Guillain–Barré syndrome. Respiratory failure and death may ensue. Ticks may be removed by various methods, but should never be plucked off as body fragments

may be left behind. Accepted techniques include covering the area with nail polish, mineral oil or petrolatum, cryotherapy with liquid nitrogen, heating the area with an extinguished match, and application of a few drops of chloroform or ether.

Ticks may transmit a number of systemic diseases with dermatologic manifestations, particularly *Rocky Mountain spotted fever* (RMSF) and *Lyme disease*. RMSF is an acute exanthematous illness caused by *Rickettsia rickettsii* that is most prevalent in the southeastern United States. The rash begins after 3 to 4 days on the extremities (including the palms and soles) and spreads to the trunk and abdomen as erythematous maculopapules that become hemorrhagic. Other features include fever, headache, conjunctivitis, nausea, and myalgias. Complications include cardiovascular collapse, gangrene, hepatosplenomegaly, disseminated intravascular coagulation, and visceral hemorrhage. Early diagnosis of RMSF is crucial and may be obtained by demonstration of the pathogen by direct immunofluorescence microscopy of skin biopsy sections. Antibodies to Proteus OX-19 or OX-2 appear in the second or third week of the illness. The differential diagnosis includes viral exanthems, meningococcemia, and typhoid fever. Tetracycline and chloramphenicol are the preferred antibiotics and should be administered as early as possible.

Lyme disease is caused by a spirochete (*Borrelia burgdorferi*) that is transmitted by ticks. The disorder usually begins in the summer or early autumn with the multiple expanding, erythematous annular lesions of erythema chronicum migrans. Constitutional symptoms, nausea, vomiting, myalgias, arthralgias, eye pain, conjunctivitis, and lymphadenopathy may accompany the cutaneous annular lesions. Weeks to months later, the erythema chronicum migrans disappear, but patients may have neurologic and cardiac abnormalities and migratory polyarthritis or chronic arthritis. Serologic testing with indirect immunofluorescence or the enzyme-linked immunoabsorbent assay (ELISA) confirms the diagnosis. The preferred treatment is tetracycline in teenagers and penicillin in younger children.

Although the black widow spider is a significant cause of morbidity, only the *brown recluse spider* causes notable dermatologic features. The brown recluse spider is distinguished by a dark violin-shaped band on its thorax. The spider's venom contains hemolytic, necrotizing, and spreading factors. Local burning or pruritus occurs after the bite, followed within hours by a painful hemorrhagic blister. Finally, the central portion becomes ulcerated and gangrenous and may not heal for months. Systemic reactions are common in children and include malaise, chills, nausea, vomiting, myalgias, a generalized erythematous or purpuric maculopapular eruption, thrombocytopenia, hemolysis, hemoglobinuria, shock, and coma. Management includes systemic corticosteroids, antihistamines, antibiotics for secondary bacterial infections, and surgical removal of the necrotic area.

INSECTA

Lice are small, wingless insects that proliferate readily through the production of eggs (nits) and depend on a blood meal for survival. When the lice feed, they release a toxin into the skin that produces tiny purpuric macules and later pruritic papules and wheals as a hypersensitivity reaction. Three forms of lice cause infections (pediculosis): the head louse, body louse, and pubic or crab louse.

Children are most susceptible to *pediculosis capitis*, caused by the head louse. Infestation results from direct contact with an infested individual or contact with hats or combs. The nits are attached to the hair shaft and resemble dandruff, but cannot be easily removed. Scalp pruritus and eczematization with secondary infection is common. The diagnosis may be confirmed by viewing the nits attached to the hair under the microscope. A single application to the scalp of gamma benzene hexachloride or pyrethrins (Rid) shampoo for 10 minutes is the preferred treatment. Malathion 0.5% applied for 12 hours and 10% crotamiton used for 24 hours are also effective. Soaking of the hair with vinegar facilitates the removal of nits with a fine-toothed comb. Combs, brushes, bedclothes, and headgear should be washed with hot water or soaked for an hour in alcohol. Contacts should be examined for lice and treated if affected.

Pediculosis corporis is caused by the body louse, which lives in the seams of clothing or bedding. The primary lesions are tiny red macules, papules, or wheals with a hemorrhagic central punctum, but are usually obscured by secondary eczematization associated with intense pruritus. Body areas under belts, collars, and underwear are usually affected, with sparing of sites not covered with clothing. The diagnosis should be confirmed by finding the nits in the seams of clothing. Laundering of all clothing and bedding with hot water or dry cleaning and good hygiene are appropriate and usually adequate therapy. Contacts must also be examined carefully.

Pediculosis pubis is caused by the crab louse, which infests the skin and hair of the genital area, thighs, lower abdomen, and axillae. The crab louse may also infest the eyelashes (*pediculosis palpebrarum*), especially in prepubertal children. The louse is transmitted by sexual contact in the adolescent and by close contact with infested adults in the prepubertal child. Rarely, the crab louse is transmitted by clothing and bedding. Pruritus is often the initial symptoms, followed by secondary eczematization or infection. With severe infestations, blue macules (*maculae caeruleae*) are occasionally noted on the thighs and lower abdomen. The diagnosis of crab louse infection is made by demonstrating the nits on affected hairs. For pubic lice, the area should be washed with gamma benzene hexachloride shampoo for 10 minutes and the nits removed, as in pediculosis capitis. Clothes and bedding should be washed. Pediculosis of the eyelashes should not be treated with pediculocides. The application of petrolatum (Vaseline) three times daily for a week with removal of nits is the preferred therapy. Contacts should be sought and treated as well.

Mosquitoes are the most common cause of insect bites in children. The bites occur in warm weather on the exposed areas of skin. Erythematous papules and urticaria result, but regional adenopathy and fever are not associated unless secondary infection occurs. Occasionally, chronic papules and nodules develop that may resemble lymphoma by a histologic examination of skin biopsy specimens. The prevention of bites with insect repellents is the best management, although calamine lotion, oral antihistamines, and topical corticosteroids may be of limited value.

Flea bites are a frequent problem of children with cats and dogs. Since fleas may live as long as 2 years and survive for months without a blood meal, children without pets may develop flea bites after moving into a home that is infested with fleas because of pets in the home previously. Fleas live in upholstery, carpeting, and debris in corners and floor cracks. Flea bites are usually located on exposed areas or on body sites where clothing is snug. The lesions are irregularly grouped urticarial papules with a central hemorrhagic punctum. This *papular urticaria* is usually due to flea bites, but has also been described following bites by mosquitoes, bedbugs, and other insects. The lesions may occasionally be vesicular, pustular, or bullous. Generalized flea bites may resemble chickenpox. Therapy includes the elimination of the fleas by treating animals and by the spraying of carpets, upholstery, floor, and corners with gamma benzene hexachloride dust, malathion, or DDT powder. Calamine lotion, topical corticosteroids, and oral antihistamines may also be helpful.

Bedbugs cause pruritic lesions that are first noted in the morning. They live in the seams of mattresses and bed frames, but may also be found on the floor and wallpaper near the bed. Grouped urticarial papules with a central punctum develop on exposed sites. Bedbugs can survive for up to a year without a meal. Extermination is the preferred therapy. *Fire ant* bites affect children in the southeastern United States. Painful wheals develop on exposed areas (especially the feet), followed by vesicles and pustules with a central punctum. Lesions are self-limited but often leave scarring. Systemic urticarial reactions may require systemic antihistamines and epinephrine. *Caterpillar dermatitis* is due to contact with hairs and spines. The reactions may range from a localized dermatitis with discrete pruritic maculopapules to painful wheals with vesicular or necrotic centers. Occasionally, marked local swelling, fever, nausea, headache, muscle cramps, seizures, and shock may be associated. The hairs travel through air or by way of clothing to cause widespread dermatitis. The

hairs can be seen by microscopic examination of skin scrapings, facilitating the diagnosis. Tape may be applied to the lesions to remove the offending hairs. Antihistamines, analgesics, ice packs, and systemic corticosteroids may be beneficial.

HELMINTH INFESTATIONS

Swimmer's itch and *seabather's eruption* are due to an immune response to schistosomal cercariae. Seabather's eruption is usually acquired on the coast of Florida or in the Caribbean and manifests as pruritic urticarial papules on sites beneath the swimsuit. Children with seabather's eruption may have systemic reactions, with fever, malaise, nausea, vomiting, and headaches. Swimmer's itch develops after exposure to cercariae in fresh water, especially on the shores of Wisconsin and Michigan. The urticarial papules are usually located on exposed sites. Both reactions subside spontaneously after 1 to 2 weeks, often with transient residual hyperpigmentation. Therapy consists of antipruritic lotions and antihistamines.

Cutaneous larva migrans (*creeping eruption*) is a distinctive cutaneous eruption that results from the migration of larval hookworms (*Ancylostoma*

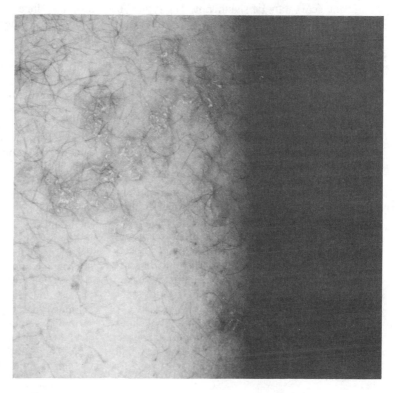

Figure 70-2. Serpiginous eruption of cutaneous larva migrans.

braziliense) through the skin. The infestation is usually acquired from the sands of the Atlantic Ocean and Gulf of Mexico. The eruption begins with pruritus at the site of penetration, usually the buttocks, feet, lower legs, or hands. The lesions are slightly elevated pink or flesh-colored serpentine tracts that progress slowly (Fig. 70-2). Vesicles or bullae may appear along the tract. The eruption may not begin for weeks to months after larval penetration. Systemic eosinophilia may be associated. The rash is self-limited and usually clears after 1 to 4 weeks, but may last as long as 6 months. Treatment consists of oral thiabendazole (25 mg/kg administered twice daily for 2 to 4 days) or topical 10% thiabendazole suspension applied four times daily for 7 days. Topical corticosteroids may alleviate the pruritus.

ANNOTATED BIBLIOGRAPHY

Honig PJ: Bites and parasites. Pediatr Clin North Am 30:563–581, 1983 (Comprehensive summary of bites and infestations in children.)

Hurwitz S: Erythema chronicum migrans and Lyme disease. Pediatr Dermatol 2:266–274, 1985 (Review of Lyme disease and its cutaneous manifestations.)

Orkin M, Maibach HI: This scabies pandemic. N Engl J Med 298:496–498, 1978 (Review of the diagnosis and management of scabies infections.)

Rasmussen JE: Pediculosis and the pediatrician. Pediatr Dermatol 2:74–79, 1984 (Current review of lice infestations and their therapy.)

Riley HD J: Rickettsial diseases and Rocky Mountain spotted fever. Curr Probl Pediatr XI:4–46 (Part 1);3–37 (Part 2), 1981 (Excellent review for the pediatrician of Rocky Mountain spotted fever.)

71
Acne
AMY PALLER

Acne is one of the most common problems of teenagers; although it is not a serious medical problem, the psychological effects of inflammation and disfiguring scars may be significant. The typical lesions of acne vulgaris are blackheads, whiteheads, and localized areas of inflammation.

PATHOPHYSIOLOGY

Many factors appear to influence the occurrence and severity of acne. These include (1) increased sebum production by sebaceous glands during and after puberty, (2) bacteria, (3) partial obstruction of the pilosebaceous canal, (4) hormonal influences, and (5) genetics.

The pilosebaceous follicles contain multilobulated sebaceous glands that discharge their contents (*i.e.*, sebum, at the skin surface). Under the influence of androgenic hormones, sebum production by sebaceous glands increases at the time of puberty. At this time the skin becomes oily and the early lesions of acne begin. The role of sebum in the pathogenesis of acne, however, is poorly understood. In the pilosebaceous canal, the triglycerides of sebum are cleaved into free fatty acids by lipase from the anaerobic bacterium *Propionibacterium acnes*, an organism that also increases dramatically at the time of puberty. These free fatty acids, as well as prostaglandins and other bacterial products, are irritating and chemotactic. Sebum, however, is not the only participant in the formation of acne lesions, since its production continues without change in content or quantity throughout adulthood, despite the disappearance of acne lesions.

Partial obstruction of the follicle also contributes to the formation of lesions. The precursor lesion of acne, the comedo, forms in the lower portion of the hair follicle or infrainfundibulum. Rather than the normal disintegration and shedding of horny cells to the surface of the hair follicle, the cells of patients with acne adhere to each other to form the plug of the comedo. The mixture of sebum, horny cells, and *P. acnes bacteria* distends the hair follicle and attracts inflammatory cells. Although the hair follicle is distended, there is not enough pressure to rupture, thus leakage of inflammatory materials, including free fatty acids, results.

Androgens, especially free testosterone and its tissue product dihydrotestosterone (DHT) and the androgenic adrenal steroid dihydroepiandrosterone sulfate (DHEAS) increase the size of sebaceous glands and the production and lipid content of sebum. Finally, genetic factors are involved in determining the occurrence and extent of acne. Identical twins are usually concordant for the expression of acne and offspring tend to follow the pattern of their parents.

CLINICAL PRESENTATION

Patients with acne vulgaris (common acne) may have several types of lesions, any of which may predominate: These include open and closed comedones, inflammatory papules and pustules, and nodulocystic lesions. In early adolescence, acne is usually comedonal and confined to the face. By mid-adolescence, inflammatory acne with papules and pustules is the most common form, and the chest and back become more readily involved.

The microcomedo, the initial lesion of acne, represents the hair follicle distended by the accumulated horny cell material, lipids, and bacteria. The closed comedo or whitehead is a skin-colored slightly palpable lesion (1 mm to 3 mm) without a readily visible central pore. Closed comedones have been called "the time bombs of acne" because they often enlarge to form the inflammatory papules or pustules. Alternatively, they may remain quiescent for months or evolve into open comedones. Open comedones or blackheads have a wide pore opening filled with black material. This material is melanin and oxidized lipids, not dirt. These open comedones tend to be more stable than the closed comedones and rarely become inflamed.

The papules and pustules of inflammatory acne develop in distended, partially obstructed follicles following the increased permeability of the follicular wall and the influx of inflammatory cells. Although papules and pustules may be superficial and resolve quickly, deeper lesions that form in the lower portion of the hair canal often take weeks to heal. Nodulocystic lesions are warm and tender abscesses. They occur most commonly along the jawline, earlobes, and neck, and result from the fusion of adjacent deep pustules. Acne cysts require 2 to 3 months to heal by granulation tissue formation and scarring.

Acne scars are the outcome of inflammatory acne. The closed and open comedones may resolve as accentuated pores, but they do not leave scars unless secondary inflammation occurs. The scars may vary in shape and extent. Ice pick scars are small, deep pits that result from inflammatory papules and pustules. Nodulocystic lesions may leave larger disfiguring scars. The most common reason for scarring of superficial lesions is self-inflicted trauma from scratching, squeezing lesions, and extracting them with fingernails (Fig. 71-1). This self-induced trauma tends to leave small, irregular, and often linear scars. Keloids may develop, especially

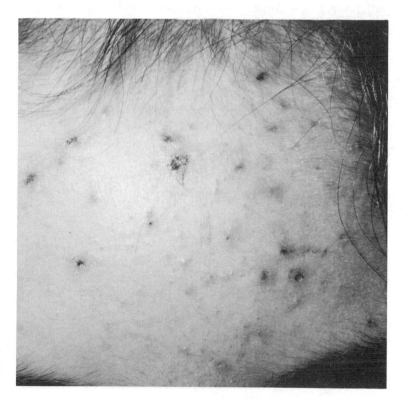

Figure 71-1. Excoriated acne lesions that became scars in a teen-aged girl with otherwise mild comedonal acne.

in black teenagers, on the anterior chest, back, neck, and occasionally on the face. Rarely, calcification of scars occurs as small blue nodules that may eventually resolve by extrusion of the calcific material.

In dark-skinned individuals, inflammatory lesions often resolve with hyperpigmentation. This postinflammatory hyperpigmentation tends to clear spontaneously after months to years, but may be exacerbated by the continued development of inflammatory lesions and sun exposure.

SPECIAL CLINICAL FORMS OF ACNE

Acne conglobata is a form of severe nodulocystic acne that occurs in 3% of white male adolescents. Multiple nodules fuse, forming large, irregular tender purple nodules that discharge purulent material from the resultant sinus tracts. Nontender large multipored open comedones cluster amidst these draining nodules and sinuses. The back is the typical site of acne conglobata, but the face, upper arms, thigh, and buttocks are also frequently involved. Pustules and cysts may form as well. Acne conglobata often remains active into the third decade of life and leaves severe scarring.

Acne fulminans is a rare form of acne associated with fever, polyarthritis, leukocytosis, and anemia. Large necrotic nodules that drain a gelatinous material are found on the back and upper chest and resolve as deep ulcerations.

Acne neonatorum manifests as tiny yellow papules on the forehead, cheeks, and nose of neonates due to sebaceous gland hyperactivity under the influence of maternal hormones. Papules and pustules are occasionally present. The acne resolves spontaneously when the maternal hormones disappear after 1 or 2 months.

Infantile acne develops after the first 3 months of life and usually resolves spontaneously by 18 months of age. Most commonly, boys with a strong family history of severe acne are affected. Typical lesions are comedones and papules on the cheeks, and occasionally pustules are present. Excessive use of oils and lotions applied to the infant's skin must be considered if there is a predominance of comedones. The pathogenesis of infantile acne is unknown, but a transient increase in gonadal production of testosterone has been postulated. An underlying endocrinologic abnormality should be considered if numerous pustules are present. Therapy is usually not required, and only mild keratolytic agents should be used if the acne is extensive.

Cosmetic acne is caused by oily moisturizers, foundations, and hair preparations. The lesions that result are closed comedones that may become inflammatory papulopustules. Most moisturizers are comedogenic, but cocoa butter is a common cause of comedogenic acne. Makeups that have an oily base and moisturizers will usually cause acne on the cheeks, whereas hair preparations tend to stimulate the formation of acne lesions on the forehead (pomade acne). This form of acne can be puzzling, because patients often use a variety of oily preparations during a period of time and lesions are slow to develop. Cosmetic acne may take 6 to 8 months to resolve following the discontinuation of the inciting agent.

Occlusion-induced acne (*mechanical acne*) is the exacerbation of mild acne by mechanical factors that rub and occlude. Acne on the chin may be aggravated by resting the chin on the hand while studying or by chin straps. Forehead lesions may become inflamed by sweatbands, hats, or excessive combing of the hair. Neck lesions may be aggravated by shirt collars or turtle-neck sweaters. Clusters of lesions in a particular pattern may suggest this type of acne.

Occupational acne is prevalent in teenagers who work at fast-food restaurants or as car mechanics. Comedonal acne tends to develop from working over frying oils or contact with greases from car lubricants or other petroleum products. *Chloracne* has rarely developed in children following exposure to chlorinated hydrocarbons at toxic waste dumps near industries.

Drug-induced acne most commonly occurs from the use of oral or fluorinated topical corticosteroids. Within a few weeks after therapy begins, crops of papulopustules without comedones appear. Androgens, gonadotropins, and adrenocorticotropins may produce lesions more typical of the mixed pattern of acne vulgaris. Other drugs that induce or aggravate acne are lithium, phenobarbital, phenytoin, trimethadione, isoniazid, rifampin, iodides, and bromides. Drug-induced acne tends to appear suddenly; it may be characterized by large numbers of lesions and involves unusual areas, such as the upper arms and lower back.

Gram-negative folliculitis develops in patients who have taken oral broad-spectrum antibiotics for long periods of time. As a result of changes in bacterial flora, pustules and cysts appear that do not respond to increased doses of antibiotics. Gram-negative organisms are most common, especially *Klebsiella*, *Enterobacter*, and *Proteus*.

DIFFERENTIAL DIAGNOSIS

The lesions of acne are easily recognizable; the underlying factors that exacerbate the acne may be more difficult to determine. Occasionally, patients with tuberous sclerosis and adenoma sebaceum may be mistakenly thought to have acne. Patients with unusual or severe forms of acne may have endocrinologic abnormalities; other signs include hirsutism, precocious puberty, irregularities in menses and those of Cushing's disease.

EVALUATION

Patients with acne should be questioned about the duration and typical severity of their acne, and the effect and duration of medications that have been tried in the past, including over-the-counter medication. Possible use of other oral and topical medications must be elicited, especially oral contraceptives and topical fluorinated corticosteroids. Knowledge of the use of moisturizers, makeup, and hair pomades is important for the pediatrician. Finally, the history of other medical abnormalities and menses of adolescent girls should be ascertained. A physical examination may be limited to the face, neck, chest, and back, unless the history suggests an underlying problem that requires a more extensive examination. The predominant lesional types will direct management. Routine laboratory testing is unnecessary. Other evidence of androgenic effects should prompt the evaluation of adrenal and gonadal function.

TREATMENT

Several misconceptions about acne must be dispelled. First, dietary factors including chocolate and carbohydrates are probably insignificant. If a patient believes, however, that a particular food aggravates the acne, it is best to eliminate that food. Second, although topical therapeutic agents cause dryness, they are more effective than harsh soaps, scrubs, and frequent washing. The use of scrubs should be discouraged in order to lower the risk of irritation by prescribed topical agents and prevent the risk of transformation of comedones into inflammatory lesions. Finally, moisturizers and oil-based makeups exacerbate acne by plugging the follicles and encouraging comedo formation. Patients should be advised to use water-based makeup or none at all. Noncomedogenic lotions, such as Nutraderm lotion, may be used for excessive dryness without causing increased comedonal acne.

Treatment regimens should be directed towards (1) altering the pattern of keratinization, (2) decreasing sebum production, (3) decreasing the population of P. acnes, and (4) producing an anti-inflammatory effect. *Benzoyl peroxide* preparations are the most commonly used acne medications. Benzoyl peroxide is an oxidizing agent with bacteriostatic properties. As a primary irritant, it also increases blood flow to the lesional skin and accelerates healing. In addition, benzoyl peroxide is keratolytic and decreases the adherence of follicular horny cells. As a result, benzoyl peroxide is useful for both comedonal and inflammatory acne. Benzoyl peroxide causes contact allergy in 2.5% of patients, resulting in pruritus, erythema, and periorbital edema. The most common reaction is an irritant reaction, which often causes postinflammatory hyperpigmentation in black patients. Improvement in acne may be seen within 1 to 3 weeks.

Retinoic acid, a metabolite of vitamin A, is an exfoliant and irritant that also increases blood flow to the skin. It is best used as a comedolytic agent; it increases the turnover of pilosebaceous epithelial cells and prevents the adherence of horny layer cells. Not uncommonly, pustules may develop as comedones are expelled 3 to 4 weeks after the onset of therapy; this is not an indication to stop the agent. Secondary hyperpigmentation may result in black and oriental patients. Patients using retinoic acid may be more susceptible to sunburn and should be advised to use sunscreens during sun exposure. Good results are seen in up to 70% of patients within 3 months.

Other keratolytic agents, such as 5% to 10% salicylic acid or 3% to 6% sulfur preparations, may be helpful for patients who cannot tolerate benzoyl peroxide or retinoic acid. The effect of sunlight is mostly keratolytic, although lesions may be obscured by the resultant erythema and pigmentation. The routine use of ultraviolet light to treat acne is not indicated in view of the potential carcinogenic effect.

Topical and systemic antibiotics are helpful for inflammatory acne as antibacterial and anti-inflammatory agents. Topical antibiotics should be used for patients with mild to moderate inflammatory acne and for patients who cannot tolerate systemic antibiotics. Topical preparations of clindamycin, erythromycin, and tetracycline are available. The only significant side effect of topical preparations is dryness, especially due to those in alcohol bases. The risk of pseudomembranous colitis from topical clindamycin is remote. Topical tetracycline produces a yellow fluorescence under black light.

Systemic antibiotics should be introduced for moderate to severe inflammatory acne. Tetracycline, erythromycin, and minocycline accumulate in the pilosebaceous canal, decrease the population of *P. acnes*, and inhibit neutrophil chemotaxis. Side effects are usually gastrointestinal intolerance and vaginal candidiasis. Unusual side effects of minocycline include dizziness and hyperpigmentation. Tetracycline and minocycline should not be prescribed for pregnant adolescents. Systemic antibiotics must be given for 2 to 3 months before effectiveness is determined. The dosage should be tapered after this time.

Isotretinoin (Accutane) use should be restricted to patients with recalcitrant cystic acne. Accutane causes involution of sebaceous glands, lowers the colonization by *P. acnes*, and limits keratinization of the follicle. Patients are generally treated for 4 months at doses of 0.5 to 2 mg/kg/day. Facial cysts tend to respond first, often within the first month; truncal lesions usually require 3 to 4 months of medication. The effect of Accutane continues, often indefinitely, after discontinuation of the drug. The major side effects are dose-related and include dry skin and lips, epistaxis, conjunctivitis, and, occasionally, musculoskeletal complaints, rashes, increased photosensitivity, peeling of the palms and soles, and headache. Triglyceride levels become elevated in 25% of patients; they may be diminished by a low-fat diet and avoidance of alcohol; and they return to normal following cessation of Accutane. Laboratory parameters should be checked monthly while taking the drug. Accutane is absolutely contraindicated in pregnancy due to its teratogenicity. Fertile female patients should be tested for pregnancy and use an effective form of contraception while taking Accutane and for at least 1 month following its discontinuation.

Doses of >50 μg of ethinyl estradiol or its equivalent suppress sebum production and diminish acne after 2 to 3 months. Therefore, the administration of oral contraceptives with higher amounts of estrogen (*e.g.*, Enovid-E, Ovulen) may be considered for patients who require birth control or adolescent girls with severe, recalcitrant acne. Antiandrogens, such as spironolactone and cyproterone acetate, have controlled acne in women with elevated androgen levels. Dapsone is an anti-inflammatory agent that has proved useful for severe cystic acne or acne conglobata, but is too toxic to use before other treatment modalities. Finally, oral zinc sulfate may be a useful adjunctive agent for inflammatory acne.

Several physical modalities are helpful in the management of acne and its sequelae. Severely inflamed papular and cystic lesions respond within 48 hours to intralesional injection of triamcinolone acetonide. Atrophy rarely results, if the amount injected is less than 0.5 mg per cm^2. The superficial scarring of acne may be treated with chemical peels, such as trichloracetic acid. Deeper scars may be eliminated by dermabrasion, in which the epidermis and upper dermis are removed to the level of the scar. Side effects include erythema, milia, pigmentary alterations, and hypertrophic scarring. Finally, bovine collagen may be injected into deep, ice pick scars to raise them to skin level.

INDICATIONS FOR REFERRAL

Most patients with acne of mild severity will respond to topical agents. Patients who require long-term systemic antibiotics, isotretinoin, or other systemic agents or physical modalities of treatment are best referred to a dermatologist.

ANNOTATED BIBLIOGRAPHY

Esterly NB, Furey NL: Acne: Current concepts. Pediatrics 62:1044–1055, 1978 (Review with good descriptions of clinical lesions.)

Matsuoka LY: Acne. J Pediatr 103:849–854, 1983 (Current review, including treatment modalities.)

Stern RS, Rosa F, Baum C: Isotretinoin and pregnancy. J Am Acad Dermatol 10:851–854, 1984 (Good review of the congenital anomalies associated with isotretinoin use during the first trimester of pregnancy.)

Tunnessen WW Jr.: Acne: An approach to therapy for the pediatrician. Curr Probl Pediatr XIV(5):6–36, 1984 (Well written, general review.)

The assessment of a child with abnormalities of the hair and nails requires a detailed history and a careful clinical examination, often including a microscopic examination of hair and fungal cultures of hair and nails (see the box, Assessment of the Child with Hair Loss). The hair texture, style, length, and the distribution of hair loss should be noted. The pattern and extent of nail changes should also be determined. Any child with hair and nail abnormalities should also be questioned and examined carefully for other defects, especially ectodermal defects.

HAIR DEFECTS

In order to understand hair disorders, it is important to review the three phases of the human hair growth cycle. *Anagen* is the period of hair growth that lasts 2 to 6 years and includes 90% of hairs. *Catagen* is a transition state that lasts a few days. *Telogen* is a resting phase that lasts about 3 months and includes 10% of hairs. The resting hair is shed as the new anagen hair emerges. The normal scalp has 100,000 hairs and hair grows at a rate of 1 cm each month. The hair growth cycle is not synchronized and it is normal to lose 50 to 100 hairs a day, especially with shampooing. Before hair loss becomes clinically evident, 25% to 50% of hair must be lost.

There are two forms of physiologic hair loss: shedding of the newborn and temporal recession at puberty. *In utero*, silky hair called lanugo hair develops over the entire fetus. Lanugo hair is shed *in utero* and replaced during the sixth to eighth month gestation by vellus hair, except on the scalp, eyebrows, and eyelashes, where lanugo hair is replaced by terminal hair. This hair is shed during the first year of life and is replaced by thicker, darker hair. The other physiologic form of hair loss is due to the increase in androgen levels in both boys and girls at puberty that changes the hairline from a straight line to an "M" shape, with vellus hairs taking the place of terminal hairs.

Most hair loss in children is acquired, due to fungal infections, trauma, or alopecia areata. Fungal infections are usually characterized by focal or

---

Assessment of the Child with Hair Loss

HISTORY

Duration of hair loss, pattern, breakage *vs* "by the roots"

Past health, use of medications, topical preparations, and diet

Use of hair care products and hair treatments

Other abnormalities of skin, nails, teeth, sweating, and so forth

Family history of hair problems and ectodermal abnormalities

EXAMINATION

Pattern of hair loss

Underlying scalp abnormalities

Hair texture, breakage, lengths, and hair tips

"Pull test"

Hirsutism elsewhere, acne, and virilization

Other ectodermal defects by examination

MICROSCOPIC EXAMINATION OF HAIR

KOH (and culture) if tinea capitis is suspected

Mount to examine for hair shaft defects

SCALP BIOPSY

For scarring alopecia and some nonscarring alopecia (may help to diagnose trichotillomania, alopecia areata)

OTHER LABORATORY TESTS

Sweat quantitation and dental radiographs for ectodermal dysplasia

Thyroid hormones and complete blood count for telogen effluvium

Thyroid homones and antibodies if indicated with alopecia areata

---

diffuse hair loss with underlying scalp scaling and erythema (see Chap. 65). If the diagnosis of tinea capitis is considered, KOH examination and fungal cultures should always be performed. Excessive traction on the hair from tight ponytails or braiding (especially "corn-rowing") often results in hair loss

323

at the sites of maximal traction, such as at the margins of the hairline, at the part line, or scattered throughout the scalp. The hair usually regrows if the traction is eliminated, unless chronic traction produces fibrosis and permanent injury. Similarly, hair may be lost by friction (usually rubbing the occipital scalp on the bedsheets in infants) that results in hair breakage or by avulsion of clumps of hair by playmates. Chemical or physical trauma to the hair from hair dyes, straighteners, permanent wave treatments, and ironing the hair may cause hair breakage or contact dermatitis of the scalp, resulting in hair loss that may take years to resolve. Occasionally, children compulsively pull out hairs of the scalp, eyelashes, or eyebrows, a condition called *trichotillomania*. The patches of hair loss are irregular in shape with short hairs of various lengths. On the scalp, the occipital hair is usually spared. The disorder may be confused with alopecia areata and a scalp biopsy may be required to differentiate the conditions. The histopathologic features of trichotillomania include evidence of follicular trauma, such as hemorrhage, increased numbers of catagen hairs, soft keratin material within the follicles, and minimal inflammation. Many cases resolve spontaneously, but it is important to make the proper diagnosis and to explain to the parents that the disorder is due to a habit. Children who are severely affected should be referred for a psychiatric evaluation.

Alopecia areata is a common disorder characterized by the sudden onset of well-circumscribed patches of nonscarring alopecia (Fig. 72-1). Ten to 20% of affected individuals have a positive family history of alopecia areata. The cause of alopecia areata is unknown, but it is suspected to be an autoimmune disorder because of the high incidence of associated autoantibodies, especially antibodies against thyroglobulin, parietal cells, and the adrenal gland, and of associated autoimmune disorders.

The typical pattern of alopecia areata is the sudden development of one or more round patches of alopecia with an underlying scalp that is normal. At the margin of the patches, short hairs with an attenuated bulb ("exclamation mark" hairs) may be found. Disease activity can be assessed by the "pull test" in which hair at the periphery is grasped and pulled. Hair comes out easily if the disorder is active at that area. The patches of alopecia usually occur on the scalp, but can appear in any hair-bearing area. Alopecia areata totalis is alopecia of the entire scalp and alopecia areata universalis is the

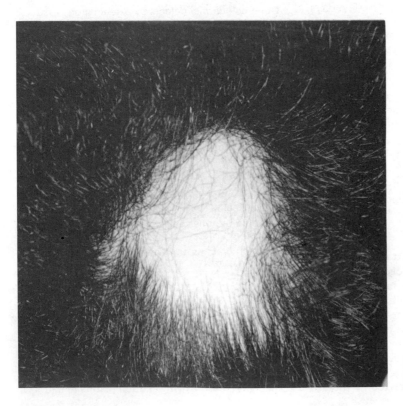

Figure 72-1. Well-demarcated patch of alopecia areata with normal underlying scalp.

complete loss of all body hair as well. The ophiasis pattern of alopecia areata is alopecia that extends from the occipital area around the sides of the scalp to the front in a band. Rarely, diffuse thinning of the scalp hair occurs and may be confused with telogen effluvium. Nail pitting may develop in 10% to 20% of patients with alopecia areata, but the dystrophy is rarely severe.

The diagnosis of alopecia areata is usually based on the clinical appearance. The disorder may be confused occasionally with the black dot form of tinea capitis or with trichotillomania. A KOH examination, fungal culture, and scalp biopsy aid in distinguishing these disorders. A histopathologic examination of the scalp biopsy of alopecia areata shows small atrophic hair follicles, sometimes with inflammatory cell infiltrates surrounding the hairbulbs. Children with alopecia areata should be examined for the concurrent possibility of Hashimoto's thyroiditis, vitiligo, and collagen vascular disease.

The course of alopecia areata is unpredictable. Most patients show hair regrowth within 1 to 2 years after the onset, especially with the limited forms of alopecia. Children with alopecia areata need encouragement and, at times, psychologic counseling. The suggestion of a wig may immediately improve the appearance and prevent children from being teased while the disorder resolves or persists. There are no clearly effective forms of therapy, but efficacy may be difficult to assess in view of the high rate of spontaneous resolution. For younger children, moderate to high potency topical steroids under occlusion or topical anthralin preparations are the available treatments. At least 6 months of therapy are often necessary. In older children, intralesional triamcinolone is most effective if the disease is limited to a few patches. Systemic steroids should not be used. Other possible treatment modalities for older children include the induction of contact allergic dermatitis with dinitrochlorobenzene or squaric acid dibutylester, psoralens and ultraviolet A light (PUVA), inosiplex (an immunostimulant), and topical minoxidil.

Anagen effluvium and telogen effluvium are conditions of diffuse hair loss that affect anagen hairs and telogen hairs, respectively. Cancer chemotherapy is the most common reason for loss of anagen hairs in children with loss of 80% to 90% of the hair occurring 7 to 14 days after use of the drugs. Telogen effluvium occurs 2 to 4 months after injury. The causes in children for later telogen effluvium include high fever, severe infection, illness or psychological stress, surgery, hypo- or hyperthyroid-

ism, pernicious anemia, and nutritional deficiency. In addition, several medications may cause telogen effluvium, such as anticonvulsants, anticoagulants (as in rat poison), retinoids, and hormones. The numbers of telogen hairs increase from 10% to between 30% and 50% in children with telogen effluvium. The hair loss of both anagen and telogen effluvium resolves after the underlying cause is eliminated.

Several congenital disorders are associated with hair loss. The hair may be totally absent (alopecia) or sparse (hypotrichosis). Many of these disorders are due to hair shaft abnormalities, and the diagnosis may be made by an examination of the hair under the microscope. Hair anomalies associated with hair shaft fragility include monilethrix, trichorrhexis nodosa, trichorrhexis invaginata, pili torti, and trichothiodystrophy. Hair shaft abnormalities without associated hair fragility include pili annulati, pseudopili annulati, woolly hair, and the uncombable hair syndrome.

Monilethrix or beaded hair is usually an autosomal dominant condition. The hair is sparse and breaks easily, so that the scalp is covered by short hairs. The scalp tends to have a rough appearance, especially at the occiput, due to follicular hyperkeratosis. Microscopic examination of hair shafts shows uniform beading along the shaft with fractures in internodal areas. Patients may improve spontaneously at puberty. There is no effective treatment.

Trichorrhexis nodosa or trichoclasis is characterized clinically by white nodules on the hair shafts. The condition is usually acquired as a result of trauma, and responds to the elimination of vigorous grooming habits. Patients may have friable, brittle hair that shows the nodules of trichorrhexis nodosa. By microscopy, the hair shafts of trichorrhexis nodosa show brush-like fractures. Trichorrhexis nodosa is seen in patients with arginosuccinic aciduria.

Trichorrhexis invaginata (bamboo hair) is a hair defect characterized by joint-like deformities of the hair shaft. The hair is short, dry, dull, and sparse. The defect tends to be present by infancy and usually persists. This type of hair defect is associated with Netherton's syndrome, an autosomal recessive disorder with nonbullous ichthyosiform erythroderma or ichthyosis linearis circumflex, nail dystrophy, and atopy with eczema, urticaria, angioneurotic edema, asthma, and rhinitis.

Pili torti or twisted hairs is a hair condition characterized by hair shafts that are twisted 180° on their own axes at irregular intervals. The defect is usually present by early infancy, and the hairs are typically fragile. As an isolated defect, pili torti is inherited as an autosomal dominant disorder. Pili torti has also been described in association with Menkes' syndrome.

Trichothiodystrophy (also called low sulfur hair syndrome and BIDS—*B*rittle hair, *I*ntellectual impairment, *D*ecreased fertility, *S*hort stature) is an autosomal recessive neuroectodermal defect with sparse and brittle scalp hair, eyebrows, and eyelashes. Amino acid analysis of hairs shows a low concentration of the sulfur-containing amino acid cystine. The fingernails and toenails of patients are often brittle and dystrophic, with spoon-shaped deformities (koilonychia). Amino acids analysis of these abnormal nails also shows a gross deficiency in cystine. Associated features include mental and physical retardation, congenital nonbullous ichthyosiform erythroderma with palmoplantar keratoderma, atopic-like eczema, congenital cataracts, neurosensory hearing loss, central nervous system abnormalities, ultraviolet B light photosensitivity, and decreased fertility with primary testicular failure.

Pili annulati or ringed hair is an autosomal dominant defect of hair noted shortly after birth. The hair shaft is not fragile, and bands of hair appear to be highlighted. By microscopy, the hair has alternating light and dark bands, due to air-filled cavities within the cortex and medulla of the hair shaft. There is no effective therapy. *Pseudopili annulati* is a variant in which light bands are seen at irregular intervals along the hair shaft, especially in blond individuals, due to twisting of the hair shaft and variations in cross-sectional diameter.

Woolly hair is a defect involving the entire scalp with fine, dry, curly hair. This hereditary defect must be differentiated from the woolly hair nevus, which is a localized patch of curly hair and is not a hereditary disorder. The *uncombable hair syndrome* (pili trianguli canaliculi, spun glass hair syndrome) appears soon after birth as thick bundles of hair that grow in all directions and cannot be arranged by combing. The hair is light in color and dry, and has a characteristic sheen, but it grows normally and is not fragile. The main differential diagnosis of the uncombable hair syndrome is woolly hair.

Generalized hair loss may also be due to metabolic abnormalities. *Multiple carboxylase deficiency* is a group of autosomal recessive disorders involving the enzymes that metabolize branched chain amino acids, including propionyl CoA carboxylase, beta-methyl crotonyl CoA carboxylase,

and pyruvate carboxylase. All of these enzymes require biotin as a cofactor. Patients with the infantile form exhibit cutaneous manifestations, including sparse hair, periorificial dermatitis, and severe mucocutaneous candidiasis. Other features include progressive ataxia, seizures, psychomotor retardation, keratoconjunctivitis, and lactic acidosis. Urine testing for organic acids reveals elevated levels of substrate metabolites. Serum biotin is decreased or normal, and patients may have hypoglycemia and hyperammonuria. The administration of biotin in doses of 10 mg to 40 mg daily corrects the immunologic abnormalities and promotes normal hair growth. Alopecia may also be a feature of acrodermatitis enteropathica and arginosuccinic aciduria.

All of the disorders discussed are nonscarring types of alopecia. Scarring alopecia is unusual in children and may be due to developmental defects (such as aplasia cutis congenita), physical injury, infection, lichen planus, lupus erythematosus, scleroderma, sarcoidosis, and neoplasm. *Aplasia cutis congenita* is a rare congenital defect characterized by the absence of circumscribed areas of skin and appendages. The lesion(s) of aplasia cutis are present at birth, usually as a solitary, well-circumscribed hairless area at the midline of the scalp by the vertex or near the sagittal suture. Less commonly, the lesions are located elsewhere on the scalp, and rarely on the face, trunk, or limbs. Lesions on the trunk or limbs are commonly multiple, extensive, and symmetric. The skin usually appears ulcerated with crusting, but may be bullous, membranous or be healed at the time of birth. As the aplasia heals, it is replaced by a smooth, atrophic, gray parchment-like scar. Although aplasia cutis is usually an isolated abnormality, 20% of patients have a defect of the underlying cranial bone and 13% have limb malformations.

Aplasia cutis congenita is most easily confused with trauma, usually due to a fetal monitor or to forceps injury. Occasionally, other traumatic injuries due to chemical or thermal burns or scarring from needles or amniocentesis must be distinguished. The well-circumscribed hairless lesion of aplasia cutis can also resemble the congenital hairless sebaceus nevus of Jadassohn. A histopathologic examination of skin biopsy sections allows the diagnosis to be made. The healed, scarred lesions of aplasia cutis must also be contrasted with those of discoid lupus erythematosus, morphea, and the more widespread congenital erosive and vesicular dermatosis.

NAIL DISORDERS

The nails grow continuously throughout life and are not normally shed. The rate of nail growth varies from 0.5 mm to 1.2 mm per week, with the growth rate of toenails almost one half that of fingernails. Dystrophic nails may result from congenital disorders, such as the nail–patella syndrome and pachyonychia congenita, or may be due to acquired disorders, such as eczema, infections, psoriasis, lichen planus, alopecia areata, or twenty nail dystrophy. Only the disorders that are not discussed elsewhere in the text are considered below.

The *nail–patella syndrome* (osteo-onychodysplasia, nail–patella–elbow syndrome) is an autosomal dominant defect that is characterized by the absence or hypoplasia of the patella and nails, subluxation of the radial heads, and renal dysplasia with chronic glomerulonephritis. Less common findings are thickened scapulae, iliac horns, and hyperextensible joints. Triangular lunulae are the most characteristic nail abnormality, although softening, spoon nails, discoloration, and narrowing of nails are common as well. The renal abnormalities include proteinuria, hematuria, and decreased renal clearance; these changes are generally asymptomatic and the prognosis is usually good.

Pachyonychia congenita or the Jadassohn–Lewandowsky syndrome usually follows an autosomal dominant inheritance pattern. The nails show marked subungual hyperkeratosis with thickening of the distal part of the nail so that the nail is lifted off of the nailbed. These changes are progressive and often begin as yellowing of the nail or recurrent nail loss at birth or during the first year of life, but have been reported to begin as late as the teenage years. All of the nails tend to be involved. Paronychial inflammation may precede or accompany the nail changes. Associated abnormalities include hyperhidrosis and thickening of the palm and soles, follicular keratoses that resemble keratosis pilaris, blisters of the hands and feet, hypotrichosis and multiple cysts (steatocystoma multiplex). Later in childhood, lesions may appear on the trunk, axillae, neck, scalp, and face. Leukokeratosis of the tongue or buccal mucosa is common, and dental and eye anomalies have occasionally been reported in patients with pachyonychia congenita. The nail thickening is persistent and management may be difficult. Most patients keep the nails short and file the nails down to a more normal thickness for ease of fine manipulation with the fingers and for cosmetic reasons.

Twenty nail dystrophy is an idiopathic nail disorder of childhood that is characterized by whitening and ridging of all twenty nails. The condition is self-limited and resolves within a few years. Therapy is not usually helpful. Other diagnoses, such as psoriasis, lichen planus, and alopecia areata, should be considered. Nail biopsy is traumatic for a child and without other evidence of these mucocutaneous disorders, the diagnosis of twenty nail dystrophy should be made.

DISORDERS OF BOTH HAIR AND NAILS: ECTODERMAL DYSPLASIAS

Ectodermal dysplasia is a term for a number of syndromes that show alterations of ectodermal structures and function, including the skin, hair, nails, teeth, and eccrine glands. Ectodermal dysplasias must be congenital and affect at least two tissues of ectodermal origin. The most common forms of ectodermal dysplasia are *hypohidrotic ectodermal dysplasia* and *hidrotic ectodermal dysplasia*. Hypohidrotic (anhidrotic) ectodermal dysplasia is the most easily recognizable of the ectodermal dysplasias. The majority of individuals that show the complete syndrome are male, with an inheritance pattern consistent with an X-linked recessive mode. Children with hypohidrotic ectodermal dysplasia have a characteristic combination of defective dentition, hypotrichosis, and a typical facies that is so easily recognizable that these affected children more closely resemble one another than they do their own siblings. The most serious feature in affected infants is the inability to sweat adequately due to deficient numbers of eccrine glands. As a result, infants have recurrent high fevers and cutaneous erythema, especially in hot weather following exercise. Febrile convulsions may be associated with the high fevers. The hair is sparse, fine, lighter in color than that of other family members and often unruly. Complete alopecia is unusual. The nails are usually normal, but the teeth are typically decreased in number and anomalous, with conical or peg-shaped teeth, discolored incisors, and malocclusion. The facial features include frontal bossing, prominent supraorbital ridges, wrinkling and hyperpigmentation of periorbital skin, a depressed nasal bridge (saddle nose deformity), a small nose with hypoplastic alae nasi, underdeveloped maxilla, pointed chin, protruberant lips and ears that are low-lying, anteriorly placed and pointed. Ectodermal glands other than eccrine glands are also hypoplastic, leading to atrophic rhinitis, dry mouth, pharyngitis, dysphagia, otitis media, recurrent respiratory tract infections, chronic laryngitis, and defective lacrimal gland function. Children with hypohidrotic ectodermal dysplasia have an increased frequency of atopic dermatitis.

The classic form of hidrotic ectodermal dysplasia (Clouston syndrome) is an autosomal dominant disorder. The major clinical features are dystrophic nails, hypotrichosis, and palmoplantar keratoderma. Sweating is quantitatively normal and dental abnormalities are rare.

ANNOTATED BIBLIOGRAPHY

Goldsmith LA: An approach to the diagnosis of genetic hair disorders. Prog Dermatol 18:1–7, 1984 (Differential diagnostic approach to hair disorders.)

Mitchell AJ, Krull EA: Alopecia areata: Pathogenesis and treatment. J Am Acad Dermatol 11:763–775, 1984 (Current review of alopecia areata and its management.)

Norton LA: Nail disorders. J Am Acad Dermatol 2:451–467, 1980 (Review of nail disorders.)

Reed WB, Lopez DA, Landing B: Clinical spectrum of anhidrotic ectodermal dysplasia. Arch Dermatol 102:134–143, 1970 (Good discussion of the problems of hypohidrotic ectodermal dysplasia.)

Solomon LM, Keuer EJ: The ectodermal dysplasias. Arch Dermatol 116:1295–1299, 1980 (Review of the various forms of ectodermal dysplasia.)

Stroud JD: Hair loss in children. Pediatr Clin North Am 30:641–657, 1983 (Current review of causes of alopecia in children.)

10

Endocrinologic Problems

73

Neonatal Screening for Thyroid Disease

ROBERT Z. KLEIN

The importance of neonatal screening for hypothyroidism has been firmly established. It allows the diagnosis of infantile hypothyroidism before there are sufficient physical signs to suggest a clinical diagnosis. The resultant early treatment prevents the brain damage so common after clinically diagnosed infantile hypothyroidism. Intelligence quotients of the patients are normal. The relatively few of these children who have gone through the third grade in school have demonstrated no neuropsychologic or learning problems.

In addition to primary, permanent, infantile hypothyroidism, the following conditions may be diagnosed as a result of neonatal screening: transient hypothyroidism, permanent or transient compensated thyroid disease (euthyroidism with consistently elevated thyrotropin [TSH] and normal thyroxine [T4] concentrations), hypothyroidism secondary to hypopituitarism which in turn may be secondary to hypothalamic dysfunction, hypothyroxinemia due to thyroid binding globulin (TBG) deficiency, and transient hypothyroxinemia due to interference in T4 binding.

SCREENING PROCEDURES AND NEONATAL THYROID PHYSIOLOGY

The ideal screening method would measure the concentrations of both TSH and T4 in the filter paper blood samples obtained at 3 to 5 days of age for screening for disorders of amino acid metabolism. At present, assaying for both T4 and TSH in all newborns is too expensive so that either TSH

or T4 is measured alone and the second hormone is measured only when the first is abnormal. Thus, whenever the T4 is 2 standard deviations or more below the normal mean or the TSH is similarly above the normal mean, the alternate hormone is also measured on the same filter paper blood specimen. In New England, a T4 of 6 μg/dl and a TSH of 20 μU/ml have been taken as convenient approximations of 2 standard deviations below and above their respective means. In North America, screening is usually done measuring T4 first, whereas TSH is the primary measure in the rest of the world. There are advantages and disadvantages to both methods without either being clearly superior. No matter what method is used, some patients cannot be diagnosed in the newborn period because their circulating concentrations of both T4 and TSH are normal for weeks or months.

Changing normal values for thyroid related hormones and binding globulins for the newborn period and later are presented in Table 73-1. The first are necessary to understand the bases for diagnosis suggested by screening and the latter are critical for proper treatment of the patient with permanent infantile hypothyroidism. The infant's T4 concentration at birth is higher than that of his mother even though maternal T4 concentrations are higher than those of nonpregnant adults because of the increase in TBG stimulated by the increased estrogen concentrations of pregnancy. The maternal free T4 is at normal adult concentrations. The newborn also has a slightly higher TBG concentration than older children and adults but this increase is too slight to

Table 73-1. Circulating Concentrations of Thyroid Related Factors

AGE	T4 μg/dl	FREE T4 ng/dl	TSH μg/dl	T3 ng/dl	TBG mg/L
Birth	12 ± 3 (SD)		20	50 ± 20	
1 hour			90–160		
24 hours	15 ± 2.5		17 ± 3	300 ± 150	
2–7 days	11 ± 2.7	2.6 ± 0.9	<20	200 ± 100	26 ± 8
4–12 weeks	11 ± 2	1.6 ± 0.46	<15	150	24 ± 7
1 year	9.5 ± 2		<10	134 ± 22	
Adolescents and adults	7.5 ± 1.75	0.9–2.4	<5	130 ± 25	21 ± 2.5

account for the elevated T4 concentrations. As would be expected from this, the free T4 concentrations are also significantly elevated in the first weeks of life. Part of the marked rise in 3,3′,5 triiodothyronine (triiodothyronine or T3) is the result of the rapid change in deiodinating enzyme activities from those of fetal metabolism. In the fetus, most of the deiodination of thyroxine occurs at the 5 position (inner ring) leading to the formation of 3,3′,5′ triiodothyronine (reverse T3) which has no known activity. Towards the end of gestation there is increasing activity of the enzyme deiodinating at the 5′ position so that slightly more T3 is formed. At birth, the activity of the latter enzyme increases even more and the activity of the enzyme producing reverse T3 declines to minimal levels unless illness or starvation supervenes. Teleologically, it may be considered that the diversion of T4 metabolism from production of the metabolically active T3 to reverse T3 in these situations is protective by lessening energy requirements. The rest of the rapid rise in T3 is due to the postnatal thyrotropin surge. The latter is caused in part by the sudden exposure of the infant to cooler ambient conditions. The magnitude of the TSH surge precludes the use of primary TSH screening in the first 48 hours of life.

CATEGORIES OF RESULTS OF SCREENING

1. A presumptive diagnosis of hypothyroidism, permanent or transient, is made when the screening T4 concentration is low and the TSH concentration is high.
2. A presumptive diagnosis of compensated thyroid disease is made when the concentration of TSH is high and the T4 is in the normal range in a primary TSH program.
3. If the screening T4 concentration is low but the

TSH concentration is not increased, further testing is required before even a presumptive diagnosis can be made. The first tests to be done are measurement of TBG and then of free T4. Since most screening laboratories are not yet capable of these measurements on filter paper blood samples, further discussion will be presented in the section on confirmatory diagnostic measures.

CAVEAT. These distinctions are oversimplified. The physician must remember that clinical hypothyroidism can develop in infants whose screening T4 and TSH concentrations had been normal. The progressively deteriorating hypofunction of the thyroid gland postnatally has been well documented. More commonly, infants are discovered who had low T4 concentrations with normal TSH concentrations on screening. The TSH may require as much as 1 to 3 months to reach diagnostic elevations. It is not known whether such patients have low screening free T4 concentrations. Furthermore, the filter paper screening methods are less precise than the diagnostic serum methods and borderline values have to be reassessed frequently. Premature infants introduce further problems of interpretation.

CONFIRMATORY DIAGNOSTIC MEASURES

1. *After screening values suggestive of hypothyroidism*

Confirmation of the diagnosis of permanent hypothyroidism is made by finding a serum TSH concentration over 40 μU/ml or values over 20 μU/ml in two serum specimens with T4 concentrations below 6 μg/dl. Repeat determinations are advised before diagnosis and treatment when the first serum

TSH is between 20 and 40 μU/ml because 80% to 85% of patients with such hormonal concentrations are eventually found to have transient disease. Conversely, the TSH concentration of 50% of patients with transient hypothyroidism is over 40 μU/ml. Some patients with transient hypothyroidism will not be able to be differentiated from those with permanent hypothyroidism in the first months of life. They will require treatment with l-thyroxine to avoid the risk of delaying treatment in a patient with permanent hypothyroidism. In New England, only about 3% of patients treated for permanent hypothyroidism for more than a month or two eventually were proven to have transient disease.

If the serum TSH concentration is elevated but the T4 concentration is normal, the patient has compensated thyroid disease.

If the serum concentrations of both T4 and TSH are normal, a diagnosis of transient hypothyroidism can be made with one reservation. The diagnosis is not certain if the screening TSH was between 20 and 40 μU/ml on blood obtained in the first 48 hours of life since it is conceivable that the TSH concentration might merely have represented slow clearance of the hormone following the neonatal surge. Indeed, for this reason, many European workers will not accept a diagnosis of transient hypothyroidism unless an elevated TSH concentration is found in the serum as well as in the screening blood.

2. *After screening values suggestive of compensated thyroid disease*

Confirmation of compensated thyroid disease is made when the serum TSH is also high but the T4 is normal. This condition, too, may be transient. Transiency is diagnosed when the serum TSH becomes normal and is suggested when the serum TSH is significantly less than the screening concentration. Compensated thyroid disease may also continue with the same degree of dysfunction or may progress to hypothyroidism during or after infancy. Patients developing hypothyroidism after the age of 3 years have never been shown to be at risk of brain damage. Since they obviously have significant amounts of remaining functioning thyroid tissue, once a transient condition has been excluded, patients with compensated thyroid disease are usually treated with thyroxine to prevent the development of a goiter.

3. *After screening demonstrating isolated hypothyroxinemia*

The most commonly identified cause of a consistently low T4 concentration with a normal TSH concentration is TBG deficiency. This is tested for first by a direct assay of TBG concentration. A few screening laboratories are able to perform this assay on the original filter paper specimen, but more often this is done after the confirmatory serum specimen shows that this combination of hormonal values still pertains. In either event, if the concentration of binding globulin is low, nothing further needs to be done for the child. The family is reassured that this condition is benign at the time the inheritance of the condition is explained. If the TBG assay is normal, an assay of free T4 should be performed. Once again, a few screening laboratories can do this on the filter paper screening blood specimen. This is the ideal. If the free T4 concentration is normal, interference with protein binding of T4 is suggested. This is a transient condition although it frequently persists for months but rarely for over a year. Again, there is no evidence that this has any clinical significance.

If the free T4 is low in the screening specimen or thereafter and the TSH still is not increased in the serum specimen, an attempt to confirm the diagnosis of hypopituitarism must be made at once since newborn hypopituitarism is often fatal. The classically described hypopituitarism is associated with breech and traumatic deliveries and becomes clinically manifest after the middle of the first year of life although there may be low screening concentrations of T4 and TSH. Diagnosis of these patients is less urgent. In either case, the diagnosis is made by standard means such as demonstrating failure of ACTH or cortisol concentrations to increase in response to clinical hypoglycemia or metyrapone administration or serum growth hormone concentration to rise after spontaneous hypoglycemia or administration of pharmacologic agents such as l-dopa, glucagon, and so forth. The induction of hypoglycemia with insulin administration is dangerous in these patients. If the pituitary hypofunction is primary, the patient will not respond to thyrotropin-releasing hormone with a rise in serum TSH concentration or a rise in growth hormone following administration of growth hormone releasing factor.

Hypopituitarism is suggested clinically by hypoglycemic attacks, history of low maternal estriol concentrations, diabetes insipidus, micropenis, small testes, and by the following frequently associated conditions: septo-optic dysplasia, holoprosencephaly, single central incisor, postaxial polydactyly sometimes with imperforate anus or cardiac lesions, and micro- or macrocephaly.

FEATURES OTHER THAN HORMONAL CONCENTRATIONS SUGGESTING TRANSIENCY OF HYPOTHYROIDISM

A diagnosis of transient hypothyroidism or transient compensated thyroid disease is clearly suggested when it becomes known that an infant's mother had been treated during pregnancy with iodides for asthma or with antithyroid drugs (thiourea derivatives or less frequently ^{131}I) or had circulating antithyroid antibodies as a result of thyroiditis. A family history of pseudohypoparathyroidism or hypocalcemic fits also strongly suggests transiency of hypothyroidism since the thyroid dysfunction associated with this condition frequently manifests itself with low T4 and elevated TSH concentrations on screening and confirmatory tests. The infants do not develop clinical signs of hypothyroidism but the TSH concentration may remain mildly elevated for several years.

Whereas 66% to 75% of patients with permanent hypothyroidism are females, 65% of those with transient hypothyroidism are males. By itself, however, gender is not of great value in suggesting which patient may have transient hypothyroidism.

65% of patients with transient hypothyroidism not associated with maternal disease or treatment are premature infants. The incidence of prematurity among infants with permanent hypothyroidism is 6% (the same as it is in the total newborn population). Fifty percent of premature infants weighing less than 1500 grams have been shown to have subclinical episodes of transient hypothyroidism marked by slight depression of T4 and elevation of TSH concentrations in the first weeks of life. Presumably, if blood samples were obtained frequently enough, the incidence would be closer to 100%. Premature infants are more susceptible both to iodine deficiency and to iodine excess, either of which causes transient hypothyroidism.

The incidence of transient hypothyroidism is highest in areas of iodine deficiency so that the incidence in Europe with pockets of marginal iodine intake or frank deficiency is 1:8000 births. In New England, 1:19,000 newborn infants were recognized to have transient hypothyroidism. The actual incidence is higher than this since blood specimens are not repeatedly obtained from small preterm infants. Lavish bathing of neonates with povidone iodine as well as administration of iodinated dyes in x-ray contrast studies have been shown to increase the incidence of transient hypothyroidism.

MANAGEMENT OF INFANTILE HYPOTHYROIDISM

The goal of treatment of infantile hypothyroidism is to prevent brain damage and to assure normal physical growth and development. Between 20% and 25% of patients treated as a result of screening are not at risk of brain damage. Most of these have compensated thyroid disease and would develop clinical hypothyroidism only after the period in which the developing brain is vulnerable to thyroid hypofunction or never would develop clinical hypothyroidism. As stated, some patients with transient hypothyroidism are also treated since treatment could not be delayed safely in order to differentiate them from those with permanent disease. Thus, one in 4500 to 5000 newborns is treated for hypothyroidism but only one in 6000 is actually at risk of brain damage from hypothyroidism. In Europe, one newborn in 3000 is treated for hypothyroidism. The number of infants included who have transient or compensated disease is not reported.

Treatment should be begun in patients with low screening T4 concentrations and TSH concentrations over 40 μU/ml before results of confirmatory serum assays are known. It seems safe to wait for the confirmatory results before treating the remaining patients. Since the experience antedating newborn screening suggested that delay in treatment had a deleterious effect, the first dictum is that at least those with the more severe thyroid hypofunction should be treated as soon as possible.

There is no consensus on whether to do thyroid imaging with ^{123}I at the time of diagnosis. The question is whether being able to give genetic counselling to the parents of the roughly 20% of hypothyroid patients with dyshormonogenesis outweighs the risk of administering 10 μC to 15 μC of the radioactive iodine to 2- to 4-week-old infants. If the parents do not intend to have more children, the decision is easy. If genetic counseling of the patient with dyshormonogenesis is desired, the imaging can be done many years later when presumably the unknown risk would be less. The joint committee on neonatal thyroid screening of the American Thyroid Association and the American Academy of Pediatrics was unable to reach a consensus on this matter. Each family and physician will have to come to their own decision.

Treatment is initiated with 1-thyroxine by mouth in a dose of 10 μg/kg of body weight. In practice, the dose is rounded off to the nearest 12.5 μg, one half a standard 25-μg tablet. Thereafter, the dose of thyroxine is altered to maintain the serum concentration of T4 between 10 to 15 μg/dl in the first year and over 10 μg/dl thereafter. The maintenance of these concentrations requires frequent serum T4 and TSH assays. With improved assay methods, the measurement of free T4 will probably replace that of total T4 since free T4 is the active moiety of serum thyroxine, but this is unlikely to alter management guidelines substantively. The infant should be examined and blood specimens for hormonal analyses obtained 2 and 6 weeks after initiating therapy, 4 weeks after any change in dosage, and routinely at 3,6,9,12, and 18 months of age, and on each subsequent birthday. Careful monitoring is necessary because it has been shown that infants with serum T4 concentrations of less than 8 μg/dl for significant periods in the first year of life had lower IQs than did patients whose serum T4 concentrations remained in the desired range. This inadequate treatment still permitted normal physical growth and development.

The average doses of thyroxine found to maintain serum T4 concentrations in the upper half of the normal range are as follows:

Until the child weighs 6 kg, 10 μg/kg of weight at the start of treatment
From 6 kg to 10 kg, 6 μg/kg of current weight
From 10 kg to 20 kg, 60 μg plus 2 μg to 3 μg for each kg above 10
Over 20 kg, 80 μg to 90 μg plus 1 μg for each kg above 20

If the patient is receiving much less than the average dose and still has T4 concentrations in the desired range, transiency of disease should be considered unless it is known that the patient has an ectopic gland or goiter. If the child is receiving significantly larger doses, it is worth making sure that he is actually ingesting the prescribed doses. Similarly, failure of serum T4 to reach 8 or 9 μg/dl 2 weeks after initiation of treatment or over 10 μg/dl on the next blood specimen raises the possibility of inadequate prescription or compliance. Failure of TSH concentration to decrease to below 20 μU/ml within 6 weeks of treatment need not be due to improper dose or failure of compliance since 10% to 15% of patients will have slightly elevated TSH concentrations for as long as a year unless serum T4 concentrations are raised to 15 μg/dl to 17 μg/dl. Such failure, however, or any subsequent elevation of TSH even with normal T4 concentrations should

serve to alert the physician that the child may not be receiving adequate thyroxine regularly and both dose and compliance should be checked. Transient elevations of T4 concentrations well above the normal range have not had discernible adverse effects. To make compliance easier and anxiety less, it may be suggested to parents that they set out a week's supply of pills each Sunday so that they can make sure they have not missed a dose. Parents can then give a missed dose with the next day's dose. This also lessens anxiety if the infant vomits and cannot take the thyroxine for a day or two. If intake of the proper dose of thyroxine is assured but the TSH has not become normal and the serum T4 concentration is in the desired range, it is not necessary to raise the serum T4 to 15 μg/dl to 17 μg/dl to suppress TSH secretion. On the other hand, if the physician suspects noncompliance (*e.g.*, suspects that the infant might have been inadequately treated until just before his appointment so that T4 was normal but TSH was elevated), the parents should be carefully reeducated and the baby tested again in 2 weeks. If the TSH is then normal on the same dose, the suspicion of poor compliance is strengthened.

INDICATIONS FOR REFERRAL

The patient with neonatal hypopituitarism should be seen in consultation immediately by a pediatric endocrinologist. Consultation is also advisable when the distinction between permanent and transient hypothyroidism is difficult. It is not necessary in the classic case of infantile hypothyroidism diagnosed as a result of neonatal screening provided that the following conditions are met:

1. The primary physician has access to a certified laboratory for hormonal monitoring.
2. He is willing to spend the time required for educating the parents about the disease and the importance of adequate treatment and for genetic counseling in cases of dyshormonogenesis.
3. He, in addition to monitoring the clinical course, must be willing to obtain the specimens for frequent monitoring of hormonal values.

Consultation, however, can help in increasing the chance of adequate compliance by reenforcing the education, genetic counseling, and reassurance provided shortly before by the primary physician. Consultation becomes a necessity when hormonal concentrations deviate from the desired range and the physician cannot determine the cause on re-examination 2 weeks later.

PROGNOSIS

The ultimate IQ of infants whose hypothyroidism is diagnosed as a result of neonatal screening but before a clinical diagnosis is possible and who are adequately treated is unaffected by their hypothyroidism. Their mean IQ and distribution of IQs are normal. It is possible that the prognosis may not be as good for the rare patient whose intrauterine thyroid hypofunction was severe enough for long enough that the infant was born with obvious classic stigmata of hypothyroidism. These patients, amounting to less than 1% of patients with infantile hypothyroidism, are too few to resolve the question of prognosis. They may, however, have irreparable brain damage akin to that of endemic cretins who frequently have become euthyroid by the time of delivery. The patients who are less than optimally treated do have lower IQs than other patients but their IQs are in the normal range of distribution. In the New England study, the hypothyroid children did fully as well as their euthyroid siblings through the third grade in school.

ANNOTATED BIBLIOGRAPHY

Glorieux J, Dussault JH, Morissette J et al: Follow-up at ages 5 and 7 years on mental development in children with hypothyroidism detected by Quebec Screening Program. J Pediatr 107:913,1985 (Second largest cohort followed for same period as the New England study, but with slightly different results.)

Klein RZ: Infantile hypothyroidism then and now: The results of neonatal screening. Curr Probl Pediatr 15:1,1985 (Most recent complete review of infantile hypothyroidism.)

Naruse H, Ire M (eds): Neonatal Screening. Amsterdam, Excerpta Medica, 1983 (Reports of proceedings of the second international conference on neonatal thyroid screening and of the international symposium on neonatal screening for inborn error of metabolism, Tokyo, August 1982.)

New England Congenital Hypothyroidism Collaborative. Neonatal hypothyroidism screening: Status of patients at 6 years of age. J Pediatr 107:915,1985 (Largest cohort with longest follow up results.)

Root AW, Rettig K, Vargas A, Reiter E: The thyroid: Recent advances in normal and abnormal physiology. In Barness LA (ed): Advances in Pediatrics. Chicago, Year Book Publ 26:441, 1979 (Reviews all forms of thyroid disease as well as physiology.)

74
Short Stature
LYNNE L. LEVITSKY

Three of every hundred normal children are by definition at or below the third percentile for height. Most have either genetically programmed decreased adult height potential or delayed physiologic maturation. In order to appropriately evaluate short children and identify those requiring medical therapy, as well as those requiring counseling because of untreatable very short stature, it is important to understand the pattern of normal and abnormal growth.

PATTERNS OF NORMAL GROWTH

The length and weight at birth depend on the sufficiency of intrauterine nutrition and blood gas exchange, as well as other poorly understood maternal and fetal factors. The growth rate in normal children in the first 2 postnatal years reflects the transition from the intrauterine to the intrinsic growth pattern. Growth rates in children with fa-

milial or "constitutional" short stature and those with delayed maturation may decrease precipitously. A period of stable growth at a lower centile then ensues, with a gradually declining height velocity to levels as low as 3.7 cm/year in slow-growing boys and 4.2 cm/year in slow-growing girls for a short time just before puberty. The only interruption to that decline is the modest increase in height velocity between 6 and 8 years occasioned by the onset of adrenarche, the earliest increase in adrenal androgen production. When plotted on a standard growth curve, children are shown to maintain their growth along the same percentile lines from the ages of 2 to 3 years until the onset of puberty. Children who are delayed in puberty may appear to change growth centiles at the time of normal puberty because they do not experience the sex steroid-induced pubertal growth spurt noted in the youngster with an average age at puberty. During puberty, children once again have accelerated growth, causing them to shift centiles. The longer and more intense growth spurt in the boy leads to an average greater final height in males compared to females.

CLINICAL PRESENTATION

Three of every 100 children do not need an extensive laboratory evaluation because of their small size. The decision to pursue an evaluation beyond the physical examination and history should be based on evidence of growth failure (growth rate less than the third percentile for age) or very short stature (height more than 3 SD below the mean for age) even if evidence for growth failure is not available. Rough figures used to define the abnormal are growth rates of 5 cm/year or less before 5 years and of 4 cm/year or less between the ages of 5 and puberty.

DIFFERENTIAL DIAGNOSIS

Before birth, growth is affected by fetal pathology and by placental function. Children with placental dysfunction tend to be underweight compared to height (decreased ponderal index) and usually display catchup growth when removed from their inhospitable intrauterine environment. Children with intrinsic fetal disorders (*e.g.*, infection or exposure to drugs inhibiting cell replication) tend to be proportionately small and display other dysmorphic stigmata typical of these disorders. The capacity for postnatal growth is variable.

Postnatal growth depends on genetic endowment and environment. Normal genetic endowment may be associated with transient short stature if delayed maturation is significant. The boy with delayed maturation is on the average 5 cm shorter than his early maturing peers by the age of 5 years. A multifactorial inheritance of familial short stature may lead to short stature during childhood and decreased final adult height. Abnormal genetic endowment often leads to short stature. Disorders affecting bone and cartilage as well as other disorders of multiple organ systems may adversely affect growth. The major chromosomal abnormalities with the exception of the XYY syndrome and Klinefelter's syndrome adversely affect growth. Genetic information on the short arm of the X chromosome is necessary for the expression of normal height potential in girls.

Adequate nutrition is essential for good linear growth. In affluent Western societies restricted intake leading to poor linear growth may be related to food faddism, unusual elimination diets, child abuse, or mechanical difficulties in intake because of abnormalities of the oropharynx and upper gastrointestinal tract. Malabsorption may lead to decreased linear growth as may inborn errors of intermediary metabolism leading to decreased use of metabolic substrate.

Some chronic illnesses may interfere with appetite, inhibiting linear growth because of undernutrition. The mechanism of growth inhibition in other chronic illnesses is not entirely understood. Inflammatory bowel disease may be recognized because of growth inhibition before the onset of clinically recognizable gastrointestinal signs and symptoms. Renal tubular acidosis may also produce asymptomatic growth failure.

Many severely mentally retarded individuals suffer from slow growth and short adult stature. In the majority, the underlying insult producing the mental retardation also affected cell multiplication and final height potential. In some the cause is an inability to take in adequate calories, and in others disordered growth hormone regulation has been implicated. A fascinating neuroendocrine dysfunction associated with delayed growth is seen in deprivation dwarfism (psychosocial dwarfism or emotional hypopituitarism). These are emotionally and sometimes physically abused children with the clinical features of slight underweight for height, potbellies, unusual eating and gorging behaviors, large malabsorptive stools, and disturbed interpersonal relationships. When tested initially, they manifest growth hormone deficiency and diminished cortisol and thyroid hormone levels. After a brief period of hospitalization or removal to a more favorable environment, all neuroendocrine function returns to normal.

Drug therapies may affect growth rate. Both glucocorticoids and sex steroid analogues may affect ultimate height. Glucocorticoids induce exogenous hypocortisolism, antagonizing the peripheral effects of growth hormone. Sex steroids initially induce a rapid growth increment, but by inducing premature epiphyseal function they may decrease the final adult height. Drugs used for hyperactivity may act as appetite suppressants and lead to a decrement in linear growth rate in susceptible individuals.

A host of endocrine disorders can alter growth. Hypothyroidism is the most common acquired endocrine disease of childhood, after diabetes mellitus. It is associated with remarkable growth arrest, a bone age that may be more delayed than the height, weight usually greater than height, and, rarely, sexual precocity in females. The spectrum of growth hormone deficiency is presently being expanded. Classical growth hormone deficiency, both congenital and acquired, is diagnosed by deficient growth hormone response to challenge by hypoglycemia, intravenous arginine, L-dopa, or other stimuli. However, we now recognize slow growing children with normal growth hormone responses to these stimuli who may grow better with exogenous growth hormone (growth hormone dependency), and children with growth hormone insensitivity (Laron dwarfism) who have normal or high growth hormone responses but an inability to generate somatomedins, the tissue mediators of growth hormone action. Further, children may have partial growth hormone deficiency or decreased growth hormone release over 24 hours but normal growth hormone response to pharmacologic studies. These disorders of growth hormone release may be transient or permanent.

The first sign of excess cortisol production is a diminution in growth rate. Cortisol has an inhibitory effect on growth even in physiologic amounts. Children with aldosterone deficiency and salt loss may have a decreased growth rate or frank failure to thrive. Sexual precocity, except when associated with hypothyroidism, initially induces rapid growth. The high levels of sex steroids, however, leads to a discordant advance in epiphyseal maturation and often to short stature in adult life. Diabetes mellitus can have a deleterious effect on growth rate if poorly controlled. Circulating somatomedin inhibitors are generated in the insulin-deficient state and decreased levels of somatomedins have been reported.

WORK-UP

The laboratory evaluation of the patient with short stature and growth failure can be appropriately directed and economically carried out only if preceded by a careful history and physical examination.

History

The prenatal history is important in determining if intrauterine or intrapartum events have contributed to the growth disorder. Children with intrauterine growth retardation may have associated anomalies leading to continuing slow growth and should not fail to have further evaluation just because of inappropriately low birth weight for gestational age. A history of maternal medication use, illicit drug or alcohol abuse may define an etiology for the child's growth disorder. Perinatal difficulties such as breech presentation or intracranial hemorrhage may be associated with hypothalamic pituitary disorder.

The growth pattern is important. Shifts from established growth curves after the first 2 to 3 years of life and until puberty suggest pathophysiology. When growth data are not available from physician's records, school records and clothing sizes may be used as an indicator of annual growth. The growth pattern of common disorders leading to short stature is graphically depicted in Figure 74-1. Physiologic maturation can be assessed in part by inquiry about maturation of secondary dentition and age at onset of signs of puberty. Past illnesses, difficulty in feeding and dietary intake, unusual bowel habits, or other signs and symptoms of physical illness should be identified.

The family history is also important. Heights, weights, and ages at puberty of family members should be obtained. This serves a dual purpose: It supplies the physician with necessary diagnostic information and allows the family of the normal but slow-growing child the opportunity to review the familial nature of this phenomenon and gain reassurance through the review. A history of children with similar problems and of chronic illness or endocrine disease in other family members should be assessed.

The social history is important. This may point the way to the diagnosis of psychosocial dwarfism or suggest the need for counseling because short stature has become a focal disruption in a child's life or in the family organization.

Physical Examination

Measurement of the child's height should not be carried out casually using an inaccurate office scale. The most accurate device is a carefully calibrated scale such as a Harpendon Stadiometer. However, careful measurement against a wall using a T-square with a built-in level is an adequate substitute. Length measurements should be used on the National Center for Health Statistics Charts until the age of 3 years. Height should be used thereafter. Standing height is always slightly less than length because of compression of intervertebral spaces in the standing position. Other measurements that can prove useful include head circumference, span, and lower segment in order to compute an upper/lower

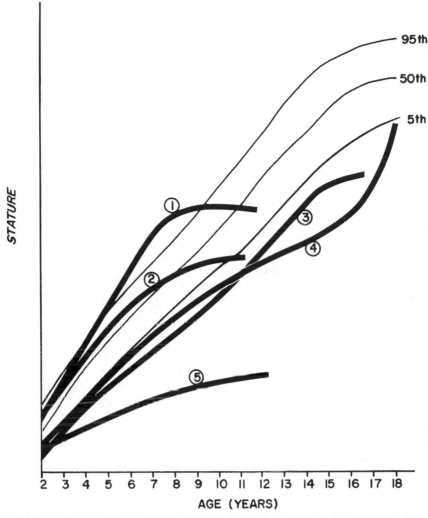

Figure 74-1. Patterns of abnormal growth: (1) sexual precocity with early epiphyseal fusion; (2) acquired growth failure (*e.g.,* acquired hypothyroidism, renal disease, or glucocorticoid therapy); (3) genetic short stature; (4) delayed maturation; (5) congenital growth disorder (*e.g.,* congenital hypopituitarism, achondroplasia, or cystinosis) (Adapted from Levitsky LL, Edidin DV: Growth disorders in children. Comp Ther 6:22–29, 1980)

segment ratio. An abnormal head circumference might suggest a central nervous system disorder. Arm span should approximate height. A short arm span, measured fingertip to fingertip with the arms outstretched might suggest a congenital disorder of bone or cartilage. The upper/lower segment ratio (lower segment measured from the top of the symphysis pubis to the heel is subtracted from height to obtain the upper segment) averages 1.7 at birth and decreases to 1 in the average white adult, re-

flecting a decreasing trunk to leg length ratio. If this ratio remains greater than one, one should consider severe hypothyroidism or a disorder of bone or cartilage as a possible diagnosis.

The general physical examination should be taken as an opportunity to search for dysmorphic signs such as a high arched palate or unusual ears or hands. An assessment of adequacy of nutrition and general physical well-being should be made. Signs of chronic illness should be noted. Finally, physical maturation should be assessed by examining dental age and pubertal status. The Tanner rating system for pubertal maturation should be employed in the initial assessment and follow-up.

Laboratory Tests

Minimum screening evaluation for children growing significantly below the third percentile or demonstrating growth failure should include a complete blood count, erythrocyte sedimentation rate, thyroid function studies and biochemistry screening to include electrolytes, CO_2, BUN and creatinine, total protein, calcium and phosphorus, a liver function test, and urinalysis with pH measurement. These screening studies will point to most occult chronic illnesses. A bone age roentgenogram permits the assessment of physiologic maturation and a prediction of adult height. Growth arrest lines suggest a past illness or psychosocial dwarfism. In all short girls, a test for Turner syndrome should be obtained. Buccal smears may not be reliable and usually will not identify mosaic Turner syndrome. Gonadotropins (LH and FSH) are clearly elevated in the presence of gonadal failure if the bone age is 11 or greater and may serve as a screening study after that time. The definitive study is an examination of chromosomal morphology. Unfortunately, this is an expensive test. Further, some girls with mosaic Turner syndrome may have normal peripheral blood chromosomes and elevated gonadotropins.

The somatomedin C assay is useful as a screening device for growth hormone deficiency. Its limitations, however, must be recognized. Children under the age of 5 tend to have low somatomedin levels that cannot be clearly differentiated from children with growth hormone deficiency. Undernourished children tend to have low somatomedin C values. Some children with growth hormone deficiency have somatomedin C levels within the normal range. Randomly obtained plasma growth hormone levels do not serve a useful purpose because they are rarely elevated into a range that will permit differentiation of normal from growth hormone deficiency.

Most children with severe growth failure will offer clues from the history and physical examination as to which studies will be most productive. For instance, short girls with other clear stigmata of Turner syndrome might have chromosomes obtained immediately. The child with disproportionate measurements might undergo a skeletal radiologic examination to help with the diagnosis. A palpable thyroid gland might encourage the examiner to obtain antithyroid antibody titers. A history of urinary tract infection might provoke more investigation of the genitourinary tract. Gastrointestinal symptoms or underweight might lead to an evaluation for malabsorption or inflammatory bowel disease.

TREATMENT AND MANAGEMENT

If the history, physical examination, and basic laboratory examination clearly delineates an etiology for short stature, management depends on the nature of the disorder. If no etiology can be ascertained with certainty, a period of 4 to 6 months of observation and remeasurement is often useful. Children with clear growth failure following such careful observation may then require further evaluation including definitive studies of growth hormone release. Specific treatment of disorders of growth is often possible. However, most children seen with short stature do not have a pathophysiologic etiology. They suffer from familial short stature or delayed maturation or a combination of the two. Adjuvant medical therapy to enhance growth rate and final height is sometimes requested for these children. In the boy with severely delayed maturation (no signs of puberty at 14 years) a short course of androgen therapy may be useful to improve self-esteem. Our usual treatment course is 100 mg of a depot testosterone preparation monthly for three doses. This causes the development of a small amount of pubic hair, some increase in phallic size, and a slight growth spurt. The growth rate usually drops below normal after the effect of the last injection of testosterone dissipates. On rare occasions a second course of testosterone may be given several months later. This treatment schedule neither enhances nor decreases final height. Continued treatment with androgen likely would adversely affect final height and should be avoided. Growth hormone, available as an expensive biosynthetic agent, may have limited use in high doses in girls with Turner syndrome and in some children with normal growth hormone release but abnormal growth rates. Its role in the treatment of short normal children is unclear and probably even more limited. Large quantities of biosynthetic growth hormones would likely be necessary to induce an increase in adult height. The potential risks and required therapeutic regimens have not yet been fully evaluated. Further, the expense of such pharmacologic plastic surgery is presently exorbitant.

INDICATIONS FOR REFERRAL

Children growing steadily at a normal rate each year rarely require subspecialist evaluation. Children with growth failure always require a full evaluation of their disorder and referral to the appropriate subspecialist if the generalist pediatrician feels uncomfortable dealing with the management of the specific problem. At the present time, because of rapid changes in management and philosophy, growth hormone therapy should probably remain within the province of the endocrinologist.

PATIENT EDUCATION

The Human Growth Foundation, a national group composed of parents and friends of children with short stature, has excellent educational materials available and can be a source of support for children with short stature and their families. The address of the national headquarters is:

4607 Davidson Drive
Chevy Chase, MD 20815

The Little People of America is an excellent resource organization for people with very short stature. Their address is:

Box 126
Owatonna, MI 55060

Growing Up Small, by KG Pfieffer, makes good reading for families of children with short stature. The address of the publisher is:

Paul S. Eriksson
Middlebury, VT 05753

ANNOTATED BIBLIOGRAPHY

Bayley N, Pinneau SR: Tables for predicting adult height from skeletal age. Revised for use with the Greulich–Pyle Hand Standards. J Pediatr 40:423, 1952 (amended 41:371, 1952) (These are the easy to use height prediction tables that allow adult height predictions.)

Horner JM, Thorsson AV, Hintz RL: Growth deceleration patterns in children with constitutional short stature: An aid to diagnosis. Pediatrics 62:529, 1978 (Shifting growth patterns in the first several years of life are described.)

Schaff–Blass E, Burstein S, Rosenfield RL: Advances in diagnosis and treatment of short stature with special reference to the role of growth hormone. J Pediatr 104:801–813, 1984 (This review describes the evaluation and management of the child with growth disorders and the use of growth hormone.)

Smith DW: Growth and Its Disorders: Basics and Standards, Approach and Classifications, Growth Deficiency Disorders, Growth Excess Disorders and Obesity. Philadelphia, WB Saunders, 1977 (This book is a classic and should be used as a reference in the understanding of normal growth patterns and disorders of growth.)

Tanner JM: Growth at Adolescence, 2nd ed. Oxford, Blackwell Scientific Publications, 1962 (All you ever wanted to know about pubertal staging and growth may be found in this monograph. For the generalist, the stages of puberty as defined by Tanner may be found in any standard pediatric endocrinology text.)

Tanner JM, Davies PSW: Clinical longitudinal standards for height and height velocity for North American children. J Pediatr 107:317–329, 1985 (These are the gold standards for the determination of linear growth in North American children.)

75

Delayed Puberty

M. JOAN MANSFIELD AND
JOHN F. CRIGLER, JR

Secondary sexual characteristics normally begin to develop between ages 8 and 13 in girls and ages 9 and 14 in boys. Breast budding is the first sign of development in 85% of girls followed by the development of sexual hair, then growth acceleration, and menarche occurring at an average age of 12.8 years, after peak height velocity has passed. Some normal girls show sexual hair as the first sign of development. The first sign of development in boys is usually an enlargement of the testes to more than 2.5 cm in length at an average age of 11.6 years. This subtle physical change is followed by phallic enlargement, the development of pubic and axillary hair, and ultimately by an increase in growth rate with peak height velocity being reached about 2.5 years after the onset of development.

Delayed development is defined by the absence of breast budding by age 13 in girls or the lack of testicular enlargement by age 14 in boys, both 2.5 standard deviations beyond the normal age of onset of these developmental changes. Delayed menarche is the absence of menarche by age 16, or 4 years after the onset of breast development.

PATHOPHYSIOLOGY

The physical changes of puberty are a response to rising levels of sex steroid hormones. In the normal sequence of events, the rise in adrenal androgens known as adrenarche occurs by about age 8 and is followed several years later by a reappearance of hypothalamic gonadotropin-releasing hormone (GnRH) pulsations that trigger the synthesis and release of luteinizing hormone (LH) and follicle stimulating hormone (FSH) from the pituitary. LH and FSH stimulate gonadal production of sex steroid hormones and development of germ cells. The absence of puberty may be the result of a failure at any point along the hypothalamic-pituitary-gonadal axis. The challenge of evaluating the child with delayed puberty is to differentiate between constitutional delay of puberty and organic disease such as chronic illness, caloric deficiency, tumor, or primary endocrinopathy associated with delayed pubertal development.

CLINICAL PRESENTATION

Although delayed development occurs in both males and females, most patients who present for an evaluation of delayed development are high-school-aged males who are concerned about their short stature as well as their lack of muscular and secondary sexual development, which put them at a disadvantage among their peers. Most of these boys have constitutionally delayed development; however, the clinical presentation of the patient with constitutional delay may be indistinguishable from that of the patient whose pubertal delay is the result of an organic lesion. Patients with constitutional delay of puberty have often been slow growers throughout childhood, their growth curves following or being below the third percentile. Growth may slow even further as these children reach the age when puberty would normally occur since growth velocity decreases in the absence of the normal sequence of hormonal changes that characterize adrenarche and gonadarche. Growth velocity increases into the normal range when these children enter puberty. Patients with constitutional delay may have a family history of delayed growth and development in relatives. Children with constitutional delay of puberty eventually enter puberty spontaneously. Although they have a longer time

to grow before their epiphyses fuse, they tend to have a less exuberant growth spurt than earlier developers so that their final height is shorter than average.

DIFFERENTIAL DIAGNOSIS

Functional Causes of Delayed Puberty

GnRH secretion can be inhibited centrally by inadequate nutrition, chronic disease, environmental stress, intensive athletic training, hypothyroidism, and drugs such as opiates. Eating disorders associated with self-imposed restriction of caloric intake have become increasingly frequent in adolescents. Although anorexia nervosa most typically develops in girls in midadolescence who have already entered puberty, young adolescent boys or girls who are dieting because of fear of obesity may present with the complaint of delayed development. Crohn's disease or celiac disease likewise may present with delayed development and poor growth as the major symptom. Since adolescence is normally a period of rapid growth and weight gain, failure to gain or small amounts of weight loss may be manifestations of significant nutritional inadequacy.

Hypothalamic Causes of Delayed Puberty

The ability of the hypothalamus to secrete GnRH may be damaged by local tumors (gliomas, germinomas, or craniopharyngiomas), infiltrative lesions such as CNS leukemia or histiocytosis, CNS irradiation, or by mass lesions such as brain abscesses or granulomas due to sarcoidosis or tuberculosis. Congenital defects in the ability to secrete GnRH may be associated with midline facial defects or olfactory defects (Kallmann's syndrome) and may be familial. Other congenital syndromes of delayed or abnormal puberty presumed to be on a hypothalamic basis include Prader–Willi syndrome (massive obesity, mental retardation, and small hands, feet, and genitalia), and Lawrence–Moon–Biedl syndrome (retinitis pigmentosa and polydactyly).

Pituitary Causes of Delayed Puberty

Puberty may not be initiated or may fail to proceed if the pituitary cannot respond to GnRH with LH and FSH production. This may be due to a pituitary tumor, an infiltrative lesion such as hemochromatosis, or due to congenital or acquired hypopituitarism. Excessive prolactin production by a pituitary adenoma (prolactinoma) may halt or prevent puberty by interfering with gonadotropin production. Galactorrhea is present in only half of the patients with prolactinomas.

Gonadal Failure

If the gonads are unable to respond to LH and FSH, puberty will not proceed. The most common cause of gonadal failure is gonadal dysgenesis, occurring in association with abnormalities of sex chromosomes (Turner's syndrome). The gonads fail to develop and become rudimentary streaks. These patients are phenotypic females with normal female genitals. They are classically short with a final height under 58 inches. Other identifying features of Turner's syndrome are low-set ears, a webbed neck, a trident hairline, an increased carrying angle of the lower arms, and short fourth and fifth fingers and toes. Renal and cardiovascular congenital anomalies are common. Half of these patients have 45-XO leukocyte karyotypes whereas the rest are mosaics with various X-chromosome abnormalities. Pure gonadal dysgenesis presents with absent puberty in patients with normal karyotype (XX or XY), normal stature, and female phenotype.

The causes of gonadal failure with normal karyotype include radiation, chemotherapy with certain agents such as cyclophosphamide, autoimmune oophoritis, or orchitis often in association with multiple endocrine abnormalities, viral orchitis or oophoritis, the resistant ovary syndrome, and gonadal failure associated with other diseases such as congenital galactosemia, ataxia telangiectasia, or sarcoidosis. Enzymatic defects, such as 17-α hydroxylase deficiency that render the gonads unable to produce estrogens or androgens are another rare cause of primary gonadal failure. No cause for the gonadal failure can be found in some cases.

In males who are cryptorchid, the testes may fail to function, particularly if they remain intraabdominal beyond infancy. Bilateral testicular torsion resulting in testicular destruction (anorchia) is another cause of gonadal failure in males. In the "vanishing testis syndrome," the testes are absent in a phenotypic male, presumably as the result of destruction *in utero*.

Primary amenorrhea with normal secondary sexual development may be due to an anatomic abnormality of the reproductive tract such as an imperforate hymen, vaginal septum, or vaginal, cervical or uterine agenesis. An XY karyotype individual who lacks the ability to respond to androgens (androgen resistance or insensitivity) presents as a phenotypic female with breast development and primary amenorrhea with an absent uterus and upper vagina.

WORK-UP

History

A detailed history and physical examination will help to focus and minimize the laboratory testing needed in the evaluation of the child with delayed development. The neonatal history should include maternal ingestion of hormones, previous maternal miscarriages, and congenital lymphedema (Turner's syndrome). The past medical history should focus on any history of chronic disease, congenital anomalies, previous surgery, radiation exposure, chemotherapy, or drug use.

Past growth measurements that are plotted on appropriate developmental charts for both height and weight are important in evaluating the child with delayed puberty. The overall pattern of growth and changes in that pattern often leads to a diagnosis. The child whose delayed puberty is associated with a nutritional deficiency due to an eating disorder, inflammatory bowel disease, or other chronic disease will show a greater decline in weight gain than in height. In contrast, the child who has delayed puberty on the basis of an endocrinopathy such as acquired hypothyroidism or gonadal dysgenesis will tend to have greater slowing of linear growth than of weight gain.

In the review of systems, special attention should be paid to weight changes, dieting, environmental stress, exercise and athletics, gastrointestinal symptoms, headaches, and neurologic symptoms including peripheral vision and ability to smell, and the symptoms suggestive of thyroid disease.

The family history should include the heights, weights, and timing of secondary sexual development and fertility of family members, a history of anosmia, and a history of endocrine disorders.

Physical Examination

The physical examination should include measurements of height and weight and vital signs. A search should be made for congenital anomalies including any midline facial defects. The patient should be examined for any evidence of secondary sexual development that may be quantified by Tanner staging of breasts and pubic hair in girls, and genitalia and pubic hair in boys. Dimensions of areolae and any glandular breast tissue in girls can be measured as an indicator of past or present estrogen effect. In boys, measurements of the testicular volume or length and width, midshaft diameter, and stretched length of the penis are useful in assessing the presence and progression of sexual development. Pubic hair may be present although the genitalia are prepubertal in a boy who has normal adrenarche but who lacks gonadal activation. Any evidence of heterosexual development, such as clitoromegaly or hirsuitism in girls or gynecomastia in boys should be noted.

The examination of the external genitalia in girls should focus on obvious congenital anomalies and an assessment of estrogen effect. A pale pink vaginal mucosa with white secretions indicates current estrogen exposure. A pelvic examination is not necessary as part of the initial work-up of a girl with delayed secondary sexual development but should be done to rule out gynecologic congenital anomalies in the patient who has normal pubertal development but delayed menarche.

The neurologic examination should include visual fields by confrontation and olfactory testing.

Laboratory Tests

Initial laboratory studies include a bone age and a complete blood count, erythrocyte sedimentation rate, LH, and FSH, DHEAS, and testosterone or estradiol. A radiograph of the left hand and wrist for bone age is useful in assessing how much linear growth remains in the patient with short stature and delayed development. A predicted height can be obtained using the Bayer and Bayley tables in the atlas of skeletal maturation by Gruelich and Pyle. The patient who has hypothyroidism will have a bone age that lags behind height age whereas, in the patient with constitutional delay, bone age and height age are usually equally delayed.

A complete blood count and erythrocyte sedimentation rate are helpful as a screen for chronic illness such as inflammatory bowel disease.

Endocrine studies can begin with the measurement of serum LH and FSH. If the LH and FSH are elevated, the patient has primary gonadal failure. A further laboratory evaluation would include a buccal smear and leukocyte karyotype searching for a chromosomal abnormality. If the chromosomes are normal in the patient with gonadal failure, antigonadal antibodies may be obtained looking for autoimmune gonadal damage. Certain causes of ovarian failure such as the resistant ovary

syndrome may reverse in time offering some chance of fertility. An ovarian biopsy to document the presence or absence of follicles is usually postponed until the patient wishes definitive information about her fertility.

In most patients with delayed puberty, the LH and FSH are in the normal prepubertal range. A further evaluation would then include a prolactin level, thyroid function tests, a lateral skull roentgenogram, and if there is a suspicion of a CNS tumor, a cranial CT scan. If there is a question of multiple pituitary hormone defects, the patient may be referred to an endocrinologist for pharmacologic and physiologic tests of neuroendocrine functions.

Breast budding and vaginal maturation in girls and penile and testicular enlargement in boys are more sensitive indicators of neuroendocrine-gonadal function than a single daytime measurement of serum gonadotropins, estradiol, or testosterone. Testosterone or estradiol levels, however, may be valuable in following the patient whose puberty is not progressing normally by clinical assessment of growth and secondary sexual development.

If a patient with delayed puberty does not have any midline facial defects, olfactory defects, or family history to suggest Kallmann's syndrome, it may be difficult to differentiate a constitutional pubertal delay that will eventually progress to normal function from a permanent abnormality in GnRH secretion that will not correct with time.

TREATMENT AND MANAGEMENT

Prior to age 14 in girls and age 16 in boys, if there is no evidence of underlying disease or neurologic abnormality and the initial work-up reveals normal prepubertal hormonal levels, the patient can be seen at 6-month intervals for measurements of growth, assessment of pubertal status by physical examination, and reassurance if progression of secondary sexual development is evident. After the first signs of testicular or breast enlargement are observed, follow up at regular intervals is desirable to reassure the patient and parents that puberty is progressing. Since the testes begin to enlarge in males before increased testosterone production and associated increased growth velocity occur, support and guidance in dealing with the frustrations of delayed puberty are important even after there is evidence that secondary sexual development has begun.

If the evaluation reveals primary gonadal failure, cyclic estrogen and progestin therapy in girls or testosterone therapy in boys will be necessary.

In girls, treatment with conjugated estrogens (Premarin) can be begun at a dose of 0.3 mg orally/day for the first year of treatment or until linear growth slows and increased thereafter to 0.625 mg/day for the first 25 days of each month with 10 mg of medroxyprogesterone (Provera) added at days 13 to 25. Patients who have been on estrogen replacement for 4 to 5 years should have regular Pap smears and should be referred to a gynecologist for an endometrial biopsy if irregular bleeding develops. The timing of initiation of sex steroid therapy in order to achieve maximum height depends on the patient's chronologic and skeletal age and current height velocity.

In boys with constitutional delay of puberty, 6-month courses of intramuscular injections of hCG or testosterone enanthate can be used to initiate secondary sexual development. Exposure to hCG or testosterone may speed the onset of the patient's own puberty. Since sex steroids cause fusion of epiphyses, care must be taken in the timing and monitoring of these therapies so that final height is not compromised. These patients should therefore be referred to an endocrinologist for treatment. In both males and females whose delayed puberty is due to abnormalities in hypothalamic GnRH secretion that do not correct with time, fertility has been achieved in research programs using a small pump to deliver pulses of GnRH intravenously or subcutaneously for weeks or months. Some GnRH deficient males will achieve spermatogenesis with hCG alone or in combination with human menopausal gonadotropin (Pergonal). Ovulation can also be induced by hMG and hCG in GnRH deficient females.

PATIENT EDUCATION

Young adolescents are preoccupied with their physical appearance. Any variation from the normal timing of sexual development is a major source of embarrassment to them and evokes feelings of personal inadequacy. A review of a patient's progress in pubertal growth and sexual development using developmental charts can help to reassure him that his growth is proceeding in a pattern that is normal for him. For those patients who have a permanent defect in reproductive function, counseling and support from both the primary health care provider and medical specialist can be helpful in enabling the patient to establish a positive self-image of himself as a capable adult. Further counseling by a mental health specialist may be necessary. Questions about fertility should be answered as they arise with emphasis on the patient's ability to function normally as a marriage partner and as a parent of adopted children.

ANNOTATED BIBLIOGRAPHY

Finkel DM, Phillips JL, Snyder PJ: Stimulation of spermatogenesis by gonadotropins in men with hypogonadotropic hypogonadism. N Engl J Med 313:651–655, 1985 (Describes the use of HCG and human menopausal gonadotropin to stimulate spermatogenesis in males with hypogonadotropic hypogonadism.)

Gruelich WW, Pyle SI: Radiographic Atlas of Skeletal Development of the Hand and Wrist, 2nd ed. Stanford, CA, Stanford University Press, 1950–1959 (Includes the Bayley and Pinneau tables for height prediction.)

Hoffman AR, Crowley WF Jr: Induction of puberty in men by long-term pulsatile administration of low-dose gonadotropin releasing hormone. N Engl J Med 307:1237–1241, 1982 (Report of induction of puberty using a portable pump to deliver intermittent GnRH in males with central hypogonadism.)

Rosenfeld RG, Northcraft GB, Hintz RL: A prospective, randomized study of testosterone treatment of constitutional delay of growth and development in male adolescents. Pediatrics 69:681–687, 1982 (Testosterone enanthate given to males with a constitutional delay for 3 months produced increased height velocity without excessive bone maturation.)

Styne DM, Grumbach MM: Puberty in the male and female: Its physiology and disorders. In Yen SSC, Jaffe R (eds): Reproductive Endocrinology, pp 313–384. Philadelphia, WB Saunders, 1986 (Complete review of normal, precocious, and delayed puberty including Tanner staging and an extensive list of references.)

Tanner JM, Davies PSW: Clinical longitudinal standards for height and height velocity for North American children. J Pediatr 107:317–329, 1985 (Most useful in evaluating growth during puberty.)

76

Precocious Puberty

M. JOAN MANSFIELD AND
JOHN F. CRIGLER, JR.

Puberty is a series of interrelated hormonal, physical, and behavioral changes that transform the child into a fully grown adult capable of mature reproductive function. The first sign of female secondary sexual development is usually breast budding, which begins between the ages of 8 to 13 in 98.8% of American girls. The average age of onset of breast development in girls in the United States is 11 years, with peak height velocity being reached by 12 years, and menarche at 12.8 years. Puberty occurs about 6 months earlier in black girls. In 98.8% of boys, secondary sexual development begins between the ages of 9 and 14. The first sign of development is testicular enlargement, which occurs at an average age of 11.6 years. Peak height velocity is attained at 14 years in boys, 2 years after the maximum height velocity in girls. Precocious puberty is defined as the onset of development 2.5 SD earlier than the mean age of entering puberty. By this definition, a girl who has breast development or pubic hair before age 8 or a boy with genital enlargement before age 9 has precocious secondary sexual development which should be evaluated.

PATHOPHYSIOLOGY

In normal children, the hypothalamic-pituitary-gonadal axis is active transiently *in utero* and in infancy causing sex steroids to be produced by the gonads. Pulsatile hypothalamic secretion of GnRH is then suppressed by the age of 6 months in boys and 2 to 4 years in girls and subsequently released from inhibition in late childhood allowing puberty to proceed. The mechanism of this normal suppression and reactivation of gonadotropin-releasing hormone (GnRH) secretion in childhood is not known.

Central precocious puberty is the result of premature secretion of GnRH by the hypothalamus activating the production and release of the pituitary gonadotropins luteinizing hormone (LH) and follicle stimulating hormone (FSH) that cause the gonads to make sex steroids. In the case of idiopathic central precocious puberty, no specific cause for this shortened period of inhibition of GnRH secretion in childhood can be identified. Less commonly, central precocious puberty can be attributed to a central nervous system insult such as a local mass lesion, hydrocephalus, anoxic damage, head trauma, radiation, or infection that presumably damages inhibitory pathways in the hypothalamus. This is known as *neurogenic precocity*.

CLINICAL PRESENTATION

Premature sexual development is more common in girls than in boys. Although most girls have idiopathic central precocious puberty, most boys with premature sexual development have an identifiable cause of their precocity such as tumor, congenital adrenal hyperplasia, or familial gonadotropin-independent precocity.

In true precocious puberty, sexual maturation (breast development in girls and testicular and phallic enlargement in boys) is accompanied or preceded by an increase in the rate of linear growth and weight gain and by acceleration of skeletal maturation leading to premature epiphyseal fusion and a final adult height below genetic height potential. In girls, pubarche (the development of pubic hair), a white vaginal secretion (leukorrhea), and menarche may accompany or occasionally precede breast development. Ovulatory menstrual cycles have been documented as early as the first year of life, although cycles are more often anovulatory and irregular. Rarely, isolated vaginal bleeding may be the first sign of precocious puberty, although in these cases, local vaginal lesions as a cause of bleeding should be ruled out by direct visualization. Emotional lability, high energy levels, and increased appetite are symptoms of precocity often noted by parents. Patients with neurogenic precocity may have other neurologic symptoms and signs such as headaches with increased intracranial pressure, changes in vision, and seizures. Central precocity can occur in patients with neurofibromatosis, with or without identifiable CNS optic gliomas. Patients with acquired hypothyroidism occasionally present with early sexual development that often ceases to progress when the hypothyroidism is treated, suggesting that the changes in neuroen-docrine-gonadal function are secondary to hypo-thyroidism.

DIFFERENTIAL DIAGNOSIS

The evaluation of a child with sexual precocity is directed toward separating the incomplete or self-limited forms of sexual development such as premature thelarche (breast development) or ad-renarche from true precocious puberty and toward excluding the correctable and possibly life-endan-gering causes of precocity such as tumors and in-born errors of steroidogenesis.

The most common limited form of premature sexual development is premature thelarche. Breast enlargement, galactorrhea, or vaginal bleeding are not uncommon in the neonatal period in response to withdrawal of estrogens of fetal-placental origin. In addition, isolated breast development sometimes accompanied by white vaginal secretions may occur later in infancy in response to transient ovar-ian estrogen production possibly as a result of in-termittent neuroendocrine-gonadal activity. This process is self-limited and is not associated with accelerated growth, progressive skeletal matura-tion, or pubic hair development.

Children occasionally have transient or inter-mittent precocious puberty in which secondary sex-ual development and acceleration of growth progress and then subside spontaneously. These episodes may recur.

Premature pubarche or sexual hair development before age 8 is not uncommon, particularly in black or Hispanic girls, and is usually associated with early maturation of androgen secretion by the ad-renal gland (adrenarche). In the patient with pre-mature adrenarche, linear growth and skeletal mat-uration are usually not significantly accelerated. Other evidence of adrenarche such as axillary hair or odor and acne, however, may be present.

The term *pseudoprecocity* is sometimes used to describe early sexual development that is not due to premature activation of the neuroendocrine-gon-adal system. Autonomous ovarian cysts and an-drogen or estrogen secreting tumors of the adrenals or gonads can cause premature sexual development without gonadotropins. In boys, untreated congen-ital adrenal hyperplasia may present as pseudopre-cocity due to excessive adrenal androgen secretion. Similarly, premature pubarche without virilization can be seen in girls with the attenuated forms of congenital adrenal hyperplasia. Pseudoprecocity may also be caused by rare gonadotropin secreting tumors such as hCG-secreting hepatoblastomas that activate steroid production by the gonads. Cases of precocious puberty in boys have been de-scribed in which testicular production of testoster-one occurs in the absence of pituitary LH or FSH secretion. These boys often have a family history of precocious puberty limited to males. The mech-anism of this gonadotropin independent form of precocity is not understood. Similar gonadotropin independent ovarian activity has been reported in girls with McCune–Albright syndrome (bone cysts, pigmented lesions of the skin, and precocity).

WORK-UP

History

The sequence and time course of sexual devel-opment, growth acceleration, and behavioral changes should be reviewed carefully. Sex steroid producing tumors often produce sudden, rapid sex-ual development, whereas idiopathic precocious puberty more closely approximates the timing of normal pubertal progression. The possibility of an external source of sex steroid hormones such as foods, cosmetics, or oral contraceptives should be investigated.

A past medical history should include a review of perinatal events that might have caused anoxic damage, a history of serious head trauma, congen-ital infection, meningitis or encephalitis, and CNS tumor or irradiation in the past. A history of neu-rologic symptoms such as seizures, headaches, or visual field defects should be sought.

Family history should include the timing of sex-ual development and final height in family mem-bers, and family history of neurofibromatosis or congenital adrenal hyperplasia.

Physical Examination

On physical examination, measurements of height or length and weight should be made. Mea-surements of current and past growth data plotted on developmental charts for height and weight are valuable in determining the duration and extent of precocity. The skin should be examined for evi-dence of café-au-lait spots suggesting neurofibro-matosis (multiple small brown macules with smooth edges) or McCune–Albright syndrome (one or more large brown macules with irregular borders). These lesions may emerge over time in the child who ini-tially presents with precocity. Acne, axillary odor, or axillary hair suggests maturation of the adrenal gland. Hypothyroidism as a cause of precocity might be suggested by changes in hair or skin, enlargement of the thyroid, slowing of pulse, a growth chart showing a slowing of linear growth, and an even greater delay in skeletal maturation. A neurologic examination should include an assessment of the fundi and visual fields in addition to an assessment of development.

In the girl with premature development, the dimensions of areolae and glandular breast tissue should be measured and Tanner staging of the breasts and pubic hair recorded. The external genitalia should be examined for evidence of estrogenization. Under the influence of estrogen, the labia minora becomes mature, and the vaginal mucosa becomes thicker and a paler pink, often with white secretions. Ovarian tumors often present as large abdominal masses in young children. A rectoabdominal examination with the child in frog-leg position is useful in the search for an ovarian mass. In the normal child, a button of cervical tissue can be felt in midline position. This may be larger than normal in the patient with precocious puberty as the uterus enlarges under the influence of estrogen. Masses that are not in the midline suggest ovarian tumors or cysts.

In boys, measurements of the dimensions of the testes and the midshaft diameter and stretched length of the penis can be helpful in documenting the progression of puberty. Testicular asymmetry or mass suggests a testicular tumor. Testes inappropriately small for the degree of phallic development are seen in boys with hCG-producing tumors or lesions of the adrenals (tumor or hyperplasia).

Heterosexual development, that is gynecomastia in a male or virilization in a female (*e.g.*, clitoromegaly, hirsutism, deepening of the voice) suggests the presence of a tumor secreting inappropriate sex steroids. Congenital adrenal hyperplasia usually presents with signs of virilization in a female.

Laboratory Tests and Indications for Referral

In the girl who has breast enlargement beyond early infancy in the absence of acceleration of growth or other evidence of precocity, a physical examination including growth measurements, measurements and staging of breast tissue, a rectoabdominal examination, and a roentgenogram of the left hand and wrist for bone age are usually sufficient initial procedures. A pelvic ultrasound may be obtained to rule out an ovarian mass lesion if the rectoabdominal examination is unsatisfactory. A vaginal smear obtained with a cotton swab and fixed immediately can be used to assess estrogen effect. Vaginal cells change from immature parabasal cells toward intermediate and finally to superficial squamous cells under the influence of estrogen. Since serum estradiol levels are often below the sensitivity of immunoassays in patients with precocious puberty, the vaginal maturation index is the most sensitive indicator of whether the child is in active puberty at the time of the examination. If the external genital examination and vaginal smear show little estrogen effect, and growth rate and bone age are normal, the patient can be followed at 3- to 6-month intervals without further studies watching for progression of sexual development or acceleration of growth.

If the patient has accelerated growth with advancing bone age and progressive sexual development, she should be referred to a pediatric endocrinologist for a more complete evaluation of the cause of the precocity. Initial laboratory evaluation would include an LH, FSH, and estradiol.

An LH and FSH can be helpful in making the diagnosis of central precocious puberty or a gonadotropin-secreting tumor. However, gonadotropin pulses are often only secreted during sleep in early puberty, so that prepubertal LH and FSH values do not exclude an active hypothalamic-pituitary-gonadal axis. A GnRH stimulation test or nocturnal monitoring for gonadotropins can confirm the diagnosis of central precocity, but it is not necessary as an initial screen.

A pelvic ultrasound can be obtained to investigate the possibility of an ovarian tumor or cyst. Pelvic ultrasound will often show multiple small ovarian cysts in patients with central precocious puberty; these are evidence of anovulatory ovarian activity. A single ovarian cyst is often seen in the patient with McCune-Albright syndrome. These cysts often resolve spontaneously, sometimes recurring multiple times. If the diagnosis of McCune–Albright syndrome is suspected, a skeletal survey is in order to search for bone lesions.

If the child has evidence of central precocious puberty, a cranial CT scan with contrast should be obtained to rule out CNS tumor, mass lesion, or hydrocephalus. Small hypothalamic hamartomas may cause precocious puberty and can be seen with the new CT scanners.

A boy who has genital enlargement should be referred to a pediatric endocrinologist without delay since there is a high probability of a specific cause of the precocity such as tumor or congenital adrenal hyperplasia. An initial examination would include a morning measurement of LH, FSH, hCG, adrenal and gonadal sex steroid levels, and a hand and wrist roentgenogram for bone age. A cranial CT scan with contrast should be obtained for any male with central precocious puberty. If there is evidence of a testicular mass or asymmetry on the physical examination, a testicular biopsy or tumor removal should be undertaken. The diagnosis of congenital adrenal hyperplasia is made by the serum hormonal analysis sometimes including a Cortrosyn stimulation test. If an adrenal tumor is strongly suspected, an abdominal CT scan is more useful in assessing the possibility of an adrenal mass than is an adrenal ultrasound.

In the child who presents with premature pubic hair development without evidence of other premature sexual development, growth data should be plotted carefully and a bone age should be obtained. If the child has premature adrenarche, the bone age is generally appropriate for height. Pubarche with rapid acceleration of growth and skeletal maturation would suggest precocious puberty or an androgen secreting lesion that should be evaluated by a pediatric endocrinologist. In simple premature adrenarche, the DHEAS will be in the adrenarchal range (100 to 280 µg/dl), and other sex steroid hormone levels are normal for the stage of development. A normal dehydroepiandrosterone level for stage of development excludes an androgen secreting tumor. The attenuated form of congenital adrenal hyperplasia (21 hydroxylase deficiency) can be identified by an elevated early morning or ACTH stimulated serum 17-α hydroxyprogesterone.

TREATMENT AND MANAGEMENT

Medroxyprogesterone acetate (Depo-Provera) and cyproterone acetate have been used previously to suppress puberty in children with precocious sexual development. Both drugs produce incomplete suppression of gonadarche and, therefore, do not increase final height. Studies over the past 5 years have demonstrated that complete suppression of gonadarche can be achieved using long-acting agonist analogues of GnRH. These analogues are thought to paradoxically suppress the pituitary-gonadal axis by down regulation of GnRH receptors of pituitary gonadotrophs. In these investigations, GnRH analogues have been shown to completely suppress gonadotropin and gonadal sex steroid secretion when given in adequate doses by daily subcutaneous injection. The suppression of gonadal activation by GnRH analogues appears to be specific, reversible, and safe. A halting or regression of breast development and a cessation of menses occur in girls and a regression in testicular size and muscular development occurs in boys during GnRH analogue treatment. Patients treated for 1 to 4 years have shown greater slowing of bone maturation than linear growth, thereby increasing predicted adult height. Whether these improvements will translate into actual gains in final height achieved has not yet been established. Adrenarche is not blocked by GnRH analogue therapy so that pubic hair may progress in adrenarchal patients. Although GnRH analogue therapy is currently available only through investigational protocols since the long-term benefits and risks have not been completely defined, it does appear to offer the only means of treatment that can completely and selectively suppress puberty with the potential long-term benefit of restoring the genetic potential for adult stature.

When sexual precocity is due to an organic lesion, initial treatment should be appropriate therapy for the lesion. Patients with congenital adrenal hyperplasia require treatment with glucocorticoids. Tumors of the adrenals and gonads, which are rare, can often be surgically removed preserving as much normal tissue as possible.

If high levels of sex steroids have been present for a long time in a patient with pseudoprecocity due to a tumor or congenital adrenal hyperplasia, central precocious puberty may develop following the elimination of the sex steroid source. Such patients as well as those with CNS tumors causing central precocity may be appropriate candidates for GnRH analogue therapy.

PATIENT AND PARENTAL EDUCATION

Parents of the child with premature thelarche or premature adrenarche may be reassured that the problem is self-limiting and has no long-term effects on growth and development. In the child with central precocious puberty, once a careful evaluation has excluded a tumor or other specific cause of precocity, the parents can be told that the puberty that the child is experiencing is a normal process except for its age of onset; thus, final sexual development and reproductive function should be normal although adult height may be shorter than the child's genetic potential due to premature epiphyseal fusion. Best estimates of final adult height in children with precocity are obtained using the Bayley–Pinneau tables with skeletal maturation determined using the Gruelich and Pyle atlas. It is important to know, however, that estimates of final height may decrease with the progression of sexual development because skeletal maturation advances more rapidly than linear growth.

In untreated patients, behavior and school problems may occur due to emotional lability and high-activity levels or poor self-image. Cognitive and psychological development are usually commensurate with chronologic age, not with physical appearance.

With the exception of familial gonadotropin independent precocity in males, and specific syndromes such as neurofibromatosis that are occasionally associated with precocity, other siblings or offspring of affected patients are not at increased risk for precocity.

ANNOTATED BIBLIOGRAPHY

Boepple PA, Mansfield MJ, Wierman ME et al: Use of a potent, long acting agonist of gonadotropin releasing hormone in the treatment of precocious puberty. Endocr Rev 7:24–33, 1986 (Five-year experience in 74 children.)

Gruelich WW, Pyle SI: Radiographic Atlas of Skeletal Development of the Hand and Wrist, 2nd ed. Stanford, CA, Stanford University Press, 1950–1959 (Includes the Bayley and Pinneau tables for height prediction.)

Styne DM, Grumbach MM: Puberty in the male and female: its physiology and disorders. In Yen SSC, Yaffe R (eds): Reproductive Endocrinology, pp 313–384. Philadelphia, WB Saunders, 1986 (Very complete review of normal, precocious, and delayed puberty including illustrations of Tanner staging.)

77
Gynecomastia

M. JOAN MANSFIELD AND
JOHN F. CRIGLER, JR.

Gynecomastia is a common accompaniment of male puberty. Two thirds of normal boys develop subareolar breast enlargement averaging 2 cm to 2.5 cm in diameter in mid-puberty. This common type of physiologic self-limited pubertal gynecomastia is usually readily distinguished from gynecomastia occurring with primary testicular disorders, estrogen-producing tumors, liver dysfunction, or medications.

PATHOPHYSIOLOGY

Underlying all gynecomastia is an abnormality in the normal male ratio of androgens to estrogens, a relative excess of estrogens resulting in breast duct proliferation. Acinae do not develop at the ends of the breast ducts in males, because this requires the synergistic action of estrogen and progesterone. If hormonal stimulation is prolonged, fibrous tissue develops which will not regress when the hormonal imbalance is corrected. Several studies have found a testosterone to estradiol ratio that is lower than normal (less than 100:1 with the normal adult ratio being in the range of 140:1) in males with pubertal gynecomastia. It has been hypothesized that the stimulation of the immature testis early in puberty results in transient excessive testicular estradiol secretion that decreases as the testis matures. Excessive levels of estrogens created by peripheral conversion of adrenal androgens may also be a cause of pubertal gynecomastia. Since adrenarche precedes gonadarche, peripheral conversion of adrenal androgens to estrogens at a stage in puberty where testosterone production by the testis has not yet reached mature levels could result in a temporary relative estrogen excess. Prolactin levels have been found to be transiently elevated just prior to the onset of pubertal gynecomastia in longitudinal studies. This increase in prolactin appears to be secondary to estrogen excess and is not thought to be causally related to gynecomastia.

CLINICAL PRESENTATION

The average age of onset of physiologic pubertal gynecomastia is 13.2 ± 0.8 years. Gynecomastia may develop at genital Tanner stages II, III, or IV and usually lasts 12 to 18 months. Breast enlargement often begins unilaterally but usually becomes bilateral. Pathologic gynecomastia may develop in the prepubertal, pubertal, or postpubertal male.

DIFFERENTIAL DIAGNOSIS

All causes of true gynecomastia share a common basis of a relative excess of estrogen. The source of this estrogen may be an excessive production by the testes or adrenal glands, excessive conversion of androgens to estrogens by extraglandular metabolism, or exposure to environmental estrogens. Gynecomastia, which occurs in childhood prior to the normal time of puberty, is rare: It is always pathologic and is usually accompanied by other evidence of precocious sexual development. Childhood gynecomastia may be caused by environmental exposure to topical or ingested estrogens, or by estrogen-secreting tumors.

Leydig cell tumors of the testis secrete estrogen and can present with gynecomastia that will be accompanied by precocious puberty if the tumor is present in childhood. Testicular development may be asymmetric and a mass may be present, although in some cases, these tumors are too small to palpate. hCG-secreting germ cell tumors may present with gynecomastia and precocious puberty, because both androgen and estrogen production by the testes is stimulated by hCG. Feminizing adrenal adenomas or carcinomas that secrete sex steroid hormones are another rare cause of gynecomastia in childhood.

Pathologic gynecomastia in the pubertal male may be due to any of the causes of gynecomastia in childhood, but also may be caused by excessive peripheral conversion of androgens to estrogens, primary testicular disorders with or without chromosomal abnormalities, androgen resistance, liver dysfunction, or drugs.

Gynecomastia is a frequent presenting complaint in obese males at puberty. Fatty tissue in the breast area may mimic true gynecomastia in many of these individuals. True gynecomastia may also be more common in obese males due to an excessive conversion of androgens to estrogens in adipose tissue.

Patients with suboptimal testicular function from various causes may present in puberty with gynecomastia. Altered testicular function can be associated with a chromosomal abnormality such as Klinefelter's syndrome, which occurs in one in every 400 males. One third of patients with Klinefelter's syndrome (XXY) have gynecomastia. Elevated gonadotropins drive the hyperplastic testicular Leydig cells to secrete estrogen as well as androgens. XXY patients with gynecomastia have a risk of breast cancer similar to that of normal females, far in excess of that of normal males with or without gynecomastia.

If the patient with gynecomastia has incompletely masculinized genitalia with hypospadias or cryptorchism, he may have a chromosomal abnormality or the syndrome of androgen resistance. Patients with mixed gonadal dysgenesis or true hermaphroditism may develop gynecomastia during puberty. During puberty these patients develop breasts and may also have cyclic bleeding through a penile urethra or urogenital sinus. Patients with partial androgen resistance on the basis of decreased testosterone receptor function or 5 α-reductase deficiency may also present with gynecomastia during puberty.

Causes of partial testicular failure resulting in gynecomastia with normal male karyotype include congenital anorchia (these patients may have testicular remnants that secrete some androgens and estrogens), damage due to radiation or chemotherapy, viral orchitis, and infiltrative lesions of the testis. Enzymatic defects in testosterone production are another unusual cause of gynecomastia.

Prolactinomas are a rare cause of secondary hypogonadism in males. Excessive prolactin levels produced by a pituitary adenoma may suppress gonadotropin release and thereby depress testicular function. Excessive prolactin may cause galactorrhea, but does not directly stimulate breast tissue proliferation. Gynecomastia does not usually develop in males with prolactinomas.

Gynecomastia may occur in pubertal or postpubertal males with thyrotoxicosis (Graves' disease). Sex-steroid-binding globulin is increased in the presence of thyroid hormone excess resulting in a decrease in the ratio of free biologically active testosterone to free estradiol. There is also an increase in the peripheral conversion of androgens to estrogens in hyperthyroidism. The diagnosis is usually clinically obvious with the presence of thyroid enlargement and symptoms of thyroid hormone excess.

Gynecomastia also occurs in patients with significant liver dysfunction, presumably due to an alteration in sex steroid hormone metabolism. Breast enlargement occurs in some males recovering from starvation, perhaps due to temporary liver dysfunction. Gynecomastia can also be seen as the nutritional state improves during the treatment of a chronic illness associated with malnutrition.

Drugs that have been associated with gynecomastia include spironolactone, cimetidine, digitalis, metronidazole, and chemotherapeutic agents toxic to the testis. Spironolactone and cimetidine cause gynecomastia by interfering with the androgen receptor function. Heavy use of alcohol resulting in liver dysfunction may result in gynecomastia. There is some evidence that frequent use of marijuana may cause gynecomastia.

Tumors of the breast are an unusual cause of a

breast mass in males during childhood and adolescence. As in women, bloody nipple discharge, irregular fixed masses, and axillary adenopathy are suggestive of possible malignancy. Benign masses such as neurofibromas may be seen occasionally in the breast area in males and may be confused with gynecomastia.

WORK-UP

History

The age of onset of gynecomastia, its progression, and its duration should be determined. The relationship of breast enlargement to other pubertal events, and the progression of puberty should be reviewed. A rapid progression of gynecomastia in the absence of genital changes suggests an environmental or tumor source of estrogen. A family history of other males with marked gynecomastia suggests pubertal macromastia on a genetic basis.

Physical Examination

On physical examination, measurements of height, weight, arm span, and staging of sexual development with determination of testicular size and consistency are important. In addition, a testicular examination should be done looking for masses or asymmetry suggestive of a Leydig cell or other testicular tumors. Hypospadias and incomplete testicular descent suggest a syndrome of incomplete masculinization. The testes in fully developed males with Klinefelter's syndrome are small (2 cm to 2.5 cm in length) and firm due to the occurrence of tubular fibrosis. Early in pubertal development, the testes of a patient with Klinefelter's syndrome may be difficult to differentiate from normal. The testes may also be small in other causes of hypogonadism. An evaluation of the breast enlargement should include a measurement of the dimensions of glandular tissue and areolae. Some obese patients may have pseudogynecomastia, which consists of smooth fatty tissue only. True glandular tissue has a more firm consistency and is palpable as a mobile symmetric mass embedded in fat underlying and extending out from under the areola. Nipple discharge, fixed asymmetric masses, and axillary adenopathy should be sought. Signs of thyroid hormone excess as a cause of gynecomastia would include thyromegaly, rapid pulse, and diaphoresis. Evidence of liver dysfunction might include hepatomegaly, jaundice, or spider angiomata.

Laboratory Tests

Laboratory testing should be determined on the basis of the clinical presentation of the patient. If the patient is in mid-puberty with normal testicular volume for stage of development, and has Tanner II breast development (less than 3 cm of glandular tissue), laboratory testing is usually not necessary since the patient has pubertal gynecomastia. If breast development has occurred in a prepubertal boy without genital changes or if genital abnormalities exist (small testes with penile enlargement, hypospadias, or incomplete testicular descent), the patient should be referred to an endocrinologist. A laboratory evaluation would include measurements of serum levels of LH, FSH, testosterone, and estradiol as a minimum and other sex steroid hormone metabolites if an adrenal abnormality is suspected. If the genitals are abnormal or gonadotropins are elevated, a karyotype and buccal smear should be obtained. A serum β-hCG can be included to rule out an hCG-producing tumor. If there is evidence of liver disease, liver function tests can be obtained to evaluate hepatic dysfunction. Thyroid function tests should be done if there is a clinical suspicion of thyroid hormone excess. Thermography and testicular ultrasound can be useful in evaluating the patient suspected of having a testicular tumor too small to be definitely palpated. If there is a strong clinical suspicion of a feminizing adrenal tumor, an abdominal CT scan should be obtained.

TREATMENT AND MANAGEMENT

If the patient has physiologic pubertal gynecomastia, he can be reassured that transient breast enlargement is a normal part of male puberty and should resolve within 2 years. A follow-up at 6-month intervals is usually helpful to provide support and reassurance. Although most pubertal gynecomastia resolves spontaneously within 2 years, the patient with Tanner III or more breast development is likely to be left with residual fibrous tissue even if the hormonal imbalance returns to normal. This patient may benefit from prompt referral for surgical correction. In counseling these boys, it is important to get a sense of the impact of the gynecomastia on the patient's life-style and self-image. A teenage boy will often refuse to go swimming, take off his shirt, or participate in school sports due to his concern about breast enlargement. In this case, if reassurance and support do not suffice, surgical referral may be appropriate. Medical approaches to the treatment of gynecomastia have included the use of antiestrogens (clomiphene), and aromatase inhibitors such as Teslac. Although these medications can temporarily decrease breast tissue, they are not used routinely in pubertal gynecomastia.

INDICATIONS FOR REFERRAL

The patient should be referred to an endocrinologist for an evaluation of breast enlargement if gynecomastia begins in childhood, or after puberty is complete, if it persists beyond 2 years, if it is unusually prominent (Tanner III or more), or if it is accompanied by abnormal genital development.

ANNOTATED BIBLIOGRAPHY

Berkovitz GD, Guerami A, Brown TR et al: Familial gynecomastia with increased extraglandular aromatization of plasma carbon-19 steroids. J Clin Invest 75:1763–1769, 1985 (Increased extraglandular aromatase activity in familial macromastia.)

Carlson HE: Gynecomastia. N Engl J Med 303:795–800, 1980 (General review of gynecomastia in all ages with an extensive list of references.)

Lee PA: The relationship of concentrations of serum hormones to pubertal gynecomastia. J Pediatr 86:212–215, 1975 (Longitudinal study of pubertal gynecomastia showing changes in estradiol and prolactin levels preceding the onset of breast enlargement.)

Moore DC, Schlaepfer LV, Paunier L, Sizonenko PC: Hormonal changes during puberty: V. transient pubertal gynecomastia: Abnormal androgen-estrogen ratios. J Clin Endocrinol Metab 58:492–499, 1984 (Androstenedione to estrone ratios are abnormal in pubertal gynecomastia.)

Wilson JD, Aiman J, MacDonald PC: The pathogenesis of gynecomastia. Adv Intern Med 25:1–32, 1980 (General review focusing on the endocrinology of gynecomastia.)

78
Diabetes Mellitus
HERBERT BOERSTLING

Diabetes mellitus is a heterogeneous group of chronic metabolic disorders with one common denominator—hyperglycemia. It is the most common of the pediatric endocrine diseases, with a prevalence of 2:1000 children, and an annual incidence of 16 new cases per 100,000 children.

Primary type 1 insulin dependent diabetes mellitus (IDDM) is the most prevalent form of diabetes among children. Since it is a disease of absolute insulin deficiency, all patients require insulin to control hyperglycemia and ketoacidosis. Primary type 2 noninsulin dependent diabetes mellitus (NIDDM) is a heterogeneous group of disorders manifesting diminished insulin effect, due to decreased or defective receptor sites, or abnormal insulins with diminished activity. Obese adolescents may have this form of diabetes. Secondary diabetes mellitus develops in patients with diminished pancreatic tissue or with endocrine diseases that interfere with insulin action.

PATHOPHYSIOLOGY

IDDM tends to develop in patients who have the genetic predisposition (specific HLA antigens) and who may have experienced an environmental insult (*e.g.*, rubella, mumps, or Coxsackie infection) that provoked the progressive autoimmune destruction of the insulin-producing cells, resulting in the progressive diminution of insulin.

Insulin is an anabolic hormone released in bursts during food intake to promote glucose entry into cells, and glycogen, lipid, and protein synthesis. During periods of fasting, insulin release decreases to a basal level and counter-regulatory or stress hormones such as epinephrine, glucagon, growth hormone, and cortisol are released. This results in increased glucose production by glycogenolysis and glyconeogenesis from protein catabolism, while fats are broken down to fatty acids and ketones for additional energy requirement.

In insulin deficiency, unrestrained glucose production and decreased peripheral glucose utilization result in hyperglycemia. When the renal threshold for glucose reabsorption is exceeded (around 160 mg/dl), an osmotic diuresis is created, causing polyuria with the loss of water and electrolytes. This may result in dehydration and hyperosmolality. Insulin deficiency also results in lipolysis, which produces hyperlipidemia and the conversion of free fatty acids to ketones. Urinary excretion of ketones causes further water and mineral loss. These ketoacids accumulate when production exceeds excretion, resulting in metabolic acidosis.

With increasing hyperglycemia, dehydration, hyperosmolality, and ketoacidosis, consciousness becomes progressively impaired and may lead to a diabetic coma.

During the initial "honeymoon" phase of treatment, which can occur from weeks to months after the onset of diabetes, about three quarters of these children will exhibit some recovery of β cell function, often leading to near normoglycemia. This phase may last weeks to months. Eventually, the β cell function deteriorates permanently, resulting in total dependence on exogenous insulin.

The pathophysiology of long-term diabetic complications, while not fully understood, is related to chronic metabolic imbalance. Longstanding diabetes mellitus damages the microvasculature, partly due to glycosylation, causing retinopathy and nephropathy. Joint contractures may be due to increased glycosylation of the joint collagen. An accumulation of the sugar alcohol, sorbitol, in the lens leads to cataract formation, and in the nerve fibers to neuropathy. Macrovascular disease may result from insulin deficiency, glycosylation, and a high fat/cholesterol diet.

CLINICAL PRESENTATION

Most children with diabetes are diagnosed early in their disease. They usually present with increased thirst and polydypsia secondary to dehydration, and weight loss due to significant loss of calories from glucosuria, which also results in polyuria and nocturia. Nocturnal enuresis may occur in a previously toilet-trained child. Fatigue, weakness, and listlessness are common complaints; polyphagia is less common. Severe diabetic ketoacidosis, with Kussmaul respiration, fruity odor to the breath (from acetone), and impaired consciousness, is an uncommon presentation.

DIFFERENTIAL DIAGNOSIS

Glucosuria without hyperglycemia occurs in renal tubular disease. Polyuria and polydypsia, in the absence of hyperglycemia, suggest diabetes insipidus or psychogenic polydypsia. Kussmaul respiration and metabolic acidosis but without hyperglycemia may be seen in salicylate overdose. On rare occasions, children with Cushing's syndrome, pheochromocytoma, or acromegaly may present with hyperglycemia and glucosuria; however, the underlying endocrinopathy is usually apparent. An infant or toddler with severe dehydration from gastroenteritis may have hyperglycemia and glucosuria. A child in diabetic ketoacidosis may mimic an acute surgical abdomen.

WORK-UP

A child presenting with the aforementioned symptoms should be tested for diabetes mellitus. Hyperglycemia confirms the diagnosis. The physical examination of a child with early IDDM is usually unremarkable. The child with serious diabetic ketoacidosis will have dehydration, Kussmaul respirations, and a decreased level of consciousness.

Before initiating treatment, obtain a complete blood count (CBC), blood sugar and ketones, glycosylated hemoglobin, electrolytes, blood pH, blood urea nitrogen (BUN), creatinine, and urine analysis.

A newly diagnosed nonketoacidotic diabetic may be treated as an out-patient if the pediatrician has the time and experience to adequately teach the principles of diabetes management; otherwise, the patient should be hospitalized. A very young diabetic or a diabetic in moderate to severe acidosis must be hospitalized.

PRINCIPLES OF MANAGEMENT

Optimal long-term diabetes management provides the diabetic child and family with the knowledge and tools not only to attain normal growth and development and a healthy emotional adjustment to the chronic disease, but also to forestall the development of the long-term complications of diabetes. Specific goals for the patient and family include an understanding of the causes of diabetes mellitus, the rationale for the use of the different types of insulin, the methods for monitoring diabetes care, and the inter-relationship of diet and exercise on diabetes care. Patients must also learn to recognize and treat the acute complications of diabetes.

Insulin Regimen

Human insulin or purified pork insulin is recommended because of their lower incidence of lipodystrophic and allergic reactions. The insulin is administered subcutaneously, rotating injection sites on the upper arms, thighs, buttocks, and abdomen.

A newly diagnosed diabetic, without ketonuria, may start at 0.25 unit of insulin per kilogram of body weight per day; a new diabetic with mild ketonuria may need 0.5 unit/kg/day. Established diabetics

Table 78-1. Key Characteristics of the Three Most Frequently Used Insulins

INSULIN NAME	INSULIN ACTIVITY		
	Onset	Peak	Duration
Short acting			
Regular	½ hr	2–4 hr	6–8 hr
Intermediate			
NPH	2	4–12	24
Lente	2	8–10	24

To avoid reactions, meals and snacks must be consumed at intervals to coincide with these characteristics.

usually take 1.0 unit/kg/day. The insulin dosage usually increases during adolescence to 1.2 to 1.5 units/kg/day, and returns to 1.0 unit/kg/day after the pubertal growth spurt. It should be emphasized that the doses are approximations and must be individualized.

A twice daily injection of a combination of intermediate-acting (either NPH or Lente) and short-acting (regular) insulins is usually recommended because it best approximates the physiologic insulin release in the nondiabetic state. Table 78-1 illustrates the key characteristics of the insulins. The ratio of intermediate-acting to short-acting insulin is about 2:1, or two thirds NPH/Lente and one third regular insulin. Younger children may require less regular insulin. Two thirds of the total daily insulin is given before breakfast and the remaining one third before dinner. A careful adjustment of the insulin dose must be made in concert with responses obtained by blood glucose tests.

Monitoring of Diabetes Control

Because the semiquantitative double voided urine test is unreliable and results correlate poorly with simultaneous blood sugar, it has largely been replaced by blood glucose determinations. Home monitoring of blood glucose is reliable and enables insulin doses to be accurately adjusted to preprandial blood glucose, anticipated changes in activity or diet, and management of diabetes during illness. Those diabetics who rely on urine sugar monitoring should be encouraged to switch. All diabetics must check their urine for ketones whenever the blood sugar is over 240 mg/dl and during illnesses.

The short-acting (i.e., regular) insulin dose administered before breakfast must be adjusted to bring the prelunch blood sugar to the normal range (80 to 120 mg/dl). If the blood sugar before lunch is elevated, the morning regular insulin may be pro-

gressively increased every 2 to 3 days by 1 to 2 units or up to 10% of that regular insulin dose. The morning intermediate insulin should likewise be titrated to bring the predinner blood sugar to the normal range. The short-acting insulin given before dinner regulates blood sugar at bedtime and should be titrated so that the bedtime blood sugar is normal. The before dinner intermediate insulin regulates the next morning's prebreakfast blood sugar. This intermediate-acting insulin dose must be adjusted cautiously because the blood sugar level of the diabetic patient tends to be lowest between 2 AM and 4 AM. The rapid blood sugar rise after 4 AM, the so-called *dawn phenomenon*, is probably due to the early morning surge of either ACTH and cortisol or growth hormone. The tendency is to increase the predinner intermediate insulin when the morning blood sugar is elevated (over 140 mg/dl). However, raising the predinner intermediate insulin dose should be done only if the blood sugar at 3 AM is over 70 mg/dl. If it is less, the excess insulin administered may cause hypoglycemia, followed by rebound hyperglycemia, often with ketonuria. This is the *Somogyi reaction*. Patients often do not have specific symptoms when this occurs; occasionally, they may complain of headaches on awakening, nightmares, night-sweats, or even nocturnal enuresis. The treatment is to reduce the evening intermediate-acting insulin dose. Similarly, in the event of daytime hypoglycemia, the responsible insulin dose must be reduced by 10% daily until the blood sugar is over 70 mg/dl.

It should be emphasized that tight control, with preprandial blood glucose under 120 mg/dl, may be hazardous and unrealistic for many diabetic children because of increased potential for reactions and more restricted life-style. Some experts feel that a more realistic goal is to aim for blood glucose to be under 180 mg/dl for young diabetics and under 140 mg/dl for adolescent diabetics most of the time.

Diet

Balanced nutrition, total daily calories appropriate for the age of the child, and a consistent eating schedule are crucial for the management of diabetics. The child's dietary adjustment is facilitated if the entire family adopts this routine.

Children require approximately 1000 calories plus 100 cal/yr of age daily. Of the total calories, 50% to 60% should be derived from carbohydrates, 30% from fats, and the remainder from proteins. Most of the carbohydrates should be in the form of complex carbohydrates, and foods with refined or simple sugars should be avoided. The use of polyunsaturated fats such as margarine or vegetable oil should be encouraged; substituting poultry, veal, and fish for red meats and eggs lowers the saturated fats and cholesterol.

Because the daily insulin doses are based on meals and snacks at regular intervals to coincide with the onset and peak action of the two insulins, the daily eating pattern must be fairly consistent in both the time and in the calories or content (especially the carbohydrate content) per meal/snack. Younger children usually have three meals and three snacks daily, with the total calories divided into 2:10 for breakfast, 2:10 for lunch, and 3:10 for dinner, and 1:10 for each of the three snacks at midmorning, midafternoon, and at bedtime. Older children often skip the midmorning snack; these calories can be added to their breakfast or lunch. The bedtime snack should not be missed.

Both the diabetic child and the parents should learn the basic principles of diet exchange; it allows increased flexibility in preparing meals and helps to minimize the sense of restriction. The pediatrician should work closely with a nutritionist and the family to plan meals based on the family's eating habits.

Exercise

Exercise, either unstructured play or participation in competitive sports, should be encouraged. It enhances both the peer relationship and a sense of well-being. The benefits from exercise far outweigh the risks of hypoglycemic reactions that may occur during or shortly after sports. These reactions are easily avoided if the diabetic plans ahead by an additional carbohydrate exchange consumed ½ hour before sports. It is important to inform coaches of the child's diabetes and to have glucose readily available. Diabetics are also encouraged to wear Medic–Alert tags.

Psychosocial Aspect

Diabetes mellitus imposes strains and restrictions on the family. Activities must be planned in regard to insulin administration. Parental fears of reactions and feelings of guilt contribute to their tendency to overprotect the child, and the diabetic child quickly learns to manipulate the parents. Adolescent concerns regarding altered body image, regulated life-style, and peer acceptance often become a hindrance to good diabetes care.

The pediatrician must be supportive and provide guidance. Families with diabetic children should join local diabetic groups to foster understanding and adjustment. Diabetic camps are excellent places for children to learn self-care and to realize that with a little planning, they can live normal lives. A referral for counseling should be considered when the diabetic family is overly stressed.

Management of Complications

Hypoglycemia, especially when mild, is the most common complication. It may occur suddenly when there is a rapid release of epinephrine in response to true hypoglycemia (blood sugar less than 60 mg/dl) or to a rapid drop in blood sugar, but still in the normoglycemic range. Shakiness, sweating, and restlessness are common symptoms of epinephrine response. Hunger, headache, confusion, coma, or seizures are signs of CNS glycopenia. If possible, document hypoglycemia with a blood sugar test, and immediately give concentrated simple sugars, such as a nondietetic soft drink, juice with extra sugar, or premade Instant Glucose. Glucagon, 0.5 mg for a child or 1.0 mg for the adolescent should be given if the patient is unresponsive or unable to swallow. Since hypoglycemia is potentially serious, the cause of the reaction should be investigated and efforts made to prevent recurrences.

Ketoacidosis usually develops over a period of hours to days of poor control. It usually coincides with persistent hyperglycemia, due to inadequate insulin dosage or to illness. Additional insulin is needed to correct moderate to high ketones, even if the blood sugar is not elevated. Short-acting insulin, between 5% to 10% of the total daily dose, is administered in addition to the usual insulin dose for a child with moderate ketonuria. With large ketonuria, give an additional 10% to 15% of the total daily insulin dose as regular insulin. Repeat this insulin dose every 3 to 4 hours until ketosis resolves. If the blood sugar is less than 120 mg/dl, additional calories must be provided to prevent hypoglycemia. Frequent blood sugar monitoring along with close phone contacts with the pediatrician are crucial in managing the ketoacidosis.

Although there are no conclusive data showing that good diabetes control delays long-term complications, there are short-term data suggesting that poor diabetes control accelerates complications and that improved control ameliorates some of the existing complications. Therefore, it is incumbent on the pediatrician to help delay or prevent the development of these life-threatening chronic complications by striving for "realistically" tight control.

OFFICE FOLLOW-UP

The frequency of office visits is based on the needs of the family and the medical condition of the child. A stable, well-controlled diabetic should be followed every 3 months. Office visits should provide an opportunity to review diabetes education and management. A careful interval history with specific focus on the family's adjustment to the demands of diabetes as well as the child's adjustment to peer and school routine should be discussed. The child's general health and well-being should be assessed. Insulin doses, injection sites, and glucose monitoring results must be carefully reviewed. Patients must document test results in a notebook; comments, such as possible explanations for reactions or high test results, should also be recorded. Families without a reflectance meter should bring the blood test reagent strips of the previous 3 days with them to assess the accuracy of their readings. Parents are also requested to bring a 3-day dietary history log so that overall nutrition may be reviewed. A review of systems should focus on illnesses that might interfere with diabetes control.

A thorough physical examination should be done at each office visit. Because heights and weights are critical parameters in a diabetic child, growth charts must be maintained. The examination should focus on those organs affected by the complications of diabetes. Attention should be paid to the possibility of other autoimmune endocrinopathies often associated with IDDM (*e.g.*, hypothyroidism).

Yearly laboratory studies should include urine analysis and culture, blood tests for BUN, creatinine, cholesterol, and triglycerides. A yearly ophthalmologic visit is recommended.

At the every 3-month visit, a glycosylated hemoglobin level should be obtained because it provides objective evidence of the quality of control over the preceding 2 to 3 months. The degree of control is excellent if the glycosylated hemoglobin is less than 8% (normal range 6.0% to 9.5%). A level between 8% and 10% is good and 10% to 12% is considered fair control. Any level over 12% is indicative of poor control.

The pediatrician can assess the overall quality of diabetes care by (1) the major variables that affect diabetes control, such as insulin dosage, diet, and exercise; and (2) the objective parameters of care: home blood sugar monitoring, glycosylated hemoglobin, the frequency of hypoglycemic reactions or ketoacidosis requiring intensive medical attention, and the rate of growth in height and weight. Efforts must be made to achieve the best control possible without risking serious reactions and with as few minor reactions as possible. The frequency of testing may need to be increased (preprandial and bedtime, as well as 2-hour postprandial and 3 AM blood sugar levels) to provide data to allow fine tuning of insulin dosage.

INDICATIONS FOR REFERRAL AND ADMISSION

At any point the primary care physician can refer the diabetic child to an endocrinologist, particularly if there is a problem with control, or to a mental health specialist for psychological problems. A child with a poor growth rate, recurrent significant reactions, and deteriorating glycosylated hemoglobin level, despite intensified efforts, must be referred. A child with vomiting and diarrhea, who is dehydrated with moderate or severe acidosis, or has an altered level of consciousness must be admitted for treatment.

ANNOTATED BIBLIOGRAPHY

Castello S (cd): Juvenile diabetes mellitus. Pediatr Clin North Am June 1984 (Superb up-to-date symposium on the etiology and treatment of IDDM. Tamborlane's article on "Insulin Infusion Pump Therapy of Type 1 Diabetes" provides the rationale and potential benefits for the use of the pump.)

Chase P: Avoiding the short- and long-term complications of diabetes. Pediatr Rev 7(5): 140, 1985 (Excellent review of the current management of diabetes in children, including an annotated bibliography of the chronic complications of diabetes.)

Geffner MKE, Kaplan SA, Lippe BM, Scott M: Self-monitoring of blood glucose levels and intensified insulin therapy: Acceptability and efficacy in childhood diabetes. JAMA 249(21): 2938, 1983 (Effectiveness of home monitoring of blood glucose in improving diabetes care, and the ready acceptance by children of the intensified diabetes management is documented.)

Ginsberg–Fellner F, Witt M, Franklin B et al: Triad of markers for identifying children at high risk of developing insulin-dependent diabetes mellitus. JAMA 254(11):1469, 1985 (Detailed longitudinal study of siblings of diabetic children, identifying the markers [HLA antigens, anti-islet cell antibodies, and decreasing insulin response to glucose challenge] that predict the development of diabetes among the siblings.)

Schneider AJ: Starting insulin therapy in children with

newly diagnosed diabetes: An out-patient approach. Am J Dis Child 137:782, 1983 (Excellent article detailing 8 years of experience treating newly diagnosed diabetics as out-patients.)

Travis LB: An Instructional Aid on Insulin Dependent Diabetes Mellitus. Galveston, TX, The University of Texas Medical Branch, 1985 (Excellent and "classic" instructional aid in pictorial form, easy to understand by both parents and children, detailing diabetes and its management. Each section is followed by a short test emphasizing the important facts; answers are provided.)

11

Ear, Nose, and Throat Problems

79
Diseases of the External Ear
HOWARD G. SMITH

Otitis externa refers to an inflammatory disease of the external structures of the ear including the auricle or pinna and its surrounding skin, and both the cartilagenous and the osseous portions of the external auditory canal. The inflammatory process may be produced by primary tissue infections due to bacteria, fungi and yeasts, viruses, or parasites. Inflammation with or without secondary infection may also be produced by various types of trauma or epithelial hypersensitivity reactions. These conditions may produce exquisite pain and tenderness.

PATHOPHYSIOLOGY

Infections of the auricle and periauricular tissues are usually caused by streptococci or staphylococci and are initiated by a traumatic epithelial breakdown that permits the entry of microorganisms. This trauma may be produced by the penetration of foreign objects or by pressure of prosthetic devices such as hearing-aid molds. The resultant infection may be a generalized cellulitis or infection of an obstructed sebaceous gland in the pinna. In either case, the infection may proceed to abscess formation.

Both the auricle and the external ear canal may be injured or invaded by insects. Enzymes, toxins, or microorganisms released by the insect injure the skin directly and may permit other microorganisms to enter and produce secondary infections.

Four factors make variable contributions to the development of external canal infections:

1. The loss of the protective, hydrophobic, acidic cerumen, and lipid epithelial coatings following exposure of canal linings to moisture during periods of high environmental temperature and relative humidity or during periods of skin immersion in water
2. Local penetrating trauma by fingernails or other implements such as cotton-tipped applicators
3. Contamination of the ear canal by pathogenic gram-negative bacteria
4. The immunologic competence of the host

In the cartilagenous outer portion of the external canal, streptococci and staphylococci may invade channels surrounding the hair follicles and produce folliculitis or furunculosis. In more medial portions of the canal, infection is produced by gram-negative organisms such as pseudomonas and proteus species, mycoplasma, fungi such as aspergillus or monilia species, or viruses such as herpesviruses. Rarely, the external ear may be invaded by mycobacterial organisms. The infections produced by each class of microorganism have certain unique clinical characteristics.

Habitual scratching of the skin with a fingernail, hairpin, or toy will cause pruritus and a characteristic neurodermatitis of the auricular and external canal skin. This sequence of events may signal the presence of significant psychological problems that are themselves in need of treatment.

Reactions to chemical or physical agents may occur on the skin of the auricle or the external

357

canal. Chemicals such as cerumenolytic agents (*e.g.*, Cerumenex drops), detergents, or organic solvents will produce an irritant dermatitis after repeated or prolonged exposure. Allergic contact dermatitis may occur after exposure to hair sprays and tinting compounds, pigments used in clothing or linen dyes, metallic compounds containing nickel and chromium, and certain plastic or rubber compounds contained in earphones or hearing-aid ear molds. Some agents require light as a catalyst to initiate the reaction.

CLINICAL PRESENTATION

Diseases of the external ear become apparent to the patient with the onset of otic pain, a sensation of fullness in the ear, and a hearing loss. Other clinical characteristics such as local tissue changes, exudates, and systemic symptoms and signs may develop depending on the site of disease, the etiologic agent, and host resistance factors.

Ear pain or otalgia may begin gradually or suddenly and progress rapidly. The sensation of *fullness* in the affected ear occurs early in the disease process due to stimulation by the inflammatory process of pressure sense receptors. This perception may continue well after the disease process has clinically resolved.

Hearing loss associated with external ear disease may be conductive or sensorineural. Edematous tissues or canal debris may produce a mild to moderate conductive hearing loss. Viruses such as the herpesvirus varicella-zoster may attack the cochlea, producing sensorineural hearing losses varying in severity from mild to profound.

Local tissue changes include erythema, edema, and tissue sensitivity. Abscess formation in the external canal is accompanied by fluctuance and spontaneous purulent drainage. Tissue inflammation in the osseous external canal is often accompanied by exudate formation and sometimes by epithelial breakdown and granulation formation.

Systemic symptomatology such as fever, chills, and myalgias is uncommon except in cases of extensive disease, often involving multiple sites. Fatigue is common in both patients and parents due to the sleep deprivation caused by otalgia.

WORK-UP

History

Important historical information to elicit from parent and child includes:

- Site of initial pain, discomfort, fullness, and direction of subsequent spread
- Presence of contributory acute or chronic disease such as upper respiratory infection or diabetes mellitus
- Exposure to potential vectors such as contaminated swimming water or insects
- History of recent ear trauma, including penetrating, blunt, thermal
- History of cotton-tipped applicator use or habitual insertion of foreign bodies including fingers
- Occurrence of bleeding or purulent exudate
- Status of hearing in the affected ear
- History of previous episodes of similar disease
- History of middle ear disease, particularly that associated with tympanic membrane perforation
- History of dermatologic disease, particularly eczema, psoriasis, or contact dermatitis due to shampoos or metallic products such as earrings

Physical Examination

The clinician should assume that the ear is exquisitely tender. The auricle and periauricular soft tissues should be inspected and palpated looking for signs of inflammation. The infraauricular cervical lymph nodes should be examined for evidence of lymphadenitis.

Viewing the canal with the electric otoscope may require use of a smaller than normal speculum because of tissue edema. Epidermal and exudative debris that obstruct the canal must be removed, usually by suction under direct vision using an operating otoscope head. Clinicians without access to otic microsuctions may substitute 18- or 20-gauge plastic intravenous catheters. Gentle irrigation with isotonic saline or topical antibiotic solution may be used to cleanse the canal. The canal epithelium should be examined for evidence of vesiculation, bulla formation, or granular epithelial degeneration, the latter indicating severe underlying disease in the temporal bone.

The tympanic membrane should be observed and manipulated using the pneumatic otoscope. Inflammation of the epithelium covering the tympanic membrane layer may obscure ossicular landmarks and reduce the translucency of the eardrum, but it is possible to determine the presence or absence of a middle ear disease.

Laboratory Tests

The laboratory evaluation includes a study of inflammatory exudates obtained from sites of disease and the evaluation of a patient's systemic response to the disease. Although most cases of otitis externa are initially managed empirically, a thorough microbiologic evaluation is imperative for patients with a disease resistant to initial management. Cultures should be obtained using microswabs designed specifically for use within the ear canal. Exudates or tissue obtained should be cultured and examined microscopically after staining to demonstrate bacterial and fungal organisms.

Routine hemograms or blood cultures are unnecessary for most patients with external ear disease. Patients with advancing external ear disease and those with evident systemic toxicity should have a white blood cell count determination and a differential as well as have blood cultures.

Audiometry is recommended for those patients who have a persistent hearing loss after the resolution of disease. Testing should be delayed for at least 1 month after all signs of acute disease have disappeared. All patients who have had a herpes infection of the external ear should also have auditory testing during convalescence because the virus may cause permanent damage to portions of the cochlea.

MANAGEMENT

Auricular Disease

Primary cellulitis of the auricle should be treated aggressively with systemic antibiotics. It is critical to prevent the spread of infection from the epithelial layers to the auricular cartilage to avoid dissolution of the cartilage and irreversible loss of the auricular skeleton. Antibiotics useful for treatment include dicloxacillin, erythromycin, cephalosporins, clindamycin, and trimethoprim-sulfamethoxazole. The presence of perichondritis and chondritis, either primary or secondary, signals the need for adequate gram negative antibacterial coverage. An application of moist local heat and elevation of the head are adjunctive measures. Fluctuant regions of cellulitic auricles should be promptly incised and drained. Any necrotic tissue, including cartilage fragments, should be removed. A drain is placed and slowly removed as the perichondrium reattaches to the underlying cartilage.

Viral infections should be treated symptomatically to avoid secondary bacterial infection by the use of topical antibiotic ointments containing bacitracin, polymyxin, or neomycin.

Disease of the auricle is often initiated by trauma, and an innocent but firm bump on the ear may produce a hematoma beneath the perichondrium. If undrained, the hematoma may become organized by fibrous tissue producing a characteristic "cauliflower" ear deformity. Partially drained hematomas may become infected, leading to abscess formation and ultimate deterioration of the underlying auricular cartilage.

Hematomas of the auricle should be promptly drained. Needle aspiration followed by the application of an auricular pressure dressing may be sufficient. Prophylactic treatment with a broad-spectrum, antistaphylococcal antibiotic should be given. Reaccumulation of blood or serum indicates the necessity for incision and placement of a drain, usually under general anesthesia.

Bacterial Otitis Externa

The best treatment is prevention. Children and adolescents with a history of recurrent otitis externa should regularly use an acidifying-antiseptic solution such as 5% boric acid in ethanol after swimming or during hot, humid weather. An antibiotic-steroid topical solution (Cortisporin otic suspension [TM]) may also be used as prophylactic treatment.

Prompt treatment is necessary once infection begins. During the otologic examination, all canal debris must be removed. If edema of the canal skin would prevent passage of antibiotic drops, a small wick composed of either gauze or absorbent sponge should be inserted into the external canal to carry a topical antibiotic-steroid solution into the ear canal.

The antibiotic-steroid topical solution may contain polymyxin or colistin, neomycin, and hydrocortisone. Patients who develop a cutaneous hypersensitivity to neomycin should use commercial preparations without this antibiotic (Pyocidin otic solution). The patient or parent should insert 4 drops 4 times a day. If a wick is inserted, the patient places the drops on the wick for the first 2 days. The wick is removed thereafter and the ear drops are continued for an additional 8 days. The child should be examined after the treatment is concluded.

External otitis is painful, and the child should be treated with analgesics, using narcotic compounds sparingly. The ear must also be kept dry. Swimming is not permitted. During showers and shampoos, the affected ear is protected using cotton coated with petrolatum jelly. Ear plugs that are inserted into the canal should be avoided.

More severe disease requires careful monitoring, and additional suctioning may be required. It may be necessary to reinsert a wick. If the disease spreads to adjacent soft tissue and presents clinically as periauricular cellulitis, a broad spectrum antibiotic such as cephalosporin should be added to the regimen.

Fungal Otitis Externa

Fungal microorganisms are suspected as the primary etiologic agents or as secondary invaders if the external canal is filled with exudate or a membrane covered by black or white filamentous material. Opportunistic fungi such as *aspergillus niger* may grow in an ear canal during bacterial infections or after prolonged use of antibiotic-steroid drops. Pathogenic fungal organisms such as *trichophyton, microsporum*, and *candida* species may cause a primary infection.

If there is colonization or superficial infection with minimal epithelial breakdown, 5% boric acid in ethanol may be instilled into the cleansed ear canal as an antiseptic and drying agent. Otherwise, antimycotic agents such as clotrimazole (Lotrimin and miconazole (Monistat–Derm Lotion) in solution may be instilled alone or in conjunction with topical antibiotic-steroid solutions, if an accompanying bacterial infection is suspected or if the use of a topical corticosteroid is desirable. Patients responding to treatment should be followed at 1- to 2-week intervals, with removal of external canal debris as necessary.

Eczematoid Otitis Externa

Chronic inflammatory changes of the external canal skin are usually accompanied by chronic pruritus. This disease entity occurs in older adolescents, and hypersensitivity to ingredients in shampoos or cosmetics should be suspected.

If there is infection, treatment should begin with an antibiotic-steroid solution. After the infection has resolved, a solution of 0.1% betamethasone valerate in ethanol (Valisone Lotion) may be used up to three times a day. After 7 to 10 days of intense treatment, the use of this fluorinated steroid should be tapered to a dose that controls the pruritus.

Bullous or Vesicular Otitis Externa and Myringitis

This disease is characterized by the sudden onset of excruciating otalgia relieved as serous fluid escapes from the ear canal. Bullous myringitis accompanies or follows upper respiratory infections and is thought to be caused by viruses or myco-

plasma. An examination of the ear shows multiple hemorrhagic bullae on the medial external canal wall and on the posterior aspect of the tympanic membrane.

The external walls of bullae should be punctured with either an otic suction or with a spinal needle to relieve pain. Extended treatment includes the instillation of an antibiotic-steroid topical suspension three times a day, the administration of a broad-spectrum systemic antibiotic (*e.g.*, an erythromycin-sulfa combination (Pediazole), and the use of adequate analgesics including narcotics for older children and adolescents. The antibiotic should have activity against most gram-positive organisms, *Hemophilus influenzae*, and mycoplasma.

Careful follow-up is necessary since bleb formation continues during the first week after disease onset and periodic cleansing of the external canal is necessary. As the disease regresses, it is important to reexamine the patient to confirm resolution of tympanic membrane and middle ear disease.

Malignant Otitis Externa

This necrotizing infection may develop in a child with diabetes mellitus or immunosuppression due to chronic illness or chemotherapy. Beginning as granular, diffuse otitis externa caused by *Pseudomonas aeruginosa*, the infection rapidly spreads to the underlying temporal bone and the vital structures contained within it, including the facial nerve. The osteitis and secondary osteomyelitis readily spreads to involve the skull base, and sepsis damages cranial nerves IX through XII, the sigmoid sinus, and the jugular vein. Preterminal events include progressive cranial neuropathies, jugular vein, and sigmoid sinus thrombosis, meningitis, and brain abscess.

Susceptible children with external canal disease should be referred to an otolaryngologist for an immediate evaluation. Disease unresponsive to antibiotics alone requires surgical debridement of severely infected or necrotic soft tissue and bone.

INDICATIONS FOR REFERRAL

Children should be referred to an otologist or otolaryngologist if difficulty is encountered in completely cleansing and visualizing the external canal or if the clinician has difficulty inserting a wick to carry topical medication along the length of an infected canal. Referral is also recommended if a child fails to satisfactorily respond to therapy or has a marked progression of disease. Children with diabetes mellitus or immunologic depression due to chronic disease or treatment with chemotherapeutic agents should be immediately referred to an otolaryngologist for treatment of otitis externa.

ANNOTATED BIBLIOGRAPHY

Doroghazi RM, Nadol JB Jr, Hyslop NE Jr et al: Invasive external otitis. Report of 21 cases and review of the literature. Am J Med 71:603–614, 1981 (Recent, comprehensive review of the pathophysiology and treatment of malignant otitis externa in both adult and pediatric patient groups.)

Hawke M, Wong J, Krajden S: Clinical and microbiological features of otitis externa J Otolaryngol 13:289–295, 1984 (Describes the results of a prospective study of both acute and chronic forms of otitis externa. The patient demography, predisposing factors, clinical features, and microbiology are discussed.)

Horn KL, Gherini S: Malignant external otitis of childhood. Am J Otol 2:402–404, 1981 (Case report and review of the problem of malignant otitis externa in the pediatric population.)

Ichimura K, Hoshino T, Yano J, Nozue M: Neutrophil disorders in a child with necrotizing external otitis. J Otolaryngol 12:129–133, 1983 (Case history of a 2-year-old child with congenital neutropenia who developed malignant otitis externa and was successfully treated using a combination of medical and surgical modalities.)

Mugliston T, O'Donoghue G: Otomycosis: A continuing problem. J Laryngol Otol 99:327–333, 1985 (Retrospective clinical review of fungal otitis external in over 1,000 patients of varying ages.)

Senturia BH, Marcus MD, Lucente FE: Diseases of the External Ear: An Otologic Dermatologic Manual. New York, Grune and Stratton, 1980 (Comprehensive treatise discussing the theoretical and practical aspects of external canal disease.)

80
Acute Otitis Media
MICHAEL MACKNIN

Acute otitis media, also called suppurative or purulent otitis media, is characterized by the rapid onset of signs and symptoms of inflammation of the middle ear. Middle ear disease is the most common reason for office visits to pediatricians, accounting for one third of all visits. By the age of 3, 71% of children will have experienced one or more episodes of otitis media, and one third of children will have had three or more episodes.

PATHOPHYSIOLOGY

Eustachian tube dysfunction is the major predisposing factor of acute otitis media. The normal eustachian tube protects, drains, and ventilates the middle ear. Children have shorter, more horizontal, and "floppier" eustachian tubes than adults. Viral infections, particularly with respiratory syncytial virus, influenza virus (types A or B), and adenovirus confer an increased risk of developing otitis media by presumably impairing eustachian tube function. Despite the documented increased risk of developing acute otitis media with an antecedent viral illness, most studies have failed to isolate viruses from acute otitis media in more than 5% of cases. Bacteria are the major organisms isolated in acute otitis media, and *Streptococcus pneumoniae* is the most common organism isolated at any age. Nontypable hemophilus influenza is an important pathogen throughout childhood and in adults. *Branhamella catarrhalis* is the third most common isolate in acute middle ear effusions. Other organisms such as *group A β-hemolytic streptococcus* are isolated in less than 5% of cases. *Mycoplasma pneumoniae* is an infrequent cause of acute otitis media and bullous myringitis. Bullous myringitis is generally caused by the same organisms that cause acute otitis media. Neonates, particularly infants with a complicated neonatal course in a neonatal intensive care unit, can have acute middle ear infection with a wide variety of organisms including gram negative enteric rods and *group B β-hemolytic streptococcus* in addition to the more usual organisms.

Risk factors for the development of recurrent otitis media include male sex, American Indians and Eskimos, white race more than black race, enrollment in day care, family history of otitis, siblings at home, low socioeconomic class, possibly bottle vs breast-feeding, bottle propping, atopic history in patient or siblings, previous positive history of otitis, winter season, cleft palate, and Down's syndrome. The precise role of allergy in acute otitis media is poorly defined.

CLINICAL PRESENTATION

The most consistently present abnormalities in acute otitis media are a full or bulging tympanic membrane, absent or obscured bony landmarks due to opacification of the tympanic membrane, and decreased or absent mobility of the tympanic membrane by pneumatic otoscopy due to middle ear effusion. Erythema of the ear drum is an inconsistent finding. By definition, one or more of the following symptoms are present: otalgia (ear pulling in the young infant), fever, or the recent onset of irritability.

DIFFERENTIAL DIAGNOSIS

The classic case of acute otitis media seldom poses a problem in differential diagnosis. Ear pain, however, is not a universal finding in acute otitis media, and there are many causes of ear pain other than acute otitis media. Ear pain may be caused by a furuncle on the external ear or by otitis externa. These conditions usually present with visible inflammation of the external ear or external auditory canal with pain on manipulation of the pinna or tragus. Temporomandibular joint dysfunction can be detected by palpating the tender joint with a finger in the external auditory canal during opening and closing of the mouth. Cervical lymphadenopathy, pharyngitis, trauma, negative middle ear pressure, tooth infections, foreign bodies, parotitis, sinusitis, tumors, infected sinus tracts or cysts, and mastoiditis can cause ear pain, but can generally be diagnosed by a careful history and physical examination.

WORK-UP

History

Patients often complain of otalgia (ear pulling in the young infant). Ear pain, however, is absent in approximately 20% of patients with acute otitis media. Fever is also an inconsistent finding, present in approximately 50% of patients with acute otitis media. Fevers over 40°C occur in less than 5% of cases of isolated acute otitis media. Young children with acute otitis media are often irritable. Hearing loss is generally present in most cases of acute otitis media, but is most commonly noted on history in cases of bilateral disease. Dizziness, unsteady gait, and tinnitus are less frequent complaints. Loose stools and vomiting may occur as a systemic response to acute otitis media. A history of middle ear disease and other infections including sinusitis and pneumonia should be obtained. Risk factors previously outlined under pathophysiology should be discussed.

Physical Examination

The key to the diagnosis of acute otitis media is the physical examination. The tympanic membrane is abnormally full or bulging. Pneumatic otoscopy shows decreased or absent mobility due to middle ear effusion. It is difficult to overemphasize the importance of properly performed pneumatic otoscopy in the evaluation of middle ear disease in children. The bony landmarks are obscured or absent due to opacification of the tympanic membrane. Erythema of the tympanic membrane is an inconsistent finding, as it may also be caused by vascular engorgement due to fever or by crying.

Critical to performing a proper physical examination are (1) proper equipment including a hermetically sealed otoscopy with a pneumatic attachment. Most otoscopes manufactured prior to 1983 do not maintain a seal adequate for pneumatic otoscopy. The seal can be checked by first squeezing the insufflator bulb, covering the speculum tip with your finger, releasing the pressure on the bulb and checking to see if the bulb remains deflated. A well-charged battery with a bright white, not dull yellow, light source is also essential. (2) The patient must be still: This can be achieved preferably through gentle persuasion. Some helpful hints are: In a young child demonstrate that looking at ears is not painful by first checking the child's doll, an older sibling, or parent. You may distract a young infant by gentle talking or soft whistling. Give the older child a sense of control by asking, "Which ear should I look at first?" Never ask, "May I look at your ears now?" If the child says "no" you lose all credibility and trust when you insist on looking. Emphasize the positive, never say, "This won't hurt." When doing pneumatic otoscopy, let the patient know that, "I will be blowing in your ears and this is going to tickle. Try not to laugh too much, because when you laugh you wiggle and it's hard for me to see your ears." If gentle persuasion fails, the child must be restrained. A young child can sit upright facing to the side on a parent's thigh. The child's legs can be restrained between the parent's thighs. The parent can hold the child's head against the parent's chest with one hand on the child's temple. The parent's other hand can be wrapped around the child's trunk to restrain both arms. If this does not work, the child can have head, arms, and legs restrained (at or above knees and not just at ankles to avoid wiggling) while laying on the examination table. (3) The external auditory canal must be cleared of cerumen prior to the examination of the tympanic membrane. If the drum is not perforated, this can be accomplished by irrigation with lukewarm water (not too hot or cold to avoid performing calorics) using a water pick or a butterfly with the needle cut off attached to a syringe. Hydrogen peroxide or colace may be instilled in the ear prior to irrigation to facilitate the removal of cerumen. Flushing the ear with water often causes erythema of the tympanic membrane and cerumen may also still obscure some of the drum surface. This makes pneumatic otoscopy particularly important for an accurate assessment of the tympanic membrane, because the normal appearance of the drum is obscured. Cerumen can also be removed by using a curette. This technique can be safely used only under direct visualization.

Many mistakes are made in performing pneumatic otoscopy. The most common one is not obtaining an adequate seal. It is important to use an ear speculum that is large enough to obtain an airtight seal with the external auditory canal. The seal should be made with the cartilagenous outer one third of the external auditory canal. The bony inner two thirds of the external canal is exquisitely sensitive to pain and should not be touched by the speculum. Soft-tip speculae, although not essential to performing a pneumatic otoscopy, have been specifically designed to achieve a comfortable airtight seal with the external auditory canal. All portions of the drum should be checked for mobility. A bulging drum is already maximally stretched toward the examiner and thus will not move when negative pressure (the collapsed bulb is released) is applied in the external auditory canal. Conversely, a retracted drum will not move when positive pressure (a full bulb is squeezed) is applied. Whether a bulging drum will show decreased or no mobility on positive pressure, and whether a retracted drum will show decreased or no mobility on positive pressure, depends on the forces exerted on the drum. Occasionally, particularly with a thinned drum, a hypermobile area may be detected. The large speculum needed to obtain an adequate seal often makes it difficult to completely visualize the entire tympanic membrane simultaneously. Therefore, it will often be necessary to reposition the otoscope to observe multiple segments of the drum to determine the complete appearance of the tympanic membrane.

Laboratory Tests

Laboratory tests are seldom needed in uncomplicated acute otitis media. Indications for performing tympanocentesis for culture and sensitivity of the middle ear effusion in unusual cases of acute otitis media include: (1) systemically toxic patients, (2) patients with a suppurative complication of otitis media such as mastoiditis, (3) immune compromised hosts such as patients on chemotherapy with neutropenia, (4) patients with severe pain unresponsive to oral analgesics and topical Auralgan, (5) neonates with otitis who do not appear entirely well or who have not had uncomplicated neonatal courses or in whom an excellent follow-up is not assured, and (6) patients already on "appropriate" antimicrobial therapy or patients who have just completed recent courses of antimicrobial therapy. Gram stain of middle ear effusion obtained at tympanocentesis can be helpful in guiding initial therapy.

Recurrent acute otitis media alone is seldom a presentation of immune deficiency. However, recurrent otitis media in association with other recurrent infections may be indicative of abnormal body defenses. Sinusitis or pneumonia associated with recurrent acute otitis media are among the most common infections associated with detectable immune deficiencies. An initial laboratory work-up for patients with multiple well-documented episodes of acute otitis media and sinusitis or pneumonia should include a complete blood count with differential, sweat test, quantitative IgG, IgA, IgM, IgE, and quantitative IgG subclasses. A biopsy of nasal mucosa for ciliary abnormalities might also be considered.

TREATMENT AND MANAGEMENT

The preferred treatment for acute otitis media is antibiotic therapy. The major pathogens beyond the neonatal period are *Streptococcus pneumoniae*, nontypable *Hemophilus influenzae, and Branhamella catarrhalis*. The choice of antimicrobial agents should be influenced by the geographic prevalence of β-lactamase producing *H. influenzae* and *Branhamella catarrhalis* causing otitis media. Up to 30% of nontypable *H. influenzae* and 75% of *B. catarrhalis* produce β-lactamase. Many practitioners, however, find that amoxicillin 40 mg/kg/day divided tid is still an effective first line drug. Ampicillin need not be used because it offers no advantage over amoxicillin. The drugs have an identical spectrum of activity, comparable cost, but ampicillin causes more diarrhea and must be given four instead of three times a day and on an empty stomach.

Trimethoprim sulfamethoxazole (Bactrim, Septra) 8 mg/kg/day and 40 mg/kg/day, respectively (1 ml/kg/day) has the advantages of a bid schedule and low cost. It is not active against β streptococcus group A and has the disadvantage of the allergic reactions caused by sulfa drugs.

Erythromycin sulfisoxazole (Pediazole) 50 mg/kg/day and 150 mg/kg/day, respectively divided qid is another good choice for treating acute otitis media. It has a good spectrum of activity. It is more expensive than amoxicillin or trimethoprim sulfamethoxazole and must be given qid.

Cefaclor (Ceclor) 40 mg/kg/day divided tid has excellent in vitro activity against major middle ear pathogens. Despite adequate clinical response, there is a poor in vivo bacteriologic response of *Hemophilus influenzae* in the middle ear. However, increasingly stable forms of this drug may be developed. Ceclor's high cost is also a negative factor in prescribing this drug.

Amoxicillin and clavulanate (Augmentin) 40 mg/kg/day of amoxicillin divided tid has a broad spectrum of activity. Although it has theoretical advantages over amoxicillin in eradicating β lactamase producing organisms, a clear clinical superiority has yet to be demonstrated. Augmentin causes a high incidence of diarrhea and is expensive.

Analgesics are often important in the initial therapy of acute otitis media until antibiotic therapy can eradicate the infection and decrease pain. Acetaminophen 10 to 15 mg/kg/dose every 4 hours is usually effective. Aspirin, 10 mg/kg/dose every 4 hours, may be used instead of acetaminophen as long as the patient does not have chickenpox or influenza (illnesses in which aspirin use is associated with Reye's syndrome). Codeine, 0.5 to 1.0 mg/kg/dose every 4 to 6 hours not to exceed 3 mg/kg/day, may sometimes need to be given with acetaminophen or aspirin for a few doses. Topical Auralgan, which should be used only in the absence of perforation, may also help relieve the ear pain of acute otitis media.

When acute otitis media is effectively treated, symptomatic relief can be expected within 2 to 3 days. Standard treatment continues for 7 to 10 days. If a patient does not respond within several days, but is not systemically toxic, antibiotics can gen-

erally be safely and effectively switched without performing tympanocentesis for culture and sensitivity. Changing to any of the discussed antibiotics is usually effective. If there is not an acceptable response to a second drug, tympanocentesis to obtain cultures and sensitivities should be performed.

Middle ear effusion commonly persists even after acute otitis media has been effectively treated. Effusion is present in 70% of cases at 2 weeks, 40% at 4 weeks, 20% at 2 months, and 10% at 3 months. Because of the common persistence of middle ear effusion in the first 2 months after an acute infection, follow-up ear checks to ensure complete resolution of middle ear effusion can be scheduled for 2 months after an episode of acute otitis media. Waiting for follow-up for 2 months is appropriate only if the patient can be relied on to return sooner if symptomatic, and to keep a 2-month follow-up appointment even if asymptomatic. Patients who have recurrent ear infections should probably have their first follow-up visit scheduled near the end of therapy to ensure an adequate initial response to treatment.

Recurrent episodes of acute otitis media are common. In about 25% of the cases, infections occurring within 30 days of the original infection are with the same organism as caused the initial infection. Therefore, it is reasonable to empirically use a different antibiotic for a recurrence within 1 month. After 30 days, the infection is usually with another organism, and the infection can probably be treated as an event separate from the initial infection.

Antihistamines and decongestants probably do not help prevent acute otitis media or promote the resolution of acute otitis media. The *Hemophilus influenzae* type B vaccine is not helpful in preventing acute otitis media because most *H. influenzae* causing otitis are nontypable. The pneumococcal vaccine helps prevent some type specific pneumococcal otitis media. The pneumococcal vaccine, however, does not dramatically decrease the total number of episodes of acute otitis media and the vaccine is not recommended for routine prophylaxis against ear infections. Myringotomy relieves pain in acute otitis media; however, it has not been proven to promote the resolution of the infection. Gamma globulin may prove effective in preventing recurrent ear infections in young children, but it should be used only in carefully controlled clinical trials until its safety and possible efficacy are clearly defined.

Antibiotic prophylaxis is effective in preventing

acute otitis media. Children with multiple episodes of acute otitis media who clear their middle ear effusions between episodes are ideal candidates for antimicrobial prophylaxis. Criteria for consideration of antimicrobial prophylaxis are three episodes of acute otitis media in 6 months, or 2 episodes before 6 months of age. Effective antimicrobial choices include Sulfisoxazole 75 mg/kg/day divided bid, and once daily doses of Amoxicillin 20 mg/kg/day, or trimethoprim-sulfamethoxazole 4 mg/kg/day and 20 mg/kg/day. Prophylaxis may be up to 6 months and the duration is often based on the child's history of seasonal variation of symptoms. Usually winter, when respiratory infections are most prevalent, is the most common period for using antimicrobial prophylaxis. Because middle ear effusion can persist without symptoms of acute otitis media, children on chemoprophylaxis should be examined approximately every 2 months.

INDICATIONS FOR REFERRAL
OR ADMISSION

Complications and sequelae of otitis media often necessitate ear, nose, and throat (ENT) referral, and less commonly, admission. Hearing loss, particularly bilateral ≥20 dB for more than 3 months, is an indication for otology referral for possible myringotomy and tube placement. Recurrent episodes of otitis unresponsive to medical management is also an indication for referral, as are the less frequent complications of chronic tympanic membrane perforation, chronic suppurative otitis media, retraction pocket, cholesteatoma, adhesive otitis media, ossicular discontinuity, ossicular fixation, mastoiditis, petrositis, labyrinthitis, facial paralysis, and cholesterol granuloma.

Intracranial suppurative complications of otitis media and mastoiditis include meningitis, extradural abscess, subdural empyema, focal otitic encephalitis, brain abscess, lateral sinus thrombosis, and possibly otitic hydrocephalus. These are immediate indications for admission.

PATIENT EDUCATION

Patients should be taught to seek medical care for ear pain. The use of home remedies such as "sweet oil" should be discouraged. Bottle propping may predispose children to recurrent episodes of otitis media and should be avoided. Patients and families should know that acute otitis media means an infection on the inside of the ear drum and that swimming without diving will probably not precipitate or exacerbate acute otitis media with an intact ear drum. A common misbelief that may need to be dispelled is that going outside in the cold without ear muffs causes acute otitis media. The importance of follow-up examinations to document clearing and to rule out persistent middle ear effusion and hearing loss should be stressed. Parents should know that there will probably be some degree of hearing loss until the ear infection is clear. People who speak to the child, therefore, should face the child and perhaps gently touch the child's shoulder to be sure that the child knows someone is speaking. Until the middle ear effusion is resolved, the child should have preferential seating at the front of the classroom. Parents should be encouraged to stop smoking because of data suggesting that exposure to smoke prolongs the presence of a middle ear effusion after episodes of acute otitis media.

ANNOTATED BIBLIOGRAPHY

See references at end of Chapter 81.

81
Otitis Media with Effusion
MICHAEL MACKNIN

Relatively asymptomatic middle ear effusion has many synonyms such as "secretory," "nonsuppurative," or "serous" otitis media, but the most acceptable term is *otitis media with effusion* (OME). The mobility of the tympanic membrane by pneumatic otoscopy is decreased. The appearance of the tympanic membrane, however, may vary from bulging, opaque, with no visible landmarks to retracted, translucent, with visible landmarks and a clear air fluid level. Most commonly on otoscopy, the tympanic membrane is opaque making assessment of the type of effusion (*i.e.*, serous, mucoid, or purulent) impossible. The most important distinction between OME and acute otitis media is that signs and symptoms of acute infection such as otalgia or fever are lacking in OME. Because of the imprecision over the definition of terms used to describe otitis media, the terminology used to describe otitis media must be defined clearly and used correctly.

OME is the most common cause of hearing loss in childhood. The fluctuating hearing losses associated with OME have been linked by some investigators to language and speech delays and poor school performance. Developing an organized approach to the management of OME is essential to the office practice of pediatrics.

PATHOPHYSIOLOGY

Otitis media with effusion most commonly results from eustachian tube dysfunction (ETD). ETD can result from various causes including antecedent viral illnesses, anatomic abnormalities such as cleft palate, barotrauma, and possibly allergies. ETD can result in the development of relatively asymptomatic middle ear effusion without the initial development of the acute inflammatory response seen in acute otitis media.

One series of pathologic events leading to the development of OME begins with ETD. This leads to the sequence of metaplasia of the middle ear mucosa from a ciliated respiratory epithelium with goblet cells and seromucinous glands to a predominantly secretory mucosa with numerous additional mucous glands formed. Mucous production subsequently arises from goblet cells and transudation occurs from middle ear blood vessels. The effusion may become increasingly viscous and glue-like as the middle ear mucosa absorbs the effusion's watery component. Resolution can begin with mucous plugging of the glandular tubules with degeneration and the transformation of the secretory epithelium back to the nonsecretory respiratory epithelium.

Another series of pathologic events leading to the development of OME begins with ETD, which then develops into acute otitis media. It is the natural history of acute otitis media that middle ear effusion will be present for 2 weeks in 70%, 1 month in 40%, 2 months in 20% and 3 months in 10%.

Otitis media with effusion had previously been thought of as a collection of sterile and relatively asymptomatic middle ear fluid. Research has shown, however, that approximately half of all these effusions in children contain pathogenic bacteria such as nontypable *Hemophilus influenzae, Branhamella catarrhalis*, and *Streptococcus pneumoniae*. The precise role of these organisms in the pathogenesis of OME is poorly understood.

CLINICAL PRESENTATIONS

By definition, OME is relatively asymptomatic. The most common symptoms are hearing loss, minor ear discomfort or fullness in the ear, tinnitus, the sensation of water rushing or popping in the ear, and occasionally impaired balance or dizziness. It is commonly revealed that days or weeks earlier there was a brief episode of ear pain or fever resolving spontaneously. Otitis media with effusion is often discovered during a routine physical examination with no contributory antecedent history.

DIFFERENTIAL DIAGNOSIS

The differential diagnosis for hearing loss in children is extensive and well outlined in standard otology and otolaryngology texts. The diagnosis of OME, however, is best made by pneumatic otoscopy, and if present, the differential diagnosis is vastly narrowed. In older adolescents and adults, unilateral OME must indicate possible nasopharyngeal carcinoma. Recurrent or persistent middle ear effusion must alert the practitioner to possible anatomic abnormalities.

WORK-UP

History

The history should include the occurrence of previous middle ear disease as well as the presence of risk factors for recurrent otitis media as outlined under acute otitis media in Chapter 80.

Physical Examination

The principles of pneumatic otoscopy as outlined under acute otitis media apply to OME (see pp 362, 363). The only consistent finding on physical examination in OME is impaired mobility of the tympanic membrane by pneumatic otoscopy. It is impossible to accurately diagnose OME by otoscopy without performing pneumatic otoscopy. The appearance of the drum may vary from bulging and opaque to retracted and translucent.

A careful examination of the head and neck should be done to rule out anatomic abnormalities associated with the development of OME. Cleft palates are easy to detect. A submucosal cleft should be looked for. The normal soft palate forms an arc at its junction with the hard palate. With a submucosal cleft palate, this junction is V-shaped and can be examined easily by palpation. In the uncooperative patient, the examiner can safely palpate by using a stack of tongue blades to prevent the patient from biting down.

Laboratory Tests

Laboratory tests are not always necessary in the diagnosis and treatment of OME. However, confirmatory objective tests for the diagnosis of middle ear effusion and hearing acuity are often helpful in the management of OME (see Chap. 82 for a more detailed discussion).

Tympanometry assesses the change in tympanic membrane compliance as air pressure is varied in the ear canal. The results are plotted on a chart called a tympanogram, which graphically displays compliance as a function of air pressure. This valuable tool can be used to objectively follow the status of a patient's middle ear. The correlation of the tympanogram with the clinical condition of the middle ear, however, has been validated by findings at myringotomy for only a few of the many tympanometers. Thus, the practitioner would be well advised to ask the manufacturer if the clinical validity of the machine has been tested as a prerequisite to purchasing it.

Audiograms can be performed on children of all ages by qualified personnel. A child is never too young to have a hearing test. The specific methods employed at each age group are beyond the scope of this review. The pediatrician, however, should be able to interpret a conventional audiogram. The audiogram reports hearing threshold for the left and right ear and for air and bone conduction in decibels at different frequencies. Decibels are a log scale with 0 decibels representing normal adult hearing threshold levels. Many children have better than normal adult hearing threshold levels and therefore may have a negative hearing threshold levels, such as -5 decibels. Twenty decibels is about as loud as a whisper. Forty decibels is about the normal loudness of speaking. Ninety decibels can become painful. The hearing threshold in decibels on the ordinate is reported at various frequencies given on the abscissa. The normal speaking frequencies of the human voice range from about 250 Hz to 4000 Hz.

The symbols for air and bone conduction and left and right ear are always reported on the audiogram. Bone conduction reflects sensorineural hearing. Air conduction reflects conductive hearing, and it is typically adversely affected by OME.

An air bone gap (*i.e.*, bone conduction better than air conduction) in the same ear at the same frequency of 15 dB or more represents a significant conductive abnormality. Normally, air and bone conduction are similar. A hearing threshold level of 20 dB or more represents a significant hearing loss in a child. (The exact level of dB loss representing a "significant" hearing loss is controversial.)

If air and bone conduction hearing threshold levels are similarly decreased, there is no air bone gap and the hearing loss is sensorineural. If bone conduction is normal and air conduction is impaired, there is an air bone gap and conductive hearing is abnormal. A conductive hearing loss is typical of OME. Combined sensorineural (with impaired bone conduction) and conductive (with an air bone gap) hearing losses may be present occasionally with OME. The sensorineural component is thought to be due to increased tension and stiffness of the round window membrane. When the OME is resolved, the hearing generally returns to normal. Rarely, permanent sensorineural hearing loss may result from chronic otitis media.

Additional methods of assessing hearing such as electrocochleography and auditory brain stem response are beyond the scope of this review. The auditory brain stem response (ABR) is preferred over electrocochleography (ECOCHG) by most clinicians because a surgical procedure under general anesthesia for placing the active electrode is not required for ABR as it is for ECOCHG. Candidates with OME for ABR as outlined by Fria in Bluestone and Stool's text are as follows: (1) Infants with recurrent acute otitis media or persistent OME, or both and (2) children with significant mental retardation, emotional disturbances, or both.

Acoustic reflectometry is a newer method of detecting middle ear effusion and is based on the principle of partial cancellation of incident sound by sound reflected back from the tympanic membrane. It is easy to perform, but its exact accuracy and role in clinical medicine have not yet been completely determined.

TREATMENT

The treatment of OME is controversial. Treatment can be subdivided into medical and surgical.

I suggest that all patients with newly diagnosed OME be given a 14-day course of a systemic antibiotic appropriate for acute otitis media (see Chap. 80). This recommendation is based on the frequently documented presence of pathogenic bacteria in OME. It should be noted, however, that the efficacy of antibiotic treatment of OME is not as well documented as for acute otitis media.

The patient should be scheduled for a follow-up

visit in 2 months or sooner if symptomatic. Meanwhile, the patient should be given preferential seating in school and every effort should be made to have the child face people when they are speaking.

If the effusion is resolved at the 2-month follow-up visit, the patient should be seen again only for routine well-child visits or if symptoms occur. If the effusion persists, another 14-day course of a different antibiotic should be given and the child scheduled for follow-up in 1 month (*i.e.*, 3 months after initial presentation). The efficacy of treating children 2 to 5 years old with a minimum 6-week history of middle ear effusion with a 1-month course of trimethoprim sulfamethoxazole (8 mg/kg and 40 mg/kg, respectively, per 24 hours in two divided doses) has also been demonstrated.

Many other medical therapies of OME have been tried. None of the therapies discussed below are of any proven benefit. Antihistamines and decongestants probably do not help the resolution of OME. Nasal steroids and systemic steroids with antibiotics have been shown in some studies to be helpful in promoting the resolution of middle ear effusion. The use of nasal and systemic steroids to treat middle ear effusion should be used only in carefully controlled clinical trials until their safety and possible efficacy are established. Controlled middle ear inflation by forcing air up the eustachian tube has no proven long-term efficacy. The role of mucolytic agents is also unsettled. In summary, antibiotics are probably helpful in clearing some OME, but no medical therapy for OME is of proven benefit in most cases of OME. Time is often the best healer.

INDICATIONS FOR REFERRAL

If effusion persists 3 months after initial presentation, an audiogram should be obtained. The precise criteria for referral to an otolaryngologist for possible myringotomy and tube placement are controversial. I would suggest a bilateral air bone gap of greater than or equal to 20 dB as criteria for referral to an otolaryngologist. Other important factors that should be considered include the child's language development, seasonal pattern, an associated permanent conductive or sensorineural hearing loss, and the number of previous infections. A child with language delay may most need the rapid return of normal hearing acuity which usually results from myringotomy and tube placement. A child who is most prone to ear infections in the winter and is usually clear during the warm months should preferentially have a myringotomy and tube

placement for persistent effusion in October rather than in March. Severe pain, ossicular fixation, mastoiditis, labyrinthitis and vertigo, facial paralysis, cholesterol granuloma, cholesteatoma, chronic tympanic membrane perforation, adhesive otitis media, ossicular discontinuity, and retraction pockets are also indications for referral to an otolaryngologist. The immediate efficacy of myringotomy and tube placement in improving hearing is documented, although the long-term balance of the risks and benefits of myringotomy and tube placement has not yet been clearly defined. Children with persistent middle ear effusion for several months without significant hearing loss, language delay, or the other aforementioned complications can be safely followed by their primary care provider. Repeat examinations and hearing screens should be performed at least every 1 to 2 months to monitor for the need for referral.

A tonsillectomy and an adenoidectomy are other surgical interventions used to treat OME. A tonsillectomy probably has no role in the treatment of middle ear disease. Adenoidectomy probably does afford some benefit to selected patients with recurrent middle ear problems. Unfortunately, it is difficult to prospectively identify the minority of patients with recurrent middle ear disease who would benefit from adenoidectomy.

PATIENT EDUCATION

Families with children who have OME should know that there is often a hearing loss associated with this condition. The importance of follow-up examinations to document clearing and to rule out persistent middle ear effusion and hearing loss should be stressed. Families should be reassured that with time, most cases of OME will resolve without any long-term adverse effects on hearing.

ANNOTATED BIBLIOGRAPHY

Bluestone CD, Klein JO (eds): Controversies in antimicrobial agents for otitis media. Pediatr Ann 13:361–421, 1984 (Summary of symposium organized to clarify the present state-of-knowledge concerning antimicrobial agents for otitis media.)

Bluestone CD, Fria TJ, Arjona SK et al: Controversies in screening for middle ear disease and hearing loss in children. Pediatrics 77:57–70, 1986 (Experts in pediatrics, infectious disease, otolaryngology, epidemiology, audiology, and biostatistics assess the current status of screening for otitis media in infants and children.)

Bluestone CD, Klein JO, Paradise JL et al: Workshop on

effects of otitis media on the child. Pediatrics 71:639–652, 1983 (Workshop providing summary of experts from pediatrics, otolaryngology, infectious disease, audiology, speech, linguistics, and psychology. An outstanding summary.)

Cantekin EI, Mandel EM, Bluestone CD et al: Lack of efficacy of a decongestant-antihistamine combination for otitis media with effusion (''secretory'' otitis media) in children. N Engl J Med 308:297–301, 1983 (The classic paper proving the lack of efficacy of a decongestant and antihistamine combination in treating otitis media with effusion.)

Lim DJ, Bluestone CD, Klein JO, Nelson JD (eds): Recent Advances in Otitis Media with Effusion. Philadelphia, BC Decker, 1984 (Collection of papers providing an excellent overview of the direction of otitis media research and current knowledge. Refer to Healy's paper on 1 month of antibiotic treatment for persistent OME.)

Mandel EM, Rockette HE, Bluestone CD et al: Efficacy of amoxicillin with and without decongestant–antihistamine for otitis media with effusion in children. N Engl J Med 316:432–437, 1987 (Excellent double-blind, randomized trial showing amoxicillin treatment increases to some extent the likelihood of resolution of OME. The addition of a decongestant-antihistamine to amoxicillin treatment increased side effects without increasing resolution of OME.)

Marchant CD, Shurin PA: Therapy of otitis media. Pediatr Clin North Am 30:281–296, 1983 (Another excellent review of therapy.)

Paradise JL: Otitis media in infants and children. Pediatrics 65:917–943, 1980 (Outstanding review article covering all aspects of otitis media.)

The Ear and Related Structures. In Bluestone CD, Stool SE (eds): Pediatric Otolaryngology, pp 85–646. Philadelphia, WB Saunders, 1983 (Detailed summary of all aspects of ear disease in the standard pediatric otolaryngology test.)

82

Testing Hearing and Middle Ear Function

HOWARD G. SMITH AND MARILYN WARREN

Communication using spoken language requires the reception, processing, and production of a specific subset of sounds called *speech*. The physical study of sound, called *acoustics*, defines and describes sounds by their intensities or apparent loudness and by their frequencies or group of frequencies.

The human ear and its supporting neural structures represent an ultrasensitive, ultra-high-fidelity sound processing system. The ear can detect both a whisper and a sound one million times more intense, such as the roar of a jet engine. A logarithmic unit called the *decibel* (dB) is used to quantify given sound levels. The human ear detects sounds in the frequency range from 20 to 20,000 cycles/sec (*i.e.*, Hertz or Hz), but has a different sensitivity to various sound frequencies. The ear is most sensitive to sounds in the range between 1000 Hz to 6000 Hz, the speech frequency range.

Hearing acuity is usually tested by exposing the subject to various calibrated sound and by measuring either behavioral or physiologic responses produced by the subject. Tones of specific frequency, called pure tones, are presented in octave intervals at frequencies from 125 Hz to 8 kHz.

The level of hearing or, conversely, that of hearing loss, is a threshold level or average threshold level measured in dB referring to dB HL or dB relative to normal hearing threshold. A normal hearing ear demonstrates a threshold for hearing near 0 dB. An ear with a profound hearing loss has a threshold exceeding 90 dB. Such an ear would barely hear a sound presented at the 95 dB level.

The severity of a hearing loss is determined by the threshold hearing level and is categorized according to one of many hearing impairment scales (Table 82-1).

The fidelity or lack of sound distortion decreases with increasing hearing thresholds. Children with sensorineural hearing losses have difficulty understanding and differentiating words that they hear. This situation limits the practical use of even the most powerful hearing aids for children with severe to profound hearing losses.

Pure tones are used to test the neuronal connections from the cochlea to the brainstem and beyond. Other testing routines can determine the integrity of the middle ear sound conduction system.

Table 82-1. Typical Hearing Loss Scale

HEARING IMPAIRMENT	HEARING THRESHOLD (dB)	FIDELITY (Discrim)
None	$-10-25$	Excellent
Mild	26–40	Very good
Moderate	41–55	Good
Moderate to severe	56–70	Fair
Severe	71–90	Fair to poor
Profound	Above 91	Poor to none (0–50%)

TESTING TECHNIQUES

Behavioral Audiometry

Behavioral audiometry requires that the child be willing and able to give reliable and reproducible responses to sounds generated by calibrated equipment and presented within a sound-isolated room. To decide whether or not a child is making a definite behavioral response to sound requires the professional skill of an audiologist experienced in the testing of children, particularly in the case of infants and toddlers. Sounds are presented through either loudspeakers or through earphones and bone conduction phones depending on the age of the child. For younger children, testing is performed with the parent and often with a second audiologist in the test room to facilitate observation.

The usual audiometric battery includes a determination for each ear of (1) a hearing threshold for sounds transmitted through the air of the ear canal and middle ear space called the *air conduction threshold*; (2) a hearing threshold for sounds transmitted directly to the temporal bone bypassing the air conduction system using a vibrator resting on the mastoid process called the *bone conduction threshold*; (3) the *speech reception threshold* (SRT), the lowest sound intensity at which a child can correctly identify selected words in 50% of trials; (4) the *speech discrimination score*, a measure of hearing fidelity determined by the percentage of a standardized list of monosyllabic words correctly identified if presented at a sound intensity 25 dB to 40 dB above the speech reception threshold. For infants and toddlers, the goal of the audiometric evaluation is to determine a *sound detection level* or *minimal response level* and to decide whether the child's responses to sound are within the normal range.

The air conduction and bone conduction thresholds are determined and plotted on a standard graphic form called an audiogram (Fig. 82-1). The hearing levels are plotted on the vertical axis using an inverse linear scale and the test frequencies are plotted on the horizontal axis using a logarithmic scale. All audiograms have legends that indicate the symbols used for plotting the data. If color is used, the right ear is drawn in red and the left ear in blue. The audiogram shows the hearing of a child with a bilateral mixed hearing loss. The bone conduction threshold is 30 dB. Most of this loss is likely due to cochlear malfunction and the attendant sensorineural hearing loss, but middle ear pathology may also raise the bone conduction threshold adding to the apparent sensorineural hearing loss. The air conduction thresholds are in the 60-dB to 70-dB range, indicating an overall hearing loss in the moderate to severe range, with a 30-dB to 40-dB potentially treatable conductive hearing loss as a component of the total hearing loss. The SRT usually approximates the average of the pure tone air conduction thresholds at 500 Hz, 1000 Hz, and 2000 Hz, which is a useful internal check on the test results.

If one ear has significantly better hearing than the other, it is often necessary to mask the hearing of the better ear to prevent it from interfering with accurate testing of the poorer hearing ear. This is accomplished by presenting either white noise, sound including a broad range of frequencies, or narrow band noise at a sufficiently intense level to the better hearing ear.

The speech discrimination scores indicate the fidelity of the hearing in each ear. Scores normally diminish along with general auditory acuity. Unusually low or asymmetric scores, particularly in a child with a unilateral or an asymmetric sensorineural hearing loss, may indicate a neural lesion and the need for further work-up.

Evoked Response Audiometry

Several techniques are available for measuring the electrophysiologic response of the auditory system to sound. All techniques share common technical features. Sound is delivered to the ear through an earphone, loudspeaker, or through a bone conduction device. Measuring electrodes are positioned on the child's head. Repetitive sound stimuli are delivered to the patient, and faint electrical signals produced within the auditory pathways after each stimulus are amplified and channelled into a signal averaging computer. The averaging computer is time-locked to the stimulus so that as the signal

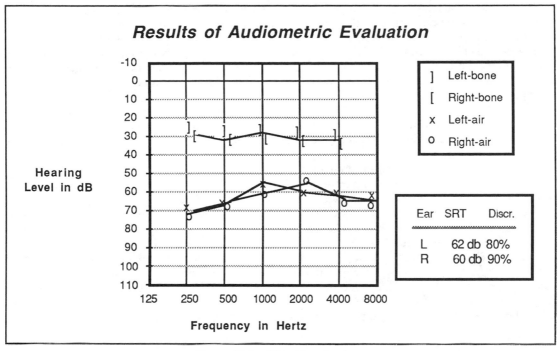

Figure 82-1.   Mixed hearing loss.

averaging takes place, the random background electrical noise is averaged out. Sound stimuli such as tone bursts may be presented at varying intensities and frequencies. Speech is not used as a stimulus for clinical threshold measures.

The auditory evoked response measure in most frequent clinical use today is called *brainstem evoked response* (BSER) or *auditory brainstem response* (ABR). This technique measures the initiation of sound-induced electrical signals in the cochlea and their propagation along the auditory nerve into the brainstem during the first 15 to 20 milliseconds (msec) after the sound stimulus. The stimuli used are clicks or tone bursts of varying intensities and frequencies delivered to the cochlea by way of either air or bone conduction with the patient in a shielded sound booth. The resultant electric signals are recorded by noninvasive surface electrodes. The test is performed with infants and young children under sedation with a hypnotic agent such as chloral hydrate. A general anesthetic agent may be used, but is usually unnecessary.

With this system it is possible to selectively determine the sound intensity response thresholds for air or bone conduction in each ear at several frequencies important for speech. The results obtained seem to agree closely with those obtained using behavioral audiometric techniques. The ABR or BSER evaluation, while accepted as a routine method of hearing assessment in infants and difficult-to-test patients, does require careful interpretation in conjunction with behavioral audiometric data.

Another technique providing similar information is *electrocochleography* (ECoG). This technique is not widely used today because ABR is easier and safer to accomplish and yields more useful data.

Impedance Audiometry

Many children have ear disease that interferes with the efficient conduction of sound energy from the external ear canal through the tympanic membrane and ossicular chain. Middle ear infections and effusions as well as ossicular malformations produce *acoustic impedance*, which may be measured. Sudden intense sound should produce contraction of the stapedius and tensor tympani muscles to protect the cochlea by attenuation of ossicular mobility.

Instruments and procedures have been developed to evaluate middle ear dynamic function. The instrument used for these tests is called an *electroacoustic impedance/admittance bridge*, and current models can test several different middle ear functions. Impedance audiometry requires little cooperation from the child other than the acceptance of an appropriately sized test probe in the external ear canal.

Tympanometry is a technique that quantitates the change in tympanic membrane mobility or compliance as air pressure in the external ear canal is varied. The tympanic membrane is most compliant and able to absorb sound energy when the pressures on either side of it are equal. The test is carried out by placing a three channel probe from the impedance bridge into the ear to be tested. The probe contains (1) acoustic input tubing connected to a tone oscillator that provides a standard sound source, usually 220 Hz, (2) acoustic output tubing connected to a microphone and amplifier to measure the percentage of input sound energy that is reflected back by the tympanic membrane, and (3)

a pneumatic tube connected to an air pump that can control the air pressure within the external ear canal. As the test proceeds, the air pressure within the ear canal is varied from + 200 mm water to − 400 mm water and the sound absorbed by the eardrum is measured. A graph called a *tympanogram* is produced.

Several types of common tympanograms are shown in Figure 82-2. In the type A tympanogram, the point of peak tympanic membrane compliance or mobility is at the point where the air pressure in the ear canal varies from atmospheric pressure by less than 100 mm water. If the absolute compliance of the tympanic membrane is not within a defined normal range, ossicular pathology may exist. Uniformly low compliance may indicate that the attached ossicles are partially fixed. High compliance may suggest the presence of a partial or complete ossicular discontinuity or a recently healed tympanic membrane perforation. In a type B tympanogram, the tympanic membrane compliance is uniformly low and varies little with change in air

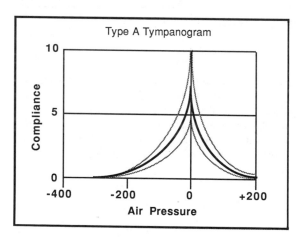

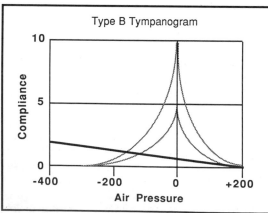

Figure 82-2. (*A*) Type A tympanogram, (*B*) Type B tympanogram, (*C*) Type C tympanogram.

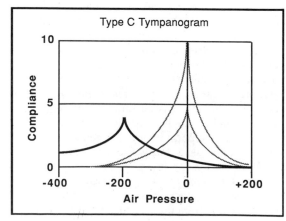

pressure within the ear canal. This condition may exist in the presence of an effusion within the middle ear space or in the case of a firm, complete fixation of the ossicles. The third general type of tympanogram is the type C, in which the point of peak compliance of the tympanic membrane occurs when the air pressure within the ear canal is reduced and falls in the -100 mm to -400 mm water range. This indicates that the air pressure within the middle ear space is similarly reduced.

The impedance bridge can calculate the physical volume of the external auditory canal by measuring the apparent canal volume from the tip of the probe to the tympanic membrane. If the volume is unusually low, the probe tip may be resting against a cerumen plug or may be misdirected toward the canal wall rather than toward the tympanic membrane. If the volume is abnormally high, there may be a perforation in the tympanic membrane secondary to a middle ear infection or trauma. The patency of tympanostomy tubes may also be determined in this way.

The impedance bridge is a useful screening tool for the objective determination of hearing loss and its possible cause. Loud sound stimuli at the 70-dB to 95-dB level normally produce a sudden contraction of the stapedius (by way of the facial nerve) and tensor tympani muscles (by way of trigeminal nerve). These muscle contractions create a momentary but measurable decrease in tympanic membrane compliance. The absence of this acoustic reflex may indicate a significant hearing loss. Such information may be valuable as an adjunct to behavioral audiometry, particularly when there is a concern about whether an older child may be simulating a hearing loss. The presence of acoustic reflexes does not rule out certain types of severe sensorineural hearing losses.

TESTING CHILDREN OF DIFFERENT AGES

Infants and Toddlers

Neonates at high risk for hearing loss are screened by either behavioral or objective audiometric techniques. The behavioral methods require the presentation of a calibrated loud sound through a speaker placed near the child's head. Tone bursts in the 2000-Hz to 4000-Hz frequency range are presented at a 90-dB level. A trained observer watches for characteristic eye and body movements or arousal responses that indicate that the child has heard the sound. The entire process has been partially automated by use of a device called a *crib-o-gram*, which electronically detects the babies motor responses to randomly presented sound stimuli and has been shown to be an effective alternative to professional observation of the behavioral responses. Such behavioral testing yields information only about a child's better hearing ear, if there is an asymmetry, and may rule out deafness but not milder hearing losses.

With increasing availability of auditory evoked response instrumentation, high-risk neonates are now commonly screened either before hospital discharge or within 3 months following discharge. Such screening is performed for each ear using clicks at 30 dB to 40 dB followed by the presentation of a higher intensity stimulus, such as 60 dB, if no response is measured. If the child fails the screen at one or both sound levels, additional threshold testing is recommended. Follow-up behavioral audiometry at 1 year of age is advisable for those children who pass an ABR screen.

The techniques useful for testing older infants and toddlers depend on the child's chronological age and cognitive developmental stage. Behavioral testing may be accomplished at any age, and the results not only indicate that the child is capable of hearing a sound of a certain frequency and intensity, but that the child is able to process the acoustic information and generate predictable behavior as a result. Behavioral test results may sometimes be difficult to interpret because of random body movements or a child's short attention span. Objective audiometric tests such as evoked response audiometry and impedance audiometry provide reliable electrophysiologic evidence that the auditory neural pathways are operative. These tests do not indicate whether a child has normal cerebral processing of the auditory information. For this reason, behavioral testing is preferred, but objective test procedures are invaluable for certain difficult-to-test individuals such as children with mental retardation, emotional, or psychiatric disorders or neuromuscular disorders.

The child's behavioral response to sound is age dependent. Children under the age of 3 are tested by listening to sounds from loudspeakers, a process denoted as *sound-field testing*. In general, younger children require pure tone or speech sounds of higher intensity to respond, and their responses are more rudimentary. During the first 4 months of life, noise or tones at the 50-dB to 70-dB level and speech at the 40-dB level should produce the *auropalpebral response* (APR), which consists of eye widening, eye blink or eye roving in the awake infant or lid tightening in the sleeping infant. Other possible responses include a Moro's startle response, awakening, sucking, facial movements, or termination of active movement. The presentation of sound and determination of response from such behaviors is called *behavioral observation audiometry*.

From 5 to 9 months the noise or tones at the 30-dB to 50-dB level and speech at the l0-dB to 20-dB level elicit a more sophisticated localizing behavioral response. Between 9 and 24 months there is a slight reduction in the sound threshold necessary to produce this localization response. Because children above the age of 4 months make visual localization responses, they may be conditioned to reliably reproduce the localization response by showing them a visually interesting "reward" when they turn in the direction of a sound. This technique is called *visual reinforcement audiometry*.

Some infants and toddlers tolerate the placement of earphones or a bone conduction oscillator during behavioral audiometry. Their responses to sounds presented in this way may permit the independent assessment of air conduction and bone conduction thresholds for each ear.

Children of any age may undergo impedance audiometric testing as a screen for the existence of middle ear disease. Some investigators feel that tympanometry is unreliable in infants below 6 months due to the increased compliance of the cartilagenous external canal.

Younger Children

Children age 3 and older accept headphones and bone conduction oscillators. This permits the reliable determination of air conduction and bone conduction thresholds for pure tones and speech in each ear rather than determination of sound and speech detection levels for the better hearing ear only. Children under the age of 5 years are often tested using a technique called *play audiometry*. The child is taught to perform a play task such as placing a peg in a pegboard whenever a tone or word is heard. Children in this age group will be able to recognize a closed set of words including body parts and common toys so that their speech reception, recognition, and discrimination may be tested. Some older children may be able to actually repeat the words, whereas others may indicate that they understand the word by pointing to an appropriate object in the sound room or by pointing to a picture of the object. Children in this age group should undergo routine impedance testing and determi-

nation of the tympanogram for each ear because of the high incidence of middle ear disease.

Other Children and Adolescents

Children above the age of 5 or 6 years will usually respond to a standard audiometric test battery including the determination of air and bone conduction thresholds, speech reception thresholds, and speech discrimination scores for each ear. Older children should also undergo impedance testing. Many children in the age group undergo routine auditory and tympanometric screening in local school screening programs. Children who fail the screening tests require a prompt otoscopic evaluation and an audiometric evaluation, including tympanometry.

Special test routines have been developed to evaluate children who are thought to have a functional hearing loss and children who have central auditory processing problems. Children with the latter problem may have difficulty attending to and understanding speech presented in noisy settings, have difficulty synthesizing a sequence of words into linguistic meaning, or having a problem with localizing sounds. Below age 7 years, central auditory processing skills are so closely allied with receptive language development that the assessment of these skills is best accomplished by a speech and language pathologist, after a hearing loss has been ruled out.

ANNOTATED BIBLIOGRAPHY

Jerger J (ed): Pediatric Audiology: Current Trends. San Diego, College–Hill Press, 1984 (Recent compendium of the theory and practice of pediatric audiology.)

Jerger J, Anthony L, Jerger S, Maudlin L: Studies in impedance audiometry. Arch Otolaryngol 99:165–171, 1974 (Discussion of principles and practice of impedance testing.)

Keith RW (ed): Audiology for the physician. Baltimore/London, Williams and Wilkins, 1980 (Excellent review of current audiologic theory and practice with additional chapters on related otologic subject matter.)

Northern J, Downs MP: Hearing in Children. Baltimore, Williams and Wilkins, 1974 (Covers all aspects of diagnostic and rehabilitative pediatric audiology.)

Simmons FB, Russ FN: Automated newborn hearing screening, the crib-o-gram. Arch Otolaryngol 100:1–7, 1974 (Description of the technique for neonatal hearing screening using automated sound stimulus and motion detection equipment.)

Supplementary statement of the Joint Committee on Infant Hearing Screening, July 1, 1972. ASHA 16:160, 1974

83
Hearing Loss
HOWARD G. SMITH

Current estimates indicate that as many as 15% of school-aged children have significant conductive hearing losses. The incidence of profound sensorineural hearing loss is approximately 1:1000 children. An older child or adolescent who experiences a hearing loss has already acquired sufficient linguistic information to permit serviceable communication using an amplification device and deductive reasoning. In contrast, infants or toddlers with undiagnosed hearing losses are faced with the difficult if not impossible tasks of deciphering and learning spoken language and the cultural rules on which it is based without the ability to hear words clearly.

The identification of a hearing loss in children requires that the clinician have a high index of suspicion and be sensitive to the concerns of parents, who are usually the first to become aware of the hearing loss. Parents of children with confirmed hearing losses often bitterly complain that their doctor unnecessarily delayed the diagnosis with comments such as: "Sara is only going through a stage. She will outgrow it."

PATHOPHYSIOLOGY

Hearing losses are characterized by *site of dysfunction* in the auditory mechanism, whether *the etiology* is genetic and hereditary or environmental and acquired, *the age at onset* of the hearing loss, and the *severity* of the loss. This latter aspect is discussed in detail in Chapter 82.

Conductive hearing losses occur due to interference with sound transmission through the external ear canal, tympanic membrane, or the ossicular chain. *Sensorineural hearing losses* are caused by malfunctions of cochlear transduction or signal transmission. *Mixed hearing losses* are the sum total of individual conductive and sensorineural losses.

Conductive Hearing Loss

Acquired conductive losses are the most common types of hearing loss in childhood. Mild to moderate fluctuating hearing losses are caused by cerumen impaction and otitis media. More significant conductive losses are produced by tympanic membrane and ossicular chain fixation, disruption or destruction by cholesteatoma or by trauma.

Hereditary conductive losses may be congenital or delayed. Congenital deformities of the auricle alone may be inherited as a autosomal dominant or a sex-linked trait. Congenital aural atresia and the partial or complete agenesis of the external auditory canal, middle ear space, or ossicles due to malformations of the first and second branchial arch components occur in 1 of 10,000 to 20,000 live births. The atresia may be unilateral or bilateral and may be inherited as an isolated finding or as part of a syndromic constellation. Aural atresia is often associated with the autosomal dominantly inherited craniofacial (Crouzon's) syndrome and the mandibulofacial (Treacher Collins Franceschetti) syndrome. Nonhereditary congenital aural atresia may also occur after fetal exposure to teratogenic pharmaceuticals such as thalidomide or as part of the congenital rubella syndrome. Children who have orofacial syndromes with associated cleft palate often have severe eustachian tube dysfunction, which itself produces secondary acquired conductive hearing losses. Another form of hereditary progressive conductive hearing loss that may first present during adolescence is otosclerosis in which there is fixation of the stapes caused by repetitive resorption and redeposition of bone in the otic capsule. Otosclerosis apparently follows an autosomal dominant hereditary pattern.

Sensorineural Losses

Acquired sensorineural losses may occur either during embryogenesis or at any time after birth. The etiologic agents implicated include microorganisms, toxic chemicals, pharmaceuticals, and metabolic products. These agents cause profound deterioration of labyrinthine structures including the peripheral auditory and vestibular sensory receptors, vascular structures, and supporting membranes. Maternal infection with microorganisms such as the rubella virus, the cytomegalovirus, the protozoan *toxoplasma gondii*, and the spirochete *treponema pallidum* may produce mid- to high-frequency hearing losses, dysequilibrium or rotatory vertigo. Hearing loss due to congenital syphilis may occur suddenly during childhood or may develop slowly during adulthood. Childhood viral infections such as measles, mumps, acute respiratory infections, and infectious mononucleosis have been strongly associated with unilateral and bilateral sudden hearing losses in preschool and school-aged children. Bacterial meningitis has been associated with significant hearing impairment in about 10% of affected children. Hearing loss is not associated with viral meningitis.

Ototoxic drugs administered either to the embryo or to the neonate may produce labyrinthine damage. The antimalarial drugs quinine and chloroquine as well as the aminoglycoside antibiotics gentamycin, kanamycin, tobramycin, and amikacin have profound ototoxic effects. Loop diuretics, such as ethacrynic acid and furosemide, also produce a hearing loss, an effect exacerbated by the concomitant use of aminoglycosides. Careful monitoring of drug blood levels as well as cochlear and vestibular function will prevent irreversible damage when these agents are used.

Acquired sensorineural hearing losses have also been associated with congenital hypothyroidism, erythroblastosis fetalis, prematurity, hypoxia, prolonged or difficult labor, maternal diabetes mellitus, and toxemia of pregnancy.

Acoustic or head trauma may cause immediate or delayed sensorineural hearing loss. Repeated intense noise, a sudden explosion, or head trauma with or without temporal bone fracture produces a characteristic high frequency hearing loss, often partially or completely reversible, that may later present as a permanent loss. An important, potentially treatable cause of *sudden acquired sensorineural hearing loss* is perilymph leakage through disrupted membranes at the oval or round windows. A high frequency hearing loss, with or without accompanying positional vertigo, usually follows vigorous physical activity, marked altitude or barometric pressure changes, or physical trauma to the ear or head. Prompt exploratory surgery and sealing of leaks with soft tissue will often prevent a progressive hearing loss and may restore serviceable hearing.

Hereditary sensorineural hearing losses represent from 20% to 50% of all cases of severe to profound sensorineural hearing losses. The estimated incidence of hereditary hearing loss is at least 1 in 4000 live births. The hearing loss, often severe to profound, may occur as an isolated finding or may occur in conjunction with other clinical features as shown in Table 83-1. Abnormalities of ocular structures, the renal system, the nervous system, and general metabolism may accompany hereditary sensorineural hearing losses.

CLINICAL PRESENTATION

Clinicians have traditionally depended on both their own and parental observations to suggest the existence of a childhood hearing loss. The lack of age-appropriate responses to sound such as eye blink, eye widening, startle response, and head turning in infants and toddlers should prompt referral to an audiologist for formal testing, but the apparent presence of these responses should not delay otherwise indicated testing. Any infant with one or more of the following factors, known to be associated with a higher than normal risk of a hearing loss, should be referred as soon as possible for comprehensive auditory testing:

1. Birth weight of 1500 g or less
2. Apgar score of 5 or less at 5 min
3. Delayed growth and development
4. More than 24 hours in a neonatal intensive care unit, with or without artificial ventilatory assistance
5. Hyperbilirubinemia (> 20 mg/100 ml) requiring prolonged phototherapy or exchange transfusion
6. Seizures or other neurologic abnormalities
7. Known physical abnormalities of the skull or the ear, nose, or throat at birth
8. History of maternal or neonatal infection or sepsis
9. History of head injury at birth or otherwise
10. Family history of hereditary hearing loss

Children of any age with a history of bacterial meningitis, encephalitis, severe head injury, or repeated episodes of otitis media should be evaluated for a possible hearing loss.

Hearing losses in preschool children are often heralded by obvious communication difficulties, excessive sound volume on the television, radio, or cassette player, and speech delay or poor speech intelligibility. Children with frequent middle ear problems, even in the absence of other evidence of hearing loss, should also be highly suspect.

School-aged children are often unaware of gradual or even sudden hearing losses. Signs of such losses include failed school screening tests, deterioration of a child's notetaking performance, development of unusual communication problems,

Table 83-1. Types of Hereditary and Genetic Sensorineural Hearing Losses (SNHL)

NAME	INHERITANCE	ONSET	ASSOCIATED FEATURES
SNHL Occurring Alone			
Michel's deafness	AD	C	Complete aplasia of cochlea
Mondini's deafness	AD	C	Partial aplasia of cochlea; associated CSF leak
Familial progressive deafness	AD	D	Partial aplasia of cochlea at basal turn
Scheibe's deafness	AR	C	NL bony labyrinth; abn of cochlear membranes
X-linked deafness	SL	C	Severe to profound hearing losses
X-linked deafness	SL	D	Moderate to severe hearing losses
SNHL and Metabolic ABN			
Waardenberg's syndrome	AD	C or D	Partial albinism; abn of tyrosine metabolism
Schafer's syndrome	AD	C	Prolinemia; MR
Tietze's syndrome	AD	C or D	Albinism; abn of tyrosine metabolism
Nelson's syndrome	AD	—	Homocystinemia; MR
Albinism	AD, AR, or SL	C	Albinism, strabismus, nystagmus
Hypophosphatasia	AR	—	Decreased bone mineralization
Hyperphosphatasia	AR	—	Dwarfism; other skeletal abn
Hurler's syndrome	AR	D	Lipochondrodystrophy, dwarfism; MR; hepatosplenomegaly
Morquio's disease	AR	—	Osteochondrodystrophy
Onychodystrophy	AR, AD	C	Abnormal nail growth
Tay–Sach's disease	AR	—	MR; ganglioside llpidosis
Pendred's syndrome	AR	C	Goiter
Wilson's disease	AR	—	Hepatic and ocular lens degeneration
SNHL and Nephropathies			
Alport's syndrome	AD	D	Glomerulonephritis; 1% of hereditary deafness
Muckle–Well's syndrome	AD	D	Nephritis; amyloidosis
Herrmann's syndrome	AD	D	Nephritis, epilepsy; DM; MR
Renal tubular acidosis	AR	D	Metabolic acidosis; failure to thrive
SNHL and Ocular Disease			
Usher's syndrome	AR, SL, or AD	C	Retinitis pigmentosa; 10% of hereditary deafness
Alstrom's syndrome	AR	D	Retinitis pigmentosa; DM; obesity
Cockayne's syndrome	AR	D	Retinitis pigmentosa; dwarfism; MR
Leber's disease	AR	—	Optic atrophy
Norrie's disease	AR, SL	D	Retinal pseudoglioma
Refsum's syndrome	AR	D	Retinitis pigmentosa; ichthyosis; polyneuritis; ataxia
SNHL and Nervous System Disease			
Huntington's chorea	AD	D	Progressive chorea
Von Recklinghausen's disease	AD	D	Neural schwannomas
Friedreich's ataxia	AR	—	Cerebellar xia
Richards–Rundle disease	AR	D	Ataxia; MR; muscular dystrophy; absent sexual development
SNHL and Heart Disease			
Jervell and Lange–Nielsen syndrome	AR	C	Prolonged QT interval, heart block
Lewis' syndrome	AR	—	Pulmonic stenosis
SNHL and Skeletal Disease			
Klippel–Feil syndrome	AR	D	Cervical fusion; spina bifida; scoliosis
Paget's disease	AR	D	Deformities of skull and long bones
Chromosomal Abnormalities			
Trisomy 13–15 (D)		C	Ext and middle ear abn; eye abn
Trisomy 18 (E)		C	Ext ear abn; micrognathia; digit abn
CHARGE association	?	C	Coloboma; cardiac abn; choanal atresia, genital abn

Mode of Inheritance—AD: autosomal dominant; AR: autosomal recessive; SL: sex-linked. *Onset time of SNHL*—C: congenital; D: delayed; —: variable.

and a change in telephone or portable stereo sound system usage patterns. Such a loss should also be suspected if a child complains of noises in the head (tinnitus) or a distortion of hearing.

DIFFERENTIAL DIAGNOSIS

Currently available behavioral testing methods and increasingly sophisticated evoked potential audiometry and impedance audiometry permit an accurate determination of the severity and site of a presumptive hearing impairment at *any* age. These techniques are described in Chapter 82.

WORK-UP

History

The historical review for a child with a suspected hearing loss begins with a review of the prenatal and perinatal periods including maternal exposure to infectious disease; use of prescription, over-the-counter, and recreational drugs; the nature of the gestational period, the labor, and the delivery of the infant including any birth trauma or hypoxia; the neonatal period including the occurrence of jaundice, sepsis, cardiopulmonary disease, and renal disease and the treatment regimens used. Other important information includes the history of the child's middle ear infections, the parent's assessment of the child's responses to sounds and listening skills, the development of communication skills, a history of head injury or acoustic trauma, and a family history of hearing loss or other otologic problems. The older child should be asked about the incidence of ear pain, changes in hearing level and quality, and signs of balance problems such as lightheadedness, clumsiness, or stomach upset.

Physical Examination

The otologic examination begins with a careful appraisal of the position and anatomy of auricular appendages, the surface anatomy of the temporal bone, the size and shape of the external canal, and the appearance of the tympanic membrane and ossicular landmarks. The mobility of the tympanic membrane and the presence or absence of middle ear air or fluid are determined with the pneumatic otoscope. (For review of technique, see under Physical Examination, Chap. 80.) An intranasal examination should be performed, and, in the newborn, a catheter or fiberscope passed to assess choanal patency. Within the oral cavity, the num-

ber, position, color, and shape of the teeth should be noted. The structure and function of the hard and soft palate are assessed, looking for evidence of complete, partial, or submucosal clefting and abnormal soft palatal motion. The cervical structures should be evaluated by inspection and palpation for evidence of sinus tracts, or embryonic cysts. The thyroid should be palpated to check for enlargement or nodules.

A complete general physical examination should be performed with particular attention to the eyes, skin, skeletal system, and the nervous system.

Laboratory Tests

Age-appropriate hearing testing should be carried out according to the principles outlined in Chapter 82 if screening tests or clinical presentation suggests the possibility of a hearing loss. To determine the etiology of a congenital sensorineural hearing loss, infants and toddlers should have serum tested in a TORCH screen to assay their IgM antibody levels to toxoplasma, rubella, cytomegalovirus, and the herpesviruses. In an older child, a routine serologic test for syphilis, the fluorescent treponemal antibody-absorption (FTA-ABS) test, and a screening heterophil test are drawn. A child with a newly diagnosed hearing loss should have radiographic imaging of the temporal bones by a polytomographic or computerized tomographic technique.

Serum chemistry tests including random blood sugar, blood urea nitrogen, creatinine, calcium, phosphate, thyroxine, triiodothyronine, and T3-resin uptake may be carried out to discover if a hearing-impaired child has an associated metabolic disorder. An ECG should be performed. If renal disease is suspected, other useful tests include a complete urinalysis, a creatinine clearance, and an abdominal or renal ultrasound. There is an increased incidence of renal disorders in children with first and second bronchial arch syndromes.

MANAGEMENT AND SPECIALIZED CARE

It is not within the scope of this discussion to provide a detailed discussion of the long-term management of hearing loss, because services must be individually tailored to the nature and severity of the hearing loss. Middle ear disease, which commonly produces reversible forms of mild to moderate conductive hearing loss, should be actively treated with medical management supplemented by surgical approaches as the longevity or the severity of the disease increases. The approach to this type of otologic disease is discussed in Chapter 81.

Unilateral hearing losses must be evaluated carefully using auditory evoked responses and radiographic imaging to rule out retrocochlear lesions such as cerebellopontine angle or internal auditory canal lesions. Careful monitoring, preferred classroom seating, and the use of appropriate amplification devices are necessary to minimize the academic impact of the hearing loss.

More severe or irreversible bilateral hearing losses, usually sensorineural, present a difficult management challenge calling for a highly organized, multidisciplinary team approach. This team has three goals: (1) to initially assess and periodically monitor the medical and psychological status of the child and his family; (2) to provide sufficient background information about deafness and the necessary emotional support for a family to accept the reality of their child's hearing loss and proceed to realistically deal with it; (3) to help the family choose suitable educational programs for themselves and their child.

A typical team is coordinated by a pediatric otologist and includes a clinical psychologist specializing in therapy and counseling for families with hearing-impaired children, a pediatrician with expertise in developmental pediatrics and genetics, a pediatric ophthalmologist, an audiologist, an educational psychologist experienced in evaluating deaf children, a speech–language pathologist, a nonvocal communication specialist, a teacher of the hearing impaired, and a professional educator of deaf children. Each child undergoes an otologic examination, complete audiologic testing and fitting with appropriate hearing aids, a developmental pediatric evaluation with consultation to a pediatric neurologist, an ophthalmic evaluation, a cognitive and psychological evaluation, and a two-part communication evaluation to assess the child's communication skills using verbal and nonverbal language techniques. Monitoring evaluations by selected clinicians are scheduled to take place every 6 months. When a family history or clinical presentation indicates the possibility of a genetic etiology, a complete family pedigree is constructed.

Supportive and therapeutic counseling sessions for family members help them cope with expected initial reactions of grief and denial as well as frequently associated situational crises such as marital strife. Such sessions also permit staff the opportunity to better understand the psychodynamics operative within the child's family. If a genetic etiology is established, genetic counseling will help family members understand the implications for other family members.

Through reading and discussions with clinicians, other parents, and deaf professionals, family members learn to accept that hearing impairment alone will not prevent their child from leading a happy, rewarding life. Information is presented to family members about the following subjects: the function of the auditory system; the causes of hearing loss; the measurement of hearing; the effect of hearing loss on child growth and development; the importance of good family communication; life as a hearing impaired child, adolescent, and adult; historical perspectives about education for hearing impaired children and local educational alternatives; differences in educational methodology; and the legal rights of the hearing impaired child. Parents are strongly urged to enroll themselves and their child in programs with expertise in educating hearing impaired children and which provide a wide variety of ancillary services.

Clinicians must be aware of the considerable influence that their factual statements and opinions have on not only the families of hearing impaired children but also on professionals and others within the community. The child's linguistic, intellectual, and emotional development must be monitored carefully to detect and solve problems. When necessary, advocacy on behalf of the child will be essential to ensure the availability and funding of services essential for hearing impaired children to learn strategies that will enable them to reach their full potential in life.

ANNOTATED BIBLIOGRAPHY

Catlin FI: Prevention of hearing impairment from infection and ototoxic drugs. Arch Otolaryngol 11:377–384, 1985 (Review of literature related to the varied causes and the prevention of acquired forms of sensorineural hearing loss.)

David LE, Johnsson LG: Viral infections of the inner ear: Clinical virologic and pathologic studies in humans and animals. Am J Otolaryngol 4:347–362, 1983 (Review article about viral-induced acquired forms of sensorineural hearing loss.)

Freeman RD, Carbin CF, Boese RJ: Can't Your Child Hear: A guide for those who care about deaf children. Baltimore, University Park Press, 1981 (Excellent book that summarizes the current body of opinion and fact about the causes and consequences of deafness. Primarily written for parents of hearing impaired children, it is of equal value for professionals beginning to learn about deafness.)

Healy GB, Friedman JM, Strong MS: Vestibular and auditory findings of perilymphatic fistula: A review of 40 cases. Trans Am Acad Ophthalmol Otolaryngol 76:1444–1450, 1972 (Long-term study of patients with hearing losses due to leakage of perilymphatic fluid.)

Konigsmark BW, Gorlin RJ: Genetic and Metabolic Deafness. Philadelphia, WB Saunders, 1976 (Encyclopedic review of syndromic constellations that include hearing loss.)

Nadol JB: Hearing loss as a sequela of meningitis. Laryngoscope 88:739–755, 1978 (Retrospective study of 547 meningitis cases comparing the hearing losses associated with bacterial vs viral meningitis.)

Proctor CA, Proctor B: Understanding hereditary nerve deafness. Arch Otolaryngol 85:23–40, 1967 (Compendium of the known hereditary syndromes associated with hearing impairment organized according to mode of inheritance.)

Schuknecht HF: Pathology of the Ear. Cambridge, MA, Harvard University Press, 1974 (Classic treatise describing the pathophysiology of otologic disease.)

84
Epistaxis
ELLEN M. FRIEDMAN

Nosebleeds, or epistaxis, are relatively common occurrences in the pediatric population. These episodes are usually infrequent, mild, and self-limited. Nevertheless, epistaxis may be quite frightening and, at times, even life-threatening. The highly vascular nasal septum and nasopharynx lend themselves to difficulty with bleeding. The fragile nasal mucosa lacks surrounding tissue to aid in compression, which may result in persistent and recurrent bleeding.

PATHOPHYSIOLOGY AND CLINICAL PRESENTATION

Epistaxis should be divided into anterior and posterior nosebleeds. Ninety percent of epistaxis in children is anterior in origin. This is fortunate because anterior nosebleeds are generally less severe and more easily controlled.

Anterior nosebleeds originate in Little's area or Hesselbach's triangle. This highly vascular area is a rich congregation of terminal blood vessels of the anterior ethmoidal artery. The hallmark of anterior epistaxis is that the blood will exit almost exclusively from the anterior nares.

Posterior epistaxis is usually more brisk and severe. Vigorous bleeding may occur, usually from a branch of the sphenopalatine artery. Most of the bleeding will be in the nasopharynx and mouth. Blood may also exit from the nares.

DIFFERENTIAL DIAGNOSIS

The most common etiology for epistaxis in childhood is trauma and inflammation. The nose is an accessible target for external trauma and the nasal mucosa is highly susceptible to the effects of nose-picking and sneezing. Inflammation from rhinitis can lead to erosion of the tiny blood vessels, and the drying effect of inspiration can further inhibit mucosal healing.

Other etiologies for epistaxis in childhood are far less common. Juvenile angiofibroma is a benign tumor that occurs in adolescent males and commonly presents with recurrent unilateral nosebleeds. These tumors may originate in the anterior wall of the sphenoid sinus and may be visualized on intranasal examination. Other nasal and sinus neoplasms, which are even less common in the pediatric population, may also be associated with epistaxis.

Intranasal foreign bodies commonly present with unilateral, foul-smelling, purulent nasal drainage. Epistaxis may occur if the foreign body has developed surrounding friable granulation tissue.

Familial hereditary telangiectasia, Osler–Weber–Rendu, is a disease with several areas of confluence of dilated arterials, venials, and capillaries. The nasal and oral mucosa are most frequently involved, although the entire gastrointestinal tract may have lesions.

Systemic disease may also have associated episodes of epistaxis. Leukemias, anemias, hepatic failure, and hypertension may result in nosebleeds. Coagulation defects are responsible for only approximately 5% of epistaxis.

WORK-UP

It is estimated that 10% of the population experience a significant nosebleed. It is helpful to bear in mind that most cases of pediatric epistaxis are readily controllable at home or by the primary health care provider. Since most cases are due to local trauma or inflammation, an extensive work-up should be reserved for those cases that are recurrent or particularly severe.

Early assessment of the severity of the blood loss is necessary. Vital signs and blood parameters, for example, a coagulation profile, should be obtained. A brief family history concerning easy bruisability and coagulopathy should be elicited. In general, it is best to control the nasal hemorrhage prior to initiating an extensive search for the underlying etiology.

If, due to the severity of blood loss or recurrent nature of the problem, an etiology other than local trauma is suspected, other tests should be performed. Specialized tests, such as computed tomographic scanning will be helpful if an intranasal tumor is suspected. If a primary coagulopathy is suspected, screening blood tests should include hematocrit, hemoglobin, PT, PTT, platelet count, and bleeding time.

TREATMENT

Many pediatric patients with epistaxis can be treated at home. The application of pressure to the anterior nasal septum will frequently result in clot formation. Vasoconstriction through topical drops (e.g., Neo-Synephrine) should be suggested. An ice pack placed around the neck or an ice cube under the lips may also aid with vasoconstriction. The treatment of a patient with severe or recurrent epistaxis will require a clinic visit. The hemorrhage may be controlled by (1) local cauterizing agents; (2) packing the nose/nasopharynx; and (3) arterial ligation.

In order to select the appropriate management, it is essential to determine if the bleeding is anterior or posterior. A nasal examination with good illumination and point suction is necessary to locate the bleeding vessels. In this manner, blood and secretions can be removed in order to completely visualize the nasal mucosa and septum.

Frequently, topical vasoconstriction, in conjunction with local pressure in Little's area, will control mild bleeding. If dilated blood vessels are easily visualized, silver nitrate cauterization may be necessary. The application of the silver nitrate stick to the dry, dilated vessels will result in the destruction and coagulation of the vessel. Although this procedure causes a stinging sensation, most children can tolerate this procedure with a preliminary explanation. Electrocoagulation should be limited in the pediatric population due to the possibility of

significant injury (e.g., septal perforation) to the mucosa or septum.

If cauterization and pressure do not control the epistaxis, anterior nasal packing is indicated. Various materials may be used. Dissolvable topical agents, such as gelfoam, topical thrombin, or microfibrillar collagen, may be applied to abraded or oozing areas (one's choice of agent is based on the ease of application). This type of packing is most successful when placed on a relatively dry field and direct pressure is immediately applied. If a prolonged compression packing is indicated, 1" Vaseline gauze strips may be positioned. It is preferable to use antibiotic-impregnated strips of gauze in order to avoid associated infection from a blocked sinus ostia. Inflatable balloon-type packs have been used in adults; however, they are of limited use in pediatrics. Compression packs should remain in position for approximately 3 days. Patients are usually placed on oral antibiotics while compression packs are in position in order to avoid sinusitis.

It is helpful to instruct the patient and family about local measures that may decrease the likelihood of further episodes of epistaxis. A bedside humidifier, the local application of petroleum jelly to the nares for lubrication, and the reduction of nasal trauma will enhance the healing of the nasal mucosa. If bacterial rhinitis is associated with the local irritation, oral antibiotics for 5 to 7 days may be indicated.

INDICATIONS FOR REFERRAL

Posterior epistaxis is more difficult to control. Cauterization and anterior nasal packing will not be useful. Compression packs positioned in the posterior nasopharynx and anterior nasal cavity are necessary. Considerable skill is required to place a posterior pack and, in a pediatric patient, sedation or general anesthesia may be indicated (see Bluestone et al, 1967 for technique). Initially, one should use a topical vasoconstrictor in the anterior nasal chamber. A soft catheter should be passed through the nostril into the mouth. A specially designed pack should be used. The antibiotic-impregnated posterior nasal pack should be tied to the catheter with the first string. The second string from the packing will be secured to the outside of the cheek at the end of the procedure and used for the eventual removal of the pack perorally. Withdrawing the catheter from the nose, the pack should be tightly positioned into the nasopharynx. While tensing the string attached to the posterior pack, an anterior nasal packing of Vaseline gauze should be placed.

In this manner, the posterior pack will be secured and appropriate pressure will be delivered to the nasopharynx. The anterior string exiting from the nose should be tied to a dental roll anterior to the columella. Patients with posterior packs require hospitalization and antibiotic therapy.

Although posterior packs in children have not been known to cause significant carbon dioxide retention, reports of respiratory depression associated with these packs in adults have caused concern. Frequent monitoring of vital signs should be performed. Daily hematocrit and hemoglobin is indicated to assure hematologic stability. If bleeding continues following the position of a posterior pack, surgical intervention may be necessary. Ligation of the internal maxillary artery may be achieved by the transantral approach.

With severe recurrent epistaxis, as associated with Osler–Weber–Rendu or hereditary hemorrhagic telangiectasia, other surgical procedures may be indicated. Septal dermoplasty may relieve the recurrent epistaxis, although GI bleeding and bleeding from the mouth may continue to be a significant problem in this disease.

If an intranasal foreign body is identified, it may be removed in the office setting by an otolaryngologist. Patient cooperation is important in order that removal will proceed smoothly and will not result in further impaction of the object or aspiration of the foreign body. General anesthesia is occasionally indicated. A referral to a pediatric otolaryngologist should also be made if an intranasal tumor is suspected. In certain settings a hematologic work-up, as well as subsequent management, may best be handled by a pediatric hematologist.

ANNOTATED BIBLIOGRAPHY

Bluestone CD, Smith HC: Intranasal Freezing for Severe Epistaxis. Arch Otolaryngol 85:445, 1967 (Excellent description of the technique of inserting nasal packing.)

Montgomery WW: Surgery of the Upper Respiratory System. Philadelphia, Lea & Febiger, 1973 (Excellent discussion concerning the anatomic and surgical considerations in epistaxis.)

85
Sinusitis
ELLEN R. WALD

Acute (<30 days duration) infections of the paranasal sinuses are seen in children and adults usually as a complication of viral upper respiratory tract infections or allergic inflammation. Chronic (at least 30 days duration) sinusitis results when the symptoms of acute sinusitis are not recognized as such, or when they are inadequately treated. Although there are few data on which to base an estimate of the frequency of these disorders, acute sinusitis is commonly encountered in clinical practice and chronic sinusitis is not rare.

ANATOMY AND PATHOPHYSIOLOGY

The anatomic relationships of the sinus cavities are shown in Figure 85-1. Three shelf-like structures, the superior, middle, and inferior turbinates, protrude from the lateral nasal wall. Beneath each turbinate is a corresponding meatus. The ostia of the maxillary, frontal, and anterior ethmoid sinuses drain into the middle meatus. The ostia of the sphenoid sinuses and the posterior ethmoid air cells drain into the superior meatus. Only the lacrimal duct empties into the inferior meatus.

The maxillary sinus develops as a lateral outpouching of the nasal cavity. As the child grows the maxillary sinus enlarges in width and height and eventually assumes a quadrilateral shape. The position of the maxillary ostium in relation to the body of the sinus is notable. The location of this outflow tract, high on the medial wall of the maxillary sinus, impedes gravitational drainage of secretions; ciliary activity is required to move secretions from the body of the maxillary sinus through the ostia to the nose. Secretions are carried from there into the nasopharynx to be either expectorated or swallowed.

The ethmoid sinuses, as seen on the coronal and sagittal sections (Fig. 85-1 A, B) are not single large cavities but are divided into 3 to 15 air cells. These air cells, separated from each other by thin bony septa, drain by individual ostia into the middle meatus. The lateral wall by the ethmoid sinus, the lamina papyracea, is a paper-thin plate of bone that may permit the direct extension of infection from the ethmoid sinus to the orbit through natural dehiscences in the bone.

The frontal sinus, seen on a sagittal section Figure 85-1B), develops either from an anterior eth-

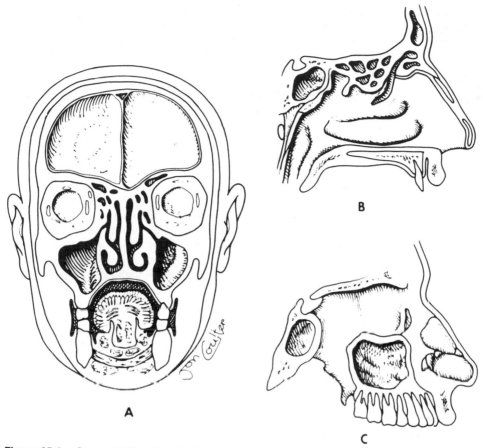

Figure 85-1. Coronal (*A*) and sagittal sections (*B* and *C*) of the nose and paranasal sinuses.

moid cell or from a separate evagination of the an-
terosuperior portion of the middle meatus. In either
case, its drainage is similar to that of the anterior
ethmoid sinuses. The sphenoid sinuses, which are
immediately anterior to the pituitary fossa, are adjacent to the posterior ethmoid air cells and drain
into the superior meatus.

The maxillary sinus is the principal site of disease in most cases of sinus infection in children.
The anatomy of the draining ostia probably accounts for its frequent involvement. In most of these
patients, the ethmoid air cells are also involved. The
drainage of the ethmoid, frontal, and sphenoid sinuses is aided by gravity; on the other hand, the narrow ostia of the ethmoid sinuses are easily obstructed by mucosal swelling, thus predisposing
them to infection. After the age of 10 years, the
frontal sinus assumes greater clinical importance
because it becomes a more common site of sinus
infection and may serve as a focus for rare but se-

rious intracranial complications. Isolated infection
of the sphenoid sinuses is uncommon; however,
these sinuses may be involved in cases of pansinusitis.

The predominant organisms of acute sinusitis
include *Streptococcus pneumoniae*, *Branhamella
catarrhalis*, and *Hemophilus influenzae*. Both *H.
influenzae* and *B. catarrhalis* may be β-lactamase-
producing and consequently ampicillin-resistant.
Staphylococcus aureus has not been isolated from
a child with acute sinusitis; anaerobic flora are also
uncommon in acute infection. Several viruses including adenovirus and parainfluenza have been recovered.

The microbiology of chronic sinusitis has been
studied less thoroughly than that of acute sinusitis.
Anaerobic bacteria appear to be the predominant
pathogens in most studies. The predominant anaerobic organisms are *Bacteroides* species, anaerobic Gram-positive cocci, *Veillonella* and *Fuso-*

bacterium species. The common aerobic organisms isolated include *Streptococcus viridans* and *H. influenzae*. *S. aureus* has occasionally been isolated.

CLINICAL PRESENTATION

Commonly recognized symptoms of sinusitis in adults and adolescents are facial pain, headache, and fever. However, children with acute sinusitis frequently have complaints that are less specific. During the course of apparent viral upper respiratory infections, there are two common clinical developments that should alert the clinician to the possibility of bacterial infection of the paranasal sinuses. The first, less common presentation is a "cold" that seems more severe than usual: the fever is high (>39.0°C), the nasal discharge is purulent and copious and there may be associated periorbital swelling and facial pain. The periorbital swelling is gradual in onset and is most obvious in the early morning shortly after awakening. The swelling may decrease and actually disappear during the day, only to reappear once again the following day. A less common complaint is headache (a feeling of fullness or a dull ache either behind or above the eyes), most often reported in children over 5 years of age. Occasionally there may be dental pain, either from infection originating in the teeth or referred from the sinus infection.

The second, more common clinical situation in which sinusitis should be suspected is when the signs and symptoms of a "cold" are protracted. Nasal discharge or daytime cough or both that continue beyond 10, but less than 30, days and are not improving are the principal complaints. Most uncomplicated viral upper respiratory infections last 5 to 7 days; although patients may not be asymptomatic by the tenth day they have usually improved. The persistence of respiratory symptoms beyond the 10-day mark, without appreciable improvement, suggests a complication of the upper respiratory infection. The nasal discharge may be of any quality (thin or thick; clear, mucoid, or purulent) and the cough (which may be dry or wet) must be present in the daytime, although it is often noted to be worse at night. A cough occurring only at night is a common residual symptom of an upper respiratory infection. When it is the only residual symptom, it is nonspecific and does not suggest a sinus infection. On the other hand, the persistence of a daytime cough is frequently the symptom that prompts medical attention. The patient may not appear very ill, and if fever is present it will usually be low grade. Fetid breath is often reported by par-

ents of preschoolers. Facial pain is not usually a prominent complaint; however, intermittent painless morning periorbital swelling may have been noted. In this case it is not the severity of the clinical symptoms but their persistence that calls for attention.

Chronic sinusitis should be suspected when there are protracted respiratory symptoms—nasal discharge, nasal congestion, or cough that has lasted for more than 30 days. Although the nasal discharge is most often purulent, it may be thin and clear. Once again, the cough should be present during the daytime, although it is usually reported to be worse at night. The patient may complain additionally of facial pain, headache, or malaise. However, unless these less specific complaints are accompanied by respiratory symptoms, they should not be attributed to sinus infection. Fever is less prominent and is found less frequently than in acute sinusitis.

DIFFERENTIAL DIAGNOSIS

The major differential considerations are uncomplicated upper respiratory infection or allergic inflammation. The former is discriminated from sinusitis by the severity or duration of symptoms. Allergic inflammation, which may give rise to nasal discharge or cough or both (and may be complicated by a secondary bacterial infection), may be suspected on the basis of family or personal history of atopy. A physical examination may demonstrate the stigmata of allergic inflammation with Denny's lines, an allergic nasal crease, and pale edematous nasal mucosa. In uncomplicated allergic rhinitis or in bronchospasm (manifested as cough) triggered by upper respiratory infection, the sinus radiographs will be normal.

WORK-UP

History

The important elements that should be included in the history are the duration and severity of respiratory complaints, the quality of nasal discharge, and the determination of frequency and timing of cough. In addition, an inquiry should be made regarding the presence or absence of malodorous breath (despite good oral hygiene), morning headaches that subside during the daytime if the patient is erect, puffiness about the eyes, dental discomfort, and an allergic history (*e.g.*, asthma, seasonal rhinitis, conjunctivitis, or eczema).

Physical Examination

The important elements of the physical examination include an assessment of the nasal mucosa, nasal septum, tonsillar and pharyngeal areas, cervical lymph nodes, and an inspection of the face for localized swelling. Intranasal instillation of a topical decongestant may shrink the nasal mucosa and permit visualization of purulent material coming from the middle meatus. This is a most helpful clinical observation.

Transillumination may be helpful in diagnosing inflammation of the maxillary or frontal sinuses. The patient and examiner must be in a darkened room. The light source, shielded from the observer, is placed over the midpoint of the inferior orbital rim. The transmission of light through the hard plate is then assessed with the patient's mouth open. In judging light transmission, light passing through the alveolar ridges should be excluded. Transillumination of the frontal sinus is accomplished by placing a high intensity light source inferior to the medial border of the supraorbital ridge and evaluating the symmetry of the blush bilaterally. Transillumination is useful in adolescents and adults if light transmission is either normal or absent. "Reduced" transmission or "dull" transillumination are assessments that correlate poorly with results of sinus aspiration. The increased thickness of both the soft tissue and bony vault in children less than 10 years of age limits the clinical usefulness of transillumination in the younger age group.

Laboratory Tests

Radiography. Radiography has been used traditionally to determine the presence or absence of sinus disease. Standard radiographic projections include an anteroposterior, a lateral, and an occipitomental view. The anteroposterior view is optimal for evaluation of the ethmoid sinuses and the lateral view is best for the frontal and sphenoid sinuses. The occipitomental view, taken after tilting the chin upward 45° to the horizontal, allows an evaluation of the maxillary sinuses. Although much has been written about the frequency of abnormal sinus radiographs in "normal" children, these studies have been flawed either by inattention to the presence of symptoms and signs of respiratory inflammation or by failure to classify abnormal radiographic findings into major (significant) and minor (insignificant) categories. One report shows, however, that significantly abnormal maxillary sinus radiographs are infrequent in children beyond their first birthday, who are without recent symptoms and signs of respiratory tract inflammation.

The radiographic findings most diagnostic of bacterial sinusitis are the presence of an air-fluid level in, or complete opacification of, the sinus cavities. An air-fluid level, however, is an uncommon radiographic finding in children less than 5 years of age with acute sinusitis. In the absence of an air-fluid level or complete opacification of the sinuses, measuring the degree of mucosal swelling may be useful. If the width of the sinus mucous membrane is 5 mm or greater in adults or 4 mm or greater in children, it is likely that the sinus will contain pus or will yield a positive bacterial culture. When clinical signs and symptoms suggesting acute sinusitis are accompanied by abnormal maxillary sinus radiographs, bacteria will be present in a sinus aspirate 75% of the time. A normal radiograph suggests, but does not prove, that a sinus is free of disease.

Sinus Aspiration. Although by no means a routine procedure, aspiration of the maxillary sinus (the most accessible of the sinuses) can be accomplished easily in an outpatient setting with minimal discomfort to the patient. The puncture is best performed by the transnasal route with the needle directed beneath the inferior turbinate through the lateral nasal wall. This route for aspiration is preferred in order to avoid injury to the natural ostium and permanent dentition. In adults, an anterior approach to the maxillary sinus is a Caldwell–Luc antrotomy. If the patient is unusually apprehensive or too young to cooperate, a short-acting narcotic agent can be used for sedation. This procedure is indicated when the infection fails to respond to the usual medical therapy or when the patient presents with intracranial or intraorbital complications of sinus infection.

Surface Cultures. It would be desirable to culture the nose, throat, or nasopharynx in patients with acute sinusitis if the predominant flora isolated from these surface cultures were predictive of the bacterial species recovered from the sinus secretions. Unfortunately, the results of surface cultures have no predictive value; therefore, these cultures cannot be recommended as a guide to the bacteriology and therapy of acute or chronic sinusitis.

TREATMENT

Antimicrobials

Medical therapy with an antimicrobial agent is recommended in patients diagnosed to have acute maxillary sinusitis. The relative frequency of the various bacterial agents suggest that amoxicillin (40 mg/kg/day, orally, in three divided doses) is an appropriate agent. Amoxicillin is usually prescribed to a maximum dose of 500 mg or 750 mg three times a day. The prevalence of β-lactamase-positive, ampicillin-resistant *H. influenzae* and *B. catarrhalis* may vary geographically. In areas where ampicillin-resistant organisms are prevalent or when the patient is allergic to penicillin or when there has been an apparent antibiotic failure, several alternative regimens are available. The combination agent sulfamethoxazole-trimethoprim (8 and 40 mg/kg/day, respectively, orally, divided into two doses) has been shown to be efficacious in acute maxillary sinusitis in adults. It is important to remember, however, that this agent may be ineffective in patients with group A streptococcal infections. Cefaclor (40 mg/kg/day, orally, in three divided doses to a maximum dose of 500 mg or 750 mg three times daily) or the combination of erythromycin-sulfisoxazole (50 and 150 mg/kg/day, orally, in four divided doses) is also suitable. Augmentin, a combination of amoxicillin and potassium clavulanate, is another potential therapeutic agent for use in patients with β-lactamase-producing bacterial species in their maxillary sinus secretions. Potassium clavulanate irreversibly binds the β-lactamase, if present, and thereby restores amoxicillin to its original spectrum of activity. Augmentin is prescribed in the same dose as amoxicillin.

Clinical improvement is prompt in almost all patients treated with an appropriate antimicrobial agent. Patients febrile at the initial encounter will become afebrile, and there is a remarkable reduction of nasal discharge and cough within 48 hours. If the patient does not improve or worsens in 48 hours, a clinical re-evaluation is appropriate. If the diagnosis is unchanged, a sinus aspiration may be considered for precise bacteriologic information. Alternatively, an antimicrobial agent should be prescribed that is effective for β-lactamase-producing bacterial species.

The antimicrobial regimens recommended to treat acute sinusitis are similar (in type and duration) to those used to treat acute otitis media. The usual duration of antimicrobial therapy is 10 to 14 days. When the patient is improved but not completely recovered by 10 or 14 days, it seems reasonable to extend the duration of the antimicrobial agent for another week.

When treating patients with chronic sinusitis, the duration of antimicrobial therapy should be 3 to 4 weeks. Most anaerobes isolated from patients with chronic sinusitis have been penicillin-sensitive. All *S. viridans* and most *H. influenzae* will be susceptible to amoxicillin. However, there is the potential for the anaerobes or *H. influenzae* to be β-lactamase producing and thereby amoxicillin-resistant. The list of appropriate antimicrobial agents for chronic sinusitis is the same as for acute sinusitis, unless the patient has already failed to respond to a particular regimen. Amoxicillin at 40 mg/kg/days, orally, in three divided doses is a reasonable choice; if the patient does not improve, an alternative antimicrobial should be selected or surgery should be considered.

Decongestants or Antihistamines

The effectiveness of antihistamines or decongestants or combination antihistamine–decongestants applied topically (by inhalation) or administered by mouth in patients with acute or chronic sinus infection has not been adequately studied.

Irrigation and Drainage

Irrigation and drainage of the infected sinus may result in dramatic relief from pain for patients with acute sinusitis. In addition, by relieving pressure in the sinus, oxygenation and blood flow improve, thus restoring compromised defense mechanisms. Drainage procedures are reserved usually for those who fail medical therapy with antimicrobials or who have a suppurative intraorbital or intracranial complication. If an episode of acute or chronic sinusitis cannot be effectively treated by medical therapy alone or medical therapy and simple sinus puncture, more radical surgery may become necessary.

INDICATIONS FOR REFERRAL AND ADMISSION

Complications of sinus disease may cause both substantial morbidity and occasional mortality. Major complications result either from the contiguous spread or from the hematogenous dissemination of infection and result in intraorbital or intracranial suppuration, either of which requires hospital admission and consultation with neurosurgeons, ophthalmologists, and infectious disease experts.

In office practice the only complication that will commonly be seen is preseptal cellulitis or, more properly, inflammatory edema. This is not an actual infection of the orbit but rather soft tissue swelling of the periorbital area caused by impedence of the local venous drainage. As such, it is a warning of a potentially serious infection within the sinus. Inflammatory edema about the eye is always associated with an ipsilateral ethmoid sinusitis. There is usually an ipsilateral maxillary sinusitis and also often a contralateral sinus infection. Frequently, there is a history of intermittent periorbital swelling, which is worse in the morning and improves during the day. The swelling is soft, nontender, and without induration but there may be prominent erythema. An examination of the globe shows no displacement and full extraocular movements. This latter finding assures the examiner that there is no orbital involvement. The management of these children must be individualized. Those children who have minimal eye swelling and minimal constitutional signs can be managed cautiously as outpatients. If a child has a high fever, or the periorbital swelling has resulted in more than 50% closure of the eye, hospital admission and parenteral antimicrobials are a reasonable treatment decision.

The youngster who presents with an involvement of the frontal sinus must be followed carefully when treatment is undertaken with oral antimicrobials on an ambulatory basis. Infection of this sinus cavity may lead to intracranial, intraorbital, or osseous complications.

ANNOTATED BIBLIOGRAPHY

Brook I: Bacteriologic features of chronic sinusitis in children. JAMA 246:967–970, 1981 (One of the few studies in children on this subject.)

Kovatch AL, Wald ER, Ledesma–Medina J: Maxillary sinus radiographs in children with nonrespiratory complaints. Pediatrics 73:306–308, 1984 (Study showing that children over 1 year of age without recent respiratory symptoms or current signs of respiratory inflammation infrequently have abnormal maxillary sinus radiographs.)

Rachelefsky G, Katz RM, Siegel SC: Diseases of paranasal sinuses in children. Curr Probl Pediatr 12:1–57, 1982 (Comprehensive review of many aspects of paranasal sinus inflammation.)

Wald ER, Chiponis D, Ledesma–Medina J: Comparative effectiveness of amoxicillin and amoxicillin-clavulanate potassium in acute paranasal sinus infections in children: A double-blind, placebo-controlled trial. Pediatrics 77:795–800, 1986 (Study showing that children with acute sinusitis treated with antimicrobials recover earlier and more often than children on placebo.)

Wald ER, Milmoe GJ, Bowen A'd et al: Acute maxillary sinusitis in children. N Engl J Med 304:749–754, 1981 (Describes the bacteriology of acute sinusitis in children as learned from maxillary sinus aspirates.)

Wald ER, Pang D, Milmoe GJ et al: Sinusitis and its complications in the pediatric patient. Pediatr Clin North Am 28:777–796, 1981 (Detailed discussion of the serious intraorbital, intracranial, and osseous complications of sinus infection.)

86
Sore Throat
L. GERARD NIEDERMAN

A sore throat is among the most common complaints seen by the pediatric practitioner, yet its optimal management is both controversial and evolving. Most of the debate focuses around the group A β-hemolytic streptococcus (GABHS). The demonstration that penicillin treatment of GABHS pharyngitis prevents rheumatic fever has been the basis for widespread diagnostic use of the throat culture for confirming GABHS tonsillitis, and guiding treatment. There has, however, been a remarkable decline in the incidence of rheumatic fever in the past 20 years. New data also suggest that early antibiotic treatment shortens the symptomatic course of streptococcal pharyngitis, which is an important issue when considering the societal cost (days lost from school and parental days lost from work) of sore throats. These considerations, as well as the increasing availability of rapid, though less perfect, diagnostic tests for GABHS have provoked a re-evaluation of the "culture and treat, depending on culture results" approach. The practitioner's task of providing a prompt, accurate diagnosis and treatment for GABHS pharyngitis, while avoiding unnecessary laboratory tests and unnecessary antibiotics for most children who have sore throats from viral or other non-GABHS agents, is both complex and challenging.

PATHOPHYSIOLOGY AND CLINICAL PRESENTATION

Pharyngitis occurs more often in the colder months similar to the seasonal pattern of other upper respiratory infections. The age-specific incidence peaks between 5 and 8 years of age; person-to-person spread of infection in schools is an important source of transmission. Tonsillar tissue increases in size during the years when acute nasopharyngeal infections are most common. It reaches maximum size between 8 and 12 years of age and then involutes during adolescence. The temporal association between tonsillitis and tonsillar hypertrophy was primarily responsible for the widespread practice of performing tonsillectomies on school-aged children.

Bacterial Pharyngitis

GABHS is responsible for about 15% of acute tonsillitis and pharyngitis. Its onset is usually acute and characterized by a sore throat (often with dysphagia), fever (often above 38.5°C), pharyngeal and tonsillar erythema, and tonsillar exudate. Anterior cervical lymph nodes, particularly the jugular-digastric nodes just beneath the angle of the mandible, are tender and enlarged. If present, the erythematous "sandpaper" rash of scarlet fever, Pastia's lines (petechiae in the flexor skin creases of joints), and an enanthem of "doughnut" lesions on the soft palate greatly enhance the likelihood of streptococcal disease. A history of streptococcal exposure also supports this diagnosis. Headache, abdominal pain, and vomiting are common with GABHS, whereas other upper respiratory symptoms such as cough, rhinorrhea, and conjunctivitis, reduce the probability of streptococcal disease. If left untreated, streptococcal pharyngitis usually resolves in 5 to 7 days, although suppurative complications such as otitis media, lymphadenitis, and peritonsillar abscess may occur.

Acute rheumatic fever (ARF) is currently a rare complication of untreated GABHS infections, although recent (*i.e.*, mid-1980s) reports indicate that it is on the rise. An attack rate of 3% was found in untreated military recruits during the 1940s. In the 1950s an attack rate of 0.4% was documented in untreated children. Even with many undiagnosed and untreated streptococcal infections, the annual incidence of ARF is below 0.5 cases per 100,000 population, making it a disease that many primary care practitioners will never diagnose.

Groups C and G β-hemolytic streptococci have also been isolated from children with symptomatic pharyngitis and have, on rare occasions, been implicated in the development of acute glomerulonephritis. Their epidemiologic and clinical importance as an endemic cause of pharyngitis is unclear.

Fusobacteria and spirochetes cause Vincent's angina, which is characterized by friable, ulcerating tonsillitis with a pseudomembranous exudate. Gingival lesions are frequently present.

Tonsillar or pharyngeal diphtheria, due to *Corynobacteria diphtheria*, is rare in an adequately immunized child. It is characterized by a gray adherent membranous exudate that bleeds when removed. A careful history of immunizations and a high index of suspicion are needed to consider this diagnosis. Gonococcal pharyngitis, seen in sexually active adolescents and sexually abused children, may present with acute inflammatory, exudative tonsillopharyngitis or with chronic sore throat.

Viral Pharyngitis

A sore throat is a common complaint with viral upper respiratory infections, and often there are no clinical features distinguishing the specific etiologic viral agent (see Chap. 159). The associated symptoms of cough and rhinorrhea strongly implicate a viral etiology, particularly in the child who is old enough to complain of a sore throat.

Adenoviruses are a frequent cause of exudative pharyngitis, especially in the child under 3 years old. Fever, nasal discharge, congestion, and cough are common; laryngobronchitis and pneumonia may occur. The duration of symptoms averages 5 to 7 days. Epidemic adenovirus pharyngitis is usually a winter/spring disease. Pharyngoconjunctival fever, also due to adenovirus, is characterized by a high fever, bulbar and palpebral conjunctivitis, and tonsillitis often with exudate. It is usually epidemic during the summer and is often associated with transmission in swimming pools.

Herpangina due to Coxsackie and ECHO viruses is an acute illness, often with temperature to 39°C or higher. There may be headache, malaise, as well as sore throat and dysphagia. The typical oral lesions are small vesicles or ulcers on the anterior tonsillar pillars and soft palate, though they may be on the tonsils, pharynx, or posterior buccal mucosa. Hand, foot, and mouth syndrome (due to Coxsackie A16) is characterized by oral ulcerative lesions often on the tongue and buccal mucosa, though not infrequently on the palate and anterior pillars of the tonsils. The vesicular and papulovesicular lesions on the dorsum and intraphalangeal areas of the hands and feet, and occasionally on the buttocks, allow a clinical diagnosis of this syndrome. Both herpangina and hand, foot, and mouth syndrome occur in the summer and early fall.

Infectious mononucleosis caused by Epstein–Barr virus may present with pharyngitis, with or without exudative tonsillitis. A fever is common, although a child rarely appears toxic. Cervical or generalized lymphadenopathy, palatal petechiae, splenomegaly, and edema of the eyelids support the clinical diagnosis of mononucleosis. A macular erythematous rash may be present, and if ampicillin is inadvertently administered, the rash may occur more frequently and be more prominent. Other viral causes of pharyngitis include herpes simplex, parainfluenza, and influenza viruses; the latter two occur more commonly during the winter.

Other Agents

Mycoplasma pneumoniae can cause pharyngitis that is clinically indistinguishable from streptococcal disease. It is uncommon in younger children, but it may account for up to 10% of pharyngitis seen in adolescents. The significance of *Chlamydia trachomatis* as a cause of pharyngitis is unclear. Candida may also cause pharyngitis accompanied by a sore throat.

DIFFERENTIAL DIAGNOSIS

A sore throat may be the presenting symptom of peritonsillar or retropharyngeal abscesses. Anaerobic bacteria, most commonly the *Bacteroides* species, peptostreptococci and fusobacteria, and also group A streptococci, *Staphylococcus aureus*, and *Hemophilus influenzae* are the most frequent organisms isolated from these abscesses. Peritonsillar abscesses are more common in older children and adolescents and usually follow an episode of tonsillitis. Sore throat, fever, dysphagia, odynophagia, and trismus are frequent complaints. The oropharynx may be difficult to examine in the child with trismus. The tonsil on the affected side is usually displaced medially. There may be edema and erythema of the soft palate contiguous to the tonsil, and fluctuance may be palpable. The tonsil itself may be without significant inflammation or exudate. Tender, anterior cervical adenopathy is present.

Retropharyngeal abscesses occur more commonly in young children. Fever, refusal to swallow, drooling, and the development of stridor are due to the abscess and its surrounding edema and cellulitis. An examination may reveal swelling of the posterior pharynx. Stiffness with flexion of the neck is common due to irritation and spasm of paravertebral muscles. Children with epiglottitis may complain of a sore throat, but the rapid onset of extreme toxicity and inspiratory stridor make confusion with uncomplicated tonsillopharyngitis unlikely (see Chap. 163).

Trauma from penetrating injuries, thermal injury, chemical injury from a caustic ingestion, foreign body, irritation from dryness and coughing, and uncommonly thyroiditis may also present with a sore throat. The rash, mucositis, and toxicity of Kawasaki's disease may be confused with scarlet fever.

WORK-UP

History

When considering the management of a child with suspected GABHS pharyngitis, important history includes streptococcal exposure at home or at school, previous rheumatic fever, and the occurrence of a community outbreak of rheumatic fever or poststreptococcal glomerulonephritis. A history of inadequate immunizations or a community outbreak of diphtheria may suggest that diagnosis. Orogenital sexual contact or sexual abuse should raise the possibility of gonococcal pharyngitis. Symptoms of cough or rhinorrhea suggest viral pharyngitis. A history of significant dysphagia or odynophagia, drooling, or an inability to open one's mouth should alert the physician to the possibility of peritonsillar or retropharyngeal abscess formation, or the possibility of epiglottitis.

Physical Examination

The physical signs of the common bacterial and viral etiologies of sore throats have been discussed above. Signs that strongly suggest GABHS are a scarletiniform rash, Pastia's lines, and a soft palate enanthem. Findings of tonsillar and pharyngeal erythema, tonsillar exudates, and anterior cervical adenitis are frequently present with GABHS tonsillitis, but may be seen with mononucleosis, adenovirus, mycoplasma, and other non-GABHS causes of pharyngitis. Ulcerative or vesicular oral lesions, conjunctivitis, or rhinitis suggest viral pharyngitis.

Trismus and displacement of the tonsil and adjacent soft palate, sometimes with palpable fluctuance, are characteristic of a peritonsillar abscess. Airway stridor, stiffness of the neck, and a visible posterior pharyngeal mass suggest a retropharyngeal abscess. Stridor, drooling, and fever in a toxic-appearing young child suggest epiglottitis.

Laboratory Tests

The diagnosis of streptococcal pharyngitis is confirmed by throat culture. Although considered the "gold standard," it is known to have up to 10% false negatives (usually the result of improper collection or transportation of the specimen) and also up to 50% false positives (carriers of streptococci who are not truly infected). The occurrence of false positive throat cultures will depend on the prevalence of streptococcal carriers, which has been shown to vary greatly among school-aged children, and also on the selection of children to be cultured. Despite these shortcomings, for children with clinical findings suspicious of GABHS or for children at increased risk for rheumatic fever, the throat culture is the most accurate test to confirm GABHS.

Office techniques for the detection of GABHS antigen from throat swabs are commercially available and offer the advantage of a rapid diagnosis and appropriate treatment while the child is still in the office. Most studies have shown high (>95%) specificity but variable sensitivity (60% to 93%). Until improvements provide a test with reliable sensitivity of at least 95%, they may be clinically useful when positive, but cultures should be performed on negative specimens.

Serology (*e.g.*, antistreptolysin O and antideoxyribonuclease B) is rarely useful in the acute management of sore throats, but may be useful for documenting recent GABHS infection when considering the diagnosis of rheumatic fever or glomerulonephritis, or when the differentiation of streptococcal carriage from infection is necessary.

Diphtheria can be confirmed with isolation of *C. diphtheriae* from the pharyngeal membrane. Fluorescent antibody techniques are available, but may be inaccurate in inexperienced laboratories. Pharyngeal gonorrhea is also confirmed by culture for *N. gonorrhoeae*. Viral cultures are not clinically useful in the management of pharyngitis, and rapid antigen detection for viral agents is currently available only in research laboratories.

A positive heterophil agglutination test when properly performed is highly diagnostic of mononucleosis. Unfortunately, the heterophil test may be negative in children under 3 years of age, and also negative early in the course of mononucleosis. The mono spot test is highly sensitive and is more rapidly performed. It may remain positive for several months, thus it may be confusing when evaluating acute or recurrent pharyngitis. More specific serologic tests to confirm EB virus infection can be performed if clinically indicated.

The complete blood count (CBC) is helpful; children with a monocytosis of greater than 40% or atypical lymphocytosis of greater than 10% should be suspected of having mononucleosis. It is also uncommon for children with GABHS pharyngitis to have a WBC under 12,500.

If a retropharyngeal abscess is suspected, a lateral roentgenogram of the neck will often reveal a posterior pharyngeal mass, sometimes with gas formation.

TREATMENT AND MANAGEMENT

Successful management of children with sore throats involves the prompt and accurate differentiation of streptococcal pharyngitis from "viral" non-strep pharyngitis. It also involves recognizing other uncommon, yet important, bacterial causes of sore throats such as diphtheria and gonorrhea, as well as recognizing the child with symptoms and signs suggesting a peritonsillar abscess, retropharyngeal abscess, or epiglottitis.

The two decisions most often faced by the practitioner managing a child with a sore throat are whether or not to obtain a culture (or rapid antigen determination) for GABHS and whether or not to begin antibiotic treatment prior to obtaining culture results. The throat culture should be used selectively when there are clinical (*e.g.*, exudate, significant erythema, adenitis, and fever) or epidemiologic (*e.g.*, exposure and epidemicity) factors to suggest streptococcal pharyngitis. As the clinical probability of GABHS increases, a positive culture is more likely to be a true positive rather than a noninfected streptococcal carrier. The decision to treat a patient with antibiotics is based on the rationale that penicillin treatment of GABHS pharyngitis prevents rheumatic fever, prevents suppurative complications, and shortens the clinical course of pharyngitis. Antibiotic treatment is indicated in the child with a past history of rheumatic fever, the toxic-appearing child, the child with clinical scarlet fever, the child with symptoms suggesting an early peritonsillar abscess, or other situations where there is a reasonably high likelihood of streptococcal disease or its sequelae. Most children presenting with sore throats will, in fact, have signs and symptoms predictive of *not* having GABHS and should not be cultured or treated. The incidence of rheumatic fever in most parts of the United States is currently so low that there *is not* justification for treating all sore throats expectantly with antibiotics.

The streptococcal carrier poses a difficult diagnostic problem. Up to 50% of children symptomatic with sore throats and culture positive for GABHS show no serologic evidence of streptococcal infection. These symptomatic carriers cannot be differentiated from true streptococcal infections by any readily available clinical tests. A second group of carriers is the asymptomatic child with a positive throat culture. Whether the carrier state poses a significant risk for subsequent rheumatic fever is unresolved. In practice, the symptomatic carrier is unrecognized and is treated with antibiotics; the asymptomatic carrier, when identified, also usually receives antibiotics. The failure rate of penicillin treatment is quite high for streptococcal carriers and, although rarely indicated, the combination of intramuscular benzathine penicillin and rifampin has been shown to be more efficacious in eradication of the spread of GABHS. Because of confusion over the carrier state, reculturing children after completing antibiotic treatment or culturing close contacts of children found with GABHS is not routinely recommended.

Recommended treatment for GABHS pharyngitis is penicillin either orally or intramuscularly. Phenoxymethyl penicillin (penicillin V) 250 mg three or four times daily (25,000 U/kg/day) for 10 days is necessary to prevent rheumatic fever, although symptomatic improvement may be complete in 24 to 72 hours. In situations where the risk of ARF is high and compliance may be questionable, intramuscular benzathine penicillin G may be preferable to oral treatment. Current recommendations for rheumatic fever prophylaxis are 600,000 units of benzathine penicillin for patients weighing under 60 lb, and 1,200,000 units for patients weighing over 60 lb. The combination of 900,000 units benzathine penicillin and 300,000 units procaine penicillin is also acceptable. Erythromycin is an effective, inexpensive alternative antibiotic for the child allergic to penicillin. The physician must weigh the relative risks of developing complications, either suppurative or nonsuppurative, following noncompliance with oral regimens against the discomfort and more serious allergic complications associated with intramuscular benzathine penicillin.

Diphtheria is treated with equine antitoxin and penicillin or erythromycin to eradicate *C. diphtheriae*. Vincent's angina is also adequately treated with penicillin.

Pharyngeal gonorrhea is treated preferably with ceftriaxone, or alternatively with the combination of either ampicillin or amoxicillin and probenecid. For children weighing more than 100 lb, ceftriaxone 250 mg can be given intramuscularly; or amoxicillin 3.0 g or ampicillin 3.5 g in combination with probenecid 1 g can be given by mouth. For children under 100 lb, ceftriaxone 125 mg intramuscularly can be given or amoxicillin 50 mg/kg with probenecid 25 mg/kg (maximum 1.0 g) (see Chap. 195). A serologic test for syphilis as well as an examination and culture for other sexually transmitted diseases is needed for the child or adolescent with oral gonorrhea. The social and psychological needs for the sexually abused child must also be addressed.

The symptoms of a sore throat can be treated with acetaminophen, lozenges, and salt water gargles alone or in combination. Many preparations of topical anethesics, such as the aqueous solution of lidocaine, are available, but their efficacy in the young child is unproven. Their use should be avoided because of systemic reactions from their absorption and allergic sensitization.

INDICATIONS FOR HOSPITALIZATION OR REFERRAL

The child with uncomplicated pharyngitis can be managed on an ambulatory basis. A child may occasionally be dehydrated or toxic-appearing and require treatment with intravenous fluids and parenteral antibiotics.

Peritonsillar abscess may complicate both GABHS and non-GABHS tonsillitis and requires immediate surgical drainage and parenteral antibiotic therapy. Tonsillectomy is usually performed several weeks after the resolution of the acute process, though some otolaryngologists prefer tonsillectomy during the acute phase. Retropharyngeal abscess is a potentially life-threatening infection, requiring hospitalization for appropriate surgical drainage and intravenous antibiotic treatment.

Recurrent tonsillitis is the most frequent and controversial reason for which tonsillectomy is performed. A small group of children do indeed have a disproportionately high incidence of throat infections, and these children will have fewer infections after tonsillectomy. Whether this warrants the risks, complications, and costs of surgery requires a decision on an individual basis. Minimally, a physician should document by examination, not by patient or parental recall, that sore throats are frequent (5 or more per year), symptomatic (fever, erythema, exudate, adenopathy), and costly (days lost from school or work, medical expenses) before considering tonsillectomy.

ANNOTATED BIBLIOGRAPHY

Breese BB, Disney FA: The accuracy of diagnosis of beta streptococcal infections on clinical grounds. J Pediatr 44:670, 1954 (In this classic study, clinical diagnosis of GABHS tonsillitis was at best 75% accurate for positive prediction and 77% accurate for predicting nonstreptococcal pharyngitis.)

Committee on Rheumatic Fever and Infective Endocarditis of the American Heart Association: Prevention of rheumatic fever. Circulation 70:1118A, 1984 (Current recommendations for rheumatic fever prophylaxis.)

Glezen WP, Clyde WA, Senior RJ et al: Group A streptococci, mycoplasmas, and viruses associated with acute pharyngitis. JAMA 202:455, 1967 (Viruses and "other agents" are the predominant etiologic agents of acute pharyngitis.)

Kaplan EL: The group A streptococcal upper respiratory tract carrier state: An enigma. J Pediatr 97:337, 1980 (The bottom line is that there is no *completely* reliable clinical method to differentiate streptococcal carriage from infection.)

Kaplan EL, Hill HR: Return of rheumatic fever: Consequences, implications and needs. J Pediatr 111:244–246, 1987 (Resurgence of ARF is discussed in this editorial; outbreaks are not isolated. See also the article in the same issue by Congeni B, Rizzo C, Congeni J et al: Outbreak of acute rheumatic fever in northeast Ohio.)

Krober MS, Bass JW, Michels GN: Streptococcal pharyngitis: Placebo-controlled double-blind evaluation of clinical response to penicillin therapy. JAMA 253:1271, 1985 (Does early treatment with penicillin favorably alter the clinical course of GABHS pharyngitis? This study says "yes.")

Land MA, Bisno AL: Acute rheumatic fever: A vanishing disease in suburbia. JAMA 249:895, 1983 (Population-based study documenting declining incidence of acute rheumatic fever.)

Pantell RH: Pharyngitis: Diagnosis and management. Pediatr Rev 3:35, 1981 (Excellent, detailed, and critical discussion of the cost and clinical effectiveness of various strategies for managing children with pharyngitis.)

Paradise JL, Bluestone CD, Bachman RZ et al: Efficacy of tonsillectomy for recurrent throat infection in severely affected children: Results of parallel randomized and nonrandomized clinical trials. N Engl J Med 310:674, 1984 (Important data that quantifies the clinical benefits of tonsillectomy in a selected group of children.)

Shulman ST (ed): Pharyngitis: Management in an Era of Declining Rheumatic Fever. New York, Praeger, 1984 (Current collection of well referenced papers by many of the leading "streptococcologists.")

87
Gingivostomatitis
ILANA KRAUS

Gingivostomatitis is not a single entity. The term encompasses several diseases that affect the oral mucosa and is broadly divided into three categories: (1) *Gingivitis* is an infection of the gingiva, the keratinized tissue between the teeth; (2) *Gingivostomatitis* is an infection of both the gingiva and any other part of the oral mucosa; and (3) *Stomatitis* is the term applied if lesions are in any part of the oral mucosa other than the gingiva.

PATHOPHYSIOLOGY AND CLINICAL PRESENTATION

Gingivitis

Gingivitis is a periodontal disease caused by bacterial plaque formation at the gingival margin. The bacterial overgrowth is noninvasive, but causes local irritation resulting in a gingival inflammatory response.

Gingivitis affects over 50% of children. The term *adolescent gingivitis* is used when it arises in prepubertal and pubertal children and it is believed that hormonal changes exacerbate this condition. On examination, the gingiva is red or bluish-purple having lost its pink appearance. The color change is due to the increased blood flow, with or without bleeding. The inflammatory response causes swelling of the gingiva. With progression, the sharp edges of the gums (papillae) become eroded and assume a stippled appearance. Minor mouth pain results, which is exacerbated by activities such as vigorous tooth brushing. A mild mouth odor (fetor oris) is frequently present.

Acute Necrotizing Ulcerative Gingivitis

Acute necrotizing ulcerative gingivitis (Vincent's infection, trench mouth), is thought to be caused by two bacterial organisms: *Bacillus fusibacterium* and a spirochete, *Borrelia vincentii*, which are normal inhabitants of the oral flora. It is hypothesized that under certain conditions such as stress, severe malnutrition, or with excessive smoking, the local bacterial balance is altered, causing an overgrowth of these two organisms. It is rarely seen in young children in the United States and is more prevalent in adolescents and young adults.

In contrast to gingivitis, these bacteria invade the gingival mucosa. The inflammation begins at the interdental papilla, which becomes swollen and red, and progresses from the papillae to the gingival margins. A necrotic pseudomembranous exudate is formed, which eventually sloughs and leaves crater-like ulcers with a gray-white base and a linear red border.

Symptoms include severe pain, severe fetor oris, and a peculiar metallic taste. General malaise and decreased appetite are common. A mild fever and local lymphadenopathy may occur.

Acute Herpetic Gingivostomatitis

Acute herpetic gingivostomatitis is caused by herpes simplex virus (HSV), mainly type I. HSV is a deoxyribonucleic acid (DNA) containing virus and causes both primary and recurrent infections. The severity of primary infections may range from unrecognized, to extremely mild, or may cause acute, painful herpetic gingivostomatitis. After the primary infection, the virus becomes dormant but is reactivated in 20% to 40% of individuals. Fever, stress, and sun exposure are frequent precipitants for viral reactivation. The most common form of recurrence is *herpes labialis* (cold sore, fever blister), with lesions at the junction of the lips. Recurrences occasionally occur intraorally. Man is the only known reservoir for the virus, and the disease is transmitted by close contact or through oral secretions. The incubation period is usually 3 to 4 days, but may last up to 2 weeks. The virus is extremely prevalent: by puberty over 50% of adolescents will have antibodies to the virus, and the rate rises to 90% by adulthood. Infection occurs most commonly in children between 1 and 5 years of age.

Primary herpetic gingivostomatitis can present with the sudden prodrome of high fever, general malaise, refusal to eat or drink, and excessive drooling. Within 24 to 48 hours, vesicles appear on any part of the oral mucosa, but rarely on the lips and circumoral skin. The vesicles rupture early, leaving 2-10 mm ulcers that are covered by a yellow-gray membrane surrounded by an erythematous base. The ulcers may coalesce to form larger ulcers. The ulcers heal within 7 to 14 days without scarring. The pain usually subsides within 5 to 7 days, before complete healing occurs. Cervical (especially submaxillary and submental) lymphadenopathy is common.

Aphthous Stomatitis

Aphthous stomatitis, or aphthous ulcers, are recurrent oral ulcerations most frequently on the labial or buccal mucosa, but may appear anywhere within the oral mucosa. The etiology of this disease remains obscure. Local injury, stress, gluten sensitivity, allergy to chocolate and nuts, B_{12}, zinc, folate or iron deficiencies, and the L form of *Streptococcus sanguinis* have all been implicated but are unproven. An autoimmune mechanism is currently believed to be the etiologic factor, but an autoantibody has not been found.

The disease is familial, and women are slightly more often affected than men. Peak onset is between 10 and 19 years of age. A burning sensation often heralds the lesion, after which a red macule appears. It progresses to form a shallow ulcer about 1 cm in diameter. Lesions are usually single, or in a cluster of up to 4 or 5 ulcers. They cause local discomfort but rarely systemic manifestations. The ulcers heal within 7 days and recurrence is the rule. If recurrence of aphthous ulcers is periodic (every 4 weeks) and persists for 5 to 8 days, it may be a manifestation of cyclic neutropenia, an obscure hematologic disorder in which cyclic maturational arrest of the granulocytes occur. A white blood count and differential count during recurrent attacks will establish the diagnosis.

DIFFERENTIAL DIAGNOSIS

Differential diagnoses usually arise when only intraoral vesicular lesions are present, and in clinical practice needs to be distinguished from HSV infections. Gingivitis and acute necrotizing ulcerative gingivitis are easily differentiated; gingivitis is a common disorder, whereas acute necrotizing ulcerative gingivitis is rare.

Acute herpetic gingivostomatitis can be difficult to differentiate from other viral infections. Herpangina, caused by a Coxsackie A virus, presents with small vesicular lesions that ulcerate in 2 to 3 days. It mainly affects children, causing a mild to high fever, mild malaise, and a sore throat. The lesions have a characteristic distribution that is the hallmark of the differential diagnosis. They are confined to the oropharynx (*i.e.*, pharynx, tonsils, anterior tonsilar pillars, and soft palate). Healing is usually within 1 week. Hand, foot, and mouth disease, also caused by a Coxsackie A virus, presents with vesicular lesions on the buccal mucosa and palate, but the gingiva is rarely involved. General symptoms of mild fever, malaise, and mild lymphadenopathy are present. The buccal lesions are most often accompanied by a maculopapular and vesicular rash of the hands and feet. Varicella (chickenpox) may present with oral vesiculoulcerative lesions, which occur most commonly on the palate and resolve in 5 to 7 days. Skin lesions almost always precede the oral lesions and are diagnostic.

Aphthous stomatitis may sometimes be confused with herpetic gingivostomatitis. However, unlike HSV infection, they usually present as single or up to four lesions. Herpes most commonly affects the gingiva, whereas recurrent aphthous stomatitis rarely does.

WORK-UP

History

A history of exposure to an individual with gingivostomatitis should be sought. Since recurrent aphthous stomatitis is familial, inquire about a family history as well as the timing of recurrence. Because both it and acute necrotizing ulcerative gingivitis are often secondary to stress and poor nutrition, explore these possibilities.

Physical Examination

A physical examination is the hallmark in the diagnosis of these entities. The appearance, location, distribution, and number of lesions will often clarify the diagnosis. Lymphadenopathy may be present and body rashes may be diagnostic.

Laboratory Tests

Occasionally, acute herpes virus infection needs to be confirmed. A stained scraping of an ulcer reveals multinucleated giant cells with intranuclear inclusions. The herpes virus can also be cultured or demonstrated by at least a fourfold increase in neutralizing antibody titers in acute and convalescent sera. If cyclic neutropenia is suspected, a complete white blood count and differential should be obtained every 2 to 3 days during recurrences.

MANAGEMENT

Gingivitis is best managed by a dentist or periodontist. Regular and proper oral hygiene is both corrective and preventive (for recurrence) and should be reinforced by the physician. With acute necrotizing gingivostomatitis, the lesions should be promptly debrided (preferably by a dentist) and vigorous oral hygiene should be initiated. Oxygenating mouth washes such as 3% hydrogen peroxide are effective in converting the anaerobic mouth condition to an aerobic environment. In severe cases, antibiotic therapy using penicillin or tetracycline 250 mg QID is indicated. Metronidazole 200 mg TID has been used with excellent results.

The dual goals in the treatment of acute herpetic gingivostomatitis are to prevent dehydration and control discomfort. Encouraging fluid intake, especially chilled beverages because they are soothing, prevents dehydration. In the older child, local anesthetics such as 1% viscous lidocaine (Xylocaine), or chloraseptic spray or lozenges containing benzocaine can be used. The parents, though, must be alerted to the danger of aspiration. In young children, a mixture of diphenhydramine (Benadryl) elixir (12.5 mg/tsp) with kaopectate 1:1 may be used as either a mouth rinse or a paste to alleviate pain.

A child with active lesions should be temporarily excluded from day care and school settings to protect other children. Older children with cold sores do not pose a great risk for spreading the infection and hence they may attend school. The major exception is children who have eczema. They are at risk of developing eczema herpeticum and should be instructed to avoid contact with children with herpetic gingivostomatitis. Acyclovir is not recommended for the child with an initial herpes gingivostomatitis infection or for those with occasional recurrences. Many authorities, however, recommend either IV or oral acyclovir in immunocompromised patients having HSV gingivostomatitis or in normal hosts having particularly severe cases to avoid hospitalization for dehydration. Hopefully, more definitive therapeutic guidelines will soon be available. Steroids should not be used as they may disseminate the virus and photodyes should be avoided because they are possible carcinogens.

The treatment of aphthous stomatitis is aimed at symptomatic relief. Oral hygiene should be reinforced and hydrogen peroxide mouth rinsing is recommended. Topical antibiotics such as 2% tetracycline mouth wash (250 mg capsule dissolved in 15 ml water) can be effective in reducing pain and promoting healing to avoid overgrowth of resistant opportunistic microorganisms. The rinse should be used sparingly and for short periods only. Topical steroids are the most effective treatment. Their anti-inflammatory properties facilitate ulcer healing and should be used in the early stages of the disease to be most effective. Twenty-five mg pellets of hydrocortisone hemisuccinate or 0.1% triamcinolone paste are recommended. Stronger steroid preparations should be avoided. Prolonged use of any steroid should also be avoided because the oral mucosa is highly absorbant and adrenal suppression may result.

INDICATIONS FOR HOSPITALIZATION

Young infants may occasionally refuse oral intake and will need intravenous rehydration therapy. An extension of herpetic stomatitis or a generalized herpetic infection is rare, but especially in young children, may cause the child to be toxic. Hospitalization is often indicated for these severe infections.

ANNOTATED BIBLIOGRAPHY

Abrams RG, Jasell SD: Common oral and dental emergencies and problems. Pediatr Clin North Am 29:681–715, 1982 (Comprehensive discussion and nice illustrations of common conditions causing gingival pain.)

Blackman JA, Andersen RD, Healy A et al: Management of young children with recurrent herpes simplex skin lesions in special educational programs. Pediatr Infect Dis 4:221–224, 1985 (Good, sensible guidelines.)

Bryson YJ: The use of acyclovir in children. Pediatr Infect Dis 3:345–348, 1984 (Helpful, though tentative, therapeutic recommendations.)

Eversole LR: Clinical Outline of Oral Pathology. Diagnosis and Treatment. Philadelphia, Lea & Febiger 1978 (Excellent illustrations and differential diagnosis.)

Tyldesley WR: Oral Medicine. New York, Oxford University Press, 1981 (Comprehensive discussion of oral medicine in Chapters 2 and 3.)

Wright JM, Taylor PP, Allen EP et al: A review of the oral manifestations of infections in pediatric patients. Pediatr Infect Dis 3:80–88, 1984 (Excellent elaboration of the differential diagnoses.)

88
Dentistry for the Pediatrician
JOAN M. O'CONNOR

Most anomalies of the oral tissues are seen by the pediatrician before the child's first dental visit, which is usually at 2 to 3 years of age. Unfortunately, a large segment of the population has no dental care. Advancements of dentistry, particularly in the fields of prevention and materials, have led to many questions from parents, which are frequently asked of pediatricians. The more common disorders of the mouth are outlined in this chapter and preventive recommendations for pediatric dentistry are reviewed.

SOFT TISSUE

(Included are disorders involving alveolar ridges, mucosa, palate, and floor of the mouth)

Eruption cysts are small, white, gray, or bluish, translucent eruptions along the crest of the maxillary and mandibular ridges, probably resulting from remnants of the dental lamina. These are usually shed shortly after birth.

Epstein's pearls are small, white, keratinized lesions found along the midpalatine raphe. Considered to be remnants of epithelial tissue trapped as the fetus grew, they are sometimes incorrectly referred to as *natal teeth*. They usually slough after birth.

In the older child, a bluish elevation of tissue is often seen in the molar region as a second primary molar or permanent first molar is about to erupt. This is known as an *eruption hematoma*. No treatment is necessary because the hematoma resolves when the tooth breaks through.

Congenital epulis of the newborn is an unusual benign, slow-growing, pedunculated tumor of the anterior maxillary (and less commonly mandibular) ridge. Ninety percent of these growths occur in female babies. Histologically, it is similar to the granular cell myoblastoma. Surgical excision is the preferred treatment and a recurrence is rare.

Tumors of the intraoral accessory salivary glands occur frequently and can occur throughout the oral cavity. Approximately one half of these tumors are malignant. The diagnosis is made by microscopic examination but clinically, the benign tumor is often nonulcerated, painless, and slow growing.

A mucocele is not a tumor, although it may resemble one. It is a common lesion of the lower lip, but it is not limited to that area. Because of the absence of salivary glands, it is not often seen on the attached gingiva or the anterior hard palate. A mucocele is thought to result from trauma that severs a minor salivary gland duct and causes the saliva to pool in the connective tissue. Since it does not contain an epithelial lining, it is not a true cyst. Superficial mucoceles appear bluish whereas deeper ones may be pink due to the thickness of the overlying mucosa. It cannot be emptied by digital pressure and the aspirant is sticky, clear, and viscous (which differentiates it from vascular lesions and superficial nonkeratotic cysts). Early mucoepidermoid tumors and mucinous adenocarcinoma must be ruled out. Thus, the clinician should inspect and palpate the base and the periphery of the site for induration, which might suggest a tumor rather than a mucocele. A complete excision and a pathologic examination is the preferred treatment.

Ranula is a mucocele of the tissue of the floor of the mouth. It often causes the tongue to be displaced forward and laterally. Surgical excision or marsupialization is recommended unless the size is so great that the displaced tongue causes obstruction. An emergency aspiration or incision and drainage is then necessary.

Hemangioma may be congenital or traumatic and may vary in size from a millimeter to several centimeters. It is often seen on the lips, buccal mucosa, and palate. As opposed to mucoceles and other cysts, it can blanch and empty with digital pressure. Blood can be aspirated with a fine needle. It is distinguished from an aneurysm and arteriovenous shunt by the absence of a pulse. Sclerosing agents, such as sodium psylliate or sodium morrhuate, used either singly or prior to surgical excision, are the preferred treatments.

THE TONGUE

Ankyloglossia (tongue tie) is a term given to any situation where a short lingual frenum extending from the tongue to the floor of the mouth or lingual gingival tissue interferes with protrusion of the tongue. Despite some opinions to the contrary, it probably has no effect on speech or nursing in most cases. Thus, no treatment is warranted if the tongue can be protruded beyond the lips. If the tongue cannot be protruded, an evaluation of the functions of the tongue is necessary to determine if any treatment is required. True ankyloglossia results when the frenum is replaced by a thick fibrous band of tissue. When the gingiva is pulled from the lingual surface of the mandibular anterior teeth by either the result of the position of the attachment of the frenum or local inflammation, surgical repair is indicated.

Migratory glossitis (geographic tongue) is a common anomaly. It is characterized by red smooth areas resulting from desquamation of the keratin layers of papilla encircled by slightly elevated gray margins and is confined to epithelium. Two to four lesions usually occur at a time and patterns may be altered daily. It usually only occurs in children, and its cause is unknown. No treatment is indicated.

Macroglossia may either be an idiopathic or a secondary condition. Lymphangioma and hemangioma are the two most common causes of macroglossia. In the tongue, a lymphangioma may present as a diffuse smooth or nodular enlargement. The enlargement is often unilateral. Its color is less blue than from a hemangioma, ranging from normal coloration to bluish but may be translucent. The aspirant is the distinguished feature between the two lesions. Treatment is not necessary unless the tongue is sufficiently large to cause disfigurement or airway interference, in which case surgical excision is performed.

A transitory tongue enlargement is often caused by angioneurotic edema from an allergic reaction. The maintenance of the airway is important.

THE TEETH

An exception to the sequence (Fig. 88-1) is the eruption of the natal or neonatal tooth. About 85% are lower primary incisors rather than supernumerary teeth. A radiograph will determine the type of tooth. Most natal/neonatal teeth are hypermobile due to the inadequate root formation. If the tooth is so mobile that aspiration is feared, it should be removed. The removal is accomplished by gauze (to reduce the chance of losing the tooth due to the small, slippery nature of these teeth) with light finger pressure. This can be done by the pediatrician rather than referring to the dentist; otherwise, the immature primary incisor will become more firm as the root develops.

A practical method of examining teeth is to divide the arches of the mouth at the midline and compare each tooth to its contralateral tooth in the arch. When examining a whole mouth, supernumerary or

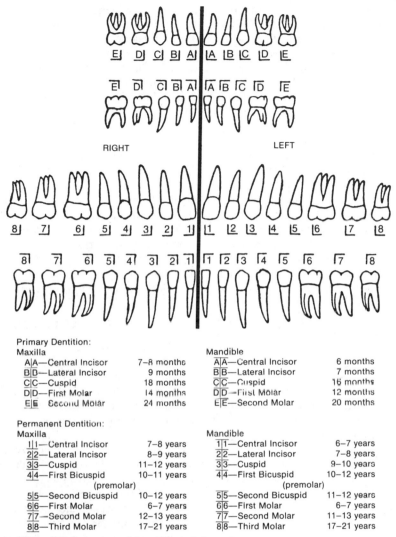

Figure 88-1. The names and locations of the primary and permanent dentition are depicted as well as their usual times of eruption.

Primary Dentition:

Maxilla			Mandible		
A|A—Central Incisor	7–8 months		A|A—Central Incisor	6 months	
B|D—Lateral Incisor	9 months		B|B—Lateral Incisor	7 months	
C|C—Cuspid	18 months		C|C—Cuspid	16 months	
D|D—First Molar	14 months		D|D—First Molar	12 months	
E|E—Second Molar	24 months		E|E—Second Molar	20 months	

Permanent Dentition:

Maxilla			Mandible		
1|1—Central Incisor	7–8 years		1|1—Central Incisor	6–7 years	
2|2—Lateral Incisor	8–9 years		2|2—Lateral Incisor	7–8 years	
3|3—Cuspid	11–12 years		3|3—Cuspid	9–10 years	
4|4—First Bicuspid	10–11 years		4|4—First Bicuspid	10–12 years	
(premolar)			(premolar)		
5|5—Second Bicuspid	10–12 years		5|5—Second Bicuspid	11–12 years	
6|6—First Molar	6–7 years		6|6—First Molar	6–7 years	
7|7—Second Molar	12–13 years		7|7—Second Molar	11–13 years	
8|8—Third Molar	17–21 years		8|8—Third Molar	17–21 years	

missing teeth are often overlooked because there is not the corresponding crowding or spacing present that might be expected; counting teeth minimizes this oversight. By looking for bilateral symmetry, teeth that have not erupted or exfoliated at approximately the same schedule as the corresponding contralateral tooth can be evaluated for pathology. If, for example, one permanent incisor has completely erupted and the corresponding incisor's predecessor has not loosened sufficiently for exfoliation, one might be suspicious of impaction, congenital absence, or the presence of a supernu-

merary tooth or odontoma. A referral should be made to a dentist if there is more than 6 months' difference between the eruption of corresponding teeth.

The congenital absence of teeth can be total (anodontia) or partial (oligodontia). Anodontia is rare and is often seen with hypotrichosis, anhidrosis, and asteatosis as a characteristic of ectodermal dysplasia. Oligodontia in the primary dentition is rare. It is more common in the permanent dentition. The most frequently missing teeth (in order of frequency) are the third molars, mandibular second bicuspids, maxillary lateral incisors, and the maxillary second bicuspids; the absence may be unilateral or bilateral. Treatment depends on the space needs of the rest of the arch and the rate of root resorption of the primary tooth. If there is insufficient space for a normal-sized replacement to be made or if crowding exists elsewhere in the arch, orthodontic movement can reposition the teeth as necessary.

The presence of a "double tooth" can be seen in either dentition but it is more likely to be seen in the primary dentition. It is usually limited to anterior teeth. A double tooth is the result of either fusion or gemination. It either reduces the count (double tooth is counted as one) by one or results in the normal amount if the fusion is between a normal and a supernumerary tooth. Gemination occurs as a result of the division of a single tooth germ leaving the count as normal. In most cases, when there is a reduction in the number, there is a corresponding absence of one or more permanent teeth. When the count is normal, there is no effect on the permanent teeth. Confirmation of congenitally absent teeth by radiographs allows for planning of proper treatment at the appropriate time.

Some abnormalities observed on clinical examination, such as delayed eruption of a permanent incisor, a large space between the maxillary central incisors, severe labial positioning or rotation of an incisor or prominent bulging of the alveolar ridge may be indicative of underlying pathology. The presence of unerupted supernumerary teeth, impacted teeth (normal teeth but diverging from the usual eruption path), or odontomas (calcified masses with some anatomic similarity to teeth) among the developing permanent teeth prevent normal eruption or alignment. Supernumerary teeth occur most commonly in the maxillary incisor region of the dentition, whereas impacted teeth are (in order of frequency) maxillary cuspids, central incisors, mandibular second bicuspids, and second molars. Odontomas can be discovered at any age or in any tooth-bearing area of the mouth. The presence of any of these abnormalities is confirmed radiographically.

Surgical removal is the preferred treatment for supernumerary teeth and odontomas whereas surgical exposure and orthodontic traction of the impacted tooth is used if its position is favorable for eruption.

Ankylosis of teeth is the abnormal bony fusion of dentin with bone. The ankylosed tooth is often identified as "submerging" due to the fact that ad-jacent areas experience continued eruption and alveolar growth while the ankylosed area is static. The second primary molar is the most common tooth in which ankylosis occurs except for anterior teeth that have been traumatized. Percussion of the tooth with an instrument usually produces a very dull, solid sound in contrast to the surrounding teeth where the intact periodontal membrane absorbs some of the blow. The treatment is varied depending on the severity. The tooth is often extracted and a space maintainer is placed until the permanent tooth erupts.

An ectopic eruption of the permanent first molar, especially in the maxillary arch, is seen frequently. It is detected radiographically or clinically. The child will sometimes complain of pain in the area as the distal root is resorbed and oral fluids irritate the pulp. Many ectopic molars will correct spontaneously, but if the mesial edge is trapped, simple orthodontic intervention is recommended.

DENTAL CARIES

The incidence of dental caries has decreased considerably with the introduction of systemic and topical fluorides and fluoride toothpastes, earlier examination of children, the application of occlusal sealants, and increased dental health education. The main agents of caries production are streptococci (*i.e., S. mutans, S. sanguis*, and *S. salivarius*). The acids that demineralize enamel are derived from carbohydrate sources that have undergone microbial degradation. If enough acid is formed and remains in contact with the enamel, demineralization occurs and the caries process is initiated. Heredity may be a factor in determining resistance or susceptibility to caries, but the environmental factors learned from parents (hygiene and diet) are of much greater significance. The anatomy of the tooth, the degree of crowding, and the presence of appliances in the mouth are also factors in the caries process. The deep developmental pits and fissures on the occlusal (biting) surfaces of molars predispose them to carious lesions. Fluoride is effective in controlling smooth surface (*i.e.,* those surfaces between the teeth in addition to the cheek and tongue sides of the tooth) caries but the chewing surface with its deep grooves receives little protection.

Occlusal sealants are organic polymers that bond to the surface of the enamel. It forms an impervious barrier to oral fluids. Clinical trials extending to 7 years indicate that prolonged wear does occur with time but that resin tags in the enamel still provide protection. They are intended for teeth with deep developmental grooves. It is probably not cost effective to seal all primary molars. The greatest benefit comes from not having to cut into tooth structure as is done with amalgam restorations once caries is present. An amalgam restoration lasts only about 8 to 10 years; at that point it must be replaced, which involves the removal of still more tooth structure. Since primary teeth may be lost before it would be necessary to replace the restoration, it may be argued to simply treat caries that develop in primary teeth and save the sealants for the permanent molars. (In addition, the primary molars usually have more shallow grooves, the material does not adhere as well to the enamel of primary teeth, and the primary molars are more accessible for good hygiene than the more posterior permanent molars.)

Nursing bottle caries is the term used to identify the pattern of carious involvement of multiple teeth following prolonged nursing (either bottle or breast) at bedtime. When the child falls asleep, the liquid pools on the teeth due to the decreased salivary flow and diminished clearance from the mouth. Multiple maxillary incisors are usually involved with occlusal surfaces of the first primary molars affected next most frequently. The mandibular incisors are rarely involved, probably because of the tongue's overlying position in nursing. By the time the second molars and cuspids erupt, the practice has usually been discontinued.

COMMON MALOCCLUSIONS

Anterior open bite is often associated with a thumb habit, tongue thrust, or abnormal tongue posture.

Because severe protrusion of maxillary anterior teeth renders teeth susceptible to fracture from trauma, early correction is often performed to minimize this risk.

Crossbite is the term applied to a malocclusion in which the maxillary tooth or teeth are positioned behind the mandibular in the anterior region or palatally in the posterior region. Crossbites are frequently seen in both the primary and mixed dentition and are quite varied according to severity. Single anterior tooth crossbites warrant immediate attention. When the teeth are closed, the maxillary incisor is trapped behind the opposing mandibular incisor(s) causing forward pressure on the mandibular incisor. As a result of this forward pressure,

the gingiva often recedes from the front surface of the mandibular incisor. There is also a possibility of space loss on the maxillary arch as a result of drifting of the adjacent incisors into the space normally occupied by the maxillary tooth. The complete crossbite of all the incisors is indicative of a possible developing mandibular skeletal discrepancy. An evaluation regarding the extent of the problem and the timing of correction should be made by an orthodontist.

Posterior crossbites can be unilateral or bilateral. The treatment is an expansion of the width of the palate.

PERIODONTIUM

The most common gingival disorders are discussed in detail in Chapter 87 and are not mentioned here.

Dilantin-induced gingivitis consists of generalized hyperplasia of the gingiva. Excellent oral hygiene should be stressed in children undergoing phenytoin therapy. Surgical removal of the excessive tissue is often done, but a recurrence is common.

Localized juvenile periodontitis is a disease that occurs in healthy pubertal patients and is characterized by severe and rapid bone loss. Particularly important is the fact that acute inflammatory gingival symptoms are absent. Treatment is best rendered by a specialist to try to minimize tooth loss as a result of the rapid bone loss. Tetracycline therapy has been used in some patients with varied success.

Gingival recession in children usually appears localized rather than generalized, as is the case in adults with advanced periodontal disease. Localized gingival recession is often seen along the labial surface of crowded mandibular incisors. This stripping of the gingiva from the root of the tooth results from pressure of the tooth against the buccal plate of bone or as the result of occlusal trauma. Tooth brush abrasion is another cause of gingival recession. Tooth brushing with a soft brush reduces this damage. Gingival grafting is necessary if the tissue loss is severe.

FLUORIDE

The usefulness of fluoride supplements to pregnant women who live in nonfluoridated areas has not been established, although no hazards have been discovered to contradict its use. However, recent studies seem to indicate that the major effect of fluoride on the primary teeth is postnatally.

Fluoride supplements are recommended for nursing infants even in fluoridated areas because human milk contains such low levels of fluoride. Once the infant begins to drink water or formula made with fluoridated water, the fluoride can be discontinued.

Many studies show that fluoridated water reduces dental caries by 35% to 65%. In nonfluoridated areas or in areas where water is obtained from wells, it is recommended that daily supplements be given systemically.

CONCENTRATION OF FLUORIDE IN DRINKING WATER

AGE (YRS)	0–0.3 ppm	0.3–0.7 ppm	0.7 ppm
0–2	0.25 mg F	0	0
2–3	0.5 mg F	0.25 mg F	0
3–16	1.0 mg F	0.5 mg F	0.25 mg F

Many schools now have children participate in topical fluoride rinse programs (usually stannous or sodium fluoride). Such programs, along with semi-annual topical application of acidulated phosphate fluoride at the dental visit and use of fluoridated toothpastes, have further decreased the caries rate in children. Care should be taken, however, to assure that the fluoride given in schools is topical rather than systemic if water is fluoridated in the community or if fluoride supplements are already prescribed. If the water supply is not fluoridated, topical treatment may be used in conjunction with, but should not substitute for, systemic fluoride.

The use of topical fluoride rinses for children under 4 years of age should be administered carefully because the child may not have full control of swallowing reflexes.

COMMON QUESTIONS ASKED OF PEDIATRICIANS AND DENTISTS

Q. When should the child's first dental appointment be?

A. Two years old is the age recommended by the Academy of Pediatric Dentistry. At this age, usually an examination only is scheduled and the child is best held by the parent during the examination. An examination will reveal any existing caries and eruption abnormalities and will provide an opportunity for oral hygiene instruction. At 3 years of age, a child is familiar with the routine, the dental office, and the staff, and is able to participate in the examination, cleaning, and fluoride treatment.

Q. With the decreased incidence of tooth decay, how often should a child visit the dentist?

A. It is still recommended that a child be seen twice a year. In the preschool child, the personality development and changes are so rapid that a child who is seen only annually often finds the visit traumatic because he has forgotten the procedure; he does not remember the staff, and so forth. Once the permanent teeth begin to erupt, semiannual examinations allow interception of developing malocclusion at an early age.

Q. When should toothbrushing begin?

A. Cleaning of the teeth should begin as soon as teeth erupt. The parent should wipe the first teeth with a gauze before bedtime each day. A soft toothbrush can be used as early as tolerated. Once a child is 2 to 3 years old, he should be allowed to brush his own teeth twice a day to encourage good hygiene habits, but at bedtime the toothbrushing should be completed by the parent. A child usually lacks manual dexterity to brush satisfactorily until he is almost 6 years old.

Q. When should toothpaste be used and what kind?

A. The greatest benefit of toothbrushing is the removal of plaque by the mechanical action of brushing. Toothpaste adds flavor, some abrasiveness for better cleaning, and fluoride for caries prevention. Toothpaste can be used once the child is mature enough not to ingest it completely. Any toothpaste with fluoride is recommended; the brand depends on acceptability. Some children do not like any flavor; it is probably wiser to forego toothpaste if brushing alone can be accomplished without a fight, rather than having every session be an ordeal.

Q. At what age should flossing start?

A. Rather than age specification, flossing should start when tight contact exists between teeth. If spaces are wide enough to allow access to all surfaces with a toothbrush, flossing is not necessary. A parent should floss for the child when indicated since children tend to lacerate their tissues.

Q. Is staining of teeth a permanent condition?

A. Extrinsic staining is usually of microbial origin except for that caused by oral iron preparations. Common stains are green (thought to be the result of chromogenic bacteria on the enamel surface); orange (often associated with poor hygiene); or black. Removal of these stains can be accomplished by the use of an abrasive pumice paste applied with rotary instruments.

Q. What is bruxism and is treatment necessary?

A. Bruxism is an oral habit consisting of grinding or gnashing of the teeth, which occurs most often at night. Severe abrasion of the teeth (through both the enamel and the dentin layers) can occur. In the primary dentition, no treatment is usually necessary but if the habit continues and wear of the permanent teeth is observed, a plastic night guard can be fabricated to lessen the damage to the teeth.

Q. At what age are braces applied to the teeth?

A. It is recommended that the occlusion should be evaluated at 7 years of age. Crossbites, ectopic eruptions, and severe incisor protrusions susceptible to fracture can be corrected at this age with limited treatment; attention can be directed toward correcting certain habits that contribute to malocclusions, such as thumb sucking and tongue thrust. Future spacing needs can be assessed and future treatment can be planned. Most appliances for complete treatment are placed in the late mixed dentition stage.

Q. What are the major indications for braces?

A. Malocclusions that interfere with function such as anterior open bite, anterior and posterior crossbites, severe protrusion of incisors that make them susceptible to fracture and those that are disfiguring causing emotional problems in development are the chief indications for orthodontic treatment.

Q. What is the role of thumb sucking in malocclusions? At what age, if any, are changes reversible?

A. Thumb sucking often results in protrusion of the maxillary incisors (sometimes accompanied by lingual inclination of the mandibular incisors) and anterior open bite (which is the more dif-ficult malocclusion to correct). Many children suffer no effects to the dentition. However, thumb sucking may have become a great family issue. Prior to the age of 4, efforts to reduce the habit are impractical because of the immaturity of the child and only result in increased stress for all concerned. As a child associates with other children in preschool programs, the habit usually stops (at least during the day). Some effects may be reversed if stopped by age 4.

If damage is such that the habit should be stopped, several methods have proven somewhat effective. If the family agrees to not interfere, to stop any nagging, and to ignore the habit, a practitioner can often speak privately with the child and ask the child to keep a record and report progress made in decreasing the habit. Appliances can be made to serve only as a reminder to the child—preferably, removable appliances, so that if emotionally necessary, the child is still able to suck his thumb.

ANNOTATED BIBLIOGRAPHY

American Society of Dentistry for Children and The American Academy of Pedodontics Pediatr Dent 5:89, 1983 (Good review of the use of pit and fissure sealants.)

Finn S: Clinical Pedodontics, 4th ed. Philadelphia, WB Saunders, 1973 (Good general pediatric dentistry textbook.)

Gellin M: The distribution of anomalies of primary anterior teeth and their effect on the permanent successors. Dent Clin North Am 28:69–80, 1972 (Detailed discussion of missing and supernumerary teeth in the primary dentition.)

McDonald R, Avery D: Dentistry for the Child and Adolescent, 3rd ed. St. Louis, CV Mosby, 1978 (Very detailed, inclusive pediatric dental textbook; well written.)

Wood N, Gooz P: Differential Diagnosis of Oral Lesions. St. Louis, CV Mosby, 1975 (Excellent oral pathology textbook, especially in the differential diagnosis as well as in descriptions of pathology.)

89
Thrush

THOMAS J. HATHAWAY

Thrush is a common superficial infection of the oral mucosa caused by the saprophytic yeast *Candida albicans*.

PATHOPHYSIOLOGY

C. albicans can frequently be cultured from asymptomatic infants and children. Colonization increases during the first weeks of life and subsequently decreases with age; rates are as high as 82% at 4 weeks of age and fall to 50% at 1 year. Colonization rates of approximately 50% have also been reported for older children and adults. Despite high colonization rates, the incidence of clinical infection is much lower. Rates range from 0.5% to 20% during infancy. Infants born vaginally to mothers with active vaginal candidal infections have higher rates of thrush. Thrush is relatively uncommon after infancy.

Local and environmental host-defense factors including the epithelial barrier, microbial competition and inhibition, and the antimicrobial properties of saliva appear important in preventing thrush. The role of humoral and cell-mediated defense in preventing clinical infection is less clear. A specific antibody against Candida can be demonstrated in saliva and serum. Serum antibody titers are usually not elevated with oral infection. Salivary antibody titers do appear to be increased in patients with oral candidiasis and may have some role in preventing local infection. Cell-mediated immunity is presumed to be important in systemic candidal disease. Its role in local infection, however, is not clear.

The factors responsible for the appearance of a clinical infection are unknown, but they are believed to include the breakdown of local host-defense factors and perhaps humoral and cell-mediated defense.

CLINICAL PRESENTATION

Thrush presents typically as areas of small, white, curd-like plaques on the buccal mucosa, tongue, and gingiva. The plaque can be scraped away, re-

vealing an erythematous base with occasionally some punctate bleeding. Infection is usually asymptomatic. Oral thrush may be associated with a monilial diaper rash.

Infants and children who are immunocompromised, malnourished, diabetic, or receiving systemic antibiotics or corticosteroids are commonly affected as are infants and children with anatomic deformities of the mouth such as cleft palate. Thrush may be seen as part of a complex of opportunistic infections in AIDS. However, these children characteristically experience more severe and refractory mucocutaneous candidiasis.

DIFFERENTIAL DIAGNOSIS

The primary entity that may be confused with thrush is milk coating the oral mucosa. This can be differentiated from thrush by a lack of adherence to the mucosa, an ease of removal, and an absence of underlying erythema.

WORK-UP

A microscopic examination of scrapings with KOH reveals typical hyphae. However, this and other tests are rarely necessary to make the diagnosis (which can be easily made on appearance alone). Culture of the lesions typically grows *C. albicans* after 1 to 2 days, although a culture is not necessary for the diagnosis in the usual case. In questionable cases, however, a KOH examination and a fungal culture may be helpful in establishing the diagnosis. A further diagnostic work-up is not usually indicated except in severe or atypical cases or those that fail to respond to therapy.

If a history or physical examination suggests an underlying predisposing condition, appropriate evaluation and intervention should be undertaken.

TREATMENT

Nystatin 200,000 units applied four times daily to the lesions is usually effective within 1 to 2 weeks. Treatment efficacy is increased by prolonged contact of the nystatin with the lesions. In the infant, 1 ml of the suspension should be swabbed on each side of the mouth with each dose. The older child can swish 4 ml to 6 ml of the suspension in the mouth before swallowing.

Alternatively, a 1% gentian violet solution applied directly to the lesions several times a day is also effective. The main disadvantage of this therapy is potential staining of skin and clothing.

Underlying immunologic, endocrine, nutritional, or metabolic disorders should be treated. A referral should be made, if necessary, to an appropriate specialist.

ANNOTATED BIBLIOGRAPHY

Epstein JB, Truelove EL, Izutzu KT: Oral candidiasis: Pathogenesis and host defense. Rev Infect Dis 6:96–105, 1984 (Review of pathogenesis and host defense.)

Jenkins WM, Thomas HC, Masson DK: Oral infections with *Candida albicans*. Scott Med J 18:192–200, 1973 (Reviews spectrum of oral Candidal infections.)

Jennison RF: Thrush in infancy. Arch Dis Child 52:747–749, 1977 (Prevalence of thrush in infancy.)

Russell C, Lay KM: Natural history of Candida species and yeasts in the oral cavities of infants. Arch Oral Biol 18:957–962, 1973 (Study of prevalence of oral Candida in infants.)

90
Neck Masses
BASIL J. ZITELLI

The differential diagnosis of neck masses in children is extensive and includes congenital lesions, lymphadenopathy, and neoplastic disorders. Fortunately, most neck masses in children are benign, with malignancies comprising only about 15% of such masses in children admitted to the hospital.

CLINICAL ANATOMY AND PRESENTATION

Anatomically, two cervical triangles are formed by structures on each side of the neck. The anterior triangle extends from the mandible edge superiorly, along the sternocleidomastoid muscle to the midline of the neck anteriorly. The posterior triangle is bounded by the sternocleidomastoid muscle, the distal two thirds of the clavicle, and the midline of the neck posteriorly. These triangles are important in the physical diagnosis of neck masses. Structures that can be palpated normally in the neck and are confused occasionally with pathologic processes include the angle of the mandible, the mastoid tip, the styloid process, the pyramidal lobe of the thyroid, the greater cornu of the thyroid, and the lateral processes of C_2 and C_6.

Certain historical and physical characteristics of common lesions may lead the clinician in the appropriate direction. Lesions present at birth suggest congenital cysts or anomalies. Congenital cysts, however, may become inflamed at a later time and may be confused easily with regional lymphadenitis. Inflammation as well as tenderness may be associated with lymphadenopathy and occasionally also malignancies. In general, lesions that progress slowly over several months are congenital and are frequently benign. A rapid growth over a few weeks, especially if inflammation is not present, suggests that a neoplastic process and malignancy must be considered. Risk factors associated with malignancies include the onset by 1 month of age, rapid and progressive growth, ulceration, a lesion fixed to or below the underlying fascia, and a lesion larger than 3 cm that is firm or hard in consistency. The older child may also exhibit symptoms of fevers, night sweats, and weight loss. Inflamed masses that become painful while eating suggest sialadenitis.

The location of the mass is important. Most masses in children lying anterior to the sternocleidomastoid muscle are benign. The exception to this rule is thyroid nodules; these should be suspected to be malignant until proven otherwise. Other malignancies are more likely to be found as a single mass in the posterior triangle or as multiple masses crossing into both the anterior and posterior triangles. Supraclavicular adenopathy is strongly associated with granulomatous or malignant disease in the mediastinum. Masses along the anterior border of the sternocleidomastoid muscle, especially if they are associated with a fistula that retracts with swallowing, are more likely to be branchial cleft anomalies.

COMMON CONGENITAL LESIONS OF THE NECK

Benign congenital lesions of the neck are almost always a thyroglossal duct cyst (72%), a branchial cleft cyst (24%), or a vascular malformation (4%) such as cystic hygroma or hemangioma.

Thyroglossal Duct Cyst

The most common congenital neck mass is the thyroglossal duct cyst, an embryologic remnant of the descent of the thyroid anlage from the base of the tongue. Most cysts and fistulas are detected before age 20. There is no sex or race prediction. Frequently, a fluctuant cystic mass ranging in size from 1 to 2 cm up to 5 to 6 cm is found in the midline just below the level of the hyoid bone. The mass may occasionally be lateral to the midline but anterior to the sternocleidomastoid muscle, making differentiation from branchial cleft cysts difficult. Other locations include the suprahyoid, suprasternal, transhyoid, and submental areas. When a sinus tract is present, drainage of mucoid material may occur, and infection may lead to acute swelling and tenderness.

The mass is best examined when the neck is hyperextended. Characteristically, because of connections with the tongue, the cyst rises with tongue protrusion and swallowing. Thyroglossal duct cysts usually do not transilluminate because of the overlying tissue and fascia.

Other diagnostic considerations include lingual thyroid, pyramidal lobe of the thyroid, sebaceous cyst, lipoma, and dermoid cyst. A failure of complete descent of the thyroid may lead to ectopic placement. This can be detected by noting absent thyroid tissue in the normal position. Sebaceous cysts do not move with tongue protrusion. Lipomas are usually more lobulated and softer than thyroglossal duct cysts, and dermoids are attached to the skin and move easily with it.

The treatment of thyroglossal duct cysts, sinuses, and fistulas consists of controlling infection with systemic antibiotics followed by complete surgical excision, which often includes resection of the midportion of the hyoid bone.

Branchial Cleft Defects

Defects of the branchial clefts may be formed from remnants of the branchial grooves and pouches being buried or failing to complete fusion. Branchial cleft anomalies may arise from any of the first four clefts. However, more than 95% of these defects arise from the second cleft, perhaps because it has the greatest depth and persists the longest. Defects of the second cleft are lateral and are usually recognized by age 30, although most are diagnosed in the early school-aged child before the age of 10. Bilateral defects occur in 2% of cases. Cysts are found approximately three times more frequently than fistulas. Although the cysts may vary in position, most are found in the carotid triangle and can be palpated anterior to the middle one third of the sternocleidomastoid muscle. The posterior border of the cyst is usually below the anterior margin of the sternocleidomastoid muscle. The mass is rounded, slightly movable, and unless acutely infected, nontender. The mass may increase in size along with surrounding lymph nodes during periods of inflammation. Sinuses, when present, may open externally and are usually found as 2-mm to 3-mm slits anterior to the lower third of the sternocleidomastoid muscle. The fistula may also extend internally to open in the peritonsillar area.

The differential diagnosis includes lymphadenopathy, cystic hygroma, dermoid cyst, neurofibroma, aberrant thyroid, hemangioma and lipoma. The fibrous tumor of congenital muscular torticollis (CMT) can also be mistaken for a second cleft cyst. However, the mass in CMT is within the belly of the sternocleidomastoid muscle and there may be an associated head tilt with the head inclined to the affected side and the chin rotated to the opposite side. A complete examination of the ear, nose, throat, and nasopharynx is essential.

The treatment of branchial cleft cysts and fistulas is complete excision of the cyst and fistulous tract.

Vascular Lesions

Cystic hygromas (cavernous lymphangiomatous tissue) and hemangiomas comprise a small portion of benign congenital neck masses and are usually easily recognized. These vascular lesions are diffuse and easily compressible, and they often enlarge during a Valsalva maneuver. While cystic hygromas can be transilluminated, hemangiomas can be recognized by their more limited size and bluish hue of the overlying skin.

Cystic hygromas arise from lymphatic sacs that develop from mesenchymal tissue or from the jugular vein. Over 90% of cystic hygromas are found in the posterior cervical triangle behind the sternocleidomastoid muscle in the supraclavicular fossa. Nearly two thirds of these lesions are noted at birth and 90% are diagnosed by the second birthday.

Cystic hygromas can compromise vital structures in the neck, or enlarge secondary to hemorrhage or infection. Surgical excision may be difficult, but remains the only effective mode of therapy. Recurrence after removal of all grossly abnormal tissue is unlikely.

Hemangiomas may not be present visably at birth, but grow rapidly within the first year of life. Similar to cystic hygromas, hemangiomas can impinge on vital structures in the neck and can cause airway obstruction. Tumor growth usually ceases after the first birthday and spontaneous regression occurs by 5 or 6 years. Therapy is not required except in cases of severe cosmetic deformities or interference of vital function, and the mass should be checked for spontaneous regression. Therapy, when necessary, may include prednisone or surgery.

LYMPHADENOPATHY

Palpable cervical lymph nodes are a common finding and may not represent an ongoing pathologic process. Nearly half of all 2-year-old children will normally have palpable cervical nodes. The percentage of children with palpable nodes increases with age as recurrent minor infections occur and the amount of lymphoid tissue increases in early childhood. Lymphadenopathy is usually defined as any nontender lymph node larger than 10 mm, except epitrochlear ($\geq$5 mm) and inguinal ($>$15 mm) nodes.

The evaluation of cervical adenopathy depends on a careful history and a detailed physical examination. The clinician should evaluate the location, size, shape, consistency, mobility, inflammation, suppuration, and skin discoloration. In addition, an examination for noncontiguous adenopathy and systemic disease should be included in the complete examination.

Viral Infections

Viral upper respiratory tract infections, by far, are the most common causes of enlarged cervical lymph nodes in children. The nodes are usually bilateral, discrete, oval, soft, and minimally tender. Most of the acute changes in the lymph node usually parallel the course of the respiratory infection or lag slightly by a few days. The size of the nodes,

however, may not fully regress to their former size. One report demonstrated persistent adenopathy for 10 months after a herpes infection. Besides the herpes viruses, adenoviruses and enteroviruses are commonly associated with cervical lymph node enlargement. In addition, Epstein–Barr virus (EBV) infection may produce fever, malaise, exudative tonsillopharyngitis, with localized cervical and often generalized lymphadenopathy including hepatosplenomegaly. The diagnosis of EBV infection may be difficult, especially in the young child because many preschoolers may not develop heterophil agglutinating antibodies. Twenty-seven to 91% of patients 2 to 5 years old with EBV infection will be heterophil positive whereas 53% to 94% of patients 6 to 10 years old and 100% of older children will be positive. A definitive diagnosis can be made by measuring specific antibody titers to the viral capsid antigen and other viral components. Despite a typical mononucleosis-like illness, nearly half of patients will be EBV negative. Cytomegalovirus infection, associated with lymphocytosis and atypical lymphocytes on peripheral blood smear, is a major cause of "EBV negative" mononucleosis as are adenovirus and *Toxoplasma gondii*. Viral infections are usually self-limited and generally require no specific therapy.

Bacterial Infection

Lymphadenitis of the head and neck is most frequently secondary to infections to the upper respiratory tract, infections of the teeth and gingiva, or infections following trauma. *Staphylococcus aureus* and *Streptococcus pyogenes* cause between 40% to 80% of cases of acute unilateral cervical adenitis. Lymph nodes range from 2 cm to 6 cm and are tender with overlying warmth and erythema. Fluctuance may develop. Young infants, usually males between 3 and 7 weeks of age, may develop lymphadenitis associated with cellulitis, otitis media, and bacteremia; *S. aureus* and group B streptococci are the most common causative agents. Increasingly, anaerobic infections are being identified as causing acute lymphadenitis. Anaerobic organisms were recovered from 40% of needle aspirates in one series and were the sole organisms isolated in 20% of patients. Rarely, *Hemophilus influenzae* has been isolated from node aspirates as well. The treatment of bacterial lymphadenitis must account for a high percentage of penicillin-resistant *S. aureus* and a semisynthetic penicillin, erythromycin, or cephalosporin should be used as initial therapy.

"Cold" Inflammatory Lymphadenitis

"Cold" inflammation (subacute or chronic inflammation) of the cervical nodes is frequently secondary to cat-scratch disease (CSD), atypical mycobacterial infection, or toxoplasmosis. CSD is a zoonotic infection following contact with a cat, a cat scratch, or a break in the skin with cat licks. A primary pustule develops 3 to 10 days after the scratch and may persist up to 8 weeks. In a small percentage of patients, the eye is the site of inoculum resulting in conjunctivitis or an ocular granuloma leading to preauricular adenopathy. Impressive regional adenopathy develops about 2 weeks after inoculation but may not occur for nearly 7 weeks. Nodes are tender; they may occur in multiple sites (40% of cases); they may range from 1 cm to 8 cm; and they may persist 2 to 4 months and rarely up to 6 to 24 months. Lymph node biopsy typically demonstrates stellate granulomas and suppurative or caseous centers. The causative agent appears to be a small pleomorphic, gram-negative rod seen with Warthin–Starry silver impregnation stains of lymph node or pustular lesions. Antibiotics generally do not hasten the resolution of CSD. The aspiration of suppurative nodes is indicated. Rarely, surgical excision is necessary when the diagnosis is in doubt, or it may delay the diagnosis of a malignancy (see Chap. 200).

Atypical myobacterial lymphadenitis predominately affects children 1 to 5 years of age with its peak incidence from 1 to 3 years of age. *M. scrofulaceum* and *M. avium-intracellulare* organisms are the most common offending organisms. Typically, the lymph node enlarges suddenly. The nodes are usually unilateral, in contrast to *M. tuberculosis* infections that are usually bilateral. Minimal pain and tenderness are present, but no constitutional symptoms develop. Several nodes in an affected area may enlarge; they may become matted together and adhere to the overlying skin. Early skin changes consist of a neovascularization (rather than diffuse erythema) that progresses from pink to purplish-red. The skin is not warm to the touch (hence "cold" inflammation). The skin becomes thinned and parchment-like, and eventually the node spontaneously suppurates after several months. Generalized adenopathy does not exist and chest radiographs are normal. A diagnosis may be difficult, but is suggested if reaction to a 5 U dose of PPD-tuberculin is between 5 mm and 10 mm of induration. A definitive diagnosis rests solely with isolation of the infecting organism. These infections have a low risk of communicability and generally do not respond to drug therapy alone. Most of the literature favors surgical excision of the infected nodes although some physicians have favored a nonexcisional approach. Isoniazid and rifampin are recommended for *M. tuberculosis* infection. Acquired toxoplasmosis most frequently presents as painless, asymptomatic cervical lymphadenopathy. Although nearly two thirds of patients have a single site of involvement, multiple sites, including the axillary and inguinal regions, may be infected. Patients with cervical adenopathy and toxoplasma infection usually have posterior triangle involvement and no associated symptoms or only mild symptoms as fever, malaise, myalgia, sore throat, cough, and anorexia. Splenomegaly, palpable only a few centimeters below the costal margin, is usually transient. A generalized, nonpruritic, maculopapular rash most marked on the trunk and proximal extremities is also briefly visible. Patients may have leukocytosis with atypical lymphocytes and eosinophils on a peripheral smear. The diagnosis of an active infection is suggested by high titers to toxoplasma as measured by the Sabin–Feldman dye test. A definitive diagnosis rests with biopsy. No specific therapy is recommended for toxoplasma lymphadenitis, although excision may be contemplated if the diagnosis is in doubt.

MALIGNANT TUMORS

Over 25% malignant tumors in children occur in the head and neck, and one of every seven children admitted with a neck mass will have a malignant tumor. For every six children with a malignant tumor of the head and neck, one will have an associated tumor of the nasopharynx. In contrast to adults who frequently develop carcinomas, tumors in children are of mesenchymal origin with lymphoid tumors predominating. The predominant tumor types are Hodgkin's disease, lymphosarcoma, rhabdomyosarcoma, fibrosarcoma, thyroid malignancies, neuroblastoma, and epidermoid carcinoma.

Age is a factor in the type of tumor that may be found. Children under 6 years of age most frequently have neuroblastoma followed by lymphosarcoma, rhabdomyosarcoma, and Hodgkin's disease. In preadolescent children, Hodgkin's disease and lymphosarcoma occur with almost equal frequency whereas thyroid cancers and rhabdomyosarcomas follow. In adolescents, Hodgkin's disease is the most frequent malignant tumor of the head and neck.

Hodgkin's disease and lymphosarcoma comprise 55% of malignant tumors of the head and neck in children. Although lymphosarcoma occurs approximately twice as frequently as Hodgkin's disease, a child with a neck mass has an equal chance of having either disease since Hodgkin's disease presents twice as frequently (80%) with a neck mass as does lymphosarcoma (40%). The mass of Hodgkin's disease is often painless, slowly enlarging, unilateral (80%), and firm. It is usually located in the upper one third of the neck, although if supraclavicular nodes are involved, a mediastinal tumor is usually found as well. Approximately 6% of patients may present with preauricular adenopathy simulating parotid swelling or even cat-scratch disease. Usually children over 5 years of age are afflicted with Hodgkin's disease and they have fewer extranodal sites of involvement compared with lymphosarcoma. In contrast, lymphosarcoma is more frequent in the younger patient, and extranodal sites such as the tonsils are up to four times more frequently involved than in Hodgkin's disease. Nodes are painless, rubbery, and discrete.

A rare benign condition that may confused with a lymphoid malignancy is sinus histiocytosis, a syndrome of massive, bilateral, painless cervical adenopathy occurring usually in blacks. Fever, leukocytosis with neutrophilia, elevated erythrocyte sedimentation rate, and diffuse hypergammaglobulinemia commonly occur. Adenopathy may persist for months to years before gradual spontaneous resolution occurs. Lymph nodes can be distinguished histologically from lymphomatous conditions. The etiology is unknown, and the disease may recur.

Rhabdomyosarcoma accounts for about 10% of malignancies involving the head and neck and represents the most common solid tumor occurring in this region. It presents usually as a painless mass virtually at any site and symptoms depend on the involved organ. The nasopharynx, middle ear, mastoid, and orbit are common sites of occurrence.

Fibrosarcoma and neurofibrosarcoma may present as a painless mass arising from the cheek, jaw, nose, or sinuses. They occur with half the frequency of rhabdomyosarcomas and have a low tendency to metastasize.

Thyroid nodules occur infrequently in children, but when they do, they have nearly an 80% chance of being malignant. This is particularly true if there is a history of radiation to the head or neck. Hence, any thyroid nodule in a child should be considered malignant until proven otherwise. The nodules are generally midline or slightly lateral and are in close proximity to the thyroid gland. Most of the tumors are of the medullary or mixed papillary and follic-

ular types. The prognosis in children with well-differentiated thyroid cancer after lobectomy and node dissection is far better than in other types of childhood cancer.

Although neuroblastoma is the most common solid tumor in childhood, it ranked sixth in frequency of malignancies involving the head and neck. Most neuroblastomas are metastatic from other sites and affect lymph nodes. A metastatic disease can be distinguished from a primary disease because neurologic signs are late occurrences as enlarged nodes impinge on neural structures. Primary neuroblastoma in the neck, on the other hand, has early onset of neurologic symptoms such as Horner syndrome.

Metastatic tumors to cervical nodes other than neuroblastoma must also be considered. They include the leukemias, thyroid malignancies, nasopharyngeal carcinoma, and other tumors that metastasize lymphatic channels.

SYSTEMIC DISORDERS

Systemic disorders may have cervical adenopathy as part of generalized lymph node enlargement. Ususual cases of cervical lymphadenopathy include histoplasmosis and cryptococcosis, although more commonly these fungi cause primary pulmonary infections. Dissemination of these organisms, especially in immune-compromised hosts, may have generalized adenopathy as part of its clinical picture. Immune deficiency syndromes, including various forms of hypogammaglobulinemia, chronic granulomatous disease, hyper IgE syndrome, as well as the acquired immune deficiency syndrome (AIDS) may be associated with enlarged lymph nodes. Nodes may be enlarged from chronic antigenic stimulation, or primary infection, often with opportunistic organisms. Lymph node enlargement can also be seen with hyperthyroidism. Sarcoidosis is virtually always associated with bilateral cervical node enlargement and may also have generalized adenopathy. Over 80% of cases will have scalene node involvement. Hilar adenopathy and other parenchymal changes on chest radiograph can also be found. Autoimmune disorders, such as systemic lupus erythematosis and juvenile rheumatoid arthritis, often exhibit lymphadenopathy during active disease. Hemolytic anemias have occasionally been associated with recurrent, nontender enlarged nodes during bouts of hemolysis. Phenytoin administration has occasionally caused generalized adenopathy, usually preceded by other signs of hypersensitivity such as fever, rash, jaundice, and eosinophilia. Other drugs such as hydralazine and allopurinol have also been implicated in causing adenopathy. Kawasaki syndrome has cervical lymphadenopathy as part of its diagnostic criteria, although nodal enlargement may occur in only 50% of white patients. Other features of Kawasaki syndrome include prolonged fever; nonpurulent conjunctivitis; extremity changes with edema, erythema, or peeling of skin; rash; and oral mucosal involvement with strawberry tongue or dry and cracked lips. Tularemia and syphilis are rare causes of cervical adenopathy.

EVALUATION AND MANAGEMENT OF THE CHILD WITH A NECK MASS

A detailed history and physical examination is mandatory in the evaluation of every child with a neck mass, and in most cases may be the only eval-uation necessary. Laboratory examinations, if indicated, should be tailored to the individual case. Visual recognition is often sufficient to diagnose certain congenital lesions. It is not necessary to identify the causative agent in infectious lymphadenitis in all cases, especially when signs and symptoms are typical for viral adenopathy or if the patient responds to empirical antibiotic therapy when bacterial adenitis is suspected. Children who present with an unusual or persistent disease, or who have progression of symptoms, may require a further evaluation and perhaps an excisional biopsy. A thorough examination of the ears, nose, and throat, especially when a malignancy is suspected, is particularly important. The algorithm on chronic lymph node enlargement has been constructed to help work through common diagnostic possibilities (Fig. 90-1). This algorithm excludes congenital and acute inflammatory neck masses and

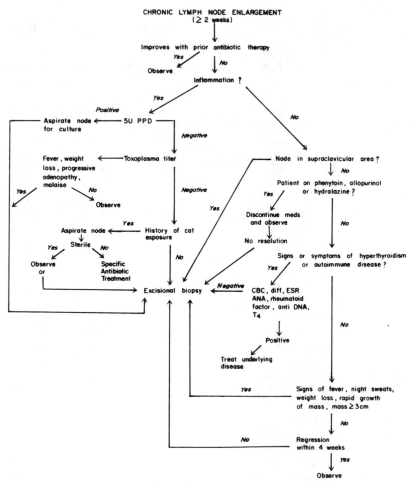

Figure 90-1.   The work-up of a child with a chronic lymph node enlargement.

is by no means all inclusive, but it provides a framework to evaluate the most dreaded diagnostic possibilities and offers suggestions such as when to biopsy the mass.

In general, a simple and directed laboratory evaluation provides the greatest yield. A complete blood count and differential, a heterophil test or titers to Epstein–Barr virus, CMV, and toxoplasma may be helpful when indicated. A chest radiograph may help determine mediastinal or pulmonary parenchymal disease. An aspiration of infected, fluctuant nodes will often identify the offending organism, and when coupled with antibiotics may be sufficient therapy for small abscesses. Large, fluctuant nodes usually require an incision and drainage. Node aspiration generally does not lead to a chronic draining fistula, except perhaps with inadequately treated infections or nodes chronically infected with mycobacteria, cat scratch, or *F. tularensis*. Acutely inflamed, fluctuant nodes rarely represent a tumor. Hence, there is almost no risk of spreading metastases by aspiration. Nodes minimally inflamed and fluctuant due to tumor necrosis may be aspirated by a direct approach that minimizes the length of the tract that may later have to be resected. A standardized 5 U PPD may be helpful in identifying mycobacterial infections, and routine serologic data might help identify an underlying autoimmune disorder.

The decision to biopsy a lesion or excise a node frequently confronts the clinician caring for a child with a neck mass. Supraclavicular lymph nodes are associated with a malignancy or a granulomatous disease involving the mediastinum and should be biopsied early in the evaluation. Other clinical features suggesting serious disease leading to early biopsy include a persistent fever or weight loss, a fixation of the node to the skin and underlying tissues. An abnormal chest radiograph is strongly associated with a granulomatous disease or a malignant peripheral lymphadenopathy. Biopsies may yield specific diagnoses in 37% to 63% of cases. Approximately one in five patients with normal histology, reactive hyperplasia, or atypical inflammation will have a specific diagnosis identified on a subsequent biopsy. In one series, patients who subsequently developed lymphoma usually had the disease diagnosed within 8 months of the first biopsy. This strongly suggests that despite a nondiagnostic initial biopsy, patients who have a persistent disease or adenopathy should be monitored closely, and a second biopsy should be considered if the clinical picture changes.

ANNOTATED BIBLIOGRAPHY

Barton LL, Feigin RD: Childhood cervical lymphadenitis: A reappraisal. J Pediatr 84:846–852, 1974 (Lymph node aspirates yielded *Staphylococcus aureus* and *Streptococcus pyogenes* as primary bacterial pathogens.)

Brook I: Aerobic and anaerobic bacteriology of cervical adenitis in children. Clin Pediatr 10:693–696, 1980 (Emphasizes the role of anaerobic organisms in infectious cervical adenitis. Anaerobic organisms were isolated in 38% of lymph node aspirates and were the sole pathogen isolated in 18%.)

Jaffe BF, Jaffe N: Head and neck tumors in children. Pediatrics 51:731–740, 1975 (Excellent review of 178 children with head and neck tumors presenting within a 10-year period.)

Kissane JM, Gephardt GN: Lymphadenopathy in childhood. Hum Pathol 5:431–439, 1974 (Retrospective review of 100 node biopsies, stating that 17% of patients with initial nondiagnostic biopsies eventually developed serious systemic disease.)

Knight PJ, Reiner CB: Superficial lumps in children: What, when, and why? Pediatrics 72:147–153, 1983 (Reviews the causes of palpable masses that were excised during an 11-year period. Reviews criteria indicative of high risk for malignancies.)

Lake AM, Oski FA: Peripheral lymphadenopathy in childhood. Am J Dis Child 132:357–359, 1978 (Reviews a 10-year experience with excisional biopsy and emphasizes the need for continued follow-up.)

Marcy SM: Infections of lymph nodes of the head and neck. Pediatr Infect Dis 2:397–405, 1983 (Excellent review and listing of infectious causes of lymphadenopathy; reviews approach to diagnosis and therapy.)

May M: Neck masses in children: Diagnosis and treatment. Pediatr Ann 5:517–535, 1976 (Excellent comprehensive review of neck masses, with many pictures and tables; superb clinical article.)

Saitz EW: Cervical lymphadenitis caused by atypical mycobacteria. Pediatr Clin North Am 28(4):823–839, 1981 (Excellent review of atypical mycobacterial adenitis and suggests a nonexcisional approach to therapy.)

Zuelzer WW, Kaplan J: The child with lymphadenopathy. Semin Hematol 12:323–334, 1975 (Classic review of both cervical and generalized lymphadenopathy in children.)

12

Ophthalmic Problems

91
Visual Testing

HENRY S. METZ

Visual testing is related directly to the age of the child being tested. As a rule, the younger the child, the more objective and less quantitative the test must be. It should be remembered that it may not be possible to get the full amount of information desired about the visual system because of infancy, developmental delay, or the presence of coexisting motor or sensory handicaps. The aim of visual testing in a child should be to get the maximum information possible. Visual testing machines offer no advantage over the considerably less expensive eye occluder and visual testing chart.

Visual acuity screening can, and should, be done on all children by the age of 3 to 3½ years old. At an earlier age, behavioral clues, such as an objection to occluding one eye during the cover test, should alert the pediatrician to investigate further or to make a referral. A Snellen chart is adequate in older children.

I believe that a specific screening test for hyperopia is unnecessary. Farsightedness often produces no problems and frequently does not require treatment. Moderate to high hyperopia will manifest itself with esotropia and symptoms of "eye strain" which, in either case, would warrant a detailed examination.

VISUAL ACUITY

- *Observation*—The examiner can often estimate a child's visual ability by observation. Does the child take an interest in his surroundings? Does the infant grasp for objects? Unsteady or wandering eye movements are a sign of subnormal vision. Parents can usually tell if their child has useful sight or behaves as if blind.

Observation of the pupillary response to light can also be useful. An active response indicates that light is able to reach the retina, the optic nerve is functioning, and the visual pathway is intact at least as far back as the full length of the optic tract.

- *Fixation*—Fixation with each eye can be determined using a colorful toy. A noisy toy can be used first to gain attention, and a silent toy substituted later in the test. Central, steady, and maintained fixation suggests good vision whereas unsteady fixation (*e.g.*, nystagmus or wandering movements) suggests reduced vision.
- *Following*—The ability to easily and smoothly follow an object of interest is evidence of at least moderate acuity. Caution should be used in interpreting the response of developmentally delayed youngsters to fixation and following tasks, as they may have little interest and thus appear visually deficient.
- *Optokinetic Nystagmus*—An optokinetic drum or tape can be rotated horizontally or vertically before the child's eyes. Nystagmus elicited in response to this stimulus indicates that the stripes on the drum or squares on the tape can be seen. Although this estimation of vision is gross, it is an objective measure and requires little cooperation or interest.
- *Allen Cards*—Before children can recognize numbers, letters, or symbols, they may be able to identify certain pictures. The Allen Cards have pictures of well-known items (*e.g.*, telephone,

410

tree, house) that can usually be recognized by 2½- to 3-year-olds. The pictures are of equal size (the size of a 20/30 letter), and the examiner moves further and further away until the picture can not longer be identified correctly. The furthest distance (in feet) that the card can be recognized is the numerator of the acuity fraction with a denominator of 30 (*e.g.*, 10/30).

- *HOTV, "E" or "C"*—The HOTV test requires the youngster to differentiate these four letters. Once this can be done, an acuity chart with these characters is used to test vision, usually at 10 ft or 20 ft. The "E" or "C" requires the child to point his finger in the same direction as the "finger" of the "E" or the opening of the "C" (up, down, left, or right). This game can be taught by parents at home prior to the doctor's examination. Charts are available to measure vision with these figures.

- *Letters or Numbers*—Once a child can read letters or numbers, acuity can easily be determined. Vision may normally be in the 20/30 to 20/40 range at age 3 or 4, and subjectively improves to 20/20 by the age of 6 or 7. Interest and cooperation are both necessary to obtain optimum visual acuity. *A difference between eyes of 2 lines or more is as important as the absolute level of acuity.*

- *Visual Evoked Response (VER), Preferential Looking*—Both techniques are in the investigative stage, but may provide an opportunity for a more quantitative visual evaluation within the first few months of life. In the VER (an objective test), a flash or an alternating black and white checker board pattern is presented. The evoked electrical response from the visual cortex is averaged and a tracing is produced that may be able to give information about acuity (without requiring fixation or accommodation for the flash stimulus). With preferential looking, the infant is presented with two disks, one gray and the other with a black and white striped pattern. In judging which disk the infant looks at, an estimate of acuity can be made as the stripe pattern is made thinner.

VISUAL FIELDS

Testing the visual field provides a measure of peripheral vision, rather than central (fovea-macular) vision. It cannot be performed in infants, although it may be estimated in young children and quantitated in older children. Visual field testing may be particularly useful in patients with suspected neurologic problems.

- *Threatening Gesture*—A threatening gesture made by a hand or finger, approaching from the periphery, can give a gross indication if vision is present in one quadrant or one half of the visual field. This should be performed one eye at a time, with the other eye being covered. The gesture should not frighten the infant, but provide only a momentary startle reaction.

- *Confrontation Fields*—The child is asked to maintain fixation straight ahead (on the examiner's eye or nose). The examiner then moves a finger in from the periphery, wiggles a finger, or asks the youngster to count the number of fingers being held up in a peripheral quadrant of the field. Although a qualitative test, quadrantic and hemianopic defects may be uncovered. This technique can prove useful between the ages of 4 and 7.

- *Tangent Screen, Perimeter*—Instrument testing of the visual field provides quantitative, reproducible measurements. The tangent screen measures the central 30° field with the blind spot, while the perimeter provides information about the peripheral field, out to 70° to 75° temporally, with a less detailed blind spot. With younger children (aged 7 to 8), fewer meridians should be investigated, because the child may become fatigued and disinterested, providing unreliable responses.

Computerized visual field testing requires long periods of attention to be performed successfully. Except for motivated teenagers, it should not be considered a procedure for most pediatric patients.

MUSCLE BALANCE

Misalignment of the visual axes, if monocular and not alternating, can cause unilateral reduction of central acuity (amblyopia). Therefore, methods to uncover strabismus are a valuable screening tool.

- *Observation*—If the deviation is large enough, above 12 prism diopters (6°), it can usually be noted by observation alone. An alternating form to strabismus will not result in amblyopia.

- *Light Reflex*—If the child is asked to fixate on a light held by the examiner, the reflex from the light will be seen on the cornea. When the eyes are straight, the reflex will be noted in the center of the pupil of each eye. With strabismus, the light reflex will be centered in one eye and off center in the other.

- *Cover Test*—When one eye is covered, the other eye is observed. If it does not move, the uncovered eye was straight. If it does move, the uncovered eye shows a deviation. The cover test is performed on each eye separately. Any objection to covering one eye and not the opposite one suggests reduced vision.

The random dot E is a test of binocularity by measuring stereo vision. Since some youngsters appreciate stereo targets easily while others do not, there is a relatively high false-positive response that makes the test of questionable acceptability

92
Visual Disturbances
HENRY S. METZ

Young children who have eye disease rarely complain. An abnormality can be determined by appearance or poor function. When only one eye is impaired, no behavioral difficulties may be noted. Only an examination of visual ability will uncover this abnormality.

Since one eye may have reduced vision while the other is normal, the eyes must be tested separately. An exception to this rule would be the patient who has latent nystagmus, which only becomes manifest when one eye is covered. With both eyes open, fixation is steady and acuity is improved.

An early diagnosis is important, as some conditions cannot be treated after a certain age. It is useful if children are examined by age 3. With a family history of eye disease (congenital cataracts, strabismus), an evaluation by 1 year of age is indicated.

PATHOPHYSIOLOGY

The eye functions much like a camera. Parallel light rays from the image are refracted by the cornea. The light then passes through the aqueous humor in the anterior chamber and is refracted by the lens. The light passes through the vitreous and stimulates the retina (inverted, as in a camera).

For the image to reach the retina undisturbed, the transparent media of the eye (*i.e.*, cornea, aqueous humor, lens, vitreous) must be clear. Opacification will impair sight (*e.g.*, corneal scar, cataract, vitreous hemorrhage).

When the image is in focus in front of the retina, the picture on the retina will be unclear. The eye is myopic (nearsighted): This can be caused by a large eye or a strong optical focusing system (lens, cornea).

When the image is in focus behind the retina, the picture will also be unclear. The eye is hyperopic (farsighted). This may be caused by a small eye or a weak optical focusing system.

If the corneal front surface or the anterior curvature of the lens is not spherical, the image will not be in focus in a single plane and will therefore not be in focus on the plane of the retina, resulting in blurred vision. This is astigmatism and can exist alone or with myopia or hyperopia.

When the image reaches the retina, a signal is initiated that travels down the optic nerve, chiasm, and optic tracts to the geniculate body. There is hemidecussation of the nerve fibers in the chiasm as information from the temporal hemiretina remains ipsilateral while that from the nasal hemiretina crosses to the opposite side. Thus, unilateral visual field defects must be due to prechiasmal pathology. From the geniculate body, the signal goes to the optic radiations and then to the visual cortex in the occipital lobe. Chiasmal and postchiasmal lesions result in bilateral field abnormalities and may be hemi- or quadrantanopic in character. As a rule, the more symmetrical the field deficit, the more posterior the pathology.

CLINICAL PRESENTATION

Complaints

Young children often do not complain. If pain is a symptom, the youngster may rub the eye. If there is light sensitivity, increased tearing and avoidance of light or squinting may be noted. When the child is older, decreased vision or discomfort may be a complaint. It is not unusual for the first indication of subnormal acuity to be noted at a school examination.

Decreased Visual Acuity

During infancy, the best estimate of vision is derived from behavior. Are targets of interest (faces, toys) fixated steadily and followed? Is reaching observed for near objects? Does the child act as if his sight is normal? Specific tests can be performed as the child grows older (see Chap. 91). The Allen cards, HOTV test, "E" game, and Snellen charts are all useful to quantitate visual ability. Acuity should be essentially equal in each eye. An objection to covering one eye or a decreased performance on any of the aforementioned tests with one eye is abnormal. By age 3 or 4, acuity is usually at the 20/30 level while at age 6, it has often reached 20/20. Squinting, which creates a pinhole aperture effect, suggests the presence of an uncorrected refractive error.

Abnormal Face or Head Position

A child holding his face or head in an abnormal position may be an indication of an eye problem. If the null position of nystagmus (location of the smallest amplitude eye movement) is not in straight ahead gaze, a head turn may be used to allow maximum visual acuity. A head or face position to allow fusion may be noted when strabismus with diplopia is present in the primary position. A superior oblique palsy might present with a head tilt to the opposite shoulder, whereas a lateral rectus palsy would show a face turn to the same side as the palsy (Fig. 92-1).

Findings

A loss of corneal transparency reduces vision. Blood (hyphema) or white cells (hypopyon) in the anterior chamber can result from trauma or inflammation. A white pupil may be due to cataract, ocular tumor, persistent hyperplastic primary vitreous, or retrolental fibroplasia. A clear lens with loss of the normal "red reflex" from the fundus can be caused by vitreous opacification due to vitreous hemorrhage or infection.

A lack of parallel alignment of the visual axes (strabismus) will often be noted if the angle of deviation is greater than 6° (about 12 prism diopters). The turn may be inward (esotropia), outward (exotropia), upward (hypertropia), or downward (hypotropia). Upper lid ptosis may accompany strabismus in some patients or may be noted as an independent finding. A decreased range of ocular motility may be seen in some congenital conditions (Duane's or Brown's syndrome) or as a result of muscle palsy. Abnormal or wandering eye move-

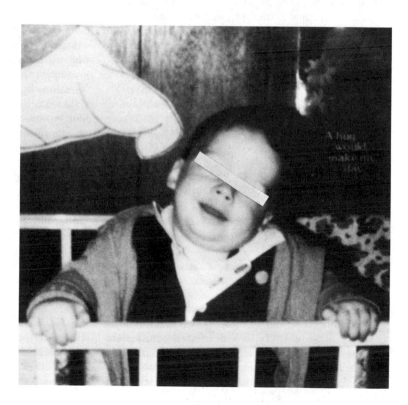

Figure 92-1. Habit head tilt to the left shoulder caused by a right superior oblique muscle palsy.

ments (nystagmus, opsoclonus) suggest reduced vision.

Proptosis of the globe is often an indicator of an orbital tumor, and thyroid ophthalmopathy is infrequent in the pediatric age group. Orbital inflammatory disease can also produce proptosis.

Conjunctival injection accompanied by discharge and tearing suggests conjunctivitis. If the engorgement of vessels is localized at the limbus (corneoscleral junction) with increased light sensitivity, iritis may be responsible. Corneal abrasions, foreign bodies, or ulcers will also produce photophobia.

If the cornea is enlarged and hazy, congenital glaucoma is likely. When an enlarged cornea is clear, congenital megalocornea is a possible etiology. A small cornea is often seen with a small globe (micro-ophthalmia) and vision is usually subnormal.

The pupillary light response is usually a good indicator of optic nerve function. The lack of a brisk or equal direct response may indicate an optic nerve or optic tract lesion or, occasionally, an efferent defect involving the motor fibers of the third nerve to the pupillary sphincter.

Fundus abnormalities are best seen with the binocular, indirect ophthalmoscope in the pediatric patient. Optic nerve abnormalities, choroidal colobomas, retinal tumors, chorioretinitis, and retinopathy of prematurity should alert the practitioner to a need for further follow-up and care.

DIFFERENTIAL DIAGNOSIS

Refractive Errors

These are common and may not fit the designation "abnormality." Vision can be improved by optical means. The trial of a pinhole aperture, which will improve acuity when the blur is due to a refractive error, is a quick and easy method to rule out more serious pathology.

Amblyopia

Amblyopia (lazy eye), reduced vision without an organic cause, can result from strabismus, anisometropia (and ametropia), or deprivation. Strabismus leads to amblyopia when unilateral and not alternating. The lack of daily, foveal fixation of the strabismic eye leads to a decreased acuity. Anisometropia, unequal refractive error in the two eyes, also reduces vision. It is due to a poorly focused image in one eye over time during early childhood. Deprivation causes the most severe form of amblyopia and may be due to cataract, ptosis, corneal opacification, or vitreous hemorrhage. Prolonged, continuous therapeutic patching of one eye can also cause deprivation amblyopia (see Chap. 99).

Trauma

Blunt trauma will often lead to ecchymoses of the lids and a subconjunctival hemorrhage. If severe, a hyphema may be noted, the orbital floor may be fractured (with possible vertical diplopia and limitation of vertical gaze), and macular edema can be seen along with scattered retinal hemorrhages. Less severe trauma may include corneal abrasions and lid and corneal foreign bodies. These are accompanied by increased tearing and conjuctival injection. Fluorescein staining generally demonstrates the defect.

Penetrating trauma is serious and threatens vision permanently. The anterior chamber may be collapsed and the globe filled with blood. Endophthalmitis secondary to infection is often catastrophic (see Chap. 97).

Infection and Inflammation

Superficial infections of the lids and conjunctiva usually present with conjunctival redness and discharge or crusting (see Chap. 93). Corneal infiltration or ulceration, appearing as a localized opacity, is more serious. Iritis is accompanied by perilimbal injection, light sensitivity, and, at times, reduced vision. Prolonged or recurrent anterior segment inflammation can lead to cataract formation.

Chorioretinitis often appears yellowish-white and may be accompanied by haze in the vitreous (vitritis). Longstanding, quiet foci are usually well circumscribed with a pigmented margin. White sclera shows through with localized areas of destruction of the retina and choroid. The causes include, but are not limited to, toxoplasmosis, lues, herpes simplex, toxocara canis, tuberculosis, and cytomegalic inclusion virus. Orbital cellulitis usually presents with proptosis, lid swelling, fever, and decreased ocular motility.

Congenital Abnormalities

An iris coloboma is seen as a defect at the 6 o'clock position of the iris and, by itself, may cause no functional difficulties. When associated with a choroidal or optic disk coloboma, there is a superior field defect and reduced vision if the macula is involved. Aniridia (absence of most of the iris) is associated with secondary glaucoma.

Congenital glaucoma may be noted soon after birth or in infancy. With increased intraocular pressure, the globe becomes enlarged and the cornea hazy. There is light sensitivity, increased tearing, and eventually optic nerve cupping.

Leukocoria (white pupil) has several causes. A congenital cataract will impair vision and will lead to deprivation amblyopia. The persistence of the hyperplastic primary vitreous will result in a white or gray pupillary reflex as will Coat's disease (an exudative retinopathy), retrolental fibroplasia (the end stage of cicatricial retinopathy or prematurity), retinoblastoma, a large choroidal coloboma, and nematode endophthalmitis (see Chap. 101).

Hypoplasia (or aplasia) of the optic nerve will cause reduced visual function. The optic nerve head will appear small and a scleral ring may be seen around the disk. This ring should not be confused with the true nerve head.

Tumors

Retinoblastoma is the most common childhood ocular malignancy. It usually presents with leukocoria and strabismus (Fig. 92-2), but may appear as an endophthalmitis with hypopyon. Calcium is usually found on x-ray studies and the family history may be positive.

Rhabdomyosarcoma is the most serious orbital tumor in the pediatric age group. It presents with sudden proptosis, decreased ocular motility, and often progresses rapidly, not infrequently leading to death. Dermoid tumors, lymphangiomas, and cavernous hemangiomas of the orbit should also be considered with proptosis in children.

Capillary hemangiomas of the lids are unsightly, but they generally improve with time. They are a problem when they are large enough to cover the visual axis, because deprivation amblyopia may result.

Vascular

The most common ocular vascular diseases of adults, diabetic retinopathy and hypertensive and arteriosclerotic vasular changes, are not seen in the pediatric population. Retinopathy of prematurity is common in infants with a birth weight under 1200 grams, and it is almost invariably present with a birth weight under 1000 grams. The peripheral retina is avascular and a demarcation line or arteriovenous ridge may be noted. If progression occurs, extraretinal vascularization is noted that can lead to traction on the peripheral retina and, finally, a localized and complete retinal detachment with cicatricial changes and blindness.

CNS Abnormalities

The eyes may appear normal, but visual function can be diminished. Field defects may be present and reduced acuity noted by behavioral clues or measurements. Wandering or jerky eye movements are evidence of decreased vision. Other neurological abnormalities can accompany the visual dysfunction, and strabismus, limited ocular motility and ptosis may be noted. An abnormal pupillary light reflex and optic atrophy are sometimes found. Papilledema is an indicator of increased intracranial pressure.

WORK-UP

History

A history should be obtained first, either from a parent or the patient, if sufficiently verbal and knowledgeable. Questions concerning the major

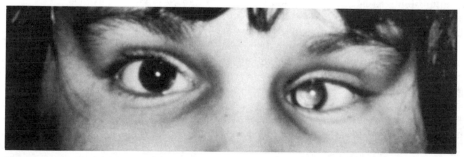

Figure 92-2. Retinoblastoma in the left eye. Leukocoria is present (white pupillary reflex) with a left esotropia.

complaint, the time of onset of symptoms, and the length of time and consistency of the problem should be asked. What has been the previous treatment and what was the response to this therapy? Is there a family history that is relevant? What is the general health of the child and what medication is presently being used? Are there any known allergies?

Physical Examination

An examination should include an estimate or measurement of visual acuity. On an external inspection, the following aspects would be noted: the appearance of the lids, conjunctiva, cornea, height and equality of the level of the upper lids, lid tumors or swelling, proptosis, injection of the conjunctiva, and localized or generalized changes in corneal transparency. The anterior chamber depth and clarity need to be considered. Pupillary shape, size, equality and reaction to light are easy to examine. The muscle balance findings can be estimated by the light reflex and the cover test. Ocular rotations, using an interesting target, are important. Ophthalmoscopy requires pupillary dilatation with a cycloplegic agent. The direct ophthalmoscope can provide a good look at the posterior pole of the fundus, including the optic disk, macula, surrounding vessels, and retina out to the equator. For more peripheral retina, for an improved stereo view, when eye movements are wandering or nystagmic and in the young child, the binocular indirect ophthalmoscope provides an excellent view.

A part of the eye examination that requires an ophthalmologist is refraction (determination of the optical error of each eye). Retinoscopy is a technique that measures the refractive error in an objective manner, whereas subjective refinement may be performed in older children. New, automated refractors can also be used in children, although not easily in infancy.

A slit lamp biomicroscopic examination of the cornea, anterior chamber, and lens is useful to reveal pathology not easily seen with unaided vision. It is especially helpful to identify flare and cells in the anterior chamber that indicate ocular inflammation.

Intraocular pressure may be difficult to measure except in older, more cooperative children. It can be determined, using a tonometer or estimated using finger palpation of the globe, although this latter method is not very accurate. The range of normal pressure is between 10 mm Hg and 20 mm Hg.

Laboratory Tests

Certain laboratory tests can help in diagnosis. X-ray studies, especially computerized tomography (CT) or magnetic resonance imaging (MRI) can be useful in suspected central nervous system abnormalities, ocular tumors, trauma, and orbital cellulitis. Ultrasound studies are similarly useful and less expensive. A complete blood count, as well as various blood chemistries and a urinalysis can be helpful when systemic disease is a consideration. Culture and sensitivity testing are often not needed for conjunctivitis, but are required in cases of corneal ulcer or endophthalmitis. The electroretinogram (ERG) and electrooculogram (EOG) can provide specific information about retinal nerve cell layer and pigment epithelial cell layer function. The visual evoked response test (VER) can provide useful knowledge about optic nerve function and integrity of the visual cortex. Visual field testing is helpful with suspected neuro-ophthalmic disorders, but can only be done well in the older pediatric patient.

TREATMENT

Optical

The simplest, most frequently prescribed treatment for reduction in visual acuity is an optical correction. This is usually in the form of glasses, although contact lenses have been used for specific problems (unilateral aphakia). A surgical technique called *epikeratophakia*, which involves sewing a preserved button of cornea on to the front surface of the child's cornea for optical purposes, has been tried, but it is too early to evaluate the success of this surgery. Myopia, hyperopia, astigmatism, and anisometropia are best treated with glasses or contact lenses.

Patching

Patching treatment for strabismic and deprivation amblyopia remains the most successful modality (Fig. 92-3). Some parents believe that patching cures strabismus, as the uncovered eye (the habitually deviating eye) appears straight. They think that patching will lead to a parallel ocular alignment and that no further treatment will be necessary. This is untrue, and it is necessary to remind parents that patching only treats the amblyopia, not the deviation.

Anti-infective Agents

Superficial ocular infections can be treated by the topical application of antibiotics, either solution or ointment, to the lids and conjunctiva. In patients

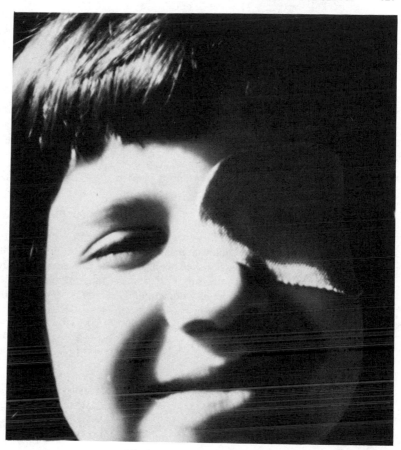

Figure 92-3. Patch over left eye.

with bacterial corneal ulcers or intraocular infection, injection into the subtenon's space has been used as well as intravitreal injection. The systemic route is useful for orbital cellulitis and endophthalmitis and in cases of penetrating ocular trauma.

Topical antiviral agents are useful for herpes simplex keratitis, but systemic use of these agents has not been found beneficial. The local instillation of antifungal agents can be helpful in culture-proven cases of fungal corneal ulcer.

Decongestants and Artificial Tears

Topical ocular decongestants are used for mild eye irritations or allergic reactions. Artificial tears assist the patient with dry eyes, although this is infrequent in children.

Corticosteroids

A mild concentration steroid eye drop is helpful in allergic conjunctivitis that is not responsive to decongestants. Iritis requires the use of more potent topical preparations, usually with cycloplegic agents. Topical steroids are contraindicated in herpes simplex keratitis, which often presents with a dendritic, branching pattern, enhanced by fluorescein staining. An intralesional injection of steroid can be used to treat large hemangiomas of the lid. Systemic steroids are indicated for an orbital pseudotumor and may be prescribed in conjuction with antibiotics in cases of orbital cellulitis. They can also be helpful in thyroid ophthalmopathy in children. The prolonged use of corticosteroids (in topical or systemic form) can cause both cataract and glaucoma; thus, this medication should be used for specific indications and for the minimum amount of time required.

Surgery

Surgery to correct strabismus is the most common ophthalmologic procedure in the pediatric population. An initial operation has a 70% to 75% success rate and may have to be repeated. Cataracts that significantly interfere with vision require early surgery to prevent deprivation amblyopia. Penetrating trauma to the globe must be repaired immediately, while orbital fractures may safely wait several days. Ptosis surgery can be done prior to entering school, unless the ptosis is so severe that the visual axis is occluded causing deprivation amblyopia. Advanced retinoblastoma generally requires enucleation, although early cases and some patients with bilateral involvement have been successfully treated with external beam irradiation, cobalt plaques, and laser therapy. Cryotherapy of peripheral, avascular retina has been tried in progressing stages of retinopathy of prematurity, but results are not yet known. Orbital rhabdomyosarcoma requires orbital exenteration to prevent spread. Goniotomy and trabeculotomy have been successfully used to treat congenital glaucoma, although repeat surgery is not uncommon. Corneal transplant operations are occasionally done in children and retinal detachment repair can be used when needed. Probing for nasolacrimal duct obstruction can relieve tearing.

INDICATIONS FOR REFERRAL

Visual Acuity

When acuity is less than 20/30 in each eye or when there is a two line difference in acuity between eyes, a referral is indicated. In the infant, young or uncooperative child, poor fixation or objection to covering one eye more than the other suggests the need for a further evaluation.

Ocular Alignment and Movements

Strabismus, at any age, deserves referral as does nystagmus. An inability to rotate one or both eyes normally should be investigated (see Chap. 98).

Pupil

Although small differences in pupil size may be physiologic, differences in response to light and accommodation are not. A pupil that is not round is unusual. A loss of the red reflex demands immediate attention.

Tearing and Light Sensitivity

Increased tearing may indicate nasolacrimal duct obstruction or congenital glaucoma and deserves attention. Sensitivity to light can also be seen in congenital glaucoma but may suggest iritis. Both conditions benefit by early recognition and treatment (see Chap. 100).

Corneal Changes

Abnormally large or small corneas, or those with a conical shape (keratoconus), can degrade vision. Opacification and vascularization can similarly reduce acuity and deserve ophthalmologic referral.

Conjunctiva

An elevated or enlarging mass should be studied. Redness, discharge, and crusting suggest external infection. An attempt can be made to treat these findings with broad spectrum, topical antibiotics. If no improvement is noted after a short time, an ophthalmologic opinion is useful.

Lids

Ptosis may be unilateral or bilateral. A referral is indicated, as it is for lumps of the lid (tumors or chalazia), lid malposition (entropion—lid margin turned inward or ectropion—lid margin turned outward), or lid coloboma.

Vitreous

Opacity of the vitreous results in loss of the red reflex and reduced vision. It can be due to blood or inflammatory debris in the vitreous and requires ophthalmologic consultation.

Retina

Although scattered retinal hemorrhages may be noted after birth, they are usually transient. Chorioretinitis, coloboma, detachment, retinopathy of prematurity, a retinal mass, or a falciform fold should all be referred.

Optic Nerve

Optic atrophy as well as papilledema deserve both an ophthalmologic as well as a neurologic evaluation. Aplastic or hypoplastic disks and cupping of the disk (especially if unilateral) require consultation.

Orbit

Proptosis may be indicative of an orbital tumor or of orbital cellulitis. Both can be life threatening and may require the help of an ophthalmologist as well as a neurosurgeon, an otolaryngologist, and an infectious disease consultant (see Chap. 95).

ANNOTATED BIBLIOGRAPHY

Gardiner PA: Vision in Children. New York, Appleton–Century–Crofts, 1982 (Vision problems in children are reviewed in a complete and understandable way. Good discussion of function and structure of visual system.)

Harley RD: Pediatric Ophthalmology, 2nd ed. Philadelphia, WB Saunders, 1983 (Encyclopedic work that is complete and well indexed. Good as a reference source on any topic.)

Helveston EM, Ellis FD: Pediatric Ophthalmology Practice. St. Louis, CV Mosby, 1980 (Written in an atlas format, this book has excellent photographs and line drawings with a good explanatory text.)

Metz HS, Rosenbaum A: Pediatric Ophthalmology—Medical Outline Series. Garden City, NY, Medical Examination Publishing Co, 1982 (Multiauthored text reviewing the major fields in pediatric ophthalmology. Written with the pediatrician and family physician in mind.)

Nelson LB, Brown GC, Arentsen JJ: Recognizing Patterns of Ocular Childhood Diseases. Thorofare, NJ, Slack and Co, 1985 (Ocular disease patterns in children are outlined in a succinct, lucid manner. Good as an easy reference source, but is not encyclopedic.)

93

Conjunctivitis

LEONARD B. NELSON AND ROBERT A. CATALANO

Conjunctival infections and inflammations are common in the pediatric population. Fortunately, few causes of conjunctivitis are severe enough to threaten vision. Therapy is often available to ameliorate symptoms and shorten the duration of clinical disease. Inappropriate therapy, however, can cause iatrogenic exacerbations and complications. This chapter will discuss the primary conjunctival disorders seen in children. Ophthalmia neonatorum is discussed in Chapter 94 and eyelid infections are discussed in Chapter 96.

PATHOPHYSIOLOGY

The conjunctiva is a thin, transparent mucous membrane that covers the globe and inner surface of the eyelids. Conjunctival epithelium is nonkeratinized. Normal flora of the eyelid margins continually spills into the tears helping to inhibit epithelial colonization by pathogenic organisms. The tears also contain lysozyme, lactoferrin, interferon, IgG, and secretory IgA. Conjunctival goblet cells produce mucin that entraps exogenous agents including microorganisms. Langerhans cells process antigens and initiate the immunologic reaction.

The first sign of conjunctival inflammation is hyperemia. The hyperemia may be localized under a foreign body or diffuse as in most conjunctivitis. Intraocular inflammations such as uveitis and acute glaucoma often cause hyperemia of the tissues of the globe itself with secondary dilatation of the overlying conjunctival vessels. It is important to ascertain the primary site of inflammation. The conjunctival vessels over the globe are fine and reticulated and bright red when inflamed. Vessels within the substance of the globe do not move with the conjunctiva; they tend to run radially from the cornea; and they are a darker violaceous color with intraocular inflammation.

Lymphatic tissue is normally present in the conjunctiva overlying the globe and in the fornix. In viral and chlamydial infections, lymphoid germinal centers called follicles may become prominent. They are yellowish to grayish white elevated avascular nodules varying between 0.2 mm to 2.0 mm in diameter.

Inflammation of the conjunctiva lining the upper eyelid is seen as regular pinkish elevations called *papillae*. They do not contain lymphoid germinal centers and each usually has a central vessel in contrast to the reticulated vascular supply seen at the base of follicles. They are usually smaller than follicles, except in vernal and giant papillary conjunctivitis, and are typically seen in atopic conditions.

The discharge seen in conjunctivitis is a mixture of transudated fluid, inflammatory cells, desquamated epithelial cells, mucin, and tears. Allergic and viral diseases usually have a watery discharge whereas a purulent discharge is characteristic of an acute bacterial infection. In certain acute conjunctival reactions, the accumulation of fibrin and inflammatory cells can result in the formation of a pseudomembrane in the cul-de-sac. Pseudomembranes are easily removed by swabbing without inducing bleeding. More chronic conjunctival reactions can lead to adherence of the coagulin to the epithelium and the proliferation of blood vessels to form a true membrane that bleeds upon scraping. Pseudomembranes and membranes are seen in bacterial (diphtheritic and streptococcal), viral (adenoviral), atopic (vernal), and chemical conjunctivitis as well as in the Stevens–Johnson syndrome.

CLINICAL PRESENTATION

Atopic Conjunctivitis

Allergic conjunctivitis is manifest by itching, redness, and swelling of the lids and conjunctiva (chemosis). It is chronic and recurrent and tends to wax and wane with or without treatment. Conjunctivitis associated with hay fever is an immediate type I hypersensitivity to airborne antigens resulting in mast cell degranulation and increased conjunctival vessel permeability.

Inflammation of the conjunctiva may also accompany *atopic dermatitis*. Conjunctival signs include chemosis, hyperemia, and papillae associated with itching. In some patients the conjunctiva may appear distinctly pale, smooth, or velvety. More typically, however, these patients are prone to develop crusting of the eyelid margins associated with a superimposed staphylococcal infection.

Giant papillary conjunctivitis (GPC) is associated with contact lenses, foreign bodies, and ocular prostheses. Giant papillae (larger than 1 mm) are seen in the conjunctiva lining the upper eyelid and are associated with erythema, mucous production, and itching.

Vernal conjunctivitis is a bilateral recurrent atopic eye disease occurring mostly in boys. The symptoms are usually worse in the spring and summer. Affected children may also suffer from asthma, eczema, or hay fever. Typically, the conjunctiva of the upper eyelids are affected with large (5 mm to 8 mm) papillae and have a cobblestone appearance. Over 80% of the children have itching and photophobia, and several times a day the child may pull a ropy, tenaceous mucoid strand from under the upper lid. Poorly healing corneal ulcers may occur in more severe cases of vernal conjunctivitis.

Bacterial Conjunctivitis

Bacterial conjunctivitis is characterized by an acute purulent or mucopurulent discharge, foreign body sensation, and matting of the eyelashes. Between the ages of 3 months and 8 years, staphylococcal, pneumococcal, and *Hemophilus* conjunctivitis predominate. *S. aureus* shows no predilection for a seasonal or geographic location whereas pneumococcus is typically seen in colder regions during the winter and *Hemophilus* in warmer areas between May and October. *Hemophilus* is toxogenic and can be accompanied by patchy conjunctival hemorrhages. Streptococcus is an infrequent cause of conjunctivitis, but the organism is invasive and is capable of causing a pseudomembrane.

Most acute bacterial conjunctivitis runs a self-limited course of approximately 10 days, but *Hemophilus* conjunctivitis occasionally can be part of a more ominous periorbital cellulitis that can lead to a bacteremia. *Neisseria* is an aggressively invasive species that can be seen in the neonate or in sexually active adolescents. It is characterized by a rapidly evolving, copiously exudative conjunctivitis associated with marked conjunctival and lid edema that can rapidly lead to corneal perforation and loss of the eye.

Viral Conjunctivitis

Viral conjunctivitis is characterized by a watery discharge, irritation, hyperemia, follicular response, and preauricular adenopathy. In children, adenovirus is the most common pathogen causing both *pharyngoconjunctival fever* (PCF) and *epidemic keratoconjunctivitis* (EKC). An incubation period of 5 to 12 days is typical for both conditions. PCF is characterized by pharyngitis, fever, and follicular conjunctivitis and is self-limited, lasting 4 to 14 days. EKC often shows asymmetric involvement initially and runs a course of 7 to 14 days. It may be accompanied by petechial conjunctival hemorrhages and membrane formation. Severe cases of EKC can involve the cornea with protracted symptoms of photophobia and decreased vision. Children remain infectious for as long as 14 days after the onset and care is necessary to prevent the transmission of this highly contagious pathogen.

Herpes simplex virus infection usually occurs early in life. Primary ocular infection may be subclinical or may present as an acute unilateral follicular conjunctivitis with regional lymphadenopathy, with or without vesicular ulcerative lesions of the eyelids and corneal involvement. The initial infection is usually self-limited but the virus remains latent in the trigeminal ganglion. A recurrent disease typically involves the cornea and is demonstrated by the staining of damaged epithelium by fluorescein dye, classically in a dendritiform pattern.

Molluscum contagiosum usually presents as an umbilicated lesion on the margin of the eyelid and rarely on the conjunctiva. The shedding of the virus onto the conjunctiva can lead to a chronic follicular conjunctivitis requiring surgical excision of the lesion.

Conjunctivitis is a common finding in childhood with *rubella* and *rubeola*, occurring in up to 70%. It is noted concomitantly with the rash and is generally mild. Keratitis is said to occur in all children with measles but is symptomatic in only 50%.

Acute hemorrhagic conjunctivitis is a relatively recently described entity caused by enterovirus 70, which has caused pandemics throughout both hemispheres in the past 15 years. Its incubation period is only 1 to 2 days and the course is short with improvement starting on the third day. It is characterized by a watery discharge, preauricular adenopathy, chemosis, and subconjunctival hemorrhages ranging from small petechiae to large blotches. No serious sequela have been reported.

Chlamydial Infections

Chlamydial organisms produce various disorders depending on the age of the affected individual and subgroup involved. *Neonatal inclusion conjunctivitis* is discussed in Chapters 191 and 195. *"Adult" inclusion conjunctivitis* presents as an acute follicular reaction with a mucopurulent discharge in sexually active young adults. This often evolves into a chronic follicular conjunctivitis. It is associated with cervicitis and urethritis and therefore systemic treatment is indicated. *Trachoma* is the result of repeated chlamydial infections transmitted by vectors, with superimposed bacterial infections. In the early stages, trachoma and inclusion conjunctivitis are similar. In the later stages of trachoma, scaring of the conjunctiva becomes prominent, which leads to eyelid abnormalities and corneal damage.

DIFFERENTIAL DIAGNOSIS

Glaucoma and iritis are the two entities most important to differentiate from conjunctivitis. The distinguishing features of these conditions are noted in Table 93-1.

The prominent signs and symptoms found in the various forms of conjunctivitis are indicated in Table 93-2.

WORK-UP

It is important to ascertain whether a child with a red eye has visual impairment, photophobia, or pain because the answers may help differentiate conjunctivitis from more serious intraocular inflammation.

History

An acute conjunctivitis with significant purulent discharge is typical of bacterial infection. Itching is a prominent sign of allergy. Itching and photophobia in a boy with a personal or family history of atopy and involvement during the summer with a ropy sticky discharge is typical of vernal conjunctivitis. A history of recent exposure to an individual with "pink-eye" or upper respiratory infection is characteristic of viral disease. A chronic mucopu-

Table 93-1. Differential Diagnosis of Red Eyes in Children

	CONJUNCTIVITIS	ACUTE GLAUCOMA	IRITIS
Vision	Normal	Markedly decreased	Decreased
Hyperemia	Superficial; brick-red color	Deep, circumcorneal violaceous color	
Phenylephrine	Blanches vessels	Deep vessels do not blanch	
Pain	Burning/itching	Severe pain	Moderate pain
Eyeball pressure	Normal	Elevated	Normal/reduced
Pupil	Normal	Mid-dilated/fixed	Small ± irregular
Cornea	Normal	Cloudy	Clear; ± precipitates posterior surface

Table 93-2.   Differential Diagnosis of Childhood Conjunctivitis

	ATOPIC	BACTERIAL	VIRAL	CHLAMYDIAL
Discharge	C	Pur	C	Mu/Pur
Cell type	P/Eos	P	M	P/M
Itching	I	−	−	−
Lymphadenopathy	−	−	+	±
Injection	+	+ +	+	+
Hemorrhage	−	+ (H)	+ (A)(E)	−
Chemosis	+	+ +	±	±
Follicles	−	−	+	+
Papillae	+	±	−	±
Pseudomembrane	−	+ (S)	+ (A)	−

C = clear; Pur = purulent; Mu/Pur = mucopurulent; P = polymorphonuclear cells; Eos = eosinophils; M = mononuclear cells; H = *Hemophilus*; A = adenovirus; E = enterovirus 70; S = *Streptococcus pyogenes*

rulent conjunctivitis in a sexually active adolescent suggests chlamydial infection. A recurrent painful red eye with apparent decreased vision and photophobia may indicate ocular herpetic disease.

Physical Examination

A physical examination includes characterizing the discharge, measuring the vision, and evaluating the clarity of the cornea. Preauricular involvement would suggest viral infection. An examination with a hand-held magnifier under good illumination may demonstrate follicles or papillae. The phenylephrine test can be performed to determine the depth of the hyperemic vessels. Phenylephrine 2.5% eyedrops will constrict conjunctival but not scleral or episcleral vessels. The hyperemia of conjunctivitis and secondary conjunctival reactions will be significantly blanched by phenylephrine administration, but the deeper hyperemic vasculature of intraocular inflammation will not. If any question of corneal involvement exists, the instillation of one drop of fluorescein dye and an examination with a Woods' lamp would vividly show corneal involvement as a bright green defect.

Laboratory Tests

When the history and clinical findings are insufficient to render a confident diagnosis or when the infection is severe and recalcitrant to treatment, conjunctival cultures and scrapings are indicated. For bacterial infections, the most widely used media are blood and chocolate agar. Thayer–Martin medium is useful when gonococcus is suspected

and Thioglycolate is used to isolate microaerophilic species. Chlamydial cultures are available at many institutions. (Precaution: wooden applicators should not be used because wood fibers inhibit chlamydial replication.) Viral cultures require special media and facilities and are generally not necessary for treatment. Immunofluorescent and immunoperoxidase techniques are available at some institutions for viral and chlamydial detection.

TREATMENT

Topical antibiotics are useful for bacterial infections. Sulfacetamide, erythromycin, and neomycin–polymyxin–bacitracin combinations are equally efficacious; however, children may develop an allergic reaction especially to neomycin. Steroids are contraindicated in bacterial conjunctivitis.

Cold compresses and oral antihistamines are often helpful in reducing the itching present in allergic conjunctivitis. If the patient is still symptomatic, a judicious use of topical antihistamines and vasoconstrictors may be beneficial. Sodium cromoglycolate 4% prevents the release of histamine and other biochemical mediators from mast cells and has been shown to be effective when used four times a day in the conjunctivitis associated with hay fever.

Topical sodium cromoglycolate is also valuable in the prophylaxis and treatment of vernal conjunctivitis. Iced compresses, dark glasses, and oral antihistamines may also give significant relief. Topical opthalmic steroids are effective, but are associated with an increased incidence of cataracts and glaucoma. The desensitization to inhalant allergens and the surgical removal of papillae have not generally been found effective.

Viral conjunctivitis is often self-limited and generally does not require more than symptomatic treatment. If molluscum is present on the lid margin, an excision of the lesion may be necessary to alleviate the conjunctivitis. A mild herpetic vesicular eruption of the eyelids without involvement of eyelid margins or conjunctiva requires no treatment. If vesicles are present on or near the lid margins, trifluridine 1% solution should be used six times per day until resolution. If conjunctival inflammation is present, the patient should be referred to an ophthalmologist for a corneal examination. Mild adenoviral conjunctivitis is self-limited and requires no therapy. Presently available ocular antiviral agents are not effective against adenovirus. Patients with adenovirus often have positive cultures for herpes simplex. Steroids, therefore, should not routinely be used for EKC. Herpes simplex keratitis may be made disastrously worse by the use of steroids.

Chlamydial infections in children should be treated with a 2-week course of systemic erythromycin. Concomitant topical therapy is unnecessary. In neonatal infections the diagnosis of chlamydial conjunctivitis places the infant at high risk for the development of chlamydial pneumonia. Systemic therapy with erythromycin may also prevent pneumonia. Alternatively, erythromycin ointment four times a day for 3 weeks may be used.

INDICATIONS FOR REFERRAL OR ADMISSION

The pediatrician should be able to comfortably treat most cases of conjunctivitis. A referral to an ophthalmologist would be appropriate if the conjunctivitis is hyperacute or recalcitrant to treatment, of if intraocular inflammation cannot be ruled out.

Any ocular infection that involves the cornea or intraocular structures should be promptly referred to the ophthalmologist. Corneal ulcers usually require hospitalization and frequent application of enriched antibiotics or antifungal agents. Intraocular inflammation warrants a complete eye examination.

Although ophthalmic steroid preparations are beneficial for many conditions, they are not without significant adverse effects. Steroid-induced cataracts and glaucoma are well recognized entities. If increased intraocular pressure persists in steroid users, the optic nerve may be damaged resulting in severe or total loss of vision. Steroid use in the presence of herpes simplex infections can lead to disastrous corneal ulcers and a loss of the eye. For these reasons, ophthalmic steroids should be used only be those specifically trained in recognizing and treating these complications. Any ocular condition severe enough to necessitate steroid treatment should probably be best referred to an ophthalmologist.

BIBLIOGRAPHY

Arentsen JJ: Disorders of the conjunctiva in children. In Harley RD (ed): Pediatric Ophthalmology. Philadelphia, WB Saunders, 1983

Fedukowicz HB, Stenson S: External Infections of the Eye, 2nd ed. New York, Appleton–Century–Crofts, 1985

Fraunfelder FT, Roy FH (eds): Current Ocular Therapy 2. Philadelphia, WB Saunders, 1985

Jones BR: Allergic disease of the outer eye. Trans Ophthalmol Soc UK 91:441–447, 1971

Matoba A: Ocular viral infections. Pediatr Infect Dis 3:358–366, 1984

Nelson LB: Pediatric Ophthalmology. Philadelphia, WB Saunders, 1984

94

Ophthalmia Neonatorum

JOHAN ZWAAN

Any conjunctivitis in infants during the first month of of life is referred to as *ophthalmia neonatorum*. The inflammation may be chemically induced by the prophylactic use of silver nitrate eyedrops or it may be infectious. Staphylococci, chlamydia, and *N. gonorrhoeae* are the more common agents involved; herpes simplex type 2 or various non-*Neisserial* bacteria are less frequently found. (For related discussions but of a broader nature, see Chaps 93, 191, and 195.)

PATHOPHYSIOLOGY

The administration of 1% silver nitrate in the conjunctival sac within 1 hour of birth to prevent venereal infection was first advocated by Crede in 1881. The chemical is only active against *N. gonorrhoeae* by binding to its surface protein and thus interfering with its metabolism. The compound needs to penetrate the microorganism to be effective. If application is delayed, or if a pregnant woman has a premature rupture of her membranes, bacteria may have time to invade the intact tissues of the neonatal eye and become inaccessible to the silver nitrate solution; thus, eradication may be incomplete. The compound is moderately irritating to the conjunctiva and often causes some hyperemia and swelling. Leukocytes migrate into the tissues and the conjunctival sac, leading to a mild purulent discharge. Theoretically, even the cornea can develop a chemical keratitis with some permanent damage as a result. This is rare, unless the percentage of the silver nitrate solution exceeds the recommended 1%.

The infectious types of ophthalmia neonatorum are thought to be the result of the passage of the baby through an infected birth canal. The transfer of microorganisms to the ocular tissues of the infant leads to conjunctivitis and occasionally keratitis.

Gonococcal ophthalmia is a hyperacute infection with a marked purulent exudate. If this infection is not treated promptly, membranes or pseudomembranes may develop. These are due to an outpouring of fibrinous exudate; condensation of fibrin on the conjunctival surfaces may lead to the formation of a translucent pseudomembrane, which can obscure the conjunctiva and cornea. Occasionally, a true inflammatory membrane will form; attempts to remove the latter will leave a raw conjunctival surface. The gonococcal organisms can penetrate cells, including intact corneal epithelium, resulting in corneal ulceration. Gram-stain negative diplococci located intracellularly in leukocytes are a typical finding when conjunctival smears are made. The almost universal use of routine prophylactic measures has made postnatal gonococcal conjunctivitis less frequent in the United States.

Chlamydia trachomatis is now the most common cause of conjunctivitis in the newborn. The inflammation is more moderate and a papillary conjunctival reaction can be seen. Follicles, membranes or pseudomembranes, micropannus (superficial vascularization of the cornea) and corneal opacities, seen in adult trachoma, are unusual. Systemic involvement, however, is common. This may consist of a typical pneumonia, otitis media, and rhinitis. Giemsa-stained conjunctival scrapings may show the presence of basophilic cytoplasmic inclusion bodies in epithelial cells (see also Chaps. 93, 191, and 195).

Herpes simplex infections in the newborn are also thought to be acquired during birth, although cases have been reported in which infection *in utero* was likely. This may occur by way of the transplacental route or across intact fetal membranes by way of the ascending route from the uterine cervix. Most cases are caused by type 2 herpes simplex; the oral strain, type 1, is found less commonly. With the increase in orogenital sex practices, the type of virus isolated can no longer be considered a useful criterion in the differentiation of in utero infection *vs* transmission from active lesions in the maternal birth canal. Herpes simplex infections in the neonate may be localized, involving the eye, skin, oral cavity or central nervous system, or they may be disseminated. The ocular infection typically starts with conjunctival redness, swelling, and moderate discharge. Pseudomembranes may develop and vesicles may be seen on the palpebral conjunctiva or skin of the eyelids. In almost half of the patients, the cornea will become involved. A punctate keratitis or a typical dendrite-shaped lesion may develop. Scrapings of the conjunctiva or cornea and smears from the vesicles show many mononucleated cells and, typically, giant multinucleated epithelial cells.

Nongonococcal bacterial infections may also be responsible for neonatal conjunctivitis. *Staphylococcus aureus* is commonly involved, but various other microorganisms can cause infection. Of greatest concern are infections due to the meningococcus; this organism can penetrate into the blood stream through the intact conjunctiva and thus cause a systemic infection.

CLINICAL PRESENTATION

It should be stressed that the clinical manifestations of the various forms of ophthalmia neonatorum are not specific enough to allow an accurate diagnosis. Although the timing and the character of the signs are somewhat typical for each type of ophthalmia, there is considerable overlap and the physician should never rely only on clinical findings. Regardless of the causative agent, ophthalmia neonatorum is characterized by redness and chemosis (swelling) of the conjunctiva, edema of the eyelids and discharge, which may be purulent. Thus, a full microbiologic work-up is essential, particularly because conjunctivitis in a neonate should be considered an emergency until proven otherwise.

Chemical conjunctivitis is characterized by its rapid onset after birth (within 24 hours), its negative cultures, and its self-limiting nature. It disappears spontaneously in 3 to 5 days. The conjunctival injection is usually mild, but some lid edema and purulent discharge may be present. Permanent damage to the cornea is rare. The incidence of chemical ophthalmia is low and can be expected to decrease even more because of the increasingly frequent practice of using 0.5% erythromycin ointment instead of silver nitrate.

Inclusion conjunctivitis due to *Chlamydia trachomatis* becomes evident from the fifth to twelfth postpartum day, although occasionally it may occur as late as 3 to 4 weeks postnatally. It is the leading cause of ophthalmia neonatorum (30%). The findings frequently involve only one eye. The inflammation is moderate, with mild conjunctival hyperemia and swelling, moderate lid swelling, and mucopurulent discharge. An inspection of the palpebral conjunctiva under magnification (slit lamp) may reveal a papillary reaction, but the follicles seen in the adult form of the disease do not occur in the neonate. Other findings are rare. Chlamydial venereal infections are common and often asymptomatic.

The next most common neonatal conjunctivitis (about 15%) is due to *Neisseria gonorrhoeae*. It starts 2 to 4 days postnatally and the clinical findings are dramatic. There is a hyperacute conjunctivitis, with a red and swollen conjunctiva and copious purulent discharge. Both eyes are usually involved. Pseudomembranes and membranes may form and, because the organism can penetrate intact epithelial cells, superficial keratitis is common. Corneal ulceration and even perforation may develop rapidly if early and appropriate treatment is not instituted. The ulceration starts typically in the periphery and extends rapidly to a ring ulcer. The ulcer deepens and may cause perforation and then endophthalmitis. It is essential to realize that *N. meningitidis* conjunctivitis presents in a similar fashion. It can also penetrate intact tissues and systemic dissemination can follow.

Staphylococcus aureus is responsible for about 10% of ophthalmia neonatorum. The conjunctivitis is similar to infection from neisseria, but its onset is slightly later (*i.e.*, from the third to seventh day). Other bacterial infections, due to various organisms, can start at any time.

Conjunctivitis caused by herpes simplex virus develops between 2 days and 2 weeks after birth. The conjunctival injection is moderately severe and there is a mucopurulent discharge. The eyelids are swollen and red, and typical herpetic vesicles appear. Pseudomembranes may be present. Keratitis may follow the conjunctivitis in about half of the babies after 1 to 4 weeks. An inspection of the cornea under magnification, preferably by slit lamp, and after an application of fluorescein will reveal punctate staining or dendritic figures. Other parts of the eye can be involved; iritis and more generalized uveitis, chorioretinitis, and occasionally cataracts may be present.

DIFFERENTIAL DIAGNOSIS

A few conditions are occasionally mistaken for conjunctivitis. Subconjunctival hemorrhages, sometimes associated with birth, are bright red and diffusely spread through the tissue. There is no discharge and they resolve in 1 to 2 weeks. Tearing and accumulation of some mucopurulent material at the nasal corner of the eye, due to nasolacrimal duct obstruction, usually do not develop until a few weeks after birth. The conjunctiva normally does not become injected. An exception may occur in the case of a congenital dacryocystocele. This occurs when mucus accumulates in the lacrimal sac of newborns due to an obstruction. A bluish swelling is noted near the nasal corner of the eye. If the lacrimal sac does not drain spontaneously or by probing to relieve the obstruction, dacryocystitis may develop with tearing, purulent discharge, and conjunctivitis. The infection may occasionally spread and cause periorbital (preseptal) cellulitis. Congenital glaucoma presents initially with excessive tearing, photophobia, and lid spasm. If the increased intraocular pressure persists, the cornea becomes hazy and its diameter enlarges. The conjunctiva, however, is generally not hyperemic.

The differential diagnosis of the types of ophthalmia neonatorum should be based on a laboratory work-up. Nevertheless, the clinical findings and the timing of the infection may be helpful in the formulation of an initial impression. The essential characteristics are listed in Table 94-1, but to repeat, there is enough overlap so that they should not be relied on exclusively.

WORK-UP

Information should be obtained about the timing of the onset of the conjunctivitis. Because of the venereal origin of most of the cases of ophthalmia

Table 94-1. Average Time of Onset and Characteristics of the Most Common Causes
of Ophthalmia Neonatorum

ETIOLOGY	ONSET (Days after Birth)	SEVERITY	NATURAL COURSE	FREQUENCY
Chlamydia	5–12	Moderate	Chronic	Common
Gonococcus	2–4	Severe	Rapid	Fairly common
S. aureus	3–7	Severe	May resolve	Fairly common
Silver nitrate	<1	Mild	Self-limited	Common
H. simplex	2–15	Moderate	Progressive	Uncommon

neonatorum, inquiries should be made about maternal exposure.

Cultures should be obtained from the conjunctival sac on blood and Thayer–Martin or chocolate agar. Antibiotic sensitivity needs to be determined. Sugar fermentation tests may be necessary to distinguish *N. gonorrhoeae* and *N. meningitidis*. If indicated, viral cultures should be requested. Chlamydia may be diagnosed from McCoy cell cultures; direct immunofluorescence of cultures may expedite the diagnosis. Scrapings of the conjunctiva are done with a blunt platinum spatula, immediately transferred to glass slides and fixed with 95% ethanol. Gram and Giemsa stains should be carried out. The first aids in the identification of bacteria, the latter allows the characterization of the cellular infiltrate. Large numbers of neutrophils are typical for bacterial infections, while monocytes may be seen in viral conjunctivitis. Basophilic cytoplasmic inclusion bodies may be found in chlamydial ophthalmia neonatorum, and multinucleated giant cells in herpetic infections. Immunofluorescence tests of the scrapings may be helpful, particularly for chlamydial infections.

TREATMENT

Chemical conjunctivitis does not require treatment. Irrigation of the conjunctival sac is not helpful and may make the eyes more irritated. Inclusion conjunctivitis is treated with topical 10% sulfacetamide, erythromycin, or tetracycline ointment, four times per day for 3 weeks. Oral erythromycin is equally effective and has the advantage of treating the nasopharyngeal colonization, which may cause reinfection, and of possibly preventing the chlamydial pneumonia syndrome. Oral tetracycline should not be used in infants or nursing mothers because of deleterious effects on growing bones and teeth.

Neisserial ophthalmia neonatorum needs to be treated with topical erythromycin or tetracycline ointment every 2 hours until the conjunctivitis begins to improve. An application can then be decreased to four times daily. Alternatively, a drop of aqueous penicillin with a strength of 10,000 U/ml to 20,000 U/ml can be used hourly for the first 12 hours and then tapered to four to six times daily. The treatment should be continued for 3 weeks. Intravenous penicillin (50,000 U/kg/day), divided to 4 to 6 doses, is given for 7 days. If gonococcal ophthalmia is suspected, the treatment should be started immediately without waiting for laboratory results.

Herpes simplex is treated with idoxiuridine or vidarabine ointment four to five times daily for up to 3 weeks. In case of severe keratitis, cycloplegia may be necessary.

Non-neisserial bacterial ophthalmia can be treated with erythromycin ointment four to six times daily. For gram-negative infections, gentamycin drops are chosen with the same frequency. *Hemophilus* is usually sensitive to tetracycline or erythromycin ointment.

INDICATIONS FOR REFERRAL AND ADMISSION

Neonates with gonococcal conjunctivitis should be hospitalized for intravenous treatment and isolation. Other infections can usually be managed on an outpatient basis, unless a systemic infection is suspected. Proper precautionary measures should be taken to prevent the spread of the infection.

All these problems are best treated by a team effort, involving the pediatrician, the infectious disease specialist, and the ophthalmologist. An early consultation is recommended. Positively identified cases of venereal types of ophthalmia and of some other infections must be reported to the local or state health department. A referral to a community health nurse may be helpful.

ANNOTATED BIBLIOGRAPHY

Armstrong JH, Zacarias F, Rein MF: Ophthalmia neonatorum: A chart review. Pediatrics 57:884, 1976 (Summarizes findings in a large series of cases with ophthalmia neonatorum, with emphasis on the percentage distribution of etiologies.)

Hutchinson DS, Smith RE, Haughton PB: Congenital herpetic keratitis. Arch Ophthalmol 93:70, 1975 (Description of a patient with congenital herpes simplex conjunctivitis and keratitis, possibly acquired *in utero*. This report is accompanied by a large review.)

Sandstrom KI, Bell AT, Chandler JW et al: Microbial causes of neonatal conjunctivitis. J Pediatr 105:706, 1984 (Reviews the causative factors in ophthalmia neonatorum.)

Tam MR, Stamm WE, Handsfield HH: Culture-independent diagnosis of chlamydia trachomatis using monoclonal antibodies. N Engl J Med 310:1146, 1984 (Description of the immunofluorescent diagnosis of chlamydia.)

95
Orbital Swelling and Infection
LEONARD B. NELSON AND
DAVID J. SEIDMAN

The orbit is a bony cavity that has the approximate shape of a quadrilateral pyramid with its base directed forward and laterally. Because the orbit is a closed space, pathologic processes tend to present with proptosis (displacement of the eyeball forward), mass effect behind the eye lids, or inflammatory signs. A detailed discussion of all of the diseases producing swelling within the orbit is beyond the scope of this chapter. Therefore, a basic overview of conditions to consider when faced with a child who shows signs and symptoms of orbital swelling or inflammation will be presented. Therapy will be discussed for the more common infections; these are the conditions in which the pediatrician is most likely to have an active therapeutic role.

PATHOPHYSIOLOGY

The orbit is bordered medially by the nasal cavity and ethmoidal air cells, posteromedially by the sphenoid sinus, superiorly by the frontal sinus and anterior cranial fossa, and inferiorly by the maxillary sinus. Anteriorly, the orbital septum separates the orbit from the subcutaneous and submuscular spaces of the eyelids. Categories of orbital disease in children include inflammation, vascular disorders, neoplasms, metabolic, and developmental anomalies.

CLINICAL PRESENTATION

In its most dramatic form, orbital disease may present with massive proptosis at birth. More commonly, it presents as a slowly enlarging mass in the orbit visible by way of mass effect behind the lids or by way of displacement of an eye away from the mass. More posterior masses may displace the eye forward and present as progressive proptosis. Rapidly progressive proptosis, with or without inflammatory signs, is another clinical presentation that is frequently seen.

The conditions leading to signs of orbital swelling or inflammation are presented in Table 95-1.

Orbital Cellulitis

Orbital cellulitis, inflammation of the orbital contents, must be distinguished from preseptal cellulitis, inflammation of the subcutaneous tissues of the eyelids, brow, and forehead. In orbital cellulitis, the infectious process extends posterior to the orbital septum. Most cases of orbital cellulitis result from the spread of infection from paranasal sinuses; the ethmoid is the most commonly involved in children. Other causes include puncture wounds that penetrate the orbital septum, surgical trauma within the orbit, acute dacryocystis (infection of the lacrimal gland), extension from intracranial or dental infections, or seeding of the orbit by a bacteremia (most commonly *Hemophilus influenzae type b*).

Fever, lid edema, and rhinorrhea are the usual early signs of orbital cellulitis. Lid tenderness, warmth, and orbital pain follow. Conjunctival chemosis, decreased ability to move the eye, and proptosis occur later. As the infection progresses, congestion of retinal veins, chorioretinal striae, and increased intraocular pressure may occur. The damage to the ocular blood supply may led to infarction of the retina and choroid. If uncontrolled,

Table 95-1. Differential Diagnosis of Orbital Swelling and Infection

Dermoid cyst	Neurofibroma
Capillary hemangioma	Optic nerve glioma
Orbital cellulitis	Fibroosseous tumors
Hemorrhage	Lymphangioma
Pseudotumor	Optic nerve meningioma
Hyperthyroidism	Histiocytosis X
Craniostenosis	Juvenile xanthogranuloma
Rhabdomyosarcoma	
Metastatic neuroblastoma	Meningoencephaloceles
	Micropthalmos with cyst
Leukemia—lymphoma	Teratoma
	Cavernous sinus thrombosis
	Metastatic Ewing's sarcoma

The left-hand column represents the more frequent problems in an approximate order of frequency. Exact frequencies are difficult to obtain because most studies are biased by the nature of the referral center involved.

the infection can spread to the cavernous sinus causing a cavernous sinus thrombosis or intracranially leading to empyema or brain abscess. The lack of response of the infection to adequate antibiotic therapy suggests the possibility that an orbital or subperiosteal abscess is present.

Dermoid Cyst

These choristomas are the most frequently encountered orbital tumors of childhood. They are nontender, circumscribed, rubbery masses most commonly located in the superior temporal quadrant of the orbit. More posteriorly located tumors may be present with proptosis without a clinically evident mass, with ptosis, or with restricted movement of the globe. If the cyst ruptures within the orbit, an inflammatory response to the released cyst contents may cause rapidly progressive proptosis and inflammatory signs similar to orbital cellulitis.

Capillary Hemangioma

Capillary hemangiomas occur during the first year of life. When the skin is involved, the lesion is commonly referred to as a strawberry nevus. An orbital hemangioma may be present with or without an associated hemangioma of the skin. In the absence of a skin lesion, an area of deep bluish discoloration underlying the lid skin, which increases

in color when the child cries, may be a clue to the underlying orbital hemangioma. They are most common in the superonasal quadrant of the orbit. Approximately one third of such tumors are noted at birth; as the tumors increase in size during the first 6 months of life, 95% are noted. This tumor regresses spontaneously in 80% of children.

Nonspecific Orbital Inflammation (Orbital Pseudotumor)

Orbital pseudotumors are a group of idiopathic orbital inflammations with an acute or subacute clinical course. In the acute form there is a sudden onset of lid edema, erythema, chemosis, proptosis, and orbital pain. Inflammation of the intraocular tissues may also be present. The presentation may be much like orbital cellulitis.

Rhabdomyosarcoma

Rhabdomyosarcoma is the most common primary orbital malignancy of children. The most common presentation is that of a unilateral proptosis, which increases rapidly. The disease may begin as a mass noted in the eyelid or the conjunctiva. The average age at onset is 7 to 8 years, although infants have been born with rhabdomyosarcoma.

Hyperthyroidism

Girls are affected more commonly than boys in a ratio of 6:1. Although proptosis occurs, it is rarely of the degree seen in adults. Lid retraction is the most common early sign and is best appreciated on the initiation of a downgaze.

Metastatic Neuroblastoma

Between one third and one half of children with neuroblastoma will develop orbital metastasis. Less than 17% of cases of neuroblastoma will present initially in the orbit. Bilateral orbital metastases occur in more than one half of the patients. The orbital disease presents with proptosis and variable signs of orbital inflammation, which sometimes simulate acute cellulitis. Bilateral eyelid ecchymosis in the absence of trauma is characteristic.

Myeloid Leukemia

Myeloid leukemia may produce a localized infiltration of neoplastic cells in the orbit and, in this form, is referred to as granulocytic sarcoma or chloroma. The orbital signs often represent the initial presentation of the disease. The median age at presentation is 7 years.

Orbital Hemorrhage

A hemorrhage may occur secondary to birth trauma and forceps injuries, blood dyscrasias, scurvy, and vitamin K deficiency. Eyelid ecchymosis usually accompanies rapid proptosis. Hemorrhage into a preexisting vascular tumor, such as capillary hemangioma or lymphangioma, may cause a sudden rapid proptosis without ecchymosis.

DIFFERENTIAL DIAGNOSIS

Rapidly progressive inflammation of periorbital tissues and orbital contents is most commonly caused by bacterial orbital cellulitis. A distinction must be made from the more common preseptal cellulitis in which infection is limited to the subcutaneous and submuscular spaces of the eyelids, brow, and forehead. Proptosis, decreased eye movement, and pain on movement are *absent* in preseptal cellulitis.

Other causes of rapidly progressive proptosis with or without inflammatory signs include (1) nonspecific orbital inflammation (pseudotumor), (2) rhabdomyosarcoma, (3) metastatic neuroblastoma, (4) rupture of a dermoid cyst, and (5) hemorrhage into the orbit or into a preexisting hemangioma or lymphangioma. Orbital cellulitis, unlike the other conditions, usually causes fever and leukocytosis greater than 15,000 wbc/ml.

The differential diagnosis of slowly progressive proptosis, stable proptosis, or orbital swelling involves the other diseases listed in the Table 95-1.

WORK-UP

History

The following information is important in differentiating the causes of orbital disease: the age at which proptosis or swelling was first noticed; the rapidity with which the proptosis progressed; associated illness; a variation in proptosis from day to day or with crying or upper respiratory infections; a history of blunt or sharp trauma to the orbit; unilateral *vs* bilateral disease; a history of sinus disease; the presence of orbital pain or pain with movement of the eye; a change in the vision of either eye; and a general medical history.

Physical Examination

An examination should be made for the following: signs of inflammation (*i.e.*, chemosis, lid edema, lid erythema, lid tenderness, or warmth); the direction in which the eye is displaced; resistance of gentle efforts by a possible mass behind the eye to displace the eye back into the orbit with palpation; pulsation of the eye; a bruit audible over the orbit; the status of extraocular movements; changes in the vision; a funduscopic examination including the optic nerve; and a general physical examination.

Laboratory Tests

Cultures are discussed under therapy and management. Plain films will delineate orbital fractures and identify sinus disease associated with an orbital process (most commonly sinusitis associated with orbital cellulitis). Computed axial tomography has become the mainstay of radiographic orbital evaluation in differentiating severe preseptal from true orbital cellulitis and in detecting orbital tumors. A pathologic examination of biopsy specimens is also important in diagnosing orbital lesions. In children with rapidly progressive proptosis not consistent with orbital cellulitis, an early biopsy must be considered. If the orbital lesion is rhabdomyosarcoma, a biopsy specimen is required for the diagnosis and planning of therapy.

THERAPY AND MANAGEMENT

Preseptal Cellulitis

The most common pathogens in preseptal cellulitis are *Staphylococcus aureus, Streptococcus pyogenes*, and in children under 5 years, *Hemophilus influenzae type b. H. influenzae* produces a characteristic blue-purple lid discoloration. Anaerobes are less common, and clostridia must be considered in cellulitis associated with dirty wounds. The conjunctiva and any purulent wound drainage should be Gram stained and cultured. If a fluctuant abscess is present, drainage should be performed near the lateral superior orbital rim. In a less severe infection, oral antibiotic therapy with a penicillinase-resistant penicillin or cephalosporin is acceptable. Intravenous therapy should be considered if the infection does not respond to oral antibiotics, if extensive lid edema develops, or if signs of orbital cellulitis develop. The Gram stain should be used as a guide to an appropriate antibiotic choice. If the Gram stain is unavailable or uninformative, penicillin G and a penicillinase-resistant penicillin should be administered. In children under 5 years of age ampicillin (or amoxicillin) should be used in place of penicillin G. If ampicillin resistance is common, cefaclor or chloramphenicol may be considered.

Orbital Cellulitis Secondary to Sinusitis

In orbital cellulitis, a Gram stain identification of organisms and a culture may be difficult unless purulent material can be found on the nasal or nasopharyngeal mucosa. If available, this material should be cultured and a smear prepared for a Gram stain. Intravenous antibiotic therapy is then guided by gram stain results. The most common organisms are *S. aureus*, *S. pyogenes*, *S. pneumoniae*, anaerobes, and, in children under 5 years, *H. influenzae type b*. Intravenous penicillin G and a penicillinase-resistant penicillin or a third generation cephalosporin as a single therapy are therefore treatments of choice in the absence of Gram stain information. In children under 5 years of age, ampicillin is substituted for penicillin. Sinus decongestion with nasal spray or oral decongestants should also be attempted. Surgical drainage of sinuses is reserved for those infections that do not respond promptly to antibiotics. The presence of an orbital abscess indicates the need for surgical drainage within the orbit.

A discussion of the management of other orbital processes are beyond the scope of this chapter and the reader is referred to the bibliography.

INDICATIONS FOR REFERRAL AND HOSPITALIZATION

Children with orbital swelling or infection should be managed by an ophthalmologist together with the pediatrician. An orbital biopsy is best performed by an opthalmologist who has experience in orbital surgery. In situations in which the sinuses are involved, an otorhinolaryngologist should be consulted.

Children with severe preseptal cellulitis or or-bital cellulitis should be hospitalized for intravenous antibiotics, and their ocular and neurologic status should be closely monitored. In other cases of rapidly progressive proptosis, hospitalization should be considered. The decision is based on an evaluation of the immediate risk to the visual system and central nervous system along with contemplated diagnostic and therapeutic approaches. This decision is best made in consultation with an ophthalmologist.

ANNOTATED BIBLIOGRAPHY

Hornblass A, Herschorn BJ, Stern K, Grimes C: Orbital abscess. Surv Ophthalmol 29:169, 1984

Jones DB: Microbial preseptal and orbital cellulitis. In Duane TD, Jaeger EA (eds): Clinical Ophthalmology, Vol 4, Chap 25. Philadelphia, Harper & Row, 1985 (Although discussion of modern orbital imaging with computed axial tomography is lacking, it is otherwise useful for those managing orbital infections.)

Jones IS, Jakobiec FA, Nolan BT: Patient examination and introduction to orbital disease. In Duane TD, Jaeger EA (eds): Clinical Ophthalmology, Vol 2, Chap 21. Philadelphia, Harper & Row, 1985 (Clinically relevant discussion of orbital anatomy, an orbital physical examination, and a review of the literature concerning the frequency of various orbital lesions in childhood.)

Kennerdel JS, Dresner SC: The nonspecific orbital inflammatory syndromes. Surv Ophthalmol 29:93, 1984 (Discussion of the various forms and therapy of orbital pseudotumor.)

Macy JI, Mandelbaum SH, Minckler DS: Orbital cellulitis. Ophthalmol 87:1309, 1980 (Detailed case report demonstrating the approach to differential diagnosis and management in an 11-year-old initially thought to have rhabdomyosarcoma.)

Nicholson DH: Tumors of the eye, lids, and orbit in children. In Harley RD (ed): Pediatric Ophthalmology, 2nd ed. Philadelphia, WB Saunders, 1983 (Includes a discussion of orbital tumors of childhood along with a discussion of other causes of proptosis.)

Weiss A, Friendly D, Eglin K et al: Bacterial periorbital and orbital cellulitis in childhood. Ophthalmol 90:195, 1983 (Recent retrospective review of the clinical features, microbiology, and therapy of 137 children.)

Chalazia, styes, and hordeola are all inflammations of the exocrine glands of the eyelids. These may be bacterial or granulomatous in nature. The various glands involved are depicted in Figure 96-1. *Hordeolum* indicates any type of inflammatory papule of the eyelids. An *external hordeolum* or a *stye*, sometimes also called an *external chalazion*, is essentially a small abscess of the sweat glands or sebaceous glands associated with the eyelashes. Thus, it is located superficially at the margin of the eyelids. An *internal hordeolum* is an infection of a meibomian gland, a large sebaceous gland inside the tarsus of the eyelid. It is deeper in the lid and is usually larger than a stye. An *internal chalazion*, commonly referred to as a *chalazion*, is a sterile lipogranulomatous inflammation of a meibomian gland. A *pyogenic granuloma* is a mass on the conjunctival surface of the eyelid. This may develop when a chalazion points to this surface and breaks through it. It is granulation tissue that tends to enlarge fairly rapidly and is fragile.

PATHOPHYSIOLOGY

Hordeola (styes) are bacterial infections that are most commonly from staphylococci. They are abscesses with pus accumulating in the lumen of the involved glands. Histologically, they present the typical picture of an acute bacterial infection, which is collections of polymorphonuclear leukocytes around the lash follicle and its associated glands.

A chalazion is induced when the orifice of the meibomian gland is obstructed and the excretion of the sebaceous product of the gland is prevented. The lipid material extravasates instead into the surrounding tarsal tissue and sets up a granulomatous foreign body reaction. Thus, the contents of a chalazion are usually sterile. There are many possible causes for the blockage such as dust, debris, or scarring from a previous infection or trauma. A chronic blepharitis or conjunctivitis may be the cause, with either the bacteria or the inflammatory response to them causing the obstruction. The pathologic appearance is that of a granulomatous re-action. There is usually a clear central area where the lipid content of the structure was dissolved during the preparation of the tissue for histology. This is surrounded by a zone with many inflammatory cells. Typically, these consist of Langerhans' giant cells and histiocytes in addition to the more common polymorphonuclear cells, plasma cells, and lymphocytes.

Pyogenic granulomas are fragile, highly vascularized masses, originating from the tarsal conjunctiva, where a chalazion has ruptured. Pyogenic granulomas consist of a loose accumulation of fibroblasts with many small blood vessels interspersed with lymphocytes and plasma cells.

CLINICAL PRESENTATION

External hordeola or styes present as localized, discrete pustules on the front part of the lid margin, usually in association with a lash. They are red, swollen, and quite tender. The pain is proportional to the amount of swelling. Internal hordeola are abscesses of the meibomian glands and are located deeper in the eyelid, in the tarsus and away from the lid margin. Their appearance is similar to that of a stye. Most point to the conjunctival side of the lid and when the latter is everted, the overlying conjunctiva is found to be red and elevated. They may extend occasionally in the opposite direction and point towards the skin. They may rupture spontaneously, releasing purulent material and granulomatous reaction products. Both types of hordeola may be complicated by cellulitis of the entire eyelid.

Chalazia are nontender, firm nodules within the tarsus. They can become fairly large and they can sometimes fluctuate in size. Acute inflammatory signs are absent. They are occasionally large enough to press on the eyeball; the induced astigmatism may cause some distortion of the vision.

Pyogenic granulomas occur on the conjunctival surface, where a chalazion has broken through the surface. They tend to become larger fairly rapidly and may be visible over the edge of the lid. They are painless and fragile and are often pedunculated.

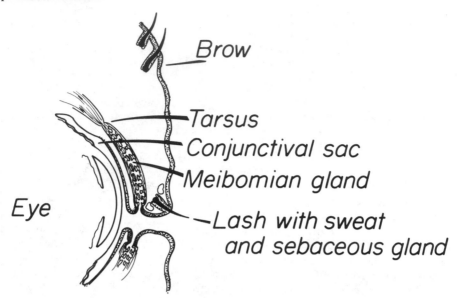

Figure 96-1. Schematic cross-section through the upper eyelid. The sebaceous and sweat glands associated with the lash are the sites of styes (*external hordeola*). The meibomian glands inside the tarsus can become infected, generally with *Staphylococcus aureus*, and they are then referred to as *internal hordeola*. Sterile lipogranulomatous inflammations are caused by an obstruction of the ostium of the glands at the posterior aspect of the lid margin and they are called *chalazia*.

Their appearance is somewhat reminiscent of a raspberry; they may bleed spontaneously.

DIFFERENTIAL DIAGNOSIS

The clinical presentation of all these lesions is typical; they can be distinguished by their location, the presence or absence or pain, and their appearance. If, in adults, a chalazion recurs repeatedly in the same location despite treatment by incision and curettage, a possible diagnosis of carcinoma of a meibomian gland needs to be entertained. However, the occurrence of such a malignancy in the pediatric age group is rare (if it occurs at all).

MANAGEMENT

No work-up is required beyond clinical observation. If a child suffers repeated recurrences of styes, however, a diminished resistance may be present; occasionally, this is seen in anemia or diabetes mellitus.

The treatment of external and internal hordeola is straightforward. The application of an ophthalmic antibacterial ointment, such as erythromycin or po-

lysporin, into the conjunctival sac should be done four or five times daily. Warm compresses for several minutes a few times daily is helpful. Systemic antibiotics are rarely necessary and should only be used if a cellulitis of the eyelid appears to be developing. The offending organism is almost always *Staphylococcus aureus* and oral dicloxacillin, erythromycin, or cefaclor is usually effective. If the infection does not begin to resolve in 48 hours, incision and drainage are indicated. This may be done under local anesthesia, but a brief general anesthesia is occasionally required for children.

Once the acute phase has passed, a recurrence may be prevented by good facial hygiene. Daily use of warm compresses and scrubbing of the eyelids once or twice daily are beneficial. For the latter, a cotton-tipped applicator is wetted with very dilute baby shampoo and is used to scrub the margin of the eyelid. The eyelids should, of course, be closed to prevent corneal irritation or abrasion.

Chalazia are treated in a similar fashion. With a combination of hot compresses and lid scrubs, followed by digital massage to stimulate drainage from the gland, many lesions will disappear during the course of 3 to 4 weeks, or will at least greatly improve. This is particularly true in the acute phase. Once the chalazion has become chronic, it will rarely subside with conservative measures. Incision and curettage become necessary. This is usually done from the conjunctival side of the eyelid. The lid is everted and a vertical incision is made through the conjunctiva into the cavity of the affected gland. This is followed by the removal of its contents, a curettage of the gland, and excision of the capsular wall. After the instillation of an antibiotic ointment, a pressure patch is applied over the eye for a few hours. On occasion, the chalazion is approached from the skin side with a linear incision parallel to the lid margin. After removal of the chalazion, the skin may be sutured; no sutures are needed in the conjunctiva.

In some cases, an intralesional injection of a small amount of steroids can be used to cure a chalazion. The injection should be done from the conjunctival side. An approach from the opposite side carries a small risk of penetration of the eye with consequent endophthalmitis.

Pyogenic granulomas should be excised.

INDICATIONS FOR REFERRAL

If there is no improvement in the condition of a stye after 48 hours of treatment with hot soaks and topical antibiotics, patients should be referred to the ophthalmologist for possible incision and drainage of the lesion.

Conservative treatment of a chalazion may be carried out for a few weeks before surgical therapy needs to be considered.

ANNOTATED BIBLIOGRAPHY

Jeffers JB, Bedrossian EH Jr: Medical and surgical treatment of chalazia, pp 97–116. In Reinecke RD (ed): Ophthalmology Annual, Vol 1. East Norwalk, CT, Appleton–Century–Croft, 1985 (Details the clinical appearance and, briefly, the pathology of various inflammations of the glands of the eyelids. Both surgical and medical treatment are discussed extensively.)

Pizzarello LD, Jacobiec FA, Hofeldt AJ et al: Intralesional corticosteroid therapy of chalazia. Am J Ophthalmol 85:818–821, 1978 (Describes how a steroid injection of chalazia can cure as many as 90% of the lesions.)

97
Acute Eye Trauma
JOHAN ZWAAN

Accidents involving the eyes of children are common, and can be frightening to patient, parent, and physician. Even relatively minor injuries, such as corneal abrasions which can be expected to heal without any sequelae, may be accompanied by severe pain and decreased vision. It is essential that a complete examination of the eye be performed to distinguish major from minor injuries, because the initial impression can be deceiving. For example, it may appear that a pellet from a BB gun has only caused a laceration of the eyelid. It may, however, have penetrated into the orbit, resulting in severe damage to the posterior aspect of the eye or to the optic nerve.

WORK-UP

A detailed history should be obtained while the initial evaluation and treatment are in progress. This should include the nature and the time of the injury, the possible administration of first aid, current symptoms, and previous eye history such as the wearing of glasses. In chemical burns, it is important to ascertain the nature of the chemical involved. Tetanus immunization should be current. If there is a possibility that the child needs an examination under anesthesia or surgery, he should not be allowed to eat or drink. The time of the last oral intake should be noted.

Care should be taken not to make the injury worse. If a penetrating wound is present, a slight pressure on the eye may lead to extrusion of intraocular tissues, with disastrous consequences. If such an injury is suspected, no attempt at a detailed examination should be made. The eye should be covered with a shield, such as a cone shaped from a piece of carton or the top of a can, which rests on the orbital bone surrounding the eye, without touching the eye itself, and the child should be referred immediately. Indeed, even though a referral may lead to a delay in the evaluation and treatment, there is no harm in this as long as the delay is moderate. One exception to this is chemical burns, which constitute a real emergency and have to be treated without any delay.

If the child has eye pain, the examination is made easier by the instillation of a topical anesthetic. As the drops take effect, blepharospasm will diminish and the patient will become more comfortable and cooperative.

An attempt should be made to record the patient's visual actuity. If no formal vision chart is available or if the child is too young to comprehend letters, a test can be improvised using readily available objects, words, or pictures in magazines. It is very reassuring if it can be established that the child can see.

The eyelids and the periorbital area should be inspected for hemorrhage, swelling, lacerations, and position. The ability to open and close the eyes needs to be established. The orbital rim should be palpated for discontinuities of the bones or masses. Tenderness should be noted.

An inspection of the eyes requires opening of the eyelids. The lids need to be separated if this is not done voluntarily. It is essential to do this without exerting any pressure on the eye. One can rest the proximal parts of the fingers on the orbital rim and use the tips to gently retract the eyelids. A penlight illuminating the eye from the side is helpful. If lacerations of the cornea or conjunctiva or prolapse of intraocular tissues are obvious, or if the pupil has a pear-shape (indicating a possible prolapse), the examination should be stopped and the patient should be referred. Otherwise, fluorescein can be applied to the eye, preferably with a dry strip rather than in solution, to check for abrasions. The use of a blue light or Wood's lamp and magnifying loupes is helpful. Defects of the iris or blood in the anterior chamber may be present.

Pupillary reactions, asymmetry, and shape should be noted. The motility of the eyes should be checked by having the child follow a small object or light.

A fundus examination requires dilatation of the pupils. Changes in the media, such as cataracts or vitreous hemorrhage may interfere, but one should attempt to at least document the status of the optic disk, macula, and retinal vasculature. Retinal hemorrhages or edema and occasionally foreign bodies may be noted. The inspection of the periphery of the retina requires the use of the indirect ophthalmoscope and is commonly left for the ophthalmologist.

If there is any question of orbital fractures or intraocular or orbital foreign bodies, appropriate roentgenograms should be ordered.

CHEMICAL BURNS

Chemical burns to the eye constitute a true emergency; seconds do count in these cases. Acids, bleach, and similar products tend to coagulate the superficial tissues of the eye, which prevents further penetration into deeper layers. These burns are somewhat self-limiting and tend to heal better and leave less scarring. Alkali, (*e.g.*, oven and toilet bowl cleaners, lye, or ammonia) on the other hand, combines with tissue lipids and causes softening. Thus, it continues to penetrate into the tissues and does progressive damage. The cornea and even the iris and lens may show severe involvement. Organic solvents and fluids such as gasoline can cause severe conjunctivitis and keratitis, but the damage is usually superficial.

In all cases, immediate irrigation of the eye should be performed using a gentle but steady stream of saline or water for 20 to 30 minutes, or even longer in the case of alkali burns. The eyelids need to be held apart, if necessary with retractors, and topical anesthetics may be applied.

After the initial flushing the child should be referred. The eye should not be patched during the transport to allow more chemicals to be washed out by the tearing of the eyes. In alkali burns, it is advantageous to continue the eye irrigation during the transfer to the referral facility.

THERMAL BURNS

Because of protective reflexes, the eye itself is rarely burned, although occasionally a cinder, part of a match, or a cigarette may hit the cornea or conjunctiva. The resulting burn is usually superficial and often heals with little or no scarring. The treatment is the same as that for a corneal abrasion. Burns of the eyelids may be small and require the application of an antibiotic ointment only, until healed. Saline soaked dressings should be applied if they are large. If eyelid closure is incomplete due to the destruction of tissue or edema, the eye must be protected from drying out by the use of artificial tears, protective ointments, or even suturing together of the upper and lower eyelids (tarsorrhaphy).

ULTRAVIOLET BURNS

Exposure to light from sunlamps or welding or to ultraviolet light reflecting from snow or sand can cause a superficial keratitis. Typically, severe pain develops several hours after the exposure in combination with blurred vision, photophobia, and a scratchy foreign body sensation. Prophylactic antibiotic ointment and a patch are applied. Systemic analgesics may be needed for intense pain. Fortunately, the cornea heals without sequelae in 1 to 2 days.

EYELID INJURIES

Contusions of the eyelids are common and result in swelling and ecchymosis. Their resolution can be expedited by the use of cold compresses. It is not unusual for a "black eye" to spread after a few days, even across the nose bridge to involve the contralateral eye. Thus, the location of the hemorrhage may not correspond to the site of the original injury. Orbital fractures and retrobulbar hemorrhages should be excluded.

Ptosis of the upper eyelid may be reflective, to protect the eye, or may be due to swelling or hemorrhage within the lid tissue. Hemorrhage within the levator muscle can also be responsible. A spontaneous resolution is the rule but may not be the case when oculomotor nerve damage has occurred.

Superficial lacerations of the lids can be repaired by the non-ophthalmologist under local anesthesia. If they are small, steristrips may allow adequate closure. Large or full-thickness lacerations, particularly those involving the lid margin or the medial area where the lacrimal drainage system is located, are best repaired in an operating room by the ophthalmologist.

ORBITAL FRACTURES

Roentgenograms need to be ordered on all patients who may have an orbital fracture. The most typical of these is a blow-out fracture. When the orbit is hit with a blunt, large object such as a tennis ball, the compression of the orbital contents increases the intraorbital pressure, which in turn blows out the weakest part of the orbital wall (*i.e.*, the floor). This may lead to a prolapse of tissue, including the inferior extraocular muscles, into the maxillary sinus. The eye may be enophthalmic and vertical diplopia can occur due to the entrapment of the inferior rectus muscle, edema, or hemorrhage. The diplopia will often resolve spontaneously and, unless severe enophthalmia is present, surgery may not be needed. It can certainly be postponed for 1 to 2 weeks to allow resorption of edema or hemorrhage.

CONJUNCTIVAL INJURIES

Subconjunctival hemorrhages can appear frightening, but they are often caused by minimal trauma or may even be spontaneous. They absorb in 1 to 2 weeks. A more serious underlying injury needs to be excluded and, if spontaneous subconjunctival hemorrhages appear repeatedly, work-up for a bleeding disorder is indicated.

Conjunctival lacerations by themselves are not very important and they rarely require suturing. However, they may indicate a penetrating injury to the eye itself, and surgical exploration is warranted if the laceration is large, or if there are other indications for possible penetrating trauma.

Chemosis or edema of the conjunctiva may be the result of insect stings. Cold packs to reduce the swelling and perhaps oral antihistamines are helpful. If the swelling accompanies other ocular or orbital trauma, it may indicate a serious injury.

CORNEA

Corneal abrasions are common. The loss of corneal surface epithelium exposes the free endings of the corneal nerve fibers, causing severe pain. Copious tearing and blepharospasm are usually present and a secondary iritis may cause a ciliary spasm and miosis. The examination is facilitated by the use of topical anesthetic drops, which give dramatic relief. Large abrasions may be seen with a penlight; more subtle ones require the use of fluorescein. One should look for foreign bodies, particularly in the conjunctival cul-de-sac and under the upper eyelid, which must be everted. They may be removed with a cotton-tipped applicator or by irrigation. If the foreign body adheres strongly, gentle scraping with a disposable injection needle or the use of a dental burr may be needed. This is best done by an ophthalmologist with the help of a slit lamp. A short-acting cycloplegic is applied, followed by an antibiotic ointment and a tight patch. The latter should be left until the next day. After the removal of the patch, a topical antibiotic may be continued for a few days, three to four times daily. Abrasions and foreign body injuries generally heal without significant scarring.

If a corneal laceration is found, the child should be kept quiet, using sedation if necessary, until the injury can be evaluated in the operating room. The eye should be covered with a shield to avoid pressure on the eye.

ANTERIOR CHAMBER

When the eye is hit with sufficient energy to cause a tear in a small ciliary blood vessel, bleeding into the anterior chamber (*i.e.*, a hyphema) results. Most are small and layer out inferiorly. The blood is absorbed in a few days. If the hyphema is large or if there is a rebleeding and the absorption takes longer, blood staining of the cornea or glaucoma may occur. A small hyphema is treated with rest; some physicians prescribe topical cycloplegics or steroids, others give no medications at all except for sedatives. The usefulness of antifibrinolytic drugs has been established. A large hyphema may require surgical evacuation to prevent complications.

An intraocular infection following injury or a sterile inflammation may lead to the accumulation of pus in the anterior chamber, called a *hypopion*. The material should be aspirated and sent for a bacteriologic work-up.

IRIS

Tears or holes in the iris may result from a penetrating trauma. Blunt injury can lead to iris sphincter rupture or to dialysis of the iris. A spastic miosis can occur even with no direct injury to the iris.

Traumatic iritis, which may follow a relatively minor injury, can only be diagnosed with certainty with a slit lamp, demonstrating the presence of leukocytes and serum proteins ("flare") in the anterior chamber. Clinically, its presence can be suspected if the child complains of photophobia and the pupil is found to be sluggishly reactive and often somewhat dilated. The accompanying injection tends to be centered immediately around the cornea and is known as a ciliary flush. Iritis is treated with cycloplegics and topical steroids.

TRAUMATIC CATARACT

Both blunt and penetrating trauma can result in the opacification of the lens. The cataract may develop rapidly or may develop after a significant delay. Less commonly, the lens may become dislocated if its suspensory ligaments are ruptured, resulting in its edge being visible in the pupil. Fragments of lens may become the focus of an inflammatory response, causing lens-induced uveitis. In all these situations, surgery to remove the lens usually becomes necessary, unless a cataract does not interfere significantly with vision.

OPTIC NERVE

Contusion injuries of the optic nerve range from swelling of the optic nerve head, similar to papilledema, to a complete avulsion. Ironically, in the latter, the optic disc at first may appear normal in the face of a severe visual deficit. The finding of a Marcus–Gunn pupil is diagnostic, with the degree of the afferent pupillary defect related to the degree of optic nerve damage.

POSTERIOR SEGMENT TRAUMA

The compression and decompression of the eye caused by a blunt force generates shearing forces between the coats of the eye and the vitreous. This may result in various injuries. A rupture of blood vessels may lead to a vitreous hemorrhage. A retinal dialysis appears as a circumferential posterior retinal break in the area where the posterior vitreous base has been detached. Similarly, an anterior dialysis may happen along the anterior vitreous base near the ora serrata. Both may lead to retinal detachments. More localized traction may result in a macular hole or retinal tears elsewhere, which can progress to detachments. Choroidal ruptures are usually curvilinear and concentric to the disc. If such a rupture involves the macula, a permanent visual impairment results. Retinal edema or a *commotio retinae* is visible as a whitish discoloration of the retina. The accompanying decrease of vision is temporary. Intra- and preretinal hemorrhages generally resolve with little or no consequences.

A penetrating trauma is equally varied. Treatment depends entirely on the type of injury. If the damage is so severe that the salvage of the eye or of vision is unlikely, enucleation may have to be performed. Two possible complications of penetrating wounds are bacterial endophthalmitis and sympathetic ophthalmia.

In endophthalmitis, the signs and symptoms are more severe than one would anticipate on the basis of the trauma alone. Pain, conjunctival edema and injection, and anterior chamber and vitreous reaction are all much greater than expected. The media may loose their clarity. All penetrating injuries should be treated prophylactically with systemic, including intravenous and topical antibiotics for at least 5 days. If evidence of infection is present, this regimen should be supplemented with periocular injections of antibiotics, vitrectomy, and an intravitreal injection of antibiotics.

Sympathetic ophthalmia is caused by an autoimmune reaction to retinal or uveal pigment antigens, secondary to injury to one eye. It results in a bilateral granulomatous inflammation, thus involving the originally non-injured eye. If left untreated, it will cause blindness of the nontraumatized eye. Initial symptoms are those of iritis, with a disproportionate decrease in visual acuity. If the exciting eye is enucleated within 2 weeks of being injured, sympathetic ophthalmia will probably not occur. Once the inflammation has started, systemic steroids or even immunosuppressants are needed to save the eye.

ANNOTATED BIBLIOGRAPHY

Crawford JS: Eye injuries in children. In Transactions of New Orleans Academy of Ophthalmology: Pediatric Ophthalmology and Strabismus, p 327. New York, Raven Press, 1986 (Reviews the mechanisms of traumatic eye injuries, including sympathetic ophthalmia and endophthalmitis.)

98
Strabismus
JOHAN ZWAAN

Strabismus is a misalignment of the eyes, resulting in a deviation of the visual axis so that they do not meet at the object being looked at. When one eye is turned in relative to the other one, it is called *esotropia* ("crossed eyes"). In *exotropia* or "wall-eyes" one eye is turned out, while a vertical deviation is a *hyper-* or *hypotropia*. A *tropia* is an overt turn of the eye, whereas a *phoria* is latent and only becomes obvious when the fusion of the images between the eyes is disrupted.

There is a major difference between young children and adults in their reactions to strabismus. Adults have diplopia if their eyes become misaligned. In children, on the other hand, the visual system of the brain is still immature and amenable to changes. The image from the deviating eye is suppressed, leading to a loss of depth perception. If this situation persists, the visual acuity of the affected eye will decrease, which is termed *amblyopia*. It is important to realize that amblyopia will not occur, as long as both eyes are being used, even if it is only intermittently.

The terms *strabismus* and *amblyopia* or "lazy eye" are often confused. The first represents a deviation of the eyes with no meaning attached concerning possible changes in visual acuity. The second indicates a decrease in visual acuity, which may be due to strabismus or to other causes, such as a congenital cataract or a large difference in refractive error between the two eyes (see Chapter 99 for a complete discussion on amblyopia).

WORK-UP

History

The history should include the time of onset of strabismus and, if appropriate, a documentation of trauma and diplopia. An inquiry should be made regarding a familial occurrence of strabismus.

Physical Examination

A detailed eye examination, including a dilated fundus examination and cycloplegic refraction or retinoscopy, is essential.

C-T scans and roentgenograms are indicated, if neurologic disease is suspected or if the strabismus is acquired following trauma.

The most useful tool for initial strabismus screening is a small penlight. The light or a small toy is moved in all cardinal directions of gaze and the child is enticed to follow it with the eyes only to determine if any restrictions of gaze are present.

Next, while the child looks at the light, the corneal light reflex is noted. The image of the light should be in the center of the pupil in both eyes, if the eyes are aligned. If one eye is turning, the image of the light will be displaced, nasally for an exotropia and temporally for an esotropia. One can even attempt an estimate of the amount of the turn. Each mm of deviation corresponds to roughly 15 diopters. Thus, because the radius of the cornea is 5 mm to 6 mm, an esotropia of around 45 diopters is present if the corneal light reflex is found halfway between the center and the edge of the cornea.

In the cover-uncover test, the child is made to fixate on an object for several seconds. This may be a mechanical toy or a cartoon at "distance" (a standard distance of 20 ft) or a handheld puppet nearby. The examiner now occludes one eye and observes possible movements of the opposite one. If the latter has to move out to take up fixation, it is esotropic. Similarly, if the eye has to move in, an exotropia is present. By placing one hand on the head of the child and thus restraining it somewhat, one can conveniently use the thumb as an occluder. The cover-uncover test should be repeated for the other eye. The alternate cover test is designed to demonstrate latent deviations or phorias. The occluder (thumb) is moved rapidly between the two eyes to prevent use of the eyes together (binocular fusion). This tends to bring out latent deviations and any movement of the eye being uncovered indicates a phoria.

TYPES OF STRABISMUS

In most cases of strabismus, the underlying pathogenetic mechanism is unknown. The central control mechanisms are probably disturbed, but the exact problem has not been pinpointed. That these mechanisms are involved is made more likely by the finding that children with cerebral palsy, trisomy 21, and so forth, have a significantly higher incidence of strabismus than the general pediatric population. Nevertheless, subtle changes of the extraocular muscles themselves cannot be excluded. The pathophysiology is easier to understand in patients with paralytic strabismus or with strabismus caused by mechanical restrictions.

Pseudostrabismus is often confused with congenital esotropia. The eyes appear to turn in, but in reality they are perfectly aligned. This false impression is created by the presence of prominent epicanthal lidfolds in many babies, which cover up some of the nasal sclera. Thus, the eye seems to be closer to the nose than it really is. Use of the corneal light reflex test or the cover-uncover test makes it easy to differentiate the pseudoform from real esotropia. With growth of the nasal bridge, the epicanthal folds become less pronounced and the "strabismus" goes away. This has given rise to the myth that esotropia may resolve spontaneously. This is not the case.

Occasionally, the optical and the anatomic center of the pupil do not coincide. Thus, the corneal light reflex is seen nasally, yet on the cover test the eye does not move at all. This effect, known as a *positive angle kappa*, can be quite deceiving. It may be particularly pronounced in infants with retrolental fibroplasia or toxoplasmosis chorioretinitis, in which the macula has been "dragged" temporally due to scarring.

Secondary strabismus can follow various eye diseases. A cataract, a large anisometropia (a difference in refractive error), particularly high myopia in one eye, or a scar in the macula can first present as strabismus, usually esotropia. Next to leukocoria, esotropia is the most common presenting sign in retinoblastoma. Thus, all children with strabismus should undergo a detailed eye examination including a dilated fundus examination.

Congenital, or preferably *infantile, esotropia* becomes noticeable 1 to 2 months postnatally. Typically, an alternating esotropia will be present and, if the turn is large, the baby tends to cross-fixate or look across the nose with the right eye to see to the left and *vice versa*. If no other problems are found, surgery is the preferred treatment. The timing of the intervention is still being debated. Some ophthalmologists prefer to operate when the infant is about 6 months old, others wait until 1 or even 2 years after birth.

In *accommodative esotropia*, the turn is related to accommodation. Accommodation is the adjustment of lens power to focus on objects. Normal eyes use this mechanism for near vision and, when the mechanism is activated, convergence or turning in of both eyes also occurs. Hyperopes need to accommodate more than average and the eyes may converge inappropriately, thus leading to esotropia. The same effect happens when the convergence response is too large for the amount of accommodation required. Thus, the ideal treatment consists of an elimination of the need to accommodate. A resolution of the esotropia should follow, and indeed, this is often the case. After a full correction of hyperopia with glasses or the prescription of bifocal lenses, the eyes may become perfectly straight. If the deviation has existed for a while, a complete resolution may not be obtained with glasses and strabismus surgery may be needed. Strong miotic drops, such as echothiophate, can occasionally be used to reduce the accommodation. Long-term use is not recommended because of the potential for significant side effects.

Exotropia can be intermittent or constant. In the intermittent type, visual functions usually develop perfectly normally. Unless the eye deviates frequently, no treatment is necessary, although some ophthalmologists do recommend surgery. Constant exotropia can lead to amblyopia, which should be treated first, usually by patching; surgery can be performed later. Interestingly, children with exotropia are often photophobic and they tend to squint or close the affected eye in bright light. This may be the first sign noted by parents.

Brown syndrome is an example of strabismus caused by a mechanical restriction. The superior oblique tendon either is short or is prevented from moving freely in its sheath at the trochlea. As a result, poor elevation is present on adduction of the eye and the eye may even dip down on going in, while elevation temporally may be normal. The child usually finds a head position in which he can use both eyes together, thus preserving binocular vision. Unless a vertical deviation is present in primary gaze, surgery is not necessary.

In *Duane syndrome*, the lateral rectus is not innervated by the sixth cranial nerve, but by the third nerve. Abduction beyond the midline does not occur and when the eye is adducted, both medial and lateral rectus muscles contract. This pulls the eye back into the orbit and as a result, the lid fissure becomes narrower on adduction. Again, headturning may be present as a compensatory mechanism and binocular vision is possible. Surgery may be done, if an esotropia is present, or if the headturn is cosmetically objectionable.

Trauma is the most common cause of an acquired or congenital palsy. If a palsy is of recent onset, a neurologic work-up is recommended to exclude brain tumor, cerebrovascular anomalies, meningitis, or hydrocephalus. A C-T scan is helpful. A relatively benign form of palsy can follow a viral infection, such as a cold. These often resolve spontaneously, but in the meantime patching may be necessary to alleviate diplopia and to prevent amblyopia. Strabismus surgery may be needed if the deviation persists for several months.

Third nerve palsies may be congenital. They are characterized by a reduced adduction, elevation, and depression of the eye. Thus, the involved eye is exotropic and hypotropic. In addition, the upper eyelid is ptotic. The pupil may be dilated and accommodation may be impaired. Amblyopia is quite common in the congenital variety. If the palsy is

acquired at a later age, severe diplopia is present, unless the ptotic eyelid acts as a patch, obscuring the visual axis of the involved eye. Acquired third nerve palsies may be due to trauma or, less frequently in children, to central nervous system abnormalities. Surgery will give a partial correction only; the goal is to have the eyes straight in the primary position with as large a range of motion as possible. The patient has to learn to adjust to the lack of eye motility by moving the head. A *sixth nerve palsy* may occasionally be present at birth. It results in a large esotropia with an inability to abduct the eye beyond the midline.

A *fourth nerve palsy* is compensated for by tilting the head to eliminate a vertical deviation. Visual development may be entirely normal. The palsy is not infrequently confused with torticollis because of the head tilt and an attempt may be made to correct the latter with a brace, exercises, or even surgery. With the loss of the compensatory head tilt, the eyes are no longer aligned and a loss of binocularity or amblyopia may be the result. In addition to the congenital form, the condition may be acquired, generally following trauma, and diplopia will be present. Mild forms may clear spontaneously, but if the deviation is large, surgery is helpful.

INDICATIONS FOR REFERRAL

All children with suspected strabismus should be referred for detailed eye examinations, if only to exclude retinoblastoma and other causes of secondary strabismus. Moreover, the treatment of strabismus is so specialized that it is best left to the (pediatric) ophthalmologist. Strabismus, in particular infantile esotropia, will not clear spontaneously and an early evaluation and treatment are essential for the prevention of vision loss due to amblyopia.

ANNOTATED BIBLIOGRAPHY

Von Noorden GK: Binocular vision and ocular motility. St Louis, CV Mosby, 1985 (Recently updated text; offers a thorough discussion of all aspects of strabismus and amblyopia.)

99
Amblyopia
ROBERT GROSS

Amblyopia is a diminution in visual acuity for which no structural cause exists. Amblyopia (also known as "lazy eye") represents an important pediatric eye problem that must be identified early in order to be properly treated and provide a good visual prognosis for the child. It is estimated to affect approximately 2% to 2.5% of the population. Amblyopia occurs in early childhood during the visual system's development, or "sensitive" period, and it may be attributed to strabismus or any cause of unequal or diminished visual input to the eyes. Amblyopia is usually unilateral, but may be bilateral in children with large amounts of refractive error in both eyes.

PATHOPHYSIOLOGY AND CLASSIFICATION

Although the precise anatomical correlate for amblyopia has yet to be determined, a basic approach to the cause of amblyopia may be summarized as asymmetric input to the retrocortical pathways. Lens opacities, strabismus, and asymmetric amounts of refractive error (anisometropia) may contribute to differences in input. Amblyopia may also occur on a psychogenic basis.

Media opacity, such as a cataract, may cause irreversible amblyopia if not treated promptly. Unilateral cataracts are best treated in the first months of life in order to provide the best opportunity for correcting the associated amblyopia.

Strabismus, a deviation of the visual axes from physiologic alignment which the individual cannot overcome, is a major cause of amblyopia. Children with deviations that are constant in all directions of gaze (comitant deviations) will have noncorresponding foveal images, because each fovea is directed towards a different object of regard. As such, an image presented to the fovea of one eye will be presented to the peripheral retina of the other eye and will likely be suppressed. Suppression occurs on a cortical level and inhibits the visual image from coming to consciousness. The area of suppression may alternate from eye to eye, depending on which eye has foveal fixation at the time. One eye may be preferred over the other; the nonpreferred eye is therefore suppressed and may become amblyopic.

As a result, strabismic amblyopia is sometimes called *suppression amblyopia* and is always unilateral (see Chap. 98 for a complete discussion on strabismus).

Babies with congenital esotropia (crossed eyes noted within the first 6 months of life) tend to have large angles of deviation (very crossed eyes) and poor abduction of the eyes (inability to move either eye laterally from the midline position). Instead of preferring one eye and ignoring the other, these babies tend to use the right eye to look "across the bridge of the nose" to the left side rather than abduct the left eye, and *vice versa*. This entity is known as *cross fixation*. As such, both eyes are used equally and amblyopia is less likely to occur in this type of strabismus.

Noncomitant deviations do not generally cause strabismic amblyopia. Children with noncomitant deviations will turn or tilt their heads in order to eliminate diplopia and fuse. For example, a child with a right sixth nerve palsy and a resultant inability to abduct the right eye will carry his head turned slightly to the right.

It is problematic to determine which comes first, the amblyopia or the strabismus. The amblyopia is traditionally thought to be due to the strabismus. However, data suggest that defects in binocular vision at birth may deprive the neonate of the appropriate visual stimulation necessary to keep the eyes straight.

Refractive amblyopia occurs most commonly in the eye with the greater amount of hypermetropia (far-sightedness) or astigmatism. A small difference in refractive error may be responsible for an acuity difference of several lines on the vision chart. Refractive amblyopia may also be caused by unilateral high myopia (near-sightedness). Bilateral amblyopia may be caused by large amounts of hypermetropia, myopia, or astigmatism. Another cause of bilateral amblyopia is congenital nystagmus.

CLINICAL PRESENTATION

Amblyopia is suspected when an acuity difference is detected between the two eyes. Although it is possible that a difference in refractive error

440

which, when properly corrected, would account for the visual asymmetry, such patients commonly have a mild underlying amblyopia based on this small difference in refractive error. For this reason, any child with better vision in one eye than the other (or less than perfect vision for age in either eye) should be referred for a further evaluation to an ophthalmologist who is familiar with pediatric eye problems.

In evaluating the visual acuity of amblyopes, it has been found that visual performance is better when tested by isolated single figures, rather than by a row of figures as on a standard vision chart. This disparity in visual performance is due to the "visual interaction" of figures in a row on a chart, making the individual figures on the row slightly more difficult to identify than the same figures presented one at a time. Although there is some sensitivity to this interaction in normal individuals, amblyopes are much more sensitive to this interaction, the *crowding phenomenon*. For this reason, if possible, children should be tested with rows of figures on a chart. Other findings in deep amblyopia include a pupillary afferent defect and subtle color vision abnormalities on the involved side.

TREATMENT

The usual sequence in the treatment of amblyopia is (1) careful ophthalmologic examination to identify or rule out an organic process contributing to poor vision; (2) cycloplegic refraction; (3) spectacle correction of any refractive error; and, if necessary, (4) *penalization* of the preferred eye to force the amblyopic eye to "work harder." Penalization may, classically, take the form of occlusion patching. Other techniques include lens occluders for the glasses, neutral density filters, and pharmacologic methods (atropine). The expectant length of treatment varies with the age of the patient; one "rule-of-thumb" is that 1 month of full-time patching is required per year of age to reverse amblyopia. As is apparent from this method of estimation, it becomes more and more difficult to maintain an effective level of therapy as children get older. Peer pressure at school is a negative influence on patch compliance, as is an unduly protracted course of therapy. On the other hand, while past teaching has suggested that children over 6 years of age are untreatable, it is sometimes possible to obtain good results in children as old as 14 years of age when both patient and parents are sufficiently motivated. A regimen requiring patching during school hours is recommended only when absolutely necessary, in order to minimize social stigmatization for the child, thereby negatively affecting motivation and compliance.

Children are followed at regular intervals to chart progress and ensure that occlusion amblyopia does not occur in the penalized eye. The sacrifice and effort on the part of the child and parents are rewarded by successful treatment yielding two healthy, visually normal eyes in adulthood.

ANNOTATED BIBLIOGRAPHY

Duane T: Clinical Ophthalmology. Philadelphia, Harper & Row, 1985 (Most complete text for clinical ophthalmology. One of its five annually revised volumes includes an authoritative section on strabismus and amblyopia by Dr. Marshall Parks.)

Helveston FM, Ellis FD: Pediatric Ophthalmology Practice. St Louis, CV Mosby, 1980 (Clear presentation of vision, amblyopia, and strabismus written for the pediatrician and general ophthalmologist. Examination techniques are included.)

Von Noorden GK: Binocular Vision and Ocular Motility, 3rd ed. St Louis, CV Mosby, 1985 (Highly comprehensive source on the theory and management of strabismus and amblyopia.)

100
Tearing
WILLIAM P. BOGER III

Tearing (or epiphora) is a common presenting symptom in both the pediatrician's and ophthalmologist's office. Tearing may be due to the overproduction of tears or due to a blockage of the lacrimal drainage apparatus. An excessive production of tears (*e.g.*, from a corneal foreign body) needs to be differentiated from an obstruction in the nasolacrimal draining apparatus. The most common cause of nasolacrimal duct obstruction is a congenital anomaly.

PATHOPHYSIOLOGY

The watery component of tears is produced by the accessory lacrimal glands in the subconjunctival tissues of the eyelids and also by the lacrimal gland, which is both within and under the lateral portion of the upper eyelid. The movements of the eyelids distribute the tears over the surface of the eye cleaning the cornea, and the movements of the eyelids also "pump" the tears into the lacrimal drainage apparatus. At the medial aspect of each lid margin, close to the nose, there is a small opening or punctum. The puncta of the upper and lower lids connect to the canaliculi which join in the common canaliculus which, in turn, enters the nasolacrimal sac. The nasolacrimal sac sits in a bony fossa in the side of the nose, and the nasolacrimal duct passes down a bony channel to open into the nostril under the inferior turbinate. The most common congenital anomaly of this system is an obstruction at the lower end of the nasolacrimal duct, which prevents tears from passing into the nostril. Tears and mucus accumulate in the nasolacrimal sac, and recurrent infections occur in the setting of this stagnation.

CLINICAL PRESENTATION

Characteristic of congenital nasolacrimal duct obstruction is a teary eye with discharge but with no conjunctival injection or photophobia. Many newborns have a brief chemical conjunctivitis following the instillation of silver nitrate at birth, and it is therefore usually difficult to be sure if a newborn has nasolacrimal duct obstruction until he tears persistently and develops recurrent episodes of discharge during the early months of life. Discharge on the lashes or lashes stuck together in the morning with a white and noninjected conjunctiva is characteristic of congenital nasolacrimal duct obstruction. There may also be true episodes of conjunctivitis (discharge and conjunctival injection) secondary to the nasolacrimal duct obstruction. The presence of a discharge and a recurrent infection indicates that the obstruction is low in the lacrimal drainage apparatus. If the obstruction is high, for example at the level of the puncta or canaliculi, the youngster will tear but will not have thick discharge or crusting.

DIFFERENTIAL DIAGNOSIS

In developing a differential diagnosis, important considerations include the age of the youngster, the presence or absence of a concomitant red eye, the character of any discharge on the lashes or in the tear film, the presence or absence of photophobia, and the presence or absence of soft tissue involvement around the eye.

Age at Presentation

Tearing that is intermittently or constantly present from birth is most likely caused by a congenital nasolacrimal duct obstruction. For an older youngster (even 1 or 2 years of age) who suddenly acquires tearing, suspect an overproduction of tearing rather than an obstruction of the nasolacrimal duct.

Tearing with a Red Eye

The differential diagnosis of tearing with a red eye includes the variety of causes of conjunctivitis (see Chap. 93) as well as corneal problems (keratitis) and intraocular inflammation (iritis). In contrast to conjunctivitis, keratitis and iritis tend to produce photophobia in addition to a red and teary eye. The nature of the injection can also be used as a differentiating characteristic. In both keratitis and iritis, the injection will be most intense around the cornea (ciliary injection) and least intense in the fornices. The red eye of conjunctivitis, in contrast, will be most intense in the fornices and least prominent near the cornea. With keratitis and iritis, tearing will occur but usually not much discharge.

A mild conjunctivitis secondary to silver nitrate *Crede* prophylaxis is common. Unfortunately, parents are sometimes inappropriately reassured over the telephone during the first week of life when, in fact, their infant is developing a serious infection. Gonococcal conjunctivitis must be eliminated in all cases of purulent conjunctivitis in the first few days of life. Because the gonococcus can rapidly penetrate the cornea, gonococcal conjunctivitis presents an urgent situation (see Chap. 94 for a complete discussion on this subject).

Chlamydial conjunctivitis usually commences 5 to 12 days after birth and differentiation from gonococcal disease can be difficult. The diagnosis is made by seeing cytoplasmic inclusions on a Giemsa stain of conjunctival scrapings. Culture techniques have only recently become available and require special media. Silver nitrate prophylaxis is ineffective against chlamydia. A long-term follow-up has indicated that poorly treated individuals may develop a trachomalike corneal pannus or corneal vascularization, which can be prevented by appropriate topical antibiotic therapy. The infant should receive topical sulfonamide, erythromycin, or tetracycline ophthalmic ointment four times a day for 3 weeks, oral erythromycin, or both (see Chaps. 93, 94, and 195).

Mild nonspecific conjunctivitis is so common and generally responds so readily to a topical antibiotic preparation that a routine culture of this condition is not necessary. A culture may be helpful if there is something unusual about the conjunctivitis, or if it is severe. An associated preauricular node suggests a viral or chlamydial etiology. Erythromycin ophthalmic ointment four times a day for at least 5 days is a satisfactory initial regimen. It is helpful to have the family call if the conjunctivitis is not significantly improved in 3 days or if it is not completely resolved in 5 days.

Itching is a prominent feature of an injected watery eye with *allergic conjunctivitis* and is common in youngsters who have allergic disorders such as hayfever and asthma. It may, however, be present in a youngster who does not have such an allergic history.

An extreme allergic response in the conjunctiva occurs in *vernal conjunctivitis*, with papillary nodules forming on the tarsal surface of the upper lids, and in "limbal" vernal conjunctivitis in which nodules form at the corneoscleral junction. Vernal conjunctivitis of the upper lid may produce such prominent, firm nodules that the roughened lid surface scratches the cornea continually. Topical corticosteroid drugs can dramatically reduce the size of the allergic nodules and make the patient comfortable. Because steroid eye drops may produce cataracts and glaucoma and may worsen corneal epithelial infections with herpes simplex, they should always be prescribed by an ophthalmologist.

Tearing with Photophobia

Keratitis and iritis must be considered. The most important causes of *keratitis* in children include the following:

- *Infantile Glaucoma* (congenital glaucoma)—It is crucial to make this diagnosis early in life before vision has been irreparably damaged or lost. It is important to maintain a high index of suspicion and to consider it routinely in the differential diagnosis of ocular problems of childhood, particularly in the newborn child with tearing.

  Tearing, photophobia, cloudy cornea, or corneal enlargement in one or both eyes are the classic signs of infantile glaucoma. These may be present at birth (truly congenital); they may develop in the newborn period; or they may develop in the first few years of life (thus the term *infantile* is more appropriate). Only one sign may be present initially, and it is important not to wait for the full constellation before undertaking a complete evaluation for glaucoma. After 2 years of age, the corneas generally do not enlarge, even if the intraocular pressure is elevated. In the childhood years, the configuration of the optic nerve cupping and asymmetry between the cupping in the two eyes is the principal early sign of glaucoma for the nonophthalmic physician.

- *Corneal Foreign Body*—Corneal foreign bodies should be removed promptly. They are painful, and significant delays increase the chance of a secondary infection. Metallic foreign bodies that have been on the cornea for a time will often leave a "rust ring" after the major foreign body has been removed.

- *Herpes Simplex*—Herpes simplex may present initially only on the eyelids. It may affect the lid margins and eyelashes (herpetic marginal blepharitis) or it may affect both the conjunctiva and the cornea (herpetic keratoconjunctivitis). Herpes simplex is a serious cause of blindness in the United States because of its tendency to leave scars in the cornea. Topical steroids may significantly worsen the course of corneal epithelial infection with herpes simplex and thus they must be avoided.

- *Ultraviolet Keratitis*—The cornea absorbs ultraviolet irradiation and may be injured by sunlamp burns, arc welding flashes, or excessive ultraviolet exposure from any source (*e.g.*, snow blindness). Characteristically, intense corneal pain develops approximately 6 hours after the exposure. Visual acuity is diminished (by corneal epithelial irregularity), and many fine punctate lesions of the cornea may be detected by fluorescein staining and a close examination with magnification. Topical erythromycin ophthalmic ointment, tight eye patches for 24 hours, and systemic analgesics are appropriate therapy.

- *Contact Lens Problems*—Contact lenses have become popular and their use is widespread. Contact lens problems bear consideration in the differential diagnosis of tearing in older children. Corneal ulcerations may threaten vision in the context of a serious ocular infection.

A red eye with little or no discharge may also be the result of *acute iritis* rather than conjunctivitis. The pupil may be somewhat smaller in the eye with iritis if the process is unilateral. For the nonophthalmic physician, the differentiation between ititis and keratitis rests on the examination of the cornea. With no apparent corneal pathology, iritis is the likely diagnosis. Since definitive diagnosis and management depend on a slit lamp examination, patients who might have iritis should be referred to the ophthalmologist.

Tearing with Significant Swelling and Erythema in the Soft Tissues Around the Eye

Congenital nasolacrimal duct obstruction may also be the underlying etiology for a severe infection of the nasolacrimal sac (dacryocystitis). Dacryocystitis presents as a red and tender swelling over the medial aspect of the eyelids on the side of the nose. The child may be severely ill. This presentation of acute dacryocystitis needs to be *differentiated* from orbital cellulitis and periorbital cellulitis (see Chap. 95 for a more complete discussion).

Orbital cellulitis denotes the infection of tissues behind the orbital septum with involvement of the retrobulbar structures producing proptosis, chemosis, limitation of the eye movement, and possibly reduction of vision. The orbit is usually infected from a contiguous structure, often from sinusitis. This is a life-threatening condition because infection may spread posteriorly to the cavernous sinus and requires emergency treatment.

Periorbital cellulitis is a facial cellulitis that involves the lids and it may produce an alarming swelling and closure of the lids. The eye itself, however, retains full range of movement; it is not proptotic and it has good visual acuity and normal pupillary reactions. Parenteral antibiotics are also indicated for periorbital cellulitis.

WORK-UP

An etiologic diagnosis of tearing can usually be made by the pediatrician in the office on the basis of a history and physical examination with careful consideration to the aforementioned differential points.

History

Congenital nasolacrimal duct obstruction alone characteristically does not present with a red eye or photophobia, and has an intermittent history from birth. One eye may remit spontaneously, and the other eye may continue to be obstructed.

Physical Examination

The presence of a nasolacrimal duct obstruction can be confirmed by digital pressure on the nasolacrimal sac. If the nasolacrimal duct is obstructed, tears and mucous accumulation in the distended nasolacrimal sac will reflux out the canaliculi and puncta. This maneuver not only confirms the diagnosis of a nasolacrimal duct obstruction, but can also occasionally be curative. Not infrequently, firm pressure over the nasolacrimal sac may result in a "popping" sensation with a release of tears and mucus into the nostril, thus relieving the nasolacrimal duct obstruction.

Laboratory Tests

Under most circumstances, the low-grade infection accompanying nasolacrimal duct obstruction can be treated satisfactorily with pressure over the nasolacrimal sac and topical antibiotic ointments (or drops). If the infection is particularly severe and is resistant to a change of antibiotics, or if a dacryocystitis exists, culturing the discharge may be helpful.

TREATMENT

Eighty to ninety percent of youngsters who have congenital nasolacrimal duct obstruction will remit spontaneously during the first 9 to 12 months of life. It becomes increasingly rare for the nasolacrimal duct obstruction to remit spontaneously after 1 year of age. The parents should be taught how to provide compression over the nasolacrimal sac and they should continue this treatment at home to keep the sac empty. During the first 6 to 9 months, it is best to prescribe direct pressure over the nasolacrimal sac (qid initially and then as frequently as necessary to keep the sac empty of mucoid material) and to prescribe antibiotic ointment or drops (*e.g.*, erythromycin ophthalmic ointment). The treatment is directed toward avoiding infection and minimizing stagnation. Topical antibiotic therapy should be started at the first sign of infection (*e.g.*, crusting or discharge on the lashes) without waiting for a full-blown conjunctivitis to develop. Many parents find it easier to instill antibiotic eye drops as opposed to eye ointment, but the blinking mechanism is so vigorous in youngsters that the antibiotic eye *drop* is quickly washed away. Because the ointment lingers longer, it is generally more effective. If the infection cannot be controlled with a particular eye drop, the pediatrician should not only change the antibiotic to one with a different spectrum, but he should also consider changing to an ointment rather than a drop.

It is helpful for each pediatrician to discuss nasolacrimal duct obstruction with the ophthalmologist or pediatric ophthalmologist who will be examining the child when a referral is made. There is a general consensus that nasolacrimal duct obstruction can be relieved in most cases by probing and irrigating the nasolacrimal duct. Although there is no controversy within ophthalmic circles with regard to the efficacy of probing, there is some variation in the recommended timing of the probing and irrigation. Some ophthalmologists, if presented with a family unhappy with a child who has a pussy, recurrently infected eye, probe at presentation regardless of age. Other ophthalmologists note that 80% to 90% of youngsters with nasolacrimal duct obstruction remit spontaneously by 9 months of life if they are treated with "massage" and antibiotics. If the discharge is minimized so that the only evidence of the nasolacrimal duct obstruction is excessive clear tearing without discharge and if the parents understand their options with regard to the timing of the probing, it would be reasonable for the pediatrician to keep following the problem until 8 or 9 months of age. It is helpful for the ophthalmologist to have the opportunity to review the options again with the parents and if the nasolacrimal duct obstruction does not remit spontaneously, a probing and irrigation can be scheduled around the first birthday.

An advantage of probing early is that youngsters are smaller and therefore weaker and require less restraint for probings done in the office. Most ophthalmologists who do office probings will tend to probe children early whereas most ophthalmologists who wait 9 to 12 months to see if the child's problem will remit spontaneously will tend to use brief general anesthetics on an outpatient basis for the probing in the older child. Endotracheal intubation is not required, thus the procedure can be done under "mask" anesthesia in an ambulatory surgery unit. Most youngsters with nasolacrimal duct obstruction are symptomatically improved after the initial probing, but if tearing persists after the initial probing, another probing is indicated. If several probings have failed, the situation is unusual and perhaps a nasolacrimal duct intubation with silastic tubing or a dacryocystorhinostomy may be required. Nasolacrimal duct obstruction in the context of craniofacial malformation or trauma to the mid-face region are settings in which these more complicated procedures are often required. It is distinctly unusual for a youngster with a normal facial structure to fail to respond to multiple probings.

Dacryocystitis should be treated with systemic antibiotics. Once the infection is cleared, the obstruction and cause of the problem may be relieved by a probing of the nasolacrimal duct. Acute dacryocystitis at any age or congenital dacryocele noted in the newborn period should be referred to the ophthalmologist as soon as the situation is recognized or even questioned.

To relieve *allergic conjunctivitis*, mild vasoconstricting agents such as naphazoline hydrochloride can be given topically as eye drops. They should not, however, be used on a continual basis. Systemic antihistamines may be helpful although their value is controversial. Topical vasoconstrictors and topical antihistamines generally do not provide a dramatic improvement. Cromolyn eye drops are more effective than the topical vasoconstrictors and topical antihistamines.

Many superficial *corneal foreign bodies* can be brushed away with a cotton-tipped applicator or a blunt spatula after a drop of local anesthetic (*e.g.*, 0.5% proparcaine) is placed in the eye. A cotton-tipped applicator may carry away more corneal epithelium and therefore leave a larger corneal abrasion, but since a cotton-tipped applicator is blunt, many physicians feel comfortable using it around the eye. A sharp needle is needed to remove embedded material. Any sharp object brought close to the eye should be kept tangential to the cornea and not perpendicular to avoid a tragedy if the youngster should suddenly get loose from their restraint or someone accidentally strikes the physician's arm or hand. A large rust ring may retard satisfactory healing. They, as well as deeply embedded corneal foreign bodies in the central cornea involving the visual axis, should be referred to an ophthalmologist for removal. Once the foreign body is removed, the remaining defect is treated like a corneal abrasion with antibiotic ointment and a tight eye patch.

If the classic branching dendritic form of an active corneal herpetic ulcer is seen with fluorescein staining, an ophthalmologist should be consulted. If the child is known to have previously had ocular herpes simplex or if it is suspected, it is best to let an ophthalmologist evaluate and treat a new episode of red eye. Although not helpful when placed topically on skin lesions, the antiviral agents IDU and ARA-A and trifluridine can be helpful when used topically on active corneal lesions from *herpes simplex*.

ANNOTATED BIBLIOGRAPHY

El-Mansoury J, Calhoun JH, Nelson LB, Harley RD: Results of late probing of congenital nasolacrimal duct obstruction. Ophthalmol 93(8):1052–1054, 1986 (104 patients with 138 blocked nasolacrimal ducts were probed after the age of 13 months. 129 (93%) were free of symptoms after the first probing.)

Paul TO: Medical management of congenital nasolacrimal duct obstruction. J Pediatr Ophthalmol Strabismus 22(2):68–70, 1985 (55 infants with 62 obstructed nasolacrimal ducts were followed prospectively using medical treatment. 89% of the nasolacrimal ducts (55/62) opened without surgical probing in the first 16 months of life.)

Petersen RA, Robb RM: The natural course of congenital obstruction of the nasolacrimal duct. J Pediatr Ophthalmol Strabismus 15(2):246–250, 1978 (50 infants with 65 blocked nasolacrimal ducts were followed prospectively with medical treatment for 8 to 13 months. 58 ducts in 54 patients opened spontaneously without probing.)

Robb RM: Probing and irrigation for congenital nasolacrimal duct obstruction. Arch Ophthalmol 104:378–379, 1986 (Primary probing continued to be an effective treatment well after 2 years of age and was successful in two 5-year-old patients.)

101
Leukocoria
JOHAN ZWAAN

When parents report that their infant has a "white pupil" or a "cat's eye," or when the pediatrician finds such an abnormality, serious concern should be raised. Leukocoria almost always indicates a serious eye disease such as a retinoblastoma. In leukocoria, the normally bright red reflex of light bouncing back from the fundus is greatly diminished or entirely absent. A white mass or a whitish reflex may be noted in the pupil.

PATHOPHYSIOLOGY

Abnormalities of the lens, the vitreous, the retina, or combinations of these may be responsible for the presence of leukocoria.

Any opacity of the lens may be termed a *cataract*, although the term is usually reserved for opacities that are dense and large enough to interfere with vision. They may be unilateral or bilateral, and they involve all or part of the lens. The cause of the opacification is often poorly understood. Cataracts involving only one eye are usually nonhereditary and are thought to be due to an abnormal developmental event. Bilateral cataracts are frequently hereditary or may be part of a generalized embryopathy, such as those related to a maternal infection during pregnancy, primarily rubella. In children with disturbances of carbohydrate metabolism, such as galactosemia, galactose kinase deficiency, or diabetes mellitus, sugar alcohols may accumulate within the lens cells. This increases the osmolarity of the cytoplasm, which draws water into the cells and causes the cells to swell, thus inducing cataract formation.

Persistent hyperplastic primary vitreous (PHPV) is a developmental anomaly involving the vitreous, as well as the lens and retina. The eye is frequently also microphthalmic. The condition is usually unilateral and sporadic. A dense white vitreous membrane or plaque is attached to the posterior aspect of the lens and blood vessels may be seen within the membrane. The membrane exerts traction and may pull the ciliary processes centrally behind the lens, where they are visible as a darkly pigmented fringe. The same mechanism can lead to retinal detachment. The cause for the anomaly is not known.

Any abnormality of the retina, in which part of it is altered enough to cause the reflection of light from it to be white rather than orange or red, can present as leukocoria.

Medullated nerve fibers consist of patches of retina in which the normally unmyelinated axons of the nerve fiber layer have become myelinated. They are occasionally confused with retinal tumors, but they are entirely benign. The cause for the myelination is unknown.

Chorioretinal colobomas are the result of a failure of the closure of the choroidal fissure early in embryonic development. Their location is always inferonasal from the optic disk, the position of the choroidal fissure on the embryonic optic stalk.

They consist of white or yellowish areas of sclera not covered, as is the case normally, by retina and choroid.

The most feared of the causes of leukocoria is a *retinoblastoma*. This potentially lethal tumor, responsible for about 1% of tumor deaths in children up to the age of 15 years, is due to a somatic mutation in about two of three patients and to autosomal dominant inheritance in the remainder. The prognosis depends on the stage at which the tumor is diagnosed. Its frequency fortunately is rare: ~ 300 new cases are diagnosed annually in the United States.

Congenital chorioretinitis due to toxoplasmosis, cytomegalic inclusion disease, or herpes simplex usually results in the presence of chorioretinal scars. These appear as irregular white lesions, often with some pigment mottling and with a hyperpigmented border. It is assumed that, in most cases, the infection is inactive or subclinical at the time of birth. Severe systemic abnormalities, particularly involving the central nervous system, may be present.

Retinal *toxocariasis* is caused by ingestion of the eggs of *Toxocara canis* or, less commonly, *Toxocara catis*. This leads to visceral larva migrans, which may affect the eye. The infestation can present as a vitreous abscess, a lesion of the posterior pole, or an inflammatory mass in the periphery of the retina with secondary vitreoretinal membranes. The lesion may be confused with retinoblastoma. It is rare for both the eye and visceral organs to be infected.

A total *retinal detachment* may lead to leukocoria. The detachment is the result of a separation of the outer layers of the retina from the retinal pigment epithelium with subretinal fluid accumulating in between the layers. Retinal detachment may be found at birth as a congenital anomaly. More commonly, it is due to a break in the retina, which allows fluid to enter the subretinal space (rhegmatogenous detachment), to traction by vitreoretinal membranes (traction detachment), or to a build-up of subretinal fluid, when exudation exceeds absorption (exudative detachment). All three mechanisms may occur in children. Breaks in the retina are commonly the result of trauma, and child abuse should be suspected. Other causes are myopia, aphakia following cataract removal, and retrolental fibroplasia. Traction detachments can be seen in diabetes mellitus, sickle cell retinopathy, and retrolental fibroplasia. Exudative retinal detachments may accompany retinoblastoma and other retinal neoplasms, uveitis, and Coats' disease.

Coats' disease is characterized by vascular dilatations on the surface of the retina and hard exudates, which progress to exudative detachments. If untreated, total retinal detachment will follow and eventually atrophy of the eye. The disease is sporadic, occurs more in males than in females, and generally affects only one eye.

Retrolental fibroplasia (RLF) or retinopathy of prematurity can progress to total retinal detachment and thus give the appearance of a white pupil. RLF occurs most frequently in premature infants who have been treated with supplemental oxygen, but it can also be seen in full-term infants or in babies who have not received oxygen. The peripheral retinal vessels are not fully developed at the end of gestation, more so on the temporal side of the retina than on the nasal side. The normal process of vasculogenesis is arrested by injury, presumably linked to oxygen exposure. A ridge of mesenchyme develops, which forms an abrupt border between the vascularized and the avascular retina. Differentiation eventually resumes in this tissue and the abnormal structure regresses in about 90% of the infants. In about 10%, neovascularization occurs and the primitive cells break through the internal limiting membrane of the retina and grow into the vitreous, along the surface of the retina. This leads to fibrovascular membrane proliferation and finally to traction retinal detachment.

CLINICAL PRESENTATION AND DIFFERENTIAL DIAGNOSIS

Leukocoria is found in such a diversity of eye abnormalities that only a detailed eye examination allows a differential diagnosis to be made. In addition to a white pupil, reduced visual acuity may be present and the eyes may be misaligned; esotropia is found more commonly than exotropia.

The lens opacities characteristic of both cataracts and PHPV are located immediately behind the plane of the iris. They may be dense and large enough to prevent any view of the fundus. PHPV is present if blood vessels or ciliary processes are seen in association with the lens opacity.

A longstanding vitreous hemorrhage (*e.g.*, from trauma, diabetes, or sickle cell disease) shows up as a yellowish discoloration behind the lens.

Medullated nerve fibers have a fluffy cotton-like appearance and often fan out from the optic nerve, following the normal course of the retinal nerve fibers. Patches may be found some distance away from the optic disk. Retinal blood vessels tend to weave in and out of the areas of myelination. Except for enlargement of the normal blind spot or the presence of additional scotomas, there is usually little, if any, effect on vision.

Colobomas present as more or less round areas of white sclera, which are fairly sharply defined and which often have a hyperpigmented border. They vary in size and are located in the inferonasal fundus, although they may be large enough to include the optic nerve or the bulk of the retina. Iris colobomas may be seen and, if the anomaly is large, microphthalmia is common. The effects on visual acuity are related directly to the extent of the lesion(s) and may range from small and difficult to detect scotomas to severe visual loss.

The presentation of *Toxocara* and retinoblastoma is similar, with a white mass (or masses) found in the retina and occasionally in the vitreous. Indeed, the differentiation is sometimes not possible based on clinical findings and may not be made until after the enucleation of the eye.

The scars of chorioretinitis are difficult to differentiate, although the ones caused by toxoplasmosis tend to be more pigmented than those due to herpes or CMV. All of these may be associated with an overlying vitreous reaction. The differential diagnosis is usually based on systemic and laboratory findings.

Retinal detachments need to be distinguished on the basis of careful indirect ophthalmoscopy. The presence of abnormal blood vessels and exudates point to Coats' disease; tears or holes in the retina are typical for rhegmatogenous detachments. The age of the child at the time of the appearance of the abnormality may be helpful in making a diagnosis. A congenital detachment is obviously present at birth. Detachments due to RLF tend to occur within the first year of life, although they may develop at a later age. Coats' disease is not manifest until the child is several years old.

WORK-UP

History

A careful gestational history should be taken, including a possible exposure of the mother to infectious disease during pregnancy. Genital herpes simplex and risk factors for infection with *Toxocara* or toxoplasmosis (presence of household pets or eating poorly cooked meat) need to be documented. A history of prematurity or trauma and the age of

the child at the time of discovery of leukocoria may yield important clues. The occurrence in family members of eye problems associated with leukocoria may allow an early tentative diagnosis.

Physical Examination

A detailed eye examination is essential. This requires that the pupil be dilated with mydriatics. In addition, the eyelids should be kept open, if necessary by the use of eyelid retractors. The head should be immobilized, preferably voluntarily or otherwise by holding the head or wrapping the child. An adequate examination often requires the use of general anesthesia. Generally, this examination is best done by a (pediatric) ophthalmologist. Ultrasonographs and CT scans are useful, particularly when the ocular media are sufficiently opaque to prevent a good view of the fundus.

Laboratory Tests

Laboratory tests need to be tailored to the suspected diagnosis. A routine urinalysis may reveal glucosuria or galactosuria, which is evidence of a disturbance of carbohydrate metabolism, sometimes responsible for cataractogenesis. Blood chemistry may show elevated serum glucose (in diabetic cataracts) or hypocalcemia, which occasionally causes cataracts. An enzymatic analysis of erythrocytes and serum allows a specific diagnosis of abnormalities of galactose metabolism. A toxoplasma, rubella, cytomegalovirus, herpesvirus (TORCH) screen is helpful for the differential diagnosis of infantile cataract and chorioretinitis. If a white mass is present in the retina or vitreous and retinoblastoma or *Toxocara* is suspected, an ELISA test for the latter is available. Chromosome analysis, including prophase banding, may be helpful in cases of retinoblastoma due to a chromosome deletion. With the isolation of the gene, whose absence may be responsible for the development of retinoblastoma, a more specific test for this disease, possibly allowing prenatal diagnosis, may soon be available. Spinal taps and bone marrows should be performed on patients with retinoblastoma to exclude metastases. Colobomas can also be associated with chromosome anomalies.

TREATMENT

The treatment of the disorders underlying the presence of leukocoria obviously differs, depending on the particular disorder. Medullated nerve fibers and colobomas usually require no treatment; exceptions depend on what associated findings are present.

Cataracts and PHPV are treated by lensectomy, sometimes in combination with vitrectomy, if they are dense enough to interfere with the formation of a sharp image on the retina. This needs to be done on an urgent basis to prevent the development of deprivation amblyopia. Even more important than the surgical therapy is a rigorous and aggressive follow-up treatment (*i.e.*, optical correction of the resulting aphakia and antiamblyopia treatment.) Without these, the visual results will be as bad as if the cataract surgery had not taken place at all.

Active chorioretinitis may require appropriate antimicrobial therapy. Toxoplasmosis is treated with a combination of pyrimethamine and sulfonamides, together with folinic acid to prevent the platelet depression caused by the first medication. Steroids are occasionally used. Systemic antiviral medications are available for chorioretinitis caused by herpes simplex.

The treatment of retinoblastoma depends on the stage of the disease. Advanced cases require enucleation to prevent metastatic disease. If both eyes are involved, an attempt will be made to save the less involved eye. Photocoagulation, cryotherapy, and radiation are commonly used modes of treatment. Chemotherapy is indicated when the tumor has become extraocular, although these cases are almost always fatal. A periodic follow-up with examinations under anesthesia is essential, because new tumors may arise in the retina several years after the original diagnosis. Additionally, it has been shown that patients with retinoblastoma have a high incidence of secondary tumors later in life, particularly osteogenic sarcoma of the orbit.

Retinal detachments, including those of RLF and Coats' disease, are treated surgically, usually with scleral buckle procedures and often in combination with vitrectomy. No specific therapy is available for *Toxocara*; depending on the extent of involvement, infected eyes may be enucleated.

INDICATIONS FOR REFERRAL

All patients with a white pupil should be referred on an urgent basis. Many of the disorders causing leukocoria need to be treated rapidly to prevent an irrevocable decrease of vision. Retinoblastoma can be life-threatening.

ANNOTATED BIBLIOGRAPHY

Beller R, Hoyt CS, Marg E et al: Good visual function after neonatal surgery for congenital monocular cataracts. Am J Ophthalmol 91:559, 1981 (Indicates that excellent visual results are possible with early cataract surgery and rigorous antiamblyopia therapy.)

Catalano J D: Leukocoria, the differential diagnosis of a white pupil. Pediatr Ann 12:499, 1983

Flynn JT: Retrolental fibroplasia: Update. In Transactions of the New Orleans Academy of Ophthalmology: Pediatric Ophthalmology and Strabismus, p. 293. New York, Raven Press, 1986 (Excellent review of RLF.)

Metz HS, Rosenbaum AL: Pediatric ophthalmology. New York, Medical Examination Publishing Co, 1982 (Paperback book with good reviews of pediatric cataracts and retinal problems in addition to other topics.)

13

Gastrointestinal Problems

W. ALLAN WALKER, Section Editor

102
Vomiting

ANNE MUNCK AND
HARLAND S. WINTER

Vomiting is a common occurrence in infancy and childhood. To identify a possible cause for this symptom, a complete history and a thorough physical examination often yield more information than any laboratory studies. The reason may be as simple as overfeeding, but several disease entities may be involved. Most frequently, treatment is directed at controlling the symptom until a cause is identified.

PATHOPHYSIOLOGY

Vomiting should be differentiated from regurgitation, rumination, and wretching. Regurgitation is an effortless expulsion of gastric contents, usually occurring in infancy. Rumination is the regurgitation of ingested food, which is then rechewed and reswallowed. Some clinicians believe that it provides a pleasant sensation to the child; that it represents self-stimulatory behavior; and that it may reflect a psychological disturbance. Rumination may also be associated with esophagitis, but somatic and psychological components may both play a role. In severe situations, a dramatic weight loss with marasmus may result. In contrast, vomiting and wretching are active processes in which a strong contraction of the abdominal muscles leads to increased intraabdominal pressure and elevation of the diaphragm into the thorax. Wretching involves voluntary attempts to empty the stomach

and uses thoracic musculature, whereas vomiting is more passive and results from compression of abdominal musculature. In addition, when someone vomits, the pyloric sphincter contracts, the cardia rises and opens so that the gastric contents are ejected forcefully by the high intraabdominal pressure. During the abdominal contraction, no active contractions are noted in the esophagus. After several seconds, peristaltic activity starts in the upper esophagus, clearing its contents into the stomach. The esophageal sphincter closes after this secondary wave. Emesis is mediated by the vomiting center in the reticular brain formation. The afferents most frequently come from the gastrointestinal tract or from the chemoreceptor trigger zone located on the floor of the fourth ventricle, but other receptors are located in the pharynx, heart, bile ducts, and respiratory tract. (This may explain the association of vomiting with biliary tract disease or pneumonia.) Efferent fibers use the sympathetic, vagal, and phrenic nerve pathways. From a clinical viewpoint, wretching is loud but vomiting is relatively silent.

CLINICAL PRESENTATION

Specific aspects of the clinical presentation should be sought to establish the cause of vomiting. Causes of vomiting in infancy may be identified by seeking information about diet and previous medication that may be related to an intolerance of a specific food or drug. A history of weight loss increases the possibility of an organic lesion or a chronic problem. An excessive weight gain may indicate overfeeding. Information on the quality and quantity of the vomitus should be obtained. The presence of bile suggests an obstruction distal to the duodenum. Undigested food may be found in disorders affecting the esophagus, such as achalasia or stricture. Mucus is often noted in infants with feeding problems or pylorospasm. Blood or hematemesis usually indicates mucosal ulceration of the esophagus, stomach, or duodenum. The relationship of vomiting to meals may help to define the cause. Early morning vomiting before eating is observed frequently in patients with intracranial hypertension (it is usually projectile) or in metabolic diseases. Vomiting that occurs when a meal is finished may lead the investigator to pursue psychological disorders or peptic ulcer. In peptic disease, vomiting frequently relieves the pain in contrast to pancreatic or biliary tract disorders in which symptoms may persist after emesis (see Chap. 111). Associated symptoms such as fever, diarrhea, jaundice, dysphagia, head trauma, or pain must be identified.

DIFFERENTIAL DIAGNOSIS

Patients may vomit for several reasons. These include inflammation of the mucosa of the gastrointestinal tract (*e.g.*, gastroenteritis), stretching of an organ or membrane (*e.g.*, bowel obstruction or otitis media), vestibular reflex (*e.g.*, seasickness), stimulation of the chemoreceptor trigger zone (*e.g.*, radiation therapy or metabolic disorders such as diabetes mellitus or salt-losing adrenogenital syndrome) and increased intracranial pressure (*e.g.*, brain tumor). In the newborn, nonsurgical causes may have presentations similar to problems requiring surgical intervention. In addition to pyloric stenosis, it is especially necessary to identify other anatomic causes of vomiting (congenital or acquired). Abdominal distention associated with the absence of passage of meconium suggests either atresia or intestinal stenosis. If bilious vomiting is present, the obstruction is below the ampulla of Vater. Meconium ileus on a plain film may imply cystic fibrosis. Abdominal distention may be absent with a partial obstruction as seen with an intestinal diaphragm because fluid and gas may pass through the lesion. Intermittent vomiting is usual in malrotation of the bowel with midgut volvulus. Although abdominal pain is often evident initially, it may resolve as the bowel undergoes ischemic ne-

crosis. The patient may have a limited time of relative well-being before presenting in septic shock.

A family history of vomiting in infancy suggests a milk protein intolerance, but the diagnosis can only be established after other etiologies have been eliminated. Immaturity of the lower esophageal sphincter usually causes regurgitation, which to some observers may be viewed as forceful emesis. Formula improperly prepared can result in emesis. Swallowed blood from an excoriation on the mother's breast may result in hematemesis, because blood is an irritant to the gastrointestinal tract. The birth history may provide important clues regarding the cause of vomiting. A difficult delivery may be associated with vomiting due to cerebral ischemia, cerebral edema, or intracranial hemorrhage.

As a manifestation of systemic disease, vomiting may be associated with a fever in acute infections or with delayed development and seizures in either meningitis, hydrocephalus, subdural effusion, or inborn errors of metabolism (*e.g.*, salt-losing adrenogenital syndrome). Other clinical features are helpful in reducing the diagnostic possibilities. Diarrhea is often associated with vomiting in gastroenteritis. When fever is present and even without localizing findings, otitis media, pneumonia, and urinary tract infections are possible. Jaundice suggests hepatitis or biliary tract obstruction as noted with cholelithiasis or choledocholithiasis.

Abdominal pain associated with emesis may be due to appendicitis, volvulus, or intussusception. If the pain is intermittent and colicky in nature or if an abdominal mass is palpable, one should consider an intussusception and perform a diagnostic as well as therapeutic barium enema. These are much less common in infants.

Migraine, abdominal epilepsy, or intracranial tumors may present predominantly with vomiting, but are usually also associated with a headache or seizure activity. Diabetic ketoacidosis is often accompanied by a history of polyphagia and weight loss. The causes for cyclic vomiting may be multifactorial, but the recurrent attacks are usually associated with headache, fever, and abdominal pain. Persistent vomiting progressing to a stuporous state suggests progressive hepatic failure as witnessed in Reye's syndrome. Some patients, however, may have a mild course without neurologic sequelae. Many of the children with "mild Reye's" have been identified as having the metabolic disorder, medium-chain acetyl-CoA dehydrogenase deficiency.

The relationship of emesis to drug therapy should be considered. Theophylline and erythromycin commonly cause vomiting. Radiation ther-

Causes of Vomiting

INFANCY

Overfeeding
Gastroesophageal reflux
Soy/milk protein intolerance
Sepsis
Pyloric stenosis
Intestinal obstruction
Subdural effusion
Metabolic disorder
Adrenal insufficiency
Neurologic damage

CHILDHOOD (in addition to those listed above)

Gastroenteritis
Peptic ulcer disease
Pneumonia
Otitis media
Diabetes mellitus
Increased intracranial pressure
Meningitis
Appendicitis
Hepatitis
Reye's syndrome
Intussusception
Migraine
Abdominal epilepsy
Ketotic hypoglycemia
Drug intolerance/toxicity

ADOLESCENCE (in addition to those listed above)

Anorexia nervosa
Bulimia
Pregnancy

apy and most drugs used for treatment of malignancy cause vomiting. Agents such as cis-platinum, nitrogen mustard, actinomycin D, and cyclophosphamide may cause more emesis than agents such as doxorubicin, methotrexate, and radiation therapy (see the box, Causes of Vomiting).

A discussion of the differential diagnosis of vomiting would be incomplete if psychological problems were not mentioned. Anorexia nervosa and bulimia must remain at the top of the list in the adolescent population and should be considered while an organic lesion is being sought. An adolescent with an unplanned pregnancy may first seek help because of vomiting. In all situations, the physician must be aware of and sensitive to the significant issues for each age group and for every individual patient.

WORK-UP

History

The evaluation of the vomiting patient is guided by the age of the child. In the neonatal period, special attention should be given to the type, amount, and method of feeding, the quantity and quality of vomitus (bilious, undigested food, blood), the child's hunger, the timing of vomiting with respect to the meals, and the concurrence of dysphagia, abdominal pain, or diarrhea. A family history of dietary protein intolerance may be relevant. Drugs prescribed prior to delivery may be important. The growth curve frequently helps to separate functional disorders from organic lesions. A history of fever or head trauma must be sought. Inquire also about seizures and abnormal movements. After the neonatal period, additional historical data such as the presence of headache, polydipsia, polyuria, muscle weakness, or drug ingestion may be more relevant. If the child has lost weight, evidence for inflammation and some determination about body image should be ascertained.

Physical Examination

As vomiting has so many causes, the physical examination should be complete and should include an evaluation of each organ system, vital signs, and assessment of the state of hydration.

In the infant, observation of the abdomen may reveal abdominal distention associated with hyperperistaltic waves. A pyloric tumor may be palpable, especially if the examination is performed immediately following a bout of emesis. A neurologic examination may reveal focal findings, delayed neurologic development, seizure activity, hypotonia, or papilledema. Signs of infection may include rales or bulging tympanic membranes. In older children, a thorough abdominal examination will include palpation in the right lower quadrant for guarding or rebound which suggests appendicitis or inflammatory bowel disease.

Laboratory Tests

Aided by the clinical work-up, diagnostic laboratory studies should help identify the etiology of vomiting. An APT test in suckling babies who vomit blood can prove that the blood was swallowed from the mother's breast. In the infant, barium enema may reveal a large bowel obstruction, whereas an upper gastrointestinal series may demonstrate esophageal stricture, intestinal stenosis or atresia, duodenal webs, pyloric stenosis, or malrotation. Abdominal ultrasound can be beneficial in establishing the diagnosis of pyloric stenosis and thereby avoiding an x-ray study. The plain film of the abdomen with an upright x-ray will guide the clinician in deciding whether to examine first the lower bowel or the upper bowel. As discussed in Chapter 103, the *p*H probe is the best way to identify pathologic reflux. A work-up for sepsis, including a complete blood cell count with differential, urinalysis, cultures of blood, stool, and spinal fluid should be performed in any child thought to be systemically ill. Liver function tests, serum glucose, ammonia, and electrolytes may be appropriate with organic and amino acids if hepatic or metabolic disease is suspected. Immunologic studies such as IgE, RAST to casein, β-lactoglobulin, or soy are usually normal even in infants with confirmed intolerance. As yet, no reliable diagnostic laboratory test can confirm suspected protein intolerance. In those children suspected of having a neurologic disease, an electroencephalogram, computerized tomography, or specialized neurologic testing may be necessary. A pregnancy test may be indicated in the ovulating female.

Laboratory studies must also be used to evaluate the complications of emesis. Acutely, three major metabolic consequences occur in association with dehydration. Potassium deficiency is caused by both a decreased food intake and a loss in the vomitus. Second, alkalosis results because of a loss of hydrogen ion, an accumulation of H^+ intracellularly, and a contraction of the extracellular fluid due to sodium depletion. Third, sodium depletion results from a loss of sodium in vomitus. Chronic complications of vomiting include metabolic disorders, aspiration pneumonia, or Mallory–Weiss syndrome in which bleeding is due to a tear at the gastroesophageal junction. In these conditions, chest roentgenograms or upper endoscopy may be useful for diagnostic purposes.

TREATMENT AND MANAGEMENT

Every pediatrician receives telephone calls from a parent concerned about a child who is vomiting. *Any child with emesis plus colicky abdominal pain should be evaluated immediately.* Generally, if vomiting or fever has persisted for over 24 hours,

the child should be examined. If the problem has started recently, the clinician should try to assess the level of dehydration. When did the child last urinate? What is the state of consciousness and activity? Are mucous membranes moist? If the child can tolerate small sips of fluid, an attempt should be made at oral rehydration. If all oral feeds are refused, the child should be evaluated by the physician. An electrolyte solution (*e.g.*, Pedialyte, Lytren, or Gatoraid) is optimal, but if this is not available a decarbonated soft drink, jello or tea can be used. An attempt should be made to provide both sodium and potassium. Should the child continue to vomit, have any changes in state of consciousness, persist with a fever, or show signs of dehydration, then he should be examined.

Steroid therapy may be life-saving if adrenal insufficiency is suspected. Once an anatomic abnormality is found, surgery may be necessary with the exception of an intussusception in which a barium enema may be both diagnostic and therapeutic. In general, no standardized approach exists for the management of vomiting because therapy depends on an identifiable etiology. One exception to this principle is the management of vomiting associated with chemotherapy. Although more severe than vomiting from acute causes, some of the treatment used for chemotherapy-induced emesis can be applied to other causes. Preparation of the child to anticipate vomiting after chemotherapy is important, but one must be careful not to place emesis basins or foods with strong aromas near the patient. These agents can act as triggers to induce vomiting. A prophylactic treatment is most helpful. If anxiety is a factor, diazepam or lorazepam may be beneficial. If vestibular symptoms are prominent, dimenhydrinate, diphenhydramine, or transdermal scopolamine may beneficial. Sucking on candy or auditory distractions may reduce sensory triggers.

Drug therapy should be initiated prior to chemotherapy. Thiethylperazine (Torecan) is one of the most effective phenothiazines and is available in a tablet, suppository, or injectable formulation. If given intravenously, it should be administered over 60 minutes to decrease extrapyramidal side effects. Diphenhydramine (Benadryl), may be given concomitantly to avoid the central nervous system side effects of the phenothiazines and also to provide additional sedation. Perphenazine (Trilafon) is another phenothiazine that can be administered either intravenously or orally. Prochlorperazine (Compazine) and Promethazine (Phenergan) are safest to use in children under the age of 5 years, but they have little antiemetic effect. Their main benefit probably results from the sedation.

Other antiemetic therapeutic agents may have a role in the refractory patient. Metoclopramide (Reglan) seems to work well in the patient receiving cis-platinum. Cannabinoid derivatives, or synthetic analogs of marijuana's active ingredient, THC, have been shown to be beneficial. Benzquinamide (Emetecon) is a nonphenothiazine that is slightly better than a placebo in controlling emesis. For the severely ill patient, high-dose steroids or intravenous nembutal sedation may be required for symptomatic relief.

INDICATIONS FOR REFERRAL OR ADMISSION

An indication for admission of a vomiting patient is either for a diagnostic evaluation or acute therapy for one of the following complications: a metabolic abnormality, an aspiration, gastrointestinal bleeding or moderate to severe dehydration. A young child with mild dehydration and continued vomiting may also warrant hospitalization. An identified underlying problem should prompt a consultation to the appropriate subspecialist.

ANNOTATED BIBLIOGRAPHY

Arthur RJ et al: Barium meal examination of infants under four months of age presenting with vomiting. A review of 100 cases. Pediatr Radiol 14(2):84–86, 1984 (Assessment of infants with regurgitation from a radiologic perspective.)

Fordtran JS: Gastrointestinal Disease: Pathophysiology and Management. Chap. 11: Vomiting, pp 127–143. Philadelphia, WB Saunders, 1975 (Pathophysiology of vomiting, its etiology in infancy and childhood, metabolic consequences.)

Hanson JS, McCallum R: The diagnosis and management of nausea and vomiting: A review. Am J Gastroenterol 3:210, 1985 (Review of the causes of vomiting and nausea.)

Hughes JG: The etiology of vomiting in infancy and childhood. Pediatr Clin North Am 2:483, 1955 (Description of the etiologies of vomiting in infants and children.)

Lichtenstain PK, Heubi JE, Daugherty CC et al: Grade I Reye's syndrome: Frequent cause of vomiting and liver dysfunction after varicella and upper respiratory tract infection. N Engl J Med 309:133–139, 1983 (Mild Reye's—now we know about medium-chain acetyl dehydrogenase deficiency.)

Sallan SE, Cronin CM: Adverse effects of treatment. In DeVita V, Hellman S, Rosenberg S (eds): Cancer—Principles and Practice of Oncology, pp 2008–2013. Philadelphia, JB Lippincott, 1982 (Discussion of the management of emesis in patients with malignancy.)

Snyder JD: From pedialyte to popsicles: A look at oral rehydration in the United States and Canada. Am J Clin Nutr 35:157–61, 1982 (Report on the practical aspects of oral rehydration therapy.)

103
Gastroesophageal Reflux

TIEN-LAN CHANG AND
HARLAND S. WINTER

Gastroesophageal reflux (GER) is defined as the effortless return of stomach contents into the esophagus. In adults, this phenomenon may cause irritation of the lower esophagus and may produce the pain sensation that is commonly referred to as *heartburn*. In the pediatric age group, especially in infants, vomiting is the most common manifestation of GER. Since there are many causes of vomiting, it is important for the pediatric practitioner to establish a differential diagnosis for each patient and to proceed with the appropriate evaluation before embarking on a specific therapy.

Gastroesophageal reflux is recognized as a common occurrence of infancy. In one report of 1100 infants studied in the first 5 days of life, 18% had forceful vomiting and 38.5% had mild spitting or regurgitation. Reflux, however, does not constitute a problem unless complications develop, and the vomiting is frequently not even brought to the attention of the pediatrician. Most of the infants with reflux improve with age. In a classic review by Carre, about 70% of patients with continued minimal symptoms at 4 years of age had clinical improvement coincident with weaning to solid foods. On the other hand, of the patients who continued to have moderate or frequent symptoms at 4 years, only 7% had any clinical improvement at the time of weaning to solid foods. Therefore, infants who persist in having reflux after weaning to solids are more likely to have pathological GER. Carre conservatively estimated that, without treatment, 60% to 65% of the patients will become asymptomatic by 2 years of age, 30% will still have some symptoms at 4 years of age, 5% will develop esophageal stricture, and less than 5% will die of either pneumonia or inanition. These estimates may not apply to all patients with GER, as his study included only patients who had hiatus hernia (a potentially higher risk group). It is more likely that a higher percentage of patients with GER will have a spontaneous resolution of reflux without any complications.

PATHOPHYSIOLOGY

In the normal esophagus, food is propelled by primary peristaltic contractions down to the stomach. The lower esophageal sphincter (LES), which is a high pressure zone above the gastroesophageal junction but has no anatomic correlate, relaxes to allow the passage of the food bolus and contracts again after it passes. In adults, the LES serves as a barrier against reflux, but other mechanical factors including an intra-abdominal segment of lower esophagus, an acute esophagogastric angle, and the phrenoesophageal membrane are also important in preventing regurgitation. The esophagogastric angle is obtuse in the infant and therefore the child relies on the intrinsic LES pressure to prevent reflux. *A low LES pressure, however, may not be the most important mechanism for reflux.* Simultaneous recordings of esophageal pH and LES pressure in adults and children have shown that reflux occurs most frequently in association with transient relaxation of LES or with an increase in the intra-abdominal pressure. Only a small percentage of children had spontaneous reflux in association with a low basal LES pressure. Hiatus hernia has been considered important in the pathogenesis of pathologic reflux because of the absence of the intra-abdominal esophageal segment. Its clinical significance, however, is unclear.

CLINICAL MANIFESTATIONS

In young infants, vomiting or regurgitation is the major symptom of reflux. It is usually effortless, but may also be forceful, and is often present in the first week of life. Reflux happens frequently after feeding, but it may occur in sleep. In some infants with pathologic reflux, vomiting or regurgitation may not be significant. Hyperirritability, refusal of feeding, or poor weight gain may be the only signs, whereas guaiac positive stools, hematemesis, or recurrent respiratory infections will lead to the suspicion of GER in others. Older children with asthma may also have GER, and some may have clinical improvement when reflux is controlled. However, GER as a cause of asthma has not been established. Apnea and near-miss sudden infant death syndrome (SIDS) patients are also found to have a significant incidence of reflux. In one study, reflux was found in 55 of 58 "near-miss" infants. However, because other risk factors are also found in these patients and because reflux is so common in this age group, a definite cause–effect relationship between GER and apnea or SIDS remains difficult to establish. For example, less than one half of patients with alleged GER-related respiratory symptoms had those symptoms witnessed during the 18- to 24-hour esophageal pH study.

DIFFERENTIAL DIAGNOSIS

Although vomiting or regurgitation is the major symptom of GER, there are many other causes of vomiting. For example, patients with anatomic obstruction, such as pyloric stenosis, achalasia, antral or esophageal web, malrotation, and mass lesions of the abdomen, may have a subtle onset of vomiting indistinguishable from that of GER; their course, however, is unrelenting and progressive. Patients with acute otitis media, urinary tract infection, or viral or bacterial gastroenteritis often have a fever or diarrhea. The vomiting is distinguishable from GER by the abrupt onset, the usually limited course, and the abnormal physical or laboratory findings. Milk or soy protein intolerance may cause diarrhea as well as vomiting, indistinguishable from GER. The stools or vomitus may be grossly blood-streaked secondary to the mucosal inflammatory response in the rectum or stomach. A diagnosis of an allergic cause is supported by the presence of eosinophils in the biopsies of the stomach or rectum and by the resolution of symptoms on an elimination diet. A confirmation of the diagnosis rests on a recurrence of symptoms following a rechallenge of the suspected substance. Eosinophilic gastroenteritis, an allergic process in which the allergies are unknown, may present with vomiting. Metabolic acidosis secondary to an inborn error of metabolism or to ingestion of a toxic substance should be considered in evaluating any child presenting with vomiting. Increased intracranial pressure from head injury, brain tumor, obstructive hydrocephalus, or Reye's syndrome may present subtly as intermittent vomiting. A careful neurologic examination should help in ruling out this group of diseases. Other possible causes of vomiting in pediatric patients that should be easily differentiated from GER by their clinical presentations include obstructive uropathy, hepatobiliary disease, and pancreatitis.

WORK-UP

A complete history and physical examination should eliminate many of the possible causes of vomiting (see Chap. 102).

History

The history should include significant events around birth, such as prematurity and perinatal stress, which might predispose to central nervous system injury. A history of apnea and the use of medications such as theophylline should be sought. The onset, frequency, and forcefulness of vomiting may be helpful in diagnosing an anatomic abnormality as GER would be an unlikely cause in a child who starts to vomit at several months of age. A review of systems should include symptoms such as headache, abdominal pain, dyspnea, fever, diarrhea, and urinary difficulty.

Physical Examination

A complete physical examination emphasizing growth parameters, neurologic development, and an abdominal examination should be performed. A child whose only symptom is regurgitation and who has grown well, has normal developmental milestones, and has a normal physical examination, can be followed prospectively. If the child has any of the complications that suggest pathologic reflux, such as failure to thrive, GI bleeding (anemia or blood per rectum), or recurrent respiratory illness, further studies are then necessary.

Laboratory Tests

Laboratory studies should include a complete blood count, differential, stool for occult blood, urinalysis, and capillary pH or serum bicarbonate. An upper GI series should be obtained to eliminate anatomic abnormalities. The esophageal pH probe study is the most sensitive test for GER. It involves placing a probe by way of the nares into the distal esophagus at a point calculated to be 87% of the distance from the nares to LES. The pH probe is connected to a monitor that records change in esophageal pH over time. A reflux episode is defined as a drop in pH to less than 4. The study can be done over a 1- to 2-hour period or over a prolonged 24-hour period. The shorter study, commonly referred to as the Tuttle test, involves placing 0.1 N HCl or apple juice into the stomach. It is adequate for some patients, but has an over 30% false positive rate. The 24-hour study, by virtue of its longer duration, is more sensitive and may enable a correlation with symptomatology such as apnea and wheezing to GER. An extensive polygraphic monitoring of chest movement, nasal air movement, heart rate, and esophageal pH monitoring may be helpful. ^{99m}Tc scintiscan involves a feeding containing the radioisotope and may detect reflux into the esophagus and aspiration of the isotope into the lungs. In addition, it can provide a quantitative measurement of gastric emptying rate. Because of its lower sensitivity in detecting reflux compared to the pH probe study and its expense, this study should be reserved for patients with suspected aspiration-induced pulmonary disease or for patients with a history suggestive of delayed gastric emptying. Esophageal manometry has been helpful in providing probable explanations for the pathogenesis of GER and reflux esophagitis in that it may reveal a low LES pressure, poor propagation of esophageal contractions, or discoordinate relaxation of the LES. It cannot assess the frequency and the duration of reflux, which are provided by the esophageal pH probe study. The role of esophageal manometry is mainly limited to preoperative evaluation of patients who have failed medical therapy and who are candidates for surgical management of GER. Patients who have poor esophageal motility may not do well with a Nissen fundoplication, because the procedure may restrict the flow of material from the esophagus. Upper endoscopy allows direct visualization of the esophagus, stomach, and duodenum. It provides visual evidence of severe inflammation or ulceration of the esophagus and guides the biopsy, but it is often inaccurate in diagnosing mild or moderate esophagitis. A "blind" esophageal biopsy by suction may provide a pathologic documentation of hyperplasia of the basal zone of epithelium, increased height of the papillae, and presence of intraepithelial eosinophils or neutrophils. However, a normal "blind" biopsy always raises the question of whether a more distal area would have been abnormal.

TREATMENT

For a young infant who has vomiting or regurgitation as the only manifestation of GER, the medical therapy should consist of frequent small feedings, burping after each feeding, and placing the infant prone, on an inclined surface at 30°. The semiupright position allows gravity to work against reflux. The prone position has been demonstrated radiologically to keep the gastroesophageal junction in a superior position relative to the liquid stomach contents. This postural treatment reduces the frequency and duration of reflux in comparison to other body positions. Contrary to previous teaching, it has been shown that placing the infant supine, semiupright in the infant seat actually leads to more reflux compared to the prone position. Thickened feedings have been part of antireflux therapy since the 1950s and may be beneficial when used in conjunction with postural treatment; however, proof of their effectiveness has not been established. The small but frequent feedings are advocated to provide adequate nutrition and reduce the possibility of overdistending the stomach. Since reflux in most infants will resolve, either because of neuromuscular maturation, transition to a more solid diet, adoption of a more upright posture with age, or because of a combination of these factors, further studies and treatment for GER are not necessary unless the symptoms persist beyond 1½ years.

INDICATIONS FOR REFERRAL

For children with possible complications of GER, and for children with vomiting persisting beyond 1½ years, a full diagnostic evaluation should be undertaken as mentioned in consultation with a (preferably pediatric) gastroenterologist. After ruling out other possibilities and establishing reflux as the diagnosis, medical management should be directed at both reflux and its complications. Several antireflux medications are now available. Bethanechol, a cholinergic agonist, increases LES tone and esophageal motility. It has been shown to decrease both reflux frequency and duration in the fasted state and to improve weight gain in patients failing to thrive secondary to reflux. Metoclopramide also increases LES tone, improves esophageal motility, and enhances gastric emptying. Its major drawbacks are central nervous system and extrapyramidal side effects, including dystonia and tardive dyskinesia. Domperidone is a new drug under investigation with purported absence of the neurologic side effects of metoclopramide. These medications are best taken a half-hour prior to a meal. Cimetidine or antacids are used for patients with esophagitis. Serial stool guaiacs may be useful for the follow-up of patients with gastrointestinal blood loss, although a negative stool guaiac does not eliminate esophagitis. Patients who have esopha-

gitis and ongoing reflux should be monitored because *Barrett's esophagus*, a metaplastic lesion where the squamous epithelium is replaced by columnar epithelium, and stricture may develop as complications. Patients with failure to thrive have been treated with supplemental nasogastric tube-feeding at night but this therapy may exacerbate the reflux. Patients with pulmonary infection and reflux should be treated with appropriate antibiotics for the infection and should be followed for new episodes of infection while being treated for reflux. A repeat esophageal pH probe study or an esophageal biopsy may help to assess the effectiveness of therapy if the patient fails to show clinical improvement after a 4- to 8-week course of therapy. Although controlled studies have shown a steady improvement in weight gain and a decreased reflux in treated patients, studies of the long-term results are inadequate.

SURGICAL TREATMENT

Before antireflux drugs were available, surgery was the only option when patients failed to respond to postural therapy and small frequent feedings. Two types of operations have been used. The gastropexy procedure involves pulling down the lower esophagus into the abdomen and anchoring the stomach either to the median arcuate ligament or to the anterior abdominal wall. The fundoplication procedure involves pulling down the lower esophagus and wrapping it either completely or partially with the fundus of the stomach. Nissen fundoplication is now the most widely used procedure. A gastrostomy for feeding may be needed in patients who swallow poorly and who are at risk for aspiration. In uncontrolled studies, the success of the operation in eliminating reflux and in improving growth has been over 90%. Success in eliminating respiratory symptoms is only 77%. Patients who have an incomplete resolution of respiratory problems are more likely to have other associated disorders, such as mental retardation, seizures, congenital heart disease, repaired tracheoesophageal fistula with or without esophageal atresia, and disorders of the laryngotracheobronchial tree. It is possible that, in some of these patients, respiratory symptoms are not due to reflux but are instead related to associated disorders. In patients whose reflux is controlled on medical treatment but whose respiratory symptoms remain unaltered, surgery may not be beneficial. Possible surgical complications include paraesophageal hernia, small bowel obstruction, pneumonia, malalignment of the wrap, and wound infections. Some authors advocate surgery in patients with coexistent apnea and GER, citing favorable statistics in the literature. In our opinion, a strong correlation between symptom and GER should be sought for each patient prior to surgical intervention. Without this evidence, a medical trial should be given.

It is hoped that, by following this approach and appropriately educating parents, much of the formula changes and use of antispasmotic agents, which are currently used widely by pediatricians for "spitting," will be avoided.

ANNOTATED BIBLIOGRAPHY

Carre IJ: The natural history of the partial thoracic stomach (hiatus hernia) in children. Arch Dis Child 34:344–353, 1959 (Classic study of a particular group of patients with GER.)

Jeffrey HE, Rahilly P, Read DJ: Multiple causes of asphyxia in infants at high risk for sudden infant death. Arch Dis Child 58:92–100, 1983 (Among other potential mechanisms of asphyxia, reflux is found in 55 of 58 "near-miss" infants.)

Keitel HG, Ziegra SR: Regurgitation in the full term infant. A controlled clinical study. Am J Dis Child 102:749–750, 1961 (Brief report on the incidence of reflux in infants less than 5 days old.)

Leape LL, Holder TM, Franklin JD et al: Respiratory arrest in infant secondary to gastroesophageal reflux. Pediatrics 60:924–927, 1977 (Report of 10 patients with apnea treated medically and surgically.)

Meyers WF, Roberts CC, Johnson DG, Herbst JJ: Value of tests for evaluation of gastroesophageal reflux in children. J Pediatr Surg 20(5):515–520, 1985 (Comparison of the tests in sensitivity and specificity for GER.)

Orenstein SR, Whitington PF, Orenstein DM: The infant seat as treatment for gastroesophageal reflux. N Engl J Med 309:760–763, 1983 (Study on the effect of position on GER.)

Werlin SL, Dodds WJ, Hogan WJ et al: Mechanisms of gastroesophageal reflux in children. J Pediatr 97(2):244–249, 1980 (Manometric study of reflux that parallels the study in adults.)

Winter HS, Madara JL, Stafford RJ et al: Intraepithelial eosinophils: A new diagnostic criterion for reflux esophagitis. Gastroenterol 83:818–823, 1982 (Presence of esophageal intraepithelial eosinophils correlated with abnormal acid clearance determined by esophageal pH probe monitoring.)

104

Acute Abdominal Pain

KENNETH E. GRANT AND
SAMUEL H. KIM

It is the frequent and often difficult task of the pediatrician to evaluate a child with sudden onset of severe abdominal pain. The differential diagnosis is large, but the pediatrician's first obligation is to decide whether a surgical emergency exists. Appendicitis, usually the parents' major concern, must also be a primary concern of the physician. In the absence of acute abdominal signs and symptoms, time is available to observe and cautiously approach diagnosis and therapy.

PATHOPHYSIOLOGY

Abdominal pain results from a complex series of physiologic processes that often make it difficult for the patient and the physician to interpret. However, clues to the disease process may be provided by the location and character of the pain.

In general, visceral pain is dull and diffuse whereas parietal pain is sharp and localized. Visceral pain fibers are located in the muscular wall of hollow viscera and the capsule of solid viscera. Many organs have common enervation with a low concentration of nerve endings, leading to poor localization of pain. The location is sensed in the path of enervation and is almost always midline. Pain from the liver, pancreas, biliary tree, stomach, and upper small bowel is generally felt in the epigastrium. The distal small bowel, cecum, appendix, and ascending colon send pain signals to the periumbilical region. The distal intestine, urinary tract, and pelvic organs are sensed in the suprapubic area. Visceral nerves are stimulated by tension and stretching rather than cutting, tearing, or crushing. Tissue congestion and inflammation tend to sensitize nerve endings and lower their threshold to stimuli. The exact mechanism by which tissue inflammation and ischemia cause visceral pain is unclear.

Parietal pain, on the other hand, is mediated by stimuli, such as acute inflammation, in the parietal peritoneum. The sensation is usually more intense and is much better localized due to the greater concentration of nerve endings in the skin. Lateralization of a process is usually possible. Referred pain has many of the characteristics of parietal pain but is felt in remote areas enervated by the same nerves as the affected organ. Pain is referred when visceral stimuli become overwhelming.

The character of a pain can sometimes be used to distinguish between diseases. A duodenal ulcer is often described as burning or gnawing; intestinal obstruction as crampy; and acute appendicitis as achy. The significance of intensity is hard to evaluate except at its extremes. The perception of painful stimuli can be modified by both central and peripheral neurologic processes. Psychological and emotional factors may also affect how pain is sensed by an individual.

CLINICAL PRESENTATION

Acute abdominal pain is a presenting feature of many diseases. The most important are conditions that will deteriorate rapidly without surgical intervention. They must be quickly differentiated from nonsurgical problems. Unfortunately, many signs and symptoms are found in both surgical and nonsurgical patients with equal frequency. It is difficult to define diagnostic criteria that are disease specific. Despite a careful evaluation, the diagnostic dilemma is often resolved only after laparotomy.

An abdomen with findings that suggest surgery will be needed is referred to as an *acute abdomen*. Generalizations can be made that will aid in the diagnosis. Symptoms are usually progressive and abdominal pain and tenderness are typically well localized, often with rebound. Nausea, vomiting, and anorexia are associated, but nonspecific, symptoms. It is characteristic of an acute abdomen that pain precedes the onset of vomiting. The onset of pain simultaneously with, or after, vomiting suggests gastroenteritis. A moderate temperature elevation is common but may also be seen in nonsurgical diseases. Acute pain that is steady for more than 6 hours is usually surgical in nature. Repeat examinations at intervals by the same observer are often the most helpful method of identifying an acute abdomen. The goal is to intervene surgically before a ruptured viscus, intra-abdominal bleeding, or strangulation ischemia develops.

DIFFERENTIAL DIAGNOSIS

Appendicitis is the most common disease requiring surgery in childhood. The true incidence is unknown, but it is estimated that between 7% and 12% of a population will develop appendicitis at some time during their lives. It may occur at any age but it is most common in the teenage and young adult years. Appendicitis is much less common under 2 years of age (less than 1% of all appendicitis) and is rare under 1 year. The classic presentation is periumbilical crampy pain progressing to constant right lower quadrant pain in a child with fever, anorexia, vomiting, and leukocytosis. The process typically evolves steadily over 12 hours. Thus, repeat examinations at 4 to 6 hours intervals often clarify uncertain diagnoses. Atypical presentations are common, particularly in the younger age groups. For example, an inflamed retrocecal appendix may display no anterior abdominal wall tenderness. An infant with appendicitis may present with only irritability, discomfort on movement, and flexed hips. It may hurt to cry so the child may be silent even though he is in pain. Appendicitis must be considered in any ill-looking child with a changing abdominal examination and no obvious alternative etiology.

A perforated viscus, an obstruction with strangulation, and a ruptured ectopic pregnancy are common surgical emergencies of the abdomen in childhood and must also be identified as quickly as possible. Other causes of acute abdominal pain are likely to evolve more slowly, allowing time for observation and evaluation.

Conditions that most often mimic an acute abdomen are gastroenteritis, urinary tract infection, and mesenteric adenitis. Gastroenteritis may present with severe abdominal pain, which is usually diffuse and crampy, but may mimic the more localized symptoms of appendicitis. Profuse diarrhea commonly differentiates gastroenteritis from appendicitis, but diarrhea is seen in a small percentage of patients with appendicitis, probably caused by irritation of the colon by the inflamed appendix. Headache, fever, and chills early in the course tend to favor a viral process.

Infections of the urinary tract may also present with severe abdominal pain and tenderness. High fever and chills point toward pain of this etiology. Acute pyelonephritis may be present without symptoms of dysuria. Differentiation from appendicitis can be difficult because an inflamed pelvic appendix may cause urinary frequency and urgency. Pyuria is a common finding in appendicitis and other diffuse intra-abdominal processes.

Mesenteric adenitis is found in approximately 11% of children treated surgically for appendicitis. Mesenteric adenitis is a diagnosis made at laparotomy and generally cannot be differentiated from appendicitis until surgery is carried out. Primary peritonitis is another diagnosis that may be made at laparotomy. However, because this is more common in a child who has other chronic illnesses such as leukemia in remission or nephrotic syndrome, a diagnostic paracentesis prior to surgery may be helpful. If the patient has gram-positive diplococci or if the fluid is nonpurulent (in contrast, fluid from secondary peritonitis is usually grossly purulent with organisms present), treatment with intravenous antibiotics and watchful waiting may be the preferred treatment. Some cases of primary peritonitis are caused by gram-negative rods, and, if found, a paracentesis would not be helpful in differentiating primary from secondary (*i.e.*, from a ruptured viscus) peritonitis. Therefore, in that situation, a laparotomy should be carried out expeditiously.

Intussusception is one of the most common causes of abdominal pain in infancy. Severe colicky pain that is paroxysmal and sometimes manifested just by screaming in the very young patient alternating with quiescent periods with or without vomiting is intussusception until proven otherwise. The pain is usually periumbilical and more severe than that seen in gastroenteritis. The classic presentation includes a right upper quandrant mass (70% cases) and current jelly stools (60%), which are, however, a late finding. Early, KUB and upright films of the abdomen may appear normal. A barium enema frequently reduces idiopathic intussusception and should be performed on an emergency basis, but only within the first 24 hours of presentation. Surgical reduction is necessary when peritonitis has developed, a pathologic lead point has been identified, or radiologic reduction has been unsuccessful.

Meckel's diverticulum can occur at any age but is also most common under 2 years of age. It usually presents as painless rectal bleeding, but rarely becomes inflamed and mimics appendicitis. A Meckel's diverticulum may serve as a lead point for intussusception and may occasionally perforate.

Several other conditions that present with acute abdominal pain are common in infancy. Incarcerated hernias do not have to have strangulation to cause symptoms. An incarcerated hernia will cause abdominal pain and a tender mass will be noted over the area of the external ring. Another cause of lower abdominal pain in boys is testicular torsion, although the usual presentation is scrotal pain (see Chap. 119). Hirschsprung's disease may cause an intermittent obstruction from retained feces and may progress to enterocolitis and perforation. Obstructive symptoms early in life may represent mid-gut volvulus. These patients are often too young to express abdominal pain. Thus, an infant who has been perfectly healthy and suddenly develops a refusal to eat, bile stain vomiting, obstipation, and abdominal distention should have a midgut volvulus secondary to malrotation ruled out immediately. Trauma and child abuse must also always be considered in the differential.

Other gastrointestinal diseases that present with acute abdominal pain include peptic ulcer disease, biliary tract disease, Yersinia enterocolitis, and, less commonly, pancreatitis, inflammatory bowel disease, and gastrointestinal tumors. Peptic ulcer disease can be seen in any age group but is most easily recognized when the child is verbal and can localize the pain and its relation to meals. In infancy, vomiting may be the only symptom (see Chap. 111). Pancreatitis presents with a steady epigastric pain that often radiates to the back. The diagnosis is difficult and remains a diagnosis of exclusion that should never serve to postpone intervention for reasonable alternatives. Cholecystitis may present with right upper quadrant or epigastric pain. Cholangitis is usually associated with jaundice. Crohn's disease during an acute flare may resemble appendicitis. However, patients usually present for an elective rather than emergent evaluation due to the chronicity of the disease. Yersinia enterocolitis may also be confused with appendicitis because fever, vomiting, and abdominal tenderness may overshadow diarrhea. A diagnosis can be made on stool culture with appropriate handling.

Many common causes of acute abdominal pain are not diseases of the gastrointestinal tract. Pneumonia is a frequently overlooked etiology. No child should be taken to surgery without an evaluation of the chest for signs of pneumonia. An examination of the lower lobes is probably the most useful role of the plain abdominal film in evaluating a child for appendicitis. Streptococcal pharyngitis and tonsillitis may also be associated with abdominal pain and fever.

Symptoms of diabetic ketoacidosis include severe abdominal pain, nausea, vomiting, and anorexia. Many newly diagnosed diabetics present mimicking appendicitis. Caution must be used with known diabetics who may develop diabetic ketoacidosis secondary to true appendicitis. Acute rheumatic fever may present with fever and abdominal pain in its early stages. Henoch–Schönlein purpura presents with gastrointestinal symptoms before the characteristic rash in 18% of patients. Hemophilia, hemolytic uremic syndrome, and sickle cell disease are other hematologic diseases that can have severe abdominal pain. Children with leukemia may have abdominal pain secondary to their disease. The development of acute appendicitis becomes a serious problem in a child who has leukemia or another immunosuppressed state. Continuing immunosuppressive therapy may mask a serious underlying abdominal illness. These children should be seen early in the course of their ailment and surgery should also be performed early.

Gynecologic disorders commonly present with acute abdominal pain in adolescent girls. Pelvic inflammatory disease can be difficult to differentiate from appendicitis. Nausea and vomiting tend to be more common in appendicitis. The symptoms of pelvic inflammatory disease usually last longer at presentation and may often begin within 1 week of menses. There may be a prior history of venereal disease. Physical findings that differentiate pelvic inflammatory disease are bilateral adnexal tenderness, bilateral peritoneal signs, and cervical motion tenderness (see Chap. 122). Ectopic pregnancy, pelvic endometriosis, corpus luteal hematoma, ovarian cyst, chronic salpingitis, and mittelschmerz must also be considered.

A rare cause of acute abdominal pain is hepatic porphyria. A first attack may consist of fever, vomiting, and epigastric or right ileac fossa pain. Symptoms rarely begin before adolescence. A diagnosis is made by finding porphyrins in the urine and stool. Pain from renal and ureteral calculi is usually in the costovertebral angle (CVA) area. When the stone migrates, the location of the pain may be expressed anywhere along this path and may extend down into the genital area.

WORK-UP

Identification of an acute abdomen is the priority in children presenting with acute abdominal pain. Reliable predictors of surgically correctable disease are localized pain, the pattern of migratory pain classically described in appendicitis, rebound tenderness on examination, and elevated polymorphonuclear white blood count. A diagnosis must be based on a careful history and physical examination.

History

A detailed history is essential to determine the timing, location, and character of the pain. The child with peritonitis will typically complain of pain excerbated by coughing, jumping, or jiggling. However, if the peritonitis has been present for a while and is walled off, the child may manifest a sense of well-being. The child with appendicitis will sometimes not be able to climb stairs or stand up straight. It should be noted whether vomiting is present and whether it preceded or followed the onset of pain. Diarrhea and urinary tract symptoms are less specific but may be important. It is crucial to identify a history of predisposing disease such as diabetes, sickle cell disease, hemophilia, inflammatory bowel disease, pancreatitis, venereal disease, pelvic inflammatory disease, pregnancy, recurrent pneumonia, or urinary tract infection. Previous abdominal surgery or trauma are important considerations and any suggestion of child abuse must be pursued.

Physical Examination

During a complete physical examination, including a rectal and pelvic examination, the physician must look for signs of peritonitis or localized tenderness. Inconclusive examinations should be repeated by the same physician in 4 to 6 hours to rule out progressive disease. Signs of acute fluid or blood loss into the abdomen require immediate surgery. A right upper quadrant mass suggests intussusception. The chest should be examined for signs of pneumonia. The inguinal and femoral areas should be inspected for evidence of an incarcerated hernia and testicular torsion.

Laboratory Tests

The laboratory evaluation must include a complete blood count with differential and urinalysis. Polymorphonuclear blood count is commonly elevated in appendicitis and other surgical emergencies. An elevated total white blood count is found in many surgical and nonsurgical diseases and is, thus, less useful. A urinalysis is essential to rule out pyelonephritis and renal calculi. Some red or white blood cells may, however, be seen in children with appendicitis. Glycosuria is an important finding suggesting that the patient has diabetes.

A radiologic evaluation should be dictated by individual presentation. Plain films are helpful in identifying intestinal obstruction, free intra-abdominal air, and pneumonia. The search for a rare calcified appendicolith does not warrant the use of an abdominal series in any child suspected of having appendicitis. Barium enemas are not diagnostic for appendicitis but may be therapeutic for intussusception. Ultrasound and intravenous pyelogram are reserved for special circumstances and are rarely needed in the routine evaluation of acute abdominal pain.

MANAGEMENT AND INDICATIONS FOR REFERRAL

A surgical exploration is indicated in any child with an acute abdomen and progressive signs of deterioration for which there is no satisfactory explanation. In children with suspected appendicitis, prolonged observation and repetition of laboratory studies serve only to increase the risk of perforation. The morbidity associated with a perforated appendix remains higher than that associated with simple appendicitis, despite modern antibiotic therapy. Expectant therapy for appendicitis is not indicated, and a referral to a pediatric surgeon should be as soon as an acute abdomen is suspected. Sedatives and analgesics should be withheld until the surgeon's first examination. Subsequently, sedation may relieve discomfort and actually improve the abdominal examination.

A suspected ruptured ectopic pregnancy must be referred to a gynecologist or surgeon immediately. A referral for a pelvic examination may be indicated in adolescent females with acute abdominal pain in whom a proper examination has not been possible and when the diagnosis is unclear.

Intussusception must be reduced as soon as possible with a barium enema. A delay may lead to a loss of bowel due to ischemia. A pediatric surgeon should be consulted quickly if the radiologist is unable to reduce the intussusception or if there are signs of peritonitis.

The prognosis for a child with an acute abdomen is excellent if treated appropriately. Overdiagnosis of appendicitis is common in most surgical practices. Fifteen to twenty percent of patients (30% of female adolescents) presenting with right lower quadrant pain have a normal appendix at surgery. The 15% morbidity associated with a negative laparotomy is accepted in an attempt to avoid the complications of a perforated appendix and peritonitis.

Therapy for acute abdominal pain of nonsurgical origin varies depending on the patient's diagnosis. A follow-up is essential to ensure that acute symptoms do not become chronic complaints.

ANNOTATED BIBLIOGRAPHY

Bongard F, Landers DV, Lewis F: Differential diagnosis of appendicitis and pelvic inflammatory disease. Am J Surg 150:90–96, 1985 (Discussion of the differential between appendicitis and pelvic inflammatory disease.)

Hatch EI: The acute abdomen in children. Pediatr Clin North Am 32:1151–1164, 1985 (Discussion of appendicitis and its differential.)

Karp MP, Caldorola VA, Cooney DR et al: The avoidable excesses in the management of perforated appendicitis in children. J Pediatr Surg 21:506–510, 1986 (Discussion of recent alternatives in the surgical care of appendicitis.)

Nauta RJ, Magnant C: Observation *vs* operation for abdominal pain in the right lower quadrant: Roles of the clinical exam and the leukocyte count. Am J Surg 151:746–748, 1986 (Good discussion of evaluation.)

Sleisinger MH, Fordtran JS: Gastrointestinal Diseases, pp 207–221, 1268–1275. Philadelphia, WB Saunders, 1983 (Standard gastroenterology text with excellent discussion of abdominal pain and the acute abdomen.)

105
Recurrent Abdominal Pain

KENNETH E. GRANT AND W. ALLAN WALKER

Recurrent abdominal pain is a common and often challenging diagnostic problem in the pediatric age group. Typically, a healthy appearing school-aged child repeatedly complains of severe abdominal pain, frustrating his parents with their inability to provide relief. Answers are sought from the physician who must carefully consider the diagnostic and therapeutic alternatives. The physician must balance the fear of missing a treatable diagnosis against clinical wisdom that suggests a low likelihood of organic disease.

Apley classically defined chronic abdominal pain as three or more episodes, severe enough to interfere with the child's activity, occurring over a 3-month period or longer. He called this presentation recurrent abdominal pain (RAP). A follow-up of children presenting with RAP identifies less than 5% to 10% who develop organic disease. Even though emotional factors are often identified to help explain the attacks, RAP remains a serious disease with a potential for long-term morbidity. The diagnosis must be confident without excess. The therapy must be compassionate, redirecting the patient's focus of attention with reassurance and support.

PATHOPHYSIOLOGY

The etiology of RAP is unknown, but the psychosomatic nature of the disease is striking. The child complaining of severe pain often appears relatively unconcerned about his problem. Commonly, children with RAP have parents who also complain of chronic abdominal pain. Abdominal pain is a means of communicating to each other that an underlying problem exists.

Stress associated with school and social performance, emotional conflicts brought on by development and changing maturity, and the real or threatened loss of a friend or family have been identified in the histories of many children with RAP. An illness may reveal a vulnerability that had previously remained hidden. Symptoms that may have been very real at first may continue supported by secondary gain. The extreme concern of either the parents or the physician serves only to reinforce the symptoms.

It remains unclear why these children respond to the stresses of growing up by complaining of abdominal pain. Most children do not. Some children may be more sensitive to painful body signals, a sensitivity that may be genetically or environmentally determined. On the other hand, the signals may be sensed normally, but stress may accentuate pains that might otherwise go unnoticed. Pain may even be the result of a malfunction of a normal physiologic process. Hyperactivity of the autonomic nervous system, noted in many children with RAP, may cause pain by altering intestinal motility. Constipation, giardiasis, and lactose intolerance also alter motility and stimulate the stretch receptors that cause pain. Each has been suggested as a cause of RAP, but an inconsistent response to therapy has made it clear that many factors must be involved.

CLINICAL PRESENTATION

RAP typically presents in children 5 to 10 years old, although the diagnosis can be considered in children between the ages of 3 and 16 years. Between 10% and 12% of school-aged children are said to be affected. The incidence is greater in women than men, particularly in the later years.

Patients usually complain of a dull colicky periumbilical pain, intermittent on a daily basis with a complete recovery in between episodes. The pain is rarely focal and localization away from the umbilicus should suggest another diagnosis. The specifics of the pain are usually presented in vague terms and no distinct association between the pain and eating, position, or time of day can be found. Behavior patterns and daily activities are interrupted by the episodes but do not always seem consistent with the severity of the pain. Abdominal pain does not awaken the patient from sleep.

Associated symptoms may include a low-grade temperature, pallor, headache, and vomiting. Constipation is also often seen. Over-the-counter medications, such as antacids and anticholinergics, do not alleviate the pain. Complex rituals including application of hot packs, careful repositioning and gentle rubbing by a parent are the sole providers of relief.

DIFFERENTIAL DIAGNOSIS

The first step in the diagnosis of RAP is to verify that the symptoms are chronic. Acute abdominal pain is discussed in Chapter 104. RAP can be distinguished from most other causes of chronic abdominal pain that present with signs and symptoms of organic disease. An ill-looking child or a child with persistent fever, weight loss, growth failure, or anemia suggests that RAP is not the correct diagnosis. Focal abdominal tenderness, pain that wakes a child at night, bilious vomiting, hematemesis, hematochezia, or melena suggest a gastrointestinal etiology. Peptic ulcer disease (see Chap. 111) and gallbladder disease, common in adults, are also seen in children, but they should be distinguishable by their presentation. Urinary tract disease is the most common organic cause of RAP and must be considered even without symptoms of dysuria and frequency.

Adolescents present their own special problems. Dramatic behavioral changes associated with abdominal pain should raise the suspicion of substance abuse. A sexual history is essential in each postpubertal patient because concern over pregnancy, venereal disease, or homosexuality may cause a healthy appearing child to complain of pain. Adolescent females may have a higher incidence of organic disease due to gynecologic disorders. Mittelschmerz, endometriosis, and pelvic inflammatory disease must always be considered.

Diagnoses difficult to distinguish from RAP based on symptoms alone are lactose intolerance, giardiasis, and constipation. Remember that a positive diagnosis does not eliminate concurrent psychosomatic illness and that treatment often fails to relieve the symptoms. Early Crohn's disease may present as RAP but is unlikely in the absence of growth failure, anemia, and blood in the stool. HSP, celiac disease, and Yersinia enterocolitis most commonly present as an acute disease but may each mimic RAP. Pancreatitis can be chronic but should be differentiated on the basis of presentation. Meckel's diverticulum and intestinal duplications almost never present with pain. Causes of abdominal pain that are often forgotten include lead poisoning, abdominal epilepsy, osteomyelitis of the spine, psoas abscess, and abdominal, inguinal, and femoral hernias. Each must be considered as the evaluation progresses.

WORK-UP

An evaluation of the child with RAP must be carefully organized from the start. A haphazard approach will destroy the family's confidence in accepting the physician's diagnosis and recommendations. Unnecessary diagnostic tests and referrals may only reinforce the already problematic symptoms.

It should be made clear early on that there is a low likelihood of finding an organic etiology and that there is no physical danger to the child. This idea is often difficult for the family to accept because the symptoms are so upsetting. The possibility that the symptoms are stress related and that counseling may be an important part of therapy should be introduced early to all patients with RAP. The physician must communicate an understanding that the symptoms are real and he must reassure the patient that they will not be ignored.

History

The initial interview should be long enough to obtain a detailed history to rule out suspicion of an underlying organic illness and to look for evidence of emotional stress or behavior problems. Routine questions including the onset, character, duration, and location of pain should be asked. Aggravating and relieving factors should be sought. A nutritional history will often help characterize the nature of the complaint. Gastrointestinal symptoms, including bowel pattern, must be examined for changes. Several commonly used medications, such as tetracy-

cline and erythromycin, can cause abdominal pain. Constant attention must be paid to the possibility of a hidden agenda throughout the interview.

Key points to look for in the history are pain that awakens the patient from sleep, pain focal in nature and referred to areas away from the umbilicus, persistent fever, weight loss or growth failure, bilious vomiting, gastrointestinal bleeding, or urinary tract symptoms. Each suggests that the etiology of the pain is more likely organic and that the diagnostic approach should be modified.

Apley described in his classic monograph several emotional factors commonly identified in patients with RAP: marital discord between parents, rigid or demanding parenting styles, a detached father, an ill or depressed mother, school problems, and a perfectionist personality in the child. A death in the family or an important upcoming examination may be elicited in the history. It is important to note the interaction between patient and parents during the interview. Commonly, the child will be eager to talk and relatively unconcerned while the parents will be overprotective and overconcerned. Conflict within the family is commonly denied. The home environment tends to discourage the child's independence.

A family history is often positive for relatives with abdominal pain. The possibility of an inherited disorder must be considered. The patient may actually have a predisposition for the disease or may have sympathetic pain.

Personal issues concerning drug abuse, sexual activity, and pregnancy must be discussed privately with the child. Time should be spent focusing on the patient's friends, interests, and goals. Behavioral or emotional problems may be more obvious in this context.

Physical Examination

The physical examination is usually nonspecific in RAP, but must be thorough to help rule out organic illness. Height and weight compared with previous growth parameters may be most important. An overall impression of wellness may give clues to the nonorganic nature of the disease. Abdominal tenderness, if any, is not usually focal in RAP. A rectal examination should be performed and stool tested for occult blood.

The patient rarely has abdominal pain during his initial examination. It is useful to reexamine the patient during an attack. Physical findings and signs will not usually match the severity of the complaints. Remember that a diagnosis of RAP does not preclude the onset of a new acute disease. Both the history and physical examination must be reviewed on each contact with close attention to changes from previous examinations.

Laboratory Tests

Laboratory tests should be kept to a minimum. Less than 5% of all cases will have an organic lesion if symptoms suggestive of organic illness are not also present. A reasonable screening includes urinalysis and culture, CBC, sedimentation rate, stool for occult blood, and stool for ova and parasites. If these tests are negative, further testing with an upper gastrointestinal series, esophagoduodenoscopy, or barium enema are rarely helpful. Extensive testing may only serve to entrench the symptoms by supporting a secondary gain or some other underlying emotional etiology. If symptoms or screening tests suggest an organic etiology for the pain, the diagnostic evaluation should depend on the specific presentation.

MANAGEMENT

The treatment of RAP is based on the reassurance that no serious organic disease exists and that the child is in no physical danger. The discussions with the family should emphasize that RAP is common and that many possible etiologies exist. Stressful events and emotional issues should be identified as possible contributory factors. Counseling should be initiated to help the child and family deal with symptoms that may not immediately disappear. Normalization of life-style, including an immediate return to school and a de-emphasis of pain episodes, is essential. A plan for follow-up and support by the physician should be outlined clearly so that the patient and family do not feel abandoned. If an organic etiology for the pain is found, treatment should, of course, be directed at the cause.

Medications are not indicated for the treatment of RAP. Sedatives and analgesics may be dangerous and may lead to either psychological or physiologic dependence. Antispasmodics offer no consistent help and may even aggravate the symptoms. Placebos will serve only to undermine the trust on which the physician–patient relationship and, therefore, RAP therapy is based.

Other therapies have been directed at the contributions of constipation, lactose intolerance, and food allergies to abdominal pain. Fiber added to the diet may improve pain symptoms by relieving constipation. A lactose-free diet may be considered, but close follow-up should continue because a recurrence of pain is frequently seen following therapy for lactose intolerance. Dietary restrictions in response to food "allergies" have not proven useful. A normal, well-balanced diet should be encouraged.

INDICATIONS FOR REFERRAL

A referral should rarely be necessary for children with RAP. If the rapport between the physician and patient is good, the family usually will not insist on looking to other physicians for other answers. A specialist may be needed when other signs or symptoms of organic illness are present.

A surgeon offers little help unless an acute abdominal problem is suspected. Chronic appendicitis should not be considered a cause of RAP. Appendectomy has failed to relieve symptoms time after time. An exploratory laparotomy without persistent fever, focal tenderness, palpable mass, or obstructive symptoms is not indicated.

Peptic ulcer disease is often considered when evaluating a child with chronic abdominal pain. Classic symptoms of epigastric pain at night and during fasting that is relieved by food may or may not be present. A referral to a gastroenterologist for an upper gastrointestinal series or an esophagoduodenoscopy should be considered only in the case of classic symptoms, a strong family history, persistent vomiting, an abnormal CBC, or stool positive for occult blood. The gastroenterologist may also offer a lactose breath hydrogen test for the diagnosis of lactose intolerance. In practice, a lactose breath hydrogen test gives no better diagnosis than a lactose-free diet trial.

Abdominal epilepsy is an often mentioned but uncommon cause of intermittent abdominal pain. It should be suspected only when pain is associated with an impairment of consciousness and postictal symptoms. A referral to a neurologist for an EEG is then indicated. This is a difficult diagnosis to make and will depend on an abnormal EEG during an episode of abdominal pain.

Hospitalization should only be necessary when the emotional environment at home has deteriorated so that observation in a neutral environment is deemed necessary. A second opinion may be indicated at this time to support the primary physician's diagnosis and management plan. The patient and family must not expect a battery of new tests. The opportunity to observe the patient alone and during an episode of pain should be taken. The length of hospital stay should be minimized to avoid fostering a dependence on the illness.

The treatment of the patient and family as a single unit is the key to success in RAP. The family must understand and believe that a problem exists even if the definitive etiology of the pain cannot be found. Despite all the reassurance and understanding that the physician can offer, symptoms of abdominal pain are likely to persist, or change somatic form, as the child moves into adulthood. RAP is a signal that all is not well and deserves immediate intervention and often long-term care.

ANNOTATED BIBLIOGRAPHY

Apley J: The Child with Abdominal Pain, 2nd ed. Oxford, Blackwell Scientific Publications, 1975 (Classic monograph.)

Apley J, Hale B: Children with recurrent abdominal pain: How do they grow up? Br Med J 3:7, 1973 (Follow-up of a classic study looking at the effect of supportive therapy.)

Farrell MK: Abdominal pain. Pediatrics (Suppl)74:955–957, 1984 (Good discussion of clinical features and counseling component of therapy.)

Levine MD, Rappaport LA: Recurrent abdominal pain in school children: The loneliness of the long-distance physician. Pediatr Clin North Am 31:969–991, 1984 (Excellent discussion of etiologies.)

Middleton AW, Banning A: Recurrent abdominal pain in children. Aust Fam Physician 13:426–427, 1984 (Brief practical approach with emphasis on the emotional makeup of the family.)

Silverman A, Roy C: Psychophysiologic recurrent abdominal pain. In Pediatric Clinical Gastroenterology, 3rd ed., pp 418–430. St. Louis, CV Mosby, 1983 (Standard pediatric gastroenterology text.)

106

Acute Diarrhea

SAMUEL NURKO AND
W. ALLAN WALKER

Diarrheal disease continues to be one of the primary causes of morbidity and mortality in the Third World. Diarrhea can be defined as an excessive loss of fluids and electrolytes in the stool. Any daily fecal loss exceeding 200 ml/sq m is considered excessive. In babies, any losses exceeding 20 ml/kg are considered significant. The transport of water across the intestinal mucosa is a passive phenomenon, and consideration of the pathophysiology of any type of diarrhea must center on the net transport of glucose, sodium, chloride, and amino acids that are the major determinants of intestinal water absorption.

PATHOPHYSIOLOGY

There are five mechanisms of diarrheal production:

1. *Osmotic*—This condition occurs when osmotically active particles are present in the intestinal lumen. Examples include the dumping syndrome, lactase deficiency, and overfeeding.
2. *Secretory Diarrhea*—This condition occurs with the inhibition of ion absorption or stimulation of ion secretion. Examples are the secretory diarrheas that occur secondary to bacterial exotoxins, or diarrheas secondary to substances produced by the body that activate secretion such as gastrin in the Zollinger–Ellison syndrome.
3. *Deletion or Inhibition of a Normal Active Ion Absorptive Process*—This can be congenital, such as in the case of congenital chloridorrhea, or acquired, such as in bile salt deficiency and pancreatic enzyme deficiencies.
4. *Inflammation*—This is usually secondary to a decrease in the anatomic or functional areas, such as occurs in mucosal diseases like celiac sprue, after bacterial invasion, or after bowel resection.
5. *Abnormal Intestinal Motility*—Abnormally reduced peristalsis may allow bacterial overgrowth; rapid motility may reduce contact time between the small bowel mucosa and its contents.

PRESENTATION AND DIFFERENTIAL DIAGNOSIS

Acute diarrhea is usually a self-limited illness lasting a few days to a week. Chronic diarrhea typically persists longer than 3 weeks and may be associated with malabsorption or malnutrition or both. Almost all acute diarrhea in children is caused by intestinal infections, although it can also be secondary to an infection outside the bowel, such as in the urinary or respiratory tracts. Other possibilities include food poisoning, inflammatory disorders (*e.g.*, Crohn's, ulcerative colitis, hemolytic uremic syndrome, Henoch–Schönlein purpura), and iatrogenic causes (*e.g.*, antibiotics, laxatives). The most common infectious agents that cause enteric infections vary around the world and consist of either viruses, bacteria, or parasites (Table 106-1). The identification of the causative agent in an episode of acute diarrhea may facilitate proper therapy. The presence of specific clinical manifestations alone is not pathognomonic of any causative agent although certain symptoms suggest specific causes. For example, bacterial organisms that invade the mucosa often cause fever, and if the colon is primarily involved, abdominal pain, tenesmus, fecal urgency, and stools with blood and mucus (*e.g.*, salmonella, shigella, and campylobacter). Patients with secretory diarrhea have abdominal cramps with the passage of a low to a moderate number of large volume stools (*e.g.*, cholera and ETEC).

WORK-UP

History

It is important to obtain a thorough dietary record (*e.g.*, breast-feeding, formulas), and changes in the diet should be correlated with stool frequency and form. A history of other family members with gastrointestinal complaints, travel, or origin from areas where there is contamination of the water system, or endemic infections, time spent in day care, or foods recently ingested are also important.

Inquiry should be made regarding previous growth, appreciating the fact that the failure to gain weight is usually secondary to hypocaloric intake. A family history should inquire about relatives with chronic diarrhea, cystic fibrosis, celiac sprue, inflammatory bowel disease, or other chronic conditions.

A careful description of the stool should be obtained, analyzing its number, consistency, odor, presence of blood or mucus, and other associated symptoms particularly fever, vomiting, or abdominal cramps. Short incubation (less than 24 hours), short duration (less than 24 hours) illnesses are usually due to the ingestion of a preformed toxin. If the duration is several days, infection with an agent that produced enterotoxin or invasion is likely. The

number of wet diapers and their dampness in the preceding 6- to 8- hour period should be quantified.

Physical Examination

The physical examination should focus initially on the hydration status of the patient, having rapidly assessed the airway and ventilation. Vital signs, particularly blood pressure and heart rate, should be monitored. Skin turgor, moistness of mucosal membranes, and tearing are useful. Weight/age and height/age should be determined to assess the nutritional status, and a careful abdominal and rectal examination should then be performed. A complete physical examination is mandatory to assure that the symptoms are not a manifestation of either a localized infection (*e.g.*, otitis) or a systemic disease (*e.g.*, hemolytic uremic syndrome), and to determine if there is systemic toxicity.

Laboratory Tests

In the child with uncomplicated diarrhea and no evidence of dehydration or toxicity, an extensive evaluation is not appropriate. However, in the toxic, dehydrated patient, additional studies may assist in determining the etiology, the hydration status, and the presumptive need for specific therapy.

The examination of the stool is the single most important step in defining the diarrheal illness. It should be observed for color, consistency, odor, and the presence or absence of blood or mucus. A stool with a yeasty or acidic odor suggests carbohydrate malabsorption; a purulent odor suggests colitis. The stool pH should be obtained, and a pH less than 6 suggests carbohydrate malabsorption. A clinitest should be performed. The presence or absence of blood should also be determined; it is more commonly found in colitic infections. An examination of the stool for fecal leukocytes is another method to narrow the diagnostic possibilities (Table 106-1).

A culture of the stool should usually be reserved for those patients in whom the results will alter the therapeutic plan. It should be performed in all children less than 1 year old who are toxic, children with severe dehydration, as well as those with underlying hemoglobinopathies or immunocompromised states. If many members are in the same family or day care, or if a member is a food handler, cultures are indicated for epidemiologic reasons. The enzyme-linked immunosorbent assay (ELISA) for rotavirus may be useful in selected cases. Specialized facilities are necessary to identify EPEC,

Table 106-1. Causes of Acute Infectious Diarrhea

AGENTS	PATHOLOGIC/ PHYSIOLOGIC		INCUBATION	AGE	DIARRHEA	DYSENTERY	BLOOD	FECAL WBC
	Toxic	Invasive						
Rotavirus	0	Villous blunting	2–3 days	Less than 5 yrs; peaks 2 yrs	Watery	0	0	12%
Norwalk	0	+	1–3 days	All	46%	0	0	0
Campylobacter fetus ss jejunum	0	+ +	2–11 days	Any; epidemic 1–5 10–29	Initially watery	+ +	90%	85%
Salmonella; gastroenteritis	0	+ +	8–48 hr	Any	Foul-smelling mucus, loose	+	80%	75%
Shigella	+	+ +	36–72 hr	Any: peak 2–10 years	Odorless mucus	+ +	+ +	84%
E. Coli								
Enterotoxigenic	+ +	0	24–48 hr	Any: peaks <1 yr	Profuse, watery	0	0	0
Enteroinvasive	0	+ +	46–72 hr	Any	Watery, mucoid	+ +	+	85%
Enteropathogenic	+ or 0	0	24–48 hr	<1 yr	Watery, severe	+	0	0
Yersinia	+	+	4–10 days	Any: peak 2 yrs	Watery	+	10%	10%– 50%
Giardia	0	Duodenum	10–21 days	Any; peaks 4 yrs	Loose, watery, foul-smelling	0	0	0

ETEC, and the invasive strains, and the test should be done in evaluating epidemics. Ova and parasitic examinations should be reserved for patients in whom there are suggestive epidemiologic and clinical data, bacterial cultures are repeatedly negative, or the diarrhea lasts more than 1 week. The value of a proctosigmoidoscopy in patients with acute diarrhea is limited. It is, however, important in the diagnosis of pseudomembranous colitis, *E. histolytica*, and in patients with chronic disorders.

TREATMENT

The therapy of acute diarrhea may be divided into two components: Specific therapy, if available (antibiotics for certain infections) (Table 106-2) and empiric (supportive) therapy.

Irrespective of the specific etiology of the diarrhea, if diarrheal losses of body water and electrolytes continue without adequate replacement, increasing dehydration, acidosis, cardiovascular collapse, and death will ensue. Children, especially infants, elderly persons, and patients with underlying conditions (*e.g.*, cystic fibrosis, diuretic therapy) are more susceptible to dehydration. The objective of the therapy should be the restoration or maintenance of adequate hydration and electrolyte balance, the avoidance of measures that could prolong the course of the disease, and the maintenance or restoration of the patient's nutritional status. The initial management must assure that the patient's condition is stable, and, if not, initial steps should be taken to stabilize the patient. The use of nonspecific therapies (*e.g.*, lactobacilli granules, yogurt, kaolin, anticholinergics, antiemetics, opiates) has not been shown to shorten the illness or change the outcome. Some have potentially serious side effects, particularly in infants, and their routine use in the management of acute diarrhea is not recommended.

ABDOMINAL PAIN	FEVER	VOMITING	EXTRAIN-TESTINAL	SEASON	DURATION UNTREATED	ROUTE	OTHER
Mild	50%–75%	90%	URI in 50%; dehydration	Winter	5–6 days	Fecal-oral; respirator	Dx by ELISA
Mild	Rare	75%	0	0	1–3 days	Fecal-oral	Explosive; epidemic nature
Severe in 60%	80%	30%	Seizures (rare); HUS; bacteria; peak July dehydration (rare)	All year; peak July	2 to 7 days	Fecal oral; food and water; person to person	Relapse 20%; neonatal transmission; FTT; chronic diarrhea
Moderate	75%	Usual	Meningitis; osteomyelitis; FTT	Warm	3–7 days	Animal or human source; food; fecal or oral	Infants at risk for invasive disease; increased risk in sickle cell dx
Severe	50%–70%	Rare	Seizures in 12% to 45% occasional bacteremia	Warm	7–14 days	Fecal; oral; rarely food	Common in day care centers; dehydration rare
Crampy	20% Low grade	Common	Dehydration	Summer	3–10 days	Oral-fecal; food and water	Leading cause of travelers' diarrhea
Moderate	Common	0	0	?	?	Oral-fecal; food	Diagnosis by guinea pig test
Mild to 0	20%	Common	Severe dehydration	Fall	7–14 days	Oral-fecal; person to person	Epidemics in nurseries
Crampy 60%	50%–80%	40%	Mesenteric adenitis; arthritis; septicemia	Winter	14–21 days	Food; animals; oral-fecal	Chronic diarrhea can occur; may mimic appendicitis; serologic evaluation useful in epidemics
Crampy	0	Common	Growth retardation; synovitis	All	4–6 weeks	Person to person; water; food; cross species	Frequent in day care centers; sprue-like syndrome

The advent of intravenous (IV) rehydration represented an important step in the management of severe diarrhea; however, since the late 1960s an alternative mode of therapy has become available, namely oral rehydration. Conventional therapy for diarrheal dehydration employs IV rehydration and fasting. When adequate hydration has been achieved by the IV route, an oral electrolyte solution is introduced, and the IV fluids are slowly weaned. Then, a period of "bowel rest" is prescribed, for 24 to 48 hours, during which time only glucose–electrolyte solutions are administered. Formula (usually lactose-free, one quarter to one half strength advancing to full strength) is usually introduced slowly over 2 to 5 days.

Oral solutions have become widely used in the world, including the United States, instead of IV fluids for the treatment of dehydration from diarrhea. This is inexpensive, highly efficacious, does not require sterile ingredients or materials, and can be administered and supervised by nonprofessional staff. An oral rehydration solution (ORS) has evolved under the auspices of the World Health Organization (WHO), and has been extensively used successfully all over the world. It contains Na-90 mEq/l, K-20 mEq/l, HCO_3-30 mEq/l, Cl 80 mEq/l and glucose 111 mM (2%), and has an osmolarity of 331 mOsm/l (Table 106-3).

Originally devised to treat the stool and electrolyte losses in patients with cholera, ORS has been shown not only to reduce the stool losses from bacterial and rotaviral diarrhea, but is equally effective in all types of diarrheas, independent of the sodium content of the stools. To address the concern about development of hypernatremia in infants, the WHO recommendation is to administer two thirds of the required volume as ORS and one third as plain water. Furthermore, the WHO recommends that following the clinical examination, the infant be classified as either mildly (less than

Table 106-2. Specific Treatment for Infectious Diarrhea

AGENT	INDICATIONS	TREATMENT	ALTERNATIVES	COMMENTS
Campylobacter	Gastroenteritis	None		
	Severe symptoms	Erythromycin 40 mg/kg q6h for 5–7 days	Clindamycin 300 mg q 6 hrs; tetracycline 250 mg q6 hrs for 5 days	Erythromycin does not change clinical course. It decreases campylobacter excretion.
	Sepsis	Gentamicin 5 mg/kg q 8 hrs 2 wk or chloramphenicol 75 mg/kg/day q 6 hrs for 2 wks		
Salmonella	Carrier	None		
	Acute gastroenteritis	None		
	Bacteremia or enteric fever	Ampicillin 200 mg/kg/day q 4 hrs 2 wks or Chloramphenicol 75 mg/kg/day IV or PO q 6 hrs for 2 wks	Trimethoprin/sulfamethoxazole TMP 10 mg/kg/day SMX 50 mg/kg/day q 12 hrs for 2 wks	Concerns that it prolongs the carrier state
	Disseminated infection	Same, but for 4–6 wks		
	Children < 3 mo with acute gastroenteritis and children with FTT	Same for 2 wks		
Shigella	All patients if symptomatic when diagnosis is made	Trimethoprin-sulfamethoxazole TMP 10 mg/kg/day SMX 50 mg/kg/day q 12 hr per 5 days Ampicillin 100 mg/kg q 6 hrs for 5 days	Tetracycline in adults 7.5 g orally in one dose	Antibiotics promptly control the infection
	Asymptomatic carriers	Treat as above if in day care or to prevent spread between family members		
E. coli				
Enteropathogenic	Life-threatening infection; nursery epidemic	Neomycin 30 mg/kg q 8 hrs for 5 days	Colistin	No controlled trials
Enterotoxigenic	Gastroenteritis	Probably none		For prevention of diarrhea doxycycline has been recommended
Enteroinvasive	Same as shigellosis	Probably none		
Yersinia	Gastroenteritis	None		
	Sepsis	Gentamicin 5 mg/kg q 8 hrs	Chloramphenicol 75 mg/kg q 6 hrs	
Giardia	All	Quinacrine 6 mg/kg q 8 hrs for 7 days Metronidazole 15 mg/kg q 8 hrs for 7 days	Furazolidone 5 mg/kg q 6 hrs for 7 days	Concerns about carcinogenesis

Table 106-3. Comparison of Solutions Used in Oral Rehydration

	Na+ (mEq/L)	K+ (mEq/L)	Cl− (mEq/L)	BASE (mEq/L)	CARBOHYDRATES (%)
Stool Losses					
ETEC/Rotavirus	30–65	18–60	26–55	HCO_3 6–18	
Cholera	90–120	30	85–120	HCO_3 30	
Solutions					
WHO–ORS	90	20	80	HCO_3 30	Gluc 2%
Hydra-lyte	84	10	59	HCO_3 30 Citrate 20	Gluc + Suc: 2%
Infalyte	50	20	40	HCO_3 30	Gluc 2%
Lytren	50	25	45	Citrate 30	Gluc 2%
Pedialyte	45	20	35	Citrate 30	Gluc 2.5%
Rehydralyte	75	20	65	Citrate 30	Gluc 2.5%
Resol	50	20	50	Citrate 34	Gluc 2%
Oral Rehydration Salts	90	20	60	HCO_3 30	Gluc 2%

5%), moderately (between 5% and 10%), or severely (more than 10%) dehydrated. All infants with moderate to severe dehydration receive 100 ml/kg ORS over 4 hours, followed by 50 ml/kg plain water over the next 2 hours. Infants with mild dehydration receive one half these volumes over 6 hours. On completion of 6 hours of oral therapy, the infant is reweighed and reexamined. If the infant is only partially rehydrated, therapy continues for 6 further hours with the fluid volumes offered based on the last assessment of severity of dehydration. If no improvement has occurred, or if the state of hydration has deteriorated, IV fluids are then initiated. In children older than 2 years, and adults, the ORS solution is administered without supplemental plain water. Using any of the aforementioned methods, oral rehydration is successful in 95% to 98% of patients and IV therapy is usually required in only 2% to 5% of cases. It has been shown repeatedly that vomiting is not a contraindication for using ORS. Oral therapy usually fails in patients who have high rates of stool loss (i.e., over 10 ml/kg/hr). Periorbital edema has been described transiently in 6% to 25% of hospitalized children who are being treated with oral rehydration; it is usually self-limited, resolves when the volume of ORS is decreased, and has not been associated with either hypernatremia or untoward consequences. The ORS WHO formula has also been used in the treatment of hypernatremic dehydration and, although a modified "slow" method has been employed successfully, further studies are necessary before oral rehydration can be recommended for this purpose.

In general, a higher sodium concentration has been advocated for rehydration solutions (75 to 90 mEq Na/l), and a lower sodium concentration for maintenance solutions (30 to 60 mEq Na/l). As can be seen in Table 106-3, several companies have marketed oral rehydration solutions for maintenance and rehydration therapy in ambulatory or hospitalized patients. The ideal solution should contain between 50 and 90 mEq/l Na, 2% to 2.5% glucose, 20 to 30 mEq/l K, and a base (bicarbonate or citrate), and should be given in frequent, small amounts, aiming to give the calculated deficit in 6 to 12 hours following the aforementioned recommendations.

It has been questioned whether fasting during an acute episode of diarrhea is necessary. The urgency of providing nutrients over and above water and solute depends somewhat on the child's initial nutritional status. The more malnourished and younger the child, the more immediate the nutritional concern should be. Many longitudinal studies from the developing countries on cohorts of children have shown that diarrhea directly causes malnutrition. The approach to diarrhea by most pediatricians in the United States and elsewhere consists of a variable period of fasting. The main arguments advanced for limited fasting are avoidance of the consequences of malabsorption, namely acidosis, excessive fluid losses, depletion of the bile acid pool, and possible mucosal injury from unabsorbed foods. Advocates of continued feeding suggest that this practice (i.e., feeding) will prevent insufficient intake of protein and calories, maintain or stimulate repair of the intestinal mucosa, and sustain breast-feeding. Few studies address specifically the impact of early feeding, but most of them show that if early feedings are introduced, the outcome is favorable.

It is difficult to make dietary recommendations with complete confidence. Nevertheless, until a definitive causal relationship between early dietary therapy and chronic malabsorption, or food allergy can be established, the only aspects of early feeding during acute diarrhea that are proven to be potentially harmful are excessive fluid loss, and increased malabsorption, particularly secondary to carbohydrate intolerance. Since those complications can easily be monitored clinically and stool characteristics can be closely followed, we think it is possible to reintroduce foods immediately after rehydration. Breast-feeding should be continued once rehydration is completed. Children who are fully weaned should receive their usual diet, and it is usually suggested that a lactose-free formula should be used, usually for 2 weeks, particularly in cases of rotaviral diarrhea, although it may also be rational to first try small amounts of the regular formula that the child usually takes, reserving the lactose-free formulas for those children who show a clinical intolerance to lactose. The consumption of complementary foods should also be encouraged. Generally, the child should determine the amount of food to be consumed, and food should not be forced on unwilling, anorectic infants; however, food should be offered to the hungry infant despite ongoing diarrhea. Once diarrhea subsides, extra food should be available to enable a recovery of any nutritional deficit imposed by the acute illness.

INDICATIONS FOR ADMISSION

All patients with circulatory insufficiency (10% to 15% dehydration), inability to drink, alteration in consciousness, and intractable vomiting should be initially rehydrated with parenteral fluids. They should be admitted to the hospital and, as soon as they are stable, they should complete the rehydration orally. Toxic-appearing patients as well as those in which the family is unable to precisely follow the oral rehydration guidelines should also be admitted.

ANNOTATED BIBLIOGRAPHY

Barkin R: Acute infectious diarrheal disease in children. J Emergency Med 3:1, 1985 (Good review of etiology.)

Brown KH, McLean VC: Nutritional management of acute diarrhea: An appraisal of the alternatives. Pediatrics 73:119, 1984 (Excellent analysis and discussion of the controversy.)

Davidson GP, Goodwin D, Robb TA: Incidence and duration of lactose malabsorption in children hospitalized with acute enteritis. Study in a well nourished urban population. J Pediatr 105:587, 1984 (Prospective study of the natural history.)

Hirschorn N: The treatment of acute diarrhea in children. An historical and physiological perspective. Am J Clin Nutr 33:637, 1980 (Thorough review of the pathophysiology and therapy.)

Levine MM, Pizarro D: Advances in therapy of diarrheal dehydration: Oral rehydration. Adv Pediatr 31:207, 1984 (Good general overview; very practical.)

SanJoaquin VH, Marks MJ: New agents in diarrhea. Pediatr Infect Dis 1:53, 1982 (Discussion of recent developments.)

Santosham M, Daum RS, Dillman L et al: Oral rehydration therapy of infantile diarrhea. N Engl J Med 306:1070, 1982 (Study comparing parenteral vs oral rehydration.)

Santosham M, Foster S, Reed R et al: Role of soy-based, lactose free formula during treatment of acute diarrhea. Pediatrics 76:292, 1985 (Compares early feedings with traditional therapy.)

107
Malabsorption Syndrome
WAYNE I. LENCER AND
W. ALLAN WALKER

Pediatricians often consider malabsorption in the differential of several common childhood syndromes such as failure to thrive, short stature, or chronic diarrhea. Malabsorption can be defined as a failure to digest or absorb dietary nutrients. It is a manifestation of a disease and not a specific entity. The clinical syndrome can range from those children with obviously voluminous large foul-smelling stools or chronic diarrhea and growth failure to relatively asymptomatic individuals with laboratory evidence of a nutritional deficiency. Practically, then, malabsorption should be considered in any patient who has a nutritional deficiency unexplained by dietary factors.

PATHOPHYSIOLOGY

All nutrients have three broad phases of digestion and absorption. The intraluminal phase comprises events that occur within the lumen of the gut. These are most sensitive to disturbances in the pancreatic and biliary functions. The intestinal phase defines those events that occur at the enterocyte surface or within the cell and are sensitive to disturbances of the intestinal mucosa itself. The removal phase refers to the transport of nutrients from the enterocyte to other organs for metabolism or storage.

The digestive processes of the intraluminal phase act to solubilize lipids in water and begin the breakdown of starch and protein. Pancreatic secretions handle the bulk of intraluminal digestion. Dietary lipids, however, require the additional presence of bile acids and thus a normally functioning liver, biliary tract, and terminal ileum. (Bile acids are reabsorbed at the terminal ileum and recycled.) Ninety percent of ingested lipids are in the form of triglyceride. These are hydrolyzed at a basic pH to free fatty acid and monoglyceride by the combination of pancreatic colipase, lipase, and bile salts. When above the critical micellar concentration, bile salts solubilize the fatty products of triglyceride hydrolysis by forming micelles. Micelles carry fatty acids and glycerol with fat-soluble vitamins and cholesterol to the enterocyte surface. Defects in these intraluminal processes tend to produce considerable fat malabsorption.

The pancreas also secretes critical enzymes for the digestion of starch and proteins. Amylase hydrolyzes amylopectin (starch) to maltose, maltotriose, or α-limit dextrans. Similarly, trypsin (activated by enterokinase at the mucosal surface) acting with carboxypeptidase and elastase (activated in turn by trypsin) hydrolyzes protein to free amino acids and short-chain peptides. The products of both starch and protein digestion move through the unstirred water layer by diffusion.

The intestinal phase begins at the enterocyte surface and serves to package lipids in a soluble form suitable for the systemic circulation; this phase completes the digestion and absorption of carbohydrates and proteins. Lipids diffuse passively through the cell membrane. The enterocyte then reforms triglyceride from absorbed fatty acids and monoglycerides adding phospholipids, apoproteins, and cholesterol to make chylomicrons. The

transportation of chylomicrons out of the cell into the lymphatics requires the specific apoprotein β-lipoprotein.

Lactase, sucrase–isomaltase, and glucoamylase contained in the brush border of the enterocyte further hydrolyze maltotriose maltose, α-limit dextrans, and ingested disaccharides (sucrose and lactose) to their component monosaccharides (glucose, galactose, and fructose). Hydrolysis of disaccharides, especially lactose, at the brush border, is the rate-limiting step.

At the mucosal surface, small peptides are either transported through the membrane on carrier proteins or are further hydrolyzed to free amino acids where other carrier proteins facilitate their absorption. Absorbed peptides are hydrolyzed within the cytosol to free amino acids. These, together with absorbed free amino acids, diffuse into the portal circulation. Defects of the intestinal phase, although almost always causing carbohydrate malabsorption, may or may not produce fat malabsorption. The degree of steatorrhea depends on the extent of mucosal injury. Viral gastroenteritis, for example, characteristically causes patchy mucosal injury that may not damage enough mucosa to cause fatty stools, whereas celiac disease causes diffuse damage and almost always steatorrhea.

The removal phase acts to carry products of absorption to the systemic circulation and is affected by diseases of the portal and lymphatic circulation.

CLINICAL PRESENTATION

The clinical presentation of malabsorption is as varied as the disease entities that cause it. Classic signs of GI tract dysfunction such as chronic diarrhea, the passage of frequent, large, pale, oily, and foul-smelling stools, increased flatus, abdominal distention, or possibly increased appetite may not be obvious. A combination of dietary, or psychosocial factors causes most nutritional deficiencies in childhood. A nutritional deficiency may, in turn, cause malabsorption. The dietary history plays a critical role in distinguishing undernutrition from malabsorption. In uncertain cases of growth failure, catch-up growth after a clinical trial of adequate nutrition in a controlled environment indicates a normal GI tract.

Growth failure is the most common sign of a nutritional deficiency in childhood and the most common presentation of malabsorption. An early detection of growth failure depends on growth monitoring. Plots of weight against height on standard curves (from the National Center for Health Statistics) provide early evidence of growth failure often before other clinical signs are evident. Plots of height against age or of height velocity will show stunting due to chronic nutritional deficiency. Other measures of nutritional status such as skinfold thickness correlate highly with anthropomorphic measurements but do not enhance the assessment of children with undernutrition beyond carefully done growth charts.

Malabsorption can present with signs of vitamin deficiency. Diseases causing defects in the intestinal phase processes will cause a deficiency of water-soluble vitamins and minerals such as folic acid, B_{12}, Fe, and other B vitamins. Pallor, fatigue, or dizziness due to anemia, cheilosis, glossitis, dermatitis, and peripheral neuropathy may be presenting signs of a malabsorption syndrome. Defects in either pancreatic or biliary processes commonly cause deficiency of the fat-soluble vitamins A, D, E, and K. This may produce hyperkeratosis of skin (vitamin A), ecchymosis and hematuria (vitamin K), and tetany, bone pain, or rickets (vitamin D).

A nutritional deficiency in older children may present as delayed puberty.

Symptoms and signs of the underlying disease process often dominate the clinical picture. For example, children who have cystic fibrosis or an immunodeficiency may present with a chronic cough or a recurrent pulmonary infection. Those who have hepatic disease may have cirrhosis and its complications, and those who have IBD may present with abdominal pain. The clinical picture in those cases suggests its own diagnostic strategy. Those children with vague symptoms or nonspecific signs such as persistent loose stools, short stature, or growth failure will benefit from a carefully done nutritional assessment, documentation of nutritional deficiency, and consideration of malabsorption in those children in whom dietary or social causes of undernutrition are not found.

DIFFERENTIAL DIAGNOSIS

The differential of malabsorption in pathophysiologic groups is listed in the box, Selected Differential Diagnosis.

Of these, acute and chronic infection, giardia, postinfectious enteritis, allergic enteritis, celiac and cystic fibrosis are the most common diseases affecting children. Neonates have physiologic steatorrhea due to decreased bile acid pools and decreased pancreatic function. This developmentally "normal" malabsorption must be differentiated from disease in the very young child.

Selected Differential Diagnosis

Intraluminal phase abnormalities

Cystic fibrosis
Chronic pancreatitis

Malnutrition

Decreased conjugated bile acids

Liver production and excretion
Neonatal hepatitis
Biliary atresia: intrahepatic and extrahepatic
Acute and chronic active hepatitis
Disease of the biliary tract
Cirrhosis
Fat malabsorption in the premature infant
Intestinal factors
Short bowel syndrome
Bacterial overgrowth
Blind loop
Fistula
Strictures—regional enteritis

Abnormalities of the intestinal phase

Mucosal diseases
Infection, bacterial or viral
Infestations
Giardia lamblia
Fish tapeworm
Hookworm
Malnutrition
Drugs: methotrexate, antibiotics
Crohn's disease
Chronic ulcerative colitis
Cow's milk intolerance and soy protein
intolerance
Secondary disaccharidase deficiency
Hirschsprung's disease with enterocolitis
Celiac disease
Circulatory disturbances
Cirrhosis
Congestive heart failure
Abnormal structural makeup of gastrointestinal
tract
Selective inborn absorptive defects
Endocrine disease

Defective delivery phase

Intestinal lymphangiectasis
Congestive heart failure
Regional enteritis with lymphangiectasis
Lymphoma
Abetalipoproteinemia

Miscellaneous

Renal insufficiency
Immunity defects
Maternal deprivation
Collagen disease
Intractable diarrhea of early infancy

(Adapted from Silverman A, Roy CC (eds): Pediatric Clinical Gastroenterology. St. Louis, CV Mosby, 1983)

WORK-UP

History and Physical Examination

The diagnostic approach depends heavily on the clinical presentation. The dietary history will identify most children with nutritional deficiency due to undernutrition. Temporal associations between symptoms and the introduction of various nutrients such as cow's milk, sucrose, or gluten-containing grains suggest food sensitivity, enzyme deficiencies, or celiac disease, respectively. Symptoms of systemic disorders associated with malnutrition, a history of abdominal surgery, or recent or past travel should be sought. The physical examination may reveal evidence of a nutritional deficiency. The height and weight plotted accurately on appropriate growth curves will identify growth failure. Sexual development should be noted. The thickness of subcutaneous tissue, skin elasticity, muscle wasting in the buttocks, thighs, and arms may indicate a recent loss of weight. Dry, fine, easily pulled out hair can be seen in protein-deficiency states. The abdomen might be distended or locally tender. Other signs of nutritional deficiency previously mentioned may be present.

Laboratory Tests

Occult blood in the stool indicates damage to the intestinal mucosa. The presence of polymorphonuclear leukocytes occurs with inflammatory diseases. Cultures will eliminate infection. Three fresh stools examined for ova and parasites will detect between 50% and 80% of those children with giardia. A fresh liquid stool sample with pH less than 5.5 and reducing substances indicates sugar malabsorption. A Hgb, Hct, U/A and sweat test should be done routinely. A bone age will assess growth potential and may show osteomalacia or rickets. The CBC, DIFF, MCV, TP/ALB, Ca, PO_4, Alk Phos, LFTs, ferritin and folate may be useful if abnormal.

In uncertain cases, the pediatrician may want direct evidence of malabsorption before proceeding with a further work-up or a small bowel biopsy. Unfortunately, the serum carotene depends heavily on dietary intake and, when reduced, does not reliably reflect the absorptive function. To demonstrate malabsorption, the D-xylose absorption and a 72-hour quantitative fecal fat collection are the most useful tests. Neither test, however, is highly sensitive. Some children with normal D-xylose and fat collection will require a further work-up including a small bowel biopsy unless a specific diagnosis

has been made by other means such as in cystic fibrosis.

D-xylose is absorbed by diffusion and on the same transport protein as glucose but with much less affinity. Its absorption reflects the available mucosal surface area and therefore the mucosal function. An oral dose of 14.5 g/M^2 followed by a 60-min blood level, will give a 20 mg/dl rise or greater in normal individuals.

Fat absorption requires normal function in all phases of digestion and absorption. This makes the 72-hr fat collection the most sensitive test for malabsorption. A positive qualitative sudan stain for stool fat, however, precludes the need to collect a 72-hr stool sample. For at least 2 days before and throughout the 72-hr collection the child must take a normal diet high in fats. Parents keep a dietary diary to quantitate fat intake. The diet diary may demonstrate inadequate nutrition, which was previously unsuspected. The amount of fat excreted in stool is normally less than 10% of intake. Beware of falsely "normal" tests from inadequate stool collection. Attempts should be made to collect all stool excreted during the collection period.

Although an abnormal 72-hr fat may reflect a defect in any phase of absorption or digestion, an abnormal D-xylose suggests that the defect lies in the intestinal phase. The tests supplement each other and direct further investigations. For example, a normal D-xylose and abnormal fat suggest a defect in the intraluminal processes such as pancreatic insufficiency, small bowel overgrowth, or liver disease. An abnormal D-xylose with a normal 72-hr fat indicates intestinal phase dysfunction such as in celiac disease or postinfectious enteritis. Abnormal tests in either case are indications for referral and consideration of small bowel biopsy. Again, the sensitivity of the tests (80%) means normal results do not necessarily rule out malabsorption. Children with nutritional deficiency *unexplained by dietary factors* should be referred to a pediatric gastroenterologist for a small bowel biopsy. Normal tests, however, in those children with nonspecific symptoms but without nutritional deficiency do *not* support further investigation unless other signs develop.

A small bowel biopsy can be done safely (mortality rate less than 0.001 to 0.0001) and with little trauma to child and family. The small bowel biopsy, however, does not establish a specific diagnosis in every case of malabsorption. Biopsies will reliably diagnose diseases that affect the mucosa diffusely and are likely to require treatment, such as celiac disease.

Diseases that produce patchy mucosal lesions, such as postinfectious enteritis and milk allergic enteropathies, are with few exceptions in the pediatric practice, transient and resolve with time. In many children, then, a normal small bowel biopsy may be followed by a period of watchful waiting. We do not place children on a gluten-free diet without a biopsy confirmation of celiac disease. The empiric treatment of children suspected of celiac disease causes undue hardship for many more families who do not have celiac disease than benefit for those who do.

In others, additional tests can be useful. Lactose and sucrose hydrogen breath tests will demonstrate a lactase or a sucrose-isomaltase deficiency with a sensitivity of 80%. Small bowel overgrowth often causes an abnormal lactulose breath test. Upper gastrointestinal (UGI) and small bowel follow through barium studies may show changes characteristic of malabsorption or anatomic defects. Sigmoidoscopy and biopsy can confirm ulcerative colitis and Crohn's disease. None of these, however, are appropriate screening tests and should be used only later in the work-up with specific aims in mind.

TREATMENT

A specific diagnosis dictates specific treatment in diseases causing malabsorption as in other syndromes. Several general principles, however, can help in management. Elemental formulas containing monosaccharides, small peptides, and MCT oil circumvent many steps of normal digestion and absorption, and can be used successfully in most children with malabsorption syndromes. Hydrolyzed proteins and MCTs are soluble in water and do not require bile salts or pancreatic enzymes. In children with severe fat malabsorption, such as cystic fibrosis or chronic liver disease, water-soluble forms of vitamins A,D,K, and E at double doses should replace their fat-soluble counterparts. Formulas containing monosaccharides do not require fragile brush border enzymes such as lactase. Finally, TPN can be used when enteral feedings of elemental diets fail.

Although discussed in greater detail in chapter 106, the treatment of common diarrhea warrants mention here. Postinfectious enteritis explains most cases of malabsorption seen by the practicing pediatrician and is the set up for the development of intractable diarrhea. The avoidance of morbidity from diarrhea depends largely on feeding practices. For almost all cases of dehydration due to diarrhea, oral rehydration solutions, such as the WHO ORS solution, will rehydrate the child, correct acidosis, and improve appetite. As soon as rehydration is achieved and in those children not initially dehydrated, feedings of breast milk, or one quarter to one half strength lactose-free formula or a diet supplemented with electrolyte solutions and free water can and should be offered immediately. The diet is advanced in strength as the appetite improves. Minor changes in stool volume or consistency bear little meaning. Lactose should be avoided routinely in the immediate postinfectious period up to 1 week. Thereafter, lactose may be empirically introduced in the diet, but lactose intolerance may last up to 6 months after infectious diarrhea. Since sucrase and isomaltase are linked membrane enzymes, the use of sucrose-free, corn syrup formulas makes little sense. This strategy will achieve a positive nutrient and fluid balance in almost all cases of diarrhea when it is so desperately needed.

ANNOTATED BIBLIOGRAPHY

Friedman HI, Nylund B: Intestinal fat digestion, absorption and transport. Am J Clin Nutr 33:1139–1180, 1980 (Excellent review of digestive physiology and supplements the pathophysiology discussed.)

Gray GM: Carbohydrate digestion and absorption. N Engl J Med 292(23):1125, 1975 (Excellent review of digestive physiology and supplements the pathophysiology discussed.)

Nutrition. Pediatr Clin North Am 32(2), April 1985 (Texts discuss malabsorption from the pediatric perspective.)

Silverman A, Roy CC (eds): Pediatric Clinical Gastroenterology, Chap. 10. St. Louis, CV Mosby, 1983 (Texts discuss malabsorption from the pediatric perspective.)

Sleisenger MH, Fordtran JS (eds): Gastrointestinal Disease, Chaps. 15, 49–51. Philadelphia, WB Saunders, 1983 (Readable and provides a comprehensive discussion of malabsorption, pathophysiology, clinical presentation, complications, and treatment.)

Sleisenger MH, Kim YS: Protein digestion and absorption. N Engl J Med 300(12): 659, 1979 (Excellent review of digestive physiology and supplements the pathophysiology discussed.)

108
Constipation

JAMES H. BERMAN AND
W. ALLAN WALKER

Constipation is, in many ways, a paradigm for pediatric disease. It represents a complex interaction of parental and cultural expectations, development, gastrointestinal physiology, and nutritional factors. Any potential diagnosis and its attendant therapy must be discussed in the context of this interaction. The large scope of the problem of constipation is evidenced in many ways. In 1982, $368 million were spent in the United States on over-the-counter laxatives. Clearly, physician visits and diagnostic tests would push this figure still higher. Constipation has been estimated to account for 4% of all pediatric office visits. These figures do not include most patients with transient symptoms who do not seek medical attention.

DEFINITION

The first task of the pediatrician in approaching constipation is to determine how the parent or patient is using the term. Constipation may be defined as an intestinal dysfunction in which the bowels are difficult or painful to evacuate. This rather broad definition will serve to reassure many parents whose children are asymptomatic although their stooling pattern does not meet some cultural or parental expectations. Defining a frequency of stooling that is abnormal is difficult because of the great influence of dietary and environmental factors. Various population surveys in adults have established a range of three times a day to three times a week. Infants taking various feedings exhibit a similar range of stooling frequency to that of adults. Defining difficulty in passing a bowel movement is more subjective and thus even more difficult to quantify than stool frequency. It is easy to recognize that the passage of pellet-like hard bowel movements is abnormal, but the passage of a soft stool that requires considerable straining may be more difficult to classify. In the infant and toddler age groups, parents often mistake the normal passage of stool (face turning red and pulling up legs) or even straining to withhold stool as a symptom of constipation. Stools flowing around a fecal impaction may be diarrheal in character.

DIAGNOSTIC EVALUATION

Fortunately, despite the high incidence of constipation, few patients with constipation have a significant organic abnormality. However, a careful history and physical examination may elicit complaints that raise more alarm. Functional constipation (no definite organic etiology) should not interfere with normal growth and development. Failure to thrive, particularly when associated with constipation, may be seen in Hirschsprung's disease, celiac disease, and various metabolic disturbances. Developmental delay and neuromuscular disorders can often present with constipation. Moderate to tense abdominal distention rarely occurs in functional constipation, but is often seen in obstructive processes, celiac disease, and Hirschsprung's disease. In the absence of an anal fissure, the presence of blood is of concern, although colitis, neoplasm, or an obstructing polyp are rare in childhood. Colicky abdominal pain may occur in functional constipation, especially while straining for stools, but abdominal tenderness is usually absent. Vomiting is not usually seen in functional constipation. Excessive milk intake, anticholinergic drugs, cathartic abuse, narcotics, and aluminum-based antacids can produce constipation. Iron-containing preparations can give rise to constipation, but whether or not iron-containing infant formulas may be constipating is questionable. Finally, constipation as a cause for fever, seizures, upper respiratory infections, otitis, or psychosis is probably more of a myth than a reality.

The presence of constipation in the newborn is always worrisome. Greater than 90% of infants will have their first stool within 24 hours after birth. Abdominal distention and vomiting are signs of functional or anatomic obstruction. Intestinal atresias and stenoses as well as meconium ileus may first present with constipation. An abdominal roentgenogram demonstrates an obstructive gas pattern and air-fluid levels. Functional ileus is usually associated with ill infants, those of low birth weight and infants with respiratory distress. The presence of hypoactive bowel sounds, distention, and feeding intolerance makes functional ileus difficult to differentiate from an anatomic obstruction. The abdominal radiograph may show diffuse dilatation of the bowel and there are generally no air-fluid levels.

Hirschsprung's disease (congenital aganglionic megacolon) merits special mention. It represents the most common cause of neonatal abdominal obstruction and is the organic cause commonly considered in the evaluation of constipation at any age. While increasing awareness of the disease has produced earlier diagnosis, one third of all cases remain undiagnosed until after 3 months of age and 15% to 25% of cases are not diagnosed until after 5 years of age. The diagnosis of Hirschsprung's disease may be particularly delayed in those cases involving only a short segment of the colon. An early diagnosis may reduce the incidence of enterocolitis (high mortality) and spare patients the morbidity of chronic constipation. Neonates who fail to pass stool in the first 48 hours of life, or who pass a meconium plug, should be observed closely. If stooling problems persist, an investigation with a mucosal rectal biopsy and a barium enema is indicated. Infants and older children, in whom Hirschsprung's disease is suspected, may be first screened with rectal manometry.

Infants may be bothered by the discomfort of passing a stool through an anal fissure. Congenital hypothyroidism, renal tubular acidosis, hypercalcemia, and diabetes insipidus are rare causes of constipation. The association of a developmental delay or sacral anomalies with constipation is suspicious for neuromuscular disorders or myelodysplasia.

The entry into the second year of life is marked by an increasing variety of foods in the child's diet and the gradual acquisition of a conscious control over defecation. Parents maintain an expectation that their offspring will soon be free of diapers, an event with implications for parental life-style as well as the child's development. Unfortunately, the low-fiber toddler diet and the complex process of toilet training can make this time of life particularly troubled by constipation. As with other newly discovered skills in this age group, the toddler with some control over defecation may choose to withhold a stool. The reason may be that he finds it uncomfortable to pass or as a gesture of independence. The parent often complains that the child will grimace and strain, then pass a small amount of stool. Other children may pass giant bowel movements infrequently. The child can spend long, unproductive sessions on the toilet. Parents often interpret these symptoms as intestinal blockage

when, paradoxically, the child is actually withholding stool. The presence of an anal fissure, which produces pain on defecation, makes the child's desire to withhold a stool understandable. Emotional stresses, such as the birth of a sibling, inconsistent or coercive toilet training, or separation from parents may also lead to withholding of stool.

Minor illnesses can produce changes in bowel patterns through several mechanisms. Febrile illness, anorexia, and vomiting produce a mild dehydration provoking constipation. Some variation in gastrointestinal motility has been suggested as a possible mechanism. Finally, a decreased dietary fiber intake during the period of illness no doubt also adds a contribution. Rarely, bacterial enteric pathogens, such as *Salmonella*, may present with fever and constipation rather than the more typical diarrhea. Once again, the presence of abdominal pain, distention, and vomiting with constipation are worrisome signs. Intussusception, volvulus, or previously undiagnosed Hirschsprung's disease are all possible in the toddler age group.

Older children enjoy the benefits of a more varied diet and other mechanisms for exerting control over their environment. Constipation may still be a problem in this age group. In fact, encopresis, or fecal soiling, may be seen in 1% to 2% of first graders. Encopresis, as defined by the passage of stool outside the toilet after 4 years of age, is associated with a high psychological morbidity (see Chap. 33).

Children with mental retardation, neuromuscular disorders, or those with surgically corrected Hirschsprung's disease may continue having difficulty passing stools. The school bathroom is a frightening or embarrassing place for many children who thus defer having a bowel movement for many hours. Active social schedules may also contribute to producing a back-up of stool in the distal colon. The consumption of "junk food," characteristically low in fiber, further aggravates the problem. As mentioned earlier, it is not uncommon for a child with Hirschsprung's disease to escape diagnosis until school age or later. In addition, acquired hypothyroidism, intestinal tumors, or even inflammatory bowel disease may present with constipation. Finally, urinary tract infections are not uncommonly associated with constipation. Patients with recurrent urinary tract infections should be questioned about their bowel habits.

TREATMENT

The treatment of constipation should be tailored to the individual patient. The mechanisms responsible for normal variations in stooling pattern should be explained to parents as completely as possible. By coping with parental and societal expectations, counseling may be the only therapy required. Parents should be cautioned that although they and the pediatrician remain concerned about the child's health, an excessive vigilance over the child's stooling and toileting behavior diminish the child's feelings of autonomy and increase the tension over what should be a normal physiologic process. At an extreme, such attention may even aggravate the constipation. The parents and child should be aware that the treatment of constipation and encopresis requires long-term, consistent intervention and follow-up. A concrete treatment plan and measurable goals to be attained aid greatly in this process. A general rule of thumb is that the constipation will take as long to reverse as the time the child has had the constipation before treatment.

Constipation during infancy generally responds to increasing the fluid intake. Osmotic agents such as Karo syrup (5 to 15ml/8-oz bottle) or malt soup extract (Maltsupex–Wallace 1 to 4 Tbl/day) have also been used. Glycerin suppositories act locally to stimulate the passage of stool.

Dietary fiber is a complex mixture of compounds including cellulose, hemicellulose, mucilages, gums, pectin, and lignins. These substances vary in their water-holding properties and effects on bacterial fermentation. Fiber has attracted much attention for its hypocholesterolemic effects and possible role in the prevention of colon and other cancers. Several national panels have advocated an increase in the intake of dietary fiber for adults. Recommendations for children have been more guarded. Concerns have been raised that a high-fiber diet may alter the mineral balance in children, but there are little clinical data to support this objection. Unfortunately, the high-fiber legumes and whole-grain products do not traditionally appeal to a child's palate. A household survey conducted by the USDA showed that a significant percentage of children consume less than the recommended daily allowance for fruits, vegetables, and cereals. Some parental education regarding the benefits of increasing fiber intake for the whole family may help alter these findings. Fiber may be conveniently added to the diet through the use of whole-grain (not whole wheat) breads. Crude bran (tasteless) may be added to prepared and baked foods at one to two teaspoons/serving. Diced prunes, dates, and raisins are less objectionable when added to cookies or sprinkled over cereal. High-fiber cereals (9 g/serving) are also useful. Although the caloric density of most fiber-rich foods is low, the child benefits from a higher intake of vitamins A and C and a reduced intake of refined sugar. These benefits appeal to many parents. The alteration in caloric density of the food can be minimized by including nuts and legumes in the diet. Commercially prepared fiber preparations (Metamucil–Searle) are frequently beneficial as a supplement in older children. One teaspoon can be added to a bottle of milk for toddlers who might not otherwise accept it. While adequate fluids should be taken with fiber products, no more than 32 oz of milk or formula should be consumed daily.

Stool softeners, like dioctyl sodium sulfosuccinate (Colace–Mead Johnson) are surface active agents increasing the penetration of stool by water. They also have some effect on GI motor and secretory functions. These agents are useful in treating simple constipation or in aiding in maintaining soft stools while weaning mineral oil. They may be most useful in the child with special needs who requires chronic stool softening without the side effects of mineral oil. Doses of 5 to 10 mg/kg/day may be required.

Lactulose (Cephulac–Merrell Dow) is a nonabsorbed carbohydrate that loosens stool by producing an osmotic load in the colon. Although it has been used to treat chronic constipation, it is expensive and may produce cramping and flatus.

Cathartic laxatives are rarely indicated in childhood. Bisacodyl (Dulcolax–Boehringer) may be useful in the evacuation of stool during the initial therapy for chronic constipation. Frequent use of cathartic laxatives may cause significant fluid and electrolyte disturbances, colonic mucosal changes, and laxative dependence.

Mineral oil (liquid petrolatum) is a hydrocarbon mixture that produces a loose, frothy stool. Although not especially palatable, it can be mixed with chocolate syrup or blenderized with fruit juice and ice cubes to make an appealing cocktail. Several flavored mineral oils are available, but some of these also contain cathartics. Doses as low as one to two teaspoons may be effective in relieving constipation, but much larger doses are generally required for chronic constipation and encopresis. One tablespoon for each 15 kg given twice daily is a good initial dose. The dose may then be increased by ½ Tbl (7.5ml) every other day until the stools produced are loose, but not runny. These stools are difficult to withhold and should eliminate straining. The passage of mineral oil through the rectum can cause unpleasant anal irritation and is generally a sign that the dose is too low with leakage occurring around impacted stool. Small amounts of mineral oil are absorbed systemically producing deposits in the liver, spleen, lymph nodes, and other tissues. Although these findings may not be clinically significant, adults chronically taking mineral oil have been reported to have, on liver biopsy, lesions resembling chronic hepatitis. An alteration in fat-soluble vitamin absorption has also been reported. Many authors suggest that a multivitamin be given daily, between mineral oil doses. Although reports of lipoid pneumonia following the aspiration of mineral oil are uncommon, its use in infants, children with severe gastroesophageal reflux, or in those with significant neurologic impairment is contraindicated. Mineral oil doses should not be given just before bedtime.

Chronic Constipation and Encopresis

Therapy for chronic constipation or encopresis requires counseling and the flexible use of the aforementioned medications since there is no universally effective remedy. Although there is considerable controversy surrounding different treatment protocols, most methods include the following aspects. First, promote normal attitudes toward bowel function as mentioned earlier. Second, assess the degree of fecal retention and remove retained feces. Third, re-educate the bowel toward normal function and finally emphasize the importance of frequent follow-up. An objective assessment of the degree of fecal retention may be achieved through physical findings (the presence or absence of a left lower quadrant mass) or an abdominal plain roentgenogram revealing the amount of feces within the colon. Serial studies can then be employed to measure progress. The reaccumulation of retained stool is frequently associated with treatment failures. Because of an overlap with the normal population, a measurement of intestinal transit time is probably not helpful. Changes in rectal manometric data with treatment are, at the moment, not a clinically proven method for following patient progress or as a prognostic tool.

Decisions regarding the initial therapy to remove retained feces must be made cautiously. Children with a less chronic course and those with less stool retention can be adequately started on oral mineral oil therapy alone. Those patients with significant stool retention may require enemas to initiate evacuation, despite the invasiveness. Normal saline enemas of 500 ml to 750 ml should be given twice daily. More than 2 days of treatment should not be required. Older children may benefit from

Bisacodyl (Dulcolax–Boehringer), one tablet given orally after the first enema. Sodium phosphate (Pediatric Fleet) enemas may be more convenient for some families, but their overaggressive use may result in electrolyte disturbances especially in those patients who retain a large portion of the enema. Hospitalization is occasionally required for "cleanout" therapy, particularly in the situation where the home environment is not able to support this therapy.

Re-education of bowel habits involves several components. The *maintenance* of soft stool ensures the ease of passage and decreases withholding. Mineral oil effectively produces the appropriate stool softness. The dose should be increased slowly until the stools are loose, but not runny; 4 to 6 oz/day may be required. Since this therapy represents some loss of control on the part of the child, a simultaneous process of enlisting the patient's help in the treatment plan is important. A comparison of bowel training with athletic training is a useful tool. Many treatment protocols include reward systems such as a star chart. The goals to be achieved should be attainable and easily measured (*e.g.*, 4 stools in the toilet = one red star, four red stars = one new toy). The reward should be for producing a stool in the toilet, not the absence of soiling. All of the child's caretakers should administer the system consistently. Toileting at specific times, when the chances of successful stooling are better, is beneficial. These times include mornings and 1 hour after meals. The possibility of needing to toilet at an inopportune moment (*e.g.*, at school or in a shopping mall) is thus also minimized. Teachers should be aware that the child may need to make an emergency visit to the toilet.

INDICATIONS FOR REFERRAL

Biofeedback techniques employing rectal manometry have thus far not proven more effective than conventional therapy, but they may benefit individual patients. Because 10% to 20% of children with refractory constipation have Hirschsprung's disease, treatment failures should be assessed with rectal manometry or rectal biopsy before continuing the treatment. A psychiatric referral can prove helpful in children with major social or family dysfunction. Older children may be particularly bothered by the embarrassment, loss of self-esteem, and social isolation associated with soiling in their pants.

ANNOTATED BIBLIOGRAPHY

Abrahamian FP, Lloyd–Still JD: Chronic constipation in childhood: Longitudinal study of 186 patients. J Pediatr Gastroenterol Nutr 3:460, 1984 (Review of manometric data and response to treatment.)

Arhan P, Devroede G et al: Idiopathic disorders of fecal continence in children. Pediatrics 71:774, 1983 (Many patients date onset of constipation from infancy.)

Barness LA, Dallman PR et al: Plant fiber intake in the pediatric diet. Pediatr 67:572, 1981 (AAP Nutrition Committee recommendations.)

Clayden GS, Lawson JN: Investigation and management of longstanding constipation in children. Arch Dis Child 51:918, 1976 (Useful management techniques for chronic constipation.)

Corazziara E, Cucchiara S et al: Gastrointestinal transit time, frequency of defecation and anorectal manometry in healthy and constipated children. J Pediatr 106:379, 1985 (Transit time cannot separate constipated from normals.)

Cummings JH: Constipation, dietary fibre and the control of large bowel function. Postgrad Med J 60:811, 1984 (Review of intestinal effects of dietary fiber.)

Kleinhaus S, Boley SJ et al: Hirschsprung's disease: A survey of Members of the Surgical Section of the American Academy of Pediatrics. J Pediatr Surg 14:588, 1979 (Large series of patients. Documents incidence of enterocolitis and missed diagnosis.)

Levine MD: The schoolchild with encopresis. Pediatr Rev 2:285, 1981 (Good review of approach to chronic constipation and encopresis.)

109
Hepatomegaly
TIEN–LAN CHANG AND RONALD E. KLEINMAN

The etiology of hepatomegaly is often determined by a complete history, a physical examination, and a few laboratory tests. However, because of the many possible causes of an enlarged liver or spleen and the potential need for specialized testing, a systematic approach is useful in differentiating the diagnosis.

DEFINITION

Hepatomegaly means enlargement of the liver. In adults enlargement of the liver is often first appreciated by palpation of the liver edge below the right costal margin. In normal children, especially in infants, the liver edge is frequently palpable below the costal margin and therefore cannot by itself be considered an abnormal finding. It has also been shown that there is no correlation between the vertical span (by x-ray) of the liver and the liver edge (by palpation) below the costal margin. An accurate estimation of the liver size is best made clinically by percussion of the upper border and palpation of the lower border of the liver at the right midclavicular line. The liver span, obtained by this method, for normal neonates is 5.9 ± 0.7 cm and for older normal children, 6.5 cm $+ 0.022 \times$ age. Eleven cm is the upper limit of normal for children 5 to 12 years of age. Measurements in different planes by ultrasound, nuclear scan, or computerized tomography will provide an accurate assessment of the liver volume. Confirmation of hepatomegaly by one or another imaging study is important because a misinterpretation of the liver size may lead to an unnecessary diagnostic evaluation and anxiety in the patient and parents. For example, Riedel's lobe is a tongue-like projection of the right lobe that increases the liver span but does not necessarily cause an increase in the total volume of the liver.

PATHOPHYSIOLOGY, CLINICAL PRESENTATION, AND DIFFERENTIAL DIAGNOSIS

Although the classification of diffuse *vs* focal processes is somewhat artificial because there are clearly disorders that produce discrete lesions found diffusely throughout the liver, we have found this to be a useful approach to the differential diagnosis of hepatomegaly.

Diffuse Enlargement of the Liver

A diffuse enlargement of the liver occurs either as a result of the excessive storage of nutrients or their metabolites or as a result of an accumulation or proliferation of red or white blood cells or macrophages.

Amyloidosis with storage of the amyloid protein in the liver rarely occurs in childhood, whether primary or secondary. In contrast, systemic α-1-antitrypsin deficiency is one of the most common causes of chronic liver disease in childhood. The PAS-positive, diastase-resistant material, which is immunologically identical with α-1-antitrypsin, accumulates in hepatocytes together with lipid. A mononuclear cell infiltrate in portal areas also contributes to the hepatomegaly. Although patients who have this disorder may be asymptomatic, some may present either with neonatal jaundice, or later in childhood with cirrhosis and its complications or chronic lung disease.

An accumulation of fat in hepatocytes is seen in malnutrition, diabetes mellitus, cystic fibrosis, obesity, Reye syndrome, Wolman disease, cholesterol ester storage disease, glucocorticoid use, and during the course of parenteral nutrition. Although fatty change is usually found diffusely throughout the liver, focal fatty metamorphosis can also occur in association with the conditions already mentioned and should be considered in the differential diagnosis of focal lesions of the liver. Fatty metamorphosis associated with hepatocellular injury is seen in drug-induced (*e.g.*, tetracycline) hepatitis, hereditary fructose intolerance, galactosemia, tyrosinemia, and Wilson disease. The storage of lipid in reticuloendothelial cells is seen in Gaucher disease (glucocerebrosidosis), Niemann–Pick disease (sphingomyelinosis), and lipoprotein lipase deficiency.

Carbohydrate accumulates in the liver in two groups of inherited metabolic disorders: glycogen storage diseases and mucopolysaccharidoses. Depending on the enzyme deficiency, the clinical presentation may be different for patients with a glycogen storage disease. In contrast, patients with mucopolysaccharidoses usually share certain clinical features that permit a provisional diagnosis. These include short stature, stiff joints, corneal clouding, deafness, hirsuitism, upper airway narrowing (resulting in respiratory insufficiency), nerve root compression, and a gradual mental deterioration.

Patients with infantile GM gangliosidosis (β-galactosidase deficiency) have an increased accumulation of both glycolipids (GM ganglioside) and mucopolysaccharides in the liver, other visceral organs, and the nervous system. These patients are hypotonic in the neonatal period and developmentally delayed thereafter. Hepatomegaly is often evident by 6 months of age.

In addition to cellular enlargement, the various types of cells within the liver may increase in number. A cellular increase resulting in hepatomegaly most commonly comes from inflammatory infiltrates, which may be due to infectious, immunologic, metabolic, or toxic causes. Along with an increase in the inflammatory cells, there may also be Kupffer cell hyperplasia as part of the reaction to injury (see Chap. 110). Periportal inflammation and ductular proliferation can also be seen in obstructive biliary diseases (*e.g.*, biliary atresia). Malignant cellular infiltrates can be seen with lymphomas, leukemias, and reticuloendothelioses (*e.g.*, histiocytosis X). Residual extramedullary hematopoiesis can be seen in normal full-term neonatal livers in the first few days of life. This fetal function may be "recalled" in conditions where the marrow space is occupied by malignant cells or metabolic products (*e.g.*, cystinosis, oxalosis) and in erythroblastosis fetalis, where the marrow erythropoiesis is inadequate to meet the demands that result from increased hemolysis.

An accumulation of blood in the liver, or hepatic congestion, is due to postsinusoidal obstruction of the portosystemic blood flow. The obstruction may occur at different levels and the principal diseases causing the obstruction include right-sided heart failure, inferior vena cava (IVC), or hepatic vein obstruction (Budd–Chiari syndrome), and veno-occlusive disease. Severe lung disease (cor pulmonale), congenital heart disease, pericardial effusion, and certain cardiomyopathies are the main reasons for right heart failure. The causes of hepatic vein thrombosis include oral contraceptives, tumorous compression or invasion of the hepatic vein or IVC, and a congenital web at the hepatic vein IVC junction. Veno-occlusive disease is most often associated with chemotherapy and radiation in patients with malignancies. Ascites is a frequent accompanying sign with all types of veno-occlusive disease.

Focal Disorders of the Liver

Diseases that produce focal or multifocal lesions in the liver can be classified as tumors, cysts, granulomas, or abscesses.

Primary malignant liver tumors in pediatric patients include hepatoblastoma, hepatocellular carcinoma, and embryonal sarcoma. Some patients with these tumors may complain of weakness, anorexia, or vomiting, but frequently these patients present with an abdominal mass with no other symptoms or complaints. Hepatoblastoma is usually clinically apparent and diagnosed before 18 months of age, whereas hepatocellular carcinoma and embryonal sarcoma are generally diagnosed in childhood. The prognosis for survival with hepatoblastoma is better than for hepatocellular carcinoma because it is less likely to have metastasized at the time of diagnosis and is more often resectable. The most common metastatic tumors in the liver in childhood are Wilm's tumor and neuroblastoma. The clinical presentation of patients with these tumors often cannot be distinguished from that of primary hepatic tumors.

Nonmalignant tumors of the liver include adenomas, focal nodular hyperplasia, hamartomas, and vascular tumors. Cavernous hemangioma is the most common type of benign tumors in adults and children. Hemangioendothelioma is usually diagnosed before 1 year of age. Most of the vascular tumors regress with age, and some tumors grow for a time before regressing. Some patients may develop high-output heart failure, and some patients may have a syndrome of thrombocytopenia, anemia, and delayed clotting resembling disseminated intravascular coagulopathy (Kasabach–Merritt syndrome).

The other benign tumors are all rare. Patients who have glycogen storage diseases and those using oral contraceptives are at increased risk for developing adenomas. Some authors consider that adenomas are premalignant because of reports of patients with adenomas who subsequently died of hepatocarcinoma.

Cystic diseases of the liver include congenital hepatic fibrosis and intrahepatic bile duct ectasia (Caroli disease). Congenital hepatic fibrosis is characterized by broad bands of connective tissue in a portal and periportal distribution, with multiple dysmorphic bile ducts lying within these bands. The liver involvement may be either complete or partial. The disease is virtually always associated with renal disease. Major causes of morbidity and mortality in these patients are renal insufficiency, cholangitis, and problems related to portal hypertension. Intrahepatic bile duct ectasia (Caroli disease) may be complicated by cholangitis and gallstone formation. Other cystic lesions include benign solitary cyst, hydatid cyst (from infection by *Echinococcus*), cyst from trauma or infarction, and cysts associated with certain rare congenital malformations.

Hepatic granulomas can occur with several infectious agents, including Mycobacteria (tuberculosis and leprosy), *Brucella, Salmonella, Leptospira, Actinomyces, Blastomyces, Histoplasma, Cryptococcus, Coccidioidomyces,* malaria, *Leishmania, Toxoplasma, Schistosoma, Fasciola, Cysticercus, Toxocara,* and *Ascaris.* Noninfectious causes include berylliosis, sarcoidosis, and certain drugs such as carbamazepine.

A hepatic abscess may originate from hematogenous dissemination, by direct extension of infection from the biliary tract, or from a contiguous site of infection. In infants and young children, the hematogenous spread of systemic infection is the most common mechanism, occurring in patients with compromised host defense mechanisms. In older children and young adults, trauma and amebae are the major causes of hepatic abscesses.

Splenomegaly

The spleen may be enlarged alone or often in association with hepatomegaly, hence its importance in the differential diagnosis of liver disease. The liver in patients with cirrhosis may be shrunken, with the result that the enlarged spleen is the first evidence of liver disease discovered during a physical examination. The major mechanisms responsible for splenomegaly are portal hypertension, lipid storage, lymphohistiocytic proliferation (*e.g.,* histiocytosis X, EBV infection), sequestration (*e.g.,* immune hemolytic anemia), extramedullary hematopoiesis, and infiltration by hematologic malignancies. Portal hypertension can be suprahepatic, intrahepatic, or prehepatic. Suprahepatic causes have already been discussed. Intrahepatic causes include any chronic liver disease leading to cirrhosis, congenital hepatic fibrosis, noncirrhotic regenerative hyperplasia, hereditary telangiectasis, and hepatoportal sclerosis. Prehepatic causes of portal vein obstruction include cavernous transformation of the portal vein, and portal vein thrombosis. Although the pathogenesis of cavernous transformation of the portal vein is unknown, umbilical vein catheterization and omphalitis have been reported as possible risk factors.

WORK-UP

History and Physical Examination

The history and physical examination provide the initial screening to eliminate many of the unlikely causes of hepatomegaly and provide clues to the diagnosis. This history should include age of onset, associated symptoms (*e.g.,* nausea, vomiting, fever, anorexia, weight loss, and so forth), duration of symptoms, environmental exposure to toxins (including drugs), exposure to persons with infections, travel to areas endemic with certain parasitic infections, and family history of inherited diseases. Growth and development should be noted in both a history and a physical examination, because failure to thrive is often an indication of a chronic metabolic or nutritional disorder. Perhaps the most helpful clues are obtained from an examination of the skin and eyes in addition to the abdominal examination. Cutaneous manifestations of liver disease include jaundice, spider angiomas, excoriations, and caput medusae. Easy bruising suggests a clotting problem. Cutaneous vascular nevi may point to the presence of hemangiomas in the liver. Possible eye findings include cataracts, macular spots, and Kayser–Fleischer rings. The liver should be palpated for tenderness, degree of firmness, smoothness, and nodularity. A pedunculated mass arising from the liver surface may be either adenoma or focal nodular hyperplasia. Both the left and right lobes should be examined, because in cirrhosis the right lobe may be normal or small whereas the left lobe is compensatorily enlarged, and in the case of hepatic tumors there may be asymmetric involvement of the lobes. The left side of the abdomen should be palpated for splenic enlargement. The enlargement of other organs and masses and the presence of ascites should be ascertained.

Laboratory Tests

The first screening tests should include CBC, differential, platelet count, sedimentation rate, and liver function tests such as prothrombin time, albumin, total protein, bilirubin, SGOT, SGPT, and alkaline phosphatase. Hematologic disorders may be suggested by anemia, thrombocytopenia, or abnormal blood smear. A bone marrow examination is usually helpful in their diagnosis. Liver function tests, however, are not helpful in the diagnosis of primary malignant liver tumors, and cirrhotic patients may have only mild changes in LFTs. Abnormal blood sugar, cholesterol, and triglyceride, though nonspecific, may suggest a metabolic basis for hepatomegaly in conjunction with other laboratory tests. Based on one's clinical suspicion, other more specific tests can be ordered, for example: α-1-antitrypsin, α-fetoprotein (for liver tumors), serum ceruloplasmin, copper, 24-hour urine copper (for Wilson disease) and serologies for infectious diseases.

Imaging Studies

Several imaging studies are now available, which not only distinguish focal from diffuse processes, but also may provide information about the nature of the lesions. A plain flat plate of the abdomen can indicate the size of the organs as well as any calcified lesions (*e.g.*, neuroblastoma, hydatid cyst). Ultrasonography (US) and computed tomography (CT) provide information regarding the size and homogeneity of the liver. US is cheaper, more easily performed, and requires little patient preparation, whereas CT is slightly more sensitive in detecting focal lesions and fluid collections. An intravenous pyelogram following hepatic imaging can identify the presence of the primary tumor and its relation to the kidney (renal or suprarenal).

Radionucleide scans provide different information depending on the agents used. ^{99m}Tc sulfur coloid is extracted by reticuloendothelial cells, so that any disturbance in the structure of the liver will cause a nonhomogeneous picture. The ^{99m}Tc IDA derivatives are taken up by the hepatocytes and excreted into bile and are useful in the diagnosis of cholestatic disorders. A delay in hepatic imaging may also indicate significant hepatocellular dysfunction. ^{67}Ga is concentrated by a tumor or an abscess. When the scans are used in combination with other studies (*e.g.*, arteriography), the type of focal lesions can often be determined prior to the tissue diagnosis. For example, a *cold* spot on the sulfur-colloid scan due to an adenoma will be normal on the IDA scan and will be highlighted on an arteriogram whereas an abscess will be *cold* on the sulfur–colloid and IDA scans, but *hot* on the gallium scan.

Magnetic resonance imaging (MRI) is a new noninvasive diagnostic technique, the full potential of which remains to be explored. This technique has potential for studying both diffuse and focal disorders. Compared to CT, it is superior in soft-tissue contrast discrimination and in identifying and defining vascular structures, such as vascular tumors, cavernous transformation of the portal vein, and collateral veins associated with portal hypertension. Its main disadvantage lies in the prolonged imaging time that leads to less sharp images because of respiratory motion.

Invasive Studies

A liver biopsy is sometimes necessary for making a diagnosis as well as for assessing the severity of the disease. In many cases a closed percutaneous needle biopsy will be sufficient for histologic, biochemical, and infectious disease studies. However, a closed biopsy may be hazardous with vascular tumors and is therefore contraindicated. An open liver biopsy, with or without arteriography, is necessary for the diagnosis of solid tumors of the liver. Cholangiography, either endoscopic or intraoperative, may also help to distinguish the nature of the lesion.

INDICATIONS FOR REFERRAL AND TREATMENT

The most common cause of hepatomegaly is acute hepatitis of viral etiology. The majority (90%) will recover without sequelae and need not be referred. All other patients with abnormalities in liver function and patients with splenomegaly with or without hepatomegaly will often be referred for an evaluation.

Patients with fulminant hepatic failure of any cause, as evidenced by a high bilirubin and a prolonged PT greater than two times normal, should be cared for in a tertiary hospital setting. In those cases in which a tumor is suspected, the evaluation is best done in a setting where surgical support is available. For many of the metabolic diseases, a multidisciplinary approach is needed for both an evaluation and management.

ANNOTATED BIBLIOGRAPHY

Alvarez F, Bernard O, Brunelle F et al: Congenital hepatic fibrosis in children. J Pediatr 99(3)370–375, 1981 (Correct clinical diagnosis can often be made based on clinical, biologic, and radiologic criteria.)

McDonald GB, Sharma P, Matthews DE et al: Venoocclusive disease of the liver after bone marrow transplantation: Diagnosis, incidence and predisposing factors. Hepatology 4(1):116–122, 1984 (Review of this iatrogenic problem.)

Pereyra R, Andrassy RJ, Mahour GH: Management of massive hepatic hemangiomas in infants and children: A review of 13 cases. Pediatrics 70(2):254–258, 1982 (30% mortality is seen in this small group of patients.)

Reiff MI, Osborn LM: Clinical estimation of liver size in newborn infants. Pediatrics 71(1):46–48, 1983 (Measurement by percussion/palpation correlated poorly with palpation of the liver edge.)

Rubin RH, Swartz MN, Malt R: Hepatic abscess: Changes in clinical, bacteriologic and therapeutic aspects. Am J Med 57:601–610, 1974 (Report of 53 patients with 3% mortality overall.)

Silberstein EB, Gilbert LA, Pu MY: Comparative efficacy of radionuclide, ultrasound and computer tomographic liver imaging for hepatic metastases. Curr Conc Diagn Nucl Med 2(3):3–9, 1985 (Concise review but has several good references.)

Stark DD, Felder RC, Wittenberg J et al: Magnetic resonance imaging of cavernous hemangioma of the liver: Tissue specific characterization. Am J Radiol 145:213–222, 1985 (MRI has a 90% accuracy in the diagnosis of hemangiomas, better than any other imaging study.)

Younoszal MK, Mueller S: Clinical assessment of liver size in normal children. Clin Pediatr 14:378–381, 1975 (Normal range of liver size for children 5 to 12 years of age is reported.)

110
Hepatitis
COLETTE DESLANDRES–LEDUC AND RONALD E. KLEINMAN

Viral infections are the most frequent cause of hepatitis in patients less than 20 years old. In one study 32% of reported cases of hepatitis in this age group were caused by hepatitis A virus (HAV), 10.3% were caused by hepatitis B virus (HBV), and 13.1% were labelled non-A non-B hepatitis. Other causes of hepatitis in infants, children, and adolescents include a wide spectrum of metabolic, toxic, ischemic, and immunologic disorders (see Chap. 190).

PATHOPHYSIOLOGY

Regardless of the mechanism leading to hepatocellular injury, one of the consequences is a loss of the selective permeability of the cellular membrane with spilling of transaminases (SGPT and SGOT) into the systemic circulation. An impaired clearance of unconjugated bilirubin from serum occurs because of a diminished uptake of bilirubin into the hepatocyte, impaired intracellular binding, and decreased conjugation. Unconjugated bilirubin then accumulates in the circulation producing icterus. High levels of free indirect serum bilirubin in the perinatal period may cause kernicterus. The excretion of conjugated bilirubin is also altered and a "regurgitation" of water-soluble conjugated bilirubin into the circulation causes icterus and dark, tea-colored urine. Clay-colored or pale stools occur because of a decrease or an absence of pigments that originate from both the diet and the bile.

With almost total hepatocyte dysfunction, a compromise of liver synthetic function becomes clinically apparent. Hepatocytes synthesize factors I (fibrinogen), II (prothrombin), V, VII, IX, and X. Factors II, VII, IX, and X require vitamin K for formation and are the most sensitive to hepatocellular disease. The prothrombin time (PT) closely reflects hepatic synthetic function because it depends on factors II, V, VII, and X. The partial thromboplastin time (PTT) will also be affected, but to a lesser degree. The liver also plays a major role in glucose homeostasis and thus, hypoglycemia may occur with a massive hepatocellular necrosis. Albumin synthesis also diminishes with the loss of hepatocyte function. Severe hypoalbuminemia contributes to the accumulation of ascites and peripheral edema.

The pathophysiology of hepatic encephalopathy is still uncertain and probably multifactorial. This neuropsychiatric syndrome is widely believed to have a metabolic basis. The various "toxins" incriminated in the development of hepatic encephalopathy include ammonia, short-chain fatty acids, mercaptans, and false neurotransmitters.

CLINICAL PRESENTATION

The prodrome of acute viral hepatitis consists of malaise, fatigue, anorexia, nausea, vomiting, low-grade fever, and abdominal pain. In 5% to 15% of cases, a triad of symptoms (Caroli's triad) similar to serum sickness occurs consisting of headaches, rash, and arthralgias. Although more commonly reported with HBV, this is also seen with HAV and non-A, non-B hepatitis. A "flu-like syndrome" can also occur with headache, fever, and myalgia.

An icteric phase often follows the prodrome and is characterized by dark urine, pale, clay-colored stools, and jaundice. With the onset of jaundice some symptoms abate whereas others worsen. The fever, arthralgias, and headaches typically disappear. Jaundice usually peaks within 5 to 10 days. Its duration varies from a few days to 6 to 7 months (an average of 1 to 3 weeks). As the jaundice increases, the other symptoms of liver disease intensify. Anorexia, fatigue, and weight loss may be severe. The first signs of recovery include the disappearance of nausea and vomiting with the return of appetite. Malaise, usually the first symptom to appear, is also the last to resolve.

Hepatitis can also present in a fulminant manner with signs of overt hepatic failure such as coagulopathy, ascites, and encephalopathy. The alteration of mental status is an early feature of fulminant hepatitis. It usually takes the form of increasing somnolence and confusion, although some patients will show agitation, violent behavior, and frank delirium. A progression to coma occurs rapidly.

Most children with viral hepatitis are asymptomatic. Indeed, in studies conducted in day-care centers only 4% to 16% of young children suspected of transmitting HAV to an older family member had symptoms of hepatitis, whereas a larger proportion of adults with HAV were symptomatic. Most HBV infections are also asymptomatic. Finally, hepatitis may be anicteric and may present only with nonspecific symptoms of anorexia, asthenia, and weight loss or in some cases with unexplained joint symptoms, colitis, and erythema nodosum.

DIFFERENTIAL DIAGNOSIS

Most cases of hepatitis are generally of viral origin. During the neonatal period, hepatitis presents with different clinical and pathologic findings and is therefore discussed separately.

Neonatal Hepatitis

In 1977, Danks and associates reported on 105 patients with neonatal hepatitis and described an incidence of 1:8000 live births. Intrauterine infections were responsible for approximately 20% of the cases: 12% CMV, 2% toxoplasmosis, 6% others, for example, rubella, *Treponema pallidum*, and enteroviruses. Alpha-l-antitrypsin deficiency was found in 11% to 15% of the cases and galactosemia in 5% of the cases. The etiology of the remaining 50% to 60% of the cases was unknown. Other known causes of neonatal hepatitis include the infectious agents herpes, HBV, adenovirus, varicella and *Listeria monocytogenes* and the metabolic disorders fructosemia and tyrosinemia. The term *neonatal hepatitis* may be used to describe all cases of "hepatitis" in neonates or may be restricted to the clinical situation in which no definable cause is found for a neonate who suffers from prolonged cholestasis, who is below 2 months of age, and whose liver biopsy displays giant cells. Such infants are more likely to be male, premature, or small for gestational age and have a positive family history (15%) for neonatal hepatitis. The mortality rate has been reported to be as high as 30%.

Postneonatal Period

Hepatitis A virus is the most frequent causal agent of hepatitis. It has an incubation period of 2 to 4 weeks. It is transmitted by the oral/fecal route predominantly by contaminated food such as shellfish or other foods washed in contaminated water. The virus can also be disseminated by food handlers responsible for the terminal preparation of food before serving. Toddlers in day-care centers are most susceptible to acquiring HAV because of the difficulty in maintaining good oral/fecal hygiene in this setting. Fortunately, children less than 2 years of age are usually asymptomatic with HAV. Chronic hepatitis does not develop after the acute illness of HAV although a small number of all patients will develop fulminant hepatitis. The estimated fatality rate from HAV is 0.14%. Reports suggest that while the incidence of HAV is declining, the incidence of HBV is increasing.

Hepatitis B has an incubation period of 3 to 10 weeks. It is transmitted through numerous body fluids including blood, saliva, tears, sweat, nasopharyngeal secretions, urine, genital secretions, and possibly human milk. In the pediatric age group, most cases are acquired through the nonparenteral route. HBV causes less than 10% of blood-transfusion hepatitis. Unlike HAV, HBV may induce a carrier state, which in the United States is estimated to be 0.1% to 0.5% of the general population. The chronic carrier rate is much higher in other parts of the world. In China, for example, 5% to 15% of the population is infected. A patient is considered a chronic carrier when hepatitis B surface antigen (HB_sAg) is present in the serum for greater than 6 months. The likelihood of developing the carrier state varies inversely with age. 70% to 90% of infants born to mothers positive for HB_eAg and HB_sAg will become infected, and up to 90% of these infected infants will become HBV carriers, whereas only 6% to 10% of acutely infected adults become carriers. Chronic carriers may be healthy or may have chronic hepatitis that may evolve to cirrhosis. Chronic HBV and the carrier state have also been associated with hepatocellular carcinoma.

The diagnosis of non-A, non-B hepatitis remains a diagnosis of exclusion because the viral agent (or agents) has not yet been identified. It accounts for about 20% of sporadic acute viral hepatitis and is the most common cause of posttransfusion hepatitis. It progresses to chronic liver disease in 23% to 46% of infected patients.

The δ agent is a distinct virus from HBV but requires HBV infection for its own replication. Thus, it will only occur in patients who are HB_sAg carriers. It can cause either an acute or chronic hepatitis. Its transmission is similar to that of HBV.

Among the other viral causes of hepatitis, mononucleosis (caused by EBV) or cytomegalovirus (CMV) should be considered. Jaundice is uncommon in mononucleosis but biochemical abnormalities demonstrating hepatocellular disease will occur in 25% to 50% of the cases. Cytomegalovirus may produce a mononucleosis-like syndrome and is a common cause of subclinical hepatitis after transfusion. CMV has been isolated from the white cells of 5% of healthy blood donors. CMV, herpes simplex, and varicella zoster can induce a severe and fulminant hepatitis in immunocompromised patients. Rubella, rubeola, mumps, and varicella zoster can cause mild elevations of serum aminotransferase activity in otherwise healthy patients.

Once viral hepatitis has been excluded, metabolic, ischemic, immunologic, and drug-induced causes of hepatitis must be considered. In the school-aged and particularly the adolescent population, Wilson disease, also known as hepatolenticular degeneration, must be included in the differential diagnosis of acute hepatitis. It is characterized by a deficiency in ceruloplasmin and abnormal deposition of copper in various tissues, including the liver, kidneys, CNS, and cornea (Kayser–Fleischer rings). Wilson disease can present as an acute fulminant hepatitis and thus mimic acute viral hepatitis. It can also present as chronic active hepatitis and cirrhosis. If left untreated, it progresses to cirrhosis and degenerative central nervous system disease.

Sickle cell disease can cause a *sickle cell hepatopathy* due to hepatic ischemia. The disorder is characterized by abdominal pain, malaise, nausea, and jaundice with markedly elevated serum aminotransferases. Thus, in a population already at risk for acquiring viral hepatitis because of numerous transfusions, the differential diagnosis of hepatitis is even more difficult.

Among the immunologic disorders that may present as an acute viral hepatitis, systemic lupus erythematous, juvenile rheumatoid arthritis, ulcerative colitis, and Crohn disease must be considered.

Several drugs commonly prescribed for pediatric patients have been associated with hepatitis or hepatocellular necrosis: aspirin, acetaminophen (at toxic levels), cimetidine, indomethacin, ketoconazole, methotrexate, phenytoin, valproic acid, and tetracyclines must be mentioned. Aspirin has been epidemiologically linked to Reye syndrome, although the pathogenesis and cause are poorly understood. Reye syndrome is characterized by an acute noninfectious encephalopathy and noninflammatory fatty infiltration of several organs, particularly the liver and the kidneys. It can present as acute fulminant hepatitis. An association has also been reported with influenza B virus and varicella.

WORK-UP

History

A complete history in a patient with suspected hepatitis will include the character of the illness and its chronicity, including the duration, onset, and possible recurrence of jaundice. Information should also be obtained about possible predisposing conditions for acquiring hepatitis. Some of these antecedents are contact with other people infected with hepatitis, travel in a developing country, shellfish ingestion, illicit IV drug abuse, blood-product transfusions, homosexual practice, medications, day-care attendance or other institutional settings, and a family history of liver disease and cirrhosis.

Physical Examination

On physical examination icterus is first seen in the sclera and will become apparent when the bilirubin is over 2.5 mg/dl. Hepatomegaly and pain on percussion over the liver may be more obvious in acute hepatitis than in cirrhosis, where the liver appears firm and may be smaller than normal. Other signs to look for include ascites, collateral circulation over the abdomen, and splenomegaly. An examination of the skin in children suffering acute HBV may reveal the Gianotti–Crosti syndrome (a papular acrodermatitis). The eye examination may reveal the typical *Kayser–Fleischer ring* of Wilson disease. Petechiae and mucosal bleeding reflect a coagulopathy. The extremities may reveal clubbing in longstanding disease. Finally, in fulminant hepatitis or decompensated chronic liver disease the patient will manifest hepatic encephalopathy which is characterized by asterixis and *fetor hepaticus*. *Fetor hepaticus* is the most specific sign of hepatic encephalopathy. It is described as a sweetish, slightly fecal smell.

Laboratory Tests

Chemical confirmation of hepatitis is provided by the measurement of serum aminotransferases, bilirubin, and alkaline phosphatase. The first indication of hepatocellular injury is an increase of the serum aminotransferases SGOT (serum aspartate aminotransferase) and SGPT (serum alanine aminotransferase). In a fulminant hepatitis, the rise in transaminases may be missed. Serum bilirubin will variably be elevated and the increase may involve both the direct and indirect fractions. Serum alkaline phosphatase and 5'nucleotidase are usually only mildly elevated. With major hepatocellular dysfunction, the prothrombin time (PT) will increase (≥ 2 seconds more than normal) as will blood ammonia.

Serologic markers of infection establish the diagnosis of hepatitis A and B. *IgM anti-HAV* is present following acute infection with hepatitis A virus and is the most useful antibody to diagnose acute HAV. IgM anti-HB$_c$Ag along with HB$_s$Ag in serum reflect acute infection with hepatitis B. With the appearance of clinical symptoms HB$_s$Ag, HB$_e$Ag, and HBV–DNA titers peak. HB$_e$Ag and HBV–DNA correlate with infectivity. Delta agent and anti-δ Ab should also be searched for in a HB$_s$Ag positive patient.

In a neonate, toxoplasma, rubella, cytomegalovirus, herpesvirus (TORCH) antibody titers, serum and urine amino acids, serum electrophoresis, Pi typing of α-l-antitrypsin, and examination of urine for reducing substances should be done. The urine may be negative for reducing substances if the patient is not ingesting enough of them and a determination of specific cellular enzyme levels will then be necessary. Older patients should be tested for Wilson disease by obtaining a serum ceruloplasmin level and a 24-hour urine collection for copper. A test for mononucleosis should be included in the evaluation of a teenager with hepatitis.

TREATMENT AND MANAGEMENT

Therapy in viral hepatitis is aimed toward minimizing the complications. Control of coagulopathy and bleeding may be obtained with the injection of vitamin K and plasma infusions. Hypoglycemia is managed by constant glucose infusion and ascites is treated by restricting salt intake to 10 mEq/m^2/day of Na$^+$ and limiting fluid intake to 1500 ml/m^2/day. Therapy focused at regulating ammonia balance is often effective in treating hepatic encephalopathy. This includes decreasing the dietary intake of protein to 0.5 g/kg/day (to decrease ammonia production) and decreasing the absorption of ammonia from the GI tract using lactulose and neomycin. Lactulose at a starting dose of 15 ml po tid will act as a cathartic and will also reduce the stool pH to <5.5, thus trapping ammonia in an acid milieu with conversion to the less diffusable ammonium. Neomycin acts by sterilizing the bowel, thus decreasing the bacterial conversion of protein to ammonia.

A specific treatment should be applied when a metabolic, immunologic, or drug-induced cause of the hepatitis is identified. Penicillamine, for example, will bind excess copper present in Wilson disease and may reverse the hepatic and central nervous system disease. In drug-related hepatic injury, the offending drug must be stopped and supportive care administered.

PREVENTION

Prophylactic measures exist to prevent HAV and HBV. Pre-exposure prophylaxis for hepatitis A for patients who plan to travel to developing countries includes a single dose of immunoglobulin (IG from 0.02 ml/kg to 0.06 ml/kg depending on the length of travel). If a patient has been exposed to HAV he should receive the IG within 2 weeks following exposure as a single dose of 0.02 ml/kg. Pre-exposure prophylaxis of HBV is administered with the hepatitis B vaccine. The following groups are at higher risks for acquiring HBV and should be protected by the vaccine: selected health workers, clients and staff of institutions for the mentally retarded, patients on hemodialysis, homosexuals, illicit drug abusers, chronic recipients of blood products, household and sexual contacts of HBV carriers, and international travelers. Hepatitis B vaccine is administered in three doses with the second and third dose given 1 and 6 months respectively after the first dose. Children under the age of 10 should receive 10 µg/dose (0.5 ml), older children should receive 20 µg/dose (1 ml). Once the patient has been exposed to HBV he should receive both the hepatitis B immune globulin (HBIG) and the vaccine. The most frequent pediatric indication for postexposure prophylaxis is for the neonate born to a Hb$_s$Ag+ mother. Such infants should receive 0.5 ml IM of hepatitis B immune globulin and 10 µg of hepatitis B vaccine IM within 12 hours of birth. Follow-up booster doses of vaccine are given at 1 and 6 months of age.

INDICATIONS FOR REFERRAL

If the biochemical evaluations of the patient with hepatitis is not helpful in making the diagnosis, a percutaneous liver biopsy should be performed. Abnormal transaminases over a 3- to 6-month period should prompt the pediatrician to refer the patient for a liver biopsy. This will help clarify the degree of chronicity of the disease process and determine the need for more aggressive treatment.

ANNOTATED BIBLIOGRAPHY

Alter MJ: Hepatitis surveillance, 1982–1983. MMWR 34:1SS, 1SS–10SS, 1983 (Review of incidence of HAV, HBV, non-A, non-B hepatitis in USA.)

Crossley IR, Wardle EN, Williams R: Biochemical mechanisms of hepatic encephalopathy. Clin Sci 64:247–252, 1983 (Review of the various "toxins" incriminated in hepatic encephalopathy.)

Danks DM, Campbell PE, Smith AL, Rogers J: Prognosis of babies with neonatal hepatitis. Arch Dis Child 52:368–372, 1977 (Review of 105 patients studied up to 10 years.)

Danks DM, Campbell PE, Jack I et al: Studies of the etiology of neonatal hepatitis and biliary atresia. Arch Dis Child 52:360–367, 1977 (Review of 105 patients with neonatal hepatitis.)

Hadler SC, Webster HM, Erken JJ et al: Hepatitis A in day care centers: A community wide assessment. N Engl J Med 302:1222–1227, (Review of HAV epidemiology in relation to day-care centers.)

Ludwig J, Axelsen R: Drug effects on the liver. An updated tabular compilation of drugs and drug-related hepatic disease. Dig Dis Sci 28:651–666, 1983 (Tabulation of adverse effects of drugs on human liver.)

Recommendations for Protection against Viral Hepatitis. MMWR 34:313–335, 1985 (Update on pre- and postexposure prophylactic measures against hepatitis A and B.)

Roche–Sicot J, Benhamou JP: Acute intravascular hemolysis and acute liver failure associated as a first manifestation of Wilson's disease. Ann Intern Med 86:301–303, 1977 (Review of three cases presenting with acute intravascular hemolysis and acute liver failure.)

111
Peptic Ulcer Disease
HARLAND S. WINTER

Peptic ulcer disease is a problem commonly faced by our colleagues in internal medicine but is a diagnosis not considered frequently in childhood. Although the condition is not rare in children, it may go unrecognized. Peptic ulcers may be primary or secondary to one of many associated underlying problems (*e.g.*, burns [Curling ulcer], intracranial lesions [Cushing ulcer], sepsis, collagen vascular diseases, immunodeficiency syndromes, lymphoma, leukemia, shock, severe stress, or medication). Frequently, secondary ulcers present as an acute medical emergency with hemorrhage or perforation, whereas primary ulcers more often may come to clinical recognition by their chronic indolent symptoms of fatigue, anemia, or abdominal pain. Individuals with a predisposition to peptic injury of the stomach or duodenum should be considered as having a chronic illness and should therefore be managed appropriately to avoid potential iatrogenic effects of long-term medication or surgery.

PATHOPHYSIOLOGY

The pathogenesis of peptic ulcer disease is usually multifactorial. Acid has long been thought to be the major culprit in the pathophysiology of peptic ulcer disease and has been the most widely studied. However, recent evidence has suggested that alterations in mucosal host-defense mechanisms may be more significant than the production of acid by the stomach. Cytoprotection is the prevention of epithelial cell injury following exposure to a noxious agent. It depends on several variables—the quantity and quality of mucus, mucosal blood flow, and epithelial cell turnover—any and all of which may be important clinically.

Two major roles for gastric acid are the conversion of pepsinogen to pepsin and the maintenance of an acidic environment to block the ability for live organisms to migrate into the small intestine. Three major endogenous secretagogues stimulate acid secretion by the parietal cell: acetylcholine, gastrin, and histamine. Acetylcholine, a neurotransmitter, is released by postganglionic vagal neurons. Gastrin, a polypeptide produced in the G cells of the antrum, is a hormone that stimulates the parietal cell to produce acid. Histamine is released from mast-like cells located in the lamina propria. This vasoactive substance diffuses across the interstitium to interact with the parietal cell. Parietal cells have specific receptors for each of these three secretagogues and therefore are under central (by way of vagal fibers), hormonal, and local (paracrine) regulatory mechanisms. The blockade of these receptors forms the basis for pharmacologic therapy of peptic ulcer disease.

In addition to secretagogue-mediated secretion of gastric acid, there is a basal secretion from the parietal cell that occurs independently of any stimulation. This basal secretion is under control of a circadian rhythm with the highest level in the evening and the lowest in the morning. Secretion by the parietal cell can also be initiated by the sight, smell, and taste of food, which is under control of the central nervous system. This phase of secretion is mediated by the vagus nerve and is obliterated following vagotomy. The introduction of food into the stomach as well as gastric distention also activates gastric acid secretion. This mechanism appears to be mediated by a vagal reflex arch from the stomach to the vagal nuclei in the brain. Finally, the absorption of nutrients, in particular amino acids, can increase gastric acid secretion.

Genetic factors may also play an important role in the pathogenesis of peptic ulcer disease (PUD). About 20% of children with PUD have a positive family history. Individuals with the gene for blood group O have a 30% increased incidence of duodenal ulcer as compared to individuals with other blood groups. In addition, those individuals who have blood group O and do not secrete ABO antigens into their gastric juice have an additional risk of developing duodenal ulcer. Pepsinogen is also genetically determined and can be divided immunochemically into two groups—pepsinogen I and pepsinogen II. The elevation of circulating pepsinogen I is inherited as an autosomal dominant trait and is found in a significant number of individuals with duodenal ulcers.

Although many epidemiologic factors may contribute to the pathogenesis of peptic ulcer disease, cigarette smoking seems to be the most important. It results not only in an increased incidence of peptic ulcer but also has an adverse effect on the healing of established ulcers.

Peptic ulcers can occur anywhere throughout the gastrointestinal tract, but most commonly they occur in the duodenal bulb or antrum of the stomach. Meckel's diverticula of the ileum may contain parietal cells that both secrete acid and pepsin and result in ulceration of the ileal mucosa. Thus, wherever acid-producing cells are located, the potential for mucosal ulceration exists.

CLINICAL PRESENTATION

In childhood, a duodenal ulcer is approximately six times as frequent as a gastric ulcer. In contrast, in the infant, primary ulcers are most likely to be gastric in location. In the neonate, the most common presentation of peptic ulcer disease is perforation and hemorrhage. The infant often presents with clinical features of septic shock. Although the premature or stressed infant is at greater risk, gastric ulcers have been reported in full-term thriving neonates.

In infancy outside the newborn period, perforation and hemorrhage are often preceded by vomiting, weight loss, or feeding difficulties; but in the preschool-aged child, vomiting and abdominal pain are more frequent. The abdominal pain is usually poorly localized and not characteristic of pain patterns identified in an adult. In the school-aged child, the clinical presentation is usually one of recurrent abdominal pain, which again is more often atypical. As the child approaches adolescence, the pain patterns become more typical of that recognized in adult patients. The classical pain pattern of ulcer disease includes well localized epigastric pain and tenderness. The timing of the pain is episodic but often occurs at night. The pain frequently occurs 1 hour after meals and is relieved briefly by food or antacids. In contrast with other causes of pain, patients with duodenal ulcer usually have intermittent pain. They may have an exacerbation several times a year that usually resolves even without treatment. Individuals with unremitting pain usually do not have uncomplicated duodenal ulcers, and the clinician should think either of some complication such as obstruction or another diagnosis such as reflux esophagitis. A patient may typically give a history that although the pain is relieved by food, it is aggravated by orange juice or aspirin. Although these pain patterns may lead the clinician to con-

sider a diagnosis of peptic ulcer, he can be misled by ruling out the diagnosis if classical findings are absent.

DIFFERENTIAL DIAGNOSIS

The causes of abdominal pain in children are numerous and are extensively discussed in Chapters 104 and 105. Briefly, the list includes functional complaints, esophagitis, inflammatory bowel disease, pancreatitis, biliary colic, gastroenteritis, appendicitis, Meckel's diverticulum, intussusception, volvulus, lead toxicity, iron and arsenic poisoning, testicular torsion, Henoch–Schönlein purpura, pneumonia, pylonephritis, and malrotation. In addition, there are other anatomic and systemic illnesses that can have abdominal pain as a component of the disease. In the infant and neonate, PUD is usually secondary to the life-saving measures that are needed to support the child. In the child who is thriving, without anemia or occult blood in the stool, the differential diagnosis is most often between a peptic disease and a functional complaint, such as irritable bowel syndrome or constipation. In the school-aged child, particularly in the black, Jewish, and Asian population, one must consider lactose intolerance as a cause of recurrent abdominal pain.

WORK-UP

History

In children under the age of 6, abdominal pain, if present, is usually located in the periumbilical region and is not related to eating or activity. In the school-aged child, recurrent abdominal pain most often will be described as having periods of exacerbation and remissions that may last many months. In contrast to adults, most children experience little relief of pain from eating and their response to antacids may also be variable.

Physical Examination

The physical examination in patients with peptic ulcer disease can vary from findings of severe shock and hypotension to a healthy appearing child. The physical examination may reveal stigmata of iron deficiency, malnutrition, or gastrointestinal blood loss with guaiac positive stools or melena. Some rare syndromes are associated with peptic ulcers: Most of these involve endocrine abnormalities in which gastrinoma is a component.

Laboratory Tests

A hemoglobin and stool guaiac are important in terms of looking for evidence of blood loss, one of the severe complications of peptic ulcer disease. In selected patients, an elevated pepsinogen I may have some value for genetic counseling. A fasting morning serum gastrin may be valuable in identifying one cause of gastric acid hypersecretion, Zollinger–Ellison syndrome. The main diagnostic studies in children, however, are the upper GI series and upper endoscopy. Certainly, an upper endoscopy is more sensitive in identifying those individuals who have mucosal lesions. It is estimated that an upper GI series will miss 25% to 30% of children with peptic ulcerations. However, the invasive nature of endoscopy in children should make the pediatrician pause before referring patients for this procedure. The thriving child with either uncomplicated recurrent abdominal pain, classical duodenal ulcer symptoms, or chronic clinically stable anemia should be evaluated primarily with an upper gastrointestinal radiograph. In contrast, the child who presents with hematemesis or melena and an acute fall in hematocrit should be considered for an endoscopy after he is hemodynamically stable. Although few studies address this specific issue, it seems clinically prudent to reserve an upper endoscopy as a first diagnostic test for those children who display evidence of an acute mucosal lesion and a severe complication (*e.g.*, anemia or shock).

TREATMENT

The treatment of ulcer disease remains controversial. A dietary restriction has not been shown to affect the incidence or healing of ulcers. Milk, which is a potent stimulant of gastric secretion, has often been used to promote healing of duodenal ulcers; however, its real benefit is unknown. Coffee, soda, and alcoholic beverages may exacerbate ulcer-like symptoms, but there is no evidence to suggest that they cause ulcer pain. It is a curious observation that in India, individuals living in the region of the country where wheat is grown have a lower incidence of duodenal ulcer than individuals living in the rice-producing area. Whether or not this is related to the higher fiber content in the wheat is unclear.

Certain medications should be avoided by patients at increased risk for developing peptic ulcers. Among the best known is aspirin, which is capable of both directly damaging the gastric mucosa as well as inhibiting the potentially cytoprotective effect of prostaglandin synthesis. Both of these factors may lead to aspirin-induced gastric ulcers.

The management of peptic ulcer disease has traditionally focused on blocking or neutralizing gastric acid secretion. The rationale for this therapy, however, is suspect; in clinical trials, up to 60% of patients with duodenal ulcers healed while taking a placebo. Nevertheless, in the child who has a peptic ulcer, some form of therapy to modify acid secretion usually improves the symptoms. Antacids, which have few side effects, neutralize intraluminal gastric acid. Magnesium-containing antacids may cause diarrhea whereas aluminum-containing products are more constipating. For these reasons, it is often valuable to alternate magnesium- and aluminum-containing antacids to minimize changes in bowel habits.

Cimetidine and ranitidine are specific histamine H_2-receptor antagonists that decrease acid stimulation induced by gastrin or acetylcholine. Cimetidine is available in a liquid formulation and is therefore more appropriate in the younger child. Because ranitidine is more potent, it is taken on a twice daily basis. This has obvious advantages for the adolescent population. Agents that block H^+-K^+-ATPase are being developed. These agents, such as omeprazole, are potent inhibitors of acid secretion and may be beneficial in the future if side effects are controlled. Anticholinergic agents such as atropine and pirenzepine may have a limited role in the refractory patient. Sulcrafate, a resin that binds to the ulcer crater, has been shown to promote healing. It has not been shown to be more beneficial than antacids or H_2 antagonists, and experience in children is limited.

INDICATIONS FOR REFERRAL

The child with an acute presentation of GI hemorrhage should be referred to a gastroenterologist or pediatric surgeon. The child who has symptoms that are refractory to standard antacid therapy and who has an ulcer demonstrable on a roentgenogram should also be referred. The child who has a recurrent abdominal pain and in whom a diagnosis is not established may be referred to a gastroenterologist after lactose intolerance, constipation, *Giardia*, and stress-related psychosomatic problems have been investigated.

The identification of potential risk factors in a child can result in appropriate anticipatory counseling and management.

ANNOTATED BIBLIOGRAPHY

Ament ME, Christie DL: Upper gastrointestinal fiberoptic endoscopy in pediatric patients. Gastroenterol 72:1244, 1977 (Discussion of the value of fiberoptic endoscopy in children suspected of having peptic ulcer disease.)

Korman MG, Hansky J, Eaves ER, Schmidt GT: Influence of cigarette smoking on healing and relapse in duodenal ulcer disease. Gastroenterol 85:871, 1983 (Shows that smoking adversely effects both the healing and the relapse rate of duodenal ulcer disease.)

Nord KS: Peptic ulcer disease in children and adolescents: Evolving dilemmas. J Pediatr Gastroenterol Nutr 2:397, 1983 (Focuses on the diagnostic value of endoscopy in children.)

Nord KS, Lebenthal E: Peptic ulcer in children; a review. Am J Gastroenterol 77:75, 1980 (Review of the epidemiology, etiology, diagnosis, and management of children with peptic ulcer disease.)

Peters MN, Richardson CT: Stressful life events, acid hypersecretion and ulcer disease. Gastroenterol 84:114, 1983 (Discussion of the relationship between severe emotional distress and ulcer disease in two patients.)

112
Gastrointestinal Hemorrhage
VICTOR L. FOX AND JOHN UDALL

Gastrointestinal bleeding is a common problem in pediatric practice. The passage of red blood in a child is sufficiently alarming to lead to immediate parental and medical attention. Reports of dark brown emesis or black stool always deserve further investigation to confirm the presence or absence of blood. In addition, stool should always be tested for occult blood whenever iron-deficient anemia is noted. Patients presenting with massive hemorrhage require immediate stablization before further diagnostic evaluation is pursued. Limited laboratory studies are necessary. Efficient use of complimentary endoscopic and radiologic techniques will, in most cases, complete the diagnostic evaluation. Most bleeding is controlled by medical therapy. The causes of bleeding are numerous and may be characterized partially by localization to the upper or lower gastrointestinal tract. The ligament of Treitz serves by convention as the dividing line between the upper and lower tract.

This chapter first discusses gastrointestinal bleeding without respect to localization and then considers upper and lower gastrointestinal bleeding as separate entities.

WORK-UP

History and Physical Examination

The characterization of the presenting hemorrhage is essential in the initial history. The description of color, consistency, and site of emerging blood may suggest the etiology and actual site of bleeding. Hematemesis refers to vomiting of either fresh blood or coffee-ground-like material representing hematin. Bleeding from sites proximal to the ligament of Treitz frequently presents with hematemesis. Melena refers to dark, tarry, or sticky stool representing blood from either the upper gastrointestinal tract or small intestine. Hematochezia is the passage of fresh blood through the rectum. This occurs with bleeding from the colon or rectum. It may rarely occur with brisk upper gastrointestinal hemorrhage and accelerated intestinal transit as seen in neonates. Delayed transit may allow proximal colonic hemorrhage to present with melena rather than hematochezia. Currant jelly stool characterizes a mixture of blood and mucus seen with ischemic or inflammatory lesions such as intestinal intussusception or acute colitis. Maroon stool describes a mixture of red and dark blood seen with bleeding from the distal small bowel or proximal colon. Formed stool with streaks or flecks of red blood along its surface generally indicates a bleeding fissure or other anorectal lesions.

Additional pertinent historical information includes significant underlying medical disorders such as chronic liver disease, use of medications such as aspirin or nonsteroidal anti-inflammatory preparations, and associated complaints such as vomiting, gastroesophageal reflux, abdominal pain, tenesmus, constipation, diarrhea, arthralgia, weight loss, or growth delay. The past medical history may reveal neonatal umbilical catheterization or a severe episode of dehydration predisposing the patient to portal vein thrombosis. A pertinent family history includes hereditary coagulopathies, familial polyposes, peptic ulcer disease, inflammatory bowel disease, Ehlers–Danlos syndrome, and telangiectasia.

Whereas vital signs provide immediate information regarding the severity of the hemorrhage, a careful examination of the nose, oropharynx, skin, abdomen, and anorectal area provide important clues to etiology. One should look for bruising, unusual pigmented lesions seen in Peutz–Jeghers syndrome and in blue rubber bleb nevus syndrome, spider nevi seen in chronic liver disease, telangiectasia seen with Osler–Weber–Rendu disease, skin hyperelasticity seen with Ehlers–Danlos syndrome, and soft tissue or bone tumors suggesting Gardner's syndrome. Liver disease or portal hypertension may be manifest as jaundice, ascites, prominent abdominal venous pattern (caput medusae), hepatosplenomegaly, or splenomegaly alone. Fissures and anorectal fistulae are often evident on careful visual inspection of the anus. Juvenile polyps are most often found in the sigmoid colon or rectum and may be palpated on digital rectal examination.

Laboratory Tests

Few laboratory studies are necessary in the initial evaluation of a child with suspected gastrointestinal bleeding (see the box, Recommended Laboratory Studies). The confirmation of blood in stool or emesis is foremost. Various food and chemical substances may resemble blood in the stool or gastric contents: tomatoes, beets, red food coloring, Jello, fruit juices, chocolate, blueberries and cranberries, iron, and bismuth subsalicylate (Pepto–Bismol) have all been implicated. Hemoccult paper may be used to detect occult blood in stool. This test uses guaiac (a colorless phenol) in combination with hemoglobin to yield a blue-colored quinone.

Recommended Laboratory Studies
for Gastrointestinal Bleeding*

If Positive

Hematocrit

Red blood cell indices

Reticulocyte and platelet count

White blood cell and differential cell count

Prothrombin and partial thromboplastin time

Bilirubin

SGOT and SGPT

Alkaline phosphatase†

Urinalysis

BUN and serum creatinine

---

* Guaiac (or suitable alternative) test for blood in stool or gastric fluid.
† If hemolytic–uremic syndrome is suspected.

False negative results may occur with a dried specimen or recent vitamin C ingestion. False positive guaiac results may occur with the ingestion of red meat or uncooked peroxidase-rich vegetables (*e.g.*, horseradish) and elemental iron. A new test called HemoQuant has been described. This test, more sensitive and more specific than Hemoccult, converts heme to porphyrins that are assayed fluorometrically. It offers the advantage of quantifying minute amounts of blood loss in stool. Gastric fluid may be tested by Hemoccult though sensitivity is poor at $pH < 3$. The test, called Gastroccult, reportedly detects blood in gastric fluid more reliably because its sensitivity is not affected by changes in pH. In the case of gastrointestinal bleeding in the newborn, fetal hemoglobin should be distinguished from adult maternal hemoglobin. Both the Apt and the Kleihauer test distinguish fetal from adult hemoglobin on the basis of greater resistance of fetal hemoglobin to pH related alteration. Both tests may be rendered unreliable by certain pretest environmental factors such as temperature and pH.

Plain radiographs of the abdomen are of limited diagnostic value. Supine and upright views of the abdomen are only indicated when there is a suspicion of intestinal obstruction, perforation, or abdominal mass.

STABILIZATION AND TRIAGE

Patients who present with a history of mild to moderate upper gastrointestinal bleeding and evidence of blood on nasogastric aspirate require hospitalization for at least 24 to 48 hours for close observation and diagnostic evaluation. Rectal bleeding, depending on the severity of presentation and associated signs and symptoms, may not require immediate hospitalization. Further diagnostic evaluation can often be performed in an outpatient setting.

The patient who presents with a massive upper or lower gastrointestinal hemorrhage requires emergency supportive care and immediate diagnostic evaluation. Vital signs should be followed at 15-min intervals. A nasogastric tube is placed to determine whether bleeding is proximal to the ligament of Treitz. The nasogastric tube should be left in place to assess ongoing losses. An aspirate negative for blood does not exclude the possibility of upper gastrointestinal source. The bleeding may have stopped, or it may arise from the duodenum and flow distally away from the tube. The presence of blood-free bile in the nasogastric aspirate more confidently excludes the possibility of ongoing bleeding proximal to the ligament of Treitz. Saline lavage should be employed when bleeding is active to more effectively remove clots and blood. Iced saline lavage offers only questionable therapeutic benefit by stimulating local vasoconstriction. Coagulation may improve at more physiologic temperatures. Furthermore, care must be taken with the young infant to avoid hypothermia. Cooling may result in even greater mucosal susceptibility to stress and ulceration.

A short, large-bore venous catheter should be placed for intravascular volume replacement. Isosmotic solutions such as normal saline or Ringer's lactate solution are initially sufficient, followed by appropriate blood products. Immediate transport to a tertiary facility should be arranged once the patient has been stabilized.

UPPER GASTROINTESTINAL BLEEDING

The diagnostic possibilities of upper gastrointestinal bleeding must be considered with respect to the patient's age (Table 112-1).

Bleeding in the newborn period may result from causes unique to this period of life, such as complications of the birthing process or those of premature birth. Past studies that review the etiology of gastrointestinal hemorrhage in the neonate have not included endoscopic evaluation, thereby failing to establish a diagnosis in as many as 50% of cases. Chang and associates, using endoscopy, established a diagnosis in 23 of 27 patients under 12

Table 112-1. Common Causes of Upper Gastrointestinal Hemorrhage

NEONATE (0–1 MO)	INFANCY–ADOLESCENCE
Swallowed maternal blood	Gastritis
Gastritis	Esophagitis
Esophagitis	
Ulcer (gastric or duodenal)	Ulcer
Coagulopathy associated with infection	Mallory–Weiss syndrome
	Varices
Vascular malformation	Gastrointestinal duplication
Hemorrhagic disease (vitamin K deficiency)	Vascular malformation
	Polyps
	Coagulopathy
	Hemobilia

months of age presenting with upper gastrointestinal bleeding. However, only two of these patients were less than 1 month old.

The newborn may swallow maternal blood while emerging from the birth canal or may later ingest small amounts of blood while nursing from an inflamed and bleeding breast nipple. Gastritis or ulcers may occur in the sick ("stressed") term or premature newborn. The etiologic role of gastric hypersecretion and circulating newborn or maternal gastrin levels has not been well studied. Coagulopathy associated with infection and resulting in prolonged clotting times or a reduction in platelet number may result in acute hemorrhage. Since the introduction of prophylactic vitamin K administration shortly after birth, the incidence of so-called hemorrhagic disease of the newborn has declined substantially. Patients who have a deficient dietary intake of vitamin K, fat malabsorption, altered bowel flora due to use of antibiotics, and breast-fed infants are at greater risk for this disease.

Beyond the first month of life, inflammatory and erosive mucosal lesions predominate as the cause of upper gastrointestinal bleeding. In the series of 27 patients reported by Chang, 9 patients had gastritis, 8 patients had duodenal ulcer(s), 5 patients had duodenal lymphoid hyperplasia, 4 patients had gastric erosions, 3 patients had esophagitis and esophageal ulcer, and 1 patient had duodenitis. Several patients had two lesions. One retrospective study by Cox and Ament reviewed upper gastrointestinal bleeding in 68 patients ranging in age from less than 1 year to 18 years. The cause of bleeding was established in 57 of 68 patients by using one or more diagnostic techniques including endoscopy, UGI roentgenographic series, and angiography. The five most common causes, in descending order of frequency, were duodenal ulcer (20%), gastric ulcer (18%), esophagitis (15%), gastritis (13%), and varices (10%).

Factors suspected to contribute to the development of erosive mucosal lesions include stress from surgery, burns, or increased intracranial pressure, pathologic hypersecretion of gastric acid, and injury or disruption of the mucosal barrier by ischemia/hypoxia, bile acids and antiprostaglandin drugs such as salicylates. Reports have implicated a Campylobacter-like organism in the pathogenesis of acid-peptic gastric and duodenal disease. Esophagitis occurs typically in the setting of chronic gastroesophageal reflux and delayed acid clearance from the distal esophagus.

Forceful vomiting and retching at any age can lead to superficial mucosal laceration at the gastroesophageal junction followed by bleeding and is known as the Mallory–Weiss syndrome. The tear usually occurs near the squamocolumnar junction of the gastric mucosa. A careful endoscopic examination may identify this lesion.

Gastric or esophageal varices arise from portal vein hypertension. This may be due to intrahepatic or extrahepatic causes. Cirrhosis represents the cause of 75% to 90% of all pediatric cases of portal hypertension. Congenital hepatic fibrosis followed by various infiltrative diseases, hereditary telangiectasis (Rendu–Osler–Weber disease), and schistosomiasis should also be considered. Extrahepatic causes of portal hypertension include prehepatic portal vein obstruction and the Budd–Chiari syndrome. Varices resulting from any of the above rarely present clinically with bleeding before 1 year of age. Variceal bleeding, however, should always be considered in the differential diagnosis of an upper gastrointestinal hemorrhage because the treatment and prognosis markedly differ from that of the more common mucosal lesions.

Work-Up

Following the stabilization and localization of bleeding to the upper gastrointestinal tract, a decision must be made for the timing and type of further diagnostic evaluation. Endoscopy is more sensitive and more specific than barium contrast radiologic studies in the identification of bleeding lesions. The sensitivity of endoscopy approaches 90%. Contrast radiography identifies approximately 50% of lesions. Air contrast barium studies enhance the sensitivity for superficial mucosal lesions but still fall short of endoscopy. Some studies indicate that duodenal ulcers may be detected equally by contrast radiology and endoscopy. Contrast studies offer the advantages of a noninvasive, easily administered and readily available test. The disadvantages include comparatively lower sensitivity, inability to distinguish innocent from active lesions in the case of coexistent varices and gastritis or ulcer, and potential interference with subsequent nuclear medicine imaging. Endoscopy permits optimal detection with visual and biopsy confirmation and potential therapeutic intervention, such as electrocoagulation, thermocoagulation (heater probe), sclerotherapy or polypectomy. Endoscopy involves the risk of an invasive procedure accompanied by drug-induced sedation. Additionally, an endoscopist skilled in pediatric procedures is not always readily accessible.

The indications for early endoscopy remain controversial. Studies in adults have shown no significant difference in outcome between patients who were or were not studied by early endoscopy. Endoscopy is recommended for children with persistent or recurrent bleeding, with suspected variceal bleeding, and with severe hemorrhage where there is urgency in making a specific diagnosis.

Angiography may be necessary in the rare instance that brisk bleeding obscures endoscopic visualization of the bleeding site. A bleeding rate in excess of 0.5 to 1 ml/min is required for adequate angiographic visualization of the bleeding site. Angiography is particularly useful in the assessment of portal hypertension and variceal bleeding and in the detection of biliary tract hemorrhage or hemobilia.

Management

Medical therapy for erosive mucosal lesions is directed toward acid reduction or neutralization. Antacids alone are indicated for patients with ongoing hemorrhage. Alternating solutions containing magnesium and aluminum hydroxides are delivered in 0.5 to 1 ml/kg doses every 1 to 2 hours to maintain gastric $pH > 5$. Histamine receptor antagonists such as cimetidine offer no proven additional benefit in the setting of active bleeding. Antacids are more effective than cimetidine in both consistently elevating gastric pH and preventing acute hemorrhage in critically ill patients.

The histamine-receptor antagonists, cimetidine and ranitidine, play an important role in the chronic outpatient treatment of duodenal ulcer. Pharmacologic reports recommend cimetidine dosage of 20 to 30 mg/kg/day administered in six divided doses, and ranitidine dosage of 1.25 to 1.9 mg/kg/day administered in two divided doses. Outpatient therapy with antacids or H2 blockers generally extends for 4 to 6 weeks to permit adequate healing (see Chap. 111).

More aggressive management of bleeding lesions includes electrocoagulation, thermocoagulation, laser therapy, transcatheter vasopressin infusion or embolization, and surgical resection or devascularization.

Variceal hemorrhage is managed acutely with intravenous vasopressin or somatostatin. Balloon tamponade using a Sengstaken–Blakemore tube is deferred whenever possible to avoid serious complications of it use. Sclerotherapy has been performed successfully in increasing numbers of children. This may be employed for both acute and prophylactic management. Other prophylactic management has included the use of propranolol. Intractable variceal bleeding may require embolization, surgical devascularization, or portosystemic vascular shunting.

LOWER GASTROINTESTINAL HEMORRHAGE

As in upper gastrointestinal hemorrhage, the causes of lower gastrointestinal hemorrhage must be considered with respect to the patient's age (Table 112-2). Swallowed maternal blood represents the most common cause of neonatal blood loss in the stool. Anal fissures, often subtle on examination, are perhaps the next most frequent source of rectal bleeding in the neonate. This problem, suspected to arise from local trauma due to the passage of frequent or hard stool, remains the most common cause of insignificant rectal blood loss in all age groups with the exception of adulthood. It is then replaced by another form of anorectal disease, hemorrhoids, which is uncommon in childhood. Necrotizing enterocolitis (NEC), a condition typically arising in the premature newborn and multifactoral in etiology, may be heralded by the presence of small amounts of blood in the stool. Intestinal malrotation with midgut volvulus together with NEC represent catastrophic ischemic events that generally present with small amounts of rectal blood loss. Whereas the latter occurs characteristically in the neonatal period, the former has been described in all ages, usually in association with intense pain and vomiting. Cow's milk protein or soy protein hypersensitivity may present as acute colitis with hematochezia. This occurs typically in the first 3 to 4 months of age and rarely beyond 1 year.

After anal fissure, infectious enterocolitis represents the next most common cause of rectal bleeding in all pediatric age groups. The typical presentation includes diarrhea and variably fever, cramping abdominal pain, and vomiting. Bacterial pathogens include *Salmonella, Shigella, Campylobacter, Yersinia entercolitica,* and *Clostridium difficile.* A cytotoxin producing serotype of *E. coli* (0157:H7) has been reported to cause sporadic cases of hemorrhagic colitis. *Neisseria gonorrhoeae* causes a proctitis that may present with hemorrhagic exudate. Patients who have unusual exposure or travel history and immunocompromised patients are at risk for less commonly found viral and parasitic pathogens. These include cytomegalovirus, herpes simplex virus, and *Entamoeba histolytica.*

Intussusception occurs most frequently between 3 months and 3 years of age. The typical clinical presentation includes abdominal distention and pain, vomiting, palpable abdominal mass in approximately two thirds of patients, and the passage of mucoid bloody stool, often described as currant jelly stool. Bleeding is rarely massive and may be occult. In contrast, bleeding from a Meckel's diverticulum generally occurs in the absence of significant pain, although the presence of large amounts of blood in the intestine may result in cramping discomfort. The blood loss can be massive. Bleeding follows ulceration of ectopic gastric mucosa in both Meckel's diverticulum and intestinal duplication.

Juvenile polyps represent a common source of rectal bleeding in childhood. They are benign hamartomatous lesions with a rich vascular supply. A digital rectal examination will identify 20% to 30% of these lesions. Bleeding is typically bright red, small in amount, and painless. The natural history

Table 112-2. Common Causes of Lower Gastrointestinal Hemorrhage

NEONATE (0–1 MO)	INFANT (1 MO–1 YR)	CHILDHOOD (1–12 YR)	ADOLESCENTS (>12 YR)
Swallowed maternal blood	Anal fissure	Anal fissure	Anal fissure
Anal fissure	UGI hemorrhage	Juvenile polyp	Idiopathic IBD
UGI hemorrhage	Intussusception	Intussusception	UGI hemorrhage
Cow's milk or soy protein allergy	Meckel's diverticulum	Meckel's diverticulum	Infectious diarrhea
Necrotizing enterocolitis	Infectious diarrhea	Infectious diarrhea	Meckel's diverticulum
Midgut volvulus	Milk protein allergy	UGI hemorrhage	Hemolytic-uremic syndrome
Coagulopathy		Hemolytic-uremic syndrome	Henoch–Schönlein purpura
		Henoch–Schönlein purpura	Angiodysplasia

is one of involution by late adolescence. Bleeding may occur in association with the passage of tissue representing an involuting, sloughed polyp. Various polyposis syndromes may present with bleeding. Histopathology, inheritance pattern, and associated lesions further identify the specific entity. A more detailed description of polyposis syndromes exceeds the scope of this discussion.

Hemolytic-uremic syndrome (HUS) and Henoch–Schönlein purpura (HSP) represent two multiorgan system, vasculitic disease entities of uncertain etiology. Both occur in childhood and are often associated with rectal bleeding. HUS is characterized by the findings of microangiopathic hemolytic anemia, thrombocytopenia, and acute renal failure. Clinical symptoms of gastroenteritis with abdominal pain, vomiting, and diarrhea (often bloody) frequently precede the illness. Acute colitis occurs in approximately 50% of cases. If not preceding the illness, it may occur concomitantly. The colitis may result from a documented bacterial enteropathogen or may prove to be idiopathic, mimicking the presentation of an ulcerative colitis. Intestinal perforation due to ischemia has been reported. Henoch–Schönlein purpura characteristically produces an urticarial rash on the buttocks and lower extremities that progresses to papular purpuric lesions. Skin edema and large joint arthralgia frequently occur. More serious complications involve renal disease (40%) and gastrointestinal symptoms (50% to 70%). Abdominal pain, vomiting, and both upper and lower gastrointestinal hemorrhages have been reported. The small intestine is primarily affected with findings resembling those of regional ileitis. Massive intestinal bleeding has been reported, although guaiac positive stool or minor gross blood loss is more the rule.

Idiopathic inflammatory bowel disease (IBD) must always be considered in the older child or adolescent presenting with rectal bleeding. Fulminant hemorrhagic colitis can occur with either ulcerative colitis or Crohn's disease. Although ileitis commonly results in occult blood loss, it does not generally cause significant gross rectal bleeding.

Rare causes of lower gastrointestinal hemorrhage include various vascular lesions. Intestinal hemangiomas may exist alone or in association with neonatal hemangiomatosis, the blue rubber bleb nevus syndrome, and Turner's syndrome. Turner's syndrome may also be complicated by telangiectasis or abnormal serosal vessels. Bleeding telangiectatic lesions commonly located in the stomach are characteristically seen in patients with Osler–Weber–Rendu disease.

Patients with Ehlers–Danlos syndrome may present with rectal bleeding presumably due to friable intestinal mucosa and anal tissue.

Work-Up

The child's age, history of illness, and specific findings on a physical examination or a laboratory evaluation will narrow the differential diagnosis.

Anal fissure can be excluded by a careful examination of slightly everted anal mucosal folds. A nasogastric aspirate is then obtained to exclude the upper gastrointestinal source. Wright stain of the stool is used to identify inflammatory cells, particularly polymorphonuclear leukocytes. The presence of inflammatory cells limits the diagnosis to causes of acute colitis. The patient's clinical status generally allows time for a careful exclusion of infectious etiologies before more invasive testing is pursued. Appropriate bacterial cultures, and where indicated, serologic testing, viral cultures, and fresh stool for ova and parasite examination should be obtained as soon as possible.

Rigid or flexible proctosigmoidoscopy is a valuable tool early in the diagnostic evaluation. Proctosigmoidoscopy and biopsy combined with external anal examination will establish the source of rectal bleeding in greater than 50% of cases. A flexible endoscopy provides the additional therapeutic option of polypectomy at the time of diagnosis. In the absence of distal findings on sigmoidoscopy, an air contrast barium enema should be performed to look for more proximally located polyps, or other mucosal or submucosal lesions. The findings on barium enema may help direct a complete colonoscopic examination. A barium enema is a useful diagnostic and therapeutic tool in the evaluation for suspected intussusception. This study must be performed cautiously where ischemia is suspected to avoid the complication of perforation. When the character of the hemorrhage suggests a bleeding Meckel's diverticulum or intestinal duplication, a technetium pertechnetate scan should be performed prior to any barium studies. An injection with pentagastrin may enhance the sensitivity of the scan. Residual barium may interfere with radioisotope detection. ^{99m}Tc-pertechnetate is selectively concentrated in gastric mucosa; this tissue is present ectopically in up to 50% of Meckel's diverticula.

When bleeding is brisk or continuous, the site of bleeding must be established as quickly and accurately as possible. ^{99m}Tc-labeled RBC scintigraphy represents a sensitive, noninvasive test that should be performed prior to angiography. Selective angiography can then be directed by the scintigraphic findings. Angiography provides precise vascular anatomic detail and the nonoperative therapeutic approach of embolization.

Management

Therapy is often supportive and directed toward the underlying disorder such as a coagulopathy or infection. It may simply require the removal of an antigenic stimulus as in milk-protein-induced colitis. Anal fissures usually heal in response to therapy for underlying constipation (when present) and local wound care. A combination of stool softener, sitz baths, and locally applied hydrocortisone-containing cream or ointment is often successful. Corticosteroids have been used to treat gastrointestinal involvement of HSP, although insufficiently controlled prospective data fuel controversy over this therapy. Alternatively, corticosteroids have proven beneficial in the treatment of Crohn's and idiopathic ulcerative colitis. Ischemic lesions are generally treated supportively. Surgery may be employed to explore and remove gross anatomic lesions compromising blood flow or to remove segments of transmurally infarcted or perforated bowel. Surgery is obviously required for the removal of a Meckel's diverticulum or ulcerated intestinal duplication. Flexible endoscopy is now used safely and routinely for polypectomy in pediatric patients. Innovations in endoscopic therapy such as electrocoagulation and laser therapy have not been evaluated for routine use in children. Successful transcatheter embolization has been reported in only a few pediatric patients. The overall safety and the rate of success is difficult to estimate.

ANNOTATED BIBLIOGRAPHY

Blumer JL, Rothstein FC et al: Pharmacokinetic determination of ranitidine pharmacodynamics in pediatric ulcer disease. J Pediatr 107:301, 1985 (One of few published reports on this drug in pediatric patients. Dosage recommendations provided for ≥90% suppression of gastric acid secretion.)

Chang MH, Wang TH, Hsu JY et al: Endoscopic examination of the upper gastrointestinal tract in infancy. Gastrointest Endosc 29:15, 1983 (Largest series of endoscopic findings in patients less than 1 year old presenting with UGI bleeding.)

Cox K, Ament ME: Upper gastrointestinal bleeding in children and adolescents. Pediatrics 63:408, 1979 (Retrospective review of UGI hemorrhage in 68 patients. Reliability of endoscopic findings is emphasized.)

Cucchiara J, Guandalini S et al: Sigmoidoscopy, colonoscopy and radiology in the evaluation of children with rectal bleeding. J Pediatr Gastroenterol Nutr 2:667, 1983 (Efficient use of current diagnostic modalities is proposed for children with rectal bleeding.)

Gryboski JD, Walker WA: Gastrointestinal bleeding. In Gastrointestinal Problems in the Infant, pp 85–121. Philadelphia, WB Saunders, 1983 (Comprehensive discussion of gastrointestinal bleeding in infancy with extensive bibliography.)

Hyams JS, Leichtner AM, Schwartz AN: Recent advances in diagnosis and treatment of gastrointestinal hemorrhage in infants and children. J Pediatr 106:1, 1985 (Discussion of most recent diagnostic and treatment modalities.)

Lloyd CW, Martin WJ, Taylor BD, Hauser AR: Pharmacokinetics and pharmacodynamics of cimetidine and metabolites in critically ill children. J Pediatr 107:295, 1985 (One of few studies examining kinetics and activity of this drug in children.)

Meyerovitz MF, Fellows KE: Angiography in gastrointestinal bleeding in children. AJR 143:837, 1984 (Retrospective review of angiographic studies in 27 patients. Discussion focuses on indications, and diagnostic and therapeutic efficacy.)

Oldham KT, Lobe TE: Gastrointestinal hemorrhage in children. Pediatr Clin North Am 32:1247, 1985 (Recent review with surgical orientation.)

Parik N, Sebring ES, Polesky HF: Evaluation of bloody gastric fluid from newborn infants. J Pediatr 94:967, 1979 (Comparison of Kleihauer and Apt tests applied to gastric fluid. Pitfalls of both tests are noted.)

Priebe HJ, Skillman JJ, Bushnell LS et al: Antacid versus cimetidine in preventing acute gastrointestinal bleeding. N Engl J Med 302:426, 1980 (Frequently quoted randomized trial demonstrating superiority of antacid prophylaxis against acute UGI hemorrhage in critically ill patients.)

Sherman NJ, Clatworthy HW Jr: Gastrointestinal bleeding in neonates: A study of 94 cases. Surgery 62:614, 1967 (Classic early review of neonatal GI hemorrhage.)

113
Groin Hernias and Hydroceles
ROBERT P. FOGLIA

A mass in the groin or scrotum of a child is a relatively common pediatric problem. This chapter reviews the embryology, anatomy, pathophysiology, evaluation, and management of the child with a hernia or hydrocele.

EMBRYOLOGY, ANATOMY, AND PATHOPHYSIOLOGY

Late in the first trimester of fetal development, a diverticulum of the peritoneum develops bilaterally at the level of the internal ring and extends in the male toward the scrotum. Beginning at about the seventh month of gestation, the testis begins to descend through the inguinal canal into the scrotum. The diverticulum of the peritoneal lining is termed the *processus vaginalis,* and normally, shortly after birth the processus vaginalis begins to close. This leaves only the most distal portion of the processus, the tunica vaginalis, surrounding the testis, patent. The major factor in the development of a hernia or hydrocele in a child is the continued patency of the processus vaginalis. The testis descends along with the processus vaginalis through the inguinal canal into the scrotum. At the time of birth in full-term males, the testes will be fully descended in 95% of babies.

Inguinal hernias are divided into two types: indirect or direct. The indirect inguinal hernia constitutes almost all (99 + %) of groin hernias in children less than 3 years of age. It is caused by a lack of obliteration of the patent processus vaginalis and is thus a congenital hernia. As the child increases intra-abdominal pressure either with crying or straining, a portion of the abdominal viscera may enter the hernia sac at the internal inguinal ring and then descends partially or completely through the inguinal canal and into the scrotum. Whether a bulge appears only in the groin, or both in the groin and the scrotum, depends on whether the processus vaginalis or hernia sac is only partly patent or fully patent into the scrotum. In contrast, as the child becomes older, the incidence of direct inguinal hernias increases. The direct hernia is usually acquired, and bowel contents can protrude into the inguinal canal through the weakened floor. A fem-oral hernia is rare in children, having an incidence in several series of only 0.2%. In a femoral hernia, the defect is inferior to the inguinal ligament and is medial to the femoral vein.

The difference between a hernia and a hydrocele is the contents of the processus. If the neck of the processus at the internal inguinal ring is wide enough to allow abdominal viscera to enter, and if abdominal viscera are present in the sac, then this is a *hernia.* If only fluid is present in the processus and if abdominal viscera have never been noted in the processus, this is a *hydrocele.* In the female, the equivalent of the processus vaginalis is the canal of Nuck; it follows the round ligament as it descends to the labia majorum. Although the small intestine is the most common structure found in a hernia sac in a boy, in the female, the hernia is more likely to contain the ovary or fallopian tube.

The presence of a patent processus vaginalis does not necessarily mean the child has or will develop a hernia or hydrocele. Although the processus is closed in most children within the first several months of life, it has been shown in adults who died with no clinical evidence of a groin hernia, that 20% had a patent processus vaginalis.

INCIDENCE

Approximately 1% of boys will develop inguinal hernias. The incidence increases in progressively more premature infants and ranges from 13% to 30%. Hernias are 6 to 15 times more common in boys, but in children less than 1 year of age this gender disparity is less pronounced. Over one third of all hernias will be diagnosed before 6 months of age and one half before the child's first birthday.

Approximately 10% to 15% of children, especially those less than 1 year of age, will have clinically apparent bilateral hernias. If only one hernia is present, it is twice as likely to be on the right side. Children with conditions that increase intra-abdominal pressure such as ventriculoperitoneal shunts, ascites, or bronchopulmonary dysplasia have a higher incidence of hernias. Children with connective tissue disorders such as Ehlers–Danlos syndrome, and the acid mucopolysaccharidoses

(Hurler–Hunter complex) also have an increased incidence of hernias.

CLINICAL PRESENTATION AND DIFFERENTIAL DIAGNOSIS

The most common finding is that the parent sees a "bulge" or "lump" in the child's groin or scrotum. The mass may be present transiently, it may come and go, or it may be present constantly. The pediatrician's major objective is to determine what caused the "bulge." The differential diagnosis includes inguinal hernia, hydrocele, undescended testis, retractile testis, inguinal lymphadenopathy or abscess, and femoral hernia. Except with incarceration and strangulation, these conditions usually occur without pain. Chapter 119 covers the causes of genital pain.

An accurate description by the parents as to where they saw the lump or bulge is helpful in making the correct diagnosis. If it were present in the inguinal region or in the inguinal region and scrotum, it is likely to be a hernia; if there was a transient swelling in the scrotum alone, it may be a hydrocele alone. The key factor is that an inguinal hernia causes a "lump" or "mass" above the inguinal ligament.

An understanding of the anatomy of the inguinal canal is helpful in making the clinical diagnosis. The examination for a hernia begins first with an inspection to determine if there is asymmetry and to see if an obvious mass is present. The examiner should ascertain if the testes are in their normal position because an undescended or retractile testis can appear as a groin mass. The child with lymphadenopathy or an inguinal abscess may have evidence of a recent infection, such as a fever or leukocytosis. The mass caused by infection is usually not directly over the inguinal canal, and it feels matted and more firm than the abdominal viscera found in a hernia. Erythema and tenderness over the inguinal region may be present with both lymphadenopathy and with a hernia having incarcerated bowel and a compromised blood supply. The findings in the child with a hernia are a sausage-shaped mass originating at the internal inguinal ring and extending a variable distance down the inguinal canal. If the processus is patent completely, the herniated viscera may extend all the way into the scrotum. A femoral hernia presents as a mass more medial than the usual hernia and may be seen as a mass high in the proximal thigh, which increases in size as the patient increased intra-abdominal pressure.

If the hernia is not identifiable, it may be helpful to have the child increase intra-abdominal pressure (*e.g.,* by crying, straining, or Valsalva maneuver) in an attempt to have the hernia protrude. A hydrocele can often be differentiated from a hernia by a history and physical examination. The parent of the child with a hydrocele will describe the boy's scrotum as being normal sized when he awakens but that during the day it increases in size. Furthermore, if the mass in the scrotum has been present for a relatively long time (over 8 hours) and if the child does not have abdominal distention, has not vomited, and is not fussy, this is much more likely to be a hydrocele rather than an incarcerated hernia. The ability to transilluminate a scrotal mass does not help differentiate a hernia from a hydrocele because an incarcerated bowel loop in a neonate easily transilluminates as does a hydrocele. Attempted aspiration of a "probable" hydrocele should not be considered because an erroneous diagnosis may lead to tragic consequences. In contrast, palpating the proximal extent of the mass may be helpful. Hydroceles will often be limited to the scrotum alone. If the examiner can palpate the pubic ramus and the cord structures exiting at the external inguinal ring and does not feel a bowel loop, then it is unlikely that the scrotal mass is a hernia. A rectal examination can be diagnostic in the child less than 1 year of age. The examiner carries out a bimanual examination with one finger in the rectum and with the other hand at the level of the internal inguinal ring. If the examiner's finger in the rectum can feel the other hand and there is no loop of bowel intervening, it is unlikely that the mass present is an incarcerated hernia. The use of an abdominal roentgenogram is also helpful because if there is air present below the inguinal ligament, this is indicative of a hernia.

HERNIOGRAPHY

It is possible to inject contrast material into the peritoneal cavity and outline a patent processus vaginalis or hernia sac if one is present. In especially problematic cases, this technique is helpful but there are several caveats involved with its use. It is an invasive procedure and carries a small but finite risk of injury to the bowel. If a patent processus is outlined, this may not constitute an indication for an operation because a patent processus is not *prima facie* evidence for a hernia. If there is an incarcerated hernia, a herniogram may give a false negative picture because no peritoneal fluid can flow down into the processus due to the bowel loop incarcerated at the internal ring.

MANAGEMENT

Inguinal hernias require operative repair. They do not resolve spontaneously, and there is no role for a truss in their management. The major risk associated with an inguinal hernia is incarceration. Approximately two thirds of all incarcerated hernias occur in children less than 1 year of age. If the child has an easily reducible hernia, an operative correction should be scheduled at the earliest convenience. The exception to this recommendation is in the premature infant. Because of the increased risk of postanesthetic respiratory problems, if the hernia is easily reducible, an elective operation may be deferred until the baby is at least 42 weeks' total gestational age.

If the hernia cannot be easily reduced, the first step in management consists of reduction; otherwise, this may lead to strangulation of the bowel, especially in males. In females, an incarcerated hernia often contains an ovary or a fallopian tube and there is less risk of strangulation.

The child with an incarcerated hernia is usually fussy, and if the bowel has been incarcerated for more than 4 to 6 hours the abdomen will be distended proximally. 95% of incarcerated hernias can be reduced. This is done by exerting steady constant pressure on the most distal portion of the hernia contents in the direction of the internal ring with one hand. Dorsal force is then directed with the other hand at the level of the internal ring. Elevation of the foot of the crib is also helpful in attempting to reduce the hernia contents. Usually, with merely maintaining steady pressure, some of the air is displaced from the incarcerated loop of bowel into the adjacent bowel proximal to the neck of the hernia. The remainder of the bowel then usually promptly reduces. If the bowel remains incarcerated, sedating the infant with Demerol or chloral hydrate, and trying again usually works. The use of ice packs over the incarcerated bowel has not been found to be helpful, and this practice is contraindicated.

If the hernia reduces easily, the child may go home and elective repair should be scheduled within the next 1 to 2 weeks. If, however, there has been any difficulty whatsoever in reducing the hernia, the child should be admitted to the hospital and maintained NPO; an IV should be started; and the child's abdomen should be examined over the next 8 hours to evaluate for any evidence of bowel ischemia. Operative repair should then be performed 24 to 48 hours later after the edema has resolved. If the hernia cannot be reduced, or if there is any question, emergency operative repair is indicated.

OPERATIVE REPAIR

Inguinal hernia repair can easily be performed on an outpatient basis. The child comes into the outpatient area in the morning; he is operated on and he is usually discharged within 2 to 3 hours. The exceptions to this practice are children with significant congenital heart disease, lung disease, a history of apnea, or children who were born prematurely. These children have a higher risk of postoperative respiratory problems, and as a rule it is preferable to have these children admitted and observed during the night following surgery.

The hernia repair is performed under general anesthesia and consists of an incision made in a skin crease, dissection down to the inguinal canal, identification of the hernia sac, freeing it from the cord structures to the level of the internal ring, and then high ligation of the sac. The distal portion of the sac should be left wide open or excised. If there is any evidence of weakness of the floor of the inguinal canal, or if the internal ring is wide open, the floor of the inguinal canal is reinforced. The use of a local anesthetic such as Bupivacaine to block the ileoinguinal nerve offers good pain relief for up to 12 hours. When the child is examined again in the office, the parents will often comment about how by the following day their child acted as though he was never operated on.

Hydroceles in children less than 1 year of age do not require an operation because many of these will resolve spontaneously with the obliteration of the patent processus. Operative repair is recommended if the hydrocele is so large that it is uncomfortable for the child or if the hydrocele is still present in a child over 1 year of age. If abdominal viscera are seen at any time in the inguinal canal or scrotum, then the child now has a true hernia and not a hydrocele, and operative repair is indicated.

CONTRALATERAL EXPLORATION

Much debate has centered about the question of exploration of the opposite asymptomatic side when a symptomatic hernia is being repaired on the other side. In children less than 2 years of age there is a 47% likelihood of a hernia present on the opposite side even if none is seen clinically. A second hernia also appears more commonly in females. A reasonable course is to explore the contralateral asymptomatic side in boys under 2 years of age, and girls less than 4 years of age.

COMPLICATIONS

The major preoperative complication is incarceration leading to bowel obstruction and potentially strangulation of the bowel. If the bowel cannot be reduced manually, emergency herniorrhaphy is required. An inspection of the bowel at operation allows the assessment of its viability, and in some cases resection of the affected bowel must be done. A testicular compromise has also been found to occur secondary to venous obstruction by the incarcerated hernia. The vas deferens is quite small in babies and there is a small risk of injury to this delicate structure during herniorrhaphy. In the female, the fallopian tube or ovary is often in the hernia sac and injury may occur to these structures unless care is taken prior to the removal of the sac.

The chance of recurrence of a hernia is small and is usually considered secondary to the lack of removal of the entire sac. Alternatively, the child may return with a direct component of an inguinal hernia after a high ligation of an indirect hernia has been performed.

ANNOTATED BIBLIOGRAPHY

Harper RG, Garcia A, Sia C: Inguinal hernia: A common problem of premature infants weighing 1000 grams or less at birth. Pediatrics 56:112, 1975 (Excellent review.)

Holder TM, Ashcraft KW: Groin hernias and hydroceles. In Textbook of Pediatric Surgery, p 594. Philadelphia, WB Saunders, 1980 (Easily readable and excellent reference.)

Rowe MI, Clatworthy HW: Incarcerated and strangulated hernias in children. Arch Surg 101:136, 1970 (Review of 2764 patients with inguinal hernias. The experience at a large children's hospital.)

Rowe MI, Lloyd DA: Pediatric Surgery, pp 779–793. Chicago, Yearbook Medical Publishers, 1986 (Most recent and comprehensive review.)

Steward DJ: Preterm infants are more prone to complications following minor surgery than are term infants. Anesthesiol 56:304, 1982 (Excellent discussion of post operative respiratory problems in infants after hernia repair.)

14

Genitourinary Problems

114
Urinary Tract Infections
JEROLD C. WOODHEAD

Most infection-related renal damage occurs during infancy and early childhood. Timely identification of urinary tract infection, appropriate treatment, detection of patients at risk for renal scarring, and prevention of recurrent infection can arrest or prevent progressive renal damage.

PATHOPHYSIOLOGY

Infection may occur at any point in the urinary tract from urethral meatus to renal parenchyma. In the newborn period, boys develop urinary tract infections more frequently than girls. Most such infections result from bacteremia or they are associated with structural abnormalities of the urinary tract, such as congenital obstruction and vesicoureteral reflux. Beyond the newborn period, most urinary tract infections occur in girls, with organisms entering by way of the urethra. Almost 90% of first infections, and 75% to 80% of recurrent infections result from entry of *Escherichia coli* into the urinary tract. Other less common organisms include *Klebsiella* species, *Proteus* species, and enterococci, although any bacterial species may cause infection. *Staphylococcus saprophyticus* has been identified as a common cause of urinary tract infection, especially in the dysuria–pyuria syndrome. The ascent of infected urine from the bladder up the ureters into the renal pelvis and parenchyma carries great risk of renal damage. Infection itself may cause edema of the vesicoureteral junction and may alter ureteral peristalsis resulting in transient reflux of mild to moderate degree. More severe and persistent reflux occurs in infants and children who have underlying abnormalities of the bladder and ureter which allow free reflux of urine, whether infected or not. Whenever urine refluxes from the bladder to the kidney, a pressure wave is transmitted. Increased pressure within the renal pelvis coupled with bacteria may produce permanent renal scarring. Children below the age of 4 or 5 years have the greatest risk of infection-caused renal scarring, because vesicoureteral reflux and other structural abnormalities occur most commonly in this age group. Approximately one half of children under the age of 5 years with urinary tract infection *and* fever will have vesicoureteral reflux. Recurrent infection in patients with persistent reflux causes scarring in over 80% of cases. Approximately 25% of end-stage renal disease in childhood results from the damage caused by infection in structurally abnormal urinary tracts.

Because the location of an infection within the urinary tract determines the risk for permanent damage to the kidney, much effort has been expended to identify clinical clues or laboratory tests that pinpoint the site of infection. Sex, age, symptoms, signs, and various laboratory tests assist in localization, but *none* reliably identifies all patients with upper tract infection. Many of the tests are unavailable to the office-based pediatrician or are impractical or too expensive for routine use.

CLINICAL PRESENTATION

Clinical clues vary with age. Infants typically present with fever, irritability, and other signs of systemic illness, including failure to thrive, vomiting, and diarrhea. In addition, signs of bladder obstruction including abdominal distention, weak urinary stream, infrequent voiding, irritability, and malodorous or discolored urine may accompany signs of sepsis. The younger the infant, the more likely are sepsis and structural abnormalities associated with, or causative of, urinary tract infection. Toddlers may complain of abdominal discomfort and demonstrate fever, altered voiding pattern, and malodorous urine. Preschool children may complain of voiding discomfort or they may develop recurrent enuresis, in addition to fever and abdominal or flank pain. School-aged children and adolescents typically have "classic" signs and symptoms (*e.g.,* dysuria, frequency, urgency, abdominal or flank pain, and fever). Diagnosis is most difficult in infancy and early childhood because clinical clues are nonspecific.

DIFFERENTIAL DIAGNOSIS

Fever occurs commonly with urinary infection in children under 1 year of age, but fever as the *only* sign of urinary infection is not common. However, a urinary tract infection should be considered when an infant has a recurrent fever without an obvious cause. Vomiting, diarrhea, and failure to thrive may accompany metabolic, gastrointestinal, cardiovascular, and neurologic disorders, as well as urinary infection.

Dysuria, frequency, urgency, and hesitancy occur with urethral and bladder mucosal irritation from infectious, chemical, or physical causes (see Chap. 115). These symptoms, accompanied by urine culture with 10^2 to 10^4 colonies/ml, occur in adult women (and probably adolescent girls) with the *dysuria–pyuria syndrome*. Cultures with such low colony counts must be considered "positive," despite past teaching that $>10^5$ colonies/ml was the diagnostic criterion for infection. Sexual abuse must be considered in children with traumatic or sexually-transmitted infectious causes for dysuria.

Abdominal pain with urinary tract infection must be distinguished from appendicitis, pelvic abscess, and pelvic inflammatory disease, which may all cause dysuria and pyuria. A vaginal discharge suggests vaginitis as the cause of dysuria and frequency. A history of sexual activity may point to one of the aforementioned conditions or may suggest a urinary infection related to intercourse. In addition to abdominal pain, constipation may cause dysuria and may predispose to urinary tract infection.

WORK-UP

Urine Collection

Collection of an uncontaminated urine specimen for urine culture presents a formidable hurdle in the diagnostic process. Even in adult women, "clean catch" voided urine may have a contamination rate of up to 20% to 30%. The contamination of voided specimens is a much greater problem for infants and young children, especially when urine bags must be used to collect the specimen. Bagged urine may be contaminated even when urine bags are applied using meticulous technique, removed immediately after the child has voided, and urine is cultured immediately. Bagged urine can only be considered valid if the culture is *sterile*. As a general rule, voided urine, including urine collected in urine bags, may be used for "screening" urinalysis or culture. A strong suspicion of urinary tract infection, especially in the presence of systemic toxicity, mandates use of a more reliable urine collection method.

When voided urines are collected for culture, a girl should have her perineum and labia cleaned gently with mild soap and water and a boy should have his penis cleaned (with the foreskin retracted if uncircumcised). Antiseptic solutions and soaps should be avoided; if they are not completely rinsed off, they may sterilize or reduce the colony count of the urine specimen. Do not attempt to "sterilize" the urethral meatus. Midstream urine specimens provide the best samples for urinalysis and culture. Cultures of voided urine with more than 50,000 colonies/ml in an asymptomatic patient or with 10^2 to 10^4 colonies/ml in a symptomatic patient *may* indicate infection, but *only when confirmed by repeat culture*, preferably obtained by suprapubic bladder aspiration or bladder catheterization.

Suprapubic aspiration of the bladder provides urine samples with low likelihood of contamination. The technique is safe and relatively easy to learn and perform. Suprapubic aspiration of the bladder can be done at any age but practical considerations restrict its use to young infants. I prefer to limit suprapubic aspiration to infants below the age of 3 months. The intra-abdominal position of the bladder in young infants permits easy palpation and increases the likelihood of a successful suprapubic tap. Complications, including "dry" taps and hematuria, may be reduced with careful attention to detail. However carefully done, though, the procedure causes some degree of discomfort to the infant and a great deal of anxiety in some parents. Urine obtained from a carefully performed suprapubic bladder aspiration should be sterile. *Any growth on culture* signifies infection. No other method of urine collection offers as much diagnostic certainty.

Catheterization of the bladder with a sterile, small-gauge, straight catheter allows the physician to obtain urine with minimal risk of contamination and minimal patient discomfort. Although not 100% free of contamination risk (because the catheter must pass through the urethral meatus which cannot be sterilized), this method provides a more reliable specimen than any voiding technique. As a rule, cultures from catheterized specimens with more than 10^2 to 10^3 colonies/ml indicate infection. A sterile No. 5 French feeding tube may be used for catheterization of newborns and young infants. A sterile technique reduces the risk of introducing infection into an uninfected urinary tract, and the restriction of the procedure to those infants and children in whom symptoms and signs strongly point to urinary tract infection further reduces the likelihood that bladder catheterization will cause complications.

Urinalysis

Traditional urinalysis has a time-honored role, but limited usefulness, in the diagnosis of a urinary tract infection. Pyuria, bacteriuria, hematuria, and proteinuria in a symptomatic patient suggest the diagnosis of urinary infection but require culture confirmation. Modifications of the standard urinalysis discussed below may increase its usefulness but cannot eliminate the need for a culture.

Pyuria, defined as more than 5 leukocytes per high-powered microscope field in a centrifuged urine specimen, is unreliable as a sign of urinary tract infection. Urine concentration, centrifugation speed and duration, and volume of sediment examined may affect microscopic quantification of pyuria. In addition, urine cultures may be positive in the absence of pyuria and urinary leukocytes may originate from causes other than infection. However, uncentrifuged urine examined with the aid of a hemacytometer shows a high correlation between the presence of more than 10 leukocytes/mm^3 and $>10^5$ colonies/ml on culture; lower colony counts in the dysuria–pyuria syndrone have a strong correlation with ≥ 8 WBC/mm^3. Thus, the use of a hemacytometer may greatly increase the value of a microscopic evaluation for pyuria.

Bacteria identified microscopically in *uncentrifuged* urine usually indicate infection. A correlation between urine culture with $>10^5$ colonies/ml and bacteria identified on uncentrifuged urine approaches 80% for unstained urine and increases to 95% when Gram stain is used. The use of the hemacytometer aids in the detection and quantification of bacteria, eliminates the need to stain urine, and has the same high correlation with positive culture as the gram-stained specimen. An examination of the centrifuged urine sediment for bacteria suffers from the same lack of standardization mentioned for pyuria.

Chemical Tests

Tests designed to detect bacteriuria include nitrite dipsticks, tetrazolium reduction, and catalase and endotoxin detection. Only the nitrite dipstick has clinical use in office-based practice. Based on the conversion of urinary nitrate to nitrite by certain types of bacteria, the dipstick detects nitrite colorimetrically. False positive tests are rare, but false negative results are common. The test can be performed reliably only on first voided morning urine since time is required for the conversion of nitrate to nitrite; it cannot be used for infants or for children with enuresis. The causes of false negative tests include an inadequate incubation time, infection with bacteria that do not reduce nitrate, and low dietary nitrate. The major use of the nitrite test is screening for infection in high risk populations. A positive nitrite test should prompt culture confirmation of infection. Used properly, the nitrite test may be performed at home by parents.

Urine Culture

Office-based physicians often avoid urine culture because of specimen handling problems, time delay, and high cost of cultures performed in microbiology laboratories. Cultures performed in the laboratory are the standard against which all other detection methods must be compared; but urine can be cultured in the physician's office with equivalent reliability, lower cost, and less inconvenience, using either standard culture methods or a commercially available "dipslide" technique. Dipslides provide culture results that compare favorably with those obtained from standard culture methods without the need for equipment or a laboratory assistant. They may even be incubated overnight at room temperature. Differential growth on the two media that coat the slide allows a preliminary bacterial identification, and a comparison of growth on the slide to pictoral standards allows an estimation of the colony count. Subculture by a microbiology laboratory provides precise bacterial identification and antibiotic susceptibility testing when needed. None of the other commercially available culture techniques offers the ease of use, reliability, and flexibility of the dipslide technique.

Proper handling of urine specimens reduces the risk of erroneous urine results. Immediate culturing of a urine specimen is optimal, but practicality often dictates a delay from collection to culture. Doubling time for urinary pathogens may be as short as 20 minutes at room temperature. Since bacterial growth is effectively arrested at 4°C, immediate refrigeration of urine specimens prevents bacterial overgrowth from contaminants and allows reliable colony counts when urine is later cultured.

Identification of bacterial species and determination of antibiotic sensitivities are *not* necessary in most *uncomplicated* cases. These procedures require the services of a hospital or commercial laboratory; they add specimen handling problems; and they increase the cost. In vitro susceptibilities do not necessarily correlate with in vivo response to antibiotics because most antibiotics achieve high concentrations in urine. Bacterial identification and susceptibility testing should be done for patients with systemic toxicity and for those who fail to respond to treatment within 2 to 3 days.

MANAGEMENT

Optimal management prevents progressive renal damage and reduces patient discomfort. Comprehensive management includes antibiotic therapy, documentation of antibiotic effectiveness, follow-up cultures, identification of children with structural abnormalities, prevention of recurrent infection in those with reflux, and patient education.

Antibiotic Therapy

Oral antibiotics effective against *E. coli* include sulfonamides (*e.g.*, sulfisoxasole—40 mg/kg/dose, qid), amoxicillin (15 mg/kg/dose, tid), ampicillin (10 to 15 mg/kg/dose, qid), trimethoprim/sulfamethoxazole (4 mg T and 20 mg S/kg/dose, bid), cephalosporin (*e.g.*, cephalexin—6 to 12 mg/kg/dose, qid), or nitrofurantoin (1 to 2 mg/kg/dose, qid). Tetracycline (250 mg qid) may be chosen for adolescents. All produce high concentration of antibiotic in urine and rapidly eradicate sensitive organisms. The dosing frequency, cost, and history of allergic or nonallergic adverse reaction (*e.g.*, severe diarrhea) affect the choice of antibiotics. Infants with fever or in whom sepsis is a consideration should

be managed in hospital, as should any child or adolescent with symptomatic pyelonephritis.

Outpatient management of urinary tract infection typically involves 10 to 14 days of antibiotics. Therapy longer than this offers no advantage. However, shorter regimens may improve compliance and may reduce inconvenience, side effects, and cost, while providing therapeutic results comparable to longer therapy. Single dose and 3-day antibiotic regimens have good efficacy in adolescent and adult women with infection localized to the bladder, but not when the upper tract (*i.e.*, kidney) is infected. In adult women, the dysuria–pyuria syndrome may be caused by a bacterial infection and responds well to single dose treatment with amoxicillin (2 to 3 g po), sulfisoxazole (1 g, po), or trimethoprim/sulfamethoxazole (2 double strength tablets, po). Such therapy may be used for adolescents with uncomplicated urinary tract infection, but 3-day treatment with trimethoprim/sulfamethoxazole (1 double strength tablet bid) may be more effective. Short-course therapy has not been shown to be reliable for infants and children and cannot be recommended.

Follow-up

Urine should be cultured 2 to 3 days after the start of standard 10-day therapy or 3 to 4 days after the completion of short-course therapy. Sterile urine demonstrates antibiotic effectiveness and obviates the need for susceptibility testing. If urine is not sterile, repeat culture should be sent for identification and susceptibility testing, a broad spectrum antibiotic should be prescribed, and urine should be recultured in 3 days to confirm antibiotic effectiveness. Once the infection has been eradicated, screen for recurrent infection with urine culture after 1 month has elapsed (or just before radiologic evaluation). Further follow-up cultures are recommended at 3-month intervals for 1 year, and then yearly for 2 to 3 years. If infection does not recur in this interval, a further recurrence is unlikely. Obviously, fever or other signs of infection mandate urine culture at any time. Dipslide cultures are ideal for follow-up. Nitrite dipsticks may replace screening culture for children who have achieved bladder control; a positive test should be confirmed with culture.

Identification of Structural Abnormalities

The most reliable technique for detection of vesicoureteral reflux is the voiding cystourethrogram (VCUG). VCUG should be done for *all children below 3 years of age* after the *first* documented urinary tract infection. In addition, *boys at any age* should have VCUG after their first urinary infection. Girls older than 3 years with systemic toxicity suggestive of pyelonephritis (*e.g.*, fever, flank pain), recurrent infection, poor growth, hypertension, or failure to respond promptly to therapy also have a strong likelihood of reflux and should be studied with VCUG. Obtain VCUG 4 to 6 weeks after completion of antibiotics. Low-dose, prophylactic antibiotics (nitrofurantoin, 1 to 2 mg/kg/dose, bid, or trimethoprim/sulfamethoxazole, 2 mg T and 20 mg S/kg/dose, once daily) will reduce the likelihood of recurrent infection until VCUG can be completed.

The renal structure must also be evaluated. This has traditionally been done by excretory urography (*e.g.*, intravenous pyelography, IVP) but in many cases ultrasonography has replaced the IVP as the preferred procedure. IVP provides both structural and functional information whereas ultrasonography only shows structure. However, IVP also has risks and discomfort not associated with ultrasonography. The choice of technique should be based on VCUG results. IVP should be done if the VCUG shows reflux. Ultrasonography without the need for IVP may be chosen if VCUG does not demonstrate reflux. IVP at the time of acute infection is indicated for children with pyelonephritis or signs of urinary obstruction after infection has been controlled by antibiotic therapy and fever and toxicity have resolved. Such patients usually require hospitalization.

The management of reflux depends on its severity. Reflux up to the renal pelvis with no or minimal distention (grades I, IIa, and IIb) spontaneously resolves in a high percentage of cases and does not require an immediate urologic evaluation. Higher grades of reflux (grades III, IV, and V) do not usually resolve and should be evaluated by a pediatric urologist. Cystoscopy and antireflux surgery may be indicated.

Prevention of Recurrent Infection

Children who have reflux demonstrated on VCUG *must* have continuous antibiotic prophylaxis to prevent renal scarring. Prophylaxis should be continued until 1 year after the resolution of the reflux. Nitrofurantoin or trimethoprim/sulfamethoxazole may be used at the doses discussed above. Reevaluate yearly with VCUG or radionuclide cystography to monitor reflux and detect the spontaneous resolution of low grades of reflux. In addition, renal growth should be monitored with an annual ultrasound or IVP, as long as the reflux persists.

Some children with normal urinary structure have recurrent infection. Although they are at minimal risk for renal damage, prophylaxis will reduce the morbidity of recurrent infection.

Methenamine (Mandelamine or Hiprex) may be useful for prophylaxis of recurrent urinary tract infections in selected cases. The dose of methenamine is 18 mg/kg/dose qid for children below age 6; for children aged 6 to 12 years the dose is 500 mg qid; children older than 12 years of age should receive 1 g qid. Maximum efficacy of this therapy is achieved when urine is acidified to pH 5.5. Cranberry juice and vitamin C will acidify urine, but large quantities of juice or vitamin C must be ingested to maintain urine pH. This therapy is difficult to maintain for long periods, although it may be valuable for patients who are allergic to antibiotics.

Teaching a child the proper wiping technique after bowel movement may reduce fecal contamination in the vaginal introitus and urethra. Similarly, the control of constipation and associated encopresis will reduce perineal soiling.

INDICATIONS FOR REFERRAL OR HOSPITALIZATION

All infants and children with symptomatic pyelonephritis, sepsis, or obstructive uropathy should be hospitalized. Infants with obstructive signs (*e.g.*, midline lower abdominal distention, flank mass, infrequent or prolonged voiding, weak or dribbling urinary stream, "thread-like" urinary stream, or ballooning of penile urethra) must be evaluated by a pediatric urologist, as should any child who has severe reflux. In addition, children who have any degree of reflux should have a urologic evaluation if there is associated hypertension, growth retardation, other structural renal abnormalities, or reduced renal function.

PATIENT EDUCATION

Parents must understand the consequences of urinary tract infections and the importance of aggressive, comprehensive management. Many adults experience urinary infection as a minor annoyance and may assume the same holds for infants and children. Physicians should avoid terms such as *cystitis* or *bladder infection* because they may lessen the importance of urinary infection in the minds of parents.

ANNOTATED BIBLIOGRAPHY

Fine JS, Jacobson MS: Single-dose versus conventional therapy of urinary tract infections in female adolescents. Pediatrics 75: 916–920, 1985 (The cure rate of UTI with single-dose antibiotic therapy in adolescents was comparable to that found with conventional 10-day therapy. Approach to treatment failure is discussed.)

Ginsburg CM, McCracken GH: Urinary tract infections in young infants. Pediatrics 69:409–412, 1982 (Presents the clinical and laboratory features of urinary tract infection in 100 infants age 5 days to 8 months.)

Hellerstein S, Wald ER, Winberg J et al: Consensus: Roentgenographic evaluation of children with urinary tract infections. Pediatr Infect Dis 3: 291–293, 1984 (Recommends evaluation of first urinary tract infections in girls below the age of 3 and boys at any age.)

Johnson CE, Shurin PA, Marchant CD et al: Identification of children requiring radiologic evaluation for urinary infection. Pediatr Infect Dis 4:656–663, 1985 (Discusses the radiologic evaluation of urinary tract infections and presents results of a prospective study de-signed to identify markers for children potentially at risk for renal damage.)

Komaroff AL: Acute dysuria in women. N Engl J Med 310:368–375, 1984 (Reviews the causes and treatment of dysuria in adult women who do not have clinical evidence of pyelonephritis; provides an updated definition of a "positive" urine culture.)

Kunin CM: Detection, Prevention and Management of Urinary Tract Infections, 3rd ed. Philadelphia, Lea & Febiger, 1979 (Extensively referenced.)

Lebowitz RL: Pediatric uroradiology. Pediatr Clin North Am 32:1353–1362, 1985 (Discusses the techniques available for evaluation of the urinary tract; describes each technique and discusses the situations in which each should be used.)

Levitt SB, Weiss RA: Vesicoureteral reflux: Natural history, classification and reflux nephropathy. In Kelalis PP, King LR, Belman AB(eds): Clinical Pediatric Urology, 2nd ed., pp 355–380. Philadelphia, WB Saunders, 1985 (Provides a comprehensive overview of vesicoureteral reflux and renal damage associated with it; 151 references.)

Todd JK: Diagnosis of urinary tract infections. Pediatr Infect Dis 1:126–131, 1982 (Describes laboratory techniques that can be used in the office laboratory to diagnose urinary tract infection.)

115
Dysuria and Frequency

ROOPA S. HASHIMOTO AND JEROLD C. WOODHEAD

Dysuria refers to painful micturition, and frequency is an increase in the number of voidings with or without increased urinary volume. Both occur commonly in children and adolescents. Accompanying symptoms include urgency, hesitancy, and urinary incontinence.

PATHOPHYSIOLOGY

Any process that irritates the mucosa of the bladder or urethra may result in dysuria, including infection, trauma, and mechanical or chemical irritation. In addition, inflamed or irritated perineal and vaginal tissue may be further irritated during urination with accompanying pain.

Frequency may result from various causes, the most common one being an increased fluid intake. In urinary tract infection, frequency results from bladder mucosal inflammation and bladder spasm. The bladder capacity is decreased by pain associated with inflammation. Excitement and stress may raise intravesical pressure and relax the detrusor muscle, thus prompting urination. Cold weather may also lead to an increased frequency and volume of urination because vasoconstriction of the peripheral circulation increases the rate of urine formation.

CLINICAL PRESENTATION

The clinical presentation of dysuria and frequency varies with age and etiology. Normally, infants and toddlers void 6 to 30 times/day, 3 to 5 year olds void 8 to 14 times/day, 5 to 8 year olds void 6 to 12 times/day, and 8 to 14 year olds void 6 to 8 times/day. Dysuria and frequency may be difficult to identify in infancy, but may be suspected if parents note crying associated with voiding, or diaper dermatitis resistant to treatment. During infancy, circumcised boys may be at increased risk of urethral meatal irritation with associated dysuria. The infant with urinary tract infection may have dysuria along with malodorous urine, failure to thrive, or signs of systemic infection. Toddlers may have dysuria noted only because of changes in voiding habits, signs of urinary tract infection, or a perineal rash and irritation. Older children and adolescents have the ability to complain of pain with urination; urinary frequency and other associated symptoms are also more evident. "Classic" signs and symptoms of urinary tract infection predominate in this age group. Sexually active adolescents with dysuria may have sexually transmitted infection. Dysuria may also be the presenting complaint in sexual abuse. Urethral prolapse presents with a painful, purple, mulberry-like mass in the perineum associated with dysuria or urinary retention.

DIFFERENTIAL DIAGNOSIS

Common infectious causes of dysuria or frequency include bacterial infection of the urinary tract (see Chap. 114), viral hemorrhagic cystitis, gonococcal and nongonococcal urethritis, herpes simplex or varicella lesions in the periurethral region, candidal dermatitis, and vulvovaginitis (see Chap. 120). All of these may cause the dysuria–pyuria syndrome, which has been identified in adult women and probably occurs in adolescent girls, especially those who are sexually active. Patients who have this syndrome have voiding symptoms and pyuria but no signs of systemic illness. Urine cultures are sterile or have low colony counts of *Escherichia coli* or *Staphylococcus saprophyticus*, although other gram-negative and positive organisms occasionally cause the syndrome. Because the dysuria–pyuria syndrome has been formally described only for adult women, its diagnosis should be made carefully, if at all, and only in adolescent girls whose urine cultures have colony counts in the range of 10^2 to 10^4/ml, or who have sterile urine and vulvovaginitis.

Trauma and irritation commonly cause dysuria. Falls, masturbation, and sexual abuse may traumatize periurethral and perineal tissues and produce painful urination. Toddlers may insert foreign bodies into the vagina or urethra. Irritant dermatitis from urine, or soap and bleach residue in diapers, and chemical urethritis from bubble bath, soap, or deodorants produce dysuria. Other causes include urethral meatal ulceration (usually in circumcised boys), urethral stricture resulting from trauma, urinary calculi (usually associated with hematuria), and pinworm infestation.

Miscellaneous causes of dysuria or frequency include appendicitis with a pelvic abscess, bladder outlet obstruction, Reiter disease, urethral prolapse, drugs, renal tuberculosis, prostatitis, and pollakiuria (*i.e.*, frequency caused by stress or excitement). Dysuria plus urinary retention may be caused by the ingestion of various drugs including amitriptyline, chlordiazepoxide, imipramine, or isoniazid. Frequency may result from the ingestion of antihistamines, carbamazepine, demeclocycline, fenfluramine, and excess vitamin D. Girls with group A, β-hemolytic Streptococcal pharyngitis may develop Streptococcal vaginitis which causes dysuria and perineal discomfort. Encopresis presumably causes frequency because fecal impaction reduces bladder capacity and also promotes relaxation of the urethral sphincter. In addition, constant fecal soiling predisposes to urinary tract infection.

WORK-UP

History

A history alone often identifies the etiology of dysuria and its frequency and avoids an excessive work-up. Chills, fever, and signs and symptoms compatible with urinary tract infection point to an infectious cause, although dysuria without a systemic illness may also be caused by an infection of the urinary tract.

A preceding viral illness followed by the acute onset of painful, frequent bloody urination suggests hemorrhagic cystitis. The physician should ask about a history of recurrent herpes lesions or current infection with varicella. A history of vaginal discharge along with dysuria and frequency in the pubertal girl suggests sexually transmitted diseases such as gonorrhea, trichomonas, chlamydia, or candida. Similar symptoms in a prepubertal girl suggest sexual abuse. Night crying in young girls may point to irritation caused by pinworm migration from the rectum to the vagina or urethra. The physician should ask about trauma including falls, masturbation, foreign body insertion into the urethra or vagina, and sexual abuse. A description of a weak urinary stream or a history of constant dribbling may provide clues that lead to the diagnosis of bladder outlet obstruction or bladder diverticulae.

An inquiry should be made about medications (both prescription and over-the-counter) and illicit drug ingestion. The use of detergents, soaps, bubble bath, or deodorants may not be mentioned by parents unless specifically asked about. Information about bowel habits including constipation, soiling, and the method used by young girls to wipe themselves after bowel movements, often proves valuable in the search for the etiology of dysuria. Causes of acute and chronic emotional stress should be sought when pollakiuria is suspected.

Physical Examination

The physical examination of a child with frequency and dysuria should be thorough. An inspection may reveal abdominal distention, rashes or evidence of perineal trauma, urethral lesions, or vaginal discharge. A vaginal examination will allow the identification of a foreign body, vaginitis, or trauma. Abdominal masses may be of renal, bladder, or bowel origin. Pain with palpation or percussion of the bladder or kidneys points to urinary tract infection. A rectal examination may disclose impacted feces or a tender pelvic abscess. Observation of the urinary stream may reveal abnormalities such as spraying or dribbling. Listening to the sound of the urinary stream may be more practical with girls.

Laboratory Tests

The most important tests in the laboratory evaluation of dysuria and frequency are urinalysis and culture of an appropriately collected specimen. At all ages, if infection appears likely, catheterization of the bladder provides the specimen with the least likelihood of contamination. Suprapubic bladder aspiration carries the risk of hematuria, which may confuse the diagnostic process. Mid-stream voided urine specimens may be adequate in older children and adolescents, but bacteriuria, pyuria, or positive urine culture on a voided specimen should be confirmed with a second specimen. (Culture criteria for the diagnosis of urinary tract infection are discussed in Chapter 114). Voided urine that is persistently sterile or has low colony counts despite voiding symptoms may signal the dysuria–pyuria syndrome, but, as mentioned, this diagnosis should be made cautiously.

Pyuria is most reliably detected in uncentrifuged urine examined with the aid of a hemacytometer. When a counting chamber is used, urine with ≥ 8 WBC/mm^3 has a high association with the dysuria-pyuria syndrome; more than 10 WBC/mm^3 correlates strongly with urine culture $>10^5$ colonies/ml. Pyuria may also be identified in centrifuged urine, but sources of error are numerous, and quantification of pyuria is much less certain than with the hemacytometer.

A suspicion of sexually transmitted infection mandates cultures for gonorrhea from the urethra, vagina, cervix, rectum, and oropharynx, depending on the patient's age and clinical history. A chlamydial culture may not be available to the office-based physician. A wet mount examination of vaginal discharge may demonstrate *Trichomonas*. KOH prep and culture may aid in the identification of candida.

If pinworms are suspected, a transparent tape test should be done during the office visit and examined for pinworm ova. If negative, parents should be taught the technique and sent home with slides to be done on 3 separate days early in the morning (before the child gets out of bed) or when night crying occurs.

Streptococcal vaginitis is identified by culture.

TREATMENT

With adequate therapy, dysuria and frequency caused by urinary tract infection resolve rapidly. Except in adolescents who fit the clinical description of the dysuria–pyuria syndrome, infection of the urinary tract accompanied by dysuria should be treated according to standard regimens (see Chap. 114). In adult women and probably in adolescent girls, the dysuria–pyuria syndrome represents bacterial infection of the urinary tract in a high proportion of cases. Single dose antibiotic therapy is known to be effective for *adult* women with this syndrome (amoxicillin, 2 or 3 g, po; sulfisoxazole, 1 g, po; or trimethoprim/sulfamethoxazole, 1 or 2 double strength tablets po). Efficacy of single dose antibiotic therapy for adolescents has *not* been well studied. One study showed that 3-day treatment with trimethoprim/sulfamethoxazole (one double strength tablet twice daily) was more effective than a single dose treatment with this antibiotic when urine culture had $>10^5$ colonies/ml. As a general rule, a short course of therapy (single dose or 3-day) has not been demonstrated conclusively to be effective in infants and children.

Dysuria associated with sexually transmitted diseases at any age responds to treatment for the specific infection. Sexually active adolescents with urethritis or vaginitis caused by *Chlamydia* may be treated with doxycycline (100 mg BID for 10 days), tetracycline (500 mg qid for 7 days), or erythromycin (500 mg qid for 7 days). Erythromycin at this high a dose may be accompanied by an unacceptable rate of gastrointestinal side effects. Gonorrhea, trichomononas, and candidal infections should be treated according to standard practice (see Chap. 195).

Pinworm infestation responds to a single 100-mg dose of mebendazole, but pruritus and dysuria may persist for several days. Physical or chemical irritation of the urethra or perineum decreases with the removal of the offending irritant and by the use of sitz baths in warm water for 20 to 30 minutes, 3 or 4 times daily. Hydroxyzine may reduce the itching of varicella. If analgesia is desired, acetaminophen (10 mg/kg/dose), or phenazopyridine (100 mg/dose) may alleviate pain. Aspirin (10 mg/kg/dose) may be used if the child does not have varicella or influenza.

INDICATIONS FOR REFERRAL OR HOSPITALIZATION

Dysuria associated with pyelonephritis may require management in hospital. Children who have evidence of bladder obstruction, urethral prolapse, abnormal urinary stream, or urethral trauma need a urologic evaluation. Sexually abused children may need hospitalization for protective reasons and *must* be referred to social services. The child who has pollakiuria may require a referral to a psychologist.

ANNOTATED BIBLIOGRAPHY

Asnes RS, Mones RL: Pollakiuria. Pediatrics 52:615–617, 73 (Reports on 4 cases and discusses the differential diagnosis of increased frequency of urination.)

Bauer SB, Retik AB et al: The unstable bladder of childhood. Urol Clin North Am 7:321–336, 1980 (Report on 110 children with symptoms of lower urinary tract dysfunction.)

Green M: Pediatric Diagnosis, Chap. 70—Symptoms referable to the urinary tract, pp 548–550. Philadelphia, WB Saunders, 1980 (Section on the characteristics of urination goes through frequency, oliguria, polyuria, the urinary stream, and incontinence, and outlines the signs and symptoms of each complaint.)

Hellerstein S: Urinary Tract Infections in Children, Chap. 7—The frequency-dysuria syndrome, pp 96–104. Chicago, Year Book Medical Publishers, 1982 (Review of the causes, diagnosis, and treatment of frequency and dysuria in patients who do not have bacteriuria.)

Hinman F: Syndromes of vesical incoordination. Urol Clin North Am 7:311–319, 1980 (Syndromes of vesical incoordination and available treatment are categorized.)

Kommaroff AL: Acute dysuria in women. N Engl J Med 310:368–375, 1984 (Reviews the causes and treatment of dysuria in adult women and provides an updated definition of "positive" urine culture. The author cautions that his discussion cannot be applied to "children of either sex or to men." However, it seems reasonable to expect that adolescent girls, especially if sexually active, would fit into most of the classifications discussed.)

Schmitt BD: Daytime wetting (diurnal enuresis). Pediatr Clin North Am 29:9–20, 1982 (Excellent review of the causes of daytime wetting, including a section on daytime frequency (pollakiuria) as well as appendix with instructions for the parent.)

Tunnessen WW Jr: Signs and Symptoms in Pediatrics, Chap. 74—Dysuria, pp 394–396. Philadelphia, JB Lippincott, 1983 (Causes of dysuria and associated signs and symptoms are discussed.)

116
Proteinuria
CRAIG B. LANGMAN

Proteinuria is one of the most common abnormalities that is frequently discovered on a routine urinalysis. It may be accompanied by other signs and symptoms of parenchymal renal disease or it may occur as the sole manifestation of an underlying nephropathy. It may also be seen in various benign or self-limited conditions that carry a uniformly good prognosis. The differentiation by the clinician of a disease state from a benign condition may be a difficult task. This chapter offers an approach to determine the etiology of proteinuria.

PATHOPHYSIOLOGY

Healthy children may excrete up to 4 mg/M^2 body surface area/hr of protein. Normal adults may excrete up to 150 mg/24 hrs. This protein consists of 40% albumin, 40% tissue proteins derived from the kidney and other urinary structures, 15% immunoglobulins, and 5% other plasma proteins.

The glomerulus normally provides a barrier to the leak of proteins into the urine when the molecular size is 40,000 or less and in a charge specific manner to exclude anionic species such as albumin. In proteinuric states the normal steric hindrance and charge selectivity of the glomerulus may be altered so that an inceased amount of protein is deposited in the urine and exceeds the tubular capacity for reabsorption.

The tubular portion of the nephron is primarily responsible for the reabsorption of small molecular weight and size proteins, such as α_2 protein, β_2 microglobulin, and smaller gamma globulins. The presumed mechanism for tubular proteinuria is the ineffective reabsorption of normally filtered proteins, although experimental and clinical evidence is scarce.

DETECTION

A commonly employed method of detection of protein in the urine is that of the citrate-buffered tetrabromophenol coloriometric ("dipstick") test. This test depends on urinary protein, especially albumin, to alter a pH sensitive dye, resulting in the characteristic deepening green appearance of the dipstick with an increasing amount of proteinuria. This test is termed *qualitative*, as the "amount" of protein detected on the dipstick is greatly affected by the specific gravity of the urine that is tested. Thus, normal amounts of urine protein may be read as positive if the urine is highly concentrated; similarly, abnormal amounts of urine protein may not be detected if the urine is sufficiently dilute. False positive urines may occur in excessively alkaline urines.

A semiquantitative test to detect the abnormal excretion of protein is the ratio of urinary protein to creatinine, both of which are determined biochemically. Normal values in children are <0.1, but may be affected by altered patterns of creatinine excretion.

The most accurate method to measure urinary protein excretion is by a timed urine collection; collection is usually 12 or 24 hours. The adequacy of such a collection may be independently assessed by the level of creatinine excretion, which should be at least 10 to 15 mg/kg/24 hrs. Protein excretion <4 mg/M^2/hr is normal, and higher values are abnormal.

DIFFERENTIAL DIAGNOSIS

Pseudoproteinuria

There are several situations in which the clinician may find that the dipstick is positive for protein, but quantitation reveals no proteinuria. Patients receiving semisynthetic penicillins excrete a breakdown product in their urine that reacts in a false-positive manner with the reagent on the dipstick. Additionally, Zephiran and some radiocontrast agents will also cause a false-positive reaction on the dipstick.

Other Benign Conditions in Which Proteinuria Occurs

There are three major entities in this category and renal function remains normal in a long-term follow-up evaluation. The first of these conditions may account for as much as 25% to 30% of proteinuria on random, in-office urinalyses, and is termed *orthostatic proteinuria*. The child excretes abnormal amounts of urinary protein (>4 mg/M^2/hr) when in the upright position but excretes normal amounts of protein when in the recumbent position. This is easily diagnosed by using two timed urine collections; that is, one from the recumbent position and one from the standing position. A protocol employed at our institution to document orthostatic proteinuria is the collection of the first morning void after the patient has emptied the bladder at bedtime the night before and has remained asleep in bed during the period of collection. The standing sample is a collection of urine following that first void for the remainder of the day and including the bedtime void that night. It is therefore essential to document *normal* protein excretion in the "recumbent" specimen. Greater than 50-year follow-up of patients with orthostatic proteinuria has documented normal renal function in all patients in whom renal function was normal at the outset.

The other entity of altered protein excretion that has a benign outlook is that of *exercise-induced proteinuria*. This entity is commonly seen in healthy adolescents and also carries an excellent prognosis. One method to detect this entity involves having the patient void, run up and down stairs for several minutes, and then void again. Commonly, the first voided urine is negative and the post-exercise urine is strongly positive for protein.

The outlook of *fever-induced proteinuria* is also excellent. Any febrile state may be accompanied by proteinuria, presumably resulting from an increased glomerular filtration rate. This proteinuria immediately disappears when the fever abates.

Proteinuria of Renal Origin

Documentation of other causes of an abnormal amount of protein is indicative of significant renal pathology. Proteinuria is usually classified as either glomerular or tubular in origin, depending on the site of entry of the protein into the urine. Several clinical pictures may be differentiated in each type of proteinuria. Protein excretion rates that are less than 40 mg/M^2/hr are compatible with proteinuria of either type, but greater amounts of proteinuria occur with glomerular protein leakage only.

The major clinical syndromes in which glomerular proteinuria occurs may be divided into three entities: acute nephritic syndrome, nephrosis, or chronic renal insufficiency.

The acute nephritic syndrome is associated with hematuria (occasionally macroscopic in nature) and often with red cell casts in the urine. Systemic hypertension and edema may be present on physical examination, and mild azotemia may be present in the blood. In contrast, 85% of children from 2 to 10 years of age who have nephrosis have a urine that only contains protein in amounts greater than 40 mg/M^2/hr. The other components of the syndrome include hypoalbuminemia and edema, often with accompaning hyperlipidemia. However, 20% of these patients may also have associated microscopic hematuria. Patients with chronic renal insufficiency, in addition to glomerular proteinuria, often have a telescoped urine sediment that consists of casts of acute and chronic nature. Hypertension is common, and azotemia is present. Growth failure may also be manifest.

Many systemic diseases have associated glomerular proteinuria. The most common in children include poststreptococcal glomerulonephritis, Henoch–Schönlein purpura, nephritis, and systemic lupus erythematosus. Essential hypertension is distinctly uncommon as the cause of proteinuria in a hypertensive child and should alert the clinician to other underlying renal pathology. Diseases intrinsic to the kidney that result in glomerular proteinuria include Berger's (IgA) nephropathy, hereditary nephritis (of which Alport's syndrome is one example) and the variants of childhood nephrosis (focal glomerulosclerosis, membranous nephropathy, and membranoproliferative glomerulonephritis).

Lastly, diabetes mellitus is a frequent cause of fixed proteinuria when the disease has been present for more than 10 years. However, children with di-

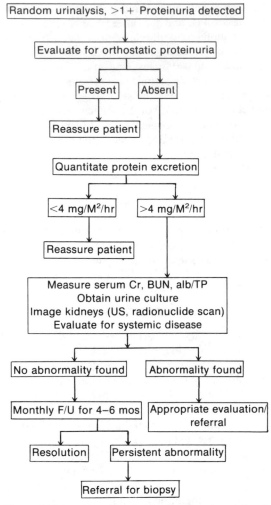

Figure 116-1. Algorithm for evaluation of proteinuria. (CR = creatinine; BUN = blood urea nitrogen; Alb = albumin; TP = total protein; US = ultrasound)

abetes less than 10 years may have exercise-induced proteinuria as an early manifestation of diabetic nephropathy, and it carries a worse prognosis only in this group of patients.

Tubulointerstitial diseases resulting in proteinuria on the urinalysis may be subdivided into acute or chronic in nature. Acute interstitial nephritis is usually secondary to immunologic disorders, drug hypersensitivity, or infections. Drug hypersensitivity, or reactions may also have accompanying hematuria and eosinophiliuria; eosinophilia may rarely be present as well. A fever and a rash may also be present. Drugs commonly associated with acute interstitial inflammation include antibiotics, especially the β-lactam classes and nonsteroidal anti-inflammatory drugs.

Immunologic disorders, including collagen vascular diseases, that cause interstitial nephritis and proteinuria are generally associated with elevated serum gamma globulins or cryoglobulins.

The tubular proteinuria that occurs in pyelonephritis generally resolves when the infection is eradicated. The persistence of proteinuria is usually indicative of either a structural abnormality, an indolent infection, or a stone. Chronic interstitial diseases are commonly the result of infections, drugs, poisonings with heavy metals, genetic diseases, or of immunologic nature.

Urinary tract malformations, especially any form of obstructive uropathy, and ureteral reflux without obstructive uropathy may also be associated with proteinuria. In a few cases, this proteinuria may reflect the earliest detectable abnormalities. It is, therefore, recommended to document normal genitourinary structure in the child who has proteinuria at the time of a bacterial urinary infection.

Chronic tubulointerstitial diseases may be associated with blood electrolyte abnormalities, and these elecrolyte changes in combination with the finding of proteinuria may be the clue to the presence of the underlying nephropathy. The electrolyte abnormalities commonly take the form of an acidosis; if proximal in origin, hypokalemia is present, and if distal in origin, hyperkalemia is seen. In addition, the inability to concentrate the urine, that is a fixed isosthenuria, may also be observed. If suspected, a water deprivation test *should not* be performed without clinical observation because of the risk of significant dehydration.

WORK-UP

Figure 116-1 depicts an easy, cost-effective way to evaluate a child with proteinuria found on routine urinalysis. If the urine specific gravity is reflective of urinary concentration (specific gravity >1.020) and trace or 1 + protein is found on dipstick testing,

the physician can reassure the patient of the likely benign nature of the finding. If a dipstick reading of >1 + is found, orthostatic proteinuria should be evaluated as the cause and, if documented, the patient should again be reassured. If testing reveals recumbent proteinuria, then a formal quantitation of urine protein excretion should be undertaken. There is no role in the usual clinical setting for fractionation of urine protein into albumin, globulins, and so forth, because most children and adults excrete, almost exclusively, only albumin. If significant proteinuria is demonsrated (>4 mg M^2/hr), an appropriate history, physical examination, and laboratory investigation (Fig. 116-1). should be planned, remembering the major clinical syndromes of proteinuria mentioned earlier.

INDICATIONS FOR REFERRAL

An abnormality in addition to the significant proteinuria demands a further evaluation or reterral. If proteinuria is the sole abnormality and persists for 4 to 6 months on monthly follow-up visits, a referral to a pediatric nephrologist is warranted for eventual renal biopsy. This will allow a histologic diagnosis that may also have prognostic implications.

ANNOTATED BIBLIOGRAPHY

Milteny M: Urinary protein excretion in healthy children. Clin Nephrol 12:216–221, 1979 (Comprehensive study of the constituents of proteinuria in children, including neonates.)

Springberg PS, Garrett LE, Thompson AL et al: Fixed and reproducible orthostatic proteinuria: Results of a 20-year follow-up study. Ann Intern Med 97:516–519, 1982 (Sixty-four patients initially studied as adolescents and restudied 20 years later remained free of functional renal impairment.)

West CD: Asymptomatic hematuria and proteinuria in children: Causes and appropriate diagnostic studies. Pediatr 89:173–182, 1976 (Classic paper by one of the best clinicians of pediatric nephrology.)

117
Hematuria
CRAIG B. LANGMAN

The appearance of macroscopic blood in the urine is one of the most frightening signs that occurs to parents and patients, although it may not portend serious disease. Alternatively, the presence of microscopic hematuria, a potentially grave sign of serious renal pathology, is often treated lightly by the physician and parent/patient. In this chapter the chronic, serious disorders associated with hematuria are separated from the disorders that may be self-limited, reversible, preventable, or, if chronic, nonthreatening to normal renal function.

PATHOPHYSIOLOGY

Red blood cells may enter the urinary tract from the level of the glomerulus to the urethral meatus and may result in either macroscopic or microscopic hematuria. Therefore, the mere presence of isolated red blood cells in the random urinalysis may not be helpful in the determination of where bleeding in the urinary tract is occurring.

The presence of blood in the urinary space is, in itself, not painful; therefore, the occurrence of painful hematuria should alert the clinician to search for an underlying cause in which hematuria also occurs.

Glomerular inflammation presumably damages the capillary basement membrane so that a diapedesis of red blood cells ensues. If the exit of red blood cells into the urinary space is brisk, gross hematuria may result in the characteristic brownish red color of the urine. However, if the leak of red cells is slower, only microscopic hematuria will be manifest. Interestingly, the degree of glomerular inflammation (assessed either pathologically or clinically) does not correlate with the presence of gross hematuria. There are no studies to document that red cell excretion is constant for any particular degree of glomerular inflammation, and thus several urines should be examined to determine the presence or absence of red blood cells.

Red blood cells that enter the urinary stream below the level of the nephron unit (glomerulus and tubules) are more likely to manifest as gross hematuria, although again the severity of such lesions does not correlate with actual red cell excretion rates.

DETECTION

Children quickly learn that the color of normal urine does not include the color red or brown. Thus, children as young as 3 years of age may report gross hematuria to their parents, or at least be able to give a historical reply to its presence when asked by the clinician. Gross hematuria often appears tea-colored, presumably because of the breakdown of heme pigments present in the hemoglobin of red blood cells.

A microscopic hematuria is easily detected in the random urinalysis with the use of the common "dipstick" examination or with a direct microscopic examination of the urinary sediment. The "dipstick" evaluation for the detection of blood relies on a chemical reaction (orthotoluidine oxidation) that detects the presence of heme pigment. The test is exquisitely sensitive, so that only 5 to 10 red blood cells per high power field may cause a positive reaction. On direct microscopic examination of the urinary sediment, 3 to 5 red blood cells per high power field may be viewed as normal in the pediatric population.

DIFFERENTIAL DIAGNOSIS

Pseudohematuria

The clinician must remain aware of the false positive findings of "hematuria" by the dipstick examination; therefore, all positive readings should be followed by the direct microscopic examination of the urinary sediment to document the degree of red cell excretion. Because the chemical reaction in the dipstick detects heme pigments, other heme-containing proteins in the urine will give a false positive reaction. The most common interfering heme pigment comes from myoglobin. Myoglobinuria, which may be either benign (after strenuous exercise) or indicative of more severe systemic pathology (*e.g.*, muscle trauma, child abuse or viral myositis), will therefore cause a false positive reaction;

however, severe myoglobinuria may itself cause a glomerular lesion and lead to red cell presence in the urine. This latter situation should be apparent from the clinical history and the physical examination. Myoglobin may be detected in the urine by a myoglobin-specific electrophoretic assay.

Free hemoglobin in the urine (hemoglobinuria) will also give a positive dipstick examination. Although hemoglobinuria may be seen clinically during transfusion reactions, or after severe burn injuries, exogenous chemicals are more common causes of the disorder. These include several toxic compounds (*e.g.*, chloroform, oxalic acid, potassium chlorate) found in household agents and compounds toxic only to patients with G6PD deficiency, such as sulfonamides and fava beans.

Exogenous substances may produce a dark brown or red urine, although red cell excretion is normal. Such substances include the aniline dyes used for coloring candy, the naturally occurring pigments of berries (elderberry and blackberry), and phenolphthalein, used in laxative preparations.

Lastly, the ingestion of several drinks containing chemical coloring agents may cause *gross hematuria* (*i.e.*, the presence of bright red urine). However, the dipstick and microscopic examination will reveal the absence of red cells. It is also important to remember that this clinical situation may be associated with *melena* or *hematochezia*.

The dipstick may occasionally be positive for blood although the microscopic examination is negative. This may be artifactual, because the exposure of red cells to dilute urine will produce hypotonic cell lysis. Thus, an examination of a freshly prepared urinary sediment will substantially reduce the likelihood of this phenomenon.

Newborn infants may have a pinkish color to their urine as the result of a large amount of urate excretion. This is easily confirmed by the presence of typical urate crystals on microscopic examination of the urinary sediment. However, red cell excretion is normal in this transient condition.

Extrarenal Hematuria

It is uncommon for urinary bleeding to be the sole manifestation of systemic bleeding disorders. However, it is common to see gross and microscopic hematuria when there is a systemic disturbance in the hemostatic process. Thus, blood in the urine has been seen with thrombocytopenia, disseminated intravascular coagulation (apart from true renal pathology, which may coexist), and in specific coagulation factor disorders (inherited and acquired).

Glomerular Hematuria

The pathognomonic finding of glomerular hematuria is red cell casts in the urinary sediment. Casts are formed from red cells embedded in a proteinaceous matrix, which has a distinct three-dimensional character under the microscope. Glomerular hematuria may be divided into acute nephritic, chronic nephritic, and nephrotic conditions.

Acute glomerulonephritis may be part of a systemic process, as in systemic lupus erythematosus, Henoch–Schönlein purpura, or hemolytic-uremic syndrome, or be isolated to the kidney, as in post-streptococcal glomerulonephritis. Generally, significant proteinuria is also present. The hematuria may be gross or microscopic.

Chronic glomerulonephritis associated with hematuria as the presenting complaint includes two important entities, Berger's disease and hereditary nephritis. Berger's disease is a chronic, relapsing cause of recurrent gross and microscopic hematuria and often, proteinuria. This entity, which is characterized pathologically by the presence of IgG–IgA immune complexes in the glomerular mesangium, is often precipitated by an innocent viral infection or strenuous physical exertion. The prognosis is uniformly good in children who present without an elevated serum creatinine or nephrotic range proteinuria. Hereditary nephritis comprises many inherited glomerular disorders, the best known of which is Alport's syndrome, in which a hearing loss is an important feature. A careful family history is important, because affected family members may only show microscopic hematuria in the early phases of the disease. Although gross hematuria is seen frequently in adult patients with polycystic kidney disease, it is not common in children with that disease.

Childhood nephrosis, in which minimal change nephrotic syndrome represents the most common histologic variety, has microscopic hematuria associated with it in 22% of cases. However, the other histologic varieties of childhood nephrosis have a higher prevalence of hematuria. The presence of either hypertension or azotemia and hematuria, in the context of childhood nephrosis, should alert the clinician to the presence of a lesion other than minimal change.

Renal vascular disorders may also be associated with hematuria. Both renal vein thrombosis and renal arterial embolus/thrombus formation have associated gross or microscopic hematuria.

The clinical history and physical examination should point to one of these possible diagnoses in which hematuria is a frequent, but not isolated, finding.

Interstitial-Tubular Hematuria

Although any tubulointerstitial disorder may be associated with microscopic hematuria, the most important condition seen clinically is that of idiopathic hypercalciuria. This inherited disorder in which excessive urinary calcium excretion occurs has been associated with the presence of gross and microscopic hematuria. It may be detected by the finding of an elevated urinary calcium to creatinine ratio (mg/mg) from randomly obtained urine (values >0.18 are abnormal) and the demonstration of an increased 24-hour excretion of calcium (to >4 mg/kg body weight). Except for several cases of Berger's disease, no other renal lesions coexist with this cause of hematuria. Hematuria in idiopathic hypercalciuria is commonly recurrent, but rarely painful as would occur if a renal stone were causing hematuria.

Extrarenal Hematuria

The entry of red blood cells into the urine beyond the tubulointerstitial area of the kidney may be the result of an abnormality in the collecting system (renal pelvis), the ureter, the bladder, and the urethra. These disorders more commonly result in bright red, rather than brownish, gross hematuria; however, either may occur in a particular patient with extrarenal hematuria.

Anatomic dilatation of the renal pelvis, seen in ureteropelvic junction obstruction, is associated with hematuria, and occasionally, proteinuria. This lesion may be silent until hematuria is discovered after otherwise innocent abdominal (or flank) blunt trauma. Diseases in which hydroureter is present (*e.g.*, reflux nephropathy) are commonly associated with hematuria.

Another important cause of hematuria secondary to dilatation of the pelvis is a Wilm's tumor. This common mesodermal tumor of childhood is generally associated with an abdominal mass and, possibly, systemic arterial hypertension.

Unilateral ureteral bleeding is seen commonly in patients with either sickle trait or sickle disease hemoglobinopathies. The exact mechanism of the ureteral bleeding is unknown, but may involve altered vascular integrity as the result of reduced oxygen tension in the renal papillae, collecting system, and ureter. Gross hematuria is the most common presentation of this condition and should be suspected in any individual with these hemoglobinopathies.

Bladder inflammation that results in hematuria is generally related to the presence of a urinary tract infection. Although a bacterial infection is the most common etiology, viral cystitis (especially adenoviral cystitis) is associated with painless gross hematuria. Other anatomic lesions of the bladder may also be associated with hematuria, although other clinical manifestations may predominate.

Isolated ureteral inflammation, as seen in tuberculosis, is an uncommon cause of hematuria. Urethral inflammation as a cause of hematuria is rare in the first decade of life, but assumes greater clinical importance in the teenager in whom sexually acquired nongonococcal urethritis is a relatively common cause of hematuria and dysuria. Frequent masturbation in men may be associated with hematuria, presumably on the basis of urethral irritation. Foreign bodies placed in the urethra commonly produce a purulent discharge, with hematuria as often a minor component of the clinical picture. Urethroprostatitis may be associated with significant hematuria in childhood. Meatal ulceration in circumcised newborns is a special situation that may cause gross hematuria.

Renal Trauma

Minor blunt trauma to the renal fossae or abdomen may be associated with microscopic hematuria. Generally, this is the result of a small renal contusion, but rarely, may be the result of significant lesions of the renal vascular or collecting systems. However, the absence of hematuria after significant trauma should not be interpreted as evidence of a lack of renal trauma; complete rupture of the kidney may not be associated with any abnormalities of the urinalysis unless the contralateral kidney is also (less severely) damaged.

Miscellaneous Causes of Hematuria

Essential hematuria is a diagnosis of exclusion, in which microscopic hematuria is not associated with any demonstrable pathology. However, because many more patients with microscopic hematuria are evaluated for the presence of idiopathic hypercalciuria, the diagnosis of essential hematuria is seldom made in the pediatric population. Familial

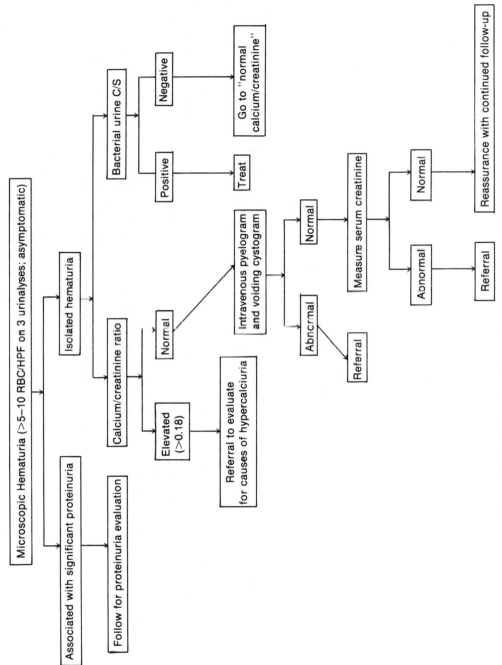

Figure 117-1. Evaluation of the patient with microscopic hematuria.

519

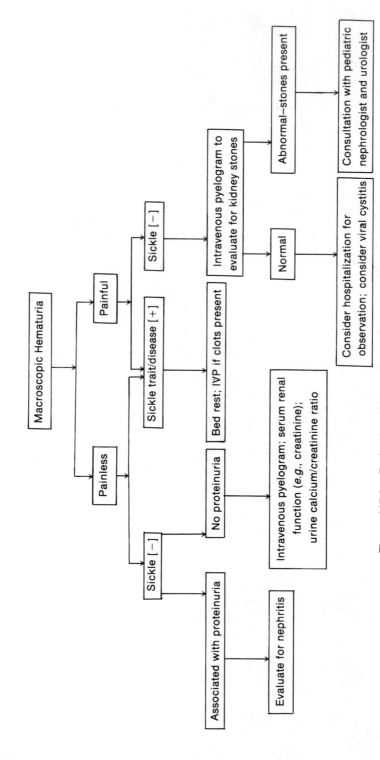

Figure 117-2. Evaluation of the patient with macroscopic hematuria.

hematuria is closely allied to both of these conditions. There is no progression to chronic renal insufficiency in either condition. Papillary necrosis may present with gross or microscopic hematuria. This disorder is seen in children with sickle cell trait and anemia, severe and chronic pyelonephritis, and secondary to chronic analgesic abuse (including acetaminophen, phenacetin, and aspirin). The condition may be associated with flank pain. On rare occasions, flank papillae or fragments can be seen in the urine.

DIAGNOSTIC EVALUATION AND INDICATIONS FOR REFERRAL

A logical approach to the evaluation of a child with hematuria may be based on the initial presentation: microscopic hematuria, painless or painful gross hematuria, as suggested in the following algorithms (Figs. 117-1 and 117-2). The demonstration of a single urinalysis with an abnormal red cell excretion (>5 RBC/HPF) should be repeated two to three more times in 7 to 14 days. The evaluation should proceed if three such urinalyses demonstrate hematuria. If subsequent urinalyses fail to demonstrate hematuria, the clinician is advised to recheck the urine in 1 month's time and, if still normal, again in 6 months, before assigning a benign outcome to the initial finding.

If only isolated microscopic hematuria is demonstrated, in the absence of a bacterial urinary infection, an evaluation for hypercalciuria is suggested. If that evaluation is normal, and the hematuria is persistent, formal anatomic studies with intravenous pyelography and voiding cystourethrography are suggested. Renal ultrasonography may be substituted for the intravenous pyelogram as an initial noninvasive study. At this time, serum renal function should be evaluated by the measurement of serum creatinine concentration. If all evaluations are normal, and the hematuria persists, a diagnosis of essential hematuria may be made.

If the child presents with painful gross hematuria, the clinician is encouraged to obtain an intravenous pyelogram, once the child is well hydrated. Consultation is almost always required for the child with painful gross hematuria. Alternatively, if painless gross hematuria occurs, and the patient is without a disorder in which hemoglobin S is present, a consultation is again suggested in pediatric nephrology if proteinuria is present and in pediatric urology if proteinuria is absent. It is also important to document the level and site of bleeding in the patient with a sickle hemoglobinopathy, and the guidance of pediatric urologists is helpful in this regard. (see Fig. 117-2 for indications for admission to the hospital.)

ANNOTATED BIBLIOGRAPHY

Northway JD: Hematuria in children. J Pediatr 78:381–396, 1971 (Although several of the known disorders of microscopic hematuria are still ill-defined in children (hypercalciuria, Berger's disease), this "oldie-but-goodie" article gives an excellent clinical and common sense approach to the evaluation of children with hematuria of diverse origin.)

Pardo V, Berian MG, Levi DF, Strauss J: Benign primary hematuria. Am J Med 67:817–822, 1979 (Convincing pathologic evidence of the benign nature of hematuria in the absence of a positive evaluation.)

Vehaskari VM, Rapola J, Koskimies O et al: Microscopic hematuria in schoolchildren: Epidemiology and clinicopathologic evaluation. J Pediatr 95:676–684, 1979 (Almost 9000 children between 8 and 15 years of age were screened for hematuria, and only 1% had increased red cell excretion in two or more urinalyses. Importantly, coexisting proteinuria alone was associated with important abnormalities on renal biopsy. Their conclusion is important to remember: low-grade hematuria, without other findings referrable to the kidneys, probably represents the upper range of the physiologic variation in red cell excretion.)

118
Undescended Testes

PETER B. H'DOUBLER, JR. AND
ROBERT P. FOGLIA

Cryptorchidism, a word derived from the Greek *cryptos* (hidden) and *orchis* (testis), is the general term used to define all forms of undescended testes. This is not an uncommon problem and causes considerable anxiety and concern for parents and patients.

EMBRYOLOGY

The development of the testis in the embryo begins in the abdomen. Testicular descent starts in the seventh fetal month, and over the subsequent weeks the testis progresses through the inguinal canal, out of the external ring, and into the scrotum. This descent is guided by the gubernaculum, a muscular cord that extends between the scrotum and testis.

Testicular descent is influenced by the presence of gonadotropic and androgenic hormones during fetal development. The failure of the testes to descend into the scrotum during fetal life may in part be related to either a lack of these hormones or the inability of the testes to respond to them. Despite this, there is no clear evidence to suggest that a cryptorchid testis with mechanical obstruction to its descent will further descend in response to exogenous or endogenous hormones.

DIFFERENTIAL DIAGNOSIS

Several types of undescended testes should be distinguished, because pathophysiology and treatment are different.

Anorchia, the complete absence of a testis, can occur on infrequent occasions. It is more common on the right side and the ipsilateral scrotum is underdeveloped. Because of their common embryologic background, agenesis of the kidney and ureter may occur in association with an absent testis.

The true undescended testis has undergone an arrest of its descent along its normal route to the scrotum. Approximately 3% of male newborns and 20% of premature male infants have undescended testes at birth. By 1 year of age, over 80% of all cryptorchid testes at birth are in the scrotum. Of those testes not in the scrotum at 1 year of age, perhaps one third are merely retractile so that a true undescended testis occurs in ~0.4% of males. Roughly 14% of boys with cryptorchidism come from families with members who have had this condition. Approximately 65% of children with an undescended testis will have a hernia sac associated with the testis and cord structures.

A retractile testis is a physiologic variation of normal and is the result of an overactive cremasteric muscular reflex and incomplete attachment of the testis to the scrotum by the gubernaculum. This results in the testis being held in a higher position during periods of muscular stimulation such as with activity or in a cold environment. The retractile testis is often bilateral. As the child gets older, the testis becomes larger and the cremasteric reflex becomes less active so that the previously retractile testis remains in the scrotum.

The examination of the child with a suspected undescended testis is begun by first ensuring that the room is warm and that the examiner's hands are not cold. The scrotum should be inspected because with a cryptorchid testis, the scrotum is usually not fully developed on the affected side. When the child is relaxed and in a supine position, the examiner's hand is then swept from the anterior superior iliac spine over the inguinal canal and towards the pubis in an attempt to palpate a testis. This procedure should be done several times and, if unsuccessful, it should also be done with the child in a cross-legged, squatting, and standing position. 85% of testes not in the scrotum will be located in this manner. The position, consistency, and size of the testis should be noted both in comparison to the contralateral testis and to the testes of boys of similar age.

If the testis is not in the scrotum, several possibilities exist. It may be *truly undescended* having suffered an arrest to its descent. The true undescended testis may be in the inguinal canal or may be in an intra-abdominal location (and not palpable). Most undescended testes are caused by a mechanical factor, a shortened spermatic artery not allowing the testis to descend into the scrotum. Alternatively, the testis may be in an ectopic position having descended through the inguinal canal, passed through the external ring, but then having come to rest in a position in the superficial inguinal space, thigh, or perineum. (Another possibility is that it is a *retractile testis*. If the testis can be palpated in the inguinal canal or in a position over the pubis and with manipulation can be brought down into the scrotum then this by definition is a retractile testis.) It is important to distinguish a retractile testis from an undescended testis because the former will function normally, will descend as the cremasteric reflex lessens, and does not require operative treatment.

The undescended testis may have become arrested in its descent, may have undergone an in utero torsion, or may be a dysgenetic testis. A careful examination of the testis at the time of operation is essential because the markedly atrophic testis should be excised; likewise, a testis that appears abnormal should be biopsied.

It is a common misconception that an undescended testis will spontaneously descend during or after puberty. This is probably due to observation of this phenomenon in patients with retractile testes. There is no evidence to suggest that pubescent changes, either hormonal or growth related, will cause the migration of a true undescended testis into the scrotum.

COMPLICATIONS OF CRYPTORCHIDISM

Spermatogenesis

Failure of the testis to descend into the scrotum leaves it subjected to a body temperature of 1.5°C to 2.5°C higher than that of the scrotum. This may severely retard the normal maturation of the gonad. Testicular growth begins at birth and proceeds continuously. Studies of testicular biopsies show that cryptorchid testes have a normal morphology and germ cell content during the first 2 years of life. However, after this time, there is a significant decrease in germ cell content, tubular growth, progressive degenerative changes, and significant dysmorphic features developing in the undescended testis of the 2- to 5-year-old. Furthermore, it has been suggested that autoantibodies may be produced by the presence of a cryptorchid testis that may cause degenerative changes in the opposite normally descended testis. Thus, an untreated undescended testis may result in the inability of one or both gonads to produce normal mature sperm.

Malignancy

There is abundant literature concerning the relationship of cryptorchidism and testicular malignancy. Approximately 3% to 12% of testicular tumors develop in a cryptorchid testis. This indicates that the chance of developing a testicular malignancy is approximatly 40 times higher in an undescended testis than in a normal testis. The chance of malignancy occurring is almost five times higher in an intra-abdominal testis when compared to an inguinal testis. Most testicular tumors are of germ cell origin, thus raising the obvious question of the correlation of dysgenesis in the cryptorchid testis and the possible functional conseqence of this, the differentiation into a testicular malignancy. Several studies have also shown an increased incidence of malignant degeneration of the contralateral normally positioned scrotal testis. This may be due to dysgenetic features or may be secondary to hormonal influences by the cryptorchid testis.

The age at which the cryptorchid testis is operated on is important. The length of time a testis is subjected to an abnormal environment appears to influence its potential for malignancy. The most common age at which a testicular tumor is diagnosed is at 25 to 30 years. This is why pediatricians rarely see or hear of a testicular tumor developing in one of their patients who has an undescended testis. The age of the child at the time of operation appears to be important. In one review, the authors found that of all patients who subsequently developed a testicular malignancy after an orchidopexy, only 3% of these children were under 10 years of age at the time of orchidopexy.

If the degree of degenerative change is related to the incidence of malignancy, then it would follow that orchidopexy should be performed sooner rather than later. The undescended testis is also significantly more difficult to examine and monitor for the development of abnormalities.

Other complications of undescended testes include the greater vulnerability to trauma, hernia, the higher incidence of gonadal loss resulting from a torsion, and finally the anxiety and embarrassment expressed by both patients and parents, especially over the possibility of sterility. Therefore, a recommendation for treating the undescended testis can be made for the child who has this condition and is over 1 year of age.

TREATMENT

The goal of treatment is to bring the testis into a low scrotal position. Two methods have been used: hormonal and operative.

Hormonal

During embryologic development, testicular descent appears to be strongly influenced by the hypothalamic-pituitary axis. Because of this, both human chorionic gonadotropic (hCG) and gonadotropin releasing hormone (GnRH) have been used to treat cryptorchidism. The parenteral use of hCG has been associated with a 15% to 40% rate of successful testicular descent, and GnRH with a rate of 50% to 80%. Much conjecture has centered on the efficacy of hormonal therapy because many of the studies have not been well controlled. This is especially true in regard to defining whether the patient had a retractile testis or an undescended testis. One double blind study resulted in a 19% testicular descent rate with GnRH and only a 6% success rate with hCG. This study carefully excluded boys with retractile testes and is probably a major factor in the results. It would seem that if most cases of undescended testes are limited by mechanical factors such as a shortened spermatic artery or hernia, then the rationale for hormonal therapy is not convincing. In selected cases, however, such as when a testis is not palpable, hormonal therapy can be helpful. It causes an enlargement of the testis and may cause partial testicular descent. Both of these effects can make the subsequent orchidopexy easier.

Operative

Orchidopexy consists of the translocation of the testis from its anomalous position to a normal position in the scrotum by means of correcting the mechanical factors limiting its descent. The procedure is usually carried out on an outpatient basis and is performed through an inguinal incision. It is accomplished by freeing the spermatic vessels and cord from the often present hernia sac, opening the floor of the inguinal canal, and changing the course of the cord structures medially through the floor of the inguinal canal to achieve sufficient length to bring the testis into the scrotum without tension on the vessels. A small pocket is then made in a dependent position in the scrotum between the skin and dartos layer, a *dartos pouch*, to hold the testis in place.

At exploration, if the testis appears normal and is not intra-abdominal, it can usually be brought down into the scrotum without difficulty. The identification of a markedly atrophic or abnormal testis would indicate that the testis probably had undergone an in utero torsion or that it is dysgenetic. In this circumstance, the removal of the testis should be carried out because the risk of a subsequent malignant degeneration in that testis is higher than the probability of normal spermatogenesis and testosterone production from the testis.

If no testis is identified, and there are no spermatic vessels and vas deferens present, an abdominal exploration is necessary to exclude the possibility of an intra-abdominal testis. It has also been suggested that, because of the high risk of malignancy in an untreated cryptorchid testis, an orchiectomy should be performed for either an intra-abdominal or inguinal testis in postpubertal boys.

Orchidopexy can be carried out at any age but it appears that elective repair after 1 year of age is most sensible. Almost all boys with an undescended testis at birth will undergo spontaneous descent before their first birthday. Histologic evidence shows dysmorphic features in cryptorchid testes after the age of 2 to 3 years. As noted previously, there appears to be some relationship between the length of time the testis was in an abnormal position, and the subsequent development of a testicular malignancy, even after orchidopexy. The success rate after orchidopexy is measured longitudinally by the rate of fertility in these patients, and it is ~80%.

COMPLICATIONS

When performed by experienced surgeons, orchidopexy has a low rate of complications. Most complications are related to injury to the delicate blood supply to the testis or vas deferens, either by torsion or by undue tension during the procedure. A testis placed in the scrotum will infrequently retract back into the inguinal canal. Since the floor of the inguinal canal is reconstructed following the mobilization of the cord structures, there is a potential for the development of a direct inguinal hernia, but this is an unusual occurrence.

ANNOTATED BIBLIOGRAPHY

Fonkalsrud EW: The undescended testis. In Welch JK, Randolph JG, Ravitch MM et al (eds): Pediatric Surgery, 4th ed. Chicago, Yearbook Medical Publishers 1986 (Excellent overview and reference.)

Hadziselimovic F: Treatment of cryptorchidism with GnRH. Urol Clin North Am 9:413, 1982 (Written by one of the experts on the subject of hormonal therapy for undescended testes.)

Martin DC: Malignancy and the undescended testis. In Fonkalsrud EW, Mengel W (eds): The Undescended Testis, pp 144–156. Chicago, Yearbook Medical Publishers. 1981 (Good review of the influence of malignancy in this group of patients.)

Mengel W, Hienz HA, Sippe WG: Studies on cryptorchidism: A comparison of histologic findings in the germinal epithelium before and after the second year of life. J Pediatr Surg 9:445, 1974 (Evidence is presented to show that dysmorphic features can occur in an undescended testis early in childhood.)

Rajfer J, Handelsman DJ, Swerdloff RS et al: Hormonal therapy of cryptorchidism. A randomized double blind study comparing human chorionic gonadotropin and gonadotropin-releasing hormone. N Engl J Med 314:466–470, 1986 (This study carefully excluded boys with retractile testes and found a relatively low success rate with hormonal therapy.)

119
Genital Pain
SAMUEL H. KIM

Inguinal hernias and hydroceles are the most common abnormalities of the lower abdomen and scrotum (see Chap. 113 for a discussion of these conditions). Because most hernias and hydroceles are asymptomatic, children who are fussy, inconsolable, vomit, or refuse to eat must be regarded as having a surgical emergency (*e.g.*, a strangulated hernia, or a twisted ovary in the hernia sac of a girl). The less common, though not rare, causes of acute genital pain are the subject of this chapter.

ACUTE SCROTUM

When a male child appears with a tender hemiscrotum, the first diagnosis that should come to mind is torsion of the testis. This is the only diagnosis that will result in the loss of a testis if the diagnosis is not made expeditiously and surgical treatment immediately performed. Fortunately, it is not the most common reason for an acute scrotum (*i.e.*, scrotal pain and swelling followed by erythema and induration). In the child or adolescent with a testicular torsion, when seen early, the testis will be exquisitely tender and somewhat higher in the scrotum than normal. This is easier to diagnose on the left side because the testis on the left is usually lower than on the right. The overlying scrotum is edematous, erythematous, and, if seen early, the twist in the cord may be apparent. When seen late, a testicular torsion will show chronic thickened induration and erythema of the overlying skin and a mildly to moderately tender mass that cannot be anatomically distinguished within the scrotum. A testicular scan will often show a bull's eye effect where there is no blood supply coming from the scrotum and tunica. Surgery is mandatory in these patients but is usually too late. An orchiectomy should be carried out and, if feasible, a testicular prosthesis should be inserted at the same time. It is mandatory that if a child has had a torsion of the testis on one side, that the other side should be fixed to the back wall of the tunica and scrotum so that it cannot twist. This should be done either at the time of the initial surgery or, if seen at a later date, as an elective surgical procedure. When a newborn male has discoloration and a hard mass in the scrotum on one side, it is likely that this is a resolving intrauterine torsion. Surgery is often too late, but the patient should have a surgical consultation.

The most common cause of an acute scrotum is a torsion of an appendage of the epididymis, the appendix epididymis. This is a small teardrop structure that is present at the superior pole of the testis attached to the epididymis. A physical examination will reveal an acutely tender scrotum and testis, but the point of maximum tenderness will be well localized to the superior pole of the testis. There will be little swelling of the testis itself, and the testis will not be retracted up toward the groin. It is essential that a testicular scan or a Doppler test measuring blood flow to the affected testis be promptly carried out. The testicular scan will show normal or increased blood flow to the affected side in all conditions except testicular torsion, where the blood supply will be markedly diminished or interrupted. If there is any question that the blood supply is dimished, surgery should be carried out immediately. If, however, the blood supply to the affected side is nomal or increased, the patient does not need surgery but should be monitored closely. The natural history of an appendage torsion is that the patient will feel sore for about 1 week and then he will feel normal. A physical examination will be normal in about 3 to 4 weeks.

Epididymitis and epididymo-orchitis are unusual in children. When present, they occur most often in the adolescent who may or may not be sexually active. This infection is self-limited and rarely needs surgery. On a physical examination, the testis or epididymis is quite swollen, with the epididymis often more so than the testis. There is exquisite tenderness of the inflamed parts. There may or may not be a history of dysuria. A urine specimen, preferably after a prostatic massage, should be sent for culture. The management of these conditions include bedrest, ambulation with the use of an athletic supporter, sitz baths, antibiotics (*e.g.*, Bactrim) and mild analgesics when indicated. Prostatitis is rare in childhood.

TUMORS

Testicular tumors are rare in children. However, the presence of a hard, nontender, solid mass in the scrotum of a child should be considered a testicular tumor until proven otherwise. This can usually only be determined at the time of surgery. Fortunately, most of these tumors are benign, and a simple removal of the testis and cord is curative in most cases. The adolescent with a testicular tumor is more likely to have the adult types of tumors and, therefore, falls into the usually worse prognostic category of *testicular tumors of adults*.

TESTICULAR TRAUMA

It is obvious that a scrotal laceration in the child requires immediate attention. An injured testes in an intact scrotum is a subtler, yet equally urgent condition. A blunt truma can cause a ruptured testis requiring an immediate operation, with evacuation of the hematoma and reconstitution of the capsule of the testis. A physical examination of these patients will often show a severely ecchymotic scrotum and perineal area with a testis that is indistinguishable from the surrounding tissues. A testicular scan will often show good blood supply going to the testis. A surgical exploration should be carried out when the testis is not easily felt or if there is a large hematoma associated with the injury.

An injury where the testis is actually protruding out through a scrotal laceration should be covered with sterile saline-soaked gauzes and then wrapped while arrangements are made for an immediate operation.

PENILE SWELLING

The two most common causes of penile swelling in infants and children are infection and trauma. In the uncircumcised infant whose foreskin has been retracted forcefully and then not reduced, the child may end up with a paraphimosis whereby the foreskin forms a constricting ring around the shaft proximal to the glans. This will result in engorgement of the head of the penis and difficulty in reducing the retracted foreskin. This condition should be examined immediately by a surgeon or a urologist and a reduction should be carried out, surgically if necessary.

An infection of the foreskin (posthitis) or glans (balanitis) or both (balanoposthitis) is usually caused by poor hygiene and will cause exquisite tenderness. Pus may sometimes be seen between the hood of the foreskin and the head of the penis. Appropriate treatment with sitz baths and antibiotics (*e.g.*, Bactrim) followed by circumcision will remedy this situation in most cases.

An infrequent though devastating problem is that of a circumferential hair or hairs twisted around the corona of the circumcised male's penis or around the shaft of an infant's penis. These foreign bodies can form a constricting ring that will erode into the surrounding tissue and eventually cause gangrene if not detected and removed.

Finally, cysts may form on the shaft of the penis in the circumcised male related to the previous circumcision suture line. These cysts should be removed because of the possibility of infection. The cysts that are frequently seen under the uncircumcised foreskin are collections of dead skin (smegma deposits) because the area cannot be cleaned properly. These will usually lead to recurrent infections. With recurrent infections and increasing phimosis, a circumcision will be necessary.

ANNOTATED BIBLIOGRAPHY

Holder TM, Ashcraft KW, (eds): Pediatric Surgery, 1st ed. Philadelphia, WB Saunders, 1980 (Authoritative reference providing a more extensive discussion on the entities presented, as well as those selectively deleted because of their rarity.)

Noronho PA, Demir RH: Differentiating the acute scrotum. Hosp Practice March, 1984, pp 216–240.(Good review with references and nice diagrams; strongest on differential diagnosis.)

Welch KJ, Randolph JD, Ravitch MM et al (eds): Pediatric Surgery, 4th ed. Chicago, Yearbook, 1986 (Authoritative reference providing a more extensive discussion on the entities presented, as well as those selectively deleted because of their rarity.)

Wilkins EW Jr et al (eds): MGH Textbook of Emergency Medicine, 2nd ed. Baltimore, Williams and Wilkins, 1983 (Authoritative reference providing a more extensive discussion on the entities presented, as well as those selectively deleted because of their rarity.)

15

Gynecologic Problems

120
Vulvovaginitis

DEBORAH E. SMITH AND
JACOB A. LOHR

Complaints of perineal itching, soreness, or vaginal discharge are common throughout childhood and adolescence. Etiology, possible diagnoses, and appropriate management depend somewhat on the age of the patient. In younger girls, a knowledge of the anatomy of the prepubertal perineum and a consideration of daily living habits are as important as an understanding of vaginal microbiology. Infections do occur in this age group, but predominate in adolescents particularly after the onset of sexual activity. A more detailed discussion of the common sexually transmitted causes of vulvovaginitis is found in Chapter 195.

PREPUBERTAL VULVOVAGINITIS

Pathophysiology

A physiologic leukorrhea is common in the newborn girl. This is a mucous vaginal discharge that may be tinged with blood. It is caused by intrauterine maternal estrogen stimulation of the vaginal mucosa and a withdrawal at delivery. The leukorrhea gradually resolves within 2 to 3 weeks.

The prepubertal child is particularly susceptible to vulvovaginitis, and indeed this occurs in almost all girls at some stage. Without estrogen stimulation, the vaginal mucosa is thin, shiny, red, and atrophic. Vaginal secretions, which are minimal, have a neutral pH. The vagina is relatively close to the anus, and the preadolescent perineum lacks the protection of thick labia and pubic hair. In addition, once the child is out of diapers, toileting is less

closely supervised and wiping techniques are usually suboptimal. Thus, contamination of the vagina with bowel flora can be expected, with or without symptoms of vulvovaginitis. Normal prepubertal vaginal flora include diphtheroids, *Staphylococcus epidermidis*, α-hemolytic streptococci, and lactobacilli. *Escherichia coli* is frequently present and, in one series, was isolated from the vaginal secretions of 90% of girls under 3 years of age. It is less common with increasing age.

Clinical Presentation and Differential Diagnosis

Typical complaints include vulvar redness with discomfort such as itching, burning, or a discharge. The presentation is often late, and chronic excoriation may lead to superinfection.

Vulvar inflammation can be caused by poor perineal hygiene and by chronic abrasion from masturbation, contact with play equipment, or sitting in sand boxes. A chemical irritation may arise from the use of harsh soaps or bubble baths. The equivalent of diaper dermatitis can be associated with the wearing of tight-fitting nylon underpants, tights, jeans, or leotards, particularly in hot weather and in the overweight girl. Nonspecific vulvovaginitis is also associated with pinworm infestation causing perianal pruritus; scratching leads to perineal excoriation and secondary vulvitis. An adult pinworm may occasionally migrate to the vagina, giving rise to a discharge. A vaginal discharge with or without vulvitis can also be caused by a foreign body.

Specific infections are associated with vulvovaginitis in the prepubertal child. These include *Neisseria gonorrhoeae*, which in this age-group usually presents with a vulvovaginitis rather than a cervicitis. Trichomonas infections and condyloma acuminata (genital warts) are also possible etiologies. Although these three infections can be caused by proximity and careless contamination from infected people, sexual abuse must be considered. Other specific infections include group A β-hemolytic streptococcus and yeast (Candida albicans). Chlamydia trachomatis is now emerging as a cause of vulvovaginitis in young girls. The presentation is similar to gonorrheal infections, and the diagnosis and treatment are discussed in the adolescent section as well as in Chapter 195. A positive diagnosis implies sexual abuse.

Systemic diseases such as chickenpox, scarlet fever, and measles can cause a vaginitis, and similar symptoms may occur with an ectopic ureter, a pelvic abscess, or a fistula. Finally, some skin conditions including atopic dermatitis, seborrhea, or psoriasis may have an associated vulvitis.

Work-Up

History. Details of the presenting symptoms must be noted, including the chronicity and a description of any discharge (*e.g.*, quantity, color, or odor). A malodorous discharge is associated with a vaginal foreign body (typically, retained toilet tissue) or, much more rarely, with a shigella vaginitis or a necrotic tumor. Blood-stained discharge suggests trauma from play (*e.g.*, bike riding or playground equipment), sexual abuse, vulvar irritation secondary to pruritus or masturbation or, rarely, a tumor. A copious, purulent discharge or a thin mucoid discharge is found with streptococcal infections, and a greenish discharge is more typical of trichomoniasis, gonorrhea, or a foreign body. The child can be asked to demonstrate her technique for perineal wiping. A review of systems is useful, as is a history of recent illnesses such as streptococcal pharyngitis in the child or mother or use of antibiotics predisposing to a yeast infection. The physician must also consider asking directly about the possibility of sexual abuse or contact with infected adults.

Physical Examination. This starts with the general observation of the child and her clothing. A full examination is needed with particular attention paid to the perineal area. This may be seen with the child supine in a frog-leg position. She should be encouraged to assist with spreading apart her labia. A knee-to-chest position allows an excellent view of the vagina and frequently the cervix. It should be used when a foreign body is suspected and also for a culture collection. To assume the knee-to-chest position, the child is instructed to kneel and then lie forwards onto her chest and folded arms, keeping her bottom up. An otoscope can be used for vaginoscopy. A rectal examination may be needed to palpate a foreign body and to check for a normal pelvic anatomy.

Laboratory Tests. Tests are indicated when a vaginal discharge is purulent or persistent. Secretions can be collected using a cotton-tipped applicator moistened with nonbacteriostatic saline, or aspirated with a sterile medicine dropper. Wet preparations may show trichomonads or yeast. Yeast is not common but, if found, a urinalysis should be done to rule out glycosuria. A Gram stain may show *Neisseria gonorrhoeae* as gram-negative intracellular diplococci. Finally, specimens should be sent for culture, including media for gonorrhea and anaerobes. A syphilis test should be done if sexual abuse is suspected and particularly if there is a diagnosis of *Neisseria gonorrhoeae*, Trichomonas, or condyloma acuminatum. The scotch tape test for pinworms may be useful, and if it is the likely cause, the mother should also check the child's anus at night for adult worms.

Treatment

General measures will improve symptoms and should be encouraged. These include good wiping techniques (gently, from front to back), cotton underpants and loose-fitting clothes, and avoidance of bubble baths and other irritants. Sitz baths are useful twice or three times a day in plain warm water for 10 to 15 minutes. The perineum should be washed with a soft cloth with or without a mild soap, patted dry, and also air dried, if possible.

The majority (up to 85%) will have a nonspecific etiology with cultures growing out gram-negative organisms such as *Escherichia coli* or normal flora. Hydrocortisone cream 1% can be used for one or two treatments. For a persistent vulvovaginitis lasting 3 to 4 weeks, use a local application of an antibacterial cream (*e.g.*, AVC cream, Vagitrol, Sultrin) or use a broad spectrum oral antibiotic (ampicillin 50 mg/kg/day divided into four doses or cephalosporin) for 10 to 14 days. If symptoms continue, an estrogen cream (*e.g.*, Premarin or Dienestrol cream) will thicken the perineal epithelium, making it more resistant to infection. This should be prescribed for local use every night for 2 to 3 weeks and then every other night for an additional 2 weeks. Caution is needed because systemic absorption may cause increased vulvar pigmentation and breast tenderness, which is reversible.

Some patients present with an acute severe edematous vulvitis. Appropriate management includes 15-minute sitz baths every 4 hours. Baking soda or saline may be added to the water, but soap should be avoided. Air drying is preferable. Witch-hazel pads (Tucks) rather than toilet paper should be used for wiping. Within 2 to 3 days, symptoms should improve, and baths can then be alternated with the application of calamine lotion. For a more pruritic vulvitis, local applications of 1% hydrocortisone cream may be used.

Specific infections should be treated appropriately in addition to the general measures as listed above. Enterobius vermicularis (pinworms) infestations are treated with mebendazole (Vermox) one 100-mg tablet as a single dose for children of all ages. *Neisseria gonorrhoeae* vaginitis treatment regimens include amoxicillin 50 mg/kg po *and* probenecid 25 mg/kg (maximum dose 1 g) taken as a single dose; or procaine penicillin G 100,000 U/kg IM and probenecid 25 mg/kg on a single occasion; or spectinomycin 40 mg/kg IM single dose; or if over 8 years old, tetracycline 10 mg/kg/day divided into 4 daily doses for 7 days. For children weighing more than 45 kg, adult doses, which are listed in Table 120-1 should be used. Trichomonas is treated with metronidazole (Flagyl) 10 to 30 mg/kg/day or 125 mg 3 times a day po for 5 to 7 days. An alternative is 1 g po as a single dose. Streptococcal vaginitis (group A β-hemolytic streptococcus or *Streptococcus pneumoniae*) is treated with penicillin 125 to 250 mg po 4 times a day for 10 days, or erythromycin 30 to 50 mg/kg/day divided into 3 or 4 doses a day for 10 days. The maximum dose is 250 mg 3 times a day. Vulvovaginitis caused by *Candida albicans* can be managed with nystatin cream (or ointment if the lesions are dry) applied locally to the vulva 3 times a day for 2 weeks. Alternatives are miconazole 2% (Monistat) or clotrimazole 1% (Gyne-lotrimin, Mycelex) creams. Persistent yeast infections may require treatment with nystatin 100,000 units/ml, 1 ml po 4 times a day or per vaginum 3 times a day for 2 weeks. Condyloma acuminata are treated with direct application of podophyllum resin 25% in tincture of benzoin, with care. This should be washed off 2 hours later; subsequent symptoms of burning can be managed with lidocaine 2% jelly or Vaseline. Repeated treatments may be necessary at weekly intervals. (For a more complete discussion on the treatment of sexually transmitted diseases, see Chap. 195.)

Long-term complications of vulvovaginitis depend on the specific etiology. It is thought that *labial adhesions* may reflect the sequence of chronic vulvar irritation, leading to erosion of the labial epithelium and subsequent adhesions. These frequently occur between the ages of 6 months to 6 years. Mild cases require no treatment; with increasing estrogen levels at puberty, the labia will separate. More extensive adhesions may occlude the vaginal oriface, impairing drainage of secretions and even of urine. Under no circumstances should forceful separation be used. Not only is this traumatic to the child, but there is also a high incidence of recurrence of the adhesions. An estrogen-containing cream such as Premarin should be applied twice a day for 2 weeks, and then nightly for an additional 1 to 2 weeks. The cream should be rubbed into the adhered area while gently separating the labia. Nightly applications of a bland ointment (*e.g.*, K-Y jelly or A and D Ointment) should then be continued for several months to prevent the reformation of the adhesions. This treatment can be extended for 1 year if there is a history of previous treatment failures.

Referral

Occasionally, when the diagnosis is unclear or the symptoms are resistant to appropriate therapy, a referral should be made. It is clearly indicated when there is any suggestion of sexual abuse.

ADOLESCENT VULVOVAGINITIS

Pathophysiology

The most common cause of discharge in the adolescent age group is a noninfectious, physiologic leukorrhea. This is a milky-white discharge that represents the shedding of the vaginal cells and endocervical mucus. It may start several months before menarche. Once the menstrual cycle is established, the discharge may show cyclic changes, being profuse and watery at midcycle and stickier and scantier in the second part of the cycle. Leukorrhea is diagnosed by direct inspection. A wet preparation with normal saline will only show epithelial cells. The treatment consists mainly of reassurance and improved general hygiene as described above. Pads may be useful, but tampon use

Table 120-1. Vulvovaginitis in Adolescents

CLINICAL PRESENTATION	CAUSE	SOURCE	DIAGNOSIS	TREATMENT
Milky discharge	Leukorrhea	Physiologic	History; saline wet preparation: epithelial cells	Reassurance, general hygiene
Foul-smelling discharge: bloody or purulent?	Foreign body usually retained tampon		History and pelvic with speculum examination	Removal of cause, irrigation of vagina with warm water General hygiene
Urethral syndrome Mucopurulent discharge	*Chlamydia trachomatis*	Sexual contact	Culture, fluorescent antibody screen Papanicolaou smear	Tetracycline 500 mg po qid × 7 days, OR Doxycycline 100 mg po qid × 7 days, OR Erythromycin 500 mg po qid × 7 days Treat contacts
Mucopurulent discharge	*Neisseria gonorrhea*	Sexual contact	Culture	Procaine penicillin G 4.8 mU IM divided into 2 injections given in 2 different sites on the same occasion and probenecid 1 g po single dose, OR Amoxicillin 3 g po and probenecid 1 g po single dose, OR Spectinomycin 2 g IM single dose, OR Cefoxitin 2 g or Cefuroxime 1.5 g or Cefotaxime 1 g IM single dose Treat contacts
White "cottage-cheese" discharge Pruritus Dysuria	*Candida albicans*	Not usually sexually transmitted Predisposing factors: diabetes mellitus, birth control pills, antibiotic use, corticosteroids, pregnancy, obesity, tight clothing	KOH preparation: budding pseudohyphae	Miconazole vaginal cream q hs. × 7 nights, OR, Clotrimazole 200 mg tablet per vaginum q hs. × 3 nights

Organism/Condition	Symptoms	Transmission	Diagnosis	Treatment
Trichomonas vaginalis	Yellow-green frothy discharge Vulvitis Ectropion Strawberry cervix	Usually sexual contact Can survive 1½ hours on wet towel	Saline wet preparation: dancing flagellated organisms	Metronidazole (Flagyl) 1.5–2 g po single dose, OR, Metronidazole 250 mg po tid × 7 days For persistent infections, rule out reinfection. Treat contacts. Note: Flagyl has antabuse effect
Gardnerella vaginalis	Profuse gray-white watery discharge Strong fish-like odor	Normal flora? Sexual contact?	Vaginal pH > 4.5 Saline wet prep clue cells = large epithelial cells coated with small refractile bacteria	Metronidazole 500 mg po bid × 7 days Treat contacts if recurrent symptoms
Condyloma acuminata (genital warts) Human papilloma virus	Pruritus, dysuria, dyspareunia	Direct contact, usually sexual	Inspection: rule out secondary syphilis with serology Papanicolaou smear	Treat any coexisting vaginitis. Podophyllin 25% in tincture of benzoin applied directly and washed off 2–4 hours later; repeat each week prn Treatment may cause burning; relieve with sitz baths or topical anesthetic jelly. Cryotherapy, cautery, laser therapy
Genital *Herpes simplex*	Pain, pruritus, dysuria, urethral or vaginal discharge Vesicles Dyspareunia Systemic symptoms	Sexual transmission	Inspection Viral culture Wright's stain of scraped lesion base: multinucleated giant cells with inclusions	Symptomatic relief: sitz baths, topical anesthetic gel For initial infection acyclovir 200 mg 5 × day × 7–10 days may be used. This does not prevent recurrences. Not recommended during pregnancy
Pediculosis pubis	Pruritus, crabs, nits (eggs on pubic hair)	Physical contact not necessarily sexual Infested clothing	Inspection	1% lindane (Kwell) shampoo single application; thorough washing of clothing Repeat in 1 week if needed.
Folliculitis *Staphylococcus aureus* or *Streptococcus pyogenes*	Bumps, *vulvar papules*		Inspection	Warm sitz baths bid–tid Topical antibacterial cream Oral antibiotics for extensive acute infections (*e.g.,* erythromycin, cephalexin)

should be restricted to menses only to minimize the risks of developing toxic shock syndrome. Daily tampon use can also be associated with vaginal ulceration.

The pattern of normal flora found in the adolescent vagina depends entirely on whether or not the adolescent has been sexually active. Before the onset of sexual activity, the normal flora closely resemble those found in the prepubertal child, with the addition of *Gardnerella vaginalis*. Vaginal colonization and infection in the sexually active adolescent show patterns similar to adults, varying somewhat in the different groups studied. Organisms can include *Ureaplasma urealyticum*, lactobacillus, *Gardnerella*, *Streptococcus* and *Staphylococcus* species, *Mycoplasma* species, yeast and pathogens such as *Neisseria gonorrhoeae*, Trichomonas, and Chlamydia.

Clinical Presentation

Complaints vary and include a vaginal discharge, localized lesions, nonspecific irritation, and the *urethral syndrome* characterized by dysuria, urinary frequency, and pyuria. Although these findings are characteristic of urinary tract infections, vulvovaginitis should also be considered in the sexually active population.

Work-Up

History. As with the prepubertal child, a history of the presenting symptoms is needed. These may include dyspareunia and pelvic pain. Symptoms may have been present for many months, as adolescents typically present late because of denial, embarrassment, or even fear of the examination. The physician should inquire about underlying disorders such as diabetes and recent or current medications (*e.g.*, antibiotics or birth control pills) as these all predispose to the occurrence of a monilia vaginitis. It is vital to know whether or not the adolescent is sexually active or if there is a history of assault. Frequently, however, the patient may not be willing to share this information. Multiple infections may coexist, and details of previous treatments or treatment failures are useful.

Physical Examination. In most cases, this must include a pelvic examination in addition to a careful inspection of the perineum. A single-digit palpation of the vagina is helpful in locating the cervix and in preparing the adolescent for the insertion of the speculum. The Huffman speculum is particularly useful because it has long, slim blades and can be inserted comfortably into most young adolescents. A bimanual examination should complete the physical assessment, noting particularly any areas with tenderness on palpation.

Laboratory Tests. Wet preparations with normal saline and potassium hydroxide are made of any discharge, looking for the presence of trichomonads, clue cells (suggestive of *Gardnerella vaginalis*), or yeast hyphae. Gram stains are less useful. A culture should be sent for gonorrhea and a chlamydia test is mandatory. This is usually a fluorescent antibody screen or a culture if available. A Papanicolaou smear showing nonspecific inflammation is also suggestive of a chlamydial infection. Syphilis serology is needed, particularly if ulcerations or condyloma are found. In a previously undiagnosed case of genital blistering or ulceration, a viral culture should be sent to confirm suspected herpes infection.

Differential Diagnosis and Treatment

Leukorrhea is the chief noninfectious cause of vulvovaginal symptoms. The details of presentation, diagnosis, and management are outlined above. The treatment of all vulvovaginal complaints should include good perineal hygiene as described in the prepubertal section. Other noninfectious causes of vulvovaginal symptoms should be considered. An allergic reaction may be associated with perfumed soaps and douches or with contraceptive creams. Skin disorders such as atopic or seborrheic dermatitis, or psoriasis may involve the vulvar region. The treatment is similar to that for lesions elsewhere on the skin. Psychosomatic vulvovaginitis has also been described.

More common are certain specific infectious etiologies: These are listed with appropriate managements in Table 120-1, but more extensive discussions of treatment are found in Chapter 195. It should be noted that some infections have significant long-term sequelae. The majority only cause a localized disease; however, gonorrhea and chlamydia infections are associated with chronic abdominal pain, pelvic inflammatory disease, and infertility. Herpes genitalis is almost always recurrent and symptoms can be debilitating; in some patients, they cause a serious psychosexual disturbance. Candida vulvovaginitis is frequently a chronic intermittent problem that can be troublesome. Finally, of particular concern to the pediatrician are those vaginal infections that may be passed to the newborn child during delivery. These include herpes, gonorrhea, chlamydia, and condyloma. (For discussions of these conditions, see Chaps. 191 and 195.)

ANNOTATED BIBLIOGRAPHY

Altchek A: Vulvovaginitis, vulvar skin disease and pelvic inflammatory disease. Pediatr Clin North Am 28:397–432, 1981 (Provides great detail on numerous conditions.)

Emans SJ, Goldstein DP: Pediatric and Adolescent Gynecology, 2nd ed. Boston, Little, Brown, 1982 (Best textbook available; excellent general resource.)

Martien K, Emans SJ: Treatment of common genital infections in adolescents. J Adolesc Health Care 8:129–136, 1987 (Broad discussion of appropriate treatments, including costs.)

STD Treatment Guidelines, Vol 34. MMWR (suppl 4S) Oct 18, 1985 (CDC's current guidelines for the treatment of sexually transmitted diseases.)

121
Vaginal Bleeding and Menstrual Problems
ODETTE PINSONNEAULT

Abnormal vaginal bleeding and dysmenorrhea are common gynecologic complaints during adolescence. These symptoms may be a tremendous source of anxiety for the young patient and her parents and should never be disregarded. Although adolescent menstrual problems, in most cases, have a dysfunctional origin, a thorough evaluation is essential to rule out an organic pathology.

Abnormal menstrual patterns, most of the time, are dysfunctional uterine bleeding, (*i.e.* unrelated to anatomic lesions of the uterus) and correct by themselves with the establishment of ovulatory menstrual cycles. In some instances, however, the bleeding aberration requires therapy because of an excessive blood loss in amount, duration, or frequency, or secondary anemia. Abnormal menstrual bleeding may also reflect an underlying gynecologic or systemic disease.

In adolescents, primary dysmenorrhea is the leading etiology of menstrual pain. The possibility of pelvic pathology should, however, be kept in mind. The early diagnosis and treatment of these conditions may save the reproductive function.

ABNORMAL MENSTRUAL BLEEDING

Pathophysiology

The first postmenarchal years are frequently characterized by anovulatory menstrual cycles, due to the immaturity of the hypothalamic-pituitary-ovarian axis resulting in acyclic release of follicle stimulating hormone (FSH) and luteinizing hormone (LH). Because of anovulation, the endometrium is subjected to continuous estrogenic stimulation, unopposed by the growth-limiting and stabilizing effect of progesterone (which should be secreted by the corpus luteum after ovulation). The endometrium, therefore, becomes hyperplastic to such a point that it cannot sustain its integrity and suffers superficial breakages. Consequently, menses are likely to be irregular, prolonged, and excessive.

Clinical Presentation

Dysfunctional uterine bleeding may present with a wide variety of clinical pictures, ranging from minor deviations from the normal menstrual cycle to life-threatening hemorrhages.

The most clinically significant presentation is *acute menorrhagia*, which is characterized by heavy vaginal bleeding lasting for many days or even weeks. This occurs, most often, after a long episode of amenorrhea and sometimes with the first menstrual period. In this situation, the adolescent may be severely anemic or hypovolemic and requires emergency therapy. Since acute menorrhagia results from anovulatory menstrual cycles, dysmenorrhea is not a characteristic feature, although the uterus contracting to expel blood clots may cause painful cramps.

Recurrent hypermenorrhea, defined as excessive but self-limiting menstrual bleeding, either in the amount or the duration, and occurring more or less regularly, is also frequent in the adolescent population. It is always difficult to accurately estimate blood loss. In general, a menstrual bleeding exceeding 7 days in duration, or the use of more than 20 moderately soaked perineal pads per period, or more than 6 well-soaked pads in any particular day, is considered to be excessive. Recurrent hypermenorrhea may also cause secondary anemia.

Polymenorrhea, or short menstrual cycles, is also a frequent occurrence in adolescents. When interpreting this complaint, the physician should obtain a detailed history, because several young patients calculate their menstrual cycles from the last day of a period to the first day of the next one. Menstrual cycles less than 22 days (from the first day of a period to the first day of the next) are abnormally short; they may lead to anemia; and certainly they interfere with the quality of life.

Oligomenorrhea (defined as menstrual cycles longer than 35 days) is also a common menstrual irregularity secondary to the physiologic anovulation in the perimenarchal patient. It does not usually cause distress, unless associated with excessive bleeding. A persistence of oligomenorrhea 5 years after menarche should be investigated, because it may be the manifestation of an endocrine dysfunction.

Differential Diagnosis

Although dysfunctional uterine bleeding is the most frequent etiology of menstrual aberrations in the adolescent, all other causes should be ruled out.

In the patient with severe or prolonged vaginal bleeding, the differential diagnosis includes *pregnancy-related complications* (*i.e.*, spontaneous abortion, ectopic pregnancy, complications of pregnancy termination procedures, and gestational trophoblastic diseases). Some *local conditions* affecting the genital tract such as vaginal, cervical, uterine, and estrogen-secreting ovarian tumors, congenital anomalies of the uterus and vagina associated with partial obstruction to the menstrual flow, pelvic inflammatory disease (PID), the presence of an intrauterine contraceptive device (IUD), traumatic lesions of the lower genital tract, and intravaginal foreign bodies should be excluded. Many *systemic diseases* may be responsible for menorrhagia, principally blood dyscrasias (*e.g.*, coagulation defects, leukemia, iron deficiency), endocrine disorders (hypo/hyperthyroidism, diabetes mellitus, adrenal diseases), and debilitating diseases (*e.g.*, renal failure and tuberculosis).

Work-Up

History. A complete medical history should be obtained for every patient with abnormal vaginal bleeding. A detailed menstrual history, including age at menarche, length of cycles, duration of bleeding, dysmenorrhea, and estimation of blood loss (*e.g.*, pads count, blood clots) often points to the diagnosis or may reveal that there is no problem at all. A notion of habitual dysmenorrhea is suggestive of ovulatory cycles and makes the diagnosis of an organic pathology more likely. A thorough endocrine questionnaire, including galactorrhea, hirsutism, symptoms of thyroid dysfunction and diabetes mellitus, is essential. The adolescent should be questioned, in a nonjudgmental manner, about sexual activity, contraception, and the possibility of pregnancy. In the patient with acute vaginal bleeding or recurrent hypermenorrhea, the history of a prior hemorrhage (gynecologic and nongynecologic) or easy bruising should be sought. Ten percent of females with a coagulation defect present with excessive menstrual bleeding as the first symptom.

Physical Examination. During the physical examination, the physician should look for signs of hypovolemia or anemia. Abdominal palpation rules out masses and peritoneal signs. A complete pelvic examination should be performed, including a speculum visualization of the vagina and cervix, and a bimanual palpation of the internal genital structures. In the young teenager with only mild symptoms, the speculum examination can be deferred, providing the uterus and adnexa are normal by rectoabdominal palpation. Tanner stages of pubertal development should be recorded, as well as any evidence of endocrine dysfunction.

Laboratory Tests. In the patient with acute menorrhagia or recurrent hypermenorrhea, a complete blood count (CBC) including platelets, prothrombin time (PT), partial thromboplastin time (PTT), bleeding time, thyroid function tests, blood sugar, and cervical cultures should be obtained. A serum β-HCG or another highly sensitive pregnancy test should be performed for every patient, even when she denies sexual activity, because adolescents do not easily volunteer this information, especially during a crisis situation. In the patient with a longstanding history of irregular menses, FSH, LH, and prolactin are necessary to rule out endocrine pathologies. A pelvic ultrasound may be useful to further define an enlarged uterus or adnexal masses, but if the pelvic examination is normal, it does not need to be performed in every case.

Management

The therapy of menstrual abnormalities depends on the severity of the bleeding aberration. When only *minor deviations from the normal menstrual cycle* exist, the best management is reassurance and observation for spontaneous establishment of ovulatory cycles. The patient should be encouraged to keep a menstrual calendar that will make a further evaluation easier.

In the patient with *acute menorrhagia*, the treatment consists of combined hormonal therapy and blood replacement as necessary. High doses of estrogens will heal endometrial bleeding sites and rapidly stop the hemorrhage. At the same time, progestational agents need to be given in order to induce endometrial stability. The most practical means to achieve both of these goals is the administration of oral contraceptives (OC) containing high doses of estrogens and a progestational agent. Preparations containing 100 µg of ethinylestradiol and 2 mg of norethindrone (Ortho Novum 2 mg or Norinyl 2 mg) can be used with the following regimen: 1 tablet every 4 hours until the bleeding stops or decreases appreciably (24 to 36 hours); then, 1 tablet every 6 hours for 24 hours, 1 tablet TID for 48 hours, and 1 tablet BID for 15 days. Since these commercial preparations are not available in all pediatric hospitals' pharmacies, it is useful to know that 2 tablets of Ortho Novum 1/50 or Norinyl 1/50 are equivalent to 1 tablet of Ortho Novum or Norinyl 2 mg. Many other therapeutic regimens have been described and work equally well. In the presence of profuse bleeding, intravenous administration of conjugated estrogens, Premarin 25 mg IV every 4 hours for 3 doses, may be added to the treatment to accelerate endometrial hemostasis.

After the completion of this initial treatment, the patient will have a withdrawal bleeding and should then be kept under progestational therapy for 3 months, using low dose OCs (less than 50 µg of estrogens). This progestational influence allows the endometrium to recover its normal height.

A failure of hormonal therapy to control the hemorrhage within 24 to 36 hours is an indication for dilatation and curettage (D & C). This surgical approach is necessary in 20% to 30% of cases and is usually curative.

Further therapy is intended to prevent a recurrence because, if anovulation persists, an hyperplastic endometrium is likely to rebuild. In the sexually active adolescent, low dose OCs are continued. When contraception is not a concern, medroxyprogesterone acetate (Provera) 10 mg/day for 10 days, is given every 6 to 8 weeks if spontaneous menses do not occur. This type of therapy has the advantage of not suppressing the hypothalamic-pituitary-ovarian axis and, therefore, does not interfere with the establishment of ovulatory cycles.

Recurrent hypermenorrhea can be treated with low dose OCs when there is concomitant birth control need. Medroxyprogesterone acetate (Provera), 10 mg/day from day 16 to day 25 of each cycle, or according to a calendar-month schedule, may also be given to induce the formation of a progestational endometrium and withdrawal bleeding. Prostaglandin synthetase inhibitors (PGSI), prescribed as for the treatment of primary dysmenorrhea, may be used to reduce the blood flow.

Polymenorrhea is best treated by the administration of medroxyprogesterone acetate, 5 mg or 10 mg/day from the 16th to the 25th days of each cycle. In the presence of short cycles (less than 18 days), the medication is given from day 11 to day 25. This will maintain endometrial stability and prevent premature shedding. Oral contraceptives are also an acceptable therapeutic alternative.

Hormonal therapy for adolescent dysfunctional uterine bleeding is continued for 3 to 6 months and the patient is then observed for a recurrence.

Indications for Referral or Admission

Profuse bleeding, signs of hypovolemia, a hematocrit lower than 28%, unreliability, and an unclear diagnosis are indications for hospitalization. Patients in whom an organic pathology is suspected and those not responding to the usual hormonal therapy should be referred to a gynecologist for further investigation and treatment.

DYSMENORRHEA

Pathophysiology

Most adolescents experiencing menstrual pain have primary dysmenorrhea, which means that there is no organic cause responsible for the symptoms. The most accepted pathophysiologic explanation for primary dysmenorrhea is an exaggerated production of endometrial prostaglandins, resulting in increased myometrial contractions, uterine ischemia, and sensitization of pain nerve terminals. Since falling progesterone levels, secondary to corpus luteum regression, initiate prostaglandin biosynthesis, primary dysmenorrhea occurs on the basis of ovulatory menstrual cycles.

Clinical Presentation

Primary dysmenorrhea usually begins 6 months to 2 years after menarche with the establishment of ovulatory menstrual cycles. The symptoms vary from mild discomfort to agonizing pain and are described as lower midabdominal cramps. Radiation of pain to the lower back, labia majora, and inner thighs is frequent. Accompanying systemic symptoms such as nausea, vomiting, headache, fatigue, nervousness, and dizziness are common. Pain usually begins within the few hours preceding or following the initiation of the menstrual flow and lasts for less than 2 days.

Differential Diagnosis

Endometriosis is probably the most frequent organic cause of dysmenorrhea. This disease is often subtle in the adolescent and does not always present with the classical physical findings. The diagnosis of endometriosis should be suspected whenever there is no response to the usual therapy of primary dysmenorrhea or when the pelvic examination reveals adnexal or uterosacral tenderness. Endometriosis should always be confirmed laparoscopically before undertaking therapy.

Acute and chronic pelvic inflammatory disease (PID) may be responsible for dysmenorrhea. In this situation, symptoms are mediated by increased prostaglandin production secondary to the inflammatory reaction. The presence of an *intrauterine contraceptive device* (IUD) is frequently a cause of menstrual pain. Increased prostaglandin secretion associated with the IUD-induced sterile endometrial inflammation is responsible for the cramping.

Obstructing malformations of the reproductive tract, such as a blind uterine horn or an obstructed hemivagina, may occasionally be a source of dysmenorrhea. These anomalies cause menstrual blood to accumulate above the obstruction and secondary endometriosis. An examination, in these patients, often reveals a vaginal or pelvic mass.

Finally, some patients have a *psychogenic* etiology. Dysmenorrhea may reflect familial, social, scholastic, and sexual maladjustment, or may be used as a pretext to obtain narcotic prescriptions.

Work-Up

History. A complete menstrual history should be obtained, with special attention to the time elapsed between menarche and the onset of dysmenorrhea. The pain should be defined in terms of its timing in relation to the beginning of the flow, location, radiation, duration, accompanying symptoms, severity and degree of disability experienced by the adolescent. Prior treatments and their efficacy should be discussed. A thorough psychosocial and familial assessment may give a clue to a psychogenic eti-

ology. The patient should be questioned about sexual activity, because it will influence the choice of therapy. The complaint of dysmenorrhea in adolescents also frequently masks the need for birth control.

Physical Examination. Besides a general physical examination, a complete pelvic examination is essential. Most of the time, it will be normal, but it is the only means to detect evidence of organic disease. Bimanual rectovaginal palpation to detect uterosacral nodularities or tenderness should be performed in every patient. Because of the early stage of the disease, the examination in adolescents with endometriosis is frequently noncontributory. The speculum examination may be deferred in the young, mildly dysmenorrheic teenager.

Laboratory Tests. Laboratory tests are not necessary when the clinical evaluation suggests primary dysmenorrhea. When PID is a possibility, a CBC and erythrocyte sedimentation rate should be obtained. A pelvic ultrasound is performed to define pelvic masses or when congenital anomalies are suspected. Laparoscopy is the only reliable diagnostic tool for endometriosis and chronic PID.

Management

The treatment of primary dysmenorrhea depends on its severity. In the patient with only mild discomfort, reassurance and analgesics, such as aspirin or acetaminophen, are all that is necessary. When the intensity of symptoms indicates more specific therapy, either PGSIs or OCs may be used, the choice depending on the birth control need.

PGSIs produce effective relief of primary dysmenorrhea in 75% to 90% of patients. Since these agents need to be taken only for the usual duration of symptoms and also because of their low incidence of side-effects, this therapeutic approach is usually well accepted by the patient. The most commonly used regimens are summarized in Table 121-1. They are all equally effective, although some patients may have a good response to one agent and not to another.

The medication should be started at the onset of menstrual bleeding and continued for the usual duration of symptoms. In patients in whom cramping precedes the flow, therapy may be initiated 24 to 48 hours before menses or, if cycles are not predictable, at the first sign of discomfort. Frequent follow-up visits or telephone contacts, in order to adjust the dosage or change the medication, assure the best compliance and results. PGSIs may also

Table 121-1. Treatment of Primary Dysmenorrhea with Prostaglandin Synthetase Inhibitors

DRUG	TRADE NAME	DOSAGE
Ibuprofen	Motrin	400–600 mg q 6 h
Naproxen	Naprosyn	250 mg q 8–12 h
Naproxen sodium	Anaprox	550 mg then, 275 mg q 6 h
Mefenamic acid	Ponstel	500 mg then, 250–500 mg q 6 h

prove useful in the treatment of IUD-induced dysmenorrhea.

An OC, prescribed as for birth control, is a good therapeutic alternative for the sexually active adolescent or when PGSIs fail to relieve primary dysmenorrhea. OCs are effective in 90% of cases. In some instances, combined therapy with both PGSIs and OCs is necessary to obtain painless menses.

Indications for Referral

Whenever an organic etiology of dysmenorrhea is suspected, the adolescent should be referred for evaluation of the need for laparoscopy or other diagnostic tests. A delay in the diagnosis and treatment of endometriosis or obstructing malformations of the reproductive tract may compromise future fertility.

ANNOTATED BIBLIOGRAPHY

Abnormal Vaginal Bleeding

Claessens EA, Cowell CA: Acute adolescent menorrhagia. Am J Obstet Gynecol 139:277–280, 1981 (Study of 59 adolescents admitted for a first episode of acute menorrhagia.)

Emans SJ, Goldstein DP: Pediatric and Adolescent Gynecology, pp 97–149. Boston, Little, Brown, 1982 (Comprehensive chapter on the evaluation and management of menstrual irregularities in adolescents.)

Gantt PA, Mc Donough PG: Dysfunctional bleeding in adolescents. In Barwin BN, Belisle S (eds): Adolescent Gynecology and Sexuality, pp 52–78. New York, Masson Publishing USA, 1982 (Excellent chapter on the differential diagnosis and management of dysfunctional uterine bleeding in adolescents.)

Pinsonneault O, Goldstein DP: Gynecologic disorders in adolescents. Part II: Dysfunctional uterine bleeding and breast masses. The Female Patient 10(12):41–44, 1985 (Discussion of the differential diagnosis and management of adolescent dysfunctional uterine bleeding.)

Dysmenorrhea

Altcheck A: Dysmenorrhea in the young patient. The Female Patient 8(9):36/7–36/28, 1983 (Discussion of the evaluation and treatment of adolescent dysmenorrhea.)

Dawood MY: Dysmenorrhea. Clin Obstet Gynecol 25:719–727, 1983 (Good review of the role of prostaglandins in primary and secondary dysmenorrhea.)

Emans SJ, Goldstein DP: Pediatric and Adolescent Gynecology, pp 167–171. Boston, Little, Brown, 1982 (Clear and concise discussion of the management of the dysmenorrheic adolescent.)

Henzl MR (ed): A new perspective on dysmenorrhea. J Reprod Med 25(suppl): 191–242, 1980 (Extensive review of dysmenorrhea.)

Pinsonneault O, Goldstein DP: Gynecologic disorders in adolescents. Part I: Pain syndromes. The Female Patient 10(11):21–27, 1985 (Discussion of the differential diagnosis and management of dysmenorrhea and chronic pelvic pain in adolescents.)

122
Pelvic Inflammatory Disease
JEAN BRODNAX

Sexual activity among adolescent females in the United States increased dramatically during the 1970s. Accompanying this increase was a rise in the occurrence of sexually transmitted diseases. Pelvic inflammatory disease (PID), or salpingitis, is the most common serious complication of sexually transmitted diseases. It is the clinical syndrome resulting from the ascending spread of microorganisms from the vagina and endocervix to the endometrium, fallopian tubes, or contiguous structures. PID is diagnosed at the highest rate during the teenage years. The younger the sexually active female, the higher is her risk of developing PID; the risk is estimated to be 1:80 for sexually active 24-year-old women but increases to 1:8 for sexually active 15-year-old girls.

PID has many medical and economic consequences. Of the one million women in the United

States treated each year for PID, 70% are less than 25 years of age. The annual cost of hospitalization and surgery resulting from PID approaches $700,000,000. The most important medical sequela is infertility. Indeed, PID is the major cause of involuntary infertility. The risk of infertility is 11% after one episode of PID, 23% after two episodes, and 54% after three or more episodes. Other medical sequelae include ectopic pregnancy, chronic pelvic pain, tubo-ovarian abscess, and dyspareunia.

Most women who have mild or moderate PID are seen in the offices of private practitioners. Those women who have more severe diseases tend to seek care in emergency room settings. Since PID occurs so frequently in adolescents and may impact on the reproductive futures of these generally healthy young women, it is crucial that the practicing pediatrician be able to recognize and appropriately treat or refer this potentially devastating disease.

PATHOPHYSIOLOGY

Possible reasons to explain why age is an important risk factor in the development of PID in adolescents include (1) lesser prevalence of protective antibody titers to involved organisms, (2) larger zones of cervical ectopy that predispose to infections by *C. trachomatis* and *N. gonorrhoeae*, (3) thinner cervical mucus resulting from the relative estrogen dominance of this age group, and (4) a greater number of sexual partners. Other risk factors include IUD use, a previous history of PID, a previous history of gonococcal disease, and multiple sexual partners. The risk of developing PID is decreased with oral contraceptive use, probably resulting from less permeable cervical mucus and a decreased menstrual flow. It is also decreased with barrier forms of contraception.

The cervical organisms most frequently associated with PID in adolescents include *Chlamydia trachomatis*, *Neisseria gonorrhoeae* and occasionally genital mycoplasmas. Endogenous vaginal aerobic and anaerobic bacteria are less common causative agents. Recent studies indicate that PID is often a polymicrobial infection. Moreover, organisms isolated from the upper genital tract by way of laparoscopy or culdocentesis do not necessarily correlate with those recovered from cervical cultures alone. *N. gonorrhoeae* and *C. trachomatis* may "pave the way" for other ascending pathogens.

N. gonorrhoeae probably produces salpingitis by direct upward extension from the cervix. Gonococcal PID occurs most commonly during, or immediately after menses, and is thought to be secondary to the loss of the protective cervical mucus plug during menses and to the excellent culture medium of blood. In addition, the endometrium normally provides a local protection against bacteria and when sloughed, protection may be lost. Ten to 17% of women who have endocervical GC will develop PID. It appears that certain auxotypes of the gonococcus are associated with the development of PID. These same auxotypes tend to cause asymptomatic disease in men.

When the gonococcus spreads to the endosalpinx, it penetrates the epithelial cells, causing cell destruction that results in a purulent exudate. If pus escapes into the peritoneum, a peritonitis will develop.

C. trachomatis also produces PID by direct upward extension from the endocervix, but is not as commonly associated with menses as is *N. gonorrhoeae*. In contrast to the gonococcus, which limits itself to the mucosal surface of the tube, *C. trachomatis* and other facultative and anaerobic bacteria may cause an infection below the basement membrane in the subepithelial connective tissue, muscularis and serosal surfaces, thereby increasing the likelihood of permanent tubal damage. In addition, chlamydia may remain in the fallopian tubes for months or years following an initial infection, causing progressive tubal damage. Mycoplasma probably spreads to the fallopian tubes by way of perivascular and perilymphatic routes. PID associated with use of an IUD is probably also mediated by lymphatic spread.

The presence of an IUD may interfere with local host defense mechanisms against cervical infection. Tailed IUDs may serve as conduits for the ascent of bacteria into the endometrial cavity. In addition, IUD users tend to have changes in their cervicovaginal flora that allow for overgrowth of anaerobes that may later be involved in an ascending infection.

CLINICAL PRESENTATION

The clinical presentation of PID is highly variable. Laparoscopic studies have shown that if the presence of the classical triad of acute pelvic pain, evidence of genital tract infection, and adnexal tenderness on bimanual examination are required to make a clinical diagnosis of PID, there will be many erroneous as well as missed diagnoses. Diagnostic accuracy is increased with the addition of other findings such as an elevated sedimentation rate, fever, or a palpable adnexal mass. Presently, laparoscopy is the only way to make an absolute diagnosis of PID.

The causative organism may vary the clinical presentation of PID. Typically, patients with gonococcal PID are acutely symptomatic, usually within a few days of menses. Chlamydial PID has a much less impressive clinical picture. It may be so insidious that many women who have tubal obstruction and evidence of prior chlamydial infection have no recollection of ever having experienced pelvic pain.

A sexually active woman presenting with pleuritic right upper quadrant (RUQ) pain, with or without evidence of PID may have the Fitz-Hugh–Curtis syndrome. This is a perihepatitis (inflammation of the liver capsule) usually associated with gonorrheal or chlamydial disease. These women are frequently misdiagnosed as having cholecystitis.

DIFFERENTIAL DIAGNOSIS

The differential diagnosis of PID includes acute appendicitis, acute pyelonephritis, twisted ovarian cyst, corpus luteum cyst bleeding, ectopic pregnancy, endometriosis, gastroenteritis, and vaginitis. Certain clinical findings may help differentiate the aforementioned disorders from PID. In acute appendicitis the sedimentation rate is usually normal with an elevated WBC and left shift, whereas in PID the sedimentation rate is usually elevated with a normal WBC. In acute pyelonephritis, CVA tenderness is usually present and urinary symptoms may be the chief complaint. A twisted ovarian cyst, bleeding corpus luteum cyst, or unruptured ectopic pregnancy typically present with unilateral pain and tenderness and WBCs are usually not present on a wet Pap smear of cervical secretions. A ruptured ectopic pregnancy commonly causes acute hypotension, tachycardia, and a falling hematocrit. Endometriosis is a frequent diagnosis in adolescents but is manifested typically by cyclic rather than constant pelvic pain. In gastroenteritis, abdominal pain and tenderness are diffuse and vomiting or diarrhea usually predominate the clinical picture. Lower abdominal pain may be seen in simple vaginitis, but true adnexal tenderness is rare. In some cases of clinically diagnosed PID, the laparoscopy will show no pelvic pathology.

WORK-UP

History

Lower abdominal pain is the most frequent complaint of patients who have PID. It is present in most cases but may notably be absent in up to 5% of patients who have disease verified by laparoscopy. In gonococcal PID, the pain is usually moderate to severe and of recent onset (3 days or less) and usually during or just after menses. A previous history of pelvic pain or diagnosed PID is uncommon. In chlamydial PID, the pain is typically mild to moderate in intensity and has usually been present for 7 or more days before the woman seeks medical attention. Patients who have nongonococcal, nonchlamydial PID also tend to have mild to moderate pelvic pain. It is important to remember that adolescents may delay seeking medical attention and may give a history of pain of longer duration than the average times stated above.

Vaginal discharge is another common complaint in PID. Seventy-five percent of patients with gonococcal or chlamydial PID will give a history of vaginal discharge of recent onset. Vaginal discharge is uncommon in nongonococcal, nonchlamydial PID.

Intermenstrual bleeding due to endometritis occurs in 40% of patients. A history of fever is elicited in less than half of the patients and is more common in gonococcal PID. Dysuria or urinary frequency may occur in a small proportion of patients. Patients who have severe disease may experience nausea and vomiting. A further history should include questions about the presence of sexual activity, the number of partners, contraceptive history, and previous episodes of sexually transmitted diseases or PID.

It must be stressed, however, that a heavy reliance on symptoms may lead to a misdiagnosis because the clinical picture in PID is so variable and nonspecific.

Physical Examination

A complete physical examination should be done on any patient with suspected PID not only to look for possible associated conditions (such as GC pharyngitis, arthritis, or rash or RUQ tenderness due to Fitz-Hugh–Curtis syndrome) but also to rule out other diagnoses.

In patients with PID, the abdominal examination is usually positive. Commonly, there is bilateral lower quadrant tenderness without an associated mass. Rebound will be present if the inflammation has extended to the peritoneal surface. RUQ tenderness, with or without signs of PID, is present in perihepatitis.

On speculum examination of the vagina and cervix, a thick endocervical discharge is present in most cases of gonococcal and chlamydial PID. On bimanual examination, cervical motion tenderness and uterine and adnexal tenderness are present. The adnexal tenderness is most commonly bilateral, although one side may be more tender than the other. Adnexal fullness or swelling may be felt in PID, but a true tubo-ovarian abscess is present in only 15% of cases.

Laboratory Tests

Routine hematologic blood tests have poor diagnostic value in PID. The WBC and hematocrit are usually normal. The sedimentation rate is elevated above 15 mm/hr in only 75% of women; thus, a normal value does not rule out the diagnosis.

A microscopic examination of cervical secretions is frequently helpful. Increased numbers of white cells (5 or more per HPF) are almost always seen on a normal saline wet preparation and are diagnostic of cervicitis. A Gram stain may show gram-negative intracellular diplococci in gonococcal PID, but it is positive in only two thirds of women with positive GC cultures of the cervix.

Cultures of cervical secretions for *N. gonorrhoeae* should be taken.

Rapid diagnostic tests to identify chlamydia in cervical secretions are available. Chlamydial serology is of little diagnostic value in PID. A culture remains the most accurate way to diagnose chlamydia but this is generally not available to the office practitioner.

The experienced clinician may do a culdocentesis, and in PID this will reveal purulent fluid containing bacteria.

The aforementioned laboratory work may be helpful but by itself is not diagnostic of PID. Laparoscopy, which is the only absolute way to make the diagnosis, is impractical in most cases.

MANAGEMENT

The goals of treatment in PID are the prevention of infertility and other chronic sequelae and, to a lesser degree, the acute relief of discomfort. The incidence of sequelae has been reduced since the advent of antibiotics but, unfortunately, they still occur frequently. The fertility outlook is much better in gonococcal PID than with other forms of PID. This may be due to the acute presentation of gonococcal PID and also because historically patients have been treated for *N. gonorrhoeae* without necessarily being covered for other organisms.

Early treatment of PID may prevent chronic residua. A treatment delay, even if only several days, may lead to tubal obstruction.

Table 122-1. Drug Regimens in Pelvic Inflammatory Disease*

INPATIENTS	OUTPATIENTS
Regimen A	**Regimen A**
Cefoxitin 2.0 g IV q 6 hr	Cefoxitin 2 g IM†
+	+
Doxycycline 100 mg IV q 12 hr for at least 4 days and at least 48 hr after improvement followed by	Probenecid 1 g po followed by
Doxycycline 100 mg po bid to complete 10–14-day course	Doxycycline‡ 100 mg po bid × 10–14 days
Regimen B	**Regimen B**
Clindamycin 600 mg IV q 6 hr	Amoxicillin 3.0 qm po
+	+
Gentamicin 2.0 mg/kg IV followed by 1.5 mg/kg q 8 hr for at least 4 days and at least 48 hr after improvement; then continue clindamycin 450 mg po qid to complete 10–14-day course	Probenecid 1 g po followed by Doxycycline 100 mg po bid × 10–14 days
	Regimen C
	Ampicillin 3.5 qm po
	+
	Probenecid 1 g po followed by
	Doxycycline 100 mg po bid × 10–14 days
	Regimen D
	Aqueous procaine PenG 4.8 million U IM at 2 sites
	+
	Probenecid 1 g po followed by
	Doxycycline 100 mg po bid × 10–14 days
	Regimen E
	Ceftriaxone 250 mg IM followed by
	Doxycycline 100 mg po bid × 10–14 days

* Adapted from the 1985 CDC guidelines for treatment of sexually transmitted diseases.
† Most consider this the current preferred treatment. The other regimens are alternatives in no order of preference.
‡ Tetracycline HCL 500 mg po qid may be substituted for doxycycline but is less active against anaerobes and may be associated with poor compliance due to its frequent dosing schedule.

The antimicrobial treatment of PID is controversial due to the large number of possible organisms that may be involved and the difficulty in making a specific microbiologic diagnosis. As stated above, organisms isolated from the endocervix frequently do not correlate with those cultured from the fallopian tubes through laparoscopy. Thus, the physician is hazarding a guess as to what the microbial etiology is in a particular case. Treatment must therefore include coverage for *N. gonorrhoeae*, *C. trachomatis*, mycoplasma, and mixed aerobes and anaerobes. No single agent is active against the entire spectrum of pathogens (Table 122-1). Oral *vs* parental therapy also remains controversial. Of course, sicker patients should receive parenteral therapy.

Patients who have suspected tubo-ovarian abscesses should be hospitalized and may be managed with parenteral antibiotics for 48 to 72 hours. If no improvement occurs at that time, surgical exploration should be done, not only to attempt to preserve fertility but also to prevent rupture. A ruptured tubo-ovarian abscess is a surgical emergency.

All outpatients with PID should be reevaluated in 48 to 72 hours to assess improvement and again after the completion of antibiotic therapy.

Partners of women with PID should be examined for evidence of sexually transmitted diseases, especially gonorrhea and chlamydia, and should be treated presumptively for 7 to 10 days with an antibiotic, such as tetracycline, that treats both *N. gonorrhoeae* and *C. trachomatis*.

INDICATIONS FOR REFERRAL OR ADMISSION

Any primary care provider who suspects a diagnosis of PID in an adolescent and feels unsure of or uncomfortable with the diagnosis, should refer the patient immediately to an adolescent or gynecologic specialist.

About 75% of patients with PID are treated on an outpatient basis. Indications for hospitalization include the following:

Patient acutely ill and toxic appearing
Noncompliance with an outpatient regimen
Failure to respond to an outpatient regimen
Strong suspicion of a surgical problem in the differential
Clinical signs of peritonitis
Pregnancy
Temperature greater than 38°C
Adnexal mass

The decision to hospitalize adolescents with PID should be influenced by a possible medication noncompliance and a high failure rate for follow-up medical care.

ANNOTATED BIBLIOGRAPHY

Emans SJH, Goldstein DP: Pediatric and Adolescent Gynecology, 2nd ed. Boston Little, Brown, 1982

Eschenback D: Acute pelvic inflammatory disease. Urol Clin North Am 11(1):65, 1984 (Good review.)

International Symposium on PID. Am J Obstet Gynecol 138:845–1112, 1980 (Excellent symposium on various aspects of PID; very complete.)

1985 STD treatment guidelines. MMWR 34 (Supp): 75, 1985 (Current CDC recommendations for treatment of all STD.)

Shafer M-A, Irwin CE, Sweet RL: Acute salpingitis in the adolescent female. J Pediatr 100 (3): 339, 1982 (Detailed explanation of theories on the pathophysiology of PID; also emphasizes the importance of this disease in the adolescent.)

16

Hematologic Problems

ORAH S. PLATT, Section Editor

123

Bleeding Disorders Of Newborns

ORAH S. PLATT

One of the most anxiety-provoking clinical situations that pediatricians face is the bleeding newborn. Fortunately, most of these bleeding disorders can be quickly diagnosed using a few basic laboratory tests and they can be managed in a relatively straightforward manner. "Sick" infants bleed as a consequence of their underlying illness (*e.g.*, sepsis and hypoxia) and usually require vigorous support with blood products as well as aggressive therapy for the underlying disorder. In contrast, apparently "healthy" infants who bleed usually have primary defects of coagulation that are either hereditary or immune-mediated. Therapy for these infants is aimed at correcting the specific coagulation defect.

dent coagulation factors: Factors II, VII, IX, and X. Because deficiencies of factor II (prothrombin) and factor X prolong both the PT and the PTT, factor VII deficiency prolongs the PT, and factor IX deficiency prolongs the PTT, it is easy to understand why normal newborns have prolonged PT and PTT (up to a few seconds over normal for PT, and 10 to 15 seconds over normal for the PTT, depending on the individual laboratory norms). In term infants treated with vitamin K at birth, the PT usually approaches adult norms in the first week, while the PTT may take weeks to reach adult values. In preterm infants, the time to achieve normal values is longer.

PATHOPHYSIOLOGY

The hemostatic pathways that protect older children and adults from bleeding also apply to the newborn. The basic components are platelets and soluble coagulation factors. In newborns as well as in adults, platelets adhere to damaged endothelium and undergo a release reaction that causes the formation of a platelet plug. The soluble coagulation factors react in a relatively orderly cascade and organize fibrin into a tight clot.

Although there are no significant qualitative differences between clotting in adults and newborns, there are some quantitative differences that must be kept in mind when interpreting laboratory data. The most important quantitative differences result from a relative deficiency of the vitamin-K-depen-

CLINICAL PRESENTATION

Many normal infants with no coagulation abnormalities are born with petechiae or bruises that result from a difficult labor or delivery. These are essentially healthy babies whose bleeding symptoms are limited locally to traumatized tissue and do not persist. Interestingly, most babies born with inherited coagulation disorders, such as hemophilia, do not have any spontaneous bleeding problems and are frequently not diagnosed until later in life. However, when these babies are traumatized, significant soft tissue bleeding can occur, for example a massive subgaleal hematoma following a difficult delivery. Other infants have been diagnosed following prolonged bleeding at circumcision, although many boys with hemophilia are circumcised during the newborn period without complication.

Oozing from venipuncture sites, showering petechiae, and bloody urine or stools are common in critically ill infants with sepsis, prematurity, hypoxia, necrotizing enterocolitis, and the other serious systemic diseases of newborns. In these infants, bleeding is a complication of the underlying disorder and usually represents a complex combination of plasma factor deficiency and thrombocytopenia, usually either on the basis of consumption or defective production. In contrast, when apparently healthy babies have extensive and evolving peteciae and mucous membrane bleeding, the diagnosis is usually immune-mediated thrombocytopenia.

DIFFERENTIAL DIAGNOSIS

The differential diagnosis of bleeding disorders differs in apparently sick and apparently healthy babies. In critically ill newborns, the likely causes of bleeding are disseminated intravascular coagulation (DIC), peripheral platelet consumption, factor deficiencies associated with liver disease, accidental heparinization, and compromized vascular integrity.

Healthy newborns bleed from local trauma, immune thrombocytopenia, maternal aspirin ingestion, vitamin K deficiency, hereditary clotting factor deficiency, or rarely from decreased platelet production syndromes (thrombocytopenia absent radii [TAR] syndrome, Fanconi's anemia, Wiskott–Aldrich syndrome).

WORK-UP

History

A newborn's past medical history is obviously short. In this case the history focuses on the family and particularly on the mother. A detailed listing of the mother's drug history is crucial. Of particular interest is aspirin in the immediate prepartum period. Coumarin is not given to pregnant mothers as it is associated with fetal malformations as well as neonatal bleeding complications. Heparin, on the other hand, can be safely used in pregnancy as it does not cross the placenta.

The mother's medical history is important. Were there any previously affected pregnancies? Does or did the mother have ITP, lupus, or any other chronic disease associated with defects in immune regulation? Does mother or any other family member have any bleeding tendency (e.g., menorrhagia, prolonged nosebleeds, bleeding after dental extraction, bleeding after surgery, and hemarthroses)?

Physical Examination

A thorough physical examination will define the clinical nature of the bleeding and will categorize the infant as belonging to either the "sick" or "healthy" groups. Classically, bleeding from thrombocytopenia results in small superficial ecchymoses, sprays of petechiae, and oozing from mucosal surfaces, conjuntivae, retinas, kidneys, or the central nervous system. Soluble coagulation factor deficiencies tend to cause more soft tissue bleeding, umbilical stump bleeding, and prolonged bleeding following surgical procedures.

The upper extremity abnormalities of the TAR syndrome result in a seriously shortened and deformed arm—not just a subtle radiographic finding. Fanconi's anemia, a rare disorder itself, rarely presents with thrombocytopenia at birth. The physical anomalies of this syndrome vary considerably from patient to patient and although hand and thumb abnormalities are classic findings, they are not always present. Other anomalies that can be associated with this syndrome include congenital cardiac malformations, abnormal kidney position or shape, and microcephaly.

Laboratory Tests

The only laboratory tests that will be needed to evaluate most bleeding newborns are the platelet count, PT, and PTT. These tests need to be interpreted in the context of the normal values for age and degree of prematurity as well as the possibilities for laboratory error.

Platelet Count. The normal platelet count for a newborn is the same as for an adult—>150,000. However, thrombocytopenia is unlikely to be the primary cause of bleeding unless the platelet count is lower than 50,000. Most automated CBC machines measure platelet count directly. A fast estimate of platelet count can be done by examining the peripheral smear. Generally, count the number of platelets per high-power field and multiply by 15,000. For example, about 10 platelets per high power field is roughly a normal platelet count of 150,000. The platelet count may be seriously underestimated if the smear is made from a difficult heel stick, because the natural tendency of the platelets is to adhere to the cut heel and not to flow onto the glass slide. In the newborn with thrombocytopenia, it is essential to measure the mother's platelet count.

PT and PTT. These tests measure all of the important clotting proteins except factor XIII. As mentioned above, both the PT and PTT are affected by vitamin K deficiency and need to be age corrected. The major pitfalls in obtaining an accurate PT and PTT are too little plasma in the citrated collection tube and too much tissue trauma and time in performing the venipuncture. In an infant whose hematocrit is over 60%, the sample must be collected in a special tube with half the citrate removed. Care must be taken to do a quick and trauma-free venipuncture to avoid contaminating the needle with tissue thromboplastin. Another source of error is contamination of the sample with heparin from an IV line.

Treatment

The treatment of bleeding newborns obviously depends on the clinical situation and the overall clinical impression and results of screening laboratory data.

SICK NEWBORNS

Decreased Platelets, Increased PT, and PTT

These babies generally have DIC secondary to sepsis, acidosis, hypoxia, and so forth. The major therapy is aimed at treating the underlying condition. Blood product support includes the use of fresh frozen plasma and platelets. These infants typically need a unit of platelets every 12 to 24 hours as well as 10 to 15 ml/kg fresh frozen plasma. In severe cases where patients continue to bleed despite aggressive replacement, exchange transfusions are sometimes helpful. Heparin therapy is not advised in infants whose major clinical problem is hemorrhage. However, if the DIC is associated with thrombosis (*e.g.*, necrosing digits or skin) heparin therapy is useful.

Decreased Platelets, Normal PT, and PTT

These sick infants usually have platelet consumption without disseminated coagulation. As for the babies with frank DIC, the treatment is aimed at the underlying disorder. These babies usually require frequent platelet transfusions to maintain a relatively safe platelet count of over 50,000.

Normal Platelets, Increased PT, and PTT

These infants are likely to have compromised liver synthesis of coagulation proteins. Typically, these infants also have low albumin levels, sometimes even in the face of normal transaminases. Although parenteral vitamin K should continue to be supplied, plasma infusions are critical to maintain normal hemostasis. The half-lives of some of the coagulation proteins are quite short (hours), and thus infusions need to be repeated frequently in cases of severe liver dysfunction.

Normal Platelets, PT, and PTT

These are compromised infants who have serious intracranial or pulmonary hemorrhage even though they have no demonstrable clotting abnormality. We postulate that such gravely ill infants have compromised vascular integrity and poor tissue support as a result of their underlying disorder. In this setting, blood component therapy is not likely to make a significant clinical difference.

HEALTHY NEWBORNS

Decreased Platelets, Normal PT, and PTT

When a vigorous healthy term infant presents with isolated thrombocytopenia, the most likely diagnosis is immune thrombocytopenia. This is a passively acquired disorder in which antiplatelet antibody passes from the mother to the baby *in utero*. There are two major classes of immune platelet destruction in newborns—isoimmune thrombocytopenia and immune thrombocytopenia due to maternal idiopathic thrombocytopenic purpura (ITP).

Isoimmune thrombocytopenia is analogous to Rh incompatibility. The mother has a normal platelet count but is lacking a platelet antigen (usually PLA-1) that is present on the baby's platelets. Fetal platelets enter into the maternal circulation early in the pregnancy and have caused her to produce an antibody that crosses the placenta and destroys the baby's (but not her) platelets. Although most fetuses and babies tolerate their thrombocytopenia very well, some do suffer severe and possibly fatal hemorrhages just before or after delivery. Since most hospitals are not organized to provide emergency platelet antigen testing, the diagnosis of isoimmune thrombocytopenia rests on clinical grounds. Therapy for these infants with platelet counts less than 50,000 or with bleeding symptoms include a unit of carefully washed maternal platelets, or a random unit of platelets depending on the availability of the mother's. Prednisone (1 to 2 mg/kg/day) can be useful if the wait for platelets will be long. Intravenous gamma globulin will likely prove effective in this disorder.

Maternal ITP is an autoimmune disease of the mother in which she produces an antibody that cross-reacts with all platelets. The mother is usually thrombocytopenic, but some mothers are able to compensate for the increased platelet destruction and thus have normal platelet counts despite the presence of antiplatelet antibody in the plasma. Symptomatic or severely thrombocytyopenic infants of mothers with ITP should be treated with random platelets and prednisone. If bleeding persists, and the platelet count is unsupportable with multiple platelet transfusions, exchange transfusion should be performed. As with isoimmune thrombocytopenia, the use of intravenous gamma globulin will likely become standard therapy.

Normal Platelets, Prolonged PT, and PTT

These findings are associated with the classical hemorrhagic disease of the newborn—vitamin K deficiency. The routine use of parenteral vitamin K in the delivery room has essentially eliminated this disease. However, some infants are overlooked (especially if there is an emergency at delivery, or if the child is born outside of the hospital) and become profoundly vitamin K deficient over the first few days of life. Bleeding, if it occurs, usually appears on about the fourth day of life. The treatment involves administration of vitamin K and, if necessary, fresh frozen plasma.

Normal Platelet Count, Normal PT, and Prolonged PTT

This pattern of abnormal laboratory values usually indicates an inherited plasma factor deficiency. In a boy the likely diagnoses are the X-linked factor VIII or factor IX deficiencies, or the autosomal dominant Von Willebrand's disease. In a girl, Von Willebrand's disease is the most likely. As mentioned previously, these disorders rarely cause significant bleeding problems in newborns unless there is trauma. Therapy is usually unnecessary, but in the case of serious bleeding, fresh frozen plasma should be used.

Normal Platelets, PT, and PTT

Hemorrhages in most healthy infants with normal coagulation screening tests are likely due to local trauma or vascular anomalies. Inherited platelet abnormalities are rare, but maternal aspirin ingestion may result in a transient neonatal platelet disorder. If the infant is symptomatic, a platelet transfusion will be necessary. Factor XIII deficiency is a rare condition that results in delayed localized bleeding (*e.g.*, 1 or 2 days following circumcision or from a dry umbilical stump). This factor deficiency can be diagnosed by measuring the specific factor. The treatment is with fresh frozen plasma.

Indications for Referral

Depending on the capabilities of the local nursery, many newborns with bleeding disorders will need to be referred for intensive care management. Interpretation of coagulation data may require consultation, especially if specific factor analyses are required. The management of pregnant women at high risk for delivering infants with bleeding problems should be coordinated with an obstetrician, pediatrician, neonatologist, and hematologist.

ANNOTATED BIBLIOGRAPHY

Avery GB: Neonatology—Pathophysiology and Management of the Newborn, 3rd ed. Philadelphia, JB Lippincott, 1987 (General; provides information on almost any topic pertaining to bleeding disorders in the newborn.)

Buchanan GR: Coagulation disorders in the neonate. Pediatr Clin North Am 33:203–220, 1986 (Well presented overview of the pathophysiology and laboratory tests to evaluate bleeding disorders in the neonate.)

Glader BE (ed), Perinatal haematology. Clin Haematol 7(1) Philadelphia, WB Saunders, 1978 (General; provides information on almost any topic pertaining to bleeding disorders in the newborn.)

Oski F, Naiman JL: Hematologic Problems in the Newborn, 3rd ed. Philadelphia, WB Saunders, 1982

Zipursky, A, deSa D, Hsu E et al: Clinical and laboratory diagnosis of hemostatic disorders in newborn infants. Am J Pediatr Hematol Oncol 1:217, 1979 (Well presented overview of the pathophysiology and laboratory tests to evaluate bleeding disorders in the neonate.)

Zipursky A (ed): Perinatal hematology. Clin Perinatol 2(2) Philadelphia, WB Saunders, 1984 (General; provides information on almost any topic pertaining to bleeding disorders in the newborn.)

124
Anemia
ORAH S. PLATT

There are four common office scenarios that the pediatrician is faced with when evaluating a child for anemia. The most common is when the healthy youngster who comes for a routine well-child visit is found to have a slightly low hematocrit as part of a standard office screening procedure. The second is when a child is brought in by a parent who suspects anemia because the child seems pale, sluggish, or a "picky eater." The third is the child who is found to have an abnormal complete blood count (CBC) in the orderly process of being evaluated for failure-to-thrive, recurrent infections, chronic diarrhea, or other chronic conditions. The least common is the child who is brought in with a rather nonspecific complaint who is obviously seriously ill, extremely pale, possible jaundiced, and who needs immediate emergency management and a quick evaluation.

The common laboratory measurements that "define" anemia are the hematocrit and hemoglobin. In general, these measurements vary directly and can, therefore, be used interchangeably, knowing that the hematocrit is usually approximately three times the hemoglobin. Clinicians are usually more comfortable with one of these measurements than the other. In this chapter, *hematocrit* rather than *hemoglobin* will be used.

PATHOPHYSIOLOGY

Anemia can be strictly defined as having an hematocrit below the "lower limit of normal" for age. From a functional point of view, *anemia* means not having enough oxygen carrying capacity in the blood for a person to conduct his normal activities. The combination of these two definitions frees the practitioner from solely using published (and highly variable) "normal" values and allows room for clinical judgment. For example, two 7-year-olds come into the office the same day. One is in for a routine examination before going off to soccer camp; his hematocrit is 34%. The other child has cystic fibrosis, mainly with chronic lung disease and he is having more trouble keeping up with this classmates. His hematocrit is 37%. Comparing these two children clinically, the one with the higher hematocrit is the one who needs to be evaluated for anemia.

An individual can only become anemic in three ways: (1) by not producing red cells efficiently (ineffective-production or hypoplasia), (2) by having red cells that survive for a relatively short time in the circulation (hemolysis), or (3) bleeding. These three categories have their characteristic presentations and differential diagnoses.

CLINICAL PRESENTATION

Hypoplastic or ineffective-production anemias are common and develop gradually over long periods of time. Because of the luxury of time, these patients can make the physiologic adjustments that can result in their tolerating extremely low hematocrits with apparent equanimity. The classic example is the iron-deficient "milk baby" who, at 16 months of age, is astonishingly pale yet perfectly comfortable with an hematocrit of 15%. These patients are usually tachycardic with loud systolic murmurs and they rarely show any other physical findings.

Children who have hemolytic anemias generally fall into two categories, acute and chronic. Acute hemolysis is rare, but dramatic in presentation. These are usually children who do not have a prior history of anemia and who suddenly become profoundly anemic and jaundiced, sometimes passing wine-colored urine. An example of this situation typically occurs in May when little boys with G6PD deficiency ingest moth balls while their parents gather up the family's winter clothes. These children have not had time to gradually make physiologic adjustments to their low hematocrit and they become symptomatic with tachycardia, lethargy, sometimes with congestive heart failure, or liver or splenic enlargement.

Chronic hemolysis usually presents as a mild to moderate anemia in a child who has periodically had episodes of mild icterus or frank jaundice. These children are typically well-compensated with mild tachycardia, systolic murmurs, and often liver or spleen enlargement. These children are sometimes so well-compensated hematologically that the diagnosis is made as part of a work-up for jaundice, splenomegaly, or gallstones, and not anemia. The most important chronic hemolytic anemia to diagnose early is sickle cell anemia (see Chap. 125).

Bleeding also occurs in acute and chronic forms. Acute bleeding is obviously not usually a difficult clinical diagnosis to make unless the blood is hidden in a cryptic space, such as a psoas muscle or in a cryptic patient such as a teenager who denies blood in the stool. In addition to the usual tachycardia, systolic murmurs, and pallor, these patients may have postural hypotension. Chronic bleeding can be difficult to ferret out. Most of these patients will be more anemic from the iron deficiency that results from the loss of red cells than from the loss of the red cells themselves.

DIFFERENTIAL DIAGNOSIS

The hypoplastic or ineffective-production anemias can be caused by a long list of common and rare disorders. The single most common cause of anemia in children is **iron deficiency**. Less common are the various thalassemia syndromes, drugs such as chloramphenicol, folic acid deficiency, and chronic diseases such as TB, JRA, liver, renal, or thyroid disease. Rare disorders include the acquired and congenital bone marrow failure syndromes, leukemias, and malignancies, as well as metabolic disorders including vitamin B_{12} deficiency syndromes.

Acute fulminant hemolytic anemias are rare, but usually arise in boys with G6PD deficiency who are exposed to oxidants (*e.g.*, fava beans, antimalarials, or some viruses); patients with acute infections associated with autoantibody production (*e.g.*, infectious mononucleosis, mycoplasma pneumonia); and patients with other acute infections that lyse red cells by various methods (*e.g.*, *H. influenzae*, clostridia, and malaria). Rarely will hemolysis be the most prominent feature of the hemolytic uremic syndrome.

Chronic hemolytic anemias in children are usually either inherited hemoglobinopathies such as sickle cell disease, or inherited red cell membrane disorders such as hereditary spherocytosis. Rarely, red cell enzyme deficiencies, such as pyruvate kinase deficiency, or chronic autoimmune hemolytic anemias are encountered.

Blood loss is discussed in detail in other chapters that deal with specific problems such as gastrointestinal bleeding (see Chap. 112), hematuria (see Chap. 117), and menorrhagia (see Chap. 121).

History

The history is one of the most important parts of the work-up of an anemic child. A family history should include information on the national heritage of parents and grandparents, other family members with anemias, splenectomy, jaundice, early gallbladder disease, sickle cell trait, or thalassemia trait (minor or Mediterranean anemia). The child's nutritional history should be reviewed in detail (as well as the mother's if nursing). The child's past medical history and a review of systems is important with special attention to episodes of jaundice (including the newborn period), extremity pain, possible sites of blood loss, recent infections, exposures, drugs, or travel.

Physical Examination

A comprehensive physical examination can be helpful in evaluating an anemic child. Plotted growth parameters, vital signs, and a general assessment will help establish chronicity and a level of concern. A quick survey for the following findings can be helpful: pallor, jaundice, petechiae, bruises, frontal bossing, adenopathy, murmurs and signs of congestive failure, organomegaly, and congenital anomalies.

Laboratory Tests

First decide if the patient really warrants an anemia evaluation based on published norms and your clinical judgment. If so, the laboratory examination begins simply with a CBC, reticulocyte count, and examination of the peripheral smear. If the patient is anemic, the next step is to note the MCV (or MCH, which varies with MCV). If this information is not available, note if the smear is hypochromic and microcytic.

If the child is microcytic, it is likely that he has an iron deficiency. The best test for an iron deficiency is a therapeutic trial. If the results of the iron trial are good, the next step is to determine the cause of the iron deficiency. This may simply be a matter of reviewing the nutritional or blood loss history or it may need to be pursued more vigorously, for example with stool examination. In young children, since the possibility of coexisting lead poisoning should not be overlooked, a lead level is indicated. If the therapeutic trial is equivocal, or if compliance is questioned, iron studies such as TIBC, serum iron, and ferritin may be helpful. Each of these tests, however, has its own idiosyncracies and may not always yield a perfectly satisfying answer. If the office is equipped with an hematocrit centrifuge, a visual inspection of the spun plasma can give useful information. The plasma normally has a slight straw color. In iron deficiency, this color fades and the plasma appears colorless like water. In hemolytic anemias, the plasma will be yellow, and in some fulminant acute cases it will be brown.

If the child is microcytic but not iron deficient, he probably has a thalassemia syndrome, especially if the family is of Mediterranean, Asian, or black heritage. The next step is to examine the blood of the parents. If one of the parents is also mildly anemic and microcytic, the diagnosis is fairly secure, and no further evaluation is necessary. If both parents are microcytic, and are planning to have more children, this diagnosis needs to be pursued more fully with hemoglobin electrophoresis and possibly gene mapping to determine whether they are at risk of producing a child with thalassemia major and whether they would benefit from genetic counseling. Hemoglobin electrophoresis will identify a patient with β thalassemia trait as having an elevated hemoglobin A_2 level. Patients with α thalassemia trait have normal hemoglobin electrophoresis patterns and can be definitively diagnosed only by gene mapping.

If the child has a normal MCV and a high reticulocyte count, a careful examination of the smear may be helpful. Elongated sickle forms, target cells, and fragmented cells suggest a sickle syndrome and warrant a hemoglobin electrophoresis. A predominance of spherocytes could mean hereditary spherocytosis or an autoimmune hemolytic anemia. An examination of the parents' CBC and smear, a Coombs' test, and an osmotic fragility test will usually be diagnostic. Elliptocytes usually mean hereditary elliptocytosis, although this is almost never associated with much hemolysis. Normal morphology and no parent with reticulocyte elevation should suggest a careful search for bleeding.

If the anemic child has normal or slightly elevated MCV and a low reticulocyte count, a BUN, creatinine. LFTs, and thyroid studies may detect an underlying chronic disease.

TREATMENT

The treatment of the anemic child depends on the cause of the anemia. The most common anemia treated in the office is iron deficiency anemia. This deficiency is corrected by treating the underlying cause of the anemia (*e.g.*, altering the diet, treating the ulcerative colitis, purging the parasites, and so forth) and providing a supplementation to rebuild the iron stores. This can usually be accomplished orally by treating with 2 to 6 mg/kg/day of elemental iron for 3 to 6 months depending on the degree of deficiency and the daily dose of iron. A gastrointestinal disturbance may result in poor compliance. Many patients would rather be on a lower dose for a longer time than endure the gastrointestinal symptoms. Heme iron in the form of meat is probably the best tolerated iron preparation. Parenteral iron is reserved for the rare patient who is unable to comply with conventional therapy or who has an abnormal iron absorption.

Thalassemia trait does not require treatment. Patient and parental education, however, is important. The emphasis is on the potential genetic implications and on the remarkable resemblance between thalassemia trait and iron deficiency and the fact that iron therapy is not indicated.

Hereditary spherocytosis is usually treated (except in mild cases) by elective splenectomy after 5 or 6 years of age. This therapy effectively eliminates the anemia and the risk of gallstones, but carries with it the potential risk of an overwhelming pneumococcal sepsis. Parental and patient education is critical in the care of the splenectomized patient and in understanding the genetic implications of the disease.

The treatment of sickle cell disease is discussed in Chapter 125.

INDICATIONS FOR REFERRAL OR ADMISSION

The same general rules pertaining to admitting critically ill children apply to children who have anemia. Children with congestive failure, hypotension, and profuse bleeding obviously need to be in the hospital. In addition, even relatively comfortable children with low hematocrits (the teens) need to be hospitalized until the diagnosis is clarified; then, with appropriate therapy even with a low hematrocit, they can be managed as outpatients.

The following is a list of disturbing features in children with anemia that warrant an early discussion with a hematologist: neutropenia, thrombocytopenia, blasts or other immature myeloid elements, nucleated red cells, elevated MCV without reticulocytosis, positive Coombs' test, congenital anomalies, unexplained failure to thrive, unexplained fevers, and bone pain.

ANNOTATED BIBLIOGRAPHY

Abshire TC, Reeves JD: Anemia of acute inflammation in children. J Pediatr 103(6):868–871, 1983 (Delineation and explanation of this anemia commonly seen in children hospitalized with inflammatory diseases.)

Addrigo JE, Hurst D, Lubin BH: Congenital hemolytic anemia. Pediatr Rev, 6(7):201–208, 1985 (Clinical and laboratory approach to the child with hemolytic anemia.)

Miller DR: Anemias: General considerations. In Miller DR, Brehner Rl, McMillan CW(eds): Blood Diseases of Infancy and Childhood, 5th ed., pp 97–114. St. Louis, CV Mosby, 1984 (Detailed overview of the problem including an excellent discussion of etiologic and morphologic classifications of the anemias, as well as an understandable explanation of appropriate laboratory tests used in diagnosis.)

Reeves JD: Iron supplementation in infancy. Pediatr Rev 8(6):177–184, 1986 (Complete summary of the clinical problems and issues of iron deficiency.)

125
Sickle Cell Anemia
ORAH S. PLATT

A single sickle gene is carried by about 10% of American blacks. These asymptomatic individuals with sickle trait have no significant medical problems, and their identification is important only in terms of genetic counseling. The clinically important homozygous sickle state—sickle cell anemia—is emphasized in this chapter. Other less common sickle syndromes such as hemoglobin SC disease and sickle cell thalassemia are briefly discussed.

PATHOPHYSIOLOGY

Children who have sickle cell anemia produce no normal hemoglobin A; instead, they synthesize sickle hemoglobin (hemoglobin S), a variant of hemoglobin A that contains valine (an amino acid that decreases protein solubility in water) instead of glutamic acid (an amino acid that promotes protein solubility in water). This single amino acid substitution does not interfere with the oxygen transport properties. Normally, hemoglobin in the red cell stays dissolved even in the extremes of the body's Po_2, pH, temperature, and osmolarity. In contrast, hemoglobin S has a tendency to come out of solution—polymerize at low Po_2, low pH, low temperature, and increased osmolarity. This polymerization reaction damages the red cell and causes a chronic hemolytic anemia. Additionally, if this reaction occurs in small vessels, ischemia or infarction of the particular tissue may ensue. The clinical picture of sickle cell anemia is a combination of chronic hemolytic anemia and ischemia.

CLINICAL PRESENTATION

The sickle mutation is located in the β gene, a gene that only becomes active in the later stages of gestation. Since the fetal hemoglobin gene is unaffected, infants who have sickle cell anemia are born without anemia and without the vaso-occlusive problems that are characteristic of the disease. (However, the disease can, and should, be diagnosed in the newborn period in order to provide appropriate care even before the disease is clinically apparent.) Symptoms usually begin to emerge as the production of hemoglobin S increases in the third and fourth months of life. On routine examination, although these babies have normal growth and development, they may be noted to be pale and somewhat jaundiced and they have splenomegaly. These findings are extremely variable; they may be subtle, and they may easily go unnoticed. It is not unusual for this chronic hemolytic anemia to go undiagnosed for a few years if the blood is not examined. The hemolytic anemia is a chronic and permanent feature of the disease, which is present whether or not the patient experiences acute vaso-occlusive episodes. The physiologic adjustments to this anemia are remarkable, and therefore the anemia is usually well tolerated. These children are generally "healthy" and happy; they are able to participate fully in academic and athletic programs; and they are only periodically and unpredictably stricken by vaso-occlusive episodes.

The most common first acute presentation of the vaso-occlusive tendency of the disease is the *hand–foot syndrome*. These cranky babies present with swollen, tender, hot hand(s) or foot (feet), often a low-grade fever, and leukocytosis. If the child is not known to have sickle cell anemia, a mistaken diagnosis of trauma is common. These irritable children with ischemia of their bones respond well to oral hydration and analgesics; there is no specific therapy. The episode rarely lasts more than a few days and essentially always resolves without permanent morbidity.

As the child gets older, bone ischemia is less likely to be accompanied by signs of inflammation. These "painful crises" present as varying degrees of pain (usually in bone, but sometimes as diffuse abdominal or chest pain) with varying degrees of fever, or leukocytosis. Most of these painful episodes can be managed at home by experienced parents, with oral hydration, rest, and analgesics. These children may require hospitalization for parenteral analgesics and hydration.

Although painful crises are the most common of the acute presentations of sickle cell anemia, the most dangerous presentation is infection. The major cause of death in children with sickle cell anemia under 5 years of age is overwhelming pneumococcal sepsis. Despite splenomegaly, these children have functional asplenia with all the risks associated with splenectomy at an early age. This frequently fatal complication may present in the context of an unimpressive febrile illness. The early diagnosis of sickle cell anemia is geared to the prevention and early recognition and treatment of this complication.

DIFFERENTIAL DIAGNOSIS

Sickle cell anemia is in the differential diagnosis of any black infant whose parents either have or do not know whether they have sickle trait, and any black child with a chronic hemolytic anemia. The hemoglobin electrophoresis makes the definitive diagnosis. In infancy, the hemoglobin electrophoresis reveals only hemoglobin S and hemoglobin F; no hemoglobin A is present. In older children and adults there is little hemoglobin F, a predominance of hemoglobin S; there is no hemoglobin A. Other sickle syndromes that are associated with some degree of hemolytic anemia and vaso-occlusion are hemoglobin SC disease and sickle cell thalassemia. These syndromes can also be diagnosed on the basis of the hemoglobin electrophoresis, although in some cases of sickle cell thalassemia, family testing may need to be done for clarification.

WORK-UP

History

Because of efficient community-based screening programs that focus on genetic counseling and education of individuals with sickle cell trait, family histories may provide important information on the presence of the sickle gene in the family. In older children, the review of systems including questions about jaundice, bone pain, or abdominal pain may be helpful. However, it must be kept in mind that a negative history of symptoms does not exclude sickle cell anemia, because there is a wide variation in clinical severity with some individuals not experiencing symptoms until late in life.

Physical Examination

The newborn with sickle cell anemia has an entirely normal physical examination. By 4 months of age, slight pallor and icterus may be apparent. By 1 year of age the child usually has splenomegaly although, as noted above, this enlarged spleen is no longer functional. Splenemogaly usually disappears by 5 years of age because the spleen undergoes its process of autoinfarction. Height and weight are usually normal during the first 5 to 7 years of life, although the weight is usually below typical normal values thereafter. Signs of puberty are delayed 3 to 4 years in both boys and girls. As described in Chapter 124, the response to chronic anemia usually involves some degree of tachycardia, tachypnea, and cardiomegaly, often with loud systolic ejection murmurs.

Laboratory Tests

By about 1 year of age, the child with sickle cell anemia has developed the classical CBC findings including hematocrit in the 20s, reticulocyte count in the 20s, normal MCV, WBC in the teens, and elevated platelet count. The peripheral smear shows fragmented cells, long crescent-shaped irreversible sickled cells, target cells, Howell–Jolly bodies, and an occasional nucleated red blood cell. The indirect bilirubin and LDH are elevated. The sickle cell preparation is positive (as in the patient's sickle trait parents), and the hemoglobin electrophoresis pattern is classical with a predominance of hemoglobin S and no hemoglobin A. These findings are present regardless of whether or not the patient is experiencing a "crisis."

TREATMENT

Children with sickle cell disease must receive routine health maintenance, including the standard immunizations. These children need to be seen every few months in order to keep track of baseline laboratory data (*e.g.*, CBC, reticulocyte count) and stay abreast with intercurrent events. Prophylactic penicillin (125 mg po bid) should be given for the first 5 years of life. In addition, these children should receive pneumococcal vaccine at 2 years of age. Supplemental folic acid (1 mg/day) is particularly useful for children with little fresh green vegetables in their diets. Most importantly, the family should be aware of the importance of seeking medical attention for even "trivial" illnesses. The threat of pneumococcal sepsis is so serious in children under 5 years of age, that all complaints of fever, poor feeding, irritability and so forth, should be evaluated in person rather than by telephone.

INDICATIONS FOR REFERRAL OR ADMISSION

The following is a list of acute problems that require emergency admission or referral: fever—R/O sepsis; pneumonia; splenic sequestration crisis—lower than usual hematocrit with larger than usual spleen; aplastic crisis—lower than usual hematocrit with lower than usual reticulocyte count; severe painful crisis; stroke, seizures, or extraordinary headache; visual disturbances; priapism. The following chronic conditions merit consultation: persistent hip pain; leg ulcers; deteriorating liver, renal, pulmonary, or cardiac function; pregnancy or contraception issues.

ANNOTATED BIBLIOGRAPHY

Charache S, Dover GJ et al: Hydroxyurea-induced augmentation of fetal hemoglobin production in patients with sickle cell anemia. Blood 69(1):109–116, 1987 (Most recent clinical application of a drug used to modify the course of sickle cell anemia by augmenting the production of hemoglobin F.)

Cole TB, Smith SJ, Buchanan GB: Hematologic alterations during acute infection in children with sickle cell disease. Pediatr Infect Dis J 6:454–457, 1987 (Clinical study that illustrate the relative uselessness of white counts or band counts in diagnosing infection in children with sickle cell anemia.)

Embry SH: The clinical pathophysiology of sickle cell disease Ann Rev Med 37:361–376, 1986 (Excellent discussion.)

Gaston MH et al: Prophylaxis with oral penicillin in children with sickle cell anemia: A randomized trial. 314(25): 1593–1599, 1986 (This randomized double blind placebo-controlled clinical trial demonstrated the efficacy of penicillin prophylaxis in sickle cell anemia.)

Phebus CK, Glominger MS, Maciak BJ: Growth patterns by age and sex in children with sickle cell disease. J Pediatr 105(1):28–33, 1984 (Demonstrates the deleterious effects of sickle hemoglobinopathies on growth in 133 children and adolescents.)

Serjeant GR: Sickle Cell Disease. New York, Oxford U Press, 1985 (Extensively documented and clinically oriented tome covering genetics, prenatal diagnosis, complications, and therapies of the sickle cell syndromes in readable format.)

126
Neutropenia
ORAH S. PLATT

The normal absolute neutrophil count varies widely between 1000 and 8000 cells/mm^3, depending on age and race. In general, whites have higher neutrophil counts than blacks, and children under 10 years of age have lower counts than adults. As a rule of thumb, the lower limit of normal neutrophil count is 1500 in white children and 1000 in black children.

Most cases of neutropenia are discovered in the process of evaluating the white blood count (WBC) of a child with an acute febrile illness. Less frequently, neutropenia is identified as an incidental finding in healthy children who have a routine complete blood count (CBC). The pediatrician rarely finds neutropenia where he expects it — in a patient with recurrent bacterial infections.

PATHOPHYSIOLOGY

Neutrophils are produced in the bone marrow where they progress from the stem cell stage to the mature neutrophil stage in about 2 weeks. The marrow itself is a reservoir of mature neutrophils which eventually leave to enter the peripheral circulation either to marginate along vessel walls or be swept up with the flowing red cells. The neutrophil has a brief life span of a few hours in the circulation. The control of neutrophil production and distribution is not completely understood, but involves a complex interplay between cellular and humoral factors. Neutropenia can be caused by faulty production or maturation in the marrow, increased margination or sequestration in the reticuloendothelial system, or peripheral destruction. The clinical distinction between decreased production and increased peripheral destruction of neutrophils is difficult. There is no neutrophil equivalent of the reticulocyte, nor is there a neutrophil survival test.

The major functions of the neutrophil are to recognize, chase, engulf, and kill bacteria. The major clinical consequence of neutropenia is serious bacterial infection, a complication that is rarely encounted unless the neutrophil count is less than 500 cells/mm^3

CLINICAL PRESENTATION

Although many patients with neutropenia are entirely asymptomatic, there is a pattern of infection that should arouse the pediatrician's suspicion of neutropenia. The tissues most often infected in children with neutropenia are the vulnerable portals of entry of bacteria. These sites are the mouth, skin, lungs, and perianal areas. Gingival and oral mucosal lesions are common and can be the most painful and distressing complication of chronic neutropenia. Recurrent skin abscesses are also seen in patients with neutropenia, although the most common cause of this type of infection is repetitive exposure to *Staphylococcus aureus* in a relatively unhygienic environment. In those rare patients with cyclic neutropenia, a clear-cut pattern of recurrent infections every 2 to 3 weeks is classical.

DIFFERENTIAL DIAGNOSIS

Healthy Children

Infection. Probably the most common cause of isolated neutropenia in otherwise healthy children is infection. The mechanism can be complex—a combination of decreased production (by toxin, antibody, or direct invasion), increased margination (in active reticuloendothelium or infected tissues), and increased peripheral destruction (antibody, drug, or toxin-mediated). This type of neutropenia is seen both in viral and bacterial infections. The diagnosis is usually made by observing the resolution of the neutropenia as the infection subsides.

Toxins. Although environmental toxins such as heavy metals, organic compounds, and ionizing ra-

diation can cause neutropenia, the most likely suspects are drugs. Drug reactions causing neutropenia can be direct toxic effects of the drug, hypersensitivity reactions, or antibody-mediated. Some of the drugs that have been implicated in neutropenia that are commonly used by pediatricians are trimethoprim/sulfa, chloramphenicol, and oxacillin. In most cases the etiology of neutropenia cannot be determined precisely, especially because an intercurrent infection is usually present. However, it is always prudent to stop all medications (even over-the-counter drugs) when neutropenia is present.

Antibody Mediated. As mentioned above, drugs and infections have been implicated in provoking antibody-mediated neutropenia. Such premature destruction of neutrophils or their marrow precursors has also been described in children with chronic autoimmune disorders and immunodeficiencies. An occasional case of isoimmune neutropenia in newborns has also been described. These diagnoses are difficult to make because of the technical problems involved in determining and interpreting the presence of antineutrophil antibody.

III Children with Prolonged Neutropenia

Congenital Bone Marrow Failure Syndromes. Although not usually present at birth, some rare congential bone marrow failure syndromes may present with isolated neutropenia. Where neutrophils are still present (albeit in small numbers) the morphology is often abnormal, with decreased lobulation or dysmorphic granules. These syndromes include Kostman's syndrome, Fanconi's anemia, Schwachman–Diamond syndrome, cartilage–hair hypoplasia, Chédiak–Higashi sydrome, and dyskeratosis congenita. Many of these syndromes have characteristic congenital abnormalities, bone marrow findings, and chromosomal abnormalities.

Immune Disorders. Many of the congenital immunodeficiencies, including the various dys- and agammaglobulinemias, are associated with various degrees of neutropenia. The mechanisms can involve both peripheral destruction and decreased production. Interestingly, in some cases, the neutropenia improves with the administration of replacement gamma globulin.

Metabolic Disorders. Several aminoacidurias have been associated with neutropenia. In many of these cases, there is megaloblastic maturation reminiscent of B_{12} or folic acid deficiencies, which can also cause neutropenia in children.

WORK-UP

History

It is important to take a comprehensive family and personal history in evaluating the child with neutropenia. The nature and timing of infections in the child and in the family are critical information. Any history of bone morrow failure or chronic blood disorder in the family can be helpful clues, as a history of drug or environmental exposure.

Physical Examination

A complete physical examination is necessary in evaluating the child with neutropenia. Plotting of growth parameters and noting any congenital anomalies are important in establishing chronicity and in pointing to some of the congenital syndromes. The examination should include a careful inspection of the mouth, lungs, skin, and perianal areas, and palpation of the liver and spleen.

Laboratory Tests

The laboratory evaluation of the child with neutropenia begins with a CBC and an examination of the peripheral smear. Special attention should be paid to the MCV (if enlarged, be suspicious of bone marrow failure or megaloblastosis), and morphology of neutrophil (lobulation pattern, granule morphology). If there is no associated anemia, thrombocytopenia, or neutrophil dysmorphology, and the child appears well, the CBC can be followed two times a week for ~6 weeks to determine chronicity and possible cyclicity. If the neutropenia persists, quantitation of immunoglobulins should be done.

TREATMENT

Well Child with Incidental Neutropenia

These children must have all drugs stopped and followed carefully with twice-weekly CBCs until resolution or referral. Parents must be educated that all illnesses and fever must be reported at once.

Fever and Neutropenia

Children with neutropenia and fever are a high-risk group for fulminant sepsis. All children with fever and neutropenia should have a careful phys-

ical examination, CBC, cultures, and chest roentgenogram. Any infection that is uncovered must be treated vigorously. A close and careful observation must be maintained if no sign of infection is found. For those with absolute granulocyte counts less than 500/mm^3, parenteral broad spectrum antibiotics should be administered. White cell transfusions are helpful in selected patients (including newborns) with severe neutropenia and documented sepsis.

Management of Chronic Neutropenia

No specific therapy is available in most cases of chronic neutropenia. Bone marrow transplantation can be done under certain circumstances. Most patients, however, will be managed in a supportive fashion, with particular attention to oral, skin, and perianal hygiene, as well as prophylactic antibiotics in severe cases.

INDICATIONS FOR REFERRAL OR ADMISSION

Sorting out the cause of neutropenia can be a difficult and discouraging task. In an otherwise healthy child, the neutropenia can be monitored twice weekly for ~6 weeks after all drugs have been stopped. If the neutropenia has not resolved, a quantitative measurement of serum immunoglobulins may point to an associated immunodeficiency. This result would warrant a referral to an immunologist. However, if the immunoglobulins are normal, if a decrease in any other cell lines appear, if there is evidence of failure to thrive, or if there are associated anomalies, the patient should be further evaluated in consultation with a hematologist.

Any febrile or infected child with less than 500 neutrophils/mm^3, regardless of the cause of neutropenia, should be hospitalized for extensive culturing and administration of broad spectrum antibiotic coverage.

ANNOTATED BIBLIOGRAPHY

deAlarcon PA, Goldberg J, Nelson DA, Stockman JA: Chronic neutropenia: Diagnostic approach and prognosis. Am J Pediatr Hematol Oncol 5(1):3–9, 1983 (Detailed discussion of the work-up of the child with chronic neutropenia and a diagnostic approach of differentiating benign and serious forms of these disorders; good bibliography.)

Lange RD, Jones JB: Cyclic neutropenia. Am J Pediatr Hematol Oncol 4:363–367, 1981 (Excellent review of the clinical manifestations of cyclic neutropenia and its management.)

Oski FO: Neutropenia in children. Pediatr in Rev 3:108–112, 1981 (Succinct overview of etiologies, differential diagnoses, normal values and diagnostic work-up of childhood neutropenia.)

Sadowitz PD, Oski FO: Differences in polymorphonuclear cell counts between healthy white and black infants: Response to meningitis. Pediatrics 72(3):405–407, 1983 (Demonstrates the differences in neutrophil counts in both healthy and ill black children and white children.)

127
Thrombocytopenia
ORAH S. PLATT

Thrombocytopenia is one of the most common reasons for referring a child to a hematologist. The symptoms are dramatic, the differential diagnosis is worrisome, and parental anxiety is high.

PATHOPHYSIOLOGY

Platelets are the first line of defense against bleeding. At the first suggestion of a breech of vascular integrity, platelets adhere to the damaged endothelium, cause other platelets to aggregate at the local site, and encourage the soluble coagulation factors to form a definitive fibrin clot. When the platelet count is reduced below ~50,000/mm³, small capillary lesions (petechiae) appear, and the skin and mucous membranes become more vulnerable to minor trauma.

Normally the megakaryocytes in the bone marrow produce enough platelets to maintain the count above 150,000/mm³. A normal platelet lasts for about 5 days in the peripheral circulation. Thrombocytopenia results if the platelet survival time is reduced to hours or minutes. Under these circumstances, the platelets are usually larger in size than normal (indicating a population of young platelets), and there appear to be plenty of megakaryocytes in the marrow. On the other hand, if the marrow is affected by toxin, infiltration, or congenital defect, production will drop and thrombocytopenia will develop. These platelets tend to be small and the marrow may be infiltrated with tumor cells, storage cells, and so forth, or else have diminished numbers of megakaryocytes. Since megakaryocytic quantitation is not reliable, it is sometimes necessary to give radiolabeled platelets and determine their survival in order to determine whether thrombocytopenia is due to increased destruction or decreased production.

CLINICAL PRESENTATION

Thrombocytopenia presents as a mild to severe bleeding tendency characterized by petechiae, mucous membrane bleeding (e.g., nose, GI, GU, retina, CNS), bleeding from superficial cuts, or superficial skin hemorrhages. Menstrual bleeding can be profuse in postpubertal girls. In contrast to most of the soluble coagulation factor deficiencies, hemarthroses and deep muscle bleeds are rare.

DIFFERENTIAL DIAGNOSIS

Given the clinical presentation described above, there are four major diagnostic possibilities: (1) thrombocytopenia, (2) platelet dysfunction, (3) diffuse vasculitis, and (4) von Willebrand's disease. Although more than one of these possibilities may occur at the same time, in general, if there is platelet-type bleeding, a platelet count will distinguish between thrombocytopenia and the others.

In otherwise healthy children with the acute onset of isolated thrombocytopenia—the most common diagnosis is ITP. The major diagnosis to exclude is acute lymphocytic leukemia. In sick, febrile children, the major diagnosis to consider first is meningococcemia.

In the patient with documented thrombocytopenia, the major diagnostic considerations are conveniently classified as either an increased destruction or a decreased production. The thrombocytopenias that result from increased peripheral destruction can be antibody mediated (e.g., ITP, drug-induced), coincident with localized consumption (e.g., vascular malformation, hemolytic-uremic syndrome, vasculitis) or disseminated intravascular coagulation (DIC), associated with hypersplenism, or toxin (e.g., drug, infection). The hypoproduction thrombocytopenias include infiltrative disease including leukemia, storage diseases, and granulomatous diseases. Acquired or drug-induced aplastic anemia as well as the constitutional bone marrow failure syndromes (*e.g.*, TAR syndrome, Fanconi's anemia) are possibilities.

WORK-UP

History

The history should include a family history of bleeding or platelet disorders. A complete drug and toxin exposure history is important. The timing, distribution, and nature of the bleeding will determine the severity and the degree of chronicity. Fever or other signs of infection may indicate disseminated infection. Systemic symptoms of weight loss, sweats, or bone pain suggest the possibility of bone marrow disease.

Physical Examination

Growth parameters, vital signs, and general assessment will help in establishing the chronicity and the level of concern. The following findings should be noted: pallor, jaundice, petechiae, peripheral thromboses, bruises, fundal hemorrhages, lymphadenopathy, hepatomegaly or splenomegaly, or congenital anomalies.

Laboratory Tests

Begin with a CBC (including a platelet count and an examination of the peripheral smear), a PT, and PTT. If everything except the platelet count is absolutely normal, the child is likely to have ITP. Most clinicians would favor doing a bone marrow aspirate to exclude leukemia at this stage. The techniques for measuring antiplatelet antibody vary and are frequently not helpful in establishing a diagnosis of ITP in children. *ITP is a clinical diagnosis and does not rest on any single diagnostic test including the bone marrow examination and platelet antibody test.*

If the PT and PTT are elevated in association with thrombocytopenia, the patient is likely to have DIC and must have cultures taken immediately to facilitate therapy.

If the peripheral smear shows fragmented red cells, thrombocytopenia, but normal PT and PTT, the hemolytic-uremic syndrome is a possibility. BUN and creatinine should be sent.

The diagnosis of diseases, such as leukemia and

storage diseases, require expert help and special bone marrow examinations.

TREATMENT

In most pediatric practices, ITP is the most common thrombocytopenia that can be treated on an outpatient basis. If the platelet count is $>50,00/mm^3$ and the child is not bleeding, he should avoid contact sports and aspirin and notify the pediatrician of any bleeding episode. In the patient with less than 50,000 platelets/mm^3 who is symptomatic (and has had a bone marrow examination to rule out leukemia), a short course of prednisone (2 mg/kg/day for 10 days, then taper over 10 days) will usually decrease the bleeding tendency even though the platelet count may not change very much or have a sustained elevation. Under special circumstances such as thrombocytopenia presenting with varicella, intravenous gamma globulin therapy can be lifesaving. A small proportion ($<25\%$) of children with ITP are refractory to standard outpatient management and eventually require splenectomy.

INDICATIONS FOR REFERRAL
OR ADMISSION

Any febrile child with thrombocytopenia and petechiae (with or without elevated PT and PTT) should be hospitalized and treated for presumed sepsis. Children with any of the following complicating features should be worked up in consultation with a hematologist: symptomatic or prolonged thrombocytopenia, neutropenia, blasts on smear, anemia, bone pain, or congential anomalies. A nephrologist will be helpful in managing the hemolytic-uremic syndrome.

ANNOTATED BIBLIOGRAPHY

Buchanan GR: Childhood idiopathic thrombocytopenia purpura: How many tests and how much treatment required? (Thought provoking editorial questioning the necessity for extensive diagnostic testing, hospitalization, and therapy [prednisone and IV gamma globulin] in acute ITP.)

Bussel JB, Schulman I et al: Intravenous use of gamma globulin in the treatment of chronic immune thrombocytopenic purpura as a means to defer splenectomy. J Pediatr 103(4):651–654, 1983 (Describes the beneficial responses of 9 of 12 children with chronic ITP treated with IV gamma globulin.)

Castle V, Andrew M, Kelton J et al: Frequency and mechanisms of neonatal thrombocytopenia. J Pediatr 108(5):749–755, 1986 (Incidence and etiology data on neonatal thrombocytopenia in a study population of 807 infants admitted to an intensive care unit.)

Naiman J: Disorders of Platelets. In Oski FO, Naiman JL (eds): Hematologic Problems in the Newborn, pp 183–215. Philadelphia, WB Saunders, 1982 (Complete discussion of neonatal thrombocytopenia emphasizing diagnosis and management.)

Stuart MJ, McKenna R: Diseases of coagulation: The platelet and vasculature. In Hematology of infancy and childhood, pp 1234–1286. Nathan DG, Oski FO (eds): Philadelphia, WB Saunders, 1980 (Exhaustive discussion of thrombocytopenia in the pediatric population; pathophysiology emphasized.)

128
Lymphadenopathy
ORAH S. PLATT

Almost every child in a typical pediatric practice eventually appears with enlarged lymph nodes. Most of these children are simply reacting normally to new environmental antigens and require little more than a limited physical examination. The chapter outlines an approach to the evaluation of the child who has lymphadenopathy. Cervical lymphadenopathy and other neck masses are the subject of Chapter 90.

PATHOPHYSIOLOGY

The lymph nodes provide the optimum setting for the education and function of lymphocytes of all types. Here, antigens are presented, recognized, and responded to. This process frequently involves lymphocyte proliferation, a reaction that can cause a node to enlarge. Pathologists describe this as *reactive hyperplasia*. This is the situation in most children who have adenopathy in the setting of uncomplicated viral or bacterial illnesses. The node itself sometimes becomes infected, enlarges, and becomes exquisitely tender because it is acutely invaded by neutrophils. Lymph node enlargement can also occur when the node is invaded and destroyed architecturally by malignant cells.

CLINICAL PRESENTATION

Lymphadenopathy is usually a straightforward diagnosis presenting as a mass in a node-bearing region. Since most of these areas are easily accessible to examining fingers and eyes, masses are usually apparent. Rarely, non-lymph node masses appear in these regions and can be confusing. Some of these masses include developmental anomalies such as thyroglossal duct cysts (see Chap. 90). Other masses that can masquerade as nodes include tumors or infections of bone or soft tissue, and vascular anomalies. Enlarged nodes in the mediastinum and along the aorta become symptomatic when they impinge on other structures and require various radiographic techniques to be delineated.

DIFFERENTIAL DIAGNOSIS

Since there are so many causes of lymphadenopathy, it is convenient to classify the differential diagnosis into groups.

Generalized Adenopathy with Fever

These usually represent the classical infectious diseases of childhood including CMV, mononucleosis, chickenpox, rubella, measles, toxoplasmosis, and enterovirus infections. Acute AIDS and Kawasaki's disease should also be considered. These diseases are diagnosed based on their clinical presentation, epidemiology, clinical course, and corroborating laboratory findings.

Generalized Adenopathy Without Fever

Although a low-grade fever may be present, these children generally do not appear to have an acute infectious disease. They may have a hypersensitivity reaction such as drug allergy, collagen-vascular disease such as JRA, or neoplasm such as leukemia or lymphoma.

Localized Adenopathy with Fever

These children usually have a localized infection with enlargement of the appropriate draining node or nodes. Viral URIs account for many of these nodes, although bacteria such as Staphylococcus and Streptococcus are certainly common pathogens. The more immunocompromised the host, the more unusual the possibilities of microorganisms become.

Localized Adenopathy Without Fever

Although these children may have a rather indolent infection without an obvious local lesion, they are at risk for malignancy such as lymphoma, Hodgkin's disease, or leukemia.

WORK-UP

History

The history should clarify how long the lesion has been present, and whether it was associated with any obvious infection. It is important to note if there have been significant systemic symptoms such as weight loss, failure to gain weight, night sweats, and fatigue. Unusual exposure to animals, unpasteurized milk, or exotic travel should also be investigated.

Physical Examination

Growth parameters, vital signs, and a general assessment will help in establishing the chronicity and level of concern. All the node-bearing areas and liver and spleen should be examined, with the size, texture, and tenderness noted. For localized adenopathy, a detailed examination of the appropriate draining region should be done to find the possible source of infection. At the same time, pallor, jaundice, petechiae, or excessive bruises should be noted.

Laboratory Tests

Most children will not require any laboratory work when adenopathy is found, because the cause is usually obvious. For persistent or particularly worrisome adenopathy, a good initial screening would include a CBC with differential and platelets, an erythrocyte sedimentation rate, mono spot test, PPD, and chest roentgenogram.

TREATMENT

Most cases of adenopathy are part of a self-limited disease process that requires no treatment. Next in frequency are other common bacterial infections which are either primary such as lymphadenitis or secondary (or associated) with other infections such as pharyngitis, otitis media, or skin infections, which are easily treated with broad spectrum oral antibiotics. Penicillin may be used if Streptococcus is the likely pathogen. Otherwise, amoxicillin, dicloxacillin, erythromycin, or cefaclor offer better coverage for other organisms such as Staphylococcus. Rarely, unusual infections, malignancies, or chronic diseases will require sophisticated diagnostics and treatment. The dilemma for the pediatrician is how long to follow an entirely healthy child who has enlarged nodes without an obvious diagnosis.

INDICATIONS FOR REFERRAL OR ADMISSION

The child with an infectious etiology who appears toxic, is immunocompromised, a neonate or the infection is progressing despite outpatient management should be hospitalized and receive parenteral antibiotics.

Ultimately, sorting out the etiology of lymphadenopathy hinges on the lymph node biopsy. Children with the following characteristics should be referred for consultation, and together, a decision is made regarding the need for hospitalization:

- Persistent (usually >2 mo) undiagnosed adenopathy
- Enlarging or matted, nontender adenopathy
- Associated with worrisome signs and symptoms such as weight loss, failure to thrive, bone pain, nightsweats, and hepatosplenomegaly.
- Associated with abnormality in CBC, PPD, or chest roentgenogram
- Associated with fever of unknown etiology

It is frequently helpful to consult either an oncologist or an infectious disease specialist (depending on the clinical intuition of the pediatrician) rather than going directly to the surgeon for a biopsy. The medical specialist will be able to work with the surgeon to facilitate the special culturing and handling of the specimen in the pathology laboratory.

ANNOTATED BIBLIOGRAPHY

Altman AJ (ed): Pediatric oncology. Pediatr North Am 32(3), 1985 (Good collection of chapters describing the most common childhood cancers having associated peripheral lymphadenopathy.)

Hicks RV, Melish ME: Kawasaki syndrome. Pediatr Clinic North Am 33:1151–1176, 1986 (Comprehensive discussion of this multisystem disease in which cervical lymphadenopathy is one of the six major diagnostic criteria.)

Knight PJ, Mulne AF, Vassy, LE: When is lymph node biopsy indicated in children with enlarged peripheral nodes? Pediatrics 69:391–396, 1982 (Presents guidelines for performing a diagnostic biopsy.)

Knight PJ, Reiner CB: Superficial lumps in children: What, when, and why? Pediatrics 72:147–153, 1983 (Good discussion as to which lumps ought to be regarded as worrisome.)

Lake AM, Oski FA: Peripheral lymphadenopathy in childhood. Am J Dis Child 132:357–359, 1978 (Reviews their 10-year experience with excisional biopsy to determine if clinical features are predictive of histologic diagnosis.)

Marcy SM: Infections of lymph nodes of the head and neck. Pediatr Infect Dis 2:397–405, 1983 (Practical and comprehensive.)

129
Splenomegaly
A. STEPHEN DUBANSKY

The spleen is normally palpable in 10% of the pediatric population. Twenty to 30% of healthy newborns, 10% of normal 1-year-olds, and 1% to 3% of fit 18-year-olds may have spleens palpable ~1 cm below the left costal margin. Pathologic splenomegaly is a relatively uncommon problem. However, when it occurs, splenomegaly can represent a puzzling diagnostic problem and a source of great concern.

PATHOPHYSIOLOGY

The spleen, a major reticuloendothelial organ, consists of masses of lymphocytes, plasma cells, and macrophages (white pulp) associated with an extensive network of Billroth's cords and sinusoids (red pulp). The spleen acts as a filter, a reservoir, an important producer of humoral proteins, and an organ of erythropoiesis.

The normal spleen removes damaged, antibody or complement coated, and senescent blood cells from the circulation. It serves as a filter for intravenous particulate antigens. The spleen is a reservoir for one third of the body's platelets. Additionally, the spleen normally contains 25-ml to 50-ml of blood as well as plasma proteins such as factor VIII. When enlarged for any reason, the reservoir's capacity of platelets, erythrocytes, and, leukocytes may increase, resulting in decreases in any or all of these cell lines. The spleen has the primary role in producing antibody to intravenous particulate antigen. It is a major site of synthesis of IgM, properidine, and tuftsin, a polypeptide that stimulates neutrophil chemotaxis. When the child is afflicted by disorders such as thalassemia major or osteopetrosis, the spleen may serve as a site of extramedullary hematopoiesis.

CLINICAL PRESENTATION

First, the enlarged spleen must be differentiated from other left upper quadrant masses. Confusion arises occasionally when differentiating splenomegaly and nephromegaly (i.e., Wilm's tumor). However, careful palpation reveals that the spleen's upper extent is lost under the left costal margin, and its tip moves caudally during inspiration. A massively enlarged left hepatic lobe may sometimes be confused with an enlarged spleen. Percussion will assist in differentiating the spleen from a floating rib. Commonly, pulmonary hyperinflation and flattening of the diaphragms as seen in reactive airway disease or bronchiolitis may allow the physician to feel an otherwise normal-sized spleen. In differentiating the normal and the pathologically enlarged spleen, remember that the spleen may be palpated 1 cm to 2 cm below the costal margin in a healthy child. Pathologic spleens may also be that size, but they are commonly firm or tender to palpation.

Splenomegaly may develop suddenly or gradually. The spleen may increase, decrease, or remain unchanged in size. The child may be free of any obvious systemic symptoms or may appear acutely or chronically ill. These varying modes of presentation will help clarify the cause of the enlargement. It is most important to differentiate the acutely and transiently enlarged spleen of a viral infection from the chronic splenomegaly that requires further examination and definition.

DIFFERENTIAL DIAGNOSIS

The list of possible diagnoses is long, and is composed of common, unusual, and frankly esoteric disorders (see the box, Causes of Splenomegaly). The causes have been grouped in the following

Causes of Splenomegaly

Infectious

Viral

Mononucleosis
Rubella
Rubeola
Cytomegalovirus
Herpes
Coxsackie

Bacterial

Subacute bacterial endocarditis
Sepsis
Tuberculosis
Salmonellosis
Congenital syphilis
Tularemia

Fungal

Histoplasmosis
Coccidiomycosis

Protozoal
Malaria
Toxoplasmosis
Parasitic
Schistosomiasis
Trypanosomiasis
Visceral larva migrans
Rickettsial
Rocky Mountain spotted fever

Immunologic—Inflammatory

Juvenile rheumatoid arthritis
Systemic lupus erythematosus
Serum sickness
Sarcoidosis
Chronic granulomatous disease
Drug-induced pseudolymphoma (phenytoin)

Hematologic

Sickle hemoglobinopathy
Thalassemia major
Hereditary RBC membrane disorder
Hereditary RBC enzyme disorder
Rh and ABO diseases
Autoimmune hemolytic anemia
Iron deficiency anemia
Osteopetrosis

Congestive

Portal vein thrombosis
Congestive heart failure
Pericarditis
Chronic hepatitis
Wilson disease
Cystic fibrosis
Biliary atresia

Metabolic

Tay–Sachs disease
Gaucher disease
Niemann–Pick disease
Metachromatic leukodystrophy
Hyperlipoproteinemia, type I
Gangliosidoses
Galactosemia
Wolman disease
Fructose intolerance

Malignant

Leukemia
Lymphoma, Hodgkin's and non-Hodgkin's
Histiocytosis X

Miscellaneous

Idiopathic–normal variant
Splenic trauma
Hemangioma
Hamartoma
Cyst

---

categories: infectious, immunologic, congestive, hematologic, malignant, metabolic, and miscellaneous. A detailed discussion of the various possibilities is beyond the scope of this text. The emphasis will be placed instead on a meticulous and thorough history and physical examination, and the minimal laboratory testing usually sufficient to uncover the appropriate diagnostic category if not the specifically responsible disease.

WORK-UP

History

A careful neonatal history may reveal omphalitis or umbilical vein catheterization compatible with a subsequent portal vein thrombosis. Did the mother have an unexplained infection or rash during pregnancy indicating congenital infection (*e.g.*, TORCH)? A social history may reveal travel to endemic areas of malaria, or travel to areas of, or exposure to persons with typhoid fever, tuberculosis, histoplasmosis, or coccidiomycosis.

A positive family history is important in clarifying the diagnosis. Were there siblings with neonatal jaundice (ABO or Rh isoimmunization, or nonimmune hemolytic anemia)? Is there a family history of jaundice, anemia, early cholecystectomy, or splenectomy (hemolytic anemias)? What is the ethnic extraction (Niemann–Pick, Gaucher, Tay–Sachs children are often Jewish; Fabry's, often Scandinavian; thalassemics, often Greek or Italian)? What is the race (sickle syndromes occur commonly in blacks and people from the Mediterranean area.)? Is there a family history of neurologic disease, retardation, or early unexplained death (lipidoses)? Is there a history of progressive liver disease and neurologic abnormalities (Wilson disease)? Is there a family history of cystic fibrosis or autoimmune or collagen vascular disease (SLE, JRA)?

The past medical history is equally important. Has the child had repeated bouts of otitis media or seborrheic rashes (histiocytosis X)? Is there a history of heart disease (pericarditis, congestive failure) or mitral valve prolapse (SBE)? Has the child had hepatitis or previously unexplained jaundice (portal hypertension)? Growth and development must be carefully assessed in ruling out chronic disease in general and the metabolic diseases associated with mental retardation in particular. Has there been recent blunt abdominal trauma (subcapsular bleed)?

A careful review of systems is essential. Has there been fever, fatigue, sore throat, or rash (cytomegalovirus or EB virus)? Has there been sudden jaundice, pallor, or dark urine (autoimmune hemolytic anemia)? Have there been systemic symptoms compatible with JRA? Has there been fever, pallor, fatigue, or bone pain of a gradual onset (leukemia, lymphoma)? Unexplained abdominal or bone pains in black children may indicate Hb SC or Hb S-β thalassemia. Blood in the stool may indicate portal hypertension with varices or hemorrhoids. A history of repeated lower respiratory tract illnesses, diarrhea, and failure to thrive indicates cystic fibrosis as a possible cause. Was the spleen palpable in infancy in an otherwise asymptomatic child (cyst, cystic hygroma, or hemangioma)? Is neonatal or early childhood splenomegaly accompanied by jaundice, hypoglycemia, developmental delay, and cataracts (galactosemia)? Has the child had seizures as may be seen with congenital infection or with hypoglycemia due to fructose intolerance or storage disease?

Physical Examination

A careful examination is as important as the history. Most importantly, does the child appear acutely or chronically ill, or is the splenomegaly an incidental finding in an otherwise normal child? Is this spleen the normal, soft, 1-cm spleen that may be normally palpated in a healthy child or a child recovering from recent viral infection(s)? Vital signs and growth parameters should be graphed and any evidence of failure to thrive should be carefully noted.

Head examination may uncover puffy eyelids and pharyngitis seen in EB virus infection or chronic otitis media as seen in histiocytosis. An eye examination may reveal the conjunctival comma vessels or proliferative retinopathy seen with sickle hemoglobinopathy, the scleral icterus of liver disease or hemolytic anemia, the cataracts of galactosemia, the cherry red macula of Tay–Sachs disease, or the chorioretinitis seen in congenital infection or visceral larva migrans. Gum hypertrophy may indicate sarcoidosis or monocytic leukemia. The neck must be palpated to rule out masses or lymphadenopathy.

Cardiovascular examination should be concerned with jugular venous distention, heart sounds, murmurs, gallops, and clicks. Chest observation and percussion may reveal hyperexpansion compatible with the air trapping seen in cystic fibrosis. Auscultation may reveal the fine moist rales of failure, the more coarse rales of chronic infiltrate, or the normal breath sounds seen in a child with chronic interstitial disease (*i.e.*, histiocytosis).

The abdomen should be palpated and percussed for masses, hepatomegaly, and ascites. Hepatosplenomegaly may indicate infection, malignancy, congestive condition, storage disease, or heart failure. An anal examination should assess the presence of hemorrhoids. A thorough neurologic examination is vital, especially in diagnosing the metabolic disorders.

Generalized lymphadenopathy should be recorded. It is commonly seen in mononucleosis, histiocytosis, lymphoma, leukemia, JRA, pseudolymphoma, and sarcoidosis. Bone and joint tenderness, as well as objective signs of arthritis should be sought, and when present, JRA and leukemia should be considered.

The skin may provide a wealth of information. Pallor with or without jaundice may indicate a hemolytic anemia. Jaundice, telangiectasias, and spider angiomata indicate an underlying liver disease.

Petechiae and ecchymoses may point to thrombocytopenia associated with infection or malignancy. Venous distention on the abdomen indicates portal vein obstruction. Seborrheic rashes are seen in histiocytosis. The "blueberry muffin" rash in the newborn invariably indicates congenital infection. Acute monocytic leukemia may be associated with subcutaneous nodules. Skin hemangiomata may be evidence of an associated splenic hemangioma. Signs of nonaccidental trauma should raise concern about a splenic blood collection or cyst. Clubbing of the nails may be seen in cystic fibrosis; splinter hemorrhages, in SBE. Chronic and evanescent rashes of many descriptions are seen concomitantly with splenomegaly, and, although their presence may not be diagnostic, their absence is useful negative information.

Laboratory Tests

The aforementioned history and physical examination should both shorten the differential list and decrease the number of laboratory tests necessary to make the diagnosis. Ordering all possible laboratory tests is invariably expensive, painful, and unnecessary. A complete blood count, platelet count, reticulocyte count, sedimentation rate, carefully observed peripheral smear, Monospot or EB viral capsid IgM, SGPT, bilirubin, and chest roentgenogram are appropriate screening tests in a situation where the history and physical examination do not alone clarify the diagnosis.

The results of the preliminary screen may indicate the need for further more specific testing. CMV IgM antibody, urine culture for CMV, TORCH titers, PPD skin test, fungal serologies, blood cultures, stool culture and hematest, urine for reducing substances, full liver chemistries, ceruloplasmin, ANA, Coombs' test, sickle cell prep and hemoglobin electrophoresis, skull and long bone films, or sweat chloride may be indicated. The screening tests and the more specific laboratory work combined with a thoughtful H&P will make the diagnosis or rule out most of the possibilities.

MANAGEMENT

Mild splenomegaly in the absence of other symptoms or positive physical findings is usually related to a transient viral illness. Viral-induced splenomegaly may last for 6 to 8 weeks, but the spleen does not usually increase in size during this time. The asymptomatic child should be reexamined every 2 weeks until resolution of the splenomegaly. Any increase in spleen size, or the development of any related symptoms should prompt the physician to repeat his screening laboratory tests immediately. In the presence of moderate or massive splenomegaly, the child should refrain from contact sports, and both the child and parent should be warned about the rare complication of splenic rupture.

The child with massive splenomegaly, despite an otherwise normal history and physical examination, should have a more thorough work-up. Any child with hypersplenism (splenic trapping and destruction of one or more cellular blood elements by the enlarged spleen) also requires immediate referral. It is clear from the list of etiologies that few of the diagnoses are themselves emergent problems. However, the child with sickle hemoglobinopathy and sequestration crisis, autoimmune hemolytic anemia, sepsis, SBE, Rocky Mountain spotted fever, serum sickness, congestive failure, or acute trauma requires immediate referral or treatment.

The otherwise normal child followed for 8 weeks without resolution of mild or moderate splenomegaly also requires a further evaluation. Due to the usually chronic nature of the underlying disorder, these patients rarely require hospitalization. Their evaluations are most appropriately done by the pediatric hematologist, who is experienced in examining those few patients with diagnostic enigmas whom the generalists refer. With the aid of the specialists in metabolic and gastrointestinal disorders, the hematologist may use skin, liver, rectal, or bone marrow biopsy, upper gastrointestinal tract films, splenic ultrasound, radionucleotide liver–spleen scan, and special urine collections for metabolic disease in order to define this small number of patients with chronic and apparently isolated splenomegaly.

ANNOTATED BIBLIOGRAPHY

Boles ET, Baxter C, Newton W: Evaluation of splenomegaly in childhood. Clin Pediatr 2(4):161, 1963 (Retrospective 12-year analysis in surgical patients with splenectomy, portal hypertension, abdominal neoplasms.)

McIntyre OR, Ebaugh FG: Palpable spleens in college freshman. Ann Int—Med 66:301, 1967 (Survey of the prevalence of splenomegaly in college students.)

McNicholl B: Palpability of the liver and spleen in infants and children. Arch Dis Child 32:438, 1957 (Prevalence of splenomegaly in the general pediatric population.)

Odom L, Tubergen D: Splenomegaly in children. Postgrad Med 65(4):191, 1979 (Concise, well done review of the general problem.)

17

Musculoskeletal and Traumatic Problems

130
Congenital Dislocation of the Hip

LORIN M. BROWN

Congenital dislocation of the hip (CDH) has been traditionally divided into three major entities: (1) complete congenital dislocation of the hip, in which the femoral head is totally removed usually superiorly and posteriorly from the acetabulum; (2) dislocatable hip, in which the hip can be pushed usually superiorly and posteriorly out from under its acetabular coverage; and (3) congenitally subluxed hip in which the acetabulum is dysplastic in its formation and the femoral head is located partially out of the acetabulum. In addition, there are also instances of acetabular dysplasia without subluxation. With this deformity, the acetabulum is flattened and elevated laterally in its coverage of the femoral head but the femoral head still sits well into the anatomic socket. These cases may be undetectable at birth and have a normal physical examination. Therefore, the hips must be repeatedly checked by the pediatrician during the first 2 years of life for the late onset of presentation.

The physical signs that are described in this chapter do not have to be present at birth or, if present at birth and later disappear, can represent the same serious underlying pathology. If not detected immediately at around the time of birth, most cases of CDH can be identified by 6 months of age. In late onset dislocation of the hip, the first detectable sign of dislocaton appears many months after birth. Some cases of CDH, and especially acetabular dysplasia, cannot be physically detected

until the second year of life or even later. It is important that the correct diagnosis be made as early as possible to allow for early treatment and hence, a better end result.

PATHOPHYSIOLOGY

The reported incidence of dislocated hips varies between 1 to 11/1000 live births for dislocated hips, and between 8 to 12/1000 live births for unstable dislocatable hips at birth. After 1 week of life, the incidence of CDH is reduced to 1/1000 because most unstable and some dislocated hips stabilize spontaneously during the first few days or week of life. Females are affected 4 times as often as males, and the left hip is affected 10 times as often as the right hip.

The cause of CDH is multifactorial and is not fully understood. Heredity is an important component. As many as one third of siblings will have an unstable hip if one parent and one other child have had an unstable hip. Another major etiologic factor is intrauterine posture. A term baby born in a breech position has a 14-fold increased likelihood of having CDH. Simple capsular laxity is also believed to play a major etiologic role.

CLINICAL PRESENTATION

The infant who has a congenital dislocation of the hip will present with either an adduction contraction of the hips or more commonly, no overt physical findings. CDH has no associated pain. There may be a calcaneovarus or a calcaneovalgus posture of the feet. If the child is of walking age, a limp will be present with a complete Trendelenburg dislocation of the hip. Later in life, associated arthritis may cause an antalgic gait.

DIFFERENTIAL DIAGNOSIS

The most important diagnosis to differentiate from a congenital dislocation of the hip in the newborn is septic arthritis of the hip. Pus distends the capsule, resulting in a subluxation or dislocation of the femoral head. The clinical findings are similar to those found with CDH except that pain will also be present. A positive Barlow or Ortolani sign is often present. The infant will cry with motion of the hip (*e.g.*, during diaper changes). Other diseases or congenital anomalies such as a congenital absence of the proximal femur will increase mobility of the hip joint on examination. A discoid meniscus, generalized joint laxity about the knee, or the snapping of the tensor fascia lata over the greater trochanter may also imitate the feel or sound of a dislocating hip. Later in life, a progressive dislocation of the hips can occur with paralytic diseases such as cerebral palsy or spina bifida. In these diseases, the imbalance of the muscles about the hip will cause the hip to be progressively pulled out of the joint.

CLINICAL EXAMINATION

From birth until about the age of 3 months is the most opportune period in which to find the two classic signs of CDH; the *Ortolani sign* and the *Barlow sign*. The Ortolani maneuver is performed with the hips held in 90 degrees of flexion. Each hip is tested independently while the opposite side of the pelvis is stabilized. The hip is first gently abducted while at the same time gentle pressure is placed on the greater trochanter to push the femoral head forward into the acetabulum (*i.e.*, relocated), but when released the femoral head again moves out of the acetabulum. If a sound is audible, which is often the case, it is that of a "thump" rather than the commonly described "click." The Barlow maneuver is positive when the hips are held in 90 degrees of flexion and pressure is applied over the lesser trochanter while adducting the hip forcing the femoral head out of the acetabulum. When the pressure is released, the dislocatable hip usually returns to its acetabular position. In both supine and prone positions, the child with a complete congenitally dislocated hip may have asymmetric skin creases

of the thighs. This finding may also be seen in normal children and is thus not pathognomonic of CDH. With unilateral dislocation of the hip, the *Galeazzi sign* may be observed. With the child lying supine, the hips are flexed to 90 degrees and the knees almost completely flexed. If positive, the affected side will show an unequal shortened height between the knee joints due to shortening on the dislocated side. The femoral head is dislocated from the acetabulum (usually posteriorly), and will cause the leg on the dislocated side to appear shortened. This is termed a *positive Galeazzi test*. It is important to know that the pelvis must be held square to the table or this test is unreliable. After the age of 3 months, as the capsular tissue and ligaments about the hip tighten, there is limitation of motion about the hip. The fully mobile flexible baby becomes more like the adult with a decrease in possible range of motion of the joints. In the child with a dislocated hip, the adductor muscles become tightened and there is marked limitation of abduction of the dislocated hip. It is again stressed that absence of this sign in the young infant does not eliminate a diagnosis of dislocated hip, because without tightening of these structures there is no decrease in the limitation of motion. Moreover, as the hip becomes tighter and more limited in motion, the initial signs of Ortolani and Barlow disappear, because the hip is held rigidly in its dislocated or subluxated position. Another sign is that of *telescoping*. With congenital dislocation of the hip, the femoral head and shaft can be pushed to and fro with the hip held in 90 degrees of flexion. This motion is due to the laxity of the hip capsule.

Another important aspect of the physical examination is that of the tightness of the hamstrings. In the child with a congenitally dislocated hip, the hamstrings are lax and allow a full extension of the knee when the hip and the leg are held in flexion and abduction in external rotation. Thus, if the knee can be completely extended, it is strongly suggestive that the hip is dislocated from the acetabulum. If, however, the femoral head is in the anatomic acetabulum, the hamstrings should be firm with extension of the knees. In the congenitally lax-jointed child, there should still be some "check" to full extension of the knee by the hamstrings.

In the child over 18 months of age who is walking, *limping* is another sign of pathology. This is termed a *Trendelenburg gait*. Due to the mechanical advantage of the hip joint, which is lost by the superior displacement of the pivot from the fulcrum, the abductor muscles of the hip joint become shortened, and therefore lax and weakened. This causes the pelvis to drop on the side opposite of the dislocation. Thus, as the child stands on the dislocated hip, the pelvis tilts downwards on the opposite side due to the laxity and weakness of the abductor muscles on the dislocated side. The severity of the limp is compounded by the shortened leg. When both hips are dislocated, there is a bilateral Trendelenburg sign present without a leg length discrepancy. This results in a duck-type waddling gait. Congenital subluxation may also cause a Trendelenburg gait when the child is tired and the abductors are fatigued.

WORK-UP

The work-up for congenital dislocation or subluxation of the hip is relatively simple. Except in the immediate newborn period where a roentgenogram may be deferred if the physical findings are minor (*e.g.*, a click only), an AP pelvis roentgenogram should be used whenever there is any reason to question the physical diagnosis. This view is usually adequate to identify pathology. As radiologists gain experience with ultrasonography, its role in the screening and treatment of CDH is likely to increase. The older the child, the more reliable will be this examination. The AP roentgenogram should be taken with the hips in neutral position to demonstrate whether the femoral head lies within the acetabulum, is partially dislocated, or is completely dislocated. The acetabular index is a measure of the covering of the femoral head by the acetabulum. With dysplasia, this index will increase. Less than 28 degrees is considered normal. With varying amounts of dysplasia, the angle progresses towards 45 degrees. Other lines may be technically drawn to prove the positioning of the femoral head, but the radiographic positioning can usually be seen when the anatomy is understood without the need for drawing quadrants. Another useful sign is the *teardrop sign*: This is the distance from the medial metaphyseal side of the femoral neck to the lateral side of the medial wall of the acetabulum. This should be symmetrical between the two hips provided both hips are normal. Asymmetry indicates subluxation or complete dislocation of one hip. The frog lateral view of the pelvis is useful to determine if a subluxed or dislocated hip will reduce into the acetabulum in the abducted position. Later, with treatment, an arthrogram may be necessary to decide if there is any interposed tissue in the acetabulum. A CT scan is another useful test if the diagnosis is questionable. Under these circumstances, a MRI scan may also prove useful. Standard tomograms are occasionally useful in delineating the pathology; however, the simpler the test, the less the amount of radiation exposure the child receives. The more sophisticated tests should be reserved for the puzzling situations.

TREATMENT OF CONGENITAL DISLOCATION AND SUBLUXATION OF THE HIP

Initially treatment in the newborn nursery may consist of double or triple diapers to abduct the hips until the child can be evaluated by an orthopedist. This allows for a gentle initial stretch of the hips and adductor muscles and lessens the change for avascular necrosis. The newborn is flaccid and not much force is needed. However, once the baby has gained strength and can adduct his hips, the treatment by diapers is of no benefit. Acetabular dysplasia is treated by the orthopedic surgeon usually for an index over 28 degrees if there is asymmetry between the hips. Some prefer to wait until over 30 degrees or possibly 35 degrees if both hips are the same, but more will treat at a lower index if only one hip is involved. It is relatively easy to treat dysplasia in newborns, and waiting for a spontaneous resolution may not be wise because later, the treatment becomes more difficult and the outcome may not be as favorable. These children, as well as those with dislocated hips, may be placed in an abduction Frejke pillow or a Pavlik harness. These are both safe means of treatment, whereas the metal types of abduction splints lead to a much higher incidence of avascular necrosis of the hip. Avascular necrosis, however, may develop no matter how careful or gentle the treatment. In acetabular dysplasia and CDH, the abduction device is used to maintain a safe concentric reduction of the femoral head until the capsular tissue has contracted to maintain the hip joint with a full acetabular coverage of the femoral head.

If little or no acetabular dysplasia is present, minimal treatment is required for a simple *dislocatable* hip. Usually 2 months of bracing is sufficient to maintain a perfect reduction of the *dislocatable* femoral head. Congenital dislocation of the hip with dysplasia found at birth will require between 6 and 12 months of bracing. Almost the same amount of time is required for acetabular dysplasia to resolve, but sometimes, a period greater than 1 year is necessary. When the dislocation is found beyond the newborn period, the child will require more time in a brace. A rule of thumb is the age in months plus 9 to 12 months. After about 18 months of age, the child is usually too old for closed conservative treatment with bracing. Varying studies have shown that this age limit can be extended towards 24 to 36 months of age, but the time required in the brace or harness for resolution of the problem is significantly increased.

Children over the age of 2½ to 3 months with dislocated hips or severe subluxation require traction to stretch the ligaments and neurovascular structures first to allow for a safe reduction of the femoral head into the acetabulum without increasing the risk of avascular necrosis. This traction may take from 1 week to months depending on the situation. The hip joint should be stretched down to below the triradiate cartilage line to allow for an easy reduction of the femoral head into the acetabulum without undue stretch on the femoral vessels. The child is then taken to the operating room and placed under general anesthesia for an abductor tenotomy followed by a closed reduction and the application of a spica cast. In the spica cast, it is essential that the child be placed in the safe "human position" to maintain the femoral head in the acetabulum but not overstretch the hips into abduction. This avoids new stress and compression of the vascular structures going to the femoral head. The human position, unlike that of the frog position in which the legs are each abducted fully 90 degrees, limits the range of abduction to no more than 60 degrees.

The usual treatment for the child over the age of 1½ to 2 years is an open reduction with an innominate or femoral osteotomy to replace the femoral head into the acetabulum. It is sometimes possible to obtain a closed reduction of the hip and later proceed with only an innominate or femoral osteotomy. This is desirable if a concentric reduction is obtained because the less surgery that is done about the femoral head the better the child's chances of avoiding an avascular necrosis of the hip. In the older child, the use of an Atlantic abduction brace may be necessary to maintain abduction and allow gait.

In a child with septic arthritis that caused the dislocated hip, the pus should be drained from the joint. Aspiration of the hip joint is not adequate and

open drainage is required. Dislocations due to neuromuscular diseases such as cerebral palsy or myelomeningocele will require tendon lengthenings of the flexors and adductors as indicated or even tendon transplantations to help rebalance the muscles about the hip and try to maintain reduction of the hip if possible.

All children treated for CDH must receive regular and careful follow-up, because not only may an apparently "cured" hip redislocate or subluxate, but also the contralateral "normal" hip may, in the future, manifest joint abnormalities. Moreover, even the successfully treated hip may be prone to develop osteoarthritis.

ANNOTATED BIBLIOGRAPHY

Asher MA: Screening for congenital dislocation of the hip, scoliosis and other abnormalities affecting the musculoskeletal system. Pediatr Clin North Am 33(6), 1986 (Clinical discussion of acetabular dysplasia and its role in hip disease.)

Dunne KB, Clarren SK. The origin of prenatal and postnatal deformities. Pediatr Clin North Am 33(6), 1986 (Excellent illustrations of the Ortolani and Barlow test.)

Hensinger RN. Neonatal Orthopaedics, Chap 10. New York, Grune & Stratton, 1981 (Specific and well written.)

Post M (ed): Physical Examination of the Musculoskeletal System. Year Book Medical Publishers, 1986 Chap. 9: Examination of the lower extremities in the child, Part I, by LM Brown and WJW Sharrard. Chap. 10: Examination of the lower extremities in the child, Part II, by LM Brown and R Salter. (Detailed and illustrated text on the examination of the lower extremities in the child.)

Salter R: Textbook of Disorders and Injuries of the Musculoskeletal System, 2nd ed. Baltimore, Leon's & Welcomes, 1983 (Excellent overview text of pediatric orthopaedics.)

Sharrard WJN: Pediatric Orthopedics and Fractures, 2nd ed. Oxford, Blackwell Scientific Pub, 1979 (Complete and well documented.)

Winter RB: Pediatric Orthopaedics. Philadelphia, JB Lippincott, 1978 (Authoritative complete text on pediatric orthopaedics.)

131
The Limping Child
HELEN M. EMERY

Limping may be the presentation of many problems, varying from a spinal cord tumor to a splinter in the foot. Determining why a child has a limp and instituting appropriate treatment can be a significant challenge to the physician.

WORK-UP

An analysis of the cause of the limp begins with a careful history. It is essential to determine if the limp is acute or chronic. When did the limp begin, how long has it been going on, did it begin gradually or acutely? Evaluate preceding events (*e.g.*, a fall) but remember that trauma may be temporally associated with onset though not the real cause of the limp. Does the limp vary with the time of day or with certain activities? Is the limp painful, and if so, where? Are there any relieving factors? Limping after strenuous activity suggests a musculoskeletal etiology such as a soft tissue strain or stress fracture. Constant pain, especially if it is increasing, suggests a tumor. Pain increasing with joint motion suggests a joint problem. Are there any systemic signs or symptoms such as fever, weight loss, rashes, or arthralgias?

Careful observations of the limp and gait pattern are usually most revealing about its cause. When watching the child walk, note signs of weakness, stiffness, or pain. Does the child bear weight on the leg, yet refuse to walk, or does he insist on being carried? An antalgic gait (a shortened stance [*i.e.*, weight bearing] phase of walking) indicates pain, whereas a shortened or abnormal swing phase often suggests hip joint pathology. A waddling gait suggests that there is a weakness of the abductors, which is not uncommon in arthritis or other conditions that have caused children to be immobile. This is also characteristic of the gait seen in the child with uncorrected congenital dislocation of the hip. A fixed back suggests a spinal or abdominal pathology such as discitis or tumor in the spine. It should be remembered that pain from renal, abdominal or spinal origin may be referred to the lower extremity, or to the hip; from one site of the lower extremity to another (*e.g.*, hip disease may present as knee pain), or to sites other than the lower extremity, such as hip pathology may be referred to the groin. If the whole leg is being dragged, a neurologic cause for the gait pattern is more likely, although this can be seen occasionally with unilateral weakness. The hip held in flexion suggests intra-articular pathology within that joint. *Hip-hiking* (*i.e.*, elevation of the hip in the swing phase of gait), is seen in a child who keeps the knee in extension while walking, either because of pain on flexion, or because of instability that is improved by locking the knee. If the knee is in flexion, the ankle is commonly plantar flexed and the child walks on his toes to equalize leg lengths.

The next stage in the examination is to ask the child to climb onto the examination table. Commonly, children favor the affected leg, especially if it is painful; they will usually use their good leg to climb up onto the examination table first. The family's reaction at this time may give clues to their degree of concern and also to any inappropriate manipulative behaviors. When the child is on the examination table, examine him supine. Observe the position in which the child holds his body at rest. A spine that is held rigidly suggests pathology and usually the child avoids rolling or wiggling. Also watch for the "position of comfort" in a hip. The position of flexion and external rotation with a little abduction is common for intra-articular hip pathology. A knee held in approximately 45 degrees of flexion is in the position of comfort for that joint. Measure both legs to eliminate leg length discrepancy and examine the spine for scoliosis. Observe closely for evidence of atrophy or change in the skin and temperature over the affected area. Next it is suggested to perform a neurologic examination, including reflexes, tone, and sensation. Proprioception is also easily tested in most children, often using games like the "piggy game." Get the child to actively range the extremities, including sit-ups for the spine, observing for pain, inability to perform full range, or weakness; then, passively put the entire extremity through range of movement. After this, examine all joints for stability, and also do manual muscle strength testing, particularly to distinguish the subtle asymmetries.

DIFFERENTIAL DIAGNOSIS

The more common causes of a limp can be approached on an anatomic basis. The age of the child and chronicity of the limp are helpful in narrowing the range of diagnostic possibilities. Toxic synovitis and Legg–Calvé–Perthes disease must always be suspected in a 6-year-old child, and slipped capital femoral epiphysis should be considered in an adolescent with a limp. In most instances, trauma is the cause of an acute limp. The injury may be to bone (e.g., fracture), soft tissue (e.g., foreign body, abrasion, strain, or inflammation of a ligament or tendon) or to a joint (e.g., meniscal injury, sprain). Causes other than trauma (e.g., neuromuscular and leg length asymmetry) become more likely if the limp is chronic.

Spine

Discitis, usually from a hematogenously spread staphylococcal infection, is one of the more common causes of back problems in a child, although it is not uncommon for the child to refer the pain to the abdomen or to the hip. Look for rigidity of the spine, and resistance to forward flexion or lateral movement. The paravertebral muscles are often also in spasm. Point tenderness can often be identified in one of the disc spaces. Spinal osteomyelitis can occur in this region, but this is less common. Spinal tumors are rare in children but are often painful. Spinal cord tumors or cord compression can also present with a limp, as can tumors involving the nerve roots, and these are usually picked up by an alteration in sensation, motor function, or atrophy. (Lower cord lesions will sometimes spare the extremities but cause bowel and bladder symptoms.) Intra-abdominal pathology can also be referred to the back, and iliopsoas injuries or infections can be referred to the hip, causing children to walk with hip flexion.

Hip

Several important causes of a limp are found in the hip of the growing child. These can include soft tissue problems such as injuries to tendon insertions and ligaments; these are usually clearly activity related, and they improve with rest. As discussed in Chapter 130, limping is the sign most often present in dislocated or dysplastic hips.

Other conditions, however, need to be differentiated. In the young child, the condition of *toxic synovitis* (transient synovitis), which usually presents with no or low-grade fever and sudden onset of hip pain, is common, if not the most common condition causing limp in children. The hip must often be tapped to exclude a septic process. Radiographs of the pelvis are normal, but a technetium bone scan shows a diffuse mild uptake over the hip joint. The white blood cell count, differential, and sedimentation rate are most often normal, though the latter may be slightly elevated. It is self-limited, and with bed rest, pain is often much improved within 48 to 72 hours, although it may last for 7 to 10 days. It is unusual for the synovitis to recur. A bacterially infected hip is usually much more painful and guarded, and the child is more toxic.

The young child, especially in the age range of 4 to 8 years, is most vulnerable to idiopathic aseptic necrosis of the femoral head, *Legg–Calvé–Perthes* disease, which usually presents with limp and sometimes knee pain. The bone scan will be helpful early, while x-rays later will show patchy sclerosis and collapse in the femoral head. The temperature, CBC, and sedimentation rate are all normal.

In the older child, stereotypically the obese adolescent, *slipped capital femoral epiphysis* presents with a progressive limp and often knee pain. This condition is a surgical emergency and requires immediate non-weight bearing status to prevent further slipping, sometimes traction to relieve spasm, and surgical pinning to stabilize the femoral head. It is most easily diagnosed by an x-ray that clearly shows the alteration of the alignment of the capital femoral epiphysis. There is also a less common condition, *chondrolysis of the hip*, that may follow pinning of a slipped epiphysis, but may occur spontaneously, and may mimic an acute arthritic process in the hip. The x-ray shows joint space narrowing.

The femur is one of the more common sites for primary bone tumors, which may present with either hip or leg pain. These include primary osteogenic sarcoma, Ewing's tumor, and occasionally secondary tumors from neuroblastoma. Fortunately, these are much less common, and usually are easily detectable by x-ray. Systemic malignancies including leukemias and lymphomas may present with limping. Benign tumors such as osteoid osteomas are usually apparent on x-ray and demonstrate increased uptake on bone scan.

Knee

The knee is another common site for the origin of a limp. Several mechanical derangements of the knee related to trauma may present with limp, localized tenderness, and effusions. Meniscal injuries seldom occur before adolescence, however, and other causes must be sought in a younger child. *Osteochondritis dessicans*, which is usually detectable by x-rays especially with special sunset views, is more common in teenage boys and may cause knee locking because of loose bodies within the joint. *Chondromalacia patellae* is a common cause of knee complaints in older school-aged children, and the pattern of pain will usually be exacerbated by activities, especially those stressing quadriceps muscles. A positive patellar inhibition sign, which is pain inhibiting resisted contraction of the patella, and tenderness over the medial joint line accompanied by crepitus of the patellofemoral joint, is characteristic of this condition. As with other joints, septic processes also need to be excluded. With *Osgood–Schlatter disease*, a limp often occurs after strenous exercise. On physical examination, the tibial tuberosity will be painful and is usually swollen.

Leg

The tibia is vulnerable to stress fractures, particularly in young athletes. These are recognized by the pattern of pain after repetitive trauma, especially in athletes, and sometimes periostitis is visible on x-ray. However, these are often subtle, and a bone scan is more sensitive at demonstrating stress fractures.

Ankle

The ankle is very vulnerable to mechanical strains and sprains, particularly the medial and lateral ligaments. Most times, there is a clear cut history of injury or recurrent injuries initiating the episode of limping. Common findings are point tenderness and a characteristic toe walking gait to protect the ankle from weight bearing. Achilles tendonitis is also common in active youngsters and is often a cause of limp. The child feels more comfortable with the calf muscles flexed, placing less weight over the ankle, and avoiding stretching the tendon area. This is also a site for inflammation of tendons attaching to bones (enthesitis), which is a part of some arthritis syndromes. Heel pain is characteristic of ankylosing spondylitis and its variants and may be accompanied by evidence of spurs on the calcaneus by x-ray. The tarsus is another common site for aseptic necrosis, presenting with pain and limp, and this can usually be detected by bone scan early and later by X-ray. Another major cause of problems in this area is a coalition between tarsal

bones, either bony or fibrous. These cause an inflexible, painful flat foot and may need surgical intervention. The common familial flexible flat foot does not cause a limp.

Foot

Metatarsal phalangeal joints are commonly affected in arthritis. Involvement is often symmetrical and other objective signs of inflammation are usually present. Penetrating foot injuries, classically a child stepping onto a sharp object such as rusty nail that penetrates his shoes and socks, often cause insidious problems in soft tissue, bone, and sometimes joints. Classically, pseudomonas is one of the causative agents, but also tetanus and other unusual organisms can cause infection. By the time these are diagnosed, extensive bone or other tissue necrosis has often occurred, requiring surgical debridement for bacteriologic diagnosis and treatment.

LABORATORY TESTS

In a child with acute onset of a limp not readily explained by injury, investigation should focus on the most likely cause of the pain as determined by the history and physical examination. In general, x-rays are valuable for looking for fractures or tumors. Bone scans are much more sensitive at detecting areas of altered blood flow such as aseptic necrosis of bone in the ankle or the femoral head, or inflammation from infection, tumor, or arthritis. A sedimentation rate is useful; if elevated, it suggests an inflammatory cause. However, it is not unusual for many tumors or even some arthritic processes to have normal values. If an intra-articular process is considered, it is safer to aspirate the joint to both diagnose the cause and to relieve the risk of damage from pus under pressure inside an inflamed or infected joint. Further work-up beyond these tests is usually unnecessary.

TREATMENT AND REFERRAL

Most limps are likely to be on a mechanical basis. For the management of such problems, the reader is referred to Chapters 136, 139, and 140. However, a limp can indicate a more serious underlying cause that requires specific treatment. In evaluating a limp, the orthopedic surgeon is often one of the best resources, both because of his experience with analyzing the gait for cause of a limp and also for his understanding of many of the mechanisms underlying it. A neurologist should be consulted for the infrequent neurologic causes of a limp (*e.g.*, spinal tumors and peripheral neuropathies).

ANNOTATED BIBLIOGRAPHY

Hensinger RN: Limp. Pediatr Clin North Am 33(6):1355–1364, 1986 (Good clinical review.)

Jacobs BW: Synovitis of the hip in children and its significance. Pediatrics 47:558–566, 1971 (Thorough and still timely review.)

Renshaw TS: Pediatric Orthopedics, Major Problems in Clinical Pediatrics, Vol 28, Chap 4. Philadelphia, WB Saunders, 1986 (Good, practical discussions, especially of Legg–Calvé–Perthes disease; lists many references.)

Thompson G, Salter RB: Legg–Calvé–Perthes Disease. CIBA Clinical Symposia, Vol 38, No 1, 1986 (Lucidly presented comprehensive review.)

Tunnessen WW: Signs and Symptoms in Pediatrics, Chap 88. Philadelphia, JB Lippincott, 1983 (Excellent differential diagnosis of limp with "pearls" to direct the work-up.)

132
Juvenile Rheumatoid Arthritis
HELEN M. EMERY

Arthritis is defined as an inflammation of one or more joints, suggested by objective findings of swelling, warmth, pain, and sometimes erythema. The definition of juvenile rheumatoid arthritis (JRA) accepted by the American Rheumatism Association is (1) objective signs of inflammation of one or more joints; (2) inflammation lasting at least 6 weeks; (3) onset before the seventeenth birthday; and (4) exclusion of other underlying causes of joint problems, such as infection or malignancy. An estimated 200,000 children in the United States (~0.1% of the population) have JRA during childhood, making it the most common childhood rheumatic disease.

PATHOPHYSIOLOGY

The etiology of this condition remains unknown. Some studies have suggested that common childhood infections (*e.g.*, viruses), in an immunologically predisposed host, will allow a persistent synovial inflammatory reaction to be initiated and perpetuated, secondarily causing damage to cartilage, bone, and surrounding structures. However, much more information is needed to establish the causes and mechanisms.

CLINICAL PATTERNS

JRA is classified by the pattern of onset in the first 6 months into three major types: systemic onset, pauciarticular onset (fewer than five joints affected in the absence of classic systemic findings), and polyarticular onset (five or more involved joints, again with the absence of classic systemic signs). A child will generally stay in one classification through the course of disease.

SYSTEMIC DISEASE

Systemic disease is characterized by fever of a particular pattern, arthritis, and characteristic extra-articular manifestations. It occurs equally in both sexes and has no striking age predilection.

Fever, by definition, lasts at least 2 weeks and may continue for months with one or two daily spikes to greater than 103°F with a return to normal or subnormal temperatures between peaks. Commonly, the fever occurs in the afternoon or evening and is debilitating. Any other fever pattern is inconsistent with systemic onset disease.

An evanescent rash consisting of macules of almost fingernail size with central clearing often occurs over the trunk and extremities with the fever (or sometimes if the skin is warmed or traumatized.) This rash may be pruritic and often disappears completely when the fever subsides. Observation of this rash is helpful in confirming the diagnosis.

Almost one third of children with this variety of JRA will experience pericarditis or pleuritis. Clinical clues include tachycardia or tachypnea out of proportion to fever, splinted or shallow respiration in an effort to reduce pain from chest expansion, refusing to lie down (so pericardial or pleural fluid drains to diaphragmatic region), and abdominal pain (referred from the chest). Occasionally (in about 5%), myocarditis accompanies pericarditis.

An enlargement of the liver, spleen, and lymph nodes is common, and an anicteric hepatitis can also occur. This group also seems to be at special risk for salicylate hepatotoxicity.

While arthritis must be observed to confirm this diagnosis, it can vary from limited and mild to extensive and severe, but may be a less prominent feature of the illness than the extra-articular manifestations.

Laboratory Tests

Anemia can be quite profound in this group, and elevations of white count, platelets, and sedimentation rates can be striking. Tests for rheumatoid factor and antinuclear antibodies are always negative and there is no test that confirms the diagnosis.

PAUCIARTICULAR JUVENILE RHEUMATOID ARTHRITIS

Pauciarticular JRA can be classified into two subgroups, according to the age and pattern of joint involvement.

One group affects predominantly young girls (average age at onset 2 years; 4 girls:1 boy sex ratio) and usually affects large joints (*e.g.*, knees, ankles, wrists, elbows, neck; almost never hips). Frequent clues are morning stiffness, delayed motor milestones, or asymmetric accelerated growth around long bone epiphyses from increased vascularity. This group is at particular risk for developing asymptomatic chronic iridocyclitis, which can be diagnosed only by a slit lamp examination in its early, most treatable stages. The worst morbidity from this form of JRA is from eye complications (*e.g.*, band keratopathy, cataracts, glaucoma, and visual loss) rather than joint disease.

Laboratory tests again do not confirm this diagnosis, because only nonspecific abnormalities (*e.g.*, mild sedimentation rate elevations) occur and rheumatoid factor is absent. The test for antinuclear antibodies, however, does help identify the group at highest risk for eye complications (80% to 90% will have positive tests).

The second group with pauciarticular disease will have onset generally over the age of 8 years: this group is male predominant and frequently has a family history for ankylosing spondylitis (AS) or other diseases now known to be related to the HLA-B27 tissue type in close relatives. The joints involved are often those of the lower extremity (*e.g.*, tarsus, ankles, knees, and hips), and this disease may be a precursor to more classic ankylosing spondylitis that may take years to declare the classic

findings (evidence of sacroiliitis on roentgenogram and decreased lumbosacral mobility). These children are more at risk for the complications of AS (*e.g.*, acute iridocyclitis and aortitis) than are children in the younger onset group. Again, laboratory findings are nonspecific; these children do not have rheumatoid factor or antinuclear antibodies but more frequently carry the HLA-B27 tissue type. (It is not recommended to test for this gene because its presence or absence will not affect patient management.)

POLYARTICULAR JUVENILE RHEUMATOID ARTHRITIS

These children usually present with multiple symmetric joint involvement, especially involving hands and feet. Some children will have a low-grade fever, malaise, and weight loss, but not the characteristic systemic findings. Two distinct groups can be defined according to the presence or absence of rheumatoid factor. Those who have rheumatoid factor behave like young onset of adult rheumatoid arthritis. They are often teenagers at the time of presentation but may occasionally be very young. The disease is usually characterized by an aggressive, destructive course with all the potential complications of an adult-type disease: nodules, vasculitis, and lung complications not seen in the other childhood types. Fortunately, this kind accounts for only about 10% of all children with JRA. The children with polyarticular disease without rheumatoid factor generally are younger at age of onset. They have a milder disease and they are not at risk for the same extra-articular complications. Some of these children will prove positive for antinuclear antibodies.

DIFFERENTIAL DIAGNOSIS

Infections

Most acute infections are hematogenously carried into the musculoskeletal system (*e.g.*, bones, joints, or immediately surrounding soft tissues). However, previous infections may cause a reactive arthritis, and sometimes an arthritis may be the product of a more generalized illness.

Acute Bacterial Infections

The age of the child suggests which organisms are most likely to occur: in newborns till 3 months, staphylococcus, *group B streptococcus*, and gram-negative organisms (including gonococcus if the child was exposed during the birth process) are most likely. General signs of a septic infant (*e.g.*, temperature instability, poor feeding, jaundice) are usual, together with signs such as pseudoparalysis or pain when the infant is handled. Infections in bones and joints at this age often lead to severe growth abnormalities. Older children exhibit more acute signs including high fever, toxicity, and localized complaints of pain which begin abruptly and progress rapidly. A septic joint will usually be painful and the joint is held in a position of comfort (where maximum joint space can accommodate the pus and inflamed synovium). The child will resist using that joint with severe muscle spasm and guarding. This is in contrast to a child with osteomyelitis, who may have a sympathetic effusion in the adjacent joint but who usually shows most tenderness over the metaphysis rather than the joint itself, and also tolerates some active or passive range of movement.

The most useful tests confirm evidence of inflammation and identify the causative bacteria. For septic arthritis, aspiration of the joint is both diagnostic (white count is usually over 50,000 cells/mm^3; protein is elevated; glucose is low; and bacteria can be seen and cultured) and therapeutic. Relieving pressure from pus on cartilage to avoid further damage is especially critical in the hip. Especially in osteomyelitis, the bone scan can be helpful but may take a day or so to become positive. Apart from soft tissue changes, x-ray changes may be absent for up to 2 weeks, and if seen, reflect bone and joint damage that could have been avoided by early initiation of treatment. Situations that cause confusion include pretreatment with antibiotics, which masks acuity of joint findings; a compromised host (*e.g.*, a child on steroids or immunosuppressive therapy); and penetrating bone and joint injuries, which are often more insidious and involve unusual and often mixed organisms and require surgical debridement.

Postinfectious arthritis is often precipitated by viral (*e.g.*, rubella, ECHO viruses) or bacterial (*e.g.*, Salmonella, Yersinia) infections. These are usually self-limiting (less than 6 weeks). Arthritis may occur as a prodrome to other immune complex processes (*e.g.*, serum sickness and hepatitis).

Malignancies

About 50% of children with malignancies have musculoskeletal pain at the time of diagnosis, which may simulate arthritis. These include both localized forms (*e.g.*, osteogenic sarcoma), metastatic processes (*e.g.*, from neuroblastoma), or systemic forms (*e.g.*, leukemia or lymphoma). Useful clues are pain at night or at rest, pain out of proportion to physical findings, and systemic illness (*e.g.*, fevers, weight loss). X-rays, bone scans, and bone marrow aspiration are most useful in diagnosing these and may be positive before blood parameters are altered. Many childhood malignancies are curable if early treatment is initiated; thus, it is critical to diagnose a disease in this group.

Mechanical Noninflammatory Disorders

Benign limb pain of childhood (*growing pains*) is an inclusive term, but is a diagnosis of exclusion. Young children (often 2 to 5 years of age) wake up at night with apparent deep calf or thigh pain, often after an active day. This pain is relieved by heat, rubbing, and simple analgesics. It is nonprogressive (although the rewards of midnight crying may escalate this behavior) and the child is otherwise totally well. Reassurance is the best treatment.

Benign hypermobile joint syndrome is usually hereditary. These children will complain of pain after activity and can be identified by physical findings of diffuse ligamentous laxity including hyperextension to more than 90 degrees at metacarpophalangeal joints, more than 15 degrees at the elbows, recurvatum of the knees, and hypermobility of the spine. This may be a benign variant of Ehlers–Danlos syndrome. Such children are often encouraged in gymnastics and dance to exaggerate these tendencies and consequently increase their complaints.

Aseptic necrosis of bone most commonly occurs at the hip (Legg–Calvé–Perthes disease) but can occur at other sites. Pain is often insidious in onset, or a limp or referred pain is noted. X-rays and bone scan are the best diagnostic tools. The treatment varies with the site and severity of pain (see Chap. 131).

Trauma

Injury is the most frequent explanation of musculoskeletal pain in children, but may also be misleading, because parents may attribute the onset of symptoms to an unrelated incident. In contrast, an injury from subtle child abuse may lead to an evaluation for other causes of pain. Sports injuries (*e.g.*, little leaguer's elbow, runner's knee) must also be considered in a child with persistent pain (see Chap. 136).

Metabolic Disorders

Although these are rare in children, hematologic disorders (*e.g.*, hemophilia, sickle cell disease), immunodeficiency (IgA and IgG deficiency), gout (from inborn errors of purine metabolism pathways), and true connective tissue diseases all present with musculoskeletal pain and sometimes frank arthritis.

Systemic Inflammatory Disorders

Inflammatory bowel disease (*e.g.*, ulcerative colitis and Crohn's disease) may present with musculoskeletal pain or true arthritis before the classic gastrointestinal findings are present. Clues include a failure of linear growth, weight loss, or decreased appetite. Anemia, occult blood loss, and low serum albumin may suggest that an evaluation of the intestinal tract (by endoscopy or contrast x-rays) is needed.

Rheumatic Diseases

Any rheumatic disease may present with either arthritis or other musculoskeletal complaints.

Rheumatic fever usually has an acute migratory (*i.e.*, lasting only a few days in any one joint) polyarthritis pattern involving primarily knees, ankles, elbows, and wrists. In addition to other criteria (*e.g.*, carditis, erythema marginatum, subcutaneous nodules, or chorea), there must be either culture or antibody evidence of a preceding streptococcal infection. Arthralgia is a minor criteria, and all musculoskeletal symptoms disappear rapidly with salicylates or steroids, and are self-limited even if untreated.

Systemic lupus erythematosus has arthritis as a presenting complaint in most cases, but is usually accompanied by evidence of other systemic disease (*e.g.*, Raynaud's phenomenon, nephritis, and hematologic disorders most commonly) and almost always has a strongly positive test for antinuclear antibodies and low complement levels secondary to immune complex formation.

Dermatomyositis presents with weakness, muscle tenderness, and a classical heliotrope rash over eyelids and hands and sometimes on the trunk. The childhood variant is commonly associated with systemic vasculitis, although not with underlying malignancies. Elevated muscle enzymes usually confirm the clinical picture, although EMG and muscle biopsy may sometimes be needed.

In the absence of a classical rash, however, polymyositis may be difficult to differentiate from muscular dystrophy or other myopathic processes, and nerve conduction times, EMGs, and a biopsy are required.

Vasculitic syndromes (*e.g.*, Henoch–Schönlein purpura, Kawasaki disease, and polyarteritis nodosa are the most common in children) usually have inflammatory musculoskeletal components and can usually be recognized by the associated physical findings, but laboratory tests may be nonspecific.

WORK-UP

History and Physical Examination

The general approach to the evaluation of a child with arthritis is similar, regardless of the etiology of the swollen joint(s). There must be a careful assessment of the pattern of pain, noting particularly the location, radiation, fluctuations of symptoms either with activity or time, and duration. The progression and preceding events is the best guide to the underlying process. Furthermore, an evaluation of nonspecific findings, such as fever, malaise, or weight loss, and a complete review for evidence of involvement of other organ systems is essential.

The history is supplemented by a careful physical examination. A clinician who does not perform a complete musculoskeletal examination may miss subtle physical findings. The general principles of inspection, palpation, and moving the affected part both actively and passively, while carefully observing for evidence of pain in the child's nonverbal as well as verbal reactions, are the mainstay of the physical examination. Remember that pain is often referred distally in children (*e.g.*, a knee complaint commonly originates in the hip).

MANAGEMENT

Medications

The usual first line of treatment is salicylates in therapeutic doses (80 to 90 mg/kg/day in four divided doses for children under 20 kg; 60 to 80 mg/kg/day for older children) to achieve a level of 20 to 30 mg/deciliter. Parents need to know about the complications of salicylates (*e.g.*, easy bruising, stomach upset) and the signs of toxicity (*e.g.*, hyperventilation, decreased hearing, drowsiness or irritability, and progressive vomiting). If there is a question of toxicity, ask parents to stop the aspirin and check a salicylate level. If the child does not tolerate aspirin, a nonacetylated salicylate (*e.g.*, choline salicylate or magnesium choline salicylate) or a nonsteroidal antiinflammatory agent (*e.g.*, sodium; tolmetin in a dose of 20 to 30 mg/kg/day) can be substituted. All of these medications will take several weeks to suppress inflammation. Thus, a trial of 3 to 6 months will usually be given before deciding to add a remission-inducing drug.

The choice of a remission-inducing drug (*e.g.*, oral or intramuscular gold, D-penicillamine, hydroxychloroquine) is not always simple and should be decided only after a full discussion of side effects and anticipated outcome with the child and family. For children who have an unresponsive, destructive disease, low dose methotrexate has been used, but is regarded as experimental.

Oral corticosteroids have a limited place in the management of childhood arthritis and are used mainly for severe systemic manifestations (*e.g.*, pericarditis, pleuritis, and severe anemia). The side-effects of sustained steroids (*e.g.*, osteoporosis, increased susceptibility to infections, growth failure, risks of diabetes, and hypertension) are not warranted in light of the fact that steroids, while making the patient feel better, do not prevent (and may even hasten) joint destruction. Topical steroids (combined with mydriatics) are valuable in controlling eye disease, and occasional intra-articular steroids are used, usually in conjunction with initiation of remission-inducing drugs and an intensive therapy program.

Physical and Occupational Therapy

The goals of management are to reduce inflammation and to maintain function in joints. All children and parents with JRA should learn the normal range of movement and be alert to even a subtle loss of range. If this occurs, a therapist can show parents how to work with the child to maintain full joint range and prevent losses (*e.g.*, laying prone during television time for hip disease.) For children with morning stiffness, a hot bath in the morning followed by ranging will enable them to be more functional. Resting splints, for example for wrists or knees, will allow the joints to remain in a functional position and prevent the formation of flexion contractures.

For children with more extensive disease, especially lower extremity contractures, a more aggressive program of ranging and strengthening, gait training, and functional skill development is necessary, and outpatient or sometimes even inpatient treatment by an experienced therapist is necessary.

Management of behavior is as important as management of the disease. Both child and parent should be fully informed about what to expect in terms of taking medications and undertaking a therapy program. Parents should be encouraged to avoid overprotecting their child while under the misapprehension that inactivity will spare their child pain. In fact, moving the joint helps the child loosen up, and muscle strength will provide stability around inflamed joints. The child should be educated to respect his joints, but should not be restricted except in unusual circumstances (*e.g.*, somersaults are not encouraged in children with neck involvement). Encouraging self-esteem and appropriate assertiveness will facilitate independence and the achievement of developmental goals. Simple behavior modification techniques (*e.g.*, encouraging a child through a painful exercise instead of focusing on crying, sticker charts, and rewards to facilitate compliance with splints and medicines) are invaluable.

Ambulation is critical in a child with JRA. Once osteoporosis, weakness, and contractures are established, they are difficult to reverse. Wheelchairs should be avoided at all costs—besides the invalid image they convey, the flexion positions of hips and knees, and the weakness from inactivity undermine the therapeutic goals. The alternative is a tricycle or walker, which encourages weight bearing and use of available range and strength.

PROGNOSIS

There is great variability in outcomes for children with JRA. In general, the young onset pauciarticular group almost never have a permanent disability from their arthritis (although they may from eye disease). However, between one third to one half of children with polyarticular rheumatoid factor positive disease or systemic onset variety will have residual deformities and functional limitations. Hopefully, these figures will improve as better treatment becomes more widely available.

INDICATIONS FOR REFERRAL

All parents should be encouraged to contact their local chapter of the Arthritis Foundation—American Juvenile Arthritis Organization to obtain information on JRA, such as medication pamphlets and brochures informing schools about arthritis. Many also have parent support groups and facilitate networking between children and parents.

The following specialities are often involved in the comprehensive management of children with arthritis:

- Pediatric Rheumatologist—When the diagnosis is uncertain, remission-inducing drugs are being considered, or the child is developing flexion contractures or functional limitations, a referral is indicated for assistance in decision-making.
- Orthopedist—The role of surgery for children with JRA is limited. A fixed flexion contracture unresponsive to aggressive therapy may benefit from soft tissue release; an end-stage joint may be replaced in a child who has completed skeletal growth with marked relief of pain and improvement in function. However, only a very experienced arthritis surgeon working with a pediatric rheumatologist, therapists, and a motivated patient should undertake these procedures.
- Opthalmologist—All children with JRA should be screened annually. The highest risk group (young onset pauciarticular JRA) should be seen at 3- to 4-month intervals for a slit lamp examination.
- Social Worker/Psychologist—Financial demands of the child's illness can be a major burden to any family with a chronically ill child. Most states cover JRA under their Crippled Children's Program. A social worker can assist in deter-

mining if the family is eligible and can facilitate the referral. These professionals can also help the entire family adjust to the chronic illness and help establish behavior programs when needed.
- Physical and Occupational Therapy—Therapists should evaluate the child initially and help teach families normal range and simple exercises. Specific directions for splinting, joint protection techniques, and more aggressive range and strengthening programs should be developed with the physician as required.

ANNOTATED BIBLIOGRAPHY

Cassidy JT: Textbook of Pediatric Rheumatology. New York, Wiley, 1982 (Most comprehensive text on the subject.)

Miller ML (ed): Pediatric rheumatology. Pediatr Clin North Am 33(5), 1986 (Highlights physical and occupational therapy, psychosocial aspects, and community and school programs for children with rheumatic diseases. Also contains current and comprehensive reviews of the major childhood arthritides and Kawasaki syndrome.)

Schaller JG: Arthritis in children. Pediatr Clinic North Am 33(6):1565–1580, 1986 (Brief, yet good overview.)

133
Toeing In
and Torsional Deformities
EDWARD SILLS

Torsional deformity including, most commonly, in-toeing, must be understood in the context of the natural history, the site of involvement, the age of the child at the time of discovery, and the degree of disability.

During postnatal life, both the femur and tibia normally undergo a process of external rotation. If the normal processes of external rotation are interfered with by genetic or by environmental factors, the internal rotational postures will persist and will thus become the various deformities discussed in this chapter.

DIFFERENTIAL DIAGNOSIS

Torsional deformity of the lower extremity can occur because of an abnormality at any site between the foot and the hip. Some abnormalities are uncomplicated, occurring at a single level, whereas

others are more complex. Multiple deformities may compensate each other as in internal femoral torsion and external tibial torsion, whereas others may be additive. An example of the latter occurs when mild femoral anteversion, internal tibial torsion, and metatarsus adductus combine to produce severe in-toeing. The major challenge to the examiner is to locate the site or sites of abnormality and to assess the degree of torsional deformity at the involved level.

PHYSICAL EXAMINATION

Most torsional deformities are present at rest. A dynamic deformity due to a muscular or neuromuscular disorder occasionally appears and is evident only with muscle activity. This discussion will be limited to those that are apparent at rest.

When examining the child, the physician should

specifically assess the angle of gait, the excursion of hip rotation, the thigh–foot angle, and the shape of the foot.

The *angle of gait* is best defined as the angle between the line of progression (*i.e.*, the direction in which the child is walking and the axis of the foot). Most children and adults walk with their feet somewhat externally rotated. When there is either a persistent internal gait or an external gait angle in excess of 30 degrees, an abnormality exists. Most commonly, the problem is that of in-toeing. In-toeing tends to be more apparent in a tired child in whom fatigued mechanisms of compensation allow the underlying malrotation to become apparent.

Hip rotation is easiest to measure with the patient prone, the knees flexed to 90 degrees, and the muscles relaxed. The legs are allowed to fall into full internal rotation after which the physician can measure the maximal internal rotation of the hip, first on one side and then on the other. Internal rotation is the angle between the vertical and the axis of the tibia when the hip is maximally internally rotated. External rotation is assessed in a similar manner. In the neonate, because of both the lateral orientation of the acetabulae and the external hip rotation contracture induced by intrauterine positioning, external rotation and femoral neck anteversion are at their peak. The full-term newborn has an external rotation of close to 90 degrees. This diminishes considerably as the more adult antero-lateral positioning of the acetabulae occurs. By childhood, external rotation gradually decreases to the extent that internal and external rotation are virtually comparable. Internal rotation is normally less than 60 degrees. Femoral neck anteversion increases as the degree of internal rotation increases above normal. Once internal rotation exceeds 80 degrees, there exists a severe femoral neck anteversion.

Tibial torsion is best measured by noting the angle between the axis of the foot (a line from the second toe to the midpoint of the heel) and the axis of the thigh when the prone patient is relaxed with the knee and ankle each at 90 degrees. Medial or internal torsion of more than 10 degrees in the infant indicates internal tibial torsion. Any medial rotation after 2 years of age indicates internal tibial torsion because the normal thigh–foot angle is 10 to 20 degrees externally rotated. External rotation beyond 30 degrees connotes external tibial torsion.

The bottom of the *foot* is examined with the child prone. Any convexity of the lateral border of the foot is indicative of *metatarsus adductus* (*varus*).

METATARSUS ADDUCTUS

The most frequently diagnosed cause of in-toeing in infancy is metatarsus adductus (varus) or toeing-in of the forefoot. Metatarsus adductus (varus) is often bilateral and is usually due to abnormal intrauterine positioning. In the more common, supple form, the mild flexible deformity resolves spontaneously and requires no treatment other than passive stretching. If the forefoot is rigid and cannot be easily corrected with gentle manipulation of the forefoot with each diaper change, orthopedic assistance is usually required by 3 to 4 months of age. This persistent rigidity is often associated with internal tibial torsion and foot eversion. Rapid correction, usually in less than 1 month, can be effected by use of corrective long leg casts. This can usually be accomplished with either a single application of a cast or with two serially abducted casts. Some orthopedists believe that the correction is best maintained with the use of outflared or reversed last shoes after the casts are removed. If, following correction of the varus forefoot there is a persistent internal tibial torsion, it can be treated with Denis Browne night splints. This latter treatment should not be applied to uncorrected metatarsus varus because the valgus part of the splint is exerted on the hindfoot as well as on the forefoot. If metatarsus varus persists and is not recognized until after 2 years of age the deformity may be sufficiently "fixed" as to make attempts to correct the forefoot deformity force the heel into a skewfoot heel valgus. In such circumstances it may be appropriate to consider correctional intermetatarsal soft tissue releases. In the rare situation of a delay of diagnosis until school-age, osteotomies may be required to correct the metatarsus varus. There is no indication that simple tendon release in the pretoddler is appropriate.

INTERNAL TIBIAL TORSION

Internal tibial torsion without metatarsus adductus (varus) is the most frequently diagnosed basis of in-toeing in the child who has begun to walk. It should be observed over time inasmuch as most children self-correct over time. If the deformity is greater than 40 degrees and it persists after the child has fully ambulated for about 6 months, the commonly accepted practice is to initiate splinting. This practice is sometimes deferred because of the danger that is presented by the action of the splints, which tends to force the feet into abduction and which can cause genu valgum and can also accentuate femoral neck anteversion. The child's usual everyday shoes are attached to a small bar at bedtime, with the side or sides to be corrected set at an external rotation of 30 degrees. Treatment is discontinued once the thigh–foot angle is 10 degrees externally rotated. This usually occurs within a 9- to 15-month period. If genu valgum (knock–knee) and foot pronation are present, active night bar treatment is best deferred because this treatment tends to worsen the genu valgum and foot prona- tion. There is no indication that an initiation of night bar treatment beyond 3 years of age is beneficial. There have been no published studies to indicate that corrective shoes, wedges, or twister cables have any benefit in this disorder. A knowledge of biomechanical principles convinces me that a skep- tical attitude towards the use of these devices in this disorder is warranted.

INTERNAL FEMORAL TORSION AND FEMORAL NECK ANTEVERSION

Internal femoral torsion and excessive femoral neck anteversion is the etiology of in-toeing gait most often diagnosed after 3 years of age. Whereas the normal child has comparable internal and ex- ternal hip rotation by this age, a child with this dis- order has greater than 30 degrees more internal than external hip rotation. It is a disorder that is usually bilateral and is seen most frequently in girls. After the age 6 or 7 years, the deformity is compensated by external tibial torsion. There is absolutely no justification for the use of any devices, splints, spe- cial shoes, wedges, twister cables, or casts to treat this "disorder." Orthopedic and pediatric studies have shown that none of these approaches is as- sociated with outcomes better than the outcome of those left untreated. Although some youngsters with this condition experience quadriceps muscle cramps in the first decade and knee pain in adoles- cence, there are no data to support the contention that this condition leads to degenerative arthritis or to a functional disability. The exceedingly rare child, dysfunctional because of greater than 90 de- grees internal hip rotation and severe anteversion, can be corrected only with a major surgical dero- tational femoral osteotomy. This major undertaking was recommended for only 2 of the nearly 800 chil- dren in whom I diagnosed the presence of femoral anteversion.

The commonly offered advice to "sit like an In-

dian" or to sit "in a tailor position" is useful, not because of a direct therapeutic benefit but merely because it discourages the habit of sitting in a "W" or "reverse tailor" position that tends to maintain the soft tissue contracture that holds the hip in in- ternal rotation. Thus, this tends to increase fatigue in the responsible quadriceps muscles which may, in turn, produce a minor discomfort.

INDICATIONS FOR REFERRAL

Since most infants and young children with tor- sional deformity require no active treatment be- cause their in-toeing will resolve spontaneously, re- ferral should be judiciously infrequent. There are theoretical concerns, in fact, that unnecessary treatment may induce "overcorrection" as the self- correction is taking place. The rare youngster with persistent, rigid, nonflexible metatarsus adductus (varus) may benefit from a short course of casting, and the rare school-aged child with undiagnosed metatarsus adductus may require surgery. The child between 18 and 36 months with progressing internal tibial torsion is benefited by a night splint or bar, although overcorrection may accentuate femoral neck anteversion. The child who has internal fem- oral torsion with femoral anteversion does not ben- efit from the use of various devices. In view of the meagre evidence that, with the few exceptions noted above, any intervention provides outcomes superior to those achieved spontaneously, there should be a general reluctance to subject children to the fashionable but unproven costly and inap- propriate nonsurgical devices. The anxieties of par- ents and grandparents are better addressed with careful education than with unneeded appliance prescriptions.

ANNOTATED BIBLIOGRAPHY

Fabry G, MacEwen G, Shands A: Torsion of the femur: A follow-up study in normal and abnormal conditions. J Bone Joint Surg 55A:1726, 1973 (Comprehensive dis- cussion with a broad perspective of the major author- ities.)

Salenius P, Vankka E: Development of the tibiofemoral angle in children. J Bone Joint Surg 57A:259, 1975 (Elu- cidating guide to comprehending a dynamic process.)

Staheli L: Torsional deformities in children. J Cont Educ Pediatr 20:11, 1978 (Excellent perspective and good orientation to basic mechanisms. Illustrative photo- graphs are used effectively.)

134

Bow Legs and Knock Knees

EDWARD SILLS

In the normal course of development, infants have some degree of genu varus or bow leg until about 1 to 1½ years of age, at which time mild overcorrection spontaneously results in minimal genu valgus or knock knees. The tibiofemoral angle, as measured on a roentgenogram, is usually in excess of 15 degrees of varus at birth; it approaches 0 degrees in the mid-second year; and it proceeds to as much as 10 degrees of valgus by the third birthday. It gradually approaches the "normal" 5 degrees of valgus by school age and remains relatively unchanged thereafter. Extreme bilateral or *any* unilateral genu varus is rare. Marked valgus is less rare and is often associated with an overweight child. The child who clinically appears to exceed the limits of physiologic bowing (varus) or knock knee (valgus) should have radiographs to ascertain whether there is an underlying condition that requires treatment in order to prevent a permanent deformity. The normal developmental pattern of early bow leg, transition to knock knee, and ultimate balanced straightening should be considered before subjecting a youngster with a moderate deformity to unnecessary investigation and treatment.

BOW LEG

The two most important causes of pronounced bow leg deformity are tibia vara (Blount's disease) and rickets.

Blount's Disease

Blount's disease, also termed *osteochondrosis deformans tibiae*, occurs in two forms: the infantile, bilateral progressive form and the milder juvenile (or adolescent) type which is most often unilateral and usually appears late in the first decade. The infantile form is much more frequently encountered than the juvenile/adolescent form. Blount's disease should be ruled out in any child older than 2 years with a persistent, unilateral, or bilateral genu varus and a radiographically confirmed tibiofemoral angle in excess of 15 degrees, and in a child of *any* age

with a radiographically confirmed tibiofemoral angle in excess of 25 degrees of varus.

Infantile Blount's disease, often associated with substantial internal tibial torsion, involves a disturbance of growth in the epiphyseal and metaphyseal regions of the posterior-medial aspect of the proximal end of the tibia. The precise etiology remains uncertain. One hypothesis, albeit controversial, is that the dysplastic ossification in this region results from abnormal forces transmitted over the medial tibial femoral compartment in early walkers. On x-ray, the proximal tibia reveals varying degrees of metaphyseal fragmentation and epiphyseal depression, with the tibia bent abruptly mediad and caudad at the proximal metaphysis. Over time, a hooked spur is formed, which radiographically indicates an advanced stage of Blount's disease.

Clinically, the major manifestation is a waddling gait. Knee, ankle, or foot pain occasionally results from excessive stress caused by the deformity. Medial swelling of the proximal tibia may be palpable. There is often significant internal tibial rotation, genu recurvatum, and pes planus with foot pronation.

The causes of acquired tibia vara include proximal tibial osteomyelitis, proximal tibial epiphyseal fracture, and proximal tibial enchondroma.

Treatment. If the angle has not begun to diminish by 18 months, or if, by 24 months, it has not fallen below 15 degrees of varus, most authorities recommend treatment. If the deformity is less than 25 degrees of varus, supportive shoes with a longitudinal arch and outer sole wedges are usually recommended. In those extraordinarily infrequent instances when the tibiofemoral angle exceeds 25 degrees of varus, long leg braces with genu varus pads to provide lateral force exertion are indicated in order to prevent a permanent deformity or dysfunction. Beyond 4 years of age, tibiofemoral angles in excess of 25 degrees varus require an osteotomy to completely correct the deformity.

The juvenile or adolescent type of tibia vara is associated invariably with a shortened extremity and an attendant limp. It is believed to be caused by trauma to the medial ossification center of the proximal tibia. The treatment is surgical; the lateral proximal tibia and the proximal fibula require epiphysiodesis as do the proximal tibia and fibula of the opposite (*i.e.*, *un*involved) leg in order to prevent leg length inequality sufficient to cause scoliosis.

Rickets

Rickets may cause severe and extreme bow leg deformity. It is a condition in which the deficiency of calcium or phosphate causes inadequate mineralization of the organic matrix of bone and cartilage. The two main causes of rickets are a lack of vitamin D (type 1) and abnormal functioning of the renal tubules (type 11). Vitamin D deficiency, due either to inadequate intake (*e.g.*, from fashionable vegan or fad diets deficient in vitamin D) or inadequate absorption (as in steatorrhea), is manifested by a combination of diminished intestinal absorption of calcium and phosphate and a decreased tubular reabsorption of phosphate with resultant hypocalcemia and hypophosphatemia. Type 11 rickets is caused by a deficiency of phosphate resulting from poor or absent renal tubular reabsorption of phosphate. Type 111 rickets is an end organ resistance to 1,25-dihydroxy vitamin D_3 and is associated with a low serum calcium.

On x-ray, the metaphyseal ends of long bones are poorly ossified and frayed. The epiphyseal plate is usually widened and cupped, and the cortices are thinned. The epiphyseal widening is associated with a bending of the softened shafts of the long bones. In addition, the femur and tibia often develop an anterior convexity.

Treatment. Rickets is treated by adequate (as defined by the underlying metabolic disorder) amounts of vitamin D or its essential metabolite 1,25-dihydroxy vitamin D. Healing begins to occur promptly and the acute healing is completed in weeks. Once the metabolic abnormality has been corrected, a more reasoned decision regarding splinting, bracing, and osteotomy can be made. The basis for these decisions generally follows those guidelines previously described for the treatment of Blount's disease. However, one must be especially careful to minimize immobilization so as to reduce the risk of recurrent osteoporosis.

KNOCK KNEES

Knock knees are measured by radiographically determining the angle between the lateral aspects of the femur and tibia. The clinical method is to measure the distance between the medial malleoli when the knees are fully extended, the medial femoral condyles are pressed together, and the patellae are facing upward.

The acute appearance of valgus deformity, especially if it is unilateral, should arouse suspicion of trauma, infection, or tumor. Stimulation of the proximal tibial epiphysis by the host's response to any of the above, for example, may lead to valgus due to the tethering effect of an intact fibula.

If an epiphyseal fracture and rickets have been excluded as causes of knock knee, it is reasonable to defer diagnostic and therapeutic maneuvers in children younger than 7 years of age. If the feet are pronated in association with "physiologic" valgus, toeing-in can be promoted by using a longitudinal arch support; it should be used if the pronation causes pain. If the child with genu valgus already toes in, or if there is no foot pronation, arch support is not indicated. There is no evidence that splints, twisters, casts, or braces play any useful role in managing the child with genu valgus who is under 7 or 8 years of age.

If, in the older child, there is an intermalleolar distance of 4 inches or more, or if valgus, as measured by the tibiofemoral angle exceeds 15 degrees, operative intervention is indicated. The usual procedure is stapling or epiphysiodesis of the deformed bone (most commonly it is the medial distal femur), preferably when the epiphyses are still open so as to allow sufficient longitudinal growth to correct the deformity. Proximal tibia and fibula osteotomies are generally performed when valgus deformity is below the knee.

Indications for Referral

The tibiofemoral angle normally progresses from genu varus in the newborn to genu valgus in the toddler. Extreme excesses in this development beyond the normal or "physiologic" expectation should raise the question of rickets or Blount's disease in the child with excessive bow leg. Trauma, tumor, infection, or, rarely, rickets must be ruled out in the child with bilaterally excessive knock knee beyond 7 years of age or at any age if unilateral.

With the exception of some rare instances of genu varus, orthosis, splints, twisters, and the like are generally considered to be inappropriate for these conditions. They certainly do not play a role in the management of knock knee. Correction of the underlying cause, if one is identified, is the first priority. In most instances of bow leg and in all cases of knock knee where appliances and elaborate regimes are of little use, the primary physician has limited options: He may carefully monitor the child or he may refer to an orthopedist for either additional reassurance or for guidance in management. A referral for orthopedic expertise is mandatory when, in the unusual extreme situation, staging of a surgical osteotomy or epiphysiodesis is considered.

ANNOTATED BIBLIOGRAPHY

Blount WP: Tibia vara. J Bone Joint Surg 19:1, 1937 (Sentinel report of an impressive study of this important disorder.)

Harrison HE, Harrison HC: Disorders of Calcium and Phosphate Metabolism in Childhood and Adolescence. Philadelphia, WB Saunders, 1979 (Offers a lucid and thorough discussion.)

Howorth MD: Knock knees. Clin Orthop 77:233, 1971 (Useful clinical diagnostic and treatment perspective.)

Morley AJ: Knock knee in children. Br Med J 2:976, 1957 (Reassuring study demonstrating a normal progression.)

Salenius P, Vankka E: Development of the tibiofemoral angle in children. J Bone Joint Surg 57A:259, 1975 (Elucidating, useful, superb graphs that enhance understanding most effectively.)

Sherman M: Physiologic bowing of the legs. South Med J 53:830, 1970 (Review that allows one to broaden a perspective on normal variation and abnormal extremes.)

135
Scoliosis
DONALD M. BERWICK

Scoliosis screening in school children has become routine in many states, and the evaluation and management of lateral curvatures of the spine is now common in pediatric practice. The practitioner must be prepared both to detect significant curves and to serve as the first site of referral for children screened elsewhere. The current enthusiasm for scoliosis screening thus places the pediatrician in the position of reassuring most families, while trying to cull out the few for whom a consistent follow-up is truly advisable. Orthopedic referral is necessary for severe curves, but correctly performed scoliosis screening tests detect many curves which, though anatomically real, will never be functionally or cosmetically damaging to the child. The pediatrician must thus walk the line between costly and anxiety-provoking over-referral and potentially hazardous delay in specialty treatment of significant curves.

For the few children in a pediatric general practice who will require therapy with a brace or spine surgery, the pediatrician's role is essential. In most cases, these invasive treatments demand modifications in the life-style of children over several years and are most commonly used during those preadolescent and adolescent years characterized by rapid physical growth and psychological turmoil. To help a teenage boy or girl and family through 2 years of use of the Milwaukee brace, or through surgery with imperfect results and months of re-

habilitation, requires the deepest resources of the pediatric practitioner.

PATHOPHYSIOLOGY

Scoliosis is a lateral curvature of the spine, usually involving the dorsal or lumbar vertebrae, or both, and accompanied by rotation of involved vertebrae and (if the curve is thoracic) of the attached ribs, producing a protuberance of the posterior portion of the ribs on the side of the convexity. The intrathoracic volume on the side of the concavity of the curve is reduced, and if the scoliosis is marked, this may compromise pulmonary function. In addition, such curvatures can be associated with a measurable reduction in vital capacity, ventilatory reserve, and expiratory flow rates. Hypoventilation of basilar lung segments and restrictive lung disease can lead to cor pulmonale, and survival rates for severe scoliotics are compromised.

Curves are named for the side toward which the convexity points and may be single, double, or more complex. A child with a *right dorsal, left lumbar* curve, therefore, has two curves: a thoracic curve with the convexity (and posterior rib hump) on the right, and a lumbar curve with the convexity on the left. Curvatures have *lateral* and *rotational* components, and one or the others of these may be accentuated in particular cases; occasionally, the lateral curvature may be significant with only min-

I. Idiopathic Scoliosis—This group, which makes up about 65% of all patients seen, is subdivided according to the age at which the scoliosis is first noticed. There can be a considerable lapse between the time when scoliosis first develops and when it is first noticed. Each subdivision has certain definite characteristics that distinguish it from the others.
  A. *Infantile Scoliosis*—spinal curvature develops during first 3 years of life
    1. Progressive
    2. Resolving
  B. *Juvenile Scoliosis*—spinal curvature develops between skeletal ages of 4 and 12 years in girls and 4 and 14 years in boys
  C. *Adolescent Scoliosis*—spinal curvature develops after skeletal age of 12 years in girls and of 14 years in boys
II. Congenital Skeletal Abnormalities—This group makes up about 15% of patients seen with scoliosis, and the deformity is caused by anomalous bony development.
  A. *Vertebral Anomalies*
    1. Open vertebral canal
      a. With neurologic deficit
        (1) Myelomeningocele
      b. Without neurologic deficit
        (1) Spina bifida occulta
        (2) Myelomeningocele
    2. Closed vertebral canal
      a. With neurologic defect
        (1) Diastematomyelia
        (2) Other forms of spinal dysrhaphia
      b. Without neurologic defect
        (1) Failure of formation of vertebral elements
          (a) Wedged vertebra
          (b) Hemivertebra
        (2) Failure of segmentation of vertebral elements
          (a) Partial—vertebral bar
          (b) Complete—vertebral coalition
  B. *Extravertebral Anomalies*
    1. Rib coalition
III. Neuromuscular Abnormalities—This group makes up about 10% of patients seen with scoliosis.
  A. *Neuropathic*
    1. Upper motor neuron lesion
      a. Cerebral palsy
      b. Spinocerebellar degeneration
        (1) Charcot–Marie–Tooth disease
        (2) Friedreich's ataxia
        (3) Roussy–Lévy syndrome
      c. Syringomyelia
      d. Spinal cord tumors
      e. Spinal cord injury
    2. Lower motor neuron lesion
      a. Poliomyelitis
      b. Other types of viral myelitis
    3. Progressive spinal muscular atrophy
      a. Infantile (Werdnig–Hoffmann syndrome)
      b. Juvenile (Kugelberg–Welander syndrome)

    4. Nonprogressive juvenile spinal atrophy
    5. Dysautonomia (Riley–Day syndrome)
  B. *Myopathic*
    1. Muscular dystrophy
      a. Pseudohypertrophic muscular dystrophy
      b. Limb–girdle muscular dystrophy
      c. Facioscapulohumeral muscular dystrophy
    2. Myotonia atrophica (Steinert's disease)
    3. Myotonia congenita (Thomsen's disease)
    4. Arthrogryposis
    5. Hypotonia
IV. Scoliosis Associated with Neurofibromatosis—This group makes up about 5% of patients seen with scoliosis.
V. Mesenchymal Disorders
  A. Congenital
    1. Marfan's syndrome
    2. Ehlers–Danlos syndrome
  B. Acquired, *i.e.*, rheumatoid arthritis
VI. Trauma
  A. Fractures of the vertebral body
  B. Surgical insult
    1. Damage to vertebral growth plates
    2. Laminectomy
    3. Extraspinal—thoracoplasty
  C. Irradiation
VII. Extraspinal Contractures
  A. Postempyema
  B. Burns
VIII. Osteochondrodystrophies
  A. Diastrophic dwarfism
  B. Mucopolysaccharidoses (Morquio's disease, and others)
  C. Spondyloepiphyseal dysplasia
  D. Multiple epiphyseal dysplasia
  E. Other
IX. Infection of Bone
  A. Acute
  B. Chronic
    1. Tuberculosis
X. Metabolic Disorders
  A. Osteomalacia
    1. Rickets
  B. Osteoporosis
  C. Osteogenesis imperfecta
  D. Homocystinuria
XI. Thoracogenic Disorders
  A. Postthoracotomy
XII. Related to Lumbosacral Joint
  A. Related to spondylosis and spondylolisthesis
  B. Congenital anomalies of the sacrum and sacroiliac joint
XIII. Tumors
  A. Vertebral column
    1. Osteoid-osteoma
    2. Hemangioma
  B. Spinal cord
    1. Astrocytoma
    2. Teratoma
    3. Intermedullary cysts
    4. Lipoma
    5. Ependymoma

---

* Reprinted with permission from Riseborough EJ, Herndon JH: Scoliosis and Other Deformities of the Axial Skeleton, p 22. Boston, Little, Brown, 1975

imal rotational elements, but usually the severity of rotation parallels the severity of the lateral curve.

Scoliotic curves can be purely reactive (nonstructural) and transient, due, for example, to intraabdominal pathology and spasm of adjacent paraspinal muscles. However, structural curves, not reactive ones, are the subject of this chapter. Structural scoliosis can be secondary to diseases that affect the bones or supporting structures of the spine, including congenital malformations of the spine, neuromuscular diseases, and deformities due to trauma or infection. The conditions that may cause secondary scoliosis, as well as the various forms of idiopathic scoliosis, are categorized in the box, Classification of Structural Scoliosis. For the diseases listed, scoliosis is almost never the first or only clue, but rather a complication of a condition already known to exist.

Despite the wide array of diseases that can cause scoliosis, most curves encountered by the general pediatrician are idiopathic and are first noticed in late latency or early teenage years. The cause of idiopathic juvenile scoliosis is unknown, but familial aggregation does occur, and a genetic mechanism is therefore plausible.

CLINICAL PRESENTATION

Idiopathic scoliosis is usually asymptomatic; in fact, most children who have detectable curves are unaware of their condition prior to discovery by a health professional. Curves that progress in severity do so most quickly during periods of rapid growth, such as early adolescence, and tend to be far more stable during latency and after the growth spurt has ended. For unknown reasons, scoliotic curves showing rapid progression and requiring treatment are four times as common in girls as in boys.

The clinical consequences of scoliosis depend on the degree of curvature. Curvature can be measured radiologically according to the angle of inclination of the vertebral bodies that define the ends of the curve. With a curve of 45 degrees, for example, lines drawn parallel to the articular surfaces of the last vertebral bodies involved in the curve intersect at that angle. In fact, on a spine x-ray, the same angle is more conveniently measured at the intersection of lines drawn perpendicular to those defining the articular surfaces. This is the so-called *Cobb angle*, which is now the most widely accepted method for measuring the degree of curvature.

Severe, rare thoracic curvatures exceeding 60 or 70 degrees can produce serious compromise in appearance, functional status, and longevity. Thoracic curves of less than 65 degrees and lumbar curves of nearly any severity do not appear to cause cardiorespiratory compromise or shortened survival. Rather, the major problems for those with curves in the range of 40 to 65 degrees are cosmetic; the curves may be noticeable and damaging to social success and self-image. Marriage rates among women with scoliosis in this range are lower than normal. Although the relationship is still unproven, many believe that lumbar and thoracolumbar curves especially predispose to back pain.

Curves below 35 degrees are of little or no functional or cosmetic significance. They are potentially of interest only to the extent that they may progress to curves of greater size and consequence. The greatest threat of rapid progression is confined to the periods of growth spurts in childhood, but very slow progression occurs in a substantial minority of curves in this range even in adulthood.

EVALUATION

The appropriate evaluation of a scoliotic curve depends on its severity and on the risk of rapid progression. Most curves are discovered in screening, which is done today not only in the doctor's office, but also in schools and other settings. The signs that can be used to detect scoliosis are indicated in Fig. 135-1. Asymmetry of the shoulder levels, scapular prominence, hip levels, or distance between arms and body may be the only sign of curvature in the erect position. Severe curves may be obvious on inspection, or may become visible in tracing the posterior elements of the spine. In such cases, the occiput may also fail to line up directly over the buttocks' crease. The most sensitive test for scoliosis, however, on a clinical examination is the *forward bending test*. With no shirt on, the child is asked to bend forward at the waist, letting the arms dangle with the thumbs just touching each other. Viewing the child from behind, with eyes at the level of the child's back, the examiner may notice an elevation of one side of the thorax (the so-called *rib hump*), a consequence of the rotational component of a scoliotic curve. Viewing the child from the front, a similar deformity may be noted due to a lumbar or thoracolumbar curve.

The forward bending test is the mainstay of most large scale scoliosis screening programs. It can detect curves of only a few degrees and is therefore "positive" in many children whose curves pose no current or potential risk to them. In school-based screening programs, up to 15% of children are found

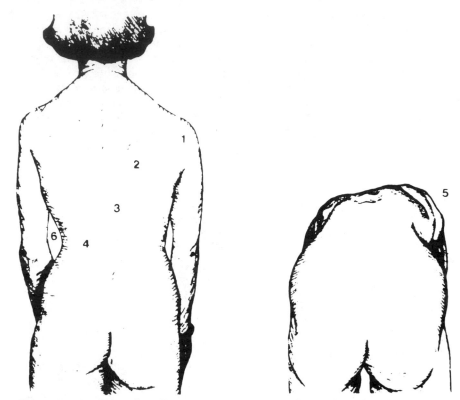

Figure 135-1. Signs of scoliosis on a screening examination include: (1) depression (or elevation) of shoulder; (2) asymmetry of scapulae; (3) visible curvature of spine; (4) sacral tilt (or asymmetry of hips); (5) rib hump (lumbar or thoracic); (6) asymmetry in distance between arms and body. In addition, failure of occiput to line up directly over buttocks' crease may be noted. (Berwick DM: Scoliosis screening. Pediatrics in Review 5:238–247, 1984)

to have positive screening examinations and up to half of these can be documented on x-ray examination to have actual curves. Most of those children, however, have curves under 10 degrees.

When a child has a positive forward bending test, the appropriate evaluation depends on the child's age, sex, and phase of growth. For the lowest risk groups (children well before their growth spurts, and those who have completed their growth) whose findings on screening are not dramatic, a simple clinical reexamination at approximately yearly intervals is adequate. Children about to enter a period of rapid growth, especially girls, may require closer follow-up. A single anteroposterior x-ray view of the spine (not multiple views) will permit measurement of the actual curvature, and, in cases exceeding 10 degrees of curvature, repeat examination (using low-dose radiologic techniques if possible) in 6 months can be used to assess the ra-

pidity of progression. A technique known as Moire topography has been developed to follow the progression of scoliotic curves without x-rays. Using this technique, ordinary light shown through a screen of closely spaced wires casts a pattern of interference "fringes" on the subject's back, and the changes in this pattern over time can be used to monitor the curve. Another rapid screening test to detect scoliosis is by use of an inclinometer (*e.g.*, Scoliometer). This instrument measures the angle of trunk rotation. An ATR angle of less than 5 degrees is generally considered as a "pass."

The overuse of x-rays to monitor scoliosis is a serious consequence of the current enthusiasm for screening. Most children with minor findings on screening probably do not require x-rays, and few children who do need x-rays require more than a single view. Extensive "spine series" of x-rays for such children should be avoided.

MANAGEMENT

Most scoliosis requires no intervention at all. In some settings, it is customary to prescribe exercises of various sorts for mild or moderate curvatures, but these exercises are of no proven benefit and may contribute to the mistaken impression of children and parents that the curve has been caused by the child's voluntary or careless "poor posture." This myth has no roots in scientific evidence. The role of exercise in more severe curves is controversial. Other therapies of no proven value include chiropractic manipulation, megavitamins, and acupuncture.

Since few of the children with scoliosis in pediatric practice will ever require a brace or surgery, the major strategies useful to the pediatrician in most cases include a cautious and parsimonious follow-up, minimizing the use of x-rays, and reassurance to the child and parents that, even though the curve be real, it poses no threat. The potential harm of overlabeling children with asymptomatic variants of normal is well-described and minimizing that form of harm is in most cases the correct goal for the pediatrician.

INDICATIONS FOR REFERRAL

Curvatures of more than 15 degrees in children entering a period of rapid growth warrant referral for orthopedic evaluation. These curves, especially in girls, are most likely to progress and to require treatment (though most will not), and early consultation may facilitate timely intervention.

Rapidly progressive curves may benefit from braces that support the spine structurally; the most commonly used of these is the Milwaukee brace. Braces are usually reserved for children with curves in excess of 25 degrees or who are judged to be at risk for rapid progression to levels of severity otherwise requiring surgery. Bracing can arrest or slow the progression of many curves and appears to have reduced the frequency of spinal surgery. In screening programs, fewer than one in every 100 children with detectable curves will ever require a brace.

As usually used, the Milwaukee brace is worn throughout the day and night during the child's period of rapid growth, for 3 to 4 years on the average. It is a significant invasion of the normal self-image and life-style of the American adolescent, and supportive counseling may be needed during its use.

Unlike exercise for the mild scoliotic (which is of no proven value), exercise is an essential component of management for the brace patient and must be scrupulously supported by the family, pediatrician, and others around the child.

Scoliosis surgery is reserved for only the most severely affected patients who are refractory or unsuitable for bracing. Barely 1:1000 children with measurable curves are potential candidates for surgery. In the past decade, surgical rates for scoliosis have fallen, probably due to innovations in bracing, and, some believe, school-based screening detecting curves in more favorable stages for bracing. The usual scoliosis surgery involves the placement of a Harrington distraction rod parallel to the convexity of the curve along with fusion of the involved vertebrae. Such surgery is followed by months of rehabilitation and by lifelong limitations in athletic activities to prevent trauma to and from the implanted device.

ANNOTATED BIBLIOGRAPHY

Berwick DM: Scoliosis Screening. Pediatr in Rev 5:238–247, 1984 (Critical review of principles of screening for scoliosis, emphasizing that few positive screenees have problems requiring intervention. Screening, if done at all, should be concentrated in age groups with rapid growth.)

Bjure J, Nachemson A: Non-treated scoliosis. Clin Orthop Rel Res 83:44–52, 1973 (Review and report on long-term consequences of severe scoliosis, emphasizing that surgical correction is indicated only in a small proportion of cases.)

Lonstein JE, Bjorklund S, Wanninger MH, Nelson RP: Voluntary school screening for scoliosis in Minnesota. J Bone Joint Surg G4-A:481–488, 1982 (Pioneering American group describes the organization and results of a state-wide screening program. Of the 3.4% with positive screens, about one third had scoliosis on follow-up evaluation.)

Rogala EJ, Drummond DS, Gurr J: Scoliosis: Incidence and natural history. J Bone Joint Surg 60-A:173–176, 1978 (Prospective epidemiologic study of idiopathic scoliosis in 1122 school children, with a 2-year follow-up of 603. Progression of curvature was observed in 6.8% of cases, and spontaneous improvement occurred in 3%.)

Torrell G, Norwell A, Nachemson A: The changing pattern of scoliosis treatment due to effective screening. J Bone Joint Surg G3-A:337–341, 1982 (Presents data suggesting that screening in Sweden may have reduced the proportion of cases ultimately requiring surgery.)

136
Sprains
and Musculoskeletal Pain

CHARLES F. SANZONE

The investigation of a musculoskeletal complaint in a child must include the complaint, its location, the time and mode of onset, and the age of the child. In circumstances suggesting trauma, the significance of osseous pain and tenderness is different from the significance of the same findings in a situation suggesting an inflammatory or infectious process. Likewise, pain in the same region of the body, and under the same circumstances, may be from different causes in children of different ages. For example, a child complains of pain in the lateral aspect of the ankle after falling. If the child has open growth plates (<13 years old), a growth plate disruption is most likely. If, however, the physes are closed, then a sprain is the most likely diagnosis.

PATHOPHYSIOLOGY

As in other parts of the body, musculoskeletal pain can be attributed to many causes. Physical factors, such as increased pressure within a closed compartment, disruption of a structure, and contusion can cause pain in bone, muscle, and fibrous tissue. Chemical derangements such as the accumulation of metabolites or prostaglandins, or ischemia may be perceived as painful. Neurogenic, viscerogenic, and vasogenic pain can be referred to parts of the musculoskeletal system. Pain may also be referred from one part of the musculoskeletal system to another. These mechanisms come into play in various situations. In the presence of neoplasm, pain may be generated by increased marrow pressure (physical), by local accumulation of prostaglandins (as in osteoid osteoma), by elevation of the periosteum, or by impending or pathologic fracture (physical).

The three components of the musculoskeletal system: bone, ligament, and the muscle–tendon unit are considered separately. The bone is the least sensitive. The periosteum investing the bone, however, is very sensitive. Any stimulation of it can be excruciating. In children, the periosteum is dense and tough, but its attachment to the surface of the bone is mediated by a thick layer of osteoprogenitor cells. Because of this arrangement, periosteal elevation occurs early in inflammatory and hemorrhagic infections. When the continuity of the bone is disrupted, it is the sensitivity of the periosteum more than the sparse free nerve endings in the bone tissue itself that gives rise to painful sensations. While elevations of marrow pressure are perceived as deep aching, rupture of abscesses into the subperiosteal space, with periosteal elevation, are acutely and sharply painful.

Ligaments are richly supplied with nerve endings as part of the proprioceptive apparatus. Pacinian corpuscles and free nerve endings are also present. Physical disruption of a ligament (sprain) and direct contusion are the only mechanisms causing pain in a ligament. In children whose growth plates (physes) are still open, sprains are rare injuries because the ligaments are usually stronger than the cartilaginous physes, when both are subjected to tension.

Muscles and tendons can be ruptured (strains, single macrotrauma episodes), injured by repetitive small stresses (microtrauma and overuse syndromes), or fatigued (accumulation of metabolites). The origins and insertions of muscles and tendons are usually mediated by cartilaginous structures similar to growth plates (apophyses). Where the structures exist, avulsions are far more common than ruptures of either the tendon or the muscle.

Injuries to nerves are not considered in this chapter.

WORK-UP

History

As with any pediatric history, it is important to note the child's age, race, sex, the nature of the complaint, and mode of onset. Acute, subacute, and chronic onsets distinguish broad diagnostic groups, as do traumatic and nontraumatic mechanisms.

In the traumatic group, fractures, sprains, and strains are of acute onset, whereas fatigue fractures and apophysitis are of subacute or chronic onset.

In the nontraumatic group, septic arthritis and osteomyelitis usually present acutely, whereas tumors present with chronic pain.

Patients who have had sports-related injuries can usually provide the examiner with an accurate description of the mechanism of injury. Even broad and unspecific mechanisms such as a "fall onto an outstretched hand" and a "twisted ankle" limit the number of diagnostic possibilities. The physician should ask if a noise was heard at the time of injury, because nearly 50% of patients sustaining a major ligament injury will report hearing a pop or a snap.

Where swelling is a part of the complaint, it is important again to determine the duration of onset. Swelling due to hemorrhage is usually of prompt onset (minutes to a few hours), whereas edema and effusion often take 6 to 12 hours to appear. This is an important point in distinguishing between traumatic effusions and acute hemarthroses.

Erythema is a late sign of most musculoskeletal inflammatory conditions, with the exceptions of superficial bursitides such as those of the prepatellar and olecranon bursae.

The significance of the ability to move an extremity or to bear weight on it varies with the age of the child. In infants pain due to any cause, but most classically pain due to septic arthritis, presents as pseudoparalysis. Toddlers may be willing to move an injured extremity, but they will almost never bear weight on an extremity that has been fractured or sprained. When the child has the power of speech, he should be able to distinguish and communicate more subtle distinctions, such as an inability to bear weight due to pain (fracture) *vs* giving way (sprains).

The physician should always seek a prodromal or pre-existing condition by inquiring after the child's health prior to the onset of the present complaint. Remember that complaints of numbness should never be ignored.

Physical Examination

No orthopaedic examination is complete without an observation of the gait and stance. A limp indicates the presence of pain, weakness, or spasticity. Specifically related to complaints of pain, the physician should look for an antalgic component in gait. In antalgic gait, the patient shortens the amount of time spent in single limb stance on the affected limb. The examiner should note a Trendelenberg lurch in gait or a positive Trendelenberg sign in any patient complaining of hip or knee pain. This will aid in distinguishing direct from referred pain, because the hip refers to the knee, and *vice versa*.

In most circumstances, it is then appropriate to continue with a detailed examination of the part in question. The alignment of the extremity should be noted. Swelling usually indicates the specific area to be evaluated. It is important to reserve maneuvers that may be painful until the end of the examination in order to maintain the patient's cooperation. Palpation for *direct bony tenderness* is most important. In the traumatic setting, direct bony tenderness indicates the presence of a fracture until proven otherwise. Similarly, in the vicinity of a joint, direct bony tenderness indicates a fracture, avulsion, or growth plate injury, rather than a sprain. In the inflammatory setting, direct bony tenderness indicates osteomyelitis until proven otherwise. Both the medial and lateral sides of the joint should be palpated. If the anatomy of the individual ligaments is known, each ligament and each component of the ligament should be palpated. Once direct tenderness has been evaluated, the examiner should test for *indirect tenderness*, confirming a disruption of the ligament in question and assessing its stability. Indirect tenderness is elicited by applying a stress without touching the structure; for example, to stress the medial collateral ligament of the elbow, one hand is placed on the lateral aspect of the joint while the other hand grasps the forearm near the wrist. Pushing the hands towards each other exerts a valgus force at the elbow, placing the medial collateral ligament on stretch. If there is a strong suspicion of instability, this should be done in the radiology suite with radiographic documentation.

No examination of a traumatized extremity is adequate unless the integrity of the skin, circulation, and neurologic function has been documented. Open fractures, traumatic arthrotomies, neurovascular disruptions, and compartment syndromes (*i.e.*, all limb-threatening emergencies) are thus ruled out.

Laboratory Tests

A radiographic examination should be made of all painful extremities. To be adequate, the examination must contain at least two views separated by 90 degrees (*i.e.*, A-P and lateral) and the entire bone in question, including the joints above and below, must be seen.

Failure to demonstrate a fracture radiographically is *not* proof that a fracture does not exist. Subtle signs of fracture include all those indicative of deep soft tissue swelling such as displacement or effacement of fatpads and soft tissue planes. If doubt exists, particularly near a joint, stress roentgenograms are indicated to differentiate sprains from physeal fracture-separations. Stress roentgenograms are also useful to classify sprains. If there is no motion with stress, a sprain is grade I, or mild. With up to 5 mm of displacement, a sprain is moderate, or grade II. Any displacement greater than 5 mm indicates that a severe grade-III sprain has occurred.

With trauma, a radiographic examination may be all that is indicated. In the nontraumatic setting, however, deep soft tissue swelling indicates infection or neoplasm. It is often useful to obtain a hemogram with a differential white cell count, erythrocyte sedimentation rate (to help rule out osteomyelitis, septic arthritis, and systemic inflammatory disease), and hemoglobin electrophoresis (to rule out sickle cell crisis). Scintigraphy and tomography may be indicated to demonstrate lesions not visible on a plain roentgenogram. Arthrocentesis of large post-traumatic effusions and all nontraumatic effusions may be diagnostic as well as therapeutic.

TREATMENT

The diagnosis and treatment of fractures and growth plate injuries are discussed in Chapter 137. Soft tissue injuries (*e.g.*, sprains and strains) of moderate severity may be treated effectively by the primary care physician.

Grade I sprains are diagnosed on the basis of direct tenderness over a ligament, indirect tenderness in the ligament on stress, and stability to stress. The treatment is aimed at the relief of symptoms. A splint, elastic wrap, or bulky dressing is used to restrict motion and prevent swelling. Range of motion exercises are instituted in a matter of days to 1 week, but weightbearing is delayed until the tenderness has subsided. *Participation in sports should be deferred until the tenderness has subsided and full range of motion has been achieved.* The truly devoted athlete may be allowed to participate provided that he understands the possibility of worsening his injury and providing that some protection in the form of a brace (not an elastic sock) or taping is provided.

Grade-II sprains (*i.e.*, those in which there is detectable instability, but in which the ligament is not totally disrupted) require some judgment. In inherently stable joints, such as the ankle, treatment consists of rigid immobilization for up to 2 weeks followed by a protected range of motion with a delay of weightbearing for 6 weeks. In complex or inherently unstable joints, such as the knee, the patient should be referred to an orthopaedic surgeon.

Grade-III sprains (*i.e.*, those in which the ligament is totally disrupted) should be referred.

Mild and moderate *strains*, diagnosed by tenderness in the muscle involved, without (grade I) or with hematoma (grade II) formation, may be treated with local compression and ice packs to control bleeding and edema. In the early phase of healing, aspirin and other non-steroidal anti-inflammatory agents are contraindicated due to their effect on platelet function. Complete muscle ruptures (grade III) are diagnosed by palpating a defect in the muscle belly and by severe weakness in the injured muscle. Complete ruptures of muscles and tendons should be referred. Complete ruptures of finger tendons should be admitted for surgical repair after consultation with a hand surgeon.

SPECIFIC INJURIES

Shoulder

The shoulder can be conceptualized as a complex of four joints: the *acromioclavicular* (AC), *glenohumeral*, *sternoclavicular*, and *scapulothoracic* joints. Injuries to the latter two components are uncommon. Injuries to the acromioclavicular joint usually result from a blow or a fall directly on the top of the shoulder. The prominence of the clavicle is easily visible in grades II and III sprains. Pain and tenderness are localized to the AC joint. Excessive motion of the AC joint is demonstrated by pushing directly on the tip of the distal clavicle, reducing the AC joint. Indirect stress, applied by pulling on the arm, causes pain. Grade-I sprains, ruptures of the AC joint capsule only, are distinguished from grade-II sprains, rupture of the capsule and elongation of the coracoclavicular (CC) ligament, and grade III, complete rupture of both structures, by a standard stress roentgenogram. Ten-pound weights are suspended from the wrists and an A-P exposure, preferably with both shoulders on the same plate, is made. If the clavicle displaces one half of its width or less on the stress roentgenogram, a grade-I sprain is diagnosed. Displacement greater than one half the width of the clavicle, but less than its full width, defines a grade-II sprain. A complete dislocation of the AC joint indicates a grade-III sprain.

There is no controversy about the treatment of grade-I sprains. Relief of stress by means of a sling and appropriate local measures such as cold packs produce uniformly good results in 2 to 3 weeks. Grades II and III sprains may be treated operatively or nonoperatively. An ordinary sling is not adequate treatment for the more severe sprains. Some means of maintaining the joint reduced while supporting the weight of the upper extremity is required. This can be accomplished by means of a sling coupled with strapping encircling the upper extremity from the elbow to a point just proximal to the coracoid process. Prefabricated splints (Kenny–Howard sling) are available. In order for such treatment to have a chance of success, the reduction must be maintained *constantly* for 4 to 6 weeks. The immobilization may lead to skin irritation and necrosis beneath the straps, maceration of the axilla, and even hydradenitis suppurativa. Patients have difficulty in cooperating with this regimen. Operative management of the injury consists of exploration of the AC joint and a repair of the CC ligament. Whichever surgical technique is selected, the complications of surgery include scarring, infection, and failure to achieve or maintain reduction. The usual management is immobilization for grade-II injuries and surgery for grade-III injuries. One study of young athletes, however, has shown that the best and most durable results in grade-II sprains were obtained with surgical management, while the quickest return to functional activity in patients with grade-III sprains was obtained by symptomatic treatment followed by early and aggressive rehabilitation.

Injuries to the intrinsic ligaments of the *glenohumeral* joint are not diagnosable by ordinary clinical means. Injuries to these ligaments lead to recurrent subluxation and dislocation of the shoulder. Dislocations are treated by prompt reduction using adequate analgesia, followed by a minimum of 4 weeks of immobilization in a sling and swathe. The *rotator cuff* is an extrinsic component of the glenohumeral joint composed of the tendons of the supra- and infraspinatus, teres minor, and subscapularis muscles. These muscles, acting in concert, initiate an abduction of the shoulder. In young patients, the rotator cuff may be torn by violent forces acting about the shoulder in abduction and external rotation. The diagnosis is based on the inability to initiate abduction of the involved shoulder and the inability to adduct the shoulder smoothly from full abduction (drop arm sign). The treatment is symptomatic, with early rehabilitation. If weakness persists beyond 6 weeks, the patient should be referred for consideration of operative repair.

Elbow

The elbow joint is intrinsically stable due to the congruency of the ulnohumeral joint. The medial and lateral collateral ligament complexes are very strong, and injuries to them are usually associated with dislocation or subluxation of the joint. Such injuries should be referred to an orthopaedic surgeon.

Avulsions of the medial and lateral epicondyles are not rare. The wrist and finger flexors originate from the medial epicondyle, as does the medial collateral ligament. The extensors originate from the lateral epicondyle. Strong varus or valgus stresses acting in conjunction with contraction of these muscle masses can produce acute avulsions. Repetitious exertion of forces of lesser magnitude over a period of time can result in apophysitis (medial = *pitcher's elbow*; lateral = *tennis elbow*). Avulsions should be referred to an orthopaedic surgeon for consideration of operative intervention, but apophysitides can be managed with rest followed by strengthening exercises. A correction of technique can also be curative for a pitcher or tennis player with apophysitis.

One elbow injury occurs with such frequency that it merits special mention: the *pulled elbow* or *nursemaid's elbow*. The injury is caused by a sudden traction on the forearm. This force causes a widening of the lateral joint space with interposition of the annular ligament of the radius between the joint surfaces, blocking spontaneous reduction. The child is irritable and often has a pseudoparalysis of the involved extremity. A roentgenogram has limited value in establishing the diagnosis, but the prompt return of function with a reduction of the radial head is diagnostic, as is the click which is usually felt on reduction. The reduction maneuver consists of gentle traction on the wrist followed by full, forced supination. No immobilization is required for first subluxations. For repeat injuries, however, a posterior splint is applied for several days.

Wrist

The ligament complexes about the wrist are composed of ligaments that are both short and stout. Consequently, wrist sprains, which are often diagnosed, rarely occur. Older children may develop instability of the wrist due to a disruption of the intercarpal ligaments. An accurate diagnosis of these injuries requires a stress series of radiographs, consisting of a true lateral and A-Ps in neutral, radial, and ulnar deviation as well as an A-P with the fist clenched. In the lateral projection, the radius, lunate, and capitate should be coaxial. In the A-P, any increase in the scapholunate distance is abnormal. Patients suspected of having ligamentous disruptions about the wrist should be referred to a hand surgeon. (For a more complete discussion, see Chap. 138.)

Hip

The capsular ligaments of the hip joint are not subject to incomplete injuries. Traumatically-induced pain about the hip is usually associated with ruptures or avulsion of the muscles originating on the pelvis. The sartorius originates from the anterior superior iliac spine, the rectus femoris from the anterior inferior iliac spine, and the hamstrings from the ischial apophysis. Direct tenderness over these points indicates avulsion injuries that are treated with rest, followed by early, gentle motion and stretching. In the healing phase these injuries can generate truly impressive amounts of callus.

Knee

Injuries to the knee may be complex and are discussed in detail in Chapter 139.

Ankle

An ankle sprain is so common in adults that early in one's training it becomes axiomatic that a tender swollen ankle in the face of negative roentgenograms is a sprain. In pediatrics, of course, this is totally wrong. First of all, most pediatric patients have open physes, making the Salter type I fracture-separation of the distal fibular physis the most common injury in that circumstance. Second, the ligaments of adolescents and young adults are so

strong that true sprains, when they occur, are relatively more serious than the same injuries in adults. It is important to palpate not only the medial and lateral collateral ligaments, but also the anterior and posterior tibiofibular ligaments and the entire length of the fibula. If doubt exists, stress radiographs should be made, and the patient should be referred to an orthopaedic surgeon for further evaluation and treatment.

The subtalar (talocalcaneal) joint can be dislocated by a forceful inversion when the ankle is in equinus. Loss of the dorsalis pedis pulse is fairly common at presentation. Immediate closed or open reduction in indicated in this injury to avoid severe vascular complications. (For a more complete discussion, see Chap. 140).

ANNOTATED BIBLIOGRAPHY

Iverson LD, Clawson DK: Manual of Acute Orthopaedic Therapeutics. Boston, Little, Brown, 1977 (Excellent and concise, with lots of solid "how-to" hints not found in other publications.)

Ogden JA: Skeletal Injury in the Child. Philadelphia, Lea & Febiger, 1982 (Scholarly tome filled with unique photographs of anatomic specimens and histologic preparations.)

Rang M: Children's Fractures, 2nd ed. Philadelphia, JB Lippincott, 1983 (Unique, folksy, and amusing presentation of the basics of pediatric orthopaedic trauma, making each chapter unforgettable; a good starting point for anyone interested in pediatric orthopaedics.)

Rockwood CA, Wilkins KE, King RE: Fractures in Children. Philadelphia, JB Lippincott, 1984 (Excellent, encyclopaedic, multicontributor textbook with excellent entries on all subjects, exhaustive listing of alternative treatments, and a statement of the author's preferred treatment for each item.)

Tachdjian MO: Pediatric Orthopaedics. Philadelphia, WB Saunders, 1972 (Massive single author text, somewhat older and far less focused on trauma. No aspect of pediatric orthopaedics is omitted.)

137

Fractures

LORIN M. BROWN

Fractures of the child's skeleton are unlike those in the adult because of the child's ongoing growth process. The child will double in size between birth and 2 years of age and again between 2 and 10 years of age. During these times of accelerated growth, the body has both a forgiving and an unforgiving

attitude toward the reshaping and future length of the remodeling skeleton. At the ends of the long bones are growth plates that connect the epiphyses to the shafts of the bones. The growth plates consist of soft cartilaginous cells structured in five specific layers. During childhood and early adolescence, these plates are softer and much more easily injured than are the tough ligaments and capsular tissue that attach to the epiphyses. Therefore, when an injury occurs, it is more likely to be a growth plate fracture than a ligamentous sprain or tear.

TYPES OF FRACTURES

The five types of fractures involving the growth plates have been categorized in the Salter–Harris classification (Fig. 137-1).

There are a few residual complications and much forgiving remodeling of the bone with a Salter I or II fracture. A Salter I fracture is usually seen on the x-ray as a rarification in the epiphyseal line. There is no displacement of the metaphysis on the epiphysis itself. Due to projection difficulties while taking x-rays, it may be that no difference in the epiphyseal width is seen. However, due to swelling over the distal epiphysis with point tenderness on the epiphysis such as the distal fibular head, the clinical diagnosis of a Salter I fracture may be made. The closer to a joint or epiphyseal line that a fracture occurs, and the younger the child at the time of the fracture, the greater will be the chance for remodeling or restructuring of that bone. Conversely, the further from a joint and the older the child, there is less chance of the bone regrowing on its own into a more suitable posture. Salter–Harris III and IV fractures have a worse prognosis. If there is displacement, an open surgical reduction will usually be required to anatomically realign the joint and the growth plates. The Salter–Harris V fracture has the worst prognosis. There is impaction and crushing of some portion or all of the growth plate, resulting in a bony bridge that will not allow further growth. If there is growth, it will occur in an angulated direction.

Other types of fractures that may be found are *simple* fractures through the metaphysis or diaphysis of the long bones. These may occur straight across and they are called *transverse* fractures. If they are at an angle, they are termed *oblique* fractures. If a twisting motion resulted in the oblique fracture, it is referred to as a *spiral* fracture, where the fracture would spiral up the bone from the torquing motion. When a transverse fracture occurs, the physician must first think of a direct blow type of trauma or a pathologic fracture. Pathologic fractures occur in various conditions ranging from a simple bone cyst to a malignancy. A fracture found in multiple pieces is termed *comminuted*. This would more likely occur with severe trauma or crushing blow. If the bone is protruding from the skin, it is referred to as a *compound* fracture. These must be surgically irrigated and reduced to prevent bone infection.

In addition to the type of fracture, the position of the fracture is important for the reduction, immobilization, and prognosis of fracture healing. The bone is angulated if it is in any way bent off its normal plane. The direction of the bend is used to describe that position. If, for example, the bone is bent at the distal radius towards the palm, it would be described as volar angulation. The outcome of these types of fractures is based on the amount of bony contact at the fracture site as well as on the alignment at the end of treatment.

Whether the fractured bone encompasses a dislocation is also important. When the bone is fractured and displaced from the joint, it is termed a *fracture–dislocation*. An example of this is if the olecranon at the elbow joint is fractured and displaced; it would be termed a fracture–dislocation of the elbow joint involving the ulna-olecranon.

CLINICAL PRESENTATION

The child presents to the pediatrician because of having fallen or in some way injured a limb. There will usually be swelling and pain. Some children, however, are more stoic than others and some fractures, such as torus-impaction types, are more stable and less painful. Joint effusion may result from intra-articular injury or epiphyseal damage. The younger child will commonly splint the limb. He will resist allowing the fractured limb from being touched and will cry when it is moved.

DIFFERENTIAL DIAGNOSIS

The differential diagnosis of fractures includes infection of the joints, sympathetic effusion from an osteomyelitis of bone juxtapositioned to the joint, synovitis, cellulitis, and soft tissue trauma. Foreign bodies, specifically in the feet and hands, must be ruled out. The older child is more likely to have a tendonitis or sprain. Portions of the ligaments around the joints can tear.

WORK-UP

History

The child or the parents of younger children should be asked how the injury occurred and also the time and onset of when the swelling or pain was first noticed. The history of a fever, recent illness, and history of prior joint swelling should be obtained. Any unusual or suspicious circumstances

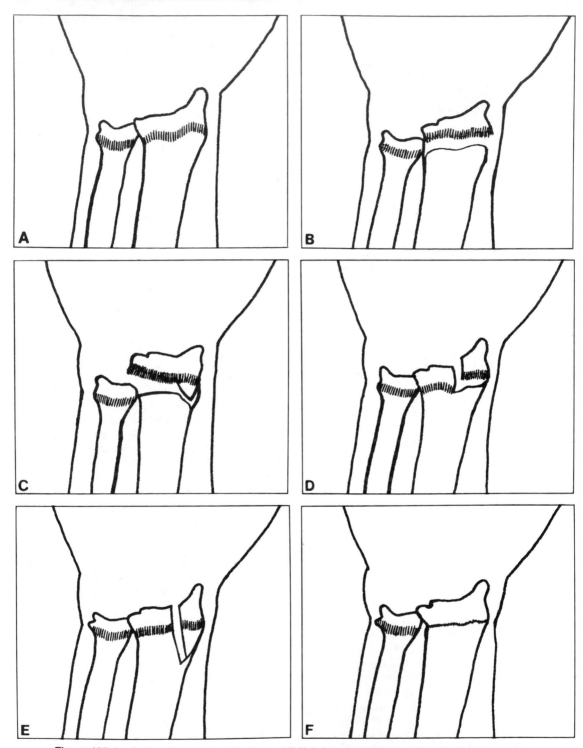

Figure 137-1.   Salter–Harris classifications: (*A*) Uninjured epiphyseal plates in the distal radius and ulna. (*B*) Type 1 epiphyseal plate injury. (*C*) Type 2 epiphyseal plate injury. (*D*) Type 3 epiphyseal plate injury. (*E*) Type 4 epiphyseal plate injury. (*F*) Type 5 compression epiphyseal plate injury. (See text for definitions of each type of fracture.)

should be carefully delineated, such as whether a new babysitter was with the child. Child abuse should also be ruled out in children with multiple fractures. The physician should inquire if other child care agencies are involved with the family.

Physical Examination

A fracture from a fall may also be accompanied by head trauma or other related fractures; therefore, the entire body should be examined for injuries including swelling. Especially in the young child, the skin should be checked for evidence of abuse or neglect, such as burns or multiple hematomas. Over approximately a 10-day period, a hematoma will resorb, turning from blue to green, and finally to yellow. Thus, the age of the bruise can be approximated. Joint swelling surrounded by an area of warmth or erythema may indicate infection. In the absence of a history of trauma, infection is more likely than a fracture. Active or passive motion produces significant pain in either condition.

Laboratory Tests

The definitive test to diagnose a fracture is the roentgenogram. Swollen joints should usually be x-rayed, because a child will rarely have "just a sprain." One does not want to overlook a displaced epiphyseal fracture that may later result in a growth disturbance, residual deformity, and arthritic problems. Roentgenograms should include the joint above and below as well as the entire shaft of the bone involved. At least two views (i.e., AP and lateral) should be taken at 90 degrees to each other. In addition, an oblique view may be useful. One specific x-ray sign noted at the elbow is termed a posterior *fat pad sign*. This is seen on a true lateral roentgenogram of the distal humerus and presents as a blackened shadow behind the humeral condyles where a bleed between the fat pad and the capsular tissue has pushed the posterior fat away from the humerus. In the absence of a grossly displaced fracture, this represents a Salter I epiphyseal fracture of the distal humerus or a nondisplaced supracondylar fracture. This finding, combined with pain about the elbow, has such a high correlation with an actual fracture that it should be considered as pathognomonic for a fracture. Selectively, tomogram x-rays (laminograms), computerized tomography, or bone scans may be helpful aids in the diagnosis and treatment of the injured child. If roentgenograms fail to reveal a fracture, appropriate laboratory tests such as a complete blood count, sedimentation rate, antinuclear antibodies, and rheumatoid factor may be ordered to evaluate for arthritis, collagen-vascular disease, or an underlying infection.

TREATMENT AND MANAGEMENT

Nondisplaced fractures of fingers are best treated by *buddy taping*. First, a stretchable type of adhesive tape may be used to fasten the fractured finger to the adjacent finger to stabilize it from rotation. They are then splintered in a position of function termed *intrinsic plus*. This holds the metacarpal-phalangeal joints at 90 degrees of flexion, 20 degrees at the proximal interphalangeal joint and 10 degrees at the distal interphalangeal joint. In this posture the ligaments are stretched to their longest and therefore have the least chance of becoming shortened causing a contracture. Maintain splinting for approximately 3 weeks, at which time guarded active range of motion is allowed for the next 3 weeks. This, however, assumes adequate healing has been obtained on x-ray examination.

When the child has caught his finger or fingers in a door or desk top (which is a common occurrence), lacerations of the nail bed must be repaired. The avulsed nail is usually discarded and the repaired nail bed covered with lubricated gauze. If there is not a partial amputation, the main concern is that an epiphyseal fracture of any type has occurred. For this reason, roentgenograms are required to rule out the need for an open reduction or a closed reduction of the fractured joint epiphysis. Fractures of the *metacarpal* bones of a child are best treated by a short arm cast. Depending on the age of the child, approximately 3 to 5 weeks of immobilization are required, followed by an additional 3 weeks of guarded active range of motion. Fractures of the capals are rare in children because these bones consist largely of cartilage and have no growth plates. In the adolescent, nondisplaced fractures of the carpal navicular bone are more common and should be treated by a short arm cast extended to include the proximal phalanx of the thumb (see Chap. 138 for a complete discussion on hand injuries).

Displaced fractures of the distal *radius* are best treated by a closed reduction, (straightening the bone without surgically opening the limb) if at all possible. Open reductions can lead to excessive callus formation and bridging across the interosseous space of the forearm. Correct alignment and angulation must be obtained to maintain a full range of motion and position. Fractures of the proximal ulna and radius, if displaced, are harder to align and may require an open reduction. Fractures of the distal humerus, if nondisplaced, should be treated initially by a posterior mold extending from the proximal humerus to the palm. Due to excessive swelling in this area, circumferential or compression bandaging which could impair the circulation should be avoided. For this reason, immediate circular casting is ill-advised unless a box configuration is used at the elbow joint. Similarly, to avoid compromising the circulation with tight casting, displaced fractures will usually either require surgical pinning or skeletal traction to obtain and maintain correct alignment. A broken shaft of the proximal humerus is best treated by means of either a hanging cast or sugar-tong splint (a long arm circular cast that hangs from the neck forming a portable traction) and swathe-type immobilization. A sugar-tong splint is similar in principle to the hanging cast. Its major advantage is that it is lighter.

Clavicular fractures are commonly seen by the pediatrician in his office. Fractures of a greenstick type should not be manipulated but rather allowed to heal and remodel on their own unless there is a significant amount of angulation. The main principle in treatment is to keep the shoulders pulled backwards in order to keep the bones within their periosteal sleeve on stretch and not allow the bone edges to rub, thereby causing pain and further bleeding. Rarely, there may be interposition of soft tissue that prevents healing of what is commonly believed to be a fracture that heals without complications. If there is a severely displaced fracture, there is also the possibility that one of the bone edges may have pierced into the lung cavity causing a partial or complete pneumothorax. The major blood vessels below the clavicle may also be torn, causing a hemothorax or subcutaneous emphysema. A child with a clavicular fracture should be immobilized for between 3 and 4 weeks by means of a figure-of-eight type shoulder hyperextension device. This may be augmented with a sling if the child is more comfortable. It is generally more comfortable for the child to sleep flat on his back with a small raise between the scapulae allowing his shoulders to fall backwards. In children with the epiphyses open, there would rarely be an acromioclavicular dislocation. If there is pain in the distal clavicle, there is probably a Salter I or II fracture of the distal clavicular epiphysis. A modified type splinting device similar to that for an acromioclavicular dislocation should be employed if there is significant displacement. Otherwise, the same treatment used for simple fractures should suffice. Pain

with apparent dislocation of the medial end of the clavicle of a growing child is rarely caused by a dislocation of the clavicle; a Salter I of the clavicle from the medial clavicular epiphysis is more likely. This fracture should be reduced onto the epiphysis as with any epiphyseal fracture and may require an open reduction to align it.

Complications from fractures of the *tibial* shaft can be insidious. A fractured tibia may bleed slowly and may develop into a compartment syndrome. This occurs because the tibial bleed is enclosed within the fascia of the lower leg muscles that envelop the tibia. There is no continuation of these compartments, especially in the anterior leg, and a significant bleed can lead to compression of the neurovascular structures of the lower extremity. Ischemic contractures with death of the muscles that move the foot and ankle may then result. Immediate circular casting for displaced tibial fractures is contraindicated without first close observation in hospital. Fractures of the *femoral* shaft usually require traction followed by a body spica cast. *Hip* fractures require traction if they are nondisplaced. More commonly, they are displaced and will require immediate open reduction with internal fixation. Fractures of the knee, foot, and ankle are covered in Chapters 139 and 140.

Children may present with low back pain, especially those who participate in athletics such as football, track, and gymnastics. This may be the result of a fracture of the pars interarticularis of the posterior ring of the lumbar vertebrae. Oblique roentgenograms aid in this specific diagnosis. A bone scan should be obtained if a lysis (break) is found in the absence of lysthesis (forward slippage of the proximal spinal column on the distal). If radioactive uptake is increased in these posterior structures without further evidence of an underlying neoplasm, a relatively fresh fracture is most likely. Immobilizing the child in a body cast from the abdomen to the ipsilateral knee for 12 weeks may result in union of the pars interarticularis. Failing union, the child is treated symptomatically by means of a custom-made lumbar-pelvis orthosis for sports or as symptomatically needed to prevent further slippage by lateral x-ray. Should there be significant movement of the vertebral bodies or intolerable back pain, operative fusion of the specific vertebral level is indicated.

INDICATIONS FOR REFERRAL

The physician should refer the child with a fracture or injury based on his training and skill in the treatment of fractures. If he does not feel confident in dealing with the undisplaced, angulated, or intra-articular fracture, it would be best to refer the child. As with all specialties, orthopedics has evolved into both general pediatric as well as anatomically regional subspecialties.

ANNOTATED BIBLIOGRAPHY

Rang M: Children's Fractures, 2nd ed. Philadelphia, JB Lippincott, 1983 (Simpler, complete volume on fractures in children.)

Rockwood C Jr, Rockwood K: Fractures in Children. Philadelphia, JB Lippincott, 1984 (Excellent authoritative book on fractures in children.)

Salter RB: Textbook of Disorders and Injuries of the Musculoskeletal System, Chaps 15, 16, 17, p 331. Baltimore, Williams and Wilkins, 1970 (Authoritative and concise.)

Sharrard WJW: Paediatric Orthopedics and Fractures, 2nd ed., Vol. 2, p 1484. Oxford, Blackwell Scientific Publications, 1979 (Complete and extremely well documented.)

138
The Injured Hand
CHARLES F. SANZONE

The hand is a uniquely human organ. Many authorities believe that the extraordinary suppleness and strength of the hand has played a major role in human evolution. The hand is also a sensory organ of exquisite sensitivity. In combining receptor and effector functions, the hand is a major channel for interaction with one's environment. Because of the primary role the hand plays in exploring and interacting with the environment, it is one of the most frequently injured body parts, especially in the curious toddler and the newly assertive adolescent. The hand is second only to the face as an expression of one's personality.

WORK-UP

History

A history taking is straightforward for most hand problems. In terms of injury, three mechanisms are particularly dangerous and deceptive: crush, bite, and injection. Crush injuries, especially those involving rollers such as are found in grocery store conveyor belts and in escalators, can cause edema out of proportion to the apparent severity of the injury. Even when the force of the injury is insufficient to cause fractures or major skin problems, the deep pressure wave caused by the roller can disrupt the muscles of the hand and forearm which are housed in tight, inelastic compartments. The resultant increase in compartment pressure can then cause ischemia and a full-blown *compartment syndrome*. Animal bites combine the dangers of penetration with those of typical bacterial flora, such as *Pasteurella multocida* and *cat bites*. Human bites are especially dangerous due to the combi-nation of penetration, introducing mixed bacterial flora, and crushing of the tissues, creating an ideal culture medium. Abrasions or lacerations incurred during fights are all potential human bites (see Chap. 141).

Physical Examination

An inspection of the hand is also straightforward and can be precisely described by reference to the many landmarks such as flexion creases, knuckle pads, and bony prominences. In most cases, a simple drawing of the hand with lesions located with respect to landmarks is the quickest and easiest way to describe a lesion on the hand. Several significant patterns of swelling may be noted. Since the volar pads are held in place by dense connective tissue septae, most edema will be apparent dorsally rather than volarly. Fusiform swelling of the digits centered on the proximal interphalangeal (PIP) joints is characteristic of rheumatoid arthritis. Flexor tendon sheath infections produce a uniform swelling of the digit. The tendon sheaths of the thumb and little finger flexors are in close proximity at the base of the palm, creating the possibility of infectious tenosynovitis of both tendon sheaths by contiguous extension and the "horseshoe abscess" which is diagnostic of it. The active and passive motion of all 15 joints can be recorded in Figure 138-1.

In cases where there is a significant question of penetration with injury to underlying structures, the hand should be inspected in the position it was in at the time of injury. An error that is made all too frequently is failing to detect an extensor tendon injury by examining the hand with the fingers ex-

Finger

Joint		Thumb	Index	Mid	Ring	Small
	DIP					
	PIP	—				
	MCP					
	MVCM		—	—	—	—

Figure 138-1. Model chart for recording the examination of all 15 joints in the hand.

tended. Palpation of the hand is mostly limited to assessing the swelling and eliciting tenderness.

Laboratory Tests

Judicious use of the laboratory is recommended to assess infections and systemic diseases that may have prominent expression in the hand (*e.g.*, rheumatoid arthritis). Roentgenography, however, is indispensible. Plain roentgenograms of the hand are difficult to read due to the multiple structures, and their superimposition on each other. Several strategies can simplify the evaluation of hand radiograms. First, order an A-P and lateral of only the part in question (*e.g.*, index finger, or carpus). Second, evaluate the parts of *least* interest first, lessening the chance of forgetting to evaluate everything on the radiogram by overconcentration on the area in question. Third, evaluate each structure on the film in turn (*i.e.*, soft tissues first, then the bones, then the joint spaces). The more sophisticated radiographic techniques are generally of little use, but in specific instances they are invaluable. Scintigraphy is useful in detecting occult fractures of the carpal scaphoid and in delineating some tumors. Magnified views can demonstrate subtle fractures of the carpus. Arthrography can demonstrate injuries to the intercarpal joints and to the triangular fibrocartilage on the ulner side of the wrist. Computed tomography is the best means of evaluating the distal radioulnar joint.

INJURIES

Fractures

The most common finger injury is the crush of the fingertip, usually by a door. A conminuted fracture of the nonarticulating portion of the distal phalanx often results. The fingernail acts as a natural splint for this fracture; thus, it should be preserved.

A protective splint is usually all that is necessary until the tenderness has subsided. The resulting subungual hematoma is a source of pain. Burning through the nail with a red-hot paperclip provides prompt relief. If the nail has been avulsed, it should be replaced under the eponychium to serve as a splint and to prevent adhesions of the eponychium to the nailbed, which result in troublesome nail deformities. Lacerations of the nailbed should be repaired with 5–0 absorbable sutures prior to replacing the nail. A blow to the tip of the finger in a longitudinal direction will result in the avulsion of the terminal tendon of the extensor apparatus. The same mechanism in a child with open physes will result in a fracture separation. If the fragment is less than 50% of the joint surface, and the joint remains reduced, this mallet (also called baseball) finger is treated with continuous splintage in extension for 6 weeks. If the joint is dislocated or subluxed, and the fragment represents a sizeable proportion of the joint surface, then a referral for operative management is indicated.

The distal articular surfaces of the proximal and middle phalanges are composed of radial and ulnar condyles. Condylar and bicondylar fractures are common athletic injuries. Nondisplaced fractures can be treated with immobilization for 10 days to 2 weeks, followed by buddy taping for 2 more weeks. Fractures of the phalangeal neck usually result from forceful hyperextension of the IP or MCP joint most often by a closing door. Closed manipulation and splinting are adequate treatment in moderately and minimally displaced fractures. Severely displaced fractures and irreducible fractures should be referred for open treatment. Transverse fractures of the shaft of the phalanges may be reduced and splinted. When the fracture is through the middle phalanx proximal to the insertion of the flexor superficialis tendon, the finger is splinted in extension; when it is distal to the flexor insertion, the finger is splinted in flexion. Oblique and spiral fractures of the shaft, however, should be referred for consideration of operative reduction and fixation. The proximal end of the phalanx is its epiphyseal end. Salter type-III injuries of this physis should be referred, but Salter type-II injuries may be reduced and splinted. Radial and ulnar angulation of proximal phalanx fractures are best corrected by placing a pencil or pen in the web space to act as a fulcrum. Fractures of the finger metacarpals are unusual in children with open physes. They are common in adolescents, however. The most common mechanism of injury is longitudinal compression, as in punching. It is, therefore, essential to inspect the knuckle to rule out penetration of the joint by a tooth in any patient presenting with a metacarpal fracture. Dorsal angulation of up to 50 degrees may be accepted in fractures of the metacarpal neck; these are treated by closed reduction and immobilization in a gutter splint for 4 weeks. The thumb metacarpal may be fractured through the metaphysis or the physis. Metaphyseal or Salter–Harris type-II injuries are treated with closed reduction and casting in a below elbow cast extending to the base of the thumbnail. Salter–Harris type III injuries, however, require accurate open reduction to avoid joint incongruity and progressive deformity. Fractures involving the proximal articular surface of the thumb metacarpal (Bennett's fractures), are rare in children with open physes. In older children, they should be referred. Fractures of the carpal bones prior to adolescence are also rare, because the relative weakness of the distal radial physis has a protective effect on the strongly supported carpus. With fusion of the distal radial physis, this protection is lost, and carpal injuries become more common.

Dislocations

The presence of open physes protects against dislocations. In the older adolescent, however, dislocations occur. IP joint dislocations are easily reduced by exaggerating the deformity, by applying longitudinal traction, and by applying thumb pressure or flexing. Dorsal dislocations are most common followed by radial and ulnar dislocations. The metacarpals dislocate dorsally, usually in association with other severe, high-energy hand injuries. Open reduction and pinning are usually required to maintain the reduction. Dislocations of the wrist are serious injuries with a high incidence of associated neurovascular injuries. Immediate neurovascular assessment, splintage, and referral are mandatory.

Sprains

As with dislocations, open growth plates protect against sprains in the young child. Older children may suffer disruptions of the intrinsic ligaments of the hand. The collateral ligaments of the IP and MCP joints are vulnerable. Instability is assessed with the IP joints in extension, but the MP joints should be stressed in 90 degrees of flexion. Treatment of even third-degree sprains is nonoperative, with splinting and buddy taping. The MP joint of the thumb is an exception. Operative repair is indicated if stress radiograms demonstrate a complete disruption of the ulnar collateral ligament. Of the intercarpal ligaments, only rupture of the scapholunate interosseous ligament is well worked out. A disruption of this ligament results in a widening of the scapholunate joint space on a regular or stress (clenched fist) radiogram. The wrist collapses into either dorsal or volar instability patterns. The treatment is surgical.

Amputations

In young children, complete or partial amputation of almost any body part is an indication for replantation of that part. The criteria for the selection of adolescents and young adults for replantation or revascularization, however, are more stringent. Replantation of the thumb, multiple digits, partial amputation of the hand through the palm or wrist, or a clean relatively transverse amputation above the wrist is indicated. Replantation of single digit amputations may be indicated if the level of amputation is above the flexor superficialis insertion (distal to the proximal third of the middle phalanx). The attending physician should make direct contact with the surgeon who will be accepting the patient. Detailed instructions for preparation of the amputated part should be obtained. This usually involves placing the amputated part in a plastic bag filled with saline and placing the bag on ice. There should be no unnecessary delay in transportation to the microvascular surgeon, because maximum allowable cold ischemia time not under the surgeon's direct supervision is about 6 hours. Fingertip amputations do not require such highly specialized intervention. Their treatment centers on three concerns: preservation of sensation, preservation of the cushioning function of the pulp, and preservation of the nail. There is little controversy that in transverse injuries with no bone exposed, healing by secondary intention provides the best results in terms of sensation and function. In amputations whose obliquity is from dorsal to volar, the main problem is a loss of digital pulp. Such complicated strategies as advancement flaps and pedicle flaps may be justified. Injuries to the nailbed should be referred to a hand surgeon. Ring avulsion injuries, in which an encircling band caught on something degloves a digit, are treated by resection of the digit and its metacarpal.

Infections

The *paronychia* is a suppurative infection of the nailfold. It occurs mainly in patients who manicure their nails. Paronychiae are diagnosed on the basis of redness, swelling, and purulent exudate. Early in the infection, prior to abscess formation, paronychia is treated by warm soaks and oral antibiotics. Surgical drainage is indicated once pus begins to accumulate. The *herpetic whitlow,* an unusual condition caused by herpesvirus, can mimic paronychia, causing swelling and erythema of the nailfold. These conditions can be differentiated on the basis of a physical examination. No frank pus is present in the whitlow. Whitlows are characterized by vesicles that may contain clear or turbid fluid, but not pus. The drainage of whitlows is contraindicated.

Felons are infections of the fingertip pulp space. Treatment is rendered difficult by the dense connective tissue septae that traverse the pulp space. There is usually a history of trauma followed by a rapidly pointing and exquisitely painful swelling. Prompt and adequate drainage is necessary to avoid osteomyelitis of the distal phalanx, suppurative flexor tenosynovitis, or necrosis of the pulp space and skin of the fingertip. Many approaches have been described for the drainage of felons. Any incision that avoids the digital nerves and does not produce a disabling scar is acceptable. All of the involved septae must be broken and all of the ne-

crotic tissue debrided. Continuous drainage is ensured by leaving a moist wick in place for 2 to 3 days.

Suppurative tenosynovitis is usually caused by a puncture through one of the flexor creases of the fingers where the skin is directly adherent to the tendon sheath. The diagnosis is made on the basis of the four signs of Kanavel: uniform swelling, tenderness over the tendon sheath, pain on passive motion, and a moderately flexed position of the finger at rest. Prompt and adequate surgical drainage is necessary in order to avoid necrosis of the tendon and extensive adhesions.

Infections of the web space have acquired the trivial name of *collar button abscesses* due to their peculiar morphology. There is usually a small intradermal abscess that communicates with a much larger deep abscess. The double configuration of the abscess predisposes to inadequate drainage by the unwary. As with all deep hand infections, a prompt referral is indicated. The palmar and thenar spaces, two other deep spaces of the hand, are prone to infection. Suppurative arthritis of the hand can arise from bites or from direct extension from nearby infections. Prompt surgical drainage is indicated. When a human bite is the suspected etiology, penicillin should be included in the perioperative regimen while awaiting culture (see Chap. 141).

ANNOTATED BIBLIOGRAPHY

Green DP (ed): Operative Hand Surgery. New York, Churchill Livingstone, 1982 (Most complete and current of the multivolume multiauthor texts. Most authors are leaders in their subspecialties.)

O'Brien ET. In Rockwood CA, Wilkins KE, King RE: Fractures in Children. Philadelphia, JB Lippincott, 1984 (Excellent resource. Treatment, bone by bone and joint by joint, is described and the author's preferences are clearly stated.)

139
The Injured Knee
LORIN M. BROWN

The child's knee is as much at risk from sports and daily accidents as is the adult knee. Damage to the epiphyseal plates of the distal femur, the proximal tibia, and the proximal fibula complicates the problems that can occur with the knee. The epi-

physeal plates, in addition to the tibial spine which is located on top of the tibial epiphysis, are easier to fracture in the growing child than it is to tear the adjacent ligaments. Epiphyseal fractures should not be overlooked as these could result in a growth disturbance later on. Towards the end of adolescence, a traumatically swollen knee is more likely to be the result of a fracture than a ligamentous tear. Later in life, the menisci, cruciate ligaments, collateral ligament, and the capsule are the first areas injured. It must be remembered, however, that any type of injury may occur at any age. The child's x-ray picture is more complicated because large portions of the joint structures in the younger child are cartilaginous and invisible. In addition, the normal laxity in the growing child's knee can confuse the picture when evaluating for ligamentous damage, especially to the anterior cruciate ligament.

PATHOPHYSIOLOGY

Injuries about the knee can occur in any type of sport or activity that the child is undertaking. Falling onto flexed knees, jumping or falling from monkey bars or other gymnastic equipment, and falling off of a bicycle are a few of the ways in which a child can injure his knee. A simple fall or a medial to lateral blow to the involved patella is sufficient to cause a displacement. There is usually an increased valgus angle to the knee as a predisposing component to the pathology as well as a generalized joint laxity. Sports activities cause adult-type injuries in the much older child. "Clipping" and "tackling" injuries cause epiphyseal separations or disruptions of the collateral and cruciate ligaments of the knee. Rotatory injuries will cause tearing and shearing of the menisci of the knee. The injuries become more related to the soft tissues and internal structures of the knee as the child's ligaments become thinned and the epiphyses fuse. A congenital deformity may present as early as 2 to 3 years of age when a congenital discoid meniscus may become symptomatic.

Osteomyelitis tends to occur about the knee due to the increased matrix of capillary flow in the metaphysis of the distal femur and proximal tibia. These form static spaces in which the bacteria grow. When the pressure becomes great enough, it may then decompress through the bone into the knee joint and be first identified as a septic joint. A hematoma from trauma may become a breeding ground for bacteria and proliferate in the same fashion. The bursae about the knee, especially the prepatellar and infrapatellar, are highly susceptible to falls and may become lacerated or otherwise inflamed from falling, sharp objects, or repeated trauma. *Osgood–Schlatter's disease* is probably either fracture or apophysitis of the tibial tubercle caused by repeated trauma and stress to the apophysitis. The degree of pain varies with the psychological and physiologic make-up of each child. The epiphyseal area becomes tender to palpation and motion because it is the site of the attachment of the patellar ligament, which is the insertion of the quadriceps mechanism. With the knee in full extension, this area is highly vulnerable to injury and stress.

Fractures of the epiphysis are described in Chapter 137. Any of the five types of fractures of the Salter–Harris classification may occur about the epiphyses of the knee. Salter I and II types are most prevalent. These types will occur in an identical biomechanical fashion as they do in adult knee injuries and result in ligamentous, meniscal, and cruciate ligament tears. A blow from the lateral side of the knee will open the epiphysis on the medial side. Depending on the angle and velocity, a force can result either in a Salter I fracture (that cannot be discerned as a fracture unless a stress roentgenogram is performed) or in a portion of the metaphysis being torn off with the epiphysis resulting in a Salter type-II injury. Forward blows directly to the knee in the child may dislocate the epiphyseal plate of the knee posteriorly or fracture the tibial spine off of the articular plateau of the proximal tibia. The analogous injury in the skeletally mature patient would be a dislocated knee or a tear of the cruciate ligaments. Other rotatory injuries that would tear the meniscal tissue in the adult may instead produce various Salter type-III and type-IV injuries, taking off portions of the epiphyses or tearing the meniscal tissue. Past puberty, the epiphyseal plates become partially bridged and injuries will most likely result in ligamentous tears and meniscal damage as seen in the adult. The worst case of all occurs with a combination injury that not only tears the soft tissue but also damages both the growth center and the articular surface of the growing joint.

CLINICAL PRESENTATION

The injured child will present with a swollen or erythematous warm knee. The history is critical since the appearance may be the same whether it is septic or traumatic. The knee will be painful and the range of motion will be limited, regardless of the etiology.

CLINICAL EXAMINATION

With a history of trauma, the child should first be examined by x-ray. This is important in that a nondisplaced tibial spine fracture or epiphyseal plate injury may become displaced by the initial physical examination of the knee. It is more important in the child than in the adult, because again the likelihood is that the injury resulted in a fracture rather than only a ligamentous or meniscal tear. After a fracture has been ruled out, the knee should be examined to ensure that there is no ligamentous tear, or Salter I injury that was not seen on the initial x-rays. The knee should be stressed with the leg in extension into both varus and valgus positions. This is accomplished by placing one palm against the distal femur and by using this palm as a fulcrum while pushing the tibia laterally, thereby placing a valgus stress on the knee. This will open the medial side of the knee if there is an epiphyseal fracture or a tear of the medial collateral ligament. With the knee in extension, the posterior capsule must also be torn for instability to occur. If the same examination is performed with the knee in 30 degrees of flexion, instability will more likely be related to just ligamentous or epiphyseal damage rather than to capsular injury. The reverse maneuver is then applied pulling the leg into varus. This will indicate whether there is a tear of the lateral collateral ligament. The fibular head may be fractured, causing laxity in the lateral collateral ligament because this is where the ligament attaches. The knee is then flexed to 90 degrees and, with pressure applied to the posterior proximal tibia, the flexed knee should be pulled forward. With the foot held stable, usually by the examiner sitting on the patient's forefoot, an increased forward laxity of the injured knee compared to the opposite knee may be found with an anterior cruciate ligament tear. Posterior stress laxity of the tibia relative to the well knee may show whether a posterior cruciate has been torn. The same maneuver can be performed with the knee at 30 degrees of flexion. In this position, it is known as the *Lachman test*. The knee that presents as "locked" in the child may not be a meniscal injury, as it is usually in the adult, because a child will "freeze" his knee more readily when it hurts than the adult. The examiner must be sure that the child is not just holding his knee stiff from a contusion. A *McMurray sign* can be elicited with a significantly torn meniscus and in the case of a discoid meniscus. For this maneuver, the child lies flat on his back with the hip and knee flexed and then, while internally or externally rotating it, the knee is pulled into extension. The knee will have a rubbery snap or popping sound if the meniscus is torn and displaced in position. If the tear is not complete, this will also elicit pain as the femoral con-

dyles are rotated and pushed onto the meniscus pulling the attached capsule with the meniscal fragment.

If the history suggests that the patella is the main cause of pain, the examination proceeds as follows. The leg is held in extension and manual force is pressed against the middle side of the patella, pushing it towards the lateral direction. If the child screams or grabs for the knee and tries to prevent this maneuver, it is termed a *positive apprehension test*. The child, having recently had the patella dislocate laterally (as is often the case), will be on guard against a recurrence and will try to prevent the examiner from reproducing the pain. In addition, if the patella was completely dislocated, the anterior-medial structures of the knee joint will be torn, swollen, and painful when palpated. If there is not a gross effusion, there may still be a mild effusion that can be detected by the *ballotment test*. The suprapatellar pouch (area proximal to the patella) is compressed, pushing any blood or effusion in this area down into the knee joint. The patella may then be pressed in an anterior to posterior manner and will ballot or bobble up and down when compressed and released.

DIFFERENTIAL DIAGNOSIS

The differential diagnosis in a young child is most often between infection and trauma. The infection considered is usually from a juxta-articular osteomyelitis, an intra-articular sepsis, or an infection of a bursa. Cellulitis overlying the knee is usually readily diagnosed although the location of infection may not always be apparent, especially if it is deep. Other causes of effusion include arthritis and, far less commonly, malignancy. Polyarthritis can result from rheumatic fever or may be a transient synovial reaction to a systemic illness (*e.g.*, bacteremia and virtually any viral illness). Osgood–Schlatter's condition is an inflammation of the tibial tubercle and it occasionally combines with a tendonitis of the patellar ligament to produce a painful prominence under the knee.

Congenital dislocations of the patella *vs* a traumatically dislocated patella is usually easily differentiated. Congenitally dislocated patellae are solidly dislocated laterally or medially. Flexion of the knee reveals the femoral condylar sulcus without a patella present. A traumatically dislocated patella is usually observed to occur by the child and is almost always associated with severe pain and immediate swelling.

WORK-UP

If trauma is not the obvious cause, a complete blood count (CBC), erythrocyte sedimentation rate, rheumatoid factor, ASO titers, and antinuclear antibodies should be ordered to try to rule out an early septic disease, juvenile rheumatoid arthritis, other arthritis, or rheumatic fever. Later, an electroencephalogram (ECG) and a slit lamp eye examination may be necessary for juvenile rheumatoid arthritis (JRA) evaluation. JRA and a septic knee can be difficult and occasionally impossible to differentiate. It may be necessary in the infant and child to perform a technesium or gallium scan to rule out infection or fracture. An infant's knee may have been injured by child abuse and trying to differentiate this from a septic knee with only regular x-rays may not be possible. One should not hesitate to repeat any tests if the clinical presentation or diagnosis remains unclear. Aspiration of the fluid from the knee joint may also be performed. A bloody effusion is usually pathognomonic for trauma, a synovial effusion more indicative of arthritis, and "pus-like" fluid could be either from a septic knee or juvenile rheumatoid arthritis. An arthrogram, which is dye injected into the knee joint to visualize the shape and contour of the menisci which are invisible on routine x-rays, may be performed if the problem does not subside with conservative treatment and if the symptoms are highly suggestive of a traumatic meniscal tear or congenital malformed discoid meniscus.

The final and ultimate examination of the knee is arthroscopy. It is much better to examine the knee with a smaller pediatric arthroscope rather than the adult-sized arthroscope. This procedure is not without its complications and more damage can occur from the unskilled arthroscopist or large arthroscopic instruments than was originally present. The knee in the young child has not had the stresses of the adult knee and the joint space itself is small. Arthrotomy, usually of a small incision size, may be necessary to remove posterior pieces of meniscus or large fragments that cannot otherwise be easily removed from the child's or adolescent's knee. Specialized procedures such as these, especially on a young child, are best performed by an experienced arthroscopist.

TREATMENT

Fractures that displace the epiphyseal plates of the distal femur or proximal tibia and that extend intra-articularly must be reduced and possibly internally fixated surgically. A displaced fracture of the tibial spine may also need to be wired into position. Some fractures of the distal femur or proximal tibia may need to be gently manipulated back into an anatomic position. General anesthesia may be required in some instances. Disruption of the tibial tubercle may likewise need a surgical reduction to reattach the tubercle. Care must be taken to avoid closure of the epiphysis or apophysis, which could cause the proximal tibia to grow into recurvatum. Furthermore, if a fracture of the cartilaginous surface of the patella causes the patellar ligament to pull off the inferior surface of the patella (sleeve fracture), a complete disruption in the extensor mechanism of the leg results.

Minor fractures, such as Salter–Harris type I, may be treated by long leg or cylinder casting whereas type II fractures of the distal femoral epiphysis usually require a body spica cast to prevent the hamstring muscles and quadriceps mechanism from redisplacing the epiphysis. Ligaments may be damaged in a child and will usually heal rapidly by casting in the appropriate position. An open repair of the collateral ligaments is rarely indicated. The reconstruction of a completely torn cruciate ligament is indicated if the child is having instability with walking. A specialized brace may be used for sports in the future. If the leg is stable and there is normal walking and running, cruciate surgical repair is purely elective. Peripheral meniscal tears will most likely heal in a child. In the young child, it is highly unlikely for a meniscus to be detached, and damage may well be the result of a congenitally malformed and biomechanically weakened discoid meniscus that will require surgical removal. Osteochondral fragments may be drilled by arthroscopy to try to hasten fusion of the fragment. Osteochondral fragments, which are found to be totally detached, are best treated by removal if there is no living osseous chondylar portion. If the surface areas are bulging or depressed and a roentgenogram shows a persistent osteochondral fragment that is clinically significant, arthroscopic drilling through the cartilage into the bony bed will possibly allow for ingrowth of bone matrix and a faster healing of the fractured fragment. Surgery, however, should be reserved for the patient with the aforementioned findings who has also effusion and pain or a persistent delayed healing time. The extent of actual articular damage can be seen directly. In addition, a septic or arthritic knee can be evaluated and fully cleansed with minimal incisions through arthroscopic surgery.

ANNOTATED BIBLIOGRAPHY

Post M (ed): Physical examination of the musculoskeletal system. In Brown LM, Sharrard WJW: Examination of the Lower Extremities in the Child. Chicago, Year Book Medical Publishers, 1987 (Complete description of the physical examination.)

Rang M: Children's Fractures, 2nd ed., Chap. 18, p 281.

Philadelphia, JB Lippincott, 1983 (Excellent general reference.)

Rockwood C, Rockwood K: Fractures in Children, Chap. 11, p 891. Philadelphia, JB Lippincott, 1984 (Excellent general reference.)

Sharrard WJW: Paediatric Orthopedics and Fractures, 2nd ed. Oxford, Blackwell Scientific Publications, 1970 (Excellent general reference.)

140

The Injured Foot

LORIN M. BROWN

The child's foot is vulnerable to injury from birth. It is the basis of the support of the body and is exposed to tremendous stress incurred by walking and running. There are multiple fractures ranging from stress fractures to compound comminuted fractures that can be acute as well as chronic problems that may last a lifetime. Thus, foot injuries should not be taken lightly and should be carefully evaluated.

PATHOPHYSIOLOGY AND CLINICAL PRESENTATION

Cuts on the foot often occur from a child stepping on glass, a pin, or a nail. A wound may be self-inflicted by a child tearing at his toe nails or by cutting the nail back in such a way that an *ingrown nail* develops. With infection, an erythematous swollen area may be seen either around the cuticle bed of the nail or on the foot. Cellulitis can rapidly develop and spread either in the streaking manner of a lymphangitis following the lymph channels proximally up the leg or the infection can pool and form a large abscess. Both can be life-threatening. Children who have juvenile diabetes must be carefully observed, because they are at greater risk for rapidly developing and chronically sustaining infections of the feet.

The foot is exposed to trauma by the child stubbing his toe against walls and other objects in the home. The likelihood of injury becomes great when the child is able to go outdoors where there are more loose items. A foreign body must always be considered as the cause of a chronic soft tissue infection. Fractures of the toes are significant when they involve an articular surface or an epiphyseal plate, especially of the great toe. As 50% of push-off occurs at the phalangeal-metatarsal joint of the great

toe, an intra-articular fracture of this joint surface must be fully treated. Fractures of the shafts of the other bones can occur in similar manners as well as dislocations of all joints of the phalanges of all toes. With the increasing popularity of athletic competition, *stress fractures* seen formally only in older adolescents are now also commonly found in the younger athlete. These fractures, although they may initially be invisible on normal x-ray, may eventually prove to be nondisplaced fractures requiring treatment.

More violent trauma can result in complete dislocations of the hind and midfoot, and occasionally may become surgical emergencies. The heel may become inflamed with constant trauma and may also develop a tendonitis at the Achilles insertion. Tendonitis may also be present over the peroneal tendons laterally, the posterior tibial tendon medially, the extensor tendons dorsally, or the flexor tendons medial and plantar. Heel pain may also be caused by an apophysitis of the posterior apophysis of the calcaneous (see also Chap. 136).

DIFFERENTIAL DIAGNOSIS

Infections of the foot must be differentiated from underlying fractures. It should be remembered that in children with paralytic conditions, such as spina bifida-myelomeningocele, what appears to be a warm erythematous infection is most likely the response pattern to a fracture.

Dislocations of the toes must be differentiated from displaced or angulated fractures. A simple toe fracture that can be treated with a minimum amount of effort leaves a less than optimal result if a dislocation of one of the phalangeal joints is overlooked. Midfoot pain may be secondary to either a fascial or tendon sprain, or it may be the result of a mid- or hindfoot bone fracture. It is essential to differentiate a septic joint from an arthritic one. A red, swollen joint is much more likely to be infected, but an underlying arthritis such as juvenile rheumatoid arthritis is possible. Pain in the foot may also be the result of an avascular necrosis. These include osteochondritis dissecans that may be present about the talus, and *Köhler's disease* which involves the tarsal navicular. *Sever's disease* is sometimes considered an avascular necrosis of the posterior calcaneal apophysis. Finally, *Freiberg's avascular necrosis* involves a flattening and arthritic degeneration of one of the phalangeal metatarsal joints. These have no known etiology and they may well be the result of trauma. Congenitally formed bars between various mid- and hindfoot bones should also be considered in the differential diagnosis of foot pain with relatively little trauma. These vary in x-ray appearance between varying amounts of partial and complete ossification.

WORK-UP

The child's foot must be carefully examined. The areas of pain or tenderness are palpated. Usually with a cellulitis, the red demarcated area will be painful over the erythematous tissue and nonpainful peripheral to this area. However, with an underlying fracture, the erythematous area may be just the surface manifestation of the fracture hemorrhage and pain may also be present over the nonerythematous areas, as the underlying bone is in continuity with the fracture. Palpation of the tendons about the foot is essential in differentiating tendonitis from ligamentous or bony involvement.

To differentiate infection and arthritis it is essential to obtain a complete blood count, sedimentation rate, c-reactive protein, rheumatoid factor, antistreptolysin-O, and antinuclear antibody titers.

Fractures must be ruled out by regular AP and lateral as well as probably oblique roentgenograms of the foot. Special views such as axial views of the calcaneous may be necessary. Failing to reveal a fracture or an infection by means of conventional x-ray, a technesium 3-phase bone scan or a gallium scan may be needed. These will show stress fractures and even show generalized stress areas in the limbs without a fracture present. They will also demonstrate an infection. Conventional tomograms or CT scans may be necessary to evaluate three dimensional fractures of the bone such as the navicular or talus, and in conditions causing pain such as the congenital fusions found between various hind- and midfoot bones. If infection is suspected,

aspiration of the area may be helpful in obtaining an organism. Often, however, nothing grows out on the culture media. Arthroscopy of the ankle joint is of limited value in the smaller child and adolescent.

TREATMENT

Fractures of the child's foot are usually of minimal consequence and most are treated by means of a short leg cast. In the more distally based fractures of the metatarsal necks and toes, it is necessary to extend the platform forward of a short leg cast to support these structures. After manipulation to the desired alignment, fractures of the individual toes may be maintained by buddy taping with stretchable tape to prevent strangulation necrosis of the distal portion of the soft tissues. As the toes may swell, especially as the child walks and the dependent position allows for increased swelling, a circumferentially applied bandage that is not made of a stretchable type of material or a spiral-type application can result in an iatrogenic amputation of the toe.

It is essential to reduce any dislocated joint to prevent an osteoarthritic deformity later. An open reduction is rarely needed unless there is a major dislocation in the position of a bone or it is an open wound. Metatarsals and phalanges, as long as they are in adequate alignment, should heal well without complications or sequelae. A fracture of the navicular passing in the longitudinal plane may require a long time for healing because it is relatively avascular and may become a non-union. Fractures of the talus are rare in children but are dangerous and should be referred immediately for emergency treatment. It may require open reduction to maintain blood supply to the involved fractured area.

Large areas of cellulitis, spreading lymphangitis, deep puncture wounds, or a systemically ill child require IV antibiotics until the infection has been arrested. Oral antibiotics can be instituted at that time, and the child can be discharged from the hospital if the parents are reliable. It is usually not necessary to decompress an early osteomyelitis with surgery, but it may occasionally be needed. A large abscess will not resolve without surgical release. Although small fragments of foreign material may become encased in the foot and may never cause a problem, certain objects (most often, pins) caught perpendicular to the planes of motion will continue to fester and will not resolve even when treated with antibiotics. These objects should be removed so that healing can occur. Osteomyelitis will require a course of treatment with IV and then oral antibiotics. Chronic infections of the toes caused by ingrown nails will likewise require systemic antibiotics and may not heal until the nail has been surgically removed.

A referral will usually be likely for most nontrivial injuries.

ANNOTATED BIBLIOGRAPHY

Brown LM, Sharrard WJW: Physical Examination of the Musculoskeletal System. Chap. 9: Examination of the lower extremities in the child, p 186. Year Book Publishers, 1987 (Complete description of the physical examination.)

Rang M: Children's Fractures, 2nd ed, Chap. 21, p 323. Philadelphia, JB Lippincott, 1983

Rockwood C, Rockwood K: Fractures in Children, Chap. 13, p 1043. Philadelphia, JB Lippincott, 1984

Salter RB: Textbook of Disorders and Injuries of the Musculoskeletal System. Baltimore, Williams and Wilkins, 1970

Sharrard WJW: Paediatric Orthopedics and Fractures, 2nd ed., Chap. 8, p 493. Oxford, Blackwell Scientific Publications, 1979 (This reference and the last 3 references are all excellent general, yet comprehensive references.)

141
Animal and Human Bites

ROBERT A. DERSHEWITZ

Animal bites occur commonly, with children being victims ~75% of the time. Although most bites are relatively minor, some result in serious infection, loss of function, disfigurement, or psychological trauma. Over one million dog bites occur each year, and the ratio of dog to cat bites is 10:1. Approximately 10 children per year, usually infants, are killed by dog attacks, usually by family or neighbors' dogs. Contrary to common belief, only 10% of bites are inflicted by stray dogs. Boys are twice as likely to be bitten by dogs than girls, whereas girls are twice as likely to be bitten by cats. Human bites are not as common as other bites, but are potentially more serious.

Although principles for treating animal and human bites are similar, the optimal management of a bite must be individualized. The type, location, time, and circumstances of the bite, and the type of animal and its condition are important considerations. Even when this information is known, a paucity of "hard" data may result in varying recommendations for treatment.

PATHOPHYSIOLOGY

Infection is the most common complication of a mammalian bite. Cellulitis and abscesses are the two most common infections. Lymphangitis and lymphadenitis also occur frequently, as does cat-scratch disease (see Chap. 200). Rabies, though rare, is the ever-present dreaded outcome of an animal bite. Rat-bite fever, osteomyelitis, and tularemia are not often encountered.

Pasteurella multocida is present as normal mouth flora in approximately half of all dogs and cats and is the causative agent in up to 50% of infections from dog bites and 80% from cat bites. The human mouth has more organisms than other animals. Infections from human bites are most often caused by *Streptococcus viridans* and *Staphylococcus aureus*. Bacteroides is the most common anaerobe found and is often recovered with other anaerobes or aerobes. *Streptobacillus moniliformis* is a common mouth flora of rats and mice and frequently causes bite infections. Other organisms that may cause infection include *Francisella tularensis, Aeromonas hydrophilia, Streptococcus viridans, Eikenella corrodens, Clostridium*, and other anaerobic species.

Although one cannot predict which bite will become infected, certain factors predispose to infection. Cat bites become infected more frequently than dog bites (20% to 50% *vs* 5% to 10%) because a cat bite usually produces a puncture, which closes quickly and is more difficult to clean and debride. Dogs may cause puncture wounds, but more typically they create lacerations. Large dogs may produce considerable crush injuries and, if not adequately debrided, these injuries are prone to infection, as are bites to relatively avascular areas. The time in seeking medical attention after the bite is another important risk factor. In one study, 59% of all infected animal bites had delays of greater than 24 hours in obtaining medical care.

A bite on the hand, especially by a human, is potentially devastating. The metacarpophalangeal joint on the dorsum of the hand is most often bitten, usually when a clenched fist hits an opponent's tooth, producing either a puncture wound or crush injury. If an extensor or flexor tendon or joint is penetrated, a rapid and fulminant closed-space infection (tenosynovitis) may develop. Any animal bite, though, may injure a tendon, periosteum, or joint space.

MANAGEMENT

Many animal bite management recommendations have differences in approach or are controversial. There is a consensus, however, on the importance of good wound care. Routine initial surveillance cultures from the bite are not recommended because of the poor correlation with cultures of infected wounds.

Wound Care. In Callaham's study, 12% of irrigated wounds became infected compared to 69% of those not irrigated. Irrigation under pressure (*e.g.,* using a 19-gauge needle or Water Pik) is more effective than soaking the wound. A saline solution is adequate, even though some authors recommend adding an antiseptic such as povidone–iodine to the solution. At least 150 ml saline should be used to irrigate the wound. Although somewhat controversial because puncture wounds close quickly and tissue damage may result from pressure irrigation, puncture bites should also be irrigated by hydrolic pressure.

All wounds, unless small and superficial, should be debrided to further reduce the risk of infection. Jagged edges should also be trimmed for a better cosmetic result.

Primary vs Secondary Healing

Puncture wounds and other bites likely to become infected (in relatively avascular areas, older than 24 hours, extensive tissue injury, and deep human bites) should not be sutured. In questionable situations, it is preferable to leave the wound open. Although increasing numbers of physicians in emergency rooms suture bites on hands, the current *written* recommendations state that bites on hands should NOT be sutured. The rationale (no adequate data exist) is that it is wiser to temporarily forego (until the scar may be revised) the better cosmetic result by primary repair than to risk infection with its resultant morbidity, including potential hospitalization. A practical but currently unproven alternative is the use of paper tape, rather than sutures, for primary closure to minimize both the scar and the risk of infection.

Prophylactic Antibiotics

Although the efficacy of prophylactic antibiotics has not been established, some authors advocate a 4- to 5-day course for all bites. A more rational approach is to restrict their use to bites that are more likely to become infected. Prophylactic antibiotics should not be given for superficial bites in well vascularized areas after adequate wound care because they are at low risk of becoming infected. Prophylactic antibiotics, however, are recommended for hand and face bites (where infection may be devastating) and for those bites that are more likely to become infected.

No single antibiotic will effectively cover all potential pathogens. For single antibiotic coverage, the most appropriate choices are penicillin or amoxicillin/clavulanate (Augmentin) for 5 days. *P. multocida* is sensitive to penicillin, but is not as susceptible to the penicillinase-resistant penicillins and cephalosporins. Amoxicillin/clavulanate (Augmentin) is especially useful in human bite wounds, where a marked number of Bacteroides strains produce β-lactamase. If *S. aureus* is of concern (*e.g.,* a human bite), one may use a penicillinase-resistant penicillin or cephalosporin with penicillin, or substitute either for penicillin. Erythromycin or, in the older child, tetracycline may be used if the patient is allergic to penicillin.

Concern Over Rabies

In the United States, rats, mice, prairie dogs, hamsters, gerbils, chipmunks, squirrels, rabbits, and hares are virtually rabies-free. If the biting animal is potentially rabid, the physician should decide if postexposure rabies prophylaxis is indicated. An ill animal, or one which behaves strangely or bites without provocation, is more likely to be rabid. If the bite was provoked and the animal can be observed, the animal should be watched or quarantined for 10 days. If the animal remains healthy during this period, no prophylaxis is required; however, if the animal behaves strangely or becomes sick, it must be sacrificed and its brain should be tested for rabies. Because of their greater chance of being rabid, bats and wild carnivores such as skunks, raccoons, foxes, coyotes, and bobcats should be killed without damaging the head. If the head cannot be delivered immediately to the Health Department, it should be stored in a refrigerator (not a freezer). If necessary, contact the State or local Health department to help in the management. Even if the biting dog or cat escaped, rabies prophylaxis may not be necessary if there have been no reported rabid dogs or cats in that geographic area.

It is safe to delay postexposure prophylaxis up to 1 week. A negative fluorescent rabies antibody test on an acceptable brain specimen obviates the need for prophylaxis. If the specimen is positive for rabies or if there is a possibility that the animal may be rabid (remember that the rabies virus may also be transmitted by licking mucous membranes, fresh wounds, or abrasions), both rabies immune globulin (RIG) and human diploid cell vaccine (HDCV) must be given. Up to half a single does of RIG (20 IU/kg) is infiltrated into the area of the wound and the rest given intramuscularly, but not at the same site as HDCV. A total of 5 intramuscular (IM) doses of HDCV, each 1ml, are given on days 0, 3, 7, 14, and 28.

TETANUS PROPHYLAXIS

Although the risk of tenanus is not great, the immunization status of the child should be determined. If the child is not completely immunized (*i.e.*, has had less than 3 doses of tetanus toxoid, or has not had a booster dose within 5 years for a contaminated wound or 10 years for a superficial bite), give 0.5 ml tetanus toxoid IM. If the child is under 6 years old and needs pertussis immunization, it may be given with DT. Only Td should be given after 6 years of age. An incompletely immunized child with a tetanus-prone injury (*e.g.*, deep, contaminated, or neglected) should also receive human tetanus immunoglobulin (TIG) 250 to 500 units IM at a separate site.

INDICATIONS FOR HOSPITALIZATION AND REFERRAL

Hospitalization is indicated if the infection is rapidly progressing; if it does not respond to antibiotics; if it is deep (*e.g.*, involves a tendon or joint space); or if it is on the hand. Most infections are uncomplicated and can be readily managed by the primary care physician. The initial choice of antibiotics(s) pending culture results should be based on a Gram's stain. For example, use a penicillinase-resistant penicillin if gram-positive cocci are seen in clusters. Combination therapy is warranted if the Gram's stain is not useful. A reasonable initial choice is penicillin and a penicillinase-resistant penicillin. The involved extremity should be elevated. If the sutured bite becomes infected, remove the sutures and, if present, drain the pus. An infectious disease consultation may be helpful, as may a surgeon, especially for wound drainage.

Human bites on the hand and any bite over a joint require a special protocol. The depth and extent of the injury must be determined since even a relatively minor closed fist injury may penetrate the tendon and joint capsule. The patient may need to be referred to an experienced surgeon because special expertise for assessing this type of wound is required. Operative repair is often required if joint involvement or tendon damage is found.

HEALTH EDUCATION

Patients or parents are instructed to observe for signs of wound infection and also lymphangitis and fever. More generally, all children should be taught how to, and when not to, approach animals because adherence to these safety rules will prevent many animal bites.

ANNOTATED BIBLIOGRAPHY

Brook I: Microbiology of human and animal bite wounds in children. Pediatr Infect Dis J 6:29–32, 1987 (Study demonstrating the polymicrobial aerobic-anaerobic nature of most human and animal bite wounds. Because Augmentin is effective against most of these pathogens, it is the current preferred drug for prophylaxis.)

Callaham ML: Treatment of common dog bites: Infection risk factors. JACEP 7:83–87, 1978 (Small and retrospective, but demonstrated that routine prophylactic antibiotics are unnecessary. The importance of good wound care is emphasized.)

Jaffe AC: Animal bites, Pediatr Clin North Am 30:405–413, 1983 (Excellent overview from the pediatric perspective.)

Lewis RC: Infections of the hand. Emerg Clin North Am 3:271–274, 1985 (Comprehensive discussion on management of [mainly human] hand bites.)

Macknin ML: Dog and cat bites. In Gerber: Pediatric Basics, pp 7–11. 1983 (Excellent overview from the pediatric perspective.)

Mann JM: Systematic decision-making in rabies prophylaxis. Pediatr Infect Dis 2(2):162–167, 1983 (Logical and practical guide in deciding which bites require rabies prophylaxis.)

Mofenson HC, Greensher J: Accident prevention. In Hoekelman RA (ed): Primary Pediatric Care, pp 237–239. St. Louis, CV Mosby, 1987 (Sound recommendations on teaching children about animals and safety rules for meeting a strange dog are enumerated.)

Rabies. MMWR 33-26S–28S, 1984 (Current and complete guide on rabies postexposure prophylaxis.)

142

Burns: The Outpatient Management

LAURIE A. LATCHAW

Each year 300,000 children are burned. Thirty thousand of these children require hospitalization and 3000 die from their injuries, but most of these children are easily cared for in an ambulatory setting.

Scald injury is the most prevalent burn seen in children and occurs typically in children less than 3 years of age. Flame burns are seen in older children, especially boys, who play with fire.

Eighty percent of all childhood burns occur in the home and are preventable by proper supervision and safety precautions.

PATHOPHYSIOLOGY AND CLINICAL PRESENTATION

A burn is caused by the transference of excessive heat energy into living tissue. The heat coagulates cell proteins and thereby destroys cellular enzyme systems. Thermal injury to skin destroys the body's protective squamous epithelium allowing warm fluids to leak out and bacteria to invade. The depth of injury determines, in part, the amount of fluid that will be lost and the wound's susceptibility to infection.

First-degree burns involve only the epidermis and are characterized by erythema, moderate pain, and edema. They heal in 5 to 10 days without the risk of scarring or infection. Sunburns and most hot water scald burns are first-degree injuries.

Second-degree burns involve the dermis and are characterized by blisters, severe pain, and edema. Second-degree burns may be superficial or deep. Superficial second-degree burns are bright red under the blister and heal in 10 to 14 days with temporary depigmentation. They may become infected if improperly cared for. Deep second-degree burns, however, are white beneath the blisters and may take up to 1 month to heal. Scarring may be severe and the risk of infection is great. Infection may destroy enough tissue to convert a deep second-degree burn to a third-degree burn. Grease burns are usually second-degree injuries. However, in small

children with relatively thin skins, even hot water scald burns can be second degree.

Third-degree burns involve the entire skin down to the subcutaneous tissue. They are white or charred in appearance and painless. Healing occurs from the burn edges at the rate of $\frac{1}{8}$ in/week. Severe scarring and contracture will occur unless skin grafts are applied. Susceptibility to both wound and systemic infection is high. Most flame injuries seen in older children are full thickness burns.

DIFFERENTIAL DIAGNOSIS

The depth and extent of a burn determines the optimal care that should be instituted.

Differentiating first-degree burns from cellulitis around an infected second-degree burn is sometimes difficult when the child presents after the first burn day. Also, differentiating a deep second-degree from a third-degree injury may be impossible. It is always safer to err toward the more serious diagnosis initially to avoid inappropriate outpatient therapy in a child who would be better served by hospitalization.

The extent of the burn should be determined by plotting all second-and third-degree areas on a Lund and Bowder chart. This chart allows for the inversely changing proportionate size of children's heads and extremities with age. First-degree burns are not considered for either hospitalization or fluid requirements.

WORK-UP

The work-up for any burned child should include a documentation of the heat source, the duration of application, and how the burn was acquired. Tetanus immunization must be documented as well as a history of congenital heart disease, implanted prosthetic material, or a recent streptococcal infection. The depth and extent of the burn should be determined as previously described. If the appearance or location of the burn is inconsistent with the history, child abuse must be suspected (see Chap. 20). Baseline laboratory tests include CBC with differential WBC, electrolytes, glucose, BUN, and a throat culture for "strep screen." Patients who have extensive burns also require arterial blood gases, serum and urine osmolalities, and carbon monoxide levels if an inhalation injury is suspected.

TREATMENT

First aid to minor burns begins with removing the heat source and cooling the injury. This is generally accomplished by placing the burned area under a briskly flowing cold water faucet. All chemicals can be safely "flushed off" with large volume, high pressure tap water because the chemical is diluted and is removed instantaneously.

Thirty minutes before outpatient burn cleansing and debriding, the child should be sedated with either codeine 1 mg/kg po or chloral hydrate 50 mg/kg po.

The burned area is cleansed gently with a sterile saline or a diluted iodine solution.

Blebs and blisters that are intact should be left as a physiologic dressing. Aspiration of the blisters to remove the fluid potentially contaminates the burn and is not recommended. Blebs and blisters that are broken or leaking should be debrided completely to ensure that bacteria are not trapped under the burned skin. Debridement can usually be done by simply wiping away the dead skin with a gauze sponge. Sharp debridement with sterile scissors is occasionally necessary. A thin coat of silver sulfadiazine is applied as a topical antibiotic. Silver sulfadiazine 1% cream is the preferred topical agent in children with burns because of its soothing quality, antipseudomonas activity, and lack of significant side-effects. The burn is wrapped with a soft, bulky dressing. Tetanus prophylaxis is given if immunizations are not current. No systemic antibiotics are prescribed unless the child has a valvular heart disease or a concomitant streptococcal infection.

The parents are instructed to increase the child's enteral fluid intake by 1% per burned body surface area, but to avoid excessive free water intake. They should return in 2 days for a dressing change or immediately if the dressing falls off or if the child's temperature exceeds 39°C.

The initial dressing change should be done in 2 days by a physician. The burn must be completely cleansed of all fibrinous debris, serous exudate, and silver sulfadiazine because this combination simulates purulence. The burn, once cleaned, must be inspected for signs of infection. Infected burns require hospitalization for systemic antibiotics and frequent dressing changes. Clean burns are redressed after an application of silver sulfadiazine. Reliable parents may be instructed to do the subsequent dressing changes at home, but the physician should inspect them once a week to ensure proper healing.

Very small burns to the face may be treated on an outpatient basis. Because dressing the burn may be difficult and excessively bulky, burns to the face are often treated open. An antibiotic ointment is applied after cleansing and debriding. Frequent reapplication of the ointment is usually necessary and the child may require "mittens" to keep the area from being touched.

Hand burns that are superficial and less than one quarter of the hand's surface area may also be cared for on an outpatient basis; however, a proper hand dressing that separates the fingers and keeps them extended must be applied. The hand should be actively or passively opened and closed during dressing changes to help maintain a full range of motion. Early tangential excision and grafting should always be considered in burn injuries to the hand.

INDICATIONS FOR REFERRAL
OR ADMISSION

The ambulatory care physician must triage the patient into one of three burn categories: critical, major, or minor.

Critically burned patients have injuries involving more than 30% of their body surface area or have inhalation or electrical injuries. These children should be transferred to a regional burn center.

A major burn injury encompasses more than 10% of the total body surface area or is composed of more than 2% third-degree injury. These children require hospitalization for their burn care and fluid resuscitation. Other criteria for hospitalization include burns in children less than 2 years of age because of increased fluid needs and burns to the face and perineum, which are often difficult to keep clean. Burns to the hands and feet in small children who are not self-sufficient do not necessarily require admission; whereas these burns in adults and older children do require hospitalization.

Minor burns cover less than 10% of the total body surface area. These burns are generally treated on an outpatient basis; however, it may be desirable to admit a child with minor burns whose family/social environment precludes proper outpatient care and follow-up.

ANNOTATED BIBLIOGRAPHY

Ahlgren L: Burns. In Gellis SS, Kagan BM (eds): Current Pediatric Therapy, 12th ed., pp 685–687. Philadelphia, WB Saunders, 1986 (Current review of pediatric burn care.)

Kiher RG, Carvagal HF, Milcah RP et al: A controlled study of the effects of silver sulfadiazine on white blood cell counts on burned children. J Trauma 17:835–836, 1977 (Study confirming silver sulfadiazine as best topical burn agent for children.)

Larkin JM, Moylar JA: The role of prophylactic antibiotics in burn care. Am Surg 42:247, 1976 (Original article throwing doubt on the prophylactic use of penicillin for burns.)

143
Trauma to the Oral Cavity
JOAN M. O'CONNOR

Trauma to the oral cavity is common. The types and extent of injury are diverse, and the emergency situation is usually stressful for both the parent and child. The pain accompanying soft tissue lacerations makes the examination uncomfortable, and the physical and psychological impact this injury will have on "the smile" produces anxiety. The most common site of injury is the maxillary central incisor. Most injuries to the primary teeth occur between 18 and 30 months, an age when the child gains independence and mobility but still lacks stability and coordination. In the permanent dentition, children who are 9 to 10 years old are in the most common group for traumatic injury. Boys sustain fractures to the permanent anterior teeth twice as often as girls.

PATHOPHYSIOLOGY AND CLINICAL PRESENTATION

The alveolar bone supporting the primary incisors is immature and pliable. Displacement, particularly intrusion, rather than fracture, is the more common injury in this dentition whereas the denser bone of the older child seems to stabilize the permanent tooth rendering it more susceptible to a fracture. The intrusion is characterized by a partial or complete disappearance into the alveolar bone. If there is a swelling of the surrounding soft tissue, the damage appears worse than it actually is. In intrusion type of displacements of the primary dentition, a risk of damage exists to the underlying permanent tooth; the extent of damage depends on the state of development of the tooth and the degree of displacement that occurs. In the permanent dentition, extrusion is a much more common type of displacement than intrusion. Extrusion is rare in the primary teeth except when the root is fractured. A partial displacement of a tooth, especially if lateral, has a better prognosis when root development is not complete. The open apex allows for hyperemia of pulpal vessels that are often strangulated in a completely formed root with a small apex. In general, a tooth traumatized but not fractured usually receives a greater shock than one that is chipped, probably because the energy of the blow is dissipated in fracturing the tooth rather than absorbing the energy internally.

When a total displacement (avulsion) occurs, the prognosis of the affected tooth or teeth is uncertain: Some reestablish normal attachment, some become ankylosed (fused to bone), and others fail completely. The primary reasons for failure are external resorption of the root and periapical abscess.

Discoloration of a tooth following trauma is usually the result of some seepage from the pulpal vessels into the dentinal tubules. A loss of vitality of the pulp is variable. If there is no resulting pulpal damage, the discoloration tends to lighten in time.

Minor crown fractures are not common in the primary dentition, probably because the stubby shape of the tooth, the thin layer of enamel, and the relatively large pulp cause fractures to involve the pulp. Coronal fractures of enamel and dentin without pulpal exposure constitute 60% to 70% of all fractures involving permanent teeth.

Root fractures should be suspected in teeth that are mobile but seem to pivot short of the apex. Successful healing may occur if fragments are in close apposition, if infection is absent, and if the fracture has occurred more closely to the root apex than the crown of the tooth.

Injury to the developing permanent tooth can occur as a sequellae to primary dentition trauma either through direct impact of the primary tooth against the permanent tooth or as a result of an infection of the primary tooth, which affects the enamel of the permanent tooth. Enamel hypoplasia (staining or rippling of the enamel), dilaceration of the root (malalignment of the long axis of the tooth occurring at the point of development that the tooth was at when the insult was felt), and cessation of root formation are common effects on the permanent tooth following trauma to the primary tooth.

Oral burns, almost exclusively the result of electrical burns, are more commonly seen in the hospital than in the pediatrician's office. Such burns can cause severe constriction, scarring, and deformation of the lip.

DIFFERENTIAL DIAGNOSIS

Child abuse should be suspected if there are signs of old wounds or if the history is inconsistent with the trauma.

WORK-UP

History

The history is significant for the following reasons:

- Age—Age will give some indication of the extent of tooth eruption and root formation/resorption. The loss of maxillary central incisors may be as simple as a bump near the time of exfoliation or a complete avulsion of teeth with fully formed roots. A severe blow to a young tooth in which root formation is incomplete has a wide apical passageway for emerging vessels. This results in a much more favorable prognosis than the tooth with advanced apical development allowing only a narrow passage for vessels. The situation in a child with a fractured tooth may look much worse than it actually is if the tooth had only partially erupted prior to the incident
- Time of Injury—Successful treatment to an injured pulp or reimplantation of avulsed teeth is inversely proportional to the time that has elapsed. Injuries to the teeth frequently involve legal or insurance claims; thus, time notation in the record is also important.
- Patient Complaints—These complaints are often invaluable in determining the extent of damage. Sensitivity to biting in a position of normal occlusion may indicate a displacement or an extrusion not initially detected. A reaction to thermal

change indicates hyperemia of a vital dental pulp and treatment is necessary.

Physical Examination

Soft Tissue Trauma. Lacerations of the lip and tongue should be examined thoroughly for internal/external (through and through) connections. The wound should also be examined for tooth fragments and particles of glass, rock, asphalt, or other puncturing objects imbedded deeply.

Hard Tissue Trauma. A direct blow to the chin or mental area may result in condylar head fractures. Particular attention should be paid to any tenderness in this area or a limited range of motion on opening or closing of the mouth. The dentition should be examined closely for missing or fractured teeth and attempts should be made to account for the missing pieces by a close examination of the soft tissue. Fractured teeth should be examined to determine the extent of damage (*e.g.*, exposure of dentin, pulp, and the presence of root fragments).

Any suspected fracture of the jaw should be x-rayed with either a panoramic or lateral jaw film. A fracture of the root can be verified by occlusal films taken by the child's dentist.

MANAGEMENT

Soft Tissue Lacerations. When treating soft tissue lacerations, local anesthetic infiltration with a 2% lidocaine solution will ease debridement with hydrogen peroxide and saline. Suturing, if necessary, can then be completed. Prophylactic antibiotic coverage should be considered if the wound is "dirty"; if it is punctured by a foreign object; or if there is skin to oral mucosal communication.

Gingival lacerations usually first appear much worse than they actually are. Displaced tissue can usually be repositioned easily after a thorough cleaning with hydrogen peroxide. If the gingiva can be repositioned (as is the case in most patients) so that it is well apposed to the surrounding tissue, healing will generally occur without any complications, since the area is so vascular. If the tissue appears greatly displaced, single sutures of resorbable gut, placed between the teeth from the labial to the palatal surface to restore the normal contour of the tissue, will ensure proper and rapid healing. Warm saline rinses and gentle swabbing with a cotton gauze are advisable for cleaning the area until healed, because the area will be too uncomfortable to clean with a toothbrush.

Hard Tissue Trauma. When intrusion-type displacements are sustained, the damage, if any, occurs at the time of impact. No further damage will occur if the affected tooth is observed closely. Re-eruption can be expected within 3 to 4 weeks. The parents must be cautioned that a severely intruded tooth frequently becomes nonvital with ensuing pulpal necrosis. When the affected tooth is a primary tooth, periapical necrosis could affect the developing permanent successor. Any tenderness on eating that develops over that tooth should be reported to the dentist and a radiograph to view the periapical area should be taken within several weeks to detect abscess formation. A tooth that fails to re-erupt should be considered for extraction, particularly in the primary dentition, to prevent interference with the normal path of eruption of the permanent tooth.

When extrusion of a primary tooth with a root fracture occurs, extraction is usually recommended. Extrusions of the permanent teeth should be referred to the dentist to rule out a fracture of the root. A root fracture that is closely apposed and does not occur in the cervical third has a good chance for successful healing if properly stabilized and if occlusal interferences are removed. Lateral displacements can often be repositioned by the parent or physician with light finger pressure. The area is often tender due to soft tissue injury; therefore, the patient will not function too heavily in this area, allowing the tooth to stabilize without any splinting. If the displacement is extreme but with minimal damage to the alveolus, it may be necessary for the dentist to apply a small acrylic splint.

Avulsion of a primary tooth is usually not replanted because of the high incidence of root resorption following such a procedure. The sequellae of possible pulpal necrosis, and attendant cost considerations must be weighed against the length of time the tooth would be expected to be a functioning component of the arch.

If a primary tooth is lost either to avulsion or extraction, the need for space maintenance must be considered. In general, if the primary cuspids have erupted (~18 months), there is little space loss in the anterior region when a tooth is lost prematurely.

Avulsed permanent teeth should be replanted in their sockets as soon as possible. If replantation occurs within the first few minutes after avulsion, root canal therapy may not be required because there is a possibility of revascularization of the blood supply to the pulp and reattachment of the periodontal membranes. Studies have shown that when a tooth is out of its socket less than 30 min-

utes, replantation is successful in 90% of cases. When the time lapsed is 30 to 90 minutes, the success rate drops to 43% and after 90 minutes, the success rate is only 7%.

If a telephone call is received from the parent, school nurse, or team coach prior to arriving at the office, the person should be instructed to have the patient spit into a cup and transport the avulsed tooth in the saliva. The tooth can also be carried in the mucosal fold of the lower lip if the patient is cautious not to swallow it.

Before replanting, the tooth should be gently washed with saline. Harsh scrubbing that may fragment the periodontal ligament must be avoided. Once the tooth has been replanted, splinting by way of orthodontic brackets or an acrylic splint is recommended. If a considerable time has elapsed, the pulp may be nonvital. A referral to the patient's dentist may be advisable for root canal treatment of the tooth prior to insertion and, if necessary, a curettage of the socket should be done to reinsert the tooth.

A tooth that is discolored by a traumatic blow should be monitored by the dentist on routine visits to ensure that no pathology of the pulp is present.

When a fracture of a tooth involving only enamel occurs, the preferred treatment (if sought at all) is minimal, requiring only a smoothing of the edges that are rough and that irritate the lips or tongue. If the pulp cannot be seen but the tooth is sensitive to cold or air, a covering of calcium hydroxide and acrylic should be applied to provide relief and protect the pulp. An application of a topical fluoride to the exposed dentin will also decrease sensitivity. When the pulpal tissue is exposed, removal of vital pulp tissue (pulpotomy), extraction of the entire pulpal chamber with replacement by a zinc oxide, eugenol and formocresol material (pulpectomy) or an extraction should be performed by the dentist after consideration of factors such as time elapsed, root development, root resorption, and the proximity to the permanent tooth. If pulpal therapy is provided, the fractured crown can then be restored by means of composite (acrylic) crowns.

INDICATIONS FOR REFERRAL

A referral for extensive lacerations of the soft tissue should be made to an emergency room or plastic surgeon or to an emergency room for electrical burns. In the case of electrical burns, an appliance with commissure posts is often made by a dentist in cooperation with the plastic surgeon to reduce the constriction and scarring that occur during healing. The appliance is worn for about 1 year and may eliminate the need for surgery or at least reduce the number of operative procedures.

A referral to a dentist should be made for any suspected fractures of the roots of teeth, exposures of the dental pulp, and when splinting is preferred.

PATIENT EDUCATION

A reduction of the incidence of oral trauma involves education of the supervising adult and the use of preventative measures and appliances.

The environment should be studied to reduce the common situations that lead to facial trauma. The young child should be restrained in an acceptable car seat while riding in a motor vehicle. The child should be taught safety precautions for the bathtub, stairways, and so forth. Electrical cords should be kept out of common traffic areas; extension cords should be eliminated wherever possible and should never be plugged in with the female end exposed (see Chap. 18 for other safety tips).

Children who have a severe protrusion of the maxillary teeth should be treated as early as possible, because these teeth are more prone to injury.

Children should be outfitted with mouthguards, either custom fitting ones, those made to fit over orthodontic appliances, or the type available in sporting goods stores that are readily molded in warm water, before participation in athletics.

ANNOTATED BIBLIOGRAPHY

Andreasen JO, Hjoring–Hansen E: Replantation of teeth I. Radiographic and clinical study of 110 human teeth replanted after accidental loss. Acta Odontol Scand 24:263–286, 1964 (The effects of trauma by one of the foremost authorities on the subject.)

Ellis RG, Davey KW: The Classification and Treatment of Injuries to the Teeth of Children. Chicago, Year Book Medical Publishers, 1970 (Excellent classification according to the extent of injury with corresponding treatment for each classification. Particularly detailed as to treatment, but probably more helpful to the dentist than the pediatrician.)

Hill C: Oral trauma to the preschool child. Dent Clin North Am 28:177–186, 1984 (Concise and practical for trauma of the primary dentition.)

McDonald R, Avery D: Management of traumatic injuries to the teeth and supporting tissues. In Dentistry for the Child and Adolescent, 3rd ed., pp 301–341. 1978 (Very thorough general text of pediatric dentistry.)

Ripa L, Finn S: The Care of Injuries to the Anterior Teeth of Children. In Clinical Pedodontics, 4th ed. pp 224–270, 1973 (Comprehensive discussion of trauma and detailed discussion, particularly of treatment. Well illustrated.)

18

Neurologic Problems

ELIZABETH C. DOOLING, Section Editor

144
Head Trauma
ELIZABETH C. DOOLING

Approximately 200,000 children are hospitalized each year in the United States because of head trauma. Boys are injured two to three times as frequently as girls. Accidents are the most common cause of death in children between 1 and 14 years of age, and many fatalities result from head injuries. The morbidity associated with head trauma is high. Many children are left with permanent disabilities and require special educational programs and ongoing rehabilitative care.

PATHOPHYSIOLOGY

The skull is covered by a fibrous sheet known as the *epicranium aponeurotica* or *galea aponeurotica*. The galea is firmly adherent to the overlying skin of the scalp but is applied only loosely to the pericranium. Fusing on each side to the temporal fascia just above the zygomatic arches, these attachments limit the spread of subgaleal effusions. Under the skull itself is the dura, which is a thick and tough bilayered membrane composed of dense collagenous tissue. The dura has the consistency of plastic wrap in the infant and waxed paper in the older child. The outer layer of the dura is fused with periosteum. The inner layer or dura proper is separate from the outer layer at certain points and forms folds that project into the cavities formed between the cerebral hemispheres, between the occipital lobes and cerebellum, and in the midline of the posterior fossa. The arachnoid, an avascular structure, lies under the dura. The CSF circulates between the arachnoid and the pia, a weblike membrane in which the blood vessels ramify. The pia is thinner over the cortex and thicker over the brainstem; thus, the cerebral tissue is protected by the bony cranium and its overlying and underlying collagenous or membranous structures.

CLINICAL PRESENTATION

Head injuries may range from superficial lacerations of the skull to penetration of foreign bodies or skull fragments through the scalp, skull, and cerebral tissue to the ventricular system. There may be a total preservation of consciousness, transient "lightheadedness," a brief loss of consciousness, or a prolonged coma, usually in proportion to the severity of the injury. The child who is struck by an automobile may sustain injuries to other major organs and may thus be further compromised by hemorrhage or shock. Usually, an acute event causes the head injury. Less commonly, a subacute or chronic course may follow trauma.

A newborn who is subjected to a traumatic delivery may present with a simple scalp swelling under which there may or may not be a skull fracture or a skull fracture associated with an epidural hematoma of arterial or venous origin. Young children most often sustain head trauma related to accidents while playing, riding in cars, or during a seizure. Other children and adolescents will incur injuries at play, at work, or while driving a car. Scalp swelling may be classified as:

- *Subgaleal hematoma* resulting from bleeding beneath the galea aponeurotica. It is the most common cause of swelling from head trauma beyond the newborn period.
- *Caput succedaneum* resulting from scalp edema due to local pressure and trauma during labor and is most easily differentiated from a cephalohematoma in that the swelling is diffuse and often crosses sutures.
- *Leptomeningeal cyst* referring to a fluid-filled space between the arachnoid and pia, and arachnoid herniation through a contiguous dural tear.
- *Cephalohematoma* or hemorrhage beneath the external periosteum of the skull, usually in the parietal region. For these conditions, surgical intervention is necessary only in the case of the leptomeningeal cyst.

If the swollen area is transilluminated, there is a diffuse increase in infants with caput succedaneum, a focal increase in a child with a leptomeningeal cyst, a diffuse decrease in a child with subgaleal hematoma, and a focal decrease overlying a cephalohematoma.

Skull fractures may be suspected clinically by direct palpation of the skull or by crepitus on palpation of the skull. Skull fractures may be classified as:

- *Linear Fractures*: About 75% of all skull fractures in children are linear. No specific treatment is usually necessary, but careful observation for 18 to 24 hours is necessary.
- *Depressed Fractures*: The outer and inner tables of the calvarium are disrupted. Tangential roentgenograms of the skull may be necessary to identify the extent of the depression. When the depression is 5 mm to 10 mm in depth, surgical elevation is indicated.
- *Compound Fractures*: Bone fragments protrude through the scalp laceration. Surgical debridement with elevation and antibiotic prophylaxis are necessary.
- *Basal Fractures*: These fractures are often not evident on plain roentgenograms but may be apparent on CT scans in the axial plane. When epistaxis, hemotympanum, or hemorrhage in the nasopharynx, mastoid, postauricular, or periorbital area occurs, a basal skull fracture is likely. Cranial nerve palsies and CSF leakage may be present.
- *Diastatic Fractures*: These fractures result from separation of the cranial bones at one or more suture sites, especially the lambdoid, and occur usually in early childhood.
- *"Growing" Fractures*: These develop within the first 6 months following linear or diastatic fractures. The parietal bone is most frequently affected. Children less than 3 years old are most susceptible. The fracture is prevented from healing because of the coexisting arachnoid cyst that prevents apposition of the bony margins.

A *cerebral concussion* is characterized by a transient loss of consciousness of varying duration (seconds, minutes, or less often, hours) and is more likely to occur when the head is not fixed at the time of blunt injury. A concussion is associated with temporary retrograde amnesia of events remotely preceding the injury, and temporary posttraumatic or anterograde amnesia that may last for several hours after the accident. The *postconcussive* syndrome is characterized by headache, dizziness, irritability, nervousness, difficulty in concentrating, and sometimes, changes in behavior or intellect. It is usually self-limited in duration, with recovery in 4 to 8 weeks but occasionally evolves into a more chronic condition.

A *cerebral contusion* or *laceration* indicates bruising or tearing respectively of brain tissue. Such lesions can cause indirect trauma to tissue directly beneath the site of blunt or penetrating injury or directly or diagonally opposite to the area of impact. These lesions are called *coup* when contiguous tissue is affected or *contrecoup* when tissue contralateral to the traumatized area is involved. These injuries are important because of their relationship to the development of post-traumatic epilepsy.

Hematomas may be *epidural* or *subdural* in location. They may result from relatively mild preceding head trauma; they may not be able to be differentiated from each other. An epidural hematoma is rarer than a subdural hematoma; it is usually unilateral; it is associated with a skull fracture; and it most often occurs in children older than 2 years. A subdural bleed usually occurs in children less than 1 year of age; it has an underlying skull fracture; it is often bilateral; the source is venous in origin; and it is more likely than an epidural hematoma to be associated with seizures. A transient period of lucidity or near-normal behavior may follow a period of depressed consciousness immediately after the injury. In the third phase, a decreased or deepening level of consciousness may supervene in a child with an epidural hematoma. Recurrent seizures, anemia, and irritability are more often seen in a child with a subdural hematoma. In either case, the hematoma is a space-occupying lesion within the fixed volume of the cranial cavity and thus produces increased intracranial pressure. Lethargy, vomiting, a full fontanel even when upright, separation of the sutures, sixth and third nerve weakness, headache, papilledema, and Cushing triad of elevated systolic blood pressure, decreased pulse, and slow respirations may be found in a child with raised intracranial pressure. Third nerve weakness and hemiparesis may develop when there is an incipient herniation of the uncus or temporal lobe. Fractures of the occipital bone in proximity to the transverse sinus and vascular tentorium may be complicated by infratentorial epidural (venous) bleeding. Patients with posterior fossa hematomas present with altered consciousness, vomiting, meningismus, ataxia, and abnormal respirations. Rarely, children who have sustained mild head trauma with lacerations may have no sequelae directly related to the injury but may have apparent unmasking of coexisting problems, such as neoplasm.

DIFFERENTIAL DIAGNOSIS

The child who has a head injury does not usually present as a diagnostic dilemma because of external evidence of trauma, and, usually, the observations of witnesses to the accident. Yet, even with a witness reporting otherwise, the possibility of child abuse, especially in a toddler, should always be considered.

A differential diagnosis must be formulated for the child found unconscious. In addition to closed head trauma—with or without external evidence of injury—other causes of coma must be considered. Most common is ingestion of drugs and poisons. Additional *nonesoteric* causes include metabolic disorders such as diabetic ketoacidosis, fulminant CNS infection, acute encephalopathy, postictal state, and rupture of a congenital vascular malformation.

WORK-UP

History

It is imperative to obtain information from the person(s) present at the scene when the child was injured. The child's behavior antecedent to the accident should be noted (*e.g.*, to exclude preceding seizure activity that may have predisposed to a fall from a bicycle). The child may be unaware of losing consciousness after an injury that produces a concussion but may be amnestic when questioned closely. A history of evolving depressed consciousness, vomiting, recurrent seizure activity, increasing weakness of arms or legs, sleepiness, or vision changes such as diplopia, dictates exclusion of an expanding intracranial lesion.

Physical Examination

Vital signs must be taken and monitored. The level of consciousness must be assessed and adequate ventilation must be maintained. A careful inspection of the scalp and body to assess abrasions, lacerations, and swellings is necessary. The nasopharynx and ears should be checked for evidence of fresh blood. The neck should be immobilized with a cervical collar before the patient is moved. The abdomen should be palpated for evidence of visceral bleeding.

Perhaps most importantly, signs of increased intracranial pressure should be systematically sought. Most commonly, these signs include a full fontanel or separated sutures, changes in the child's level of responsiveness, and changes in the pattern and rate of respirations. The most common clues in the older child are headache and papilledema. The pupillary size, equality, and reaction to light must be recorded, as must ocular movements and retinal hemorrhages. A unilateral dilated and sluggish (or fixed) pupil may represent a compression of the third nerve by a herniating portion of the temporal lobe. In the unresponsive child, the eye movements may be assessed by moving the child's head passively, or, if the eardrums are intact, by instilling ice water to stimulate oculovestibular reflexes. Abnormal or asymmetric reflexes and motor function and posture should be assessed, looking for spontaneous, normal activity of all limbs because these are often early clues of herniation. Even more ominous is decorticate posturing (characterized by flexion and adduction of the arms and extension of the legs) or decerebrate posturing (characterized by extension and internal rotation of the arms and extension of the legs).

Laboratory Tests

A hematocrit should be obtained because intracranial bleeding, especially in the neonate and young infant, may result in anemia. If there is obvious blood loss in large quantity, a sample should be sent to the Blood Bank for type and should be cross-matched in anticipation of a blood transfusion. If there is an associated neck or spine injury, the patient's head and neck should be immobilized with a cervical collar or sandbags before being moved to the x-ray department. A child with minor head trauma who is fully alert and without neurologic signs does not need skull roentgenograms. Skull roentgenograms are recommended in a child with any of the following: significant scalp swelling, localizing neurologic signs, unconsciousness for >5 min, palpable findings of a depressed or compounded skull fracture (*i.e.*, bony malalignment), signs suggestive of a basilar skull fracture, and a progressive worsening of the neurologic status. Roentgenograms of the facial bones and orbits should be obtained if facial trauma has also occurred. Computerized tomography (CT) scans should be ordered in children who have had severe head trauma or who have serious neurologic signs. A plain CT scan will disclose intracranial bleeding such as epidural or subdural hematomas, intracerebral hematomas, and posterior fossa hemorrhages, and will show areas of cerebral contusion. Mass effect and midline shifts will be readily apparent on CT scans. Fractures of the basal skull may be more easily identified on CT scans than on routine skull x-rays. CT scanning has largely eliminated the need for cerebral angiography and may supplant tomography of the base of the skull when hemotympanum, otorrhea, or rhinorrhea is present.

MANAGEMENT AND REFERRAL

If there is a fracture of a bone at its suture point, a careful follow-up including a head measurement is indicated to ensure that the fracture heals completely. If the child sustains a brief loss of consciousness (*i.e.*, 1 to 10 min), close observation for the first 24 to 48 hours is necessary. If the parents are reliable and competent, this observation may be done at home after an initial medical evaluation. Hospitalization is advised if there is any doubt about the responsibility of the child's caretakers or if there is any abnormal neurologic sign or symptom. Parents should be instructed to monitor the child's level of consciousness—how readily the child can be aroused and how coherent the child is, respiratory pattern, pupil size and reactivity, at regular intervals of 1 to 2 hours. Delayed cerebral edema from cerebral contusion may occur within 8 to 12 hours after the injury. (Maximal cerebral edema usually occurs within 48 to 72 hours after the injury.) A child with a loss of consciousness for 10 to 30 minutes or more should be hospitalized for monitoring. A child with a seizure at the onset of the injury need not be treated with anticonvulsants if the seizure is brief and generalized (*i.e.*, less than

10 min, but such a child should be hospitalized for observation). Any child with signs of increased intracranial pressure (*e.g.*, third cranial nerve palsy, Cushing's triad) requires immediate therapy to prevent brain stem herniation, with its resultant high morbidity and mortality. Similarly, the child with signs of herniation (*e.g.*, decorticate posture) or impending herniation (*e.g.*, unequal pupil) as well as the child who sustains multiple injuries or an open head injury should be admitted to an intensive care unit for close monitoring. The placement of an intracranial pressure gauge is often necessary, and additional treatment to keep the intracranial pressure below 20 Torr by using hyperventilation to reduce the P_{CO_2} to 25, mannitol or other osmotic diuretics, and fluid restriction can be implemented. Likewise, children with epidural, subdural, and intracranial hemorrhages should be admitted to an intensive care unit. With signs of increased intracranial pressure, subdural hematomas may need to be tapped. Comprehensive management of the seriously injured child requires the facilities of a pediatric tertiary center and a multidisciplinary staff.

Post-traumatic epilepsy following head trauma occurs in ~1% of all children, but in about 5% of children hospitalized for head trauma. The more serious the injury, the greater will be the chance of the child developing a learning disability and intellectual impairment (*e.g.*, memory and motor deficits and seizures). An increased incidence of neurologic sequelae occurs in those patients who are hospitalized for greater than 24 hours. Approximately 75% of patients who are in coma for more than 3 weeks are more likely to remain dependent in caring for themselves. Overall, children under 16 years of age recover more function. Memory deficits contribute greatly to dependency needs. Cognitive dysfunction and personality changes may be subtle and go unrecognized in the early convalescent stage.

Chronic seizure disorders are often associated with a poor long-term functional outcome. Three risk factors were identified by Jennett and Teasdale for development of post-traumatic seizures: (1) the occurrence of seizures within the first week of head injury; (2) the presence of an intracranial hematoma; (3) the presence of a depressed skull fracture. Seventy percent of head-injured patients who developed post-traumatic epilepsy had seizures within the first 6 months after head injury.

ANNOTATED BIBLIOGRAPHY

Berger MS, Pitts LH, Lovely M et al: Outcome from severe head injuries in children and adolescents. J Neurosurg 62:194–199, 1985 (Prospective study of mostly direct admissions to San Francisco General Hospital. Outcome was assessed ≥6 hrs; the mortality rate was 33%. Persistent elevation of ICP was usually associated with a poor prognosis.)

Bruce DA, Alavi A, Bilianuk D et al: Diffuse cerebral swelling following head injuries in children: The syndrome of malignant brain edema. J Neurosurg 54:170–178, 1981 (Diffuse brain swelling was found on 29% of CT scans of 214 patients. The authors postulate that severe cerebrovascular changes [*i.e.*, vasodilatation and initial hyperemia] are responsible for swelling, not disturbed autoregulation.)

Bruce DA, Schut L, Bruno LA et al: Outcome following severe head injuries in children. J Neurosurg 48:679–688, 1978 (Results of treatment of 53 children with severe head trauma with reference to initial grading on Glasgow Coma Scale and management with endotracheal intubation, controlled ventilation, dexamethasone, and other agents as indicated [mannitol, hypo-

thermia, pentothal]. Patients with GCS ≥5 did well. Flaccidity was a bad prognostic sign.)

Eiben CF, Anderson TP, Lockman L et al: Functional outcome of closed head injury in children and young adults. Arch Phys Med Rehabil: 65:168, 1984 (Retrospectively reviews the outcome of closed head injuries.)

Jennett B, Teasdale G: Management of Head Injuries. Philadelphia, FA Davis, 1981 (Excellent and comprehensive text addressing authors' experience with a head-injured population, mainly adult. Prognosis and objectives of care of patients are also reviewed.)

Kalinsky Z, Morrison DP, Meyer CA et al: Medical problems encountered during rehabilitation of patients with head injury. Arch Phys Med Rehabil 66:25, 1985 (Discussion of the range of problems presenting in head-injured patients and the roles of the specialists in coordinating health care.)

145
Headache
VERNE S. CAVINESS, JR.

A headache is a symptom experienced by virtually everyone at sometime in the course of one's life. A recurrent headache is the cause of sufficient disability in 20% of the population to warrant medical consultation and ranks with obesity as a principal cause of chronic morbidity among children. Most headache disorders, including the most severely disabling, are the expression of a "benign," though little understood, physiologic state. A headache may also be a symptom of a host of systemic and intracranial disorders, some of grave import. The alert physician reliably distinguishes the benign and symptomatic headache disorders on the basis of a discerning history and physical examination supplemented as appropriate by readily available diagnostic tests.

CLINICAL PRESENTATION

The most prevalent of the headache disorders are the benign forms. These may be subdivided into the following three syndromes.

Migraine

The migraine syndrome includes a remarkable spectrum of symptoms and signs. The migraine headache is typically throbbing in quality and predominantly hemicranial in distribution. Other distressing head discomforts are common. These include sensations described as aching, stabbing, squeezing, burning, tingling, or crawling. Typically, the discomfort is more intense on one side though usually not always the same side. Discomfort is generally most intense in the frontal, temporal, and orbital regions although occipital and cervical discomfort is common.

A migraine is paroxysmal in expression, reaching maximum intensity in 1 or at most a few hours. It may last no more than 1 hour. More often it continues through much of a day and may be terminated by sleep. Less commonly severe episodes of migraine may continue with declining severity over 2 or more days. The headache may be preceded by a premonitory sense of fatigue, dread, anxiety, or even excitement and is usually accompanied by light and sound intolerance or nausea and vomiting. Focal neurologic symptoms may be dramatic and when encountered for the first time, are justifiably alarming for both the patient and the physician. The most common of these symptoms are visual and may include scintillations, scotomata, or field defects. These may be unilateral or bilateral. There may be complete blindness, characteristically a sensation of "blackness." There may be "heaviness," weakness, or clumsiness of one or both extremities on a side, tingling or numbness involving variably the face, arm, and leg on one side of the body. Ophthalmoplegia, vertigo, confusional states, dysarthria or dysphasia or ataxia may also be present. Transient hemiparesis, sometimes shifting from side to side, may occur with, or at other times independently, of the headache. Typically, these focal neurologic symptoms and signs last for a short time and recovery is complete. Rarely a deficit persists. By convention, a migraine accompanied by any of these focal neurologic manifestations is designated as *classic* and those disorders without as a *common* migraine.

The focal neurologic signs and symptoms associated with a migraine are particularly prevalent in children. An ophthalmoplegic migraine is essentially a disorder of childhood and invariably has its first expression before the age of 12. The pattern of a migraine is additionally distinctive in children in that it may coexist with, and appears to be related to, the so-called *periodic syndrome*: recurrent abdominal pain, nausea and vomiting, benign vertigo or motion sickness, and high fevers. Somnambulism and syncope are also relatively prevalent among children with a migraine.

Tension Headache

The tension headache is a dull aching discomfort that is distributed typically in a band-like fashion around the head. A cervical ache and stiffness are common. The symptoms may wax and wane over many hours on a particular day or through many days. Not uncommonly a headache may persist without relief for weeks, months, or even years. Typically, a tension headache more than a migraine is more "purely" a headache disorder although it is often associated with light and sound intolerance and a queasiness in the stomach.

Cluster Headache

Pain is extreme and is described as a burning, searing, or stabbing sensation. It is concentrated in the eye or orbit and is typically associated with lacrimation, ocular injection, and rhinorrhea which are most conspicuous on the affected side. In less than 10%, ptosis and miosis are present on the same side. Pain is typically abrupt in onset and lasts from minutes to 1 or 1½ hours. In the pediatric population and in about 90% of affected adults, the attacks are clustered, occurring one or many times/day over a period of weeks to 2 or 3 months.

PATHOPHYSIOLOGY

Migraine and tension headaches appear to be closely related pathophysiologic states in that they typically co-occur in the same individual. Further, the threshold for expression of both syndromes is modulated by the same genetic, hormonal, and exogenous factors. The familial prevalence has been estimated at 50% to 90% for both syndromes. The strong prevalence of migraine and tension headaches among women, the tendency to initial expression at menarche or a strong crescendo expression in early pregnancy, at menopause, or while on birth control pills underlines the role of estrogen fluxes as a potent modulator of headache threshold. Other exogenous factors that variably lower the threshold for expression of these headache disorders include alcohol, particularly red wine, nitrates and monosodium glutamate (*e.g.*, hot dogs, Chinese food), chocolate and milk products (at times clearly an expression of lactose intolerance). Psychological stress is another critical determinant. Typically, depressive symptoms such as fatigue, nonrestful sleep, or a "down feeling" accompany or even precede a crescendo of headache. It should be emphasized, however, that a major psychiatric disturbance, including disabling neurosis or psychosis, is no more prevalent among people disabled by a headache than in the general population.

The pathophysiology of a cluster headache would appear to stand apart from that of the other two benign headache syndromes in that it is almost unique to men (90%) and has no familial predilection. There is, however, some commonality with respect to exogenous modulating factors, alcohol in particular.

The physiologic mechanisms that are modulated by genetic and other influences so as to generate the symptoms of these disorders are little understood. Experimental observations suggest that the pain arises from extracranial vessel walls and is relayed inward by the trigeminal system. Current opinion holds that substance P may be a pivotal transmitter in pain excitation and the release of this transmitter may be controlled variably by endogenous hormonal as well as extrinsic pharmacologic substances. Plausibly, the focal neurologic deficits have been ascribed to transient ischemia resulting from transient arterial spasm. Intraictal arteriography and cerebral blood flow studies have, however, been ambiguous on this point. Further, it is not at all certain that the "strokes" associated with the persisting deficit that have occurred in association with the migraine disorder are extensions of the process giving rise to the transient neurologic symptoms. Quite independent vascular occlusive mechanisms may be operating such as mitral valve prolapse, a potential source of embolus, and is four times as prevalent among young women with a migraine than in the general population.

DIFFERENTIAL DIAGNOSIS

Most headache disorders are benign. On the other hand, a headache may be a presenting manifestation of a wide variety of cranial and systemic disorders, some of which are both treatable and lethal if not treated.

A *severe headache of acute onset* in a child not subject to recurrent headache poses a different set of diagnostic possibilities than recurrent headache disorders. An acute, severe headache associated with nausea, vomiting, prostration and, not infrequently in the child, with fever, is a clinical problem regularly encountered in a hospital emergency ward. Unless there is a history of similar episodes, the history and examination may not exclude subarachnoid hemorrhage, meningitis, parameningeal infection, such as epidural abscess or other causes of increased intracranial pressure. Where gradual evolution over hours has occurred and there is meningismus with or without other evidence of systemic infection and where papilledema is not present, an immediate lumbar puncture is indicated to exclude meningitis. Where an abrupt onset is associated with meningismus and, possibly, focal neurologic signs, the initial preferred diagnostic procedure is a CT scan. This should be done primarily without contrast infusion so that blood will be recognizable. A follow-up image may be done with contrast infusion if a tumor or an abscess is suspected. A lumbar puncture may be done subsequently if the CT scan is normal and should be done especially if the question of subarachnoid hemorrhage has not been satisfactorily answered.

WORK-UP

History

In principle, the differential diagnosis of benign *vs* symptomatic *recurrent headache*, does not hinge on the character and distribution of the individual headache itself. It depends, rather on an integrated analysis emphasizing an attack pattern, family history, context of appearance, and a general medical and physical examination. Critical historical points are the attack pattern and the localization of head-

ache. Where severe headaches, separated by headache-free intervals, have recurred over 6 months or longer, the probability of an intracranial mass is low. The benign forms of headache, with only rare exceptions, are inconstant in their localization— often shifting sides and spreading across the midline. A highly localized, more or less persistent headache, lasting from a few days to a few weeks, is especially significant. This is particularly so if the pain awakens the child from sleep or is present on awakening in the morning. Pain occurring in sharply focal fashion over the eye, when associated with signs of third nerve paresis, must be assumed to be a manifestation of a posterior communicating or internal carotid artery aneurysm until proved otherwise by arteriography. Pain located in the cervical-medullary junction and associated with resistance to neck flexion, raises the possibility of posterior fossa tumor or malformation. A sinus abscess will be associated with a local point tenderness often local erythema and heat. A symptomatic temporomandibular joint will be painful when compressed or associated with decreased movement or pain on movement of the jaw.

Physical Examination

Particularly in the child, the completely normal general medical and neurologic examination may be taken as strongly reassuring. In principle, disorders caused by increased intracranial pressure, including mass lesions, hydrocephalus, and pseudotumor cerebri, will be associated with abnormal physical findings before a disabling headache leads to neurologic consultation. Lateralizing hemispheric signs, papilledema, disturbances of gaze or individual cranial nerve function, ataxia, disturbances of gait and reflex, are highly sensitive indicators. With regard to the general examination, elevation in blood pressure should alert one to the unlikely possibility of pheochromocytoma. The cutaneous lesions of the phakomatoses, visceromegaly, or large lymph nodes, or purpuric lesion, are tell-tale signs of generalized disorders that might be correlated with an intracranial mass, arterial disease or inflammatory processes. AV malformation may be suspected from the presence of cutaneous angiomata.

Laboratory Tests

It is recommended to perform readily available blood and urine studies on all patients seen in consultation for a disabling recurrent headache, even when every historical indicator and the physical examination are reassuring. The specific tests include a complete blood count, sedimentation rate, CPK, VDRL, calcium, and blood glucose. Such values, when normal, are not only diagnostically reassuring but are an essential base line starting point for several medications that might be used in the treatment of a headache.

All other diagnostic tests should be tailored to the historical and physical indications. A CT scan will be indicated in subacutely expressed headache disorders, particularly if pain is highly localized and even if other indicators are benign. A CT scan is indicated in subacute and even more chronically established headache disorders in which a neurologic examination is abnormal, papilledema is present, or the history suggests the child might be having seizures. It is only when the question of seizures is raised that an EEG is likely to be helpful diagnostically; that is, the EEG would be used in the evaluation of the seizure rather than the headache component. Plain films of the skull and sinuses, particularly if CT is unavailable, or of the TMJ may be required to clarify symptoms relating to these respective localizations.

TREATMENT AND MANAGEMENT

Where a headache is symptomatic of an underlying cranial, intracranial, or systemic disease, quite different approaches, appropriate to the underlying disease, will obviously be required. These are beyond the scope of the present discussion. The approach to therapy of benign headaches reflects the fact that young adults, aged 18 to 20, often regard the pediatrician as their primary physician and that it is among this population that many of the most disabling headache disorders are encountered.

The pediatrician should undertake three critical basic components of headache management: reassurance, identification and elimination of specific provocative factors, and pharmacologic intervention. It will also be the responsibility of the pediatrician to initiate a neurologic or psychiatric referral if warranted.

Reassurance. The importance of reassurance cannot be underestimated. Quite reasonably, the parents or the patient may seek consultation less because a headache disorder is disabling and more because they are anxious about its cause. They may be concerned specifically about the possibility of a brain tumor. It is critical that they be convinced that the physician has also considered and excluded this as well as other sinister diagnoses. It is best to discuss the evidence for and against openly. For example, the patient or family will readily get the point that a normal examination and a recurrent headache history continuing over 1 year or more make the existence of a tumor highly improbable. At least as far as the diagnosis is concerned, many will be reassured when it is brought to their attention that other members of their families have suffered similar headache disorders over years or by the observation that the headache is consistently provoked by an ingested substance. Where diagnostic uncertainty or the family's anxieties justify a CT scan, the family must be helped to understand that a normal study *does* resolve the issue and is not instead a failure to find the underlying sinister cause.

Elimination of Exogenous Substances. Frequently, exogenous substances ingested by the patient play a role in headache expression. Some items from a list provided in the initial section include alcohol, cheeses, and monosodium glutamate-containing foods. Avoidance of such offending substances may be a partial, though rarely a complete, solution. Birth control pills require particular emphasis. Used increasingly over the past two decades by adolescent girls, they have been a consistent offender and, possibly, may place a young woman who has headaches at increased risk for stroke. The physician must inquire about the use of birth control pills, which will require great tact if the parents are unaware. Where a headache crescendo is found to occur in association with use of birth control pills, the physician must make the strongest possible argument that these pills be discontinued. Further, it is completely unjustified for the physician to provide the patient with potentially toxic medications for headache provoked by birth control pills. The use of birth control pills in the management of gravely symptomatic endometriosis, which coexists with a disabling headache, is an exceptional circumstance. Here, a compromise approach such as a reduction of the estrogen dose or intermittent estrogen therapy may be worked out with the patient's gynecologist.

Pharmacologic Intervention. Rather than behavioral therapies such as biofeedback, pharmacologic intervention is the choice of most patients and physicians. (Where biofeedback is available in a community and its requirements of time and personal discipline are appropriate to patient and family, this mode of therapy should also be given consideration.

It is essentially as effective as medications in some patients and it is safe.) Mild analgesics such as aspirin or acetaminophen provide satisfactory relief for most patients who have an occasional migraine or tension headache of mild to moderate severity. Less tractable disorders require a dual strategy involving a prophylactic suppression of headache as well as treatment of the individual headaches as they occur. Cluster headache, only rarely encountered by the pediatrician, generally requires relatively extreme pharmacologic measures.

Whichever medication is chosen, several practical points are useful to keep in mind. Any drug chosen may have alarming side effects and even potential toxicities. In particular, the physician should be cautious about the use of potentially teratogenic preparations for headaches occurring in the course of a "secret" pregnancy. The patient or family should be offered reasonable expectations of the effectiveness, the potential side effects, and overall time required for medical treatment. Unexpected side effects of drugs, disappointment in the face of unrealistic expectations for relief, and an "open-ended" medication schedule without a "ground plan" are all potentially defeating sources of anxiety. Thus, the patient should be cautioned about the possibility of side effects, with emphasis on the possibility that unexpected side effects may occur. He should be cautioned that a particular preparation may not be effective.

The patient or family should understand that the development of an optimum program may require a trial of one or more preparations and that with even the optimum medication, a series of trials and errors may be required to get the optimum dose. It is well to begin each medication at a low, tolerated dose and increase only as tolerated. Several days or weeks may be required to achieve an effective dose. Patients who are frightened by the side effects of a drug advanced too quickly may refuse to use that drug in the future, even though it might be the optimum choice. Second, the tolerated drug should be used aggressively, increasing the dose as tolerated to a maximal safe dose or until the desired effect is achieved. All too often a potentially effective drug is abandoned too early without a satisfactory trial at maximum dose. Ready access to the supervising physician is essential to the success of pharmacologic therapy; the patient should not panic if the initial course of therapy does not fulfil his expectations.

A relatively large number of drugs, representing multiple, pharmacologic classes, have been varia-

bly effective in the *prophylactic* management of headaches. These include β-adrenergic receptor blockers, calcium channel antagonists, anticonvulsants, tricyclic antidepressants, phenothiazines, antihistamines, benzodiazapenes, nonsteroidal anti-inflammatory preparations, lithium carbonate, methysergide, and corticosteroids. The efficacy of each of these classes, in terms of reduction of headache frequency, has been variously estimated at 50% to 75%. In interpreting this figure, the physician should remember that the placebo effect of pharmacologic prophylaxis in benign headache disorders has been estimated to be between 40% and 50%.

Various factors will influence drug choice, including the physician's prior experience with a particular preparation, the preference of the patient or his family, the ease of administration and the experienced side effects. Propranolol and verapamil are recommended by their relative freedom from toxicity and side effects, in particular psychotropic and sedating effects. One must be alert to the appearance of bradycardia and orthostatic hypotension, generally signaled by lightheadedness. These drugs are occasionally a nuisance for the active child because of the necessity of administration several times/day. The antihistamine, cyproheptadine, and the tricyclic antidepressants may be effective choices for both migraine and tension headache disorders. The anticonvulsant, phenytoin, may be useful in migraine. These substances may be given at relatively low risk though the physician must be alert to the possibility of hematologic or hepatic toxicity. These drugs may be taken as a single dose at bed time. Among the tricyclic antidepressant preparations, desipramine is particularly reliable when, as is often the case, fatigue and sleep disturbance precede or are associated with a crescendo headache disorder. If desipramine is used, it is wise to pair it with small doses of a benzodiazepene such as diazepam (Valium) for the first week. Otherwise, an alarming agitation may bias the child against continued use of the drug.

When prophylactic medications are used, they will generally be needed for only several months. Where prophylactic treatment is required for 4 to 6 months or longer, a succession of different drugs may be required as the disorder "escapes" from an initially effective medication. For example, escape from propranolol and verapamil is "the rule," particularly when treatment must be prolonged for several months. After 1 month to 6 weeks of effective headache control, the patient should gradually taper and discontinue the drugs if headaches do not recur. When the drug classes listed above as relatively safe fail in the prophylaxis of a recurrent headache, it is possible that one of the other classes of drugs will be effective. For two reasons the pediatrician might prefer referral at this juncture. First, the other drug classes are potentially more toxic. Second, where the safer drugs fail, it is often the case that the solution will not be a pharmacologic one.

Headache Treatment. Migraine, in particular, is typically associated with nausea, vomiting, and agitation. Effective relief demands attention to these distressing symptoms as well as to the pain itself. Preparations containing butalbital, acetaminophen, caffeine, ergotamine tartrate (Fiorinal, Wigraine, Cafergot) are generally reliable choices which, for most, are well tolerated and acceptably free of risk. However, one must be alert to excessive use, signaling dependency on these preparations. Their regular use on as many as 3 to 4 days/week over several months means that an effective prophylactic program is needed. Ergotamine, when used excessively, has risks associated with arterial spasm; it may cause uterine cramps; and it is absolutely contraindicated in pregnancy.

Severe migraine headaches unresponsive to substantial doses of the aforementioned preparations are encountered regularly in medical clinics and emergency wards. These patients are usually treated by narcotic injections. They typically live in dread of headache attacks and may be fearful of traveling beyond ready access to narcotic injections. Though somewhat unorthodox, chlorpromazine, combined with Cafergot, if tolerated, may be an effective alternative. Chlorpromazine is recommended not only by its efficaciousness but by the fact that the patient or parent may give the drug at home, that it is nonaddictive, and that it is relatively well tolerated and safe when used only intermittently for episodic headache. The small risk of extrapyramidal side effects or hepatic toxicity when chlorpromazine is given intermittently is preferable to the risks, side effects, and inconvenience of narcotic injections. Relatively large doses may be required and failure to use sufficient amounts is a principal cause of an unsatisfactory response. For a teenager, depending on experience gained on several trials, 25 to several hundred milligrams may be required over 2 to 4 hours. This may be given with 2 to 4 Cafergot tablets. Suppositories are effective when severe nausea and vomiting initially preclude oral use of the drug. Metoclopramide and Tigan are other substances that may be similarly used.

Cluster Headache. This type of headache may be treated prophylactically with lithium carbonate, corticosteroids, methysergide (Sansert) or chlorpromazine, singly or in combination. Individual headaches may respond to rapidly absorbed inhalant or sublingual ergotamine preparations.

INDICATIONS FOR REFERRAL OR ADMISSION

Referral or admission to a hospital is indicated when it is established or probable that a headache is a symptom of significant intracranial or systemic disease. Indications for referral to a neurologist, specialty headache clinic, or psychiatrist may be less obvious when one is dealing with the benign headache syndromes. The following guidelines are recommended: where the diagnosis remains in doubt despite clinical analysis, CT scan, and other laboratory tests; and where the response to therapy is unsatisfactory or unexpected. Drugs with which the pediatrician is sufficiently experienced, including those which he views as acceptably free of risks, may have failed to provide satisfactory relief. Alternatively, the use of such drugs may have been associated with bizarre side effects or the patient may have been intolerant to drugs that should have helped. Extreme drug intolerance and bizarre side effects are clues that there is a substantial underlying anxiety state or other psychological disorder, and that a psychiatric consultation is indicated.

ANNOTATED BIBLIOGRAPHY

Barlow CF: Headaches and Migraine in Childhood. Philadelphia, JB Lippincott, 1984 (Excellent current review; comprehensive and thoughtful.)

Bille B: Migraine in childhood and its prognosis. Cephalalgia 1:71, 1981 (Excellent recent study of headache in children.)

Honig PJ, Charney EB: Children with brain tumor headaches. Am J Dis Child 136:121, 1982 (Abnormal physical signs are generally present when a headache is associated with a brain tumor.)

Maratos J, Wilkinson M: Migraine in children: A medical and psychiatric study. Cephalalgia 2:179, 1982 (Perspective on the relationship of psychological stresses and headache in children.)

Raskin NH, Schwartz RK: Interval therapy of migraine: Long-term results. Headache 20:336, 1980 (Although concerned with adults, the study treats well the vagaries of headache response to various medications over time.)

Sillanpää M: Changes in the prevalence of migraine and other headaches during the first seven school years. Headache 23:15, 1983 (This and the following article by Sillanpää present the epidemiology of headache among children in a northern European country.)

Sillanpää M: Prevalence of headache in prepuberty. Headache 23:10, 1983

Vahlquist B: Migraine and children. Intern Arch Allergy 7:348, 1955 (Seminal early review of the characteristics of migraine in children.)

146
Epilepsy

MOHAMAD MIKATI AND
THOMAS R. BROWNE

The International Classification of epileptic seizures divides epileptic seizures into two major categories: partial seizures and generalized seizures. Partial seizures are seizures in which the first clinical and electroencephalographic changes suggest initial activation of a system of neurons limited to part of one cerebral hemisphere. Generalized seizures are those in which the first clinical and electroencephalographic changes indicate involvement of both hemispheres. Consideration of several other factors such as age, EEG, and clinical course leads to a further delineation of several epileptic syndromes. In children, the epileptic syndromes of absence (petit mal), tonic-clonic (grand mal), infantile spasms, Lennox–Gastaut syndrome, and benign myoclonic epilepsy are included under generalized epilepsies. Simple partial (focal), complex partial (psychomotor, temporal lobe), sylvian (rolandic) seizures, and epilepsia partialis continua are considered partial epilepsies. This classification has important implications concerning the understanding and treatment of seizure disorders in children.

PATHOPHYSIOLOGY

The final common pathway of many epileptic seizures is a sudden electrical depolarization of cortical neurons that is seen on the surface EEG as a negative spike. This is frequently followed by a sustained inhibitory hyperpolarization usually seen as a slow wave on the surface EEG. In certain types of seizures, the discharges are believed to originate from single or multiple groups of *epileptic neurons*. If such a group of neurons is located in one of the cerebral hemispheres, the result is an epileptic focus with focal (partial) seizures. If, however, there is no primary epileptic focus and the epileptic discharge is manifested simultaneously in both hemispheres, a primarily generalized seizure results.

CLINICAL PRESENTATION

Generalized Epilepsies

Absence (Petit Mal) Epilepsy. This familial seizure disorder presents between the ages of 5 to 15 years with repeated episodes of unresponsiveness. Typically, there is an abrupt interruption of activity, a blank stare with unresponsiveness lasting for a mean of 10 seconds which is followed by an immediate return of full consciousness and a resumption of previous activity without a postictal period. It is associated occasionally with repeated 3-per-second (Hz) blinks or small clonic movements of the extremities. There may also be mild changes in tone (decrease or increase), automatisms (*e.g.*, chewing), or autonomic changes. Absence status is rare and, because it can manifest as a confusional state with or without blinking, it may be difficult to diagnose without the help of the EEG. The EEG of absence patients shows the typical generalized 3-Hz spike slow wave discharges. In contrast to Lennox–Gastaut syndrome, the EEG background is typically normal. Approximately 30% of patients have a positive family history of absence seizures. Most children have normal intelligence and normal neurologic examinations, but may have significant problems in maintaining attention. Prior neurologic damage and, rarely, brain tumors, may coexist with the absence seizures. These, however, are thought to act as triggers of the seizures rather than as primary etiologic agents. Approximately 50% of patients with absence seizures also manifest generalized tonic–clonic seizures. These patients generally have a less favorable prognosis than those with absence seizures alone. Ninety percent of the patients with normal IQs, no tonic–clonic seizures, and a negative family history of seizure disorder outgrow their seizures completely. The overall remission rate, however, is ~50%.

Tonic–Clonic (Grand Mal) Epilepsy. Generalized

tonic–clonic seizures are the most common type of seizure in childhood and they may start at any age. Unlike adults, most children with this disorder have primary rather than secondary generalized seizures. These children frequently have a positive family history and may manifest other associated generalized seizure types such as absence seizures or myoclonic seizures. A typical generalized tonic–clonic seizure consists of an initial short cry followed by generalized stiffening of the body (tonic phase), falling down, suppression of respiration, and cyanosis. Biting of the tongue, frothing at the mouth, and vomiting may occur and these are followed by repeated clonic jerks with intervening relaxation of muscles. This may last for a few minutes and generalized hypotonia and incontinence of urine or stools may occur. A gradual return of consciousness with varying degrees of postictal confusion, exhaustion, or sleep ensues. Approximately 50% of the patients eventually experience remissions. The interictal EEG may be normal, but typically shows bilaterally synchronous 2Hz to 6Hz spike and slow wave discharges. These frequently do not have the well formed 3Hz morphology of an absence seizure.

Some generalized tonic–clonic seizures are secondary from specific seizure foci. The clinical symptoms are essentially similar except that they may be preceded by an aura which tends to localize the seizure focus. These seizures are more difficult to control than primarily generalized seizures and frequently occur in patients who also have simple or complex partial seizures.

Infantile Spasms (West Syndrome, Saloaam Seizures, Flexor Spasms).   This is an age-dependent seizure syndrome that presents between the ages of 2 months and 1 year. The seizures consist of sudden flexion of the extremities, head, and trunk that last usually for only a fraction of a second but rarely up to 1 minute. They frequently occur in clusters of 10 to 60 spasms. Extension spasms may also occur. Accompanying phenomena may include cries, laughs, smiles, autonomic dysfunction (*e.g.*, flushing, sweating, and tachycardia), abnormal eye movements, and postictal exhaustion. Consciousness is not clearly impaired during the spasms. The disorder is relatively common and occurs in one of 4000 to 6000 births with a male predominance of 2:1.

Patients who have infantile spasms are divided into two etiologic groups: the symptomatic group (80%) and the idiopathic group (20%). The symptomatic group includes patients with known causes for their seizures such as prenatal infections, cerebral malformations, chromosomal abnormalities (*e.g.*, trisomy 21), neonatal hypoglycemia or hypoxia, icterus, aminoacidopathies, organic acidopathies, meningitis, encephalitis, hemorrhages, phacomatosis, lysosomal disorders, neuronal ceroid lipofuschinosis, mitochondrial disorders, and, rarely, Aicardi's syndrome. About 10% of the infants with infantile spasms have tuberous sclerosis. Patients in the idiopathic group generally present later and tend to do better than the symptomatic group. Up to 30% of these patients have a normal outcome in contrast to the 10% of the symptomatic group. Untreated infantile spasms can subside within 1 to 4 years of onset but are usually replaced by other forms of seizures.

The EEG picture most frequently seen in infantile spasm is hypsarrhythmia, defined as high voltage arrhythmic slow waves with multifocal spikes in waking and a burst suppression pattern in sleep. Clinical seizures are usually associated with synchronous slow waves followed by low voltage fast activity (beta seizures).

Lennox–Gastaut Syndrome (Petit Mal Variant Epilepsy, Astatic or Astatic-Myoclonic Epilepsy, Minor Motor Seizure Syndrome).   This is a seizure syndrome that typically starts between 1 to 7 years of age and manifests the following: (1) atypical absence, myoclonic, tonic and atonic seizures in various combinations; (2) typical EEG findings of slow (1.5 Hz to 2.5 Hz) spike wave discharges superimposed on an abnormal and slow background.

Unlike typical absence seizures (typical petit mal) that have less prominent changes in tone during their staring spells, patients who have Lennox–Gastaut syndrome have *atypical absence seizures* (petit mal variants) in which the staring and blinking episodes may be associated with pronounced tone changes, gradual rather than abrupt onset and resolution of the spells and irregular (rather than regular) slow (1.5 Hz to 2.5 Hz) spike and slow wave discharges. Atonic, tonic, or myoclonic seizures also occur independently. Atonic seizures include a loss of tone of the head (head drops) and of the whole body (drop attacks), which may result in limb or skull fractures and may therefore require protective helmets. Tonic seizures frequently occur in sleep. Myoclonic seizures may manifest as sudden generalized synchronous jerks (massive myoclonus) frequently preceding falls or as asynchronous, arrhythmic, asymmetrical involuntary jerks of various muscle groups (polymyoclonia). This latter form is frequently associated with CNS degenerative disease as the underlying cause of Lennox–Gastaut syndrome.

The etiology includes all the causes cited for infantile spasms. In addition, one third of the patients who develop Lennox–Gastaut syndrome have had infantile spasms. Children who have cerebral malformations, severe mental retardation, preceding CNS insults, or preceding infantile spasms have a poorer prognosis with persistent seizures and retardation. Patients who have no known etiology ($\sim 30\%$ of cases), minimal initial retardation, and late onset of the syndrome tend to have a better, though still a very guarded, prognosis.

Benign Myoclonic Epilepsies. Myoclonic seizures can occur in serious CNS diseases (*e.g.*, Lennox–Gastaut syndrome) or in developmentally and otherwise neurologically normal children who have no progressive CNS diseases (benign myoclonic epilepsies). The benign myoclonic epilepsy syndrome of Jantz starts in early adolescence or early adulthood with bilateral myoclonic jerks of the neck and shoulder muscles and with clonic–tonic–clonic seizures shortly after awakening. These patients show multiple spike slow wave discharges (4 Hz to 6 Hz) on EEG and have normal intelligence and neurologic examinations. 37% have associated absence seizures. They respond well to treatment and have a good prognosis. Other similar syndromes at younger ages have been described.

Partial Epilepsies

Sylvian Seizures (Benign Rolandic Epilepsy). This syndrome starts between the ages of 5 and 10 years and almost always disappears by the age of 15 years. A family history is frequently positive (15% of the siblings have the same syndrome). The seizures occur predominantly (75%) during sleep, usually in the early hours of the morning and typically consist of an initial oral and perioral sensation with speech arrest (when awake), salivation, tonic or clonic movements of one side of the face and the limbs. A progression of the seizures into a full-blown generalized tonic–clonic seizure frequently occurs. The EEG shows frequent spike discharges of a characteristic morphology over one or both sylvian and rolandic areas (central, midtemporal). The EEG background is normal. These seizures often alternate sides over the course of the illness. Prognosis is excellent. Most of these children outgrow their seizures by puberty or shortly thereafter.

Simple Partial Seizures (Focal Seizures). These seizures may be seen at any age and are restricted to one side of the body without impairment of consciousness. A motor seizure may sequentially involve the face, the arm, and then the leg (motor march, Jacksonian seizure) or may involve one or more of these sites at the same time. Tonic and adversive movements can also occur. Postictal (Todd's) paralysis, for minutes and rarely hours, can occur after focal motor seizures. Simple partial seizures need not be motor. Sensory phenomena such as tingling sensation, olfactory, gustatory, and visual hallucinations (*e.g.*, flashing lights in one visual field) as well as vertigo, psychic phenomena, and automatic behavior with preservation of consciousness can also occur. The location of the seizure focus determines the nature of the seizures observed. Prenatal infections, hypoxia, CNS malformation, Sturge–Weber syndrome, meningitis, cerebrovascular accidents, brain tumor, A-V malformations, lead encephalopathy and head trauma can all cause focal seizures. The prognosis of simple partial seizures is related to the etiology.

Partial Complex Seizures. These seizures were previously called *temporal lobe* or psychomotor seizures, but it is now apparent that they can also originate from foci in other sites (*e.g.*, the frontal or occipital lobes) and do not always have psychic or motor phenomena. They are distinguished from simple partial seizures by an impairment of consciousness. A typical attack starts with a motionless stare or with an aura (a simple partial seizure) that frequently gives a clue as to the site of the seizure focus (*e.g.*, olfactory: temporal lobe; visual: occipital lobe). A "rising" uncomfortable abdominal sensation is probably the most common aura. The patient may have déjà vu experiences, hallucinations, confusion, or fear. During the seizure the patient experiences impairment of consciousness and may have automatisms such as chewing, lip smacking, running in circles, fumbling with clothing, stereotyped speech, or rarely, complex behavior like riding a bicycle. Pallor and tachycardia are common. Postictally, there is amnesia, frequent exhaustion, and a gradual return to full consciousness. Partial complex seizures can also be distinguished from absence seizures by the presence of an aura, by their more gradual onset, by the presence of a postictal period, and by their usually longer duration (more than 60 sec). Automatisms can occur in both. The EEG is distinctive and shows focal spikes and sharp waves over the involved area. The causes of partial complex seizures are essentially the same as simple partial seizures. Personality and psychiatric disorders may coexist with partial complex seizures. Epidemiologic proof for such an association, however, is still lacking and in most, if not all, such cases the psychiatric disorder is independent of the seizure disorder and should be managed accordingly. Probably more than half of the patients with partial complex seizures continue to have seizures into adulthood.

DIFFERENTIAL DIAGNOSIS

Many disorders can mimic seizures. Vasovagal syncope, postural hypotension, and cardiac arrhythmias may produce a loss of consciousness followed by generalized tonic–clonic seizures due to brain hypoxia. These seizures do not necessarily imply the diagnosis of epilepsy. Breath-holding spells occur between the ages of 6 months and 6 years. These episodes often follow crying or minor painful stimuli (see Chap. 203). Narcolepsy may be misdiagnosed as a seizure disorder and cataplexy can mimic the atonic seizures. EEG (multiple sleep latency test) shows a disturbed sleep pattern with frequent rapid REM onset sleep periods in narcolepsy and cataplexy. A migraine may be episodic and may mimic focal sensory seizures (*e.g.*, tingling sensations, flashing lights) or may present as a confusional state mimicking a partial complex status or an absence status. Apnea in the newborn, sleep apnea, and night terrors may be difficult to distinguish from nocturnal seizures and may generally require prolonged EEG recordings. Ketotic hypoglycemia (typically presenting between 1.5 to 5 years of age), hypocalcemia, hypomagnesemia, and hyponatremia may also present with seizures. Infantile spasms are frequently initially misdiagnosed as spasms due to colic. Abdominal epilepsy (a rare form of partial seizures) can present as recurrent abdominal pain of unknown etiology. Pseudoseizures are seizure-like episodes of a nonorganic nature, but with a normal EEG. Simultaneous monitoring with video and EEG recordings may be required to make the diagnosis. A complicating factor, however, is that many patients with pseudoseizures also have a real seizure disorder.

WORK-UP

History

The history should identify the seizure type, its severity, and possibly its etiology. The age of onset is important because many seizure syndromes (*e.g.*, infantile spasms) are age dependent. The presence of a developmental delay should be investigated. If the child had always been delayed, a prenatal insult, a CNS malformation, or rarely a peroxisomal disorder (*e.g.*, Zellweger syndrome) is suggested. A progressive loss of milestones after an initial normal period suggests a progressive storage or degenerative disease. A detailed description of the seizures including the time of occurrence, precipitating factors, fever, the presence of aura, focal or generalized involvement of the body, cyanosis, incontinence, duration of the postictal period, frequency of the seizures and how they vary, whether there is more than one type of seizure, and associated sleep disturbances should all be documented. The physician should determine the presence or absence of prenatal distress or teratogenicity, of perinatal anoxia or hemorrhage, hypoglycemia, meningitis, head trauma, exposure to toxins and poisons, including lead encephalopathy. It is often problematic to establish which came first—the seizure or the head trauma.

A family history of seizures, febrile seizures, or degenerative storage diseases should be looked for. The ethnic background is relevant because of the predisposition of certain storage diseases to specific groups (*e.g.*, Tay–Sachs disease in Ashkenazi Jews). The social background is important in terms of assessing the ability of the family to cope with the diagnosis and to comply with the treatment. Special attention should be given to ruling out other entities that may mimic seizures (*e.g.*, syncope, breath-holding spells, narcolepsy, febrile seizures, migraine, CNS infections, and pseudoseizures).

Physical Examination

A developmental assessment to determine the presence or absence of a developmental delay is important to perform. The use of the Denver Developmental Scale or other screening tests is helpful. Macrocrania may suggest the diagnosis of hydrocephalus, or other CNS disorders. Microcephaly may be primary or secondary to an early brain injury (*e.g.*, perinatal hypoxia). In infants, transillumination of the head should be done and may suggest the presence of a porencephalic cyst.

Congenital malformations may suggest a chromosomal or malformation syndrome (*e.g.*, trisomy 21). A hemifacial hemangioma may suggest Sturge–Weber disease and café-au-lait spots (6 or more measuring at least 1.5 cm in diameter) strongly suggest neurofibromatosis. Ash leaf spots, shagreen spots, and hypopigmented lesions (seen best with a Wood's lamp) are associated with tuberous sclerosis. An intracranial bruit may signify an underlying A-V malformation. A heart examination may reveal a cardiac etiology. An extremely elevated blood pressure may signify hypertensive encephalopathy. Organomegaly may suggest storage diseases such as Tay–Sachs disease.

A complete neurologic examination should be performed. Papilledema may suggest a brain tumor, and other fundoscopic abnormalities (*e.g.*, cherry red spots) may indicate degenerative diseases. Lateralizing signs such as homonymous hemianopsia, unilateral facial weakness, hemiparesis, reflex asymmetry, facial asymmetry, limb and thumb asymmetry, or dystonia, and Babinski's sign should be sought. Subtle hemiparesis may sometimes be uncovered by having the child perform rapid movements of the hand or hop on one foot. Hyperventilation in the office may precipitate an absence spell. In acute situations, signs of meningitis, head trauma, intracranial hemorrhage, increased intracranial pressure, and possible drug intoxication should be carefully sought.

Laboratory Tests

Following the first seizure, every child should have a sleep deprived EEG, blood chemistries (*e.g.*, glucose, electrolytes, calcium, magnesium, liver and kidney function tests), and a CT scan or magnetic resonance imaging. The CT scan should be contrast enhanced if a brain tumor or an A-V malformation is suspected. A spinal tap should be performed if encephalitis, meningitis, subarachnoid hemorrhage, or a degenerative storage disease are considered. The fundi should always be checked for papilledema before the tap because herniation can occur if increased intracranial pressure is present. A sleep deprived EEG done in waking and sleep is essential. An EEG may need to be repeated because the initial EEG is occasionally normal in a patient with true epilepsy. Depending on the age, the type of seizures, and the clinical situation, an additional evaluation may include lead level, toxic screen, urine and serum amino acid chromatography, biotinidase deficiency screen, blood for lysosomal enzyme assays, urine for dolichols, an electroretinogram, skin biopsy to look for intracytoplasmic inclusions of NCL, liver or muscle biopsy to look for Lafora bodies, porphyria screen, and karyotype.

TREATMENT

The drug treatment should be based on the type of seizure. Infantile spasms are probably best treated with nonsynthetic ACTH. The dose may vary but one regimen is 110 units/sq m/day for 3 weeks followed by 70 units/sq m/day for 2 weeks followed by 50 units/sq m/day on alternate days for 3 weeks. Side effects including hypertension, electrolyte imbalances, and infections should be carefully monitored. ACTH is generally thought to offer an added advantage over prednisone, other steroids alone or the more traditional antiepileptic drugs. There is frequently an amelioration of the seizures and the EEG. Most patients, however, have a poor prognosis despite ACTH.

In Lennox–Gastaut syndrome, which is one of the most difficult seizure syndromes to treat, treatment may vary according to the preponderant type of seizures that the patient is manifesting. For tonic seizures, phenytoin with or without phenobarbital is effective and may also control the other types of seizures that the patient may have. For those patients with Lennox–Gastaut syndrome who have a preponderance of atypical absence, myoclonic and atonic seizures, ethosuximide should be the first drug to try.

Absence seizures are treated initially with ethosuximide, which is as effective as valproate but usually less toxic. Patients resistant to ethosuximide may still respond to valproate or to the combination of the two. Acetazolamide has probably the least side effects and may be tried initially, but it has the least chance of controlling the seizures and its effects are often transitory. Other medications that could be used include clonazepam, methsuximide, trimethadione, and phensuximide. Benign myoclonic epilepsies are often best treated with valproate, particularly when patients have associated grand mal seizures.

Medications effective for partial, primary, and secondary generalized tonic-clonic seizures include carbamazepine, phenytoin, phenobarbital, and primidone. In children, definitive comparative studies of these medications are lacking. In adults with partial or secondarily generalized seizures, carbamazepine and phenytoin have been shown to be more effective than phenobarbital and primidone. Carbamazepine has not been approved by the FDA for use in children less than 6 years of age, although there is a significant body of literature documenting its use in younger children. Phenytoin is approved for this age group, but has rather frequent cosmetic side effects (*e.g.*, hirsutism, gingival hyperplasia).

It is reasonable to start treatment in all children under 6 years of age with partial, primarily, or secondarily generalized seizures with phenobarbital because it has been the medication most used in this age group. If it is ineffective or if side effects (*e.g.*, hyperactivity) prohibit its use, switch to other alternative medications such as phenytoin. In children older than 6 years, it is probably best to start treatment with carbamazepine or phenytoin. Valproate is used as a secondary drug because of its potential hepatotoxic side effects, but may be the preferred drug in patients who have a combination of grand mal and absence or myoclonic seizures. Primidone is also only used as a secondary medication because of its frequent sedative side effects (Table 146-1).

Therapeutic levels should be monitored and maintained. After starting the maintenance dose or after any change in the dosage, a steady state is not reached until at least 5 half-lives, which for most antiepileptics, is about 1 week; for phenobarbital, it is 2 to 4 weeks. To achieve the therapeutic level faster, loading with twice the dose per elimination half-life may be done. Only one drug should be used initially and the dose should be increased until complete control is achieved or until side effects prohibit further increases. Another drug may then be added and the initial medication should be tapered. Control with one drug (monotherapy) should be the goal, although some patients may need to take more than one drug. The levels should be checked periodically, and on addition (or discontinuation) of a second drug, because of potential drug interactions. During follow-up, repeating the EEG may be helpful to evaluate changes in the seizure pattern. Free antiepileptic drug levels should be taken in cases of hypoalbuminemia, and in cases where drug interactions are suspected (*e.g.*, interaction of phenytoin with valproate).

Before starting treatment, baseline CBC, liver function tests, kidney function tests, and urinalysis should be obtained and repeated periodically. For

Table 146-1.   Doses and Indications of Commonly Used Antiepileptic Drugs

DRUG	DOSE	INDICATIONS	THERAPEUTIC RANGE OF SERUM CONCENTRATE
1. Phenobarbital	3–6 mg/Kg/day	Partial, primary and secondary generalized tonic–clonic seizures (probably 1st choice for ages <6 yr)	15–40 µg/ml
2. Phenytoin	4–7 mg/Kg/day	Partial, primary and secondary generalized tonic–clonic seizures; status epilepticus	10–20 µg/ml
3. Carbamazepine	10–30 mg/Kg/day	Partial, primary and secondary generalized tonic–clonic seizures	6–12 µg/ml
4. Valproate	10–60 mg/Kg/day	Combination of absence and generalized tonic–clonic seizures, resistant absence, myoclonic seizures	50–150 µg/ml
5. Ethosuximide	20–40 mg/Kg/day	Absence seizures (first choice)	40–100 µg/ml
6. Acetazolamide	15–30 mg/Kg/day	Absence seizures	
7. Clonazepam	0.01–0.2 mg/Kg/day	Resistant absence seizures, myoclonic seizures	5–70 ng/ml
8. Diazepam	0.05–0.25 mg/Kg/day	Status epilepticus*	0.6–1.0 µg/ml
9. Primidone	10–25 mg/Kg/day	Partial, primary and secondary generalized tonic–clonic seizures	5–15 mg/µl

* Note that the dosages are not for the treatment of status epilepticus, which is beyond the scope of this chapter.

carbamazepine, CBC, and platelets should be monitored more often than other drugs, especially initially. It is not uncommon (10% of patients) to encounter reversible, dose-related relative leukopenia in patients who take carbamazepine. This responds to decreasing the dose or to discontinuing the medication and should be distinguished from the much less frequent idiosyncratic aplastic anemia. Gingival hyperplasia seen with phenytoin necessitates good oral hygiene and in some cases may be so severe as to warrant a surgical reduction and a change of medication. An idiosyncratic allergic rash may occur with any medication but is probably most common with phenytoin. A Stevens–Johnson syndrome may occasionally develop. Other potential side effects are rickets from phenytoin, phenobarbital, and carbamazepine, and hyperammonemia from valproate. Irreversible hepatic injury and death are particularly feared in retarded young children who are taking valproate in combination with other antiepileptic drugs. Almost all antiepileptic drugs can produce sleepiness, ataxia, nystagmus, and slurred speech with toxic levels.

The child who has had his first seizure and who has a normal neurologic examination and a normal EEG may have a relatively low risk of recurrence of seizures, particularly if the seizure occurred in the context of an acute illness such as electrolyte imbalance, toxic encephalopathy or recent head trauma. Because only a minority of these children have further seizures (23% of those with symptomatic first seizures vs 69% of those with nonsymptomatic first seizures), it may be appropriate to delay chronic antiepileptic treatment until the second seizure occurs. Parents, however, should be informed of the risks and benefits of withholding treatment. If started, treatment should generally be maintained for a 2- to 4-year seizure-free period. Medications should always be tapered gradually and never be abruptly discontinued. Prognostic factors reported to predict a poor outcome after stopping antiepileptic drugs include an abnormal EEG, diffuse chronic encephalopathy and retardation, long duration of seizure disorder, and difficulty in initial seizure control. The overall risk of recurrence after a seizure-free period of 2 years is about 25% the first 2 years and is usually only minimally increased over the general population after that.

An important aspect of the management of a patient with epilepsy is the education of the family and the child about the disease, its treatment, and its limitations. Restriction of swimming and driving (in adolescents) is frequently necessary but is not usually needed for other sports, particularly in children with good seizure control. Counseling may frequently be helpful to support the family and to educate them about the resources available in the community. Educational and occasionally psychiatric evaluations may be necessary to evaluate possible learning disabilities or behavioral abnormalities that may coexist with the epilepsy.

INDICATIONS FOR REFERRAL OR ADMISSION

Every patient with a new onset of seizures should have an initial neurologic consultation. Day-to-day follow-up is usually best managed by the pediatrician in conjunction with the neurologist who may examine the child every few months. Earlier follow-up may be necessary if adequate seizure control is not achieved or a change in the pattern of the seizure occurs. Admission is frequently not necessary for the initial evaluation of the patient unless the child presents acutely with frequent seizures or status epilepticus, or if etiologic factors such as acute bacterial meningitis, intracranial hemorrhage, or brain tumor are suspected and further inpatient work-up and treatment are needed. Patients who have poor seizure control and who need significant modification of their drug regimen frequently benefit from admission for close monitoring and documentation of their seizures. Patients who are being considered for seizure surgery (removal of a tumor or of a seizure focus) are hospitalized for the presurgical work-up as well as the subsequent surgery.

ANNOTATED BIBLIOGRAPHY

Browne TR, Feldman RG (eds): Epilepsy, Diagnosis and Management. Boston, Little Brown, 1983 (Comprehensive and well referenced book. Detailed discussions of the choice, use, and pharmacology of antiepileptic drugs.)

Dreifuss FE: Pediatric Epileptology, Classification and Management of Seizures in the Child. Boston, Wright PSG Inc, 1983 (Comprehensive book covering all clinical aspects of pediatric epilepsy.)

Dreifuss FE: Proposal for revised clinical and electroencephalographic classification of epileptic seizures. Epilepsia 22:489, 1981 (Internationally accepted detailed classification of epileptic seizures.)

Gastaut H, Zifkin B: Classification of the Epilepsies. J Clin Neurophysiol 2 (4):313–326, 1985 (Concise clinical classification of the epilepsies.)

Gomez MR, Kloss DW: Epilepsies of infancy and childhood. Ann Neurol 12:113–124, 1983 (Concise review of aspects of epileptic syndromes in children.)

Mikati MA, Browne TR: Comparative efficacy of anti-epileptic drugs: A review. Clin Neuropharmacol (in press) (Current review of definitive comparative studies establishing the preferred drug for various epileptic seizures.)

Mikati MA, Browne TR: Generalized tonic clonic seizures. Hosp Medicine 23:19–39, 1987 (Review of the presentation and clinical features of generalized tonic–clonic [grand mal] seizures and their emergency treatment.)

Morselli PL, Pippenger CE, Pinry LK (eds): Antiepileptic Drug Therapy in Pediatrics. New York, Raven Press, 1983 (Comprehensive review of all aspects of antiepileptic therapy.)

147
Tics

PETER B. ROSENBERGER

Tics, or habit spasms, are in some form a practically universal experience in the normal population. We have all at one time or another noted minor muscular twitches, usually about the face. Their precipitation or aggravation by stress or fatigue is usually obvious.

Tics, however, are far less common among normal children. Their appearance is frequently a cause for alarm among parents and teachers and ridicule by friends and classmates. The practical problem for the pediatrician is usually not to decide whether tics are present, but whether and how to intervene.

PATHOPHYSIOLOGY

In the case of tics, unlike epilepsy, myoclonus, or tremors, formal physiologic study has added little to careful observation. Like myoclonus, as opposed to tremor, tics involve rhythmic contractions of agonist muscle groups followed by relaxation of both agonists and antagonists. Tics, like chorea, are slightly slower than myoclonus. Tics, however, differ from chorea in two important ways. First, tics are stereotyped, limiting themselves to certain muscle groups, whereas chorea moves about the body, giving the impression of a dance. Second, although not strictly under voluntary control, tics are subject to voluntary suppression, sometimes only through considerable effort. It has been shown that tics differ in their electrical properties from voluntary movements, which are usually preceded immediately by a premovement negative potential in the electroencephalogram.

When asked why they exhibit tic movements, many patients will report that "it makes something feel better."

Gilles de la Tourette's syndrome, named after the author of its definitive (although not original) description, has added a great deal to our understanding of tics. Occurring most commonly in preadolescent boys, it combines motor tics with explosive, compulsive vocalizations, usually unintelligible but occasionally in the form of obscene or scatologic language (coprolalia). It is now generally accepted that tics and Gilles de la Tourette's syndrome form a clinical continuum that frequently appear together in families. From its original description until recently, Gilles de la Tourette's syndrome was considered a primarily psychiatric disease. This view has become unfashionable since the discovery that medications with a known effect on certain neurotransmitters are therapeutically useful. Nevertheless, there is a high incidence of premorbid psychiatric difficulties in patients with Gilles de la Tourette's syndrome. Furthermore, the coprolalia is not accidental but intentional and responds to the same sort of irresistible urge as the tic.

Interest in the neuropharmacology of tics was greatly stimulated by the discovery that haloperidol, a potent antidopaminergic drug, can dramatically reduce the symptom frequency and severity in Gilles de la Tourette's syndrome. Further research has virtually confirmed the hypothesis of dopamine hyperergy in this condition. Cerebrospinal fluid levels of homovanillic acid, a principal dopamine metabolite, are reduced in the pretreatment of patients with Gilles de la Tourette's syndrome and are elevated after administration of haloperidol. These levels are also reduced by treatment with amphetamines, which are known dopamine agonists.

The genetic aspects of tic syndromes have received much recent attention. Numerous studies have shown patterns of familial association. Twin studies have shown a difference in concordance between monozygotic and dizygotic twins; thus, although precipitating influences are numerous, the basic neurochemical imbalance that favors tics is at least partly inherited.

CLINICAL PRESENTATION

The clinical presentation of tics is often insidious and is clearly a threshold phenomenon. Many more cases exist than come to clinical attention, and estimates of the date of onset by patient or parent can often be pushed back in time by careful questioning. In the case of children, peer contact on the playground or in the classroom is frequently the deciding factor in seeking medical attention.

Although tics may occur in any muscle group, the face is most commonly involved, followed by the neck and upper extremities. The movement may reflect a simple contraction of motor units, but is more often complex, frequently amounting to an expressive gesture. Movements are rarely distributed evenly in time and they usually occur in bursts. As mentioned above, the relationship to emotional stress is usually so obvious as to favor the conclusion that stress is the direct cause. As the tics themselves usually cause some degree of emotional upset, a "vicious circle" can ensue. The child will sometimes attempt to disguise the tic with a covering movement, such as scratching the face or grooming the hair.

The natural history of tics is highly variable. Although the tendency may be lifelong, the more severe forms are usually self-limited over a few years. Some change in their character (the preferred movement or gesture, or in the case of coprolalia, the word used) usually ensues eventually. This change can be insidious, with the new movement or word gradually increasing in frequency as the old one disappears.

DIFFERENTIAL DIAGNOSIS

Mention has already been made of the movement disorders with which tics can be confused. The most frequent disorder is chorea. Again, the stereotype and voluntary suppression of tics are the most useful distinguishing features. Fortunately, Huntington's chorea is rare in children and, when it does occur, it usually features rigidity and a cerebellar deficit rather than chorea. Sydenham's chorea is usually more precipitous in onset and more rapidly progressive. Paroxysmal choreoathetosis, both familial and sporadic, can involve movements similar to tics, but is usually less stereotyped and more widespread. Stuttering can include vocal mannerisms resembling Tourette's syndrome, especially when it involves precipitous changes in pitch or volume, which can also occur in chorea. In fact, there is reason at least to speculate that stuttering may resemble these disorders physiologically.

Focal motor seizures can resemble tics. They can usually be distinguished by their simpler nature, myoclonic speed, and greater frequency. Electroencephalographic abnormalities and response to anticonvulsants are helpful in differential diagnosis.

WORK-UP

History

The history should focus first on what brings the problem to attention. Although the child can offer valuable information regarding the time of onset, it is usually the parent or teacher who is the source of the complaint. Major events affecting the child's emotional stability, such as a change in school situation, a move to a new home, or the birth of a sibling, should be noted. A careful developmental and adaptive behavioral history should be taken, since attention deficits and adjustment problems are well documented premorbid features in Tourette's syndrome. Finally, a family history of motor disorders must be included.

Physical Examination

The essential physical examination in the tic work-up will frequently be completed before the child is put on the table, as a result of careful informal observation during history taking. A note should be taken of the muscle groups involved, the degree of stereotypy, and the complexity of the movement. If the movements are sufficiently frequent, a test for voluntary suppression should be performed, asking the child to concentrate hard to remain perfectly motionless for a full minute. This test can have positive therapeutic value, demonstrating to the child that control is possible, as long as the clinician indicates an understanding that such suppression is usually not worth the effort. The neurologic examination will usually be otherwise unrevealing. It is important to look for other evidence of chorea, athetosis, or rigidity.

Laboratory Tests

No specific laboratory test is essential to the diagnosis of tics, and few are helpful in differential diagnosis. If the clinical presentation is clearly ictal in nature, and especially if accompanied by some alteration in state of awareness, an electroencephalogram should be ordered. On rare occasions chorea may have an epileptic origin, and tics can occasionally be confused with focal motor seizures. If chorea is suspected, an electrocardiogram and an anti-DNAse B titer may be helpful in the diagnosis of rheumatic disease.

TREATMENT

The two cornerstones of treatment for tics are behavior management and medications. Some form of behavior intervention and counseling will be necessary in every case, even if it involves merely explaining to the child and the parent the essentially benign character of the condition. It is especially helpful in the relief of guilt for the parent to understand that tics have a neurophysiologic basis, although the clinician frequently makes the error of assuming an "either or" dichotomy, thus ignoring important environmental precipitants. It is sometimes helpful in this connection to draw an analogy with asthma and to indicate that, whereas asthma has clearly an organic basis, asthmatics in Arizona tend to wheeze less.

The physician can explain to the child that although voluntary suppression frequently involves strenuous effort, it need not be practiced all the time. A concentration on suppression can be most helpful during times of maximal public exposure. Siblings, playmates, and teachers should be informed that the movements do not indicate a serious physical or emotional disorder. Their curiosity about strange behaviors is natural, and advice to "just ignore it" are often more easily given than followed. Most can understand, however, that undue attention to the symptom merely increases the child's discomfort and sets the "vicious cycle" in motion.

The most effective of the medications for tics impair alertness and attention, and thus learning ability, especially in classroom settings. They should be reserved for more serious cases, but will usually need to be tried at some point when Gilles de la Tourette's syndrome is involved. Haloperidol is the preferred drug and is usually effective at much lower doses than needed for treatment of psychosis. The treatment is usually started at 0.5 mg once to twice a day and is increased at weekly intervals by 0.5 to 1.0 mg/day to a maximum of 0.1 mg/kg. The side effects of haloperidol, particularly akathisia, are more bothersome in children than in adults.

Clonidine is the drug of second choice, although several other drugs have been reported effective, including pimozide, lithium carbonate, propranolol, clonazepam, and imipramine.

The precipitation of tics, including the full-blown Gilles de la Tourette's syndrome, by central nervous system stimulants is now well documented. Such symptoms can persist long after the offending agent is discontinued. Dextroamphetamine, methylphenidate, and pemoline have all been implicated. This can pose a serious dilemma for the clinician, since the attention deficits and hyperactivity for which stimulants are so effective are frequent in children with tics. The frequency is well under 1% at the usual therapeutic doses of 0.3 to 0.4 mg/kg, although much higher at higher doses, and in our experience some form of dyskinesia is practically universal at 0.7 to 1.0 mg/kg. The possibility of this side effect must be mentioned whenever stimulants are prescribed. In children who show tics, stimulants in pretreatment should be used with great care and with well informed consent and only when an attention deficit is severely disabling. A recent demonstration of the effectiveness of tricyclic antidepressants for attention deficit makes these medications, particularly desipramine, a viable alternative for the treatment of this disorder in children thought to be susceptible to tics.

INDICATIONS FOR REFERRAL

Referral resources to the pediatrician for the patient with tics will commonly include the neurologist and the psychiatrist. The neurologist should be consulted if there is any doubt about the diagnosis, particularly if a progressive disease is suspected; if a simple medication trial is ineffective; if a learning disorder or attention deficit is involved. The psychiatrist can be helpful when an associated psychiatric disease is recognized in the patient or his immediate family; when behavioral or environmental precipitants are striking features of the history; or when adjustment difficulties are a prominent consequence of the motor disorder.

ANNOTATED BIBLIOGRAPHY

Cohen DJ, Shaywitz BA, Caparuo B et al: Chronic multiple tics of Gilles de la Tourette's disease; CSF acid metabolites after probenecid administration. Arch Gen Psychiatr 35:245–250, 1978 (Neurotransmitter research showing a reduced function of inhibitory seratonergic mechanisms.)

Comings DE, Comings BG: Tourette syndrome: Clinical and psychological aspects of 250 cases. Am J Hum Genet 37:435–450, 1985 (Comprehensive clinical review of the largest personal sample on record.)

Golden GS: Tics in childhood. Pediatr Ann 12:821–824, 1983 (Clinical review of the general problem of tics.)

Golden GS: Tourette syndrome: Recent advances. Pediatr Neurol 2:189–192, 1986 (Up-to-date general review, including treatment.)

Kurlan R, Behr J, Medved L et al: Familial Tourette syndrome: Report of a large pedigree and potential for linkage analysis. Neurology 36:722–776, 1986 (Most recent in a long list of such reports, with complete references to previous studies.)

Obeso JA, Rothwell JC, Marsden CD: Simple tics in Gilles de la Tourette's syndrome are not prefaced by a normal premovement EEG potential. J Neurol Neurosurg Psychiatr 44:735–738, 1981 (Convincing electrical demonstration that tics are physiologically distinct from voluntary movements.)

Shapiro AK, Shapiro E, Wayne HL: Treatment of Gilles de la Tourette's syndrome with haloperidol: Review of 34 cases. Arch Gen Psychiatr 28:92, 1973 (Reporting the clinical experience that ushered in the ''new age'' of understanding of tics as biological phenomena.)

Singer HS, Butler IJ, Tune LE et al: Dopaminergic dysfunction in Tourette syndrome. Ann Neurol 12:361–366, 1982 (Evidence supporting the hypothesis that the dopaminergic ''overactivity'' in Tourette syndrome may be a result of supersensitive receptors.)

148
Cerebral Palsy
MARGARET L. BAUMAN

Cerebral palsy is a term used to define a group of neuromotor disorders of central nervous system origin, which are nonprogressive and which probably result from many causes. The incidence of these disorders is estimated to be 1.5 to 5.0 per 1,000 live births, with a prevalence of ~400,000 living affected children in the United States. It is believed that cerebral palsy affects at least 1 of 500 school-aged children and is one of the major handicapping conditions of childhood.

PATHOGENESIS

In 1862, William J. Little first described what is now believed to be the spastic form of cerebral palsy. He was convinced that its cause was birth related. Later, however, in 1897 Freud suggested that the cause might be prenatal in onset and that obstetric difficulties might be a consequence of an underlying congenital disorder. Despite Freud's hypothesis, most modern reports pertaining to cerebral palsy have continued to place the major blame for these disorders in relationship to birth trauma and problems of delivery. In all probability, many factors contribute to the development of these neuromuscular disorders.

Evidence is mounting from retrospective and prospective studies which indicates that prenatal factors probably contribute to at least 50% of the cases of cerebral palsy. Risk factors for cerebral palsy include maternal mental retardation, third trimester proteinuria, siblings with cerebral palsy, the administration of thyroid hormone or estrogen during pregnancy, congenital malformation of the central nervous system or other body organs, recognizable syndromes, third trimester bleeding, and many dysmorphic features unassociated with a recognizable syndrome. Many of these children have been small for gestational age at the time of delivery, and all forms of cerebral palsy are represented in this group.

Evidence for perinatal causes is found in approximately one third of the children with cerebral palsy. Risk factors in this group include perinatal asphyxia, cardiorespiratory arrest, and intraventricular hemorrhage. Many of these children include babies who were small for gestational age or who were premature (<2500 g). Low birth weight appears to be one of the major risk factors in this group and may contribute to as much as 30% to 40% of the children who are later diagnosed as having spastic diplegia. A careful review of perinatal events suggests that only ~6% of birth-related factors could be considered preventable. Preventable events include asphyxia secondary to breech delivery, repeat cephalopelvic disproportion, and placenta previa.

Postnatal causes for cerebral palsy can be found in about 10% of the cases, and generally include events occurring after 7 days of age. Risk factors in this group include head trauma, largely secondary to child abuse; meningitis; anoxia related to aborted sudden infant death syndrome (SIDS); and disorders leading to acute infantile hemiplegia. It has been estimated that approximately one third of the children who later present with hemiplegia arise from this etiologic category.

Our ability to predict which children may be at particularly high risk for cerebral palsy in any individual circumstance is poor. Furthermore, we probably do not know the cause(s) for cerebral palsy.

CLINICAL PRESENTATION

Much of the difficulty encountered in understanding the causes and outcome of cerebral palsy relates to inconsistencies in definition and terminology. A functionally oriented classification was prepared by Vining and associates in 1976, and it has been used subsequently by most authors, thus improving communication and discussion among researchers and clinicians. Topographical patterns of motor dysfunction have been found to be useful in designating the spastic forms of cerebral palsy and include the following:

1. Hemiplegia—Spasticity involving two limbs on the same side of the body
2. Double hemiplegia—Spasticity involving all four extremities, with the upper limbs being predominantly affected
3. Quadriplegia—Spasticity involving all four extremities, with the lower limbs being mildly more affected
4. Diplegia—Spasticity involving all four limbs, with the lower extremities being significantly more affected

Extrapyramidal forms of cerebral palsy tend to show wide variability in many areas. Hypertonicity, where present, tends to have the quality of rigidity rather than spasticity, showing a steady increase and decrease in flexion and extension, as opposed to the sense of "give" often seen in spasticity. Abnormal movements are often seen such as chorea, dystonic posturing, athetosis, and uncommonly, tremor and ataxia. Facial grimacing, drooling, and dysarthria may also be seen.

WORK-UP

The diagnosis of cerebral palsy is primarily a clinical one, based largely on a history and a careful examination of the patient over a period of time. Experience tells us that the natural course of these disorders is associated with the evolution of signs and symptoms so that reclassification as the child develops is often necessary, and "mixed" varieties are not uncommon.

History

An evaluation of the child with suspected cerebral palsy begins with a careful review of the events relating to pregnancy, delivery, and the neonatal period. It is often helpful to review complete hospital records including obstetrical records, delivery room and nursery records, as well as nurses' notes in all settings, and potential risk factors should be sought. Information from the parents concerning the behavior of the infant in the newborn period such as abnormal levels of activity, unusual sleep patterns, feeding difficulties, and hyperirritability may be early clues.

Frequently, the earliest parental concern relates to delayed motor development, such as failure to sit, crawl, stand, or walk at the expected time.

Physical Examination

The child's length, weight, and head circumference should be noted and the growth rate since birth should be documented. Evidence of dysmorphic features should be sought. Neurologic assessment may reveal increased or decreased muscle tone, exaggerated deep tendon reflexes, possibly associated with sustained clonus, asymmetry of motor activity in one or more limbs, or increased fisting of one or both hands in a child over 3 months of age. Definite hand dominance noted prior to 12 months of age should lead to a suspicion of hemiparesis, and persistent toe-walking may be a sign of spasticity.

The persistence of primitive reflexes beyond their usual time of disappearance should be considered suspect. The tonic neck response should be essentially gone by 4 months of age, and the Moro response by 6 months. An asymmetric Moro response at an earlier age may be an early indication of hemiparesis.

Signs of choreoathetosis do not generally appear much before 12 to 18 months of age. Slow motor development, hypotonia, excessive drooling, and the retention of primitive reflexes may be seen prior to this age. Additional clues may include the presence of opisthotonic posturing, poor sucking reflex, difficulty in chewing, and poor tongue control.

Laboratory Tests

The evaluation of the child with an early motor developmental delay relies heavily on the acquisition of a good birth and developmental history and multiple physical and neurologic examinations over time. Laboratory studies can often be helpful in eliminating hereditary, metabolic, vascular, or neoplastic disorders that might present with a similar picture and that may be helpful in unraveling the possible causes of the child's motor disability.

The appearance of dysmorphic features may suggest the need for chromosomal analysis. The presence of weakness and hypotonia may lead to a determination of thyroid function, nutritional status, serum muscle enzymes, serum iron, electromyography, nerve conduction studies, and occasionally muscle biopsy. Serum and urine amino acids, and urine studies for organic acids may also be considered. Roentgenograms of the spine should be performed if the lower extremities are primarily involved. A skeletal survey by roentgenogram may be useful if child abuse is suspected. A computerized tomography (CT) scan or magnetic resonance studies (MRI) may be useful in delineating hydrocephalus, porencephaly, subdural hematoma, leukodystrophy, CNS or spinal cord vascular abnormality or tumor, or demonstrating evidence of intracranial calcification suggestive of possible cytomegalic inclusion disease, toxoplasmosis, or tuberous sclerosis.

CT scan findings in cerebral palsy may also be useful in suggesting the underlying neuropathogenetic events that resulted in the presenting clinical picture. The most common CT finding is central atrophy with ventricular enlargement. Infarction and hemiatrophy are significantly more frequent in patients with hemiplegia than with other types of cerebral palsy. Atrophy around the sella media is more frequent in children with paraplegia and in cerebral palsy attributed to prematurity.

Ultrasonographic studies of the central nervous system have also been reported. Findings in cerebral palsied children using this technique have included diffuse bilateral multiple periventricular cysts, bilateral asymmetric dilatation of the lateral ventricles following grade III intraventricular hemorrhage, and ventricular porencephaly following ipsilateral grade IV intracranial hemorrhage.

DIFFERENTIAL DIAGNOSIS

When a child with motor developmental delay under 12 to 18 months of age initially presents, a wide variety of possible diagnoses should be considered. These include global nonspecific mental retardation; muscular weakness and hypotonia secondary to a myopathy or neuropathy; spinal cord abnormality secondary to injury, tumor, or congenital defect; abnormalities of the joints or tendons; inherited syndromes such as familial spastic paraplegia, some amino acidemias, familial microcephaly, or one of the hereditary ataxias; other recognizable syndromes such as sporadic chromosomal defects or intracranial vascular malformations; possible degenerative disorders of the central nervous system; and maternal deprivation, malnutrition, or abuse. A definitive diagnosis may not be reached until the child has been repeatedly examined over a period of months and sometimes years, and laboratory studies have eliminated other possibilities.

THERAPEUTIC APPROACHES

By nature of the wide spectrum of handicaps with which the cerebral palsied child presents, a multidisciplinary approach to therapy will be needed. If available, the child should be referred to a *multidisciplinary clinic* where further diagnostic evaluation of the child's abilities and disabilities can be fully evaluated by a transdisciplinary team and a unified approach to therapy provided.

In the child less than 2 years of age, the most obvious disability is usually a motor handicap, and evaluation and intervention by a *pediatric physical therapist* should be initiated as soon as the handicapping condition is identified. In some localities, this service can be provided in the home for young children; in other areas, the child must attend a center-based facility. The aim of this therapy is initially to improve function in both upper and lower extremities, posture, and locomotion, and to prevent contractures. In order to maximize the usefulness of the therapy, the parents are taught some exercises which can be comfortably carried out daily at home and which can be altered by the therapist as the child's condition evolves and his needs change. The physical therapist also plays an important role in assisting with adaptive equipment for home and school use and in collaborating with the orthopedic surgeon.

The *pediatric occupational therapist* generally works toward the improvement of function in the upper extremities, particularly as it relates to play skills and self-help skills such as feeding and dressing. The therapist may work on improved head and trunk control, adaptive toys, equipment and clothing, and later, modified equipment for school use.

The *speech and language pathologist* will frequently become involved in the therapy of the cerebral palsied child when it becomes apparent that the function of the oral-motor musculature is poor, leading to difficulties with chewing, swallowing, and articulation. In addition, the child may exhibit delays in the ability to understand and express language, necessitating early intervention. An alternative means of communication may occasionally need to be considered, usually in conjunction with the other therapists and physicians, such as the use of sign language, a communication board or book, or an adapted typewriter or computer.

Approximately 50% to 70% of the children with cerebral palsy will show some intellectual impairment. This defect, combined with other handicapping conditions, necessitates the need for an educational program designed to meet the needs of the child while furthering independence, social and emotional growth, as well as academic and eventually vocational achievement.

The child will need to be evaluated medically by an ophthalmologist and audiologist to ensure adequate vision and hearing. Since it has been estimated that ~30% to 60% of the cerebral palsy population has seizures, management and good seizure control become a major factor in the child's care and ability to function adequately. In some centers, medications are used to alter muscular tone and improve the ease of therapy and motor function. Dantrolene sodium has been used in both athetoid and spastic children and its use as a muscle relaxant appears to be helpful in ~50% of the cases. However, diazepam has been more widely used in both athetosis and severe spasticity.

Surgical procedures may be an important aspect to the habilitation of the child with cerebral palsy. The purpose of orthopedic surgical intervention is to improve function, facilitate daily care, provide cosmetic improvement, and prevent deformity. A careful selection of patients for surgery as well as an evaluation of the child's existing functions will increase the possibility of a beneficial outcome and will prevent unnecessary or unsuccessful surgical intervention. Long-term results vary and often depend on postoperative rehabilitative efforts.

ANNOTATED BIBLIOGRAPHY

Goldkamp O: Treatment effectiveness in cerebral palsy. Arch Phys Med Rehabil 65:232, 1984 (Discussion of various therapeutic modalities and their influence on physical and social dependence.)

Graziani LJ, Pasto M, Stanley C et al: Neonatal neurosonographic correlates of cerebral palsy in preterm infants. Pediatrics 78:88, 1986 (Neuropathologic observations in children with cerebral palsy as studied by ultrasound.)

Holm VA: The causes of cerebral palsy. JAMA 247:1473, 1982 (Retrospective study looking at prenatal, perinatal, and postnatal causes of cerebral palsy.)

Lord J: Cerebral palsy: A clinical approach. Arch Phys Med Rehabil 65:542, 1984 (Discussion of diagnostic and therapeutic approaches to the child with cerebral palsy.)

Nelson KB, Ellenberg JH: Antecedents of cerebral palsy. N Engl J Med 315:81, 1986 (The cause of cerebral palsy is probably not known.)

Paneth N: Birth and the origins of cerebral palsy. N Engl J Med 315:124, 1986 (Birth asphyxia does not appear to play a central role as the cause of cerebral palsy.)

Tandorf K, Melchior JC: CT findings in spastic cerebral palsy. Neuropediatrics 15:120, 1984 (Neuroradiographic findings in children with cerebral palsy.)

Vining EPG, Accardo PJ, Rubenstein JE et al: Cerebral palsy. Am J Dis Child 130:643, 1976 (Discussion of classification of the cerebral palsy disorders and a therapeutic approach to the patient.)

149
The Floppy Infant
KALPATHY S. KRISHNAMOORTHY

Floppiness (hypotonia) is a common clinical manifestation of an underlying neurologic disorder in infancy. To some degree, hypotonia can be subjectively based on the experience of the examiner. It is strongly suspected, however, when there is a diminished resistance of the joints to passive movement; when there is an increased range of joint motion; or when the infant assumes abnormal postures. Gross motor delay is one of the indications of this condition. The parents are often the first to suspect this abnormality.

PATHOPHYSIOLOGY

The control and maintenance of muscle tone is complex. Several aspects of this function are still not well understood. Hypotonia may be due to a specific neuromuscular disorder or an associated finding of a wide variety of apparently unrelated metabolic conditions, as in malnutrition or in renal tubular acidosis. The muscle tone is maintained by suprasegmental pathways (upper motor neuron system) and their influences through the lower motor neuron system. The suprasegmental influences originate in the central nervous system through the corticospinal-corticobulbar pathways, basal ganglia, cerebellum, and some descending spinal tracts. These upper motor neuron connections exert a strong influence on the muscle tone through the motor unit. The latter, also known as the *lower motor neuron system*, includes the anterior horn cell, its axons along the peripheral nerve, the neuromuscular junction, and the innervated muscle fiber. Hypotonia may thus occur due to disorders in the integrity of the upper or lower motor neuron system.

CLINICAL PRESENTATION

The clinical picture will depend on the age of the patient, the location of the lesion, and specific features of an underlying disorder. To some extent, there are certain common features that apply to most floppy infants. In the neonatal period, poor sucking, swallowing and coordination, a weak cry, a lack of spontaneous motor activity, an abnormal posture, and respiratory distress may all raise the suspicion of a floppy infant. As they get older, floppy infants characteristically manifest a lack of normal gross motor development. They may also show feeding difficulties, recurrent aspiration pneumonia, or obvious skeletal anomalies. They usually show a delay in sitting, walking, running, and other common gross motor functions. In other instances, they may also show subnormal cognitive speech and language skills. Their neurodevelopmental skills may either remain static or deteriorate, depending on the underlying condition. Certain distinct clinical features may aid in the diagnosis, as for example fasciculations of the tongue in Werdnig–Hoffmann's disease or facial diplegia in myotonic dystrophy. Other specific abnormalities are described under the clinical examination.

DIFFERENTIAL DIAGNOSIS

The differential diagnosis is best organized around the anatomic localization of the lesion, usually proceeding in a cephalocaudal direction (Fig. 149-1). The motor development and examination of floppy infants is uniformly abnormal. This finding, with a combination of other clinical and laboratory

features, will usually aid in making a specific diagnosis. Several conditions that produce transient hypotonia as in sepsis or drug intoxications are not included in this discussion.

In some cases the examiners cannot find hard evidence for a neuromuscular disorder. A close follow-up is necessary in such instances. The term *benign congenital hypotonia* is no longer considered a tenable diagnosis.

Some of the common causes of floppy newborns include asphyxia, Werdnig–Hoffmann's disease, cerebral anomalies, metabolic disorders, myotonic dystrophy, congenital fiber-type disproportion, and congenital myopathies. In later infancy the following are some of the important considerations: atonic cerebral palsy, degenerative disorders (lipidoses), Werdnig–Hoffmann's disease, congenital structural myopathies, myotonic dystrophy, Duchenne's dystrophy, infantile botulism, Pompe's disease, and metabolic mitochondrial myopathies. Certain non-neurologic disorders may also present as hypotonia; for example, arachnodactyly, Ehlers–Danlos syndrome, renal tubular acidosis, Lowe's syndrome, and Prader–Willi syndrome.

WORK-UP

History

The clinician taking the history must focus on important additional clues to arrive at a tentative diagnosis. The parent's chief concerns need to be carefully assessed to know the severity of the situation, especially the sequence of milestones and the extent of motor delay. The physician should determine if the condition is transient or progressive; if it is a familial-genetic or a sporadic case; if the child is globally delayed or merely slow in the motor skills; and if the condition is non-neurologic.

The physician should ask the mother about her pregnancy, labor, delivery, and the neonatal period of the child. Evidence of fetal distress, difficult delivery, and low Apgar scores may all be clues for asphyxia. In the newborn, however, a primary neuromuscular disease may coexist with an asphyxial injury as in myotonic dystrophy. In the latter, the mother should always be examined carefully for evidence of myotonic dystrophy since 90% of the infants with myotonic dystrophy are born to an affected mother. These women may have a characteristic myopathic facies, a typical history of increasing muscular weakness during pregnancy, and uterine dystocia during delivery. Percussion myotonia is a characteristic finding in these women.

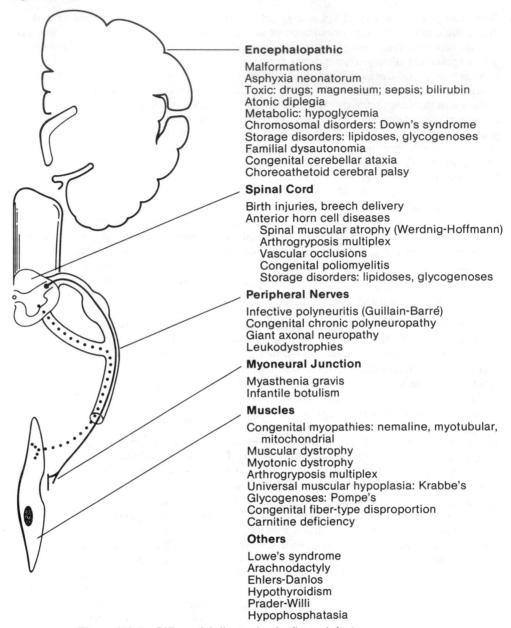

Encephalopathic

Malformations
Asphyxia neonatorum
Toxic: drugs; magnesium; sepsis; bilirubin
Atonic diplegia
Metabolic: hypoglycemia
Chromosomal disorders: Down's syndrome
Storage disorders: lipidoses, glycogenoses
Familial dysautonomia
Congenital cerebellar ataxia
Choreoathetoid cerebral palsy

Spinal Cord

Birth injuries, breech delivery
Anterior horn cell diseases
    Spinal muscular atrophy (Werdnig-Hoffmann)
    Arthrogryposis multiplex
    Vascular occlusions
    Congenital poliomyelitis
    Storage disorders: lipidoses, glycogenoses

Peripheral Nerves

Infective polyneuritis (Guillain-Barré)
Congenital chronic polyneuropathy
Giant axonal neuropathy
Leukodystrophies

Myoneural Junction

Myasthenia gravis
Infantile botulism

Muscles

Congenital myopathies: nemaline, myotubular,
    mitochondrial
Muscular dystrophy
Myotonic dystrophy
Arthrogryposis multiplex
Universal muscular hypoplasia: Krabbe's
Glycogenoses: Pompe's
Congenital fiber-type disproportion
Carnitine deficiency

Others

Lowe's syndrome
Arachnodactyly
Ehlers-Danlos
Hypothyroidism
Prader-Willi
Hypophosphatasia

Figure 149-1. Differential diagnosis of a floppy infant.

The physician should also ask if there was diminished fetal activity, which is typical of Werdnig–Hoffmann's disease (*i.e.*, spinal muscular atrophy).

During the first days or weeks of life characteristics of a floppy infant may be recognized that may later evolve into a distinct entity. Examples of such conditions include cerebral malformations, Werdnig–Hoffmann's disease, congenital myopa-thies, or myotonic dystrophy. These infants typically have feeding difficulties, lethargy, poor activity, and respiratory difficulties; later on, they exhibit characteristic findings.

A detailed survey of all of the milestones should be performed by the clinician. Additional information should be sought regarding a family history of neuromuscular disorders, hypoglycemia, enlarged liver (glycogen storage disorders), preceding viral illness (polyneuropathy), ingestion of honey and constipation (infantile botulism), hyperextensibility of the joints (Ehlers–Danlos syndrome), voracious appetite, and an abnormal increase in weight gain (Prader–Willi syndrome).

Physical Examination

This offers the most valuable information in the evaluation of floppy infants. The evaluation should include a general examination and a complete neurologic evaluation, the latter encompassing a detailed developmental assessment.

By this approach, a distinction could be made between an upper motor neuron disorder *vs* a lower motor neuron lesion. An upper motor neuron lesion is generally characterized by a lack of muscle weakness, normal muscle bulk, preserved tendon reflexes and, in some cases, evidence for cerebral dysfunction. In lower motor neuron lesions, however, there may be fasciculations, muscle atrophy, muscle weakness, and diminished or absent tendon reflexes. These children are generally appropriate in their cerebral functions as in cognitive skills and speech and language functions. It is worth emphasizing that this is only a general rule and that there are exceptions. For instance, infants with muscular dystrophy or myotonic dystrophy may show evidence for cerebral dysfunction. The physician needs to estimate the patient's overall intelligence and psychomotor development. Specific features of various conditions should then be looked for systematically.

The general examination should include the head circumference, an inspection of the face and the rest of the body, palpation of the abdomen for hepatosplenomegaly, and auscultation of the heart for cardiac murmur. This examination may disclose somatic anomalies, clues for neurometabolic disorders (*e.g.*, glycogenoses), or evidence for specific syndromes. A meticulous examination of the face may offer clues to myotonic dystrophy and myopathies. These abnormalities include facial diplegia, a tented upper lip, fish-like mouth, and a myopathic face.

During the neurologic examination the physician should especially look for the following abnormalities: ophthalmoplegia (metabolic myopathies), fasciculations of the tongue (Werdnig–Hoffmann's disease), macroglossia (glycogenosis or hypothyroidism), micro- or macrocephaly (cerebral dysgenesis; lipidoses), arthrogryposis (myotonic dystrophy), scoliosis (congenital myopa-

thy), and ptosis (congenital myopathic disorders; myasthenia gravis). The muscles should be carefully inspected. In congenital fiber-type disproportion and in Werdnig–Hoffmann's disease, atrophy is a common finding whereas pseudohypertrophy of calf muscles may be noted in Duchenne's muscular dystrophy.

It is difficult to obtain percussion myotonia in children with myotonic dystrophy but it should be attempted in the parents of a child suspected of having myotonic dystrophy. It is worth emphasizing that the diagnosis of neonatal myotonic dystrophy can almost always be established by examining the mother of the affected infant. Clinical myotonia may be elicited by a simple handshake with the mother.

The examiner should also note the characteristics of the deep tendon reflexes that are normal or increased in cerebral conditions, normal or diminished in muscle disorders, and always diminished or absent in the anterior horn cell disorders and polyneuropathy. The clinician should also elicit Gowers' sign, which is usually diagnostic of Duchenne's dystrophy.

A thorough clinical examination will also offer clues to other conditions that produce hypotonia such as in Down's syndrome, Prader–Willi syndrome, Lowe's syndrome, arachnodactyly, Ehlers–Danlos syndrome, renal tubular acidosis, Riley–Day syndrome, Leigh's disease, giant axonal neuropathy, and leukodystrophies.

Laboratory Tests

If the patient's history and physical findings suggest a cerebral cause, investigations such as a computerized tomographic (CT) brain scan, magnetic resonance imaging (MRI), electroencephalogram (EEG), and chromosomes may be useful. If a systemic metabolic cause is suspected, appropriate studies should be ordered such as thyroid screening, amino acid screening, lactate, pyruvate, serum electrolytes, and arterial ammonia.

If the clinical examination suggests a lower motor neuron disorder, the following studies may be useful.

Cerebrospinal Fluid (CSF). A lumbar puncture is indicated in postinfectious polyneuropathy in which an abnormality of the CSF protein is expected.

Serum Muscle Enzymes. The most frequently elevated muscle enzymes in muscle diseases are creatine phosphokinase (CPK), aldolase, and serum glutamic oxaloacetic transaminase (SGOT). CPK is not elevated in all muscle disorders; thus, normal values are likely in myotonic dystrophy and in most congenital myopathies. CPK is typically high in Duchenne's muscular dystrophy. Enzymes are not useful in other lower motor neuron disorders. Aldolase runs parallel to CPK in its usefulness.

Nerve Conduction Velocity (NCV). An estimation of NCV is a valuable test to investigate the disorders of peripheral nerves. The ulnar and peroneal nerves are commonly studied. NCV is abnormal in both acquired and congenital polyneuropathies associated with demyelination or failure of myelination. NCV is normal in disorders of muscles and in the early stages of the disorders of anterior horn cells.

Electromyography (EMG). The use of EMG provides valuable information about the electrical activity of muscle at every level of the motor unit. The test thus helps to localize the lesion at the anterior horn cells, peripheral nerves, axons, and the muscle fibers. Typically, EMG is useful in Werdnig–Hoffmann's disease, polyneuropathy, myopathies, muscular dystrophy (especially Duchenne's), and myotonic dystrophy. The typical EMG finding in myotonic dystrophy (dive bomber sound) is not commonly noted in infancy, although this is typical in the adult with myotonic dystrophy.

Muscle Biopsy. An examination of a biopsied muscle is the most definitive test in the evaluation of the floppy infant with a suspected lower motor neuron disorder. Besides the usefulness in establishing the diagnosis, this test helps in the determination of prognosis and in genetic counseling. Since there are difficulties in the interpretation of neonatal muscle biopsies, we propose that a biopsy be performed after the age of 2 months unless there is an emergent situation. Muscle biopsies are used to study the histology, histochemistry, and electron microscopy. The muscle biopsy is typically useful in the diagnosis of Werdnig–Hoffmann's disease, congenital structural and metabolic mitochondrial myopathies, muscular dystrophy, fiber-type disproportion, and polyneuropathy. They are obviously not useful in the upper motor neuron disorders.

Miscellaneous Tests. When myasthenia gravis is suspected, edrophonium (Tensilon) or neostigmine (Prostigmin) tests should be performed. Lysosomal enzymes, urine and white blood cell enzymes assays are all useful in suspected cases of Pompe's disease and lipid storage disorders. Blood ammo-

nia, lactate, and pyruvate are useful in some of the congenital metabolic myopathies. Stool cultures should be performed for Clostridia in suspected cases of botulism. About one half of patients with the Prader–Willi syndrome have a deletion of part of the long arm of chromosome 15, which is best detected by high resolution chromosomal banding.

INDICATIONS FOR REFERRAL AND ADMISSION

Any infant whose condition is severe or rapidly progressive should be referred for a neurologic evaluation to establish the diagnosis. If the condition is not rapidly progressive, then there is a need for at least a one-time neurologic consultation in order to help determine the etiology. In most instances, the work-up can be performed on an outpatient basis (*e.g.*, muscle enzymes, nerve conduction studies, EMG, and CT scan). However, if a muscle biopsy is necessary or if the patient's health is declining rapidly, a brief hospitalization may be necessary to complete the work-up.

MANAGEMENT

It is essential that the physician determine if the condition is static or progressive. This will enable the physician to discuss with the parents the diagnosis, their concerns, and the prognosis. Parental support is essential because there will not be a specific treatment available. The help of allied professionals such as social workers and nurse practitioners will be particularly useful for the parents to ventilate their feelings, anxiety, and depression. They should be readily accessible for the parents to provide ongoing support and counseling, especially in the early stages.

Unfortunately, many conditions are not amenable to drug treatment. The use of biotin, vitamin E, zinc, and drugs such as quinidine and dilantin have not been promising.

The children should be enrolled in a comprehensive rehabilitation program that will include physical, occupational, and speech therapists. Enrollment in the early stages often enables patients to enhance their maximal developmental potential. Furthermore, it helps the parents to deal with the situation and also provides an appropriate long-term planning for special educational needs in many of these children. The role of other professionals such as physical therapists, occupational therapists, and orthopedists cannot be underestimated in the care of these youngsters, especially on a long-term basis. Those with specific muscle diseases may be referred to the local chapter of the Muscular Dystrophy Foundation, which provides parental support groups, financial assistance, and other forms of aids for the long-term care of these children. Finally, genetic counseling is indicated in those with genetically transmitted disorders (*e.g.*, myotonic dystrophy or Duchenne's dystrophy).

ANNOTATED BIBLIOGRAPHY

Dubowitz V: The Floppy Infant. Clin Dev Med No. 31. London, Spastics International Medical Publications and Heinemann Medical Books, 1975 (Excellent monograph on floppy infants.)

Gamstrop I: Nondystrophic myopathies with onset in infancy and childhood. Acta Pediatrica Scandinavia 71:801–886, 1982 (Description of myopathic disorders.)

Gamstrop I, Sarnat HB: Progressive Spinal Muscular Atrophies. New York, Raven Press, 1984 (Textbook discussing the entire spectrum of spinal muscular atrophy.)

Hanson PA: Myotonic dystrophy and infancy and childhood. Pediatr Ann 13:123–127, 1984 (Good review of this condition.)

Parker RJ, Brown MJ, Berman PM: The diagnostic value of EMG in infantile hypotonia. Am J Dis Child 136:1057–1059, 1982 (Discusses the value of EMG.)

Salvatore DM, Edwards B et al: Mitrochondrial myopathies. Ann Neurol 17:521–538, 1985 (Current review of mitochondrial myopathies; excellent reference source.)

Swainman KF, Wright FS: Neuromuscular Disorders of Infancy and Childhood. Springfield, IL, Charles C. Thomas, 1970 (Excellent textbook on the neuromuscular diseases in infancy.)

Zellweger H: The floppy infant: A practical approach. Helv Paediatr Acta 38:301–306, 1983 (Current review on the clinical approach to this problem.)

150
Muscle Weakness
CHARLES N. SWISHER

Since weakness is a common sign of systemic disease, a careful evaluation of other systems should be undertaken before the focus narrows to the neuromuscular examination. Weakness can be either local or generalized and, depending on the location of the lesion, hypotonia rather than weakness may result. One should distinguish between muscle weakness, hypotonia, and myotonia. Muscle weakness refers to a reduction of motor power. Hypotonia refers to a reduction of muscle tone and is discussed extensively in Chapter 149. Myotonia refers to the infrequent occurrence of a pattern of sustained muscle contraction with slow relaxation that clinically presents as "stiffness" relieved by exercise. The primary emphasis of this chapter is on neuromuscular diagnosis based on the concept of the motor unit, which consists of the anterior horn cell, motor root, peripheral nerve, neuromuscular junction, and muscle fiber itself.

PATHOPHYSIOLOGY

The etiology of weakness from systemic causes other than the neuromuscular system can be any combination of infectious, metabolic, and immunologic components that results in a general pattern of debility. Several hereditary, infectious, toxic, immunologic, and metabolic conditions can act on individual components of the motor unit resulting in characteristic clinical and electrophysiologic (and in some cases biochemical) findings. For example, the anterior horn cell can be affected either by a hereditary predisposition to cell loss such as Werdnig–Hoffmann disease, or acquired infections such as poliomyelitis or Coxsackie virus. The motor root can be affected by a postinfectious immunologic process such as Guillain–Barré disease.

The lower motor neuron may be involved alone in traumatic injury and toxic neuropathy and is consistently involved in some of the progressive degenerations of the central nervous system. In the demyelinating leukodystrophies such as metachromatic leukodystrophy and Krabbe's disease, there is involvement of the peripheral nerve and slowing of the nerve conduction velocity.

CLINICAL PRESENTATION AND DIFFERENTIAL DIAGNOSIS

The clinical presentations of muscle weakness are discussed together with a differential diagnosis.

Anterior horn cell disease may be produced by various conditions. Spinal muscular atrophy refers to hereditary muscle atrophy and weakness associated with degeneration of the anterior horn cells of the spinal cord. Involvement varies from severe to mild. Various forms of anterior horn cell involvement also have a different chronologic presentation. The most severe form (*Werdnig–Hoffmann syndrome*) has an early onset, either *in utero* (reduced or absent fetal movements) or within the first 2 to 3 months of life. Due to respiratory failure, survival is rare after 1 year of age. The intermediate form usually presents after the first 6 months of life, and respiratory difficulty is later and milder, with survival to adolescence or adulthood. The mild form, *Kugelberg–Welander disease*, presents with a mild weakness after the child has begun to walk. The weakness is located primarily in the pelvic girdle, resulting in difficulty climbing stairs and limited exercise tolerance.

Lesions affecting the motor root that produce muscle weakness are predominantly acquired. The most frequent example is *Guillain–Barré disease*, in which a previously healthy child presents with an ascending pattern of progressive weakness and areflexia. The condition that usually appears a few days after a minor infection may have an associated mild sensory disturbance, such as back pain, dysesthesias, and diminished sensation.

Although focal muscle weakness can result from traumatic motor root and peripheral nerve injury such as in *Erb–Duchenne palsy* after a brachial plexus injury, some peripheral nerve lesions in childhood have a hereditary basis such as *Charcot–Marie–Tooth disease* and *Dejerine–Sottas disease*.

Disorders of the neuromuscular junction producing weakness are immunologic or toxic in nature. Immunologic disorders include the various *myasthenic syndromes*, including infants of myasthenic mothers, congenital and childhood onset myasthenia. Infants of myasthenic mothers occasionally have a transient pattern of hypotonia and weakness due to transplacental passage of maternal antibodies, responsive to prostigmin or pyridostigmine and resolving in a few days. The congenital and childhood onset forms are longstanding and require ongoing treatment with prostigmin or pyridostigmine. The classic toxin affecting the neuromuscular junction is botulism, which is associated with both palatal paralysis and nasal speech, as well as diffuse weakness and hypotonia.

Primary muscle disease can be congenital or acquired. Congenital muscle disease can either be a myopathy, with abnormal muscle fibers, or a muscular dystrophy, with progressive degeneration of skeletal muscle fibers. *Congenital muscular dys-*

trophy, in contrast to later developing forms, is most active in early postnatal life but tends to stabilize rather than progressively deteriorate with age. One cannot clinically distinguish between the various congenital myopathies, because they tend to present in a similar pattern of early hypotonia and weakness. Such weakness may be predominantly of a limb girdle pattern or may be more generalized. Electrophysiologic studies are helpful, but an appropriate diagnosis requires a muscle biopsy with histochemical studies.

The most common form of dystrophy is the *Duchenne type*, which involves the pelvic girdle; this type is severe and progressive with death late in the second or early third decade of life. The onset of weakness is noted usually between the ages of 2 and 4, and it may be associated with a learning disability or mild retardation. Characteristically, there is a pseudohypertrophy of the calves, with dystrophic calf muscle replaced with fat tissue. A later onset dystrophy, similar in clinical appearance to Duchenne but milder in degree, is the *Becker dystrophy*. Children with Becker dystrophy remain ambulatory later than 16 years of age in contrast to children with Duchenne dystrophy who are nonambulatory at that age. Both Duchenne and Becker dystrophies are inherited in an x-linked recessive manner. Carrier females may be detected by serum CPK evaluations, although the CPK level tends to drop with age. An autosomal dominant form of dystrophy is *myotonic dystrophy*, which is characterized by a slow progression, distal weakness and wasting, a variable degree of weakness, low IQ scores, joint contractures, and respiratory difficulties in infancy. An examination of other family members is helpful because the disease is frequently more striking in the adult than the child. Rarer muscular dystrophies are *limb girdle dystrophy*, which is often inherited in an autosomal recessive manner, and *facioscapulohumeral dystrophy*, which is inherited in an autosomal dominant fashion. Both conditions are relatively mild with a slow progression and presentation in adolescence or adult life.

One confusing and difficult area in the pathophysiology of weakness is the group of *periodic paralyses*, which are characterized by attacks of weakness and hypotonia, with a pattern of remission and relapse. A family history is important because these conditions are largely inherited in an autosomal dominant form. Hyperkalemic and hypokalemic forms exist as well as a normokalemic variety.

Muscle weakness can be associated with various endocrine/metabolic disorders. These disorders are important to identify because specific treatments are often available. *Hyperthyroidism* can lead to a constant or a periodic pattern of muscle weakness, or myasthenia. *Hypothyroidism* can be associated with a slowness of movement as well as easy fatigability, which is frequently associated with mental depression. *Cushing's syndrome* is associated with a weakness of the lower limbs. More commonly, muscle weakness can occur, as a result of steroid therapy, and this factor may complicate the diagnosis in the case of steroid-treated dermatomyositis, in which the primary weakness is prominent. Malnutrition may result not only in weakness, but also in associated hypotonia and hyporeflexia. Other rare causes of muscle weakness include the glycogenoses and carnitine deficiency. The latter is characterized by congestive heart failure, weakness, and hypotonia.

Inflammation can lead to muscle weakness either as a connective tissue disorder, such as dermatomyositis, or a myositis due to bacterial, viral, or parasitic involvement. Viral infection, particularly Coxsackie, has been implicated in polymyositis. In sarcoidosis, there is frequently an involvement of muscle with either localized or general weakness. Rarely, trichinosis may produce weakness and pain and should be suspected in children with eosinophilia and a history of eating undercooked pork.

WORK-UP

History

The history is important in the evaluation of a child with muscle weakness. The physician should inquire whether or not the weakness noted is proximal or distal, localized or generalized, lifelong or recent, continuous or episodic, or related to activity patterns. A family history is of particular interest in a child with apparent congenital weakness or a pattern of weakness of insidious onset. Was there exposure to infectious agents or toxins? A past history of systemic illness, malnutrition, or other contributing causes to weakness should be noted. The physician should also inquire about other or related symptoms of muscle disorder in childhood such as a delay in motor milestones, an abnormal gait, a tendency to fall, hypotonia, or muscle cramps. An inability to run or jump in a young child after the age of 3 may indicate a significant muscle weakness.

Physical Examination

The physical examination is best assessed both informally and formally. In a play setting, the child can frequently be observed to demonstrate details of gait and posture that may be inhibited in the examining room. Play activity such as handling and reaching for small toys can illustrate the presence or absence of weakness and may help to localize the pattern. The physician should test for gross motor milestones of the child. Jumping should be accomplished by 3 years of age and hopping on one foot by 4 or 5 years of age. Gowers' sign, where the child compensates for weak pelvic girdle muscles with relatively stronger distal upper extremity muscles by "climbing up himself" with the hands while attempting to move from prone to standing, is characteristic of proximal muscle disease.

Additional observations to make during the physical examination are the presence of muscle enlargement or wasting, the presence and degree of deep tendon reflexes, and a tightening of the heel cords, which may be noted in muscular dystrophies, as contrasted to the "drop foot" of the child with a peripheral neuropathy. Associated problems such as scoliosis and respiratory difficulties with a characteristic "bell shaped" chest should also be noted. Joint contractures can occur in long-standing nonambulatory children. Erythematous skin lesions involving the extensor surfaces of joints, particularly those of the fingers, are frequently seen in dermatomyositis and should be noted.

Laboratory Tests

Initial laboratory studies should complement the history and physical examination to eliminate systemic causes of weakness such as dehydration, infection, or malnutrition. These might include blood and urine electrolyte studies, thyroid studies, blood glucose and ammonia, and blood and urine cultures. In rare cases, specific biochemical studies may be definitive in degenerative disorders with weakness and a known biochemical abnormality such as the deficient urinary aryl sulfatase in metachromatic leukodystrophy or deficient leukocyte enzymes in the glycogenoses. Neuromuscular disorders should be pursued once various systemic causes have been eliminated. The three primary investigations in this area are serum enzymes, electrophysiologic studies, and a muscle biopsy. The serum enzymes (SGOT, CPK, and aldolase) are elevated when muscular dystrophy is present, and may, in the case of

Duchenne's dystrophy, precede the observation of weakness by many months. However, children who have had recent bruises, intramuscular medication, or vigorous exercise may also have elevated CPK. Isolated elevated CPK may alert the physician to potential malignant hyperthermia.

Electrophysiologic studies to determine the cause of muscle weakness include electromyography (EMG) and nerve conduction studies. EMG studies are best performed in subjects who voluntarily contract their muscles; these studies may be equivocal in young children. Nerve conduction studies are valuable in differentiating between neuropathic and myopathic weaknesses.

A muscle biopsy can be valuable in determining the etiology of muscle weakness, but it must be carefully planned in regard to biopsy technique and tissue study. A segment of muscle is removed parallel to the muscle fibers and is frozen for a histological study while separate samples are fixed for electron microscopy. Several stains are done routinely on every muscle biopsy and, when taken together, can provide information not only of morphologic features but also of individual fiber types and specialized structural and biochemical features.

MANAGEMENT

The treatment of muscle weakness resulting from systemic illness is the treatment of the underlying disease or deficiency. Dehydrated and malnourished children who are unable to lift their heads or raise to sitting can make rapid and dramatic improvement with treatment. Children with myasthenia placed on prostigmin or those with dermatomyositis placed on steroids can demonstrate gratifying recovery. Less dramatic, but no less worthy of organized and aggressive therapeutic efforts, is the treatment of many children with myopathies, neuropathies, and muscular dystrophies that are followed chronically in many pediatric practices. An accurate assessment of the current degree of motor weakness and functional disability allows efforts to be made by an interdisciplinary team of physiatrists, physical therapists, orthotists, educators, and social workers to plan for the most appropriate home and school environment for the child. For the ambulatory child, polypropylene braces and home equipment such as bathtub chairs and special handholds installed at critical areas such as stairs around the house are invaluable. A school bus taking the child to classes and a school located on one level with reasonably short distances between classes is important. Ongoing physical therapy is mandatory.

It serves a dual purpose of monitoring home exercises and assessing the current level of motor function. For the nonambulatory child, appropriate wheelchairs need to be provided and further transportation issues need to be resolved. Occupational therapy is an additional resource for maximization of independence in activities of daily living.

Just as a systemic disease can cause muscle weakness, a chronic muscle disease can cause problems in other systems. These problems need to be addressed directly as part of a therapeutic plan. Respiratory deficits are a major problem in a variety of chronic muscle disorders and result in pneumonia, which is the cause of death in most children with Duchenne muscular dystrophy and Werdnig–Hoffmann disease. Intercostal and diaphragmatic muscle weaknesses are also a problem in many other forms of myopathy and need to be managed with prompt treatment of upper respiratory infections, good respiratory toilet with suctioning, provision of adequate humidity, and postural drainage when appropriate. A difficult medical-ethical problem relates to the use of a respirator in children with chronic respiratory insufficiency resulting from motor neuron or primary muscle disease. It is best in these cases to talk with parents about the possible use or nonuse of artificial ventilation prior to the development of a crisis.

Orthopedic problems commonly accompany chronic muscle weakness and result in progressive scoliosis, heel cord shortening, and other joint contractures. Early and periodic consultation with a pediatric orthopedic surgeon can add years of ambulation to a child with muscular dystrophy and may preserve a similar function for prolonged periods of time for other children with neuromuscular disability.

Inheritance patterns for the congenital myopathies and dystrophies vary from x-linked recessive (in Duchenne dystrophy) to autosomal dominant with incomplete penetrance (myotonic dystrophy and facioscapulohumeral dystrophy). Limb girdle dystrophy is usually inherited in an autosomal recessive pattern. Thus, although the management of many congenital myopathies and dystrophies is similar, an accurate diagnosis of a particular neuromuscular condition is an essential prerequisite to genetic counseling. The aid of professional clinical geneticists should be sought whenever one is dealing with chronic familial conditions of variable or uncertain outcome, because casual or incomplete genetic counseling may lead to planned pregnancies resulting in lifelong unanticipated disability.

INDICATIONS FOR REFERRAL OR ADMISSION

The medical revolution of the 1980s has seen a proliferation of sophisticated electrophysiologic devices in outpatient settings and community hospitals. Since neuromuscular disease in childhood is a complex area, it is imperative that muscle biopsies on children be performed by laboratories skilled in this procedure and using the complex histochemical and electron microscopy available for their interpretation. EMG studies should likewise be performed by those individuals who have considerable experience in the EMG evaluation of children.

Hospitalization for children who have an acute onset of weakness is mandatory in a facility where close attention can be paid to respiratory status and appropriate action taken in case of respiratory decompensation, often seen in Guillain–Barré disease. Acute respiratory decompensation is also common in children with pre-existing muscle disease who initially have a mild upper respiratory infection. Therefore, children with a known myopathy should be hospitalized for observation whenever such an infection produces a deterioration in respiratory function. Hospitalization is indicated for those children with weakness of unknown etiology, which may be related to dermatomyositis or a metabolic or degenerative condition requiring further investigation and initial inpatient management. Hospitalization is also indicated for surgical procedures used in the management of chronic myopathic or neuropathic conditions such as heel–cord lengthening.

ANNOTATED BIBLIOGRAPHY

Downey JA, Low N (eds): The Child with Disabling Illness. Philadelphia, WB Saunders, 1974 (Practical management suggestions and discussion of pathophysiology; see especially Chap. 11: Diseases of Muscle, p 197, by A Chutorian and SJ Myers.)

Dubowitz V: The Floppy Infant, 2nd ed. Philadelphia, JB Lippincott, 1980 (Primarily a discussion of hypotonia, with many good observations on the evaluation of weakness.)

Dubowitz V: Muscle Disorders in Childhood. Philadelphia, WB Saunders, 1978 (Classic reference on muscle disorders affecting motor function.)

Dyck PJ (ed): Peripheral Neuropathy. Philadelphia, WB Saunders, 1984 (Exhaustive survey of neuropathic weakness and its clinical syndromes; see especially p 1093, *Quantitation of Muscle Contraction and Strength* by R. Edwards.)

Menkes JH: Textbook of Neurology. Chap 13: Diseases of the Motor Unit. Philadelphia, Lea & Febiger, 1985 (Clinically oriented with extensive bibliography of recent literature on the motor unit.)

Vinken PJ, Bruyn GW (eds): Handbook of Clinical Neurology, Vols 40 and 41, Diseases of Muscle. New York, Elsevier, 1979 (Exhaustive survey of clinical presentation and pathophysiology of muscle disease.)

151
Microcephaly
ELIZABETH C. DOOLING

Microcephaly or small head size refers to a head circumference that is smaller than 2 standard deviations below the 50% for the child's age. It may be classified as primary or secondary microcephaly. Primary microcephaly, sometimes called *microcephaly vera* or *microcrania*, may be inherited on an autosomal dominant or recessive basis or it may occur sporadically. Secondary microcephaly results from trauma, vascular insults, or infections to the brain that occur later in gestation to an already well-formed brain.

PATHOPHYSIOLOGY

The brain begins as a vesicular structure with large germinal centers that are composed of neuroblasts which migrate to the cortex by means of "guiding" radial fibers in two waves of migration: (1) between 6 and 12 weeks; and (2) between 16 and 24 weeks. By the end of the second trimester, the normal cortical laminar pattern has been completed and primary fissuration of the brain has occurred. The brain is sensitive to various neurocytotoxic agents including radiation, alkylating agents, alcohol, tobacco, aminoacidurias (*e.g.,* phenylketonuria), and certain viruses. Infants of mothers with diabetes and uremia may have microcephaly. A large cerebral growth spurt normally occurs after the 26th week of gestation. Secondary fissures and gyri can be recognized. The germinal matrix regresses and astrocytes, both reactive and myelinative, appear.

Primary microcephaly will result if there is a primary failure or interruption of neuronal migration. Other organs such as the eye, which are growing and developing concurrently, may be abnormal. Multiple craniofacial and somatic anomalies are also present in children with chromosomal disorders. Children who have familial microcephaly may not have associated dysmorphic features. When the infant is subjected to an intrauterine infection (viral or bacterial), ischemia, hemorrhage, or hypoxia in the late third trimester or is asphyxiated at or shortly after birth, secondary microcephaly may develop.

CLINICAL PRESENTATION

The baby with primary microcephaly has an obviously small head size at birth. The head circumference is ≤31 cm in a full-term infant while weight and length may be appropriate for the gestational age. The palpebral fissures are also short. There is a flattening of the posterior aspect of the head with underdevelopment of the normal parieto-occipital fullness. The forehead is broad and sloping. The eyes are prominent and may look frog-like. The facial features may be coarse. The ears are often posteriorly rotated. Other somatic anomalies may be readily recognized. The older child is usually also distinctive in appearance because of the small head size in proportion to a more normally developed body, although the overall stature may be small, giving a dwarf-like appearance. The child is often hyperactive and easily distractible and he may have a seizure disorder.

The baby with secondary microcephaly has a normal head circumference at birth as well as an appropriate body weight and length and normal length of palpebral fissures. As the child grows older, the slow rate of head growth becomes apparent. As the child's head circumference deviates further away from the normal curve for age, the head size sometimes conforms to the child's own percentile, over years. At other times it plateaus after 12 to 18 months of age. Developmental delay occurs and may be associated with spastic paraparesis, hemiparesis, or quadriparesis as well as sensory deficits, including blindness and deafness.

DIFFERENTIAL DIAGNOSIS

Primary microcephaly can usually be differentiated from secondary microcephaly on the basis of the prenatal and birth histories and the head circumference of the infant at birth.

Some Causes of Microcephaly

PRIMARY

Familial
  "Benign" associated with normal physiognomy and intelligence
  Associated with inferior intelligence ± seizures ± hyperactivity
Inductive-migrational disorders
  Agyria
  Pachygyria
  Microgyria
  Polymicrogyria
  Lissencephaly
  Agenesis of the corpus callosum
  Schizencephaly
  Chromosomal disorders (*e.g.*, trisomies, rings, deletions)
  Nonchromosomal disorders (*e.g.*, Smith–Lemli–Opitz, Prader–Willi, Cornelia de Lange, Hallermann–Streiff, Rubinstein–Taybi)
Toxic–metabolic
  Radiation
  Alkylating agents
  Alcohol
  Illicit drugs
  Tobacco
Infectious
  Rubella
  Mumps
  Cytomegalovirus
  Toxoplasmosis
  Syphilis
  Herpes simplex, types 1 and 2
  Listeriosis

SECONDARY

Vascular *e.g.*, asphyxia, placental separation, or septic shock resulting in:
  Porencephaly
  Hydranencephaly
  Cystic encephalomalacia
  Laminar necrosis
Metabolic (*e.g.*, maternal uremia or diabetes)

WORK-UP

History

The gestational history must be carefully reviewed to assess the occurrence of any teratogenic exposure such as alcohol, drug, and tobacco abuse, exposure to radiation, and infections in the first and second trimesters. Prenatal records should be reviewed in the event that the mother is unable to recall minor points which may be contributory. The family history should also be reviewed in depth to ascertain the range of head sizes, and, more importantly, the incidence of other affected children.

The birth records should be reviewed critically to determine whether a hemorrhage, a period of hypoxic ischemia, or sepsis occurred.

Physical Examination

The head circumference should be carefully measured with a metal or nonstretching cloth tape. The size of the anterior fontanel and eyes should be noted. The sutures should be palpated to assess their overlapping. The baby should be examined for major and minor anomalies that would suggest a chromosomal disorder or classified syndrome. Localized, discrete, or generalized vesicular eruptions, generalized petechiae, hepatosplenomegaly, jaundice, and other evidence of active viral infection should be evaluated.

Laboratory Tests

Vesicular lesions, CSF, urine, stool and throat washings should be cultured for virus in nonasphyxiated babies. TORCH titers should be drawn on the mother and baby. IgM titers of the infant should also be obtained. Chromosomes should be checked if there are associated anomalies. Roentenograms of the skull may show early fusion of the sutures caused by a failure of growth to the underlying cerebral tissue. CT scans are sensitive in detecting small areas of periventricular or intraparenchymal calcification as sequelae of an intrauterine infection.

MANAGEMENT AND REFERRAL

If the family history is clearly supportive of a familial etiology, an otherwise entirely healthy child is likely to develop and perform like other family members. Reassurance may be sufficient in such cases. If, however, the baby has microcephaly of a sporadic type, deficient intelligence may be present. Martin and Sells have found that ~7.5% of microcephalic children have normal intelligence. Sporadic cases of microcephaly should be referred to a geneticist after the basic evaluations have been completed. (For the management of microcephaly from craniosynostosis, refer to Chap. 153.)

ANNOTATED BIBLIOGRAPHY

Caffey J: Pediatric X-ray Diagnosis. Chicago, Year Book Medical Publishers, 1961 (Good basic introduction to normal and abnormal growth of the skull.)

Swaiman KF, Wright FS: The Practice of Pediatric Neurology, pp 442–444. St, Louis, CV Mosby, 1982 (Excellent textbook which gives a comprehensive tabulation of common and uncommon causes of abnormal head growth.)

152
Macrocephaly
ELIZABETH C. DOOLING

Macrocephaly or large head size refers to a head circumference that is greater than 2 standard deviations above the 50% for the child's age. It may be classified as primary or secondary macrocephaly. Primary macrocephaly, sometimes called *macrocrania*, is often inherited on an autosomal dominant basis, and, less frequently, occurs sporadically. Secondary macrocephaly may arise from conditions that cause overgrowth of the cerebral tissues, such as space-occupying lesions, or obstruction of the cerebrospinal fluid (CSF) circulation.

PATHOPHYSIOLOGY

Most of the growth and differentiation of the skull occurs during the first and second years of life. Thus, most of the features of the adult skull are present by a child's second birthday. Growth of the skull is slowest from the second year to puberty, after which the velocity of growth increases for 1 or 2 years. The skull usually attains its definitive size by the twentieth year of life.

The fontanels and sutures become smaller and narrower by the ingrowth of bone into the remnants of the fetal membranous and cartilaginous skull. This process varies from child to child and even on both sides of the skull; thus, the skull is usually asymmetric and the left side is often larger in the frontal region than the right. The anterior fontanel is usually reduced to fingertip size during the first half of the second year. The posterior fontanel may be palpable at birth but usually disappears by 2 months of age. The frontal suture begins to close in the second year but may persist throughout life in ~10% of people.

The CSF is produced in the choroid plexuses that arise from the lateral ventricles in frondlike projections from the walls of the posterior horns, and third and fourth ventricles. If the flow of the CSF is obstructed, the volume of CSF (which is produced at a regular rate of ~20 ml/hr) will not circulate normally. To accommodate the increased volume, the lateral ventricles usually expand with concomitant compaction of the adjacent central white matter of the cerebral hemispheres. When the anterior fontanel is open, it may bulge as an indicator of expanding ventricular size. The sutures may separate more widely than they normally do, and clinical signs of increased intracranial pressure may develop. Rapid head growth occurs and can be detected by careful serial measurements of the head circumference.

CLINICAL PRESENTATION

The clinical presentation of the child with macrocephaly varies according to the underlying cause of the large head size. A baby may have no dysmorphic features at birth but may have an obviously large head in proportion to his weight and length. A baby may present with multiple congenital anomalies including dysraphism with a myelomeningocele or faciopalatal clefts. In infancy, an otherwise healthy baby may have too large a head to fit a baby cap comfortably, or it may be difficult to pull a shirt over the baby's head. The head circumference should be measured regularly during routine examinations and preferably by the same person with a metal or nonstretching cloth tape to ensure precision of measurement. When a baby's head circumference falls above the 98% for age, it is necessary to measure the head circumference of both parents to determine whether they conform to similar percentiles. The child's height and weight should be plotted on growth charts to assess the proportionality of the head and body growth. The baby should be checked at intervals of 2 to 4 weeks or even weekly if necessary to determine how quickly the head is growing. The head may grow more rapidly than the body, so that a discrepancy between weight, length, and head circumference becomes apparent. When the head enlarges due to an underlying increase in the total volume of the cranial cavity (*e.g.*, from a structural malformation, blood, neoplasm, infection, or increase in volume of CSF because of obstructed CSF pathways), the child will present with signs of increased intracranial pressure (ICP). The earliest signs in a young child or infant less than 6 months of age will be a bulging or tenseness of the anterior fontanel followed by, or associated with, a change in eating or sleeping habits. The baby may be irritable and will not be comforted by feeding or rocking. Feedings may be vomited in a projectile manner, and the baby may be disinclined to nurse or suck. The baby may sleep for longer periods and may require to be woken up for feedings. There may be decreased visual responses and poor ocular fixation.

Altered feeding and sleeping habits may be more easily recognized in the older infant. If the fontanel is open, it may be tense. The cranial sutures may be palpably spread. The toddler may fall more frequently or may be content to sit and show less interest in normal activities. A sunsetting appearance of the eyes may develop due to pressure on midbrain structures that govern upward gaze and discernible broadening of the forehead with frontal bossing.

The older child may complain of having a headache or he may hold the front or sides of the head. He may vomit most frequently on awakening in the morning or after naps. A gait disturbance may become apparent. The ability to perform gross motor skills such as riding a bicycle or skating may be impaired. The child may show a disinterest in playing or may tire easily. Complaints of diplopia or blurred vision may not be made until late in the development of increased ICP. However, strabismus or changes in the child's acuity, as evidenced by holding books closer, sitting closer to the television or deterioration in school work, may suggest a decline in visuomotor function due to intracranial hypertension.

DIFFERENTIAL DIAGNOSIS

The differential diagnosis of macrocephaly is presented in the following box in order of frequency of occurrence.

---

1. Primary
    Congenital
    a. Familial
    b. Sporadic
2. Acquired
    0–6 Months
    a. Posthemorrhagic—higher in prematures
    b. Postinfectious
        i. Intrauterine
        ii. Postnatal

c. Post-traumatic
d. Malformative, *e.g.*, hydranencephaly; aqueductal stenosis
   i. Familial x-linked
   ii. Sporadic
   iii. Arnold–Chiari types I or II
e. Neoplasm
   i. Primary
   ii. Metastatic
f. Metabolic
g. Storage or neurodegenerative

6–12 Months
a. Aqueductal stenosis
b. Post-traumatic
c. Postinfectious
d. Metabolic
e. Neurocutaneous syndrome
f. Neoplasm
g. Neurodegenerative

1–6 Years
a. Post-traumatic
b. Postinfectious
c. Aqueductal stenosis
d. Neoplasm
   i. Posterior fossa
   ii. Brain stem
   iii. Cerebral hemispheres
e. Metabolic
f. Neurodegenerative

WORK-UP

History

The family history is important in the otherwise healthy child with a large head. A review of earlier medical records, including maternal infections during pregnancy and head circumference at birth, helps to determine what the rate of head growth has been, and if there has been a recent deviation from the child's curve. A history of change in eating or sleeping habits, personality, or school performance must be sought. The physician should ask about the occurrence of birthmarks in close family members to ascertain the incidence of neurofibromatosis or tuberous sclerosis, which are disorders that may be associated with a large head size or macrocephaly.

Physical Examination

A careful measurement of the head circumference in its greatest diameter is essential. The size and tension of the anterior fontanel should be assessed. The craniofacial ratio should be approximated. (The face is about one eighth of the size of the cranial vault in the infant. In adults, the face:cranium ratio is ~1:2.) A survey of the skin in bright sunlight and then with a Wood's light should be made to look for hypopigmented or café-au-lait

spots. An examination of the back for evidence of a dermal sinus may indicate underlying spinal dysraphism. Other dysmorphic features should be noted. An enlargement of the liver and spleen, chorioretinitis and other findings consistent with an intrauterine infection should also be noted. Bruits or venous distention over the cranium may reflect a vascular anomaly such as the vein of Galen malformation.

Laboratory Tests

The child with primary or familial macrocephaly can be monitored at regular intervals by his primary physician. Skull roentgenograms and CT scans are not necessary when a positive family history has been obtained or if the child is *asymptomatic* (*i.e.*, if there is no developmental delay and signs of ICP are absent). When the fontanel is still open, cranial ultrasound is useful in determining ventricular size without exposure to x-rays. If the child is *symptomatic*, the physician should assume that secondary macrocephaly is present and he should undertake appropriate studies.

The child with secondary macrocephaly requires investigation. TORCH titers should be drawn from the child and the mother. A prematurely born infant known to have had an intracranial hemorrhage may be followed with serial cranial ultrasonography for an assessment of ventriculomegaly. A midline shift of the intracranial structures and some congenital malformations such as agenesis of the corpus callosum or holoprosencephaly may be apparent on a cranial ultrasound. The delineation of processes in the subdural or subarachnoid spaces, however, cannot be made with ultrasound. Intracranial calcifications indicating an intrauterine infection or tuberous sclorsis are readily seen on CT scans. If a history of preceding infection, trauma, or seizures is obtained, a CT scan will provide information about processes such as subdural collections that necessitate prompt treatment. Although skull x-rays are helpful in assessing the chronic changes of increased ICP, the CT scan is more useful in localizing a focal abnormality and guiding surgical intervention when indicated. A plain CT scan allows the assessment of the extent and width of the cerebral mantle, ventricular size and intracranial hemorrhage, and will also show shifts of intracranial structures from the midline. A contrast-enhanced CT scan permits an assessment of the neovascularity of mass lesions and vascular malformations. A magnetic resonance imaging (MRI) scan may show a process that cannot be visualized within the resolution of the CT scan. The

MRI scanner is better suited for imaging of brain stem disorders and should be obtained in the cases where a strong suspicion of disease exists but is not confirmed by a CT scan.

INDICATIONS FOR REFERRAL

The child with uncomplicated macrocephaly needs no further evaluation in contrast to a child who has been found to have intracranial hypertension due to a space-occupying lesion, CSF flow obstruction, or a storage disorder. The latter child should be referred to a neurosurgeon and a pediatric neurologist.

ANNOTATED BIBLIOGRAPHY

Caffey J: Pediatric X-Ray Diagnosis. Chicago, Year Book Medical Publishers, 1961 (Good basic introduction to normal and abnormal growth of the skull.)

Shinnar S, Gammon K, Bergman EW et al: Management of hydrocephalus in infancy: Use of acetazolamide and furosemide to avoid cerebrospinal fluid shunts. J Pediatr 107:31–37, 1985 (Good review of the medical management of hydrocephalus.)

Swaiman KF, Wright FS: The Practice of Pediatric Neurology, pp 429–442. St. Louis, CV Mosby, 1982 (Excellent textbook which gives a comprehensive tabulation of common and uncommon causes of abnormal head growth.)

153
Craniosynostosis
BROOKE SWEARINGEN AND
　　PAUL H. CHAPMAN

Abnormalities of skull shape have been medically, socially, and cosmetically important in other centuries and cultures as well as our own. In modern pediatric practice, consideration of the diagnosis often arises from parental concern over the cosmetic deformity, but the relationship between multiple sutural fusion, intracranial hypertension, and developmental delay is an important though misunderstood question. Virchow, in his study of cretinism, first argued that premature fusion of sutures could cause a skull deformity by compensatory overgrowth of the nonfused sutures and he introduced the concept of craniostenosis reduced cranial capacity secondary to premature suture fusion. Clinical associations between craniosynostosis, papilledema, and optic atrophy were made in the late 1800s. It has since become apparent, however, that most simple single synostoses are benign conditions that require reconstruction for social and psychological as well as medical indications.

The classification of the craniosynostoses can be based on the skull shape or on the suture fused. *Scaphocephaly* or *dolichocephaly* refers to a narrow, elongated skull that is associated with fusion of the sagittal suture. *Trigonocephaly* is a narrow forehead with hypotelorism and a median supraglabellar ridge occurring with fusion of the metopic suture. Fusion of the coronal sutures bilaterally results in *brachycephaly*, which refers to a broad skull

with a high forehead. The term *oxycephaly* has been used to describe the high conically shaped head resulting from coronal with sagittal or lambdoidal synostosis. *Plagiocephaly* refers to an asymmetric skull with a sloped occiput or forehead resulting from unilateral lambdoid or coronal fusion. The cloverleaf skull (or Kleeblattschadel) may arise from multiple fusions involving the coronal, sagittal, and lambdoid sutures. Complex genetic syndromes (*e.g.*, Crouzon's or Apert's syndromes) may involve multiple premature synostoses and also other facial and skeletal abnormalities (Fig. 153-1).

PATHOPHYSIOLOGY

The factors involved in skull morphogenesis are poorly understood and involve an interaction between the brain, dura, skull base, and the developing calvaria. Sutures form over dural reflections connecting the basicranium and calvaria, which in turn reflect the underlying form of the brain. The sagittal and metopic sutures overlie the falx cerebri; the coronal overlies the dural reflection originating at the sphenoid wing; and the lambdoid overlies the transverse sinus and the tentorium cerebelli. Ossification centers form in central zones delineated by these reflective bands between the fetal ages 12 and 16 weeks. Bone forming activity normally halts at the reflective bands where a suture then forms.

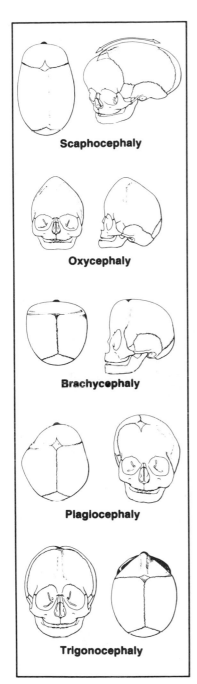

Scaphocephaly

Oxycephaly

Brachycephaly

Plagiocephaly

Trigonocephaly

Figure 153-1. The classification of the craniosynostoses based on skull shape. (Courtesy of the BNI Quarterly II(1):30, 1986)

Any underlying abnormality of the brain that has altered the normal pattern of dural reflection should also alter the pattern of suture formation. This has been found to occur in some cases of holoprosen-cephaly, craniopagus, and dicephaly. Premature fusion of sutures arises, according to one theory, when changes in the skull base alter the pattern of dural reflection. Others have emphasized the influence of local factors, with changes in the skull base as a secondary phenomenon. Sutures can be experimentally fused by transplanting the periosteum or by applying cyanoacrylate. Reports in the literature suggest that intrauterine head constraint may be contributory in isolated cases. It is interesting to note, however, that artificial skull binding, as practiced by some primitive tribes, produces skull shape abnormalities without premature synostosis.

Finally, the craniosynostoses may occur as a result of a generalized metabolic abnormality, such as rickets and hyperthyroidism.

CLINICAL PRESENTATION

Since craniosynostosis occurs during infancy, the abnormality is most often evident on inspection by the parent or pediatrician. Single fusions are usually asymptomatic. Complex multiple fusions have been associated with headaches, visual loss, and retardation. The incidence of headache varies with the age of the child and the number of sutures fused; it is most common in the older child with multiple synostoses. A loss of vision, though rare, requires further evaluation; the incidence of papilledema is 20% to 40% in those children with multiple fusions. The case for craniosynostosis as a cause of retardation is difficult to prove, but a higher incidence of retardation is apparent in those children who have multiple synostoses. This is more commonly seen with the complex deformities and only rarely with a single fusion.

DIFFERENTIAL DIAGNOSIS

The differential diagnosis of an abnormal skull shape is not extensive, and the appearance of the simple synostoses is characteristic. Multiple fusions associated with a facial abnormality should prompt a consideration of the craniofacial syndromes (*e.g.*, Crouzon's syndrome or Apert's syndrome) with their other systemic abnormalities. When primary microcephaly produces synostosis, computerized tomography may reveal an underlying loss of brain substance. Positional molding, either pre- or postnatally, may appear identical to the true premature fusion. This is particularly true for the unilateral occipital flattening that is reminiscent of lambdoidal synostosis. These infants have sutures present radiographically, but they clearly have an abnormal head shape. The abnormality can usually be corrected simply by preventing the infant from sleeping on the defect.

WORK-UP

The diagnosis is made on the basis of a physical and radiographic examination. Historical details (*e.g.*, the presence of a familial syndrome) may occasionally be important, but recognition of the characteristic appearance is essential. Palpation of the sutures in the infant may be useful, and synostosis is unlikely if the plates are clearly mobile. The entire length of the suture must be felt, because a short bony segment can prevent growth. A palpable bony ridge is often appreciated along the fused sagittal or metopic sutures. The fontanelle may provide an indication of elevated intracranial pressure. Papilledema, though usually seen only in cases of multiple fusions, is an important finding.

The most useful radiographic study is the plain skull film. The sutures should be well demonstrated; this may require oblique views. The region of bony fusion will appear as a loss of normal suture lucency with perhaps an increased density. In cases of multiple fusions, the orbit and sphenoid wing may have a characteristic appearance. Computerized tomography can be useful in cases of multiple fusion or where hydrocephalus is suspected, but it adds little to the evaluation of the simple fusions.

TREATMENT

The primary indication for surgery for a single synostosis is the desire for plastic reconstruction: the risk of developing intracranial hypertension or retardation in these children is minimal. The risk of intracranial hypertension is greater in cases of multiple suture fusion. The timing of surgery is important; better results are obtained when the surgery is performed at an early age, because skull remolding takes advantage of a rapidly growing brain in infancy. A single synostosis is generally best corrected within the first few months of life. Where there is a question of head molding rather than true synostosis (*e.g.*, unilateral occipital flattening) the physician may wish to temporize while positioning measures are tried. Such decisions should generally be made in consultation with a pediatric neurosurgeon. The child's appearance may worsen as he grows, necessitating more complex procedures.

Operating on a newborn is not necessary; deferring the procedure until the infant is 6 weeks of age allows for a larger blood volume and less anesthetic risk.

The surgical procedures currently performed involve an excision of the fused suture (strip craniectomy) sometimes with morcellation of the abnormally shaped bone. The correction of more complex fusions may involve the manipulation of a larger bone fragment such as supraorbital ridges. Surgical complications include the risk of excessive bleeding, a dural tear with resulting CSF leak and a "growing skull defect," and the ongoing risks of infection and anesthesia. Postoperatively, the child needs to be observed closely for 1 to 2 days for a continued drop in hematocrit. Significant scalp and facial edema are common for 3 to 5 days.

INDICATIONS FOR REFERRAL

The craniosynostoses are often diagnosed by the pediatrician during the newborn or well-baby examination. The parents should be informed that the deformity in simple fusions is primarily cosmetic and that the risk of intracranial hypertension is small. Reconstructive surgery can be performed at the appropriate time if the appearance is objectionable. Early neurosurgical referral is appropriate in any suspected case.

ANNOTATED BIBLIOGRAPHY

Anderson F, Geiger L: Craniosynostosis—A survey of 204 cases. J Neurosurg 22:229–240, 1965 (One of the largest early series.)

Davis CH, Alexander E, Kelly D: Treatment of craniosynostosis. J Neurosurg 30:630–636, 1969 (Description of surgical procedures for sagittal, coronal, and multiple synostosis.)

Mohr G, Hoffman H, Munro I et al: Surgical management of unilateral and bilateral coronal craniosynostosis: 21 years of experience. Neurosurg 2:83–92, 1978 (Series of 116 patients presented from the Hospital for Sick Children, Toronto.)

Moss ML: Functional anatomy of cranial synostosis. Child's Brain 1:22–33, 1975 (Describes a theory of the pathophysiology of craniosynostosis relating sutural fusion to changes in the skull base.)

Renier D, Saint–Rose C, Marchac D, Hirsch J: Intracranial pressure in craniostenosis. J Neurosurg 57:370–377, 1982 (The authors employed an epidural sensor to monitor ICP in 92 cases of craniosynostosis. ICP was found to be normal in one third, borderline in one third, and abnormal in one third, with elevations primarily in those cases of multiple fusions. A correlation was found between ICP and mental ability.)

Shillito J, Matson DD: Craniosynostosis: A review of 519 surgical patients. Pediatrics 41:829–853, 1968 (Review of the Boston Children's Hospital experience stressing the importance of early surgery.)

Whittle I, Johnston I, Besser M: Intracranial pressure changes in craniostenosis. Surg Neurol 21:367–372, 1984 (The authors propose continuous ICP monitoring as an adjunct to decide the indications for surgical therapy. Of their 20 patients, 35% (7 of out 20) had associated hydrocephalus, and 15 out of 20 had multiple sutural fusions or complex deformities.)

154
Ptosis
ELIZABETH C. DOOLING

Ptosis is defined as drooping of the upper eyelid. It may be classified as:

1. Hereditary
   a. Congenital (present at birth)
   b. Noncongenital
2. Congenital, nonhereditary
   a. Unilateral—? due to birth injury
   b. Bilateral—isolated; associated with other defects, *e.g.*, Turner's syndrome
3. Acquired
   a. Local or systemic disease—recurrent infection, *e.g.*, diphtheria, trachoma, botulism
   b. Neurologic—oculomotor or sympathetic nerve palsy
   c. Trauma
   d. Toxins—drugs, *e.g.*, morphine, cocaine

PATHOPHYSIOLOGY

Ptosis is caused by a defect in, or paralysis of, the superior levator palpebrae muscle which is innervated by the superior division of the third cranial nerve, or less commonly, by a defect in, or paralysis of, Muller's muscle which is innervated by the cervical sympathetic system. Ptosis may result from lesions at various levels in the nervous system from the cerebral cortex to the levator muscle. Unilateral ptosis caused by a hemispheric lesion without associated partial herniation is rare. Mild bilateral ptosis may occur with frontal lobe lesions. Lesions of the levator portion or caudal end of the third nerve nucleus may produce a severe, symmetric ptosis. Lesions of the peripheral third nerve are usually unilateral and are often associated with mydriasis and extraocular muscle weakness. Mechanical disruptions such as penetrating orbital injuries, fractures, or operative procedures in the posterior superior area of the orbit may cause isolated ptosis. Congenital absence of a third nerve branch to the levator muscle may occur. Sympathetic nerve lesions may produce a partial unilateral ptosis as in Horner's syndrome. Ptosis due to a lesion of the neuromuscular apparatus is usually associated with clinical evidence of involvement of other muscles, including the ocular muscles, the orbicularis oculi, facial muscle, or skeletal muscles. *Pseudoptosis* is a term describing ptosis resulting from inflammation, hemorrhage, swelling, infiltration, or other mechanical barriers to lid elevation.

CLINICAL PRESENTATION

The child with congenital ptosis usually presents with bilateral drooping lids that cover the pupils. There may be associated paralysis of the superior rectus muscles or of all the ocular muscles supplied by the third nerve. When ptosis is hereditary, it is often associated with epicanthus (a fold of skin extending vertically downward from the inner end of the brow to the side of the upper part of the nose) and other defects. Some forms of hereditary ptosis are not obvious at birth but appear later in life. Acquired ptosis is usually unilateral and neurogenic in origin, but may be related to trauma to the eyelids or levator muscle or to focal infection. When other muscles innervated by the third nerve are involved in addition to the superior levator palpebrae, the child may not be able to rotate the eye upward, downward, or medially, and he may have difficulty reading because of mydriasis and weakness of accommodation. When ptosis results from paralysis or injury of the sympathetic nerve in the neck, it is part of the triad of Horner's syndrome that includes ptosis (due to paralysis of Muller's tarsal muscle rather than the superior levator palpebrae), a constricted pupil and slight enophthalmos. Patients with bilateral ptosis not only have upper eyelid droop but also have an exaggeration of the forehead wrinkles and elevation of the eyebrows as a result of their efforts to lift the eyelids by contracting the frontalis muscles. They may throw their heads back to try to see better under their lowered lids.

The course of ptosis varies. Congenital nonhereditary forms are usually nonprogressive whereas hereditary forms generally are slowly progressive. Some acquired diseases are progressive; however, ptosis due to injury may improve partially or completely.

Ptosis is part of the uncommon jaw-winking phenomenon of Marcus Gunn. The eyelid will be raised when an infant sucks or a child opens the jaw maximally or moves the jaw from side to side. The disorder is attributed to anomalous pterygoid-lingual-levator innervations that make the levator hypofunctional unless the jaw or tongue muscles are contracted.

DIFFERENTIAL DIAGNOSIS

The differential diagnosis of unilateral ptosis includes a contralateral facial weakness that causes a widening of the opposite palpebral fissure; myasthenia gravis; encephalitis; neurofibromas of the eyelid; neoplasms of the temporal lobe, midbrain, sella, or base of brain; diabetic ischemic neuropathy; demyelinating disease; trauma and infection.

Myotonic dystrophy should be considered if ptosis is bilateral. If bilateral ptosis is progressive and nonhereditary, mitochondrial myopathies such as Kearns—Sayre syndrome or congenital fiber-type disproportion should be excluded (by muscle biopsy).

WORK-UP

History

The key points to establish are: present at birth *vs* apparent later in life; static *vs* progressive (check old photographs); unilateral *vs* bilateral; change with exercise or fatigue; associated with other anomalies or third nerve dysfunction; incidence in relatives.

Physical Examination

The following observations should be emphasized during the complete physical examination: an inspection of the eyelids for discharge, redness, or evidence of infection; an assessment of oculomotor, trochlear, and abducens nerve functions in each eye; an inspection of the face and facial movements, gag, swallowing, chewing, voice quality, handling of saliva, and bulk, alignment, and motility of the tongue. The muscle strength and tone and tendon reflexes should be checked. The skin should be checked for hemangiomas of the face and café-au-lait spots.

Laboratory Tests

No testing may be necessary in the cases of congenital unilateral, nonprogressive ptosis. When a congenital myopathy or dystrophy is suspected, muscle enzymes and electromyography will be helpful. A contrast-enhanced CT scan may exclude a mass lesion. Blood sugar and urinalysis should be obtained if diabetes may be an underlying cause.

MANAGEMENT AND TREATMENT

Children in whom ptosis obstructs vision should have surgery to prevent amblyopia due to a lack of use of the ptotic eye. A child with acquired unilateral or bilateral ptosis without a history of trauma to, or infection of, the eye should be tested with Tensilon or edrophonium chloride, 1 mg ≤ 75 lb, 2 mg ≥ 75 lb injected slowly intravenously. An obvious decrease in ptosis should be evident within 30 seconds and persist for 3 to 4 minutes. Alternatively, prostigmin or neostigmine, 0.75 mg, can be injected intramuscularly and should produce an elevation of the eyelid within 20 to 30 seconds. An EMG of extraocular muscles may be diagnostic. There is a progressive fallout or tiring as the muscle fatigues after a few voluntary contractions of the involved muscles. No improvement of ptosis occurs if the patient has myotonic dystrophy, a mitochondrial myopathy, traumatic or infectious process, or hereditary disorder. When the clinical findings are consistent with Horner's syndrome, it is appropriate to instil one drop of 10% phenylephrine into the affected eye. The pupil will dilate dramatically and the ptosis will be eliminated within 15 minutes.

INDICATIONS FOR REFERRAL OR ADMISSION

A referral to an ophthalmologist is indicated when the ptosis is so severe that vision is obscured, and there is a potential for loss of functional vision in the eye(s) with ptosis. If other muscles innervated by the third nerve are affected and strabismus is present, surgical correction can be performed concomitantly. A referral to a neurologist is indicated for an initial evaluation and treatment of myasthenia gravis, a myopathy, or a dystrophy.

ANNOTATED BIBLIOGRAPHY

Liebman SD, Gellis SD (eds): The Pediatrician's Ophthalmology, pp 182–184. St. Louis, CV Mosby, 1966 (Basic introduction to eye pathology in children.)

Miller NR: Walsh and Hoyt's Clinical Neuro-ophthalmology, pp 936–945. Baltimore, Williams & Wilkins, 1985 (Comprehensive discussion of the pathogenesis of ptosis.)

Swaiman KF, Wright FS: The Practice of Pediatric Neurology, pp 62–65. St. Louis, CV Mosby, 1982 (Excellent description of normal and abnormal eyelid innervation and function in children.)

155
Nystagmus
ELIZABETH C. DOOLING

Nystagmus designates involuntary rhythmic oscillating movements of one or both eyeballs and may occur on vertical or horizontal gaze or in both directions. It is defined by the direction of its fast component and may be rotatory, horizontal, vertical, oblique, or mixed. It may be classified as congenital or acquired and as physiologic or pathologic.

PATHOPHYSIOLOGY

Physiologic

Nystagmus can be induced in normal individuals with certain stimuli. *Voluntary* nystagmus consisting of rapid, low-amplitude, conjugate, pendular eye movements represents an exaggeration of the normal saccadic eye movements. It is likely to be seen in hysterical patients who may complain of diplopia. *Opticokinetic* nystagmus (OKN) is elicited by moving a series of objects (on a drum or strip of cloth) from side to side or up and down in front of the patient. The slow component results from following the objects out of the field of vision and an opposite fast component that results from fixating on the succeeding object. OKN is usually equal in both directions. *Vestibular* nystagmus is obtained by stimulating the semicircular canals by rotation of the patient or irrigation of the ear canal (if the drum is intact) with warm or cold water (caloric testing). *Terminal* nystagmus results at the extremes of horizontal gaze when the testing object is moved out of the patient's binocular field of vision. It is more obvious in the abducting eye, and the fast component is in the direction of the patient's gaze.

Pathologic

These types of nystagmus result from a dysfunction of normal mechanisms of ocular control of fixation and gaze, and also from vestibular dysfunction. If a child develops a severe visual defect interfering with fixation before 6 years of age (*e.g.*, from trauma, infection, tumor, or a congenital disorder such as cataracts, glaucoma, albinism, or retrolental fibroplasia), pendular nystagmus, more marked when fixation is attempted, may occur. If the visual deficit is acquired after 6 years of age, such nystagmus does not develop. Diseases of the labyrinth from ototoxic drugs such as gentamicin, the vestibular portion of the eighth cranial nerve, or the pontine vestibular nuclei will produce nystagmus. Nystagmus of vestibular origin is usually jerky. Labyrinthine and eighth nerve lesions produce a rotatory nystagmus. Disorders of gaze mechanisms most commonly result from toxic levels of phenytoin, barbiturates, tranquilizers, or antihistamines. Cerebellar and brain stem tumors, infections, and demyelinating or vascular diseases occur less frequently as the cause of gaze palsies.

CLINICAL PRESENTATION

The child with nystagmus may have ocular instability at rest or with intentional movement of the eyes. The younger child may be noted to have difficulty in fixating on faces or toys; poor visual acuity may be suspected and detected. The older child may complain of blurred vision or nausea. The child's schoolwork may deteriorate, and he may be less steady when walking or riding a tricycle or bicycle. Head tilt to one side to avoid diplopia may be noted. A child with a brain stem or cerebellar mass lesion may appear to have developed a squint, which actually represents a sixth nerve palsy from mass effect or infiltration. Disorders of gaze may precede other signs of increased intracranial pressure such as drowsiness, vomiting, lethargy, personality, or gait changes.

DIFFERENTIAL DIAGNOSIS

Congenital

Dominant
X-linked dominant or recessive

Pendular or *sensory defect nystagmus* is due to structural abnormalities that affect central vision.

Albinism
Aniridia
Cataracts
Glaucoma
Bilateral macular defects
Neonatal myasthenia gravis
Retrolental fibroplasia
Total color blindness
Arnold–Chiari malformation

Acquired

Spasmus nutans associated with head nodding and head tilt starts by 18 months of age and disappears by 3 years of age. This pendular nystagmus does not persist in sleep. On rare occasions spasmus nutans has been associated with hypothalamic tumors.

Drug intoxication
  Phenytoin
  Barbiturates
  Tranquilizers including benzodiazepines
  Antihistaminics
  Alcohol
  Aminoglycosides
  Dihydrostreptomycin
Viral mesencephalitis or encephalitis
Cerebellar or brain stem tumors including medulloblastoma, glioma, ependymoma, acoustic neuroma
Hypothalamic or diencephalic tumors including hamartoma, glioma, craniopharyngioma
Myasthenia gravis
Botulism

WORK-UP

History

The onset of the ocular motor disturbance must be determined as accurately as possible. Contributing factors must be ascertained such as prematurity, associated somatic abnormalities such as Sturge–Weber syndrome, and glaucoma due to buphthalmos, Wilms' tumor and aniridia, storage disease of the mucopolysaccharide type, and a family history of similar defects. The physician must ascertain if there is a history of treatment of seizures, allergies, or psychiatric disease.

Physical Examination

The child's eyes must be examined carefully, and the color of the irides, the opacity of the cornea and lens, and the size of the eyes should be noted. The type of nystagmus should be described: pendular, jerky, rotatory, horizontal, vertical, latent (a jerk horizontal nystagmus present only if one eye is covered), monocular, or binocular. Other signs of neurologic disability should be sought such as hearing defects, disequilibrium or ataxia to indicate vestibular dysfunction, and level of consciousness, respiratory status, and pupil size in a patient with suspected drug intoxication.

Laboratory Tests

Drug screening of blood and urine should be obtained in an afebrile child with acutely acquired nystagmus. If the child is febrile or has had an infectious contact, an examination of the cerebrospinal fluid should be made to assess encephalitis or mesencephalitis. Formal hearing tests should be obtained if a history of the use of ototoxic drugs is obtained. A CT scan with contrast may show a mass lesion in the posterior fossa, optic tracts, or optic chiasm.

MANAGEMENT AND REFERRAL

The infant who has congenital nystagmus should be examined by an ophthalmologist. A pediatric neurologic assessment should be obtained if there is any associated developmental problem that is suspected or apparent.

ANNOTATED BIBLIOGRAPHY

Cogan DG: Neurology of the Ocular Muscles, pp 184–226. Springfield, IL, CC Thomas, 1956 (Comprehensive discussion of abnormal eye movements in children.)

Liebman SD, Gellis SD (eds): The Pediatrician's Ophthalmology, pp 190–192. St. Louis, CV Mosby, 1966 (Introduction to eye pathology in children.)

Swaiman KF, Wright FS: The Practice of Pediatric Neurology, pp 65–68. St. Louis, CV Mosby, 1982 (Excellent description of ocular motility disorders in children.)

PATHOPHYSIOLOGY

Ataxia may be defined as incoordination of movement. It is associated with a dysfunction or disease of the cerebellum, although it may also result from a disease of afferent systems (sensory ataxia).

Ataxia appears in different guises in different systems: appendicular or limb ataxia, as demonstrated by tremor and dysmetria in finger-to-nose testing; truncal ataxia (with inability to support the trunk stably when sitting); and gait ataxia (inability to walk with a narrow base, as in tandem walking). Truncal and gait ataxia may be called *axial ataxia* and result from midline cerebellar disease, as opposed to *appendicular ataxia* (affecting the appendages or limbs) resulting from disease of the ipsilateral cerebellar hemisphere. Ataxia is commonly accompanied by dysarthria or nystagmus, which may be considered as ataxia of buccolingual function and of gaze mechanisms, respectively. Ataxia of sensory (afferent) systems, either peripheral nerves or dorsal columns of the spinal cord, has a dysmetric wavering quality; that associated with cerebellar outflow systems may approximate myoclonus or chorea.

Ataxia must be differentiated from chorea, which has a more writhing or dancing and quasi-purposeful or organized character; and from myoclonus or polymyoclonus, which consists of brief irregular jerky muscle movements. Weakness may simulate ataxia, whether caused by muscle disease, Guillain–Barré idiopathic polyneuropathy, or disease of cerebral hemispheres. Finally, vestibular or brain stem disease may cause dysequilibrium that simulates ataxia.

Ataxia is classified conveniently into acute, intermittent, and chronic forms. Acute ataxia is a common response of the young nervous system to many insults, especially toxic, metabolic, infectious, or epileptic. Thus, ataxia often appears before other specific neurologic dysfunctions become apparent in acute illness. Chronic ataxia presents a different clinical problem. If progressive, it is usually caused by genetic, metabolic, or degenerative systems diseases. Stable chronic ataxia may be the result of congenital encephalopathy (ataxic cerebral palsy) or brain injury (head trauma or hypoxic–ischemic insult).

Acute ataxia is a relatively common pediatric problem. Many acute ataxias will resolve spontaneously or after the withdrawal of the offending agent. Others may signal major problems other than ataxia, such as brain tumors, neuroblastoma, or metabolic disease.

CLINICAL PRESENTATION

The typical presentation of acute ataxia with unstable, veering, wide-based gait, falling, and wavering unsteadiness of arm movements will not be mistaken. On more careful examination, dysarthria and nystagmus may be evident. Other presentations in young children may be less obvious, however, and may cause ataxia to be overlooked. Toddlers with severe acute ataxia may refuse to attempt to walk or sit up, as may the child with associated lethargy, obtundation, or increased intracranial pressure. Children with posterior fossa tumors with incipient herniation may assume a fixed position (*e.g.*, prone in bed with the head turned to one side), refusing to move, thus masking ataxia. Truncal or axial ataxia may give no clue to its presence in a child examined lying in bed; it is necessary to have the child attempt to sit, stand, and walk to reveal the ataxia. Similarly, ataxia is difficult to demonstrate in a young infant until he can sit or stand holding on. Children who have brain tumors or increased intracranial pressure may have intermittent ataxia; thus, a parent's report describing ataxia should not be dismissed if the examiner finds a normal examination at first.

Chronic ataxia presents in two forms: nonprogressive and progressive. Nonprogressive ataxia may be present from early life, if caused by congenital encephalopathy or cerebral palsy; or it may be the late residual of a known insult such as a head injury or hypoxic-ischemic, or rarely hyperthermic, insult. The distinction between a stable and progressive ataxia may occasionally be obscure until the course unfolds over time. Progressive ataxia may be divided into those conditions with known genetic biochemical disorders (*e.g.*, metachromatic leukodystrophy, presenting usually in the second year, is a typical example) and those system degenerations with obscure causes (*e.g.*, the hereditary ataxias typified by Friedreich's ataxia, which has an insidious onset during the first decade).

DIFFERENTIAL DIAGNOSIS

Acute Ataxia

Acute ataxia is commonly encountered in the child as a secondary or incidental consequence of a known disease process. The commonest examples may be ataxia from excessive levels of medications, especially anticonvulsants; ataxia following seizures, especially minor motor, in the young child; ataxia following meningitis; and ataxia in the older child or adolescent from an overdose of drugs or alcohol.

Ataxia is a prominent symptom of many intoxicants, including drugs (*e.g.*, anticonvulsants, tranquilizers, sedatives, rarely lithium). The effects of these are self-limited and reversible. (Exceptions are rare intoxications with heavy metals such as organic mercury and thallium, which may have severe permanent residua.)

The most characteristic acute ataxia of childhood is acute parainfectious cerebellar ataxia, a form of parainfectious encephalomyelitis associated with patchy central nervous system demyelination. Manifestations may be essentially limited to cerebellar functions, as in the familiar postvaricella cerebellitis; or additional cerebral hemisphere, brain stem, and spinal cord involvement may occur. Severe or subacutely evolving cases may be associated with increased intracranial pressure, and a CT scan may demonstrate cerebellar swelling.

A syndrome presenting as postinfectious ataxia may be produced occasionally by a mild or slowly evolving postinfectious polyneuropathy (Guillain–Barré). This occurs in young children who cannot report sensory symptoms reliably and in whom weakness is minimal for a time.

Severe acute cerebellar encephalopathy may result in a rare syndrome of polymyoclonus and opsoclonus, which may be considered as a severe form of cerebellar ataxia. This striking syndrome, which has been called *myoclonic encephalopathy* or *dancing eyes, dancing feet* syndrome, is seen under three circumstances: (1) associated with neuroblastoma, which may be inapparent at the time the patient is first seen; (2) as a form of congenital encephalopathy; (3) in older children in relation to an acute viral illness. In such cases, it may be equivalent to severe acute parainfectious cerebellar ataxia.

Tumors of the posterior fossa must be considered in every case with the recent onset of ataxia. Papilledema, a history of headache or vomiting, or head tilt indicates a posterior fossa tumor. Sixth nerve palsy or hemiparesis suggests a brain stem tumor (pontine glioma). A posterior fossa cyst or hematoma, angioma, or Arnold–Chiari malformation occasionally presents acute or intermittent ataxia.

A basilar migraine may cause acute ataxia. It typically presents as a florid syndrome with headache, drowsiness, visual symptoms and brain stem signs and should be differentiated from a hemorrhage or other major structural disease.

Several metabolic disorders may cause an intermittent cerebellar ataxia, which is often precipitated acutely by an infectious illness and which sometimes progresses to a stupor or coma. Reye's syndrome may be an example of such a process, although the ataxic stage is brief and inconspicuous. Conditions producing such intermittent metabolic ataxias include amino acid disorders, urea cycle disorders with hyperammonemia, organic acidoses, and disorders of lactate and pyruvate metabolism. Suspected cases of recurrent metabolic ataxia should be carefully evaluated with studies of serum electrolytes, acid-base status, glucose, ammonia, lactate, pyruvate, and ketones. More specific metabolic studies should then include amino acids and organic acids. Reports describe intermittent cerebellar ataxia in an inherited biotinidase deficiency resulting in multiple carboxylase deficiencies. Affected children show immunologic defects, rash, frequent infections, acute intermittent ataxia, and lactic acidosis. The clinical manifestations are improved by pharmacologic doses of biotin. There have been rare reports of kindreds with paroxysmal intermittent ataxia without identified metabolic basis, with autosomal dominant inheritance. In one such family, attacks were completely prevented by treatment with acetazolamide.

A thiamine deficiency is an unusual cause of acute ataxia and nystagmus in children. It may occur in children with chronic illness receiving long-term intravenous therapy in which vitamin supplementation had been neglected. There is a prompt, although not always total, response to thiamine administration.

Chronic and Progressive Ataxia

Chronic progressive ataxia constitutes a different problem from that of acute ataxia. Several rare disease entities will be considered by the neurologist. Their elucidation requires a detailed clinical examination, family history, or search for specific enzymatic or metabolic disorders. The system's degenerations (spinocerebellar degeneration) may present, in addition to ataxia, some combination of spasticity, peripheral nerve disease, ocular disease, and dementia. Friedreich's ataxia, the prototype of this group, is an autosomal recessive disorder with an onset in the first decade, with ataxia, areflexia, pes cavus, and variable mental changes and heart disease. Ataxia telangiectasia has the onset of ataxia in the first 3 years of life, and later there are oculocutaneous telangiectases and sinopulmonary infections. Some neurologic degenerative and storage diseases with known biochemical disorders may present with progressive ataxia; these include Wilson's disease and some lipid storage disorders.

Vitamin E deficiency may produce ataxia, in addition to acanthocytosis, neuropathy, retinitis pigmentosa, spinal cord degeneration, and ataxia. This condition, caused by steatorrhea or liver disease with impairment of vitamin E absorption, may be halted or reversed by adequate administration of vitamin E.

WORK-UP

History

The history should elucidate the following: duration; onset; previous occurrences; drug or toxin ingestion or exposure; infection; seizures; head injury; hypoxic–ischemic or hyperthermic episode; family history; migraine; chronic illness (*e.g.*, steatorrhea, vitamin deficiency).

Physical Examination

A complete examination should be performed and particularly important aspects of the physical examination should include gait; sitting posture; arm and leg coordination (finger–nose, heel–knee shin, rapid alternating movements; looking for intention tremor, dysdiadochokinesia, dysmetria, decomposition of movements); hypotonia, decreased tendon reflexes; scanning dysarthria; nystagmus; papilledema, neck stiffness; head tilt; other neurologic abnormalities; spasticity; hemiparesis; Babinski reflexes; areflexia; weakness; obtundation; stupor; sensory deficits; hearing; retinopathy; and cranial nerves. Breath odor (*e.g.*, alcohol, ketosis, musty); somatic anomalies such as shelved posterior skull, oculocutaneous telangiectasias, and pes cavus should also be noted.

Laboratory Tests

A complete blood count (CBC), urinalysis, electrolytes, bicarbonate, BUN, blood sugar, and ammonia should usually be included in the initial laboratory evaluation of acute ataxia. Lactate, pyruvate, toxic screen, amino acids, organic acid screen, anticonvulsant levels, and EEG are ordered as indicated. Lumbar puncture should be considered if there is no papilledema. A CT scan is indicated in any patient with acute cerebellar ataxia except if a toxic or metabolic cause is suspected and ataxia promptly resolves after the cause is corrected.

In addition, for chronic progressive ataxia, obtain ceruloplasmin, immunoglobulins, vitamin E, arylsulfatase, phytanic acid, lipoprotein electrophoresis, and hexosaminidase.

TREATMENT AND MANAGEMENT

An understanding of etiology—and thus differential diagnosis—is essential for the consideration of treatment. No specific treatment for ataxia as such exists in most cases. Many acute ataxias are self-limited or will resolve after the removal of the offending agent such as a drug or toxin. Some will prove to be major problems other than ataxia (*e.g.*, brain tumor).

The question of treatment often arises in cases of parainfectious encephalomyelitis, in which the use of corticosteriods may be beneficial (dexamethasone 0.5 mg/kg/day for 7 to 10 days) and should probably be used in severe or subacutely evolving cases. With increased intracranial pressure, corticosteroids and possibly mannitol are urgently indicated. In the *dancing eyes, dancing feet* polymyoclonus syndrome, the movement disorder may respond well to ACTH. (A vigorous search for neuroblastoma should also be made.)

Epilepsy may be associated with ataxia in the young child, especially with minor motor seizures, as an ictal or postictal phenomenon. Proper treatment of the seizure disorder with valproate or clonazepam is indicated. Excess levels of anticonvulsants, of course, may also cause ataxia in the setting of epilepsy.

No useful neuropharmacologic treatment exists for ataxia. Specific agents may be useful in certain instances, such as in the treatment of thiamine deficiency or in the use of biotin in biotinidase deficiency. A discussion of the management of the rare metabolic disorders that produce ataxia is beyond the scope of this article. In established severe ataxia, the device of using weights on the wrists or ankles to reduce the amplitude of movements may afford benefit to some patients.

INDICATIONS FOR REFERRAL OR ADMISSION

It is easier to state the indications for not referring or admitting a child with acute ataxia: If the cause is evident and is self-limited, such as a medication overdose, or a postictal ataxia in a child with a known seizure disorder, or a mild postinfectious ataxia. Hospitalization is indicated when the diagnosis is uncertain, or ataxia is severe or associated with other symptoms. A neurologic or neurosurgical consultation should be obtained.

ANNOTATED BIBLIOGRAPHY

Bray PF, Ziter FA, Lahey ME, Myers GG: The coincidence of neuroblastoma and acute cerebellar encephalopathy. J Pediatr 75:983–990, 1969 (Description of neuroblastoma-associated cerebellar disease.)

Menkes JH: Textbook of Child Neurology, 2nd ed. Philadelphia, Lea & Febiger, 1980 (Standard reference.)

Pasternak JF, DeVivo DC, Prensky AL: Steroid-responsive encephalomyelitis in childhood. Neurology 30:481–486, 1980 (Good discussion of encephalomyelitis.)

Rowland L: Molecular genetics, pseudogenetics and clinical neurology. The Robert Wartenberg lecture. Neurology 33:1179–1195, 1983 (Best listing of metabolic diagnostic considerations in ataxia.)

Salam M: Metabolic ataxias. Handbook of Clinical Neurology. Vol 21: System Disorders and Atrophies, pp 573–585. New York, Elsevier, 1975 (Puts the metabolic ataxias in clinical perspective.)

Weiss S, Carter S: Course and prognosis of acute cerebellar ataxia in children. Neurology 9:711–721, 1959 (Classical clinical description of this entity.)

Weiss S, Guberman A: Acute cerebellar ataxia in infectious disease. In Vinken PJ, Bryn GW (eds): Handbook of Clinical Neurology, Vol 34, p 619. Amsterdam, North–Holland, 1978 (Comprehensive discussion of causes of ataxia in this group.)

157
Febrile Seizures

EILEEN M. OUELLETTE

Febrile seizures are defined as an event in infancy or childhood, usually occurring between 3 months and 5 years of age, which is associated with a fever but without evidence of intracranial infection or a defined cause. It is estimated that one half million children in the United States have had febrile seizures. By 5 years of age, 2% to 4.2% of children have had febrile seizures. Although most studies report that boys have a higher incidence of febrile seizures than girls, two longitudinal studies have reported no sex differences.

Younger children are more likely to have a febrile seizure: 1% to 2% are below 6 months of age; 50% are less than 2 years of age; 90% are less than 3 years of age at the time of the first febrile seizure. One to 6% of first febrile seizures occur after 5 years of age. The recurrence rate varies with age and sex, but it is generally about 33%.

PATHOPHYSIOLOGY

There is often a positive family history with febrile seizures of all types. A simple autosomal dominant inheritance with incomplete penetrance is postulated as the form of transmission.

The control of body heat depends on the integrity of the anterior hypothalamus and preoptic area (AH/POA) which contain temperature–sensitive neurons. With infection, bacterial products, known as *exogenous pyrogens* (EP) activate phagocytic leukocytes. When released into the bloodstream and cerebral ventricular system, they exert an effect on the anterior hypothalamus that results in fever. Interactions between viruses and monocytes also result in the release of EP. EP are a variety of chemicals that act as mediator substances in the production of fever and they are not believed to be normal products of thermal regulation.

Neurotransmitters of the cholinergic and monoaminergic systems are also important in temperature regulation. The fever process is also mediated in part by the release of a prostaglandin of the E series into the tissue of the brain.

Seizures are thought to be produced by the effects of neurochemicals involved in the production of fever acting on other parts of the brain; however, evidence for this hypothesis is lacking.

Clinical Presentation

The source of the fever must lie outside the central nervous system in order for a seizure to be classified as a febrile seizure. Therefore, seizures in children with meningitis, encephalitis, lead encephalopathy, seizures after immunization, or associated with marked dehydration are not considered febrile seizures, although a fever may be present.

Febrile seizures are of two types: (1) *Simple febrile seizures* are brief, lasting less than 15 minutes and generalized. Only one seizure occurs with each febrile illness. (2) *Complex febrile seizures* are prolonged, focal, or multiple within each febrile episode. Most febrile seizures occur early in the febrile illness and are often the first sign that a child is ill. They occur generally within the first 6 hours and rarely occur later than 24 hours after the onset of fever.

Most febrile seizures are simple and brief. Forty percent last less than 5 minutes; 75% last under 30 minutes; only 2% last more than 1 hour. Seizures that last longer that 30 minutes are called *febrile status epilepticus* and they carry the same risks as afebrile status epilepticus. One percent of febrile seizures occur below the age of 6 months or after 6 years. The peak age for a first febrile seizure is 13 months. The overall recurrence rate is 33%, but is higher if the first seizure occurs before 13 months of age. Prolonged seizures are more common in children under 18 months of age and in girls. About 15% are focal and 16% of children have more than 1 seizure in 24 hours.

Many children experience a postictal state of obtundation or sleep for several hours after a seizure. Focal signs, such as hyperreflexia or an extensor plantar response, may be present.

DIFFERENTIAL DIAGNOSIS

Two considerations are important in the differential diagnosis of febrile seizures: (1) to exclude disease of the central nervous system as a cause of the seizure, and (2) to determine the cause of the fever.

Bacterial and viral meningitis, encephalitis, Reye's syndrome, acute hemiplegia of infancy, and intracranial hemorrhage are all acute disorders of the central nervous system that may present with fever and seizures. More chronic diseases of the central nervous system may be manifested initially with a seizure in the context of a febrile illness. These diseases include neonatal hypoxia, congenital infections such as cytomegalovirus and toxoplasmosis, chronic subdural effusions, tuberous sclerosis, porencephaly, and other developmental defects of the brain.

Most febrile seizures are associated with common infections of childhood: pharyngitis, otitis, tonsillitis, and diarrhea. Bronchitis, pneumonia, and pyuria are less common, but are also associated with febrile seizures. Fifteen percent of children with pyuria under 5 years of age have febrile seizures. Metabolic disorders, which include hypoglycemia, hypocalcemia, hyponatremia, other electrolyte disturbances, and renal disease, must also be considered. Roseola and shigella infections have a particularly high association with febrile seizures, probably as a result of the very high fevers that occur with roseola and secondary to an endotoxin associated with shigella infections.

WORK-UP

History

Historical information should include a description of the seizure (*e.g.*, type, duration, and possible focal component). Parents generally find seizures frightening and tend to overestimate their duration. Many parents also include the postictal state in their timing of the seizure; therefore, specific questions about the actual events witnessed are important. Many parents do not witness the onset of the seizure, thus the presence of a focal component cannot be firmly established. A history of the pregnancy, perinatal period, and a developmental history of the child should be obtained to assess whether a prior neurologic abnormality was present. A history of possible trauma should be sought. A family history of seizures, both febrile and afebrile, should also be obtained.

Physical Examination

A complete general physical and neurologic examination should be performed. Signs of increased intracranial pressure should be sought by an evaluation of the level of alertness, a funduscopic examination, and the fullness of the fontanel, when appropriate. Nuchal rigidity may indicate meningitis or intracranial hemorrhage, but its absence does not preclude these diagnoses, particularly in children under 2 years of age. Focal neurologic signs should be noted. Cranial auscultation for bruits is important in diagnosing vascular malformations. In infants, transillumination of the skull may lead to the diagnosis of chronic subdural effusions, porencephaly, or other brain malformations. The skin should be examined for the presence of hypopigmented "ash-leaf spots" seen in tuberous sclerosis by observation and by carrying out a Wood's lamp examination.

Laboratory Tests

Cerebrospinal fluid (CSF) should be examined at the time of the first febrile seizure, and whenever meningitis cannot be ruled out, particularly in children under 2 years of age. In one study, 13% of 325 children with meningitis lacked meningeal signs, 50% of whom were found to have bacterial meningitis. Some children were over 2 years old. CSF pressure should be recorded and the fluid should be examined for bacteria, the number and types of cells, and the protein and glucose levels. Bacterial cultures should be obtained.

A simultaneous blood sugar should be obtained. CSF glucose should be one half to two thirds of blood glucose. Lower levels suggest meningitis or encephalitis. A white blood count and a differential count should be obtained. Serum calcium and electrolytes are often determined. Liver function tests and blood ammonia levels should be obtained when Reye's syndrome is a possibility.

Computerized tomography (CT) of the brain need not be routinely obtained. CT scans are indicated in the presence of increased intracranial pressure, focal symptoms or signs, a history of trauma, an abnormal neurologic examination, or persistent seizures.

Electroencephalograms (EEG) obtained during the acute febrile illness are inevitably abnormal and are generally not helpful, because either a fever or seizures produce slowing of the EEG for up to 10 days. Asymmetric or focal slowing may be present in the absence of a focal component to the seizure and is of little diagnostic or prognostic value. The EEG generally returns to normal 10 days after a simple febrile seizure. Persistent slowing beyond that time may be helpful in distinguishing simple from complex febrile seizures when the history is not clear or when the seizure was not witnessed.

TREATMENT AND MANAGEMENT

Acute treatment consists of a reduction of fever, treatment of the underlying cause of the fever, and treatment of the seizure(s). Elevated temperatures can be reduced by antipyretics and sponging. The cause of the fever should be treated appropriately. During the seizure, an adequate airway must be maintained and the child should be placed in a semi-prone position to reduce the risk of aspiration.

Acute anticonvulsant therapy should be given intravenously (IV) to a child who is actively seizing. Phenobarbital in a loading dose of up to 15 mg/kg of body weight can be given slowly IV. Oral phenobarbital can then be given in a dose of 3 to 6 mg/kg/24 hours while the child remains febrile. Giving oral phenobarbital without an IV loading dose is ineffective, because it requires several days to achieve a therapeutic blood level by this means.

An alternative regimen is to give diazepam IV, 0.3 mg/kg of body weight at a rate of 1 mg/minute. Both phenobarbital and diazepam are effective in stopping seizures. Diazepam acts more quickly but also wears off more quickly. It is not effective orally and cannot be used for maintenance therapy. Phenobarbital has the added advantage of having an antipyretic effect and can be used as maintenance therapy. Diazepam and phenobarbital should not be routinely used parenterally together because respiratory arrest may occur.

Long-term management of a single simple febrile seizure with continuous or intermittent anticonvulsant therapy is no longer advocated. Patients with pre-existing neurologic abnormalities or who have prolonged febrile seizures longer than 15 minutes, or whose families contain members with afebrile seizures, may be candidates for long-term therapy. Treatment is generally given for 2 years or 1 year after the last seizure, whichever is longer. The risk of recurrence of febrile seizures can be lessened with long-term continuous phenobarbital or valproic acid therapy. The long-term side effects of phenobarbital are unknown. Hepatic toxicity may occur with valproic acid treatment. These factors must be considered when assessing patients for long-term therapy.

The frequency of recurrent febrile seizures may be reduced with the prompt use of rectal diazepam at the onset of a febrile illness. Intermittent use of oral phenobarbital, however, has been shown to be ineffective in preventing febrile seizures because therapeutic levels of the drug are not achieved by this route for several days. An important preventive measure is to initiate prompt and vigorous fever control with antipyretics and sponging.

The prognosis for children with febrile seizures varies with the type of seizure and with the previous state of the child. Normal children with no history of febrile seizures have a risk of 0.9% of developing epilepsy by 7 years of age. Previously normal children with simple febrile seizures have a 1.1% to 2% risk of developing afebrile seizures by that age; if the seizure was complex, the risk is 1.7% to 3.5%. Children with a prior neurologic abnormality have a 2.8% to 3.1% risk of developing epilepsy by 7 years of age following simple febrile seizures and a 9.2% to 12.3% risk if the febrile seizure was complex.

INDICATIONS FOR REFERRAL OR ADMISSION

Children in whom central nervous system disorders cannot be excluded should be admitted to hospital. Children who have complex febrile seizures should generally be admitted to hospital to facilitate their evaluation and treatment. Children who have simple febrile seizures, whose cause of fever has been established and who have families who are competent to care for their illness, need not be admitted.

A consultation with a pediatric neurologist may be indicated for children who have abnormal neurologic examinations or when questions arise regarding diagnosis and treatment, particularly with reference to possible involvement of the central nervous system.

ANNOTATED BIBLIOGRAPHY

Consensus Statement, Conference on Febrile Seizures, NIH. Pediatrics 66:1009–1012, 1980 (Consensus statement of the significance, evaluation, and treatment of febrile seizures.)

Nelson KB, Ellenberg JH: Predictors of epilepsy in children who have experienced febrile seizures. N Engl J Med 295:1029–1033, 1976 (Comprehensive review of 1706 children with febrile seizures registered in the Collaborative Perinatal Project between 1959 and 1966.)

Nelson KB, Ellenberg JH: Prognosis in children with febrile seizures. Pediatrics 61:720–726, 1978. (Frequency of adverse outcomes and risk factors in 1706 children with febrile seizures registered in the Collaborative Perinatal Project between 1959 and 1966.)

Ouellette EM: The child who convulses with fever. Pediatr Clin North Amer 21:467–481, 1974 (Review article on febrile seizures.)

Ouellette EM: Febrile seizures. In Browne TR, Feldman RG, (eds): Epilepsy Diagnosis and Management, pp 315–323. Boston, Little, Brown, 1983 (Comprehensive review of febrile seizures, their pathophysiology, types, management, and prognosis.)

Verity CM, Butler NR, Golding J: Febrile convulsions in a national cohort followed up from birth. I: Prevalence and recurrence in the first five years of life. II: Medical history and intellectual ability at 5 years of age. Br Med J 290:1307–1315, 1985 (Report of an English series of 303 of 13,135 children followed from birth to 5 years.)

Wolf SM: Effectiveness of daily phenobarbital in the prevention of febrile seizure recurrences in "simple" febrile convulsions and "epilepsy triggered by fever." Epilepsia 18:95–99, 1977 (Report of the effectiveness of daily phenobarbital therapy on the recurrence rate of febrile seizures.)

Wolf SM et al: The value of phenobarbital in the child who has had a single febrile seizure: A controlled prospective study. Pediatrics 59:378–385, 1977 (Comparison of daily, intermittent and no long-term phenobarbital therapy on the recurrence rate of febrile seizures.)

158
Meningitis
ELIZABETH C. DOOLING

Meningitis results from an infectious process of bacterial, viral, fungal, parasitic, or protozoan origin that involves the meninges of the brain and the fluid within the spaces enclosed by the pia-arachnoid. The infection also reaches the cerebral ventricles either directly or by reflux through the foramina of the fourth ventricle. It may result from a blood-borne infection, a parameningeal infection, or dissemination from a sequestered focus such as an abscess or septic cerebral infarct. A high level of suspicion and prompt recognition, diagnosis, and initiation of treatment are mandatory in this disease because of its high morbidity and mortality.

This chapter is intended to present an overview on meningitis. Since a more detailed discussion is critical for its diagnosis and management (but beyond the scope of this book), the reader is encouraged to refer to a major textbook of pediatrics or infectious diseases for more specific "in-hospital" guidelines, especially with reference to characteristics of the cerebrospinal fluid (CSF) in the newborn and with infection, therapy, and short-term complications.

PATHOPHYSIOLOGY

In the newborn period, *group B streptococcus* and *E. coli* are the most common causes of meningitis. Unlike the older child, other gram-positive and negative organisms such as *Listeria monocytogenes*, Enterococcus, Klebsiella–aerobacter, *Staphylococcus aureus, Hemophilus influenzae*, and anaerobes must also be considered. Most cases of acute bacterial meningitis in children older than 2 months are caused by *H. influenzae* type b (~80%), meningococci, and pneumococci.

Organisms gain access into the central nervous system by direct hematogenous spread or by spread from a contiguous infected site in the cranium such as the ears, paranasal sinuses, an osteomyelitic focus in the skull, penetrating head injuries, or congenital sinus tracts in the neuraxis. The brain generally resists infections. The epidural and subdural spaces of the skull are resistant to hematogenous infections, but the spinal epidural spaces are more vulnerable. Blood-borne infections usually involve only one organism, whereas septic emboli from the lungs or sinuses, ears, or heart may include more than one organism. Hyperemia of the meningeal vessels is followed closely by a migration of neutrophils into the subarachnoid space. The subarachnoid exudate increases rapidly and extends over the base of the brain and into the sheaths of the cranial and spinal nerves, and, for a short distance, into the perivascular spaces of the cortex. Initially, polymorphs, often containing phagocytized bacteria, predominate; lymphocytes and histiocytes or macrophages become more dominant after a few days. Plasma cells subsequently appear and increase in number. In the early stages of meningitis, the ependyma and subependymal tissues are not very involved, but the subependymal perivascular spaces and tissues usually become infiltrated later in the course of the illness. The choroid plexus is initially congested but may also become covered with exudate. The presence of pus in the subarachnoid space incites an inflammatory response in the meninges and thus causes symptoms and signs similar to those caused by the presence of blood or neoplastic cells.

The neonate may become infected prenatally by transplacental infections or during passage through a purulent birth canal. A postnatal infection may be introduced through indwelling lines. In a child with congenital heart disease, especially cyanotic, or a child with valvular heart disease, seeding of infected mural or valvular vegetations may cause cerebral abscess formation. A meningitic illness results if the abscess ruptures and infective agents are distributed into the subarachnoid space or ventricular system. A parameningeal focus of infection may be caused by preceding or concurrent otitis media, sinusitis, or, less commonly, mastoiditis. CSF fistulas resulting from congenital malformations such as a sacral sinus or nasal encephalocele or trauma with dural tears may permit the introduction of pathogens. Children with sickle cell disease or postsplenectomy may be secondarily immunocompromised and may have increased susceptibility to pneumococcal infections.

CLINICAL PRESENTATION

A neonate may present with few of the classical symptoms and signs of infection. An infant who has had an intrauterine infection may have micro- or macrocephaly, rash, and hepatosplenomegaly. Lethargy, poor feeding, irritability, seizures, apnea and fever, or subnormal temperature may occur in the preterm or term infant. The infant may become ill shortly after birth in the first 24 to 48 hours or may develop symptoms and signs of sepsis after an apparently asymptomatic interval of 7 to 10 days. A baby who develops feeding or respiratory problems or becomes jaundiced without known blood incompatibility must be suspected of harboring an infection that may involve the central nervous system; a lumbar puncture must be performed.

The older infant may also present with a paucity of findings, but meningismus and a full fontanel may precede irritability, lethargy, poor feeding, vomiting, stupor or coma, and seizure. Either a low-grade fever or an elevated temperature may be present. Many children have a mild preceding respiratory illness or otitis media. In some cases, a fulminant course may be heralded by a febrile convulsion.

A young child may complain of a headache; he may develop a fever, vomiting, and meningismus; and he may be irritable, or drowsy and lethargic, confused, stuporous, or comatose. A focal or generalized convulsion may also occur. The older child usually complains of a headache; he has a stiff neck; he develops fever and vomiting; and he is hypersomnolent. He is reluctant to extend his legs fully because of meningeal irritation; thus, his gait may be affected.

DIFFERENTIAL DIAGNOSIS

The following conditions may produce a purulent CSF consistent with an infection confined to the meninges and must be considered carefully when evaluating the patient. A brain abscess, subdural empyema, or cerebral vasculitis due to septic arteritis, thrombophlebitis, or collagen-vascular disease may account for focal clinical findings such as a weakness or asymmetric pupil size and reactivity to light. A subarachnoid hemorrhage due to a ruptured vascular malformation or an aneurysm may cause a change in mental status, meningismus, and fever. A neoplasm may incidentally be accompanied by an infectious disorder. Recommended doses of phenylpropanolamine or toxic ingestions of barbiturates, tranquilizers, or illicit drugs may result in convulsions, fever, obtundation, and nuchal rigidity.

Reye's syndrome may follow a respiratory or gastrointestinal illness or varicella, and it may begin with a fever, vomiting, and an altered mental state. A child who has lead poisoning may be confused or show signs of increased intracranial pressure. Children who have metabolic disorders such as hyper- or hyponatremia, hypoglycemia, or hemolytic–uremic syndrome may be acutely febrile and unresponsive. A patient who has pseudotumor cerebri may complain of a headache or stiff neck, and he may vomit. Not all patients with Lyme disease will present with a rash nor will they recall being bitten by a tick. Osteomyelitis of the spine may be associated with fever and meningismus.

WORK-UP

History

It is important to check on recent exposure such as family contact or day care contact, preceding illness, travel to an area of endemic infections (e.g., Lyme disease), the presence of congenital defects including heart disease, spinal dysraphism, fistulas, or indwelling foreign bodies such as heart patches or valves, catheters, ventriculoperitoneal or ventriculoatrial shunts. It is equally important to inquire about concurrent diseases such as immunodeficiency states including gammaglobulinopathies, chronic renal disease, leukemia, or other illnesses that require immunosuppressant therapy. Information should be sought about recent antibiotic therapy and which drugs, if any, have been used and for how long a time.

Physical Examination

Complete vital signs must be taken. The skin and scalp must be inspected carefully to look for petechiae, rashes, pustules or vesicles, insect bites, or needle marks. A complete physical examination should include an inspection of the mouth for a gingival abscess or lead lines, auscultation of the heart and abdomen, and palpation of lymph nodes. Most importantly, an assessment should be made of neck mobility for meningismus and testing for both Brudzinski's sign (flexion of the neck causing involuntary flexion of the hips), and Kernig's sign (inability to extend the legs with the hips flexed). Mental status to determine the level of consciousness, orientation, ability to speak and follow commands, and motor strength and reflexes must also be assessed. The sinuses should be palpated and transilluminated. It is critical to check the fundi for papilledema. A neurologist or neurosurgeon should be consulted immediately and prior to the lumbar puncture if papilledema is present and a focal deficit is present or suspected.

Laboratory Tests

The following laboratory tests should be ordered: CBC; sedimentation rate; urinalysis; cultures of blood, CSF, and skin ulcers; serum electrolytes; Gram stain of CSF; CSF cell count and differential, protein and glucose determinations, ELISA, or CIE antigen determination for the three most common bacterial pathogens (i.e., H. influenzae type b, S. pneumococcus, and N. meningococcus); and glucose determination of the blood. A carefully performed complete battery of CSF tests as outlined above is mandatory in order to diagnose meningitis or to decide to presumptively initiate treatment (e.g., an abnormality of any parameter, even as subtle as a low ratio of CSF to serum glucose). If indicated, as is frequently the case, the following studies should be ordered: blood and urine samples for toxic screening and acute serologic titers; cultures of urine, pharynx, sputum, and stools; and chest roentgenogram.

Maternal toxoplasma, cytomegalovirus, herpes virus (TORCH) titers should also be obtained when a neonate is being evaluated. A determination of the serum IgM in the neonate may be helpful. Sinus roentgenograms should be obtained, if indicated, and petechiae should be gram-stained. A CT scan should be ordered if focal findings are present. If a midline shift is present, a contrast-enhanced scan may permit the identification of an abscess or the delineation of an area of vasculitis. An echocardiogram may be useful to search for valvular vegetations if a child is known to have cardiac disease. A radionuclide bone scan may localize a focus of osteomyelitis.

MANAGEMENT AND TREATMENT

The appropriate course of antibiotic therapy should be initiated as soon as the diagnosis is suspected. If any difficulty arises in performing the lumbar puncture, and the infant or child is acutely ill, it is permissible to give the first doses of antibiotics and then to obtain the CSF (Table 158-1).

Although meningitis may be caused by organisms other than bacteria, antibacterial treatment must be started immediately but may be discontinued if the CSF culture is sterile after 48 to 72 hours unless it is most likely (*e.g.*, known local epidemics) that the patient has viral meningitis. The choice of initial therapy should be based on the child's age, CIE antigen testing, and CSF Gram stain results. Therapy may need to be modified after identification of the organism and its antibiotic sensitivities. In neonates, the usual starting therapy for meningitis is similar to the treatment of sepsis and it has a broad spectrum to cover the wide range of possible organisms. Most often, intravenous ampicillin and an aminoglycoside are started initially, but individual circumstances will affect selection (*e.g.*, penicillin for documented maternal colonization with group B streptococci, or pustules on the skin requiring additional staphylococcal coverage). In the older child, intravenous ampicillin and chloramphenicol (in case of ampicillin-resistant *H. influenzae* type b) have been the standard initial therapy. The third-generation cephalosporins are rapidly modifying both the "traditional" antibiotic selection and the need for continued hospitalization for the duration of therapy.

The younger the child, the more likely is the risk for mortality and serious acute and long-term morbidity. The most serious immediate complications are shock and disseminated intravascular coagulopathy. The airway should be protected if the child's level of consciousness is depressed. The vital signs should be monitored frequently. To reduce the likelihood of the syndrome of inappropriate secretion of antidiuretic hormone (SIADH), fluid restriction should be maintained at two thirds to three quarters regular maintenance needs for the first 24 to 48 hours *if* there is no concomitant electrolyte imbalance or hyponatremia. The head circumference should be checked daily in the infant to detect hydrocephalus and subdural effusions. If the circumference is enlarging, transillumination should be performed and may need to be followed by ultrasonography or a CT scan. The monitoring of increased intracranial pressure by means of an indwelling intracranial or intraventricular bolt may be necessary to permit prompt treatment. Twenty-five to 30% of children with bacterial meningitis have seizures, with most occurring prior to treatment. Prophylactic anticonvulsant therapy is unnecessary, unless there is evidence of a focal disease such as cerebritis or phlebitis.

Because children with meningitis caused by *N. meningitidis* and *H. influenzae* type b have a high pharyngeal colonization rate that may then lead to

Table 158-1. Antimicrobial Agents for Treatment of Meningitis

	DAILY DOSE*		
	NEONATES		INFANTS AND CHILDREN
REGIMEN	*0–7 Days of Age*	*8–28 Days of Age*	
Conventional			
Penicillin G	100,000–150,000 U/kg[a]	150,000–200,000 U/kg[b,c]	250,000 U/kg[c,d]
Ampicillin	100–150 mg/kg[a]	150–200 mg/kg[b,c]	200–300 mg/kg[c]
Kanamycin	15–20 mg[a]	20–30 mg[b]	
Gentamicin†	5 mg/kg[a]	7.5 mg/kg[b]	
Tobramycin†	4 mg/kg[a]	6 mg/kg[b]	
Amikacin†	15–20 mg/kg[a]	20–30 mg/kg[b]	
Chloramphenicol†	25 mg/kg	50 mg/kg[a]	75–100 mg/kg[c]
Alternative			
Cefotaxime	100 mg/kg[a]	150–200 mg/kg[b,c]	200 mg/kg[c]
Moxalactam	100 mg/kg[a]	150–200 mg/kg[b]	200 mg/kg[c]
Ticarcillin	150–225 mg/kg[a,b]	225–300 mg/kg[b,c]	
Methicillin	100–150 mg/kg[a,b]	150–200 mg/kg[b,c]	
Oxacillin	100–150 mg/kg[a,b]	150–200 mg/kg[b,c]	
Nafcillin	100–150 mg/kg[a,b]	150–200 mg/kg[b,c]	
Vancomycin	20 mg[a]	30 mg/kg[b]	40–60 mg/kg[c]
Ceftriaxone			100 mg/kg[a]
Ceftazidime	60 mg/kg[a]	90 mg/kg[b]	125–150 mg/kg[b]

* Dosage divided and given every: [a] 12 hours, [b] 8 hours, [c] 6 hours, [d] 4 hours.
† Serum concentrations should be monitored and dosages adjusted accordingly.
(Klein JO, Feigin RD, McCracken GH Jr: Report of the Task Force on Diagnosis and Management of Meningitis. Pediatrics [Suppl] 78(5):971, 1986)

secondary cases, these patients should receive rifampin prophylaxis while they are in the hospital to reduce the spread to contacts when they return home. (For guidelines regarding rifampin prophylaxis for household and intimate contacts of children with the aforementioned organisms, see Chap. 194.)

INDICATIONS FOR REFERRAL

If the child remains febrile, has a persistent neurologic deficit, or remains obtunded during the course of the illness, and if an infectious disease expert is not available for frequent consultations, the patient may need to be transferred to a tertiary facility. Subdural effusions may be present and may require evacuation or stripping of the subdural membranes. A neurosurgical evaluation may be required if there is evidence of cerebritis or a focal collection of pus.

Up to 30% of neonates develop postinfectious hydrocephalus. There is a increased risk of neurologic deficits and seizure disorders especially in neonates, but also in older children. All children with bacterial meningitis have a high risk for mental retardation and learning disabilities. Since as many as 20% of children develop an auditory nerve dysfunction, an auditory evaluation (brain stem evoked response or audiogram) should be obtained either prior to or shortly after hospital discharge. The prognosis of children who have viral (aseptic) meningitis is considerably more favorable, although seizure, learning, and behavioral disorders may occur afterwards.

ANNOTATED BIBLIOGRAPHY

Bell WE: Current therapy of acute bacterial meningitis in children. Pediatr Neurol 1:5–11, 201–212, 1985 (Up-to-date review of bacterial meningitis in various age groups of children.)

Dodge PR, Swartz MN: Bacterial meningitis—a review of selected aspects. II: Special neurologic problems, postmeningitis complications and clinicopathologic correlations. N Engl J Med 272:898–902, 954–960, 1003–1110, 1965 (Classic article on the experience with bacterial meningitis at the Massachusetts General Hospital prior to the introduction of aminoglycosides and cephalosporins.)

Donat JF: Etiology and outcome in 42 children with acute nonbacterial meningoencephalitis. Mayo Clin Proc 55:156–160, 1980 (Prospective study with follow-up to 1 year. 19 cases of California and 8 cases of enterovirus disease were identified by CIE and culture. Morbidity and mortality in approximately one half of the cases.)

Haslam RA, Allen JR, Dorsen MM et al: Sequelae of group B hemolytic streptococcal meningitis in early infancy. Am J Dis Child 131: 845–849, 1977 (Retrospective study of 18 consecutive cases with 17% mortality. 15% severe morbidity when compared with controls [sibs or near relatives]).

Klein JO, Feigen RO, McCracken GH: Report of the Task Force on Diagnosis and Management of Meningitis. Pediatrics (Suppl) 78:959–982, 1986 (Current, concise, and complete; an ideal reference for the office-based pediatrician.)

Laxer RM, Marks MI: Pneumococcal meningitis in children. Am J Dis Child 131:850–853, 1977 (Retrospective study of 79 patients with 83 cases of pneumococcal meningitis. Increased mortality [11%, all in children ≤1 year of age] associated with pneumonia and low CSF sugar. 56% had neurological sequelae. EEGs in the acute or convalescent stage did not correlate well with the outcome.)

Nadol JB: Hearing loss of sequelae of meningitis. Laryngoscope 88:739–755, 1978 (Retrospective study of 547 patients with meningitis [235 bacterial, 304 viral]. 21% were found to have a sensorineural hearing loss during the acute and recuperative stages. Permanent hearing loss did not occur in children with aseptic meningitis.)

Schaad UB, Krucko J, Pfenninger J: Extended experience with cefuroxime therapy of childhood bacterial meningitis. Pediatr Infect Dis 3:410–415, 1984 (Prospective study of 84 children with meningitis who received cefuroxime. Mortality [first few hours] was 14%. 55% cases were *H. influenzae*. Findings indicate that cefuroxime is comparable therapeutically to other drugs.)

Swartz MN, Dodge PR: Bacterial meningitis—a review of selected aspects. I: General clinical features, special problems, and unusual meningeal reactions mimicking bacterial meningitis. N Engl J Med 272:725–731, 779–787, 842–848, 1965

19

Respiratory Problems

159
The Common Cold
ROBERT A. DERSHEWITZ

No major breakthroughs have occurred since Sir William Osler suggested that the only method to treat the common cold was with contempt. The term *cold* is a subset of, and not synonymous with, *upper respiratory tract infection* (URI). Colds are the most common infectious disease, and in children ~50% of URIs are common colds. Most children develop 3 to 8 colds/year and these colds are most prevalent in winter. Some children, for obscure reasons, are prone to more frequent respiratory infections. Preschoolers are usually responsible for spreading infections in the household, and the risk of acquiring colds is related inversely to age.

PATHOPHYSIOLOGY

Over 200 viruses cause the common cold, although occasionally, nonviruses (*e.g.*, mycoplasma) may produce "cold-like" illnesses. Rhinoviruses are the most common causative agents, which are responsible for between 30% and 50% of all colds. Coronaviruses are the next most common cause, accounting for between 10% and 20% of colds. Parainfluenza, respiratory syncytial, enterovirus, and influenza viruses are other frequent causes.

Although not firmly established, it is believed that infection is spread by inhalation and by close contact. Sneezing or coughing spreads droplets, which may then be inhaled and replicate on nasal or other respiratory epithelium. Infection is probably more commonly spread by physical contact. The virus may be transmitted from the hand of an infected person to a healthy person or from an inanimate object that may live on surfaces (*e.g.*, toys and door knobs) for up to 72 hours. The person's contaminated hand then innoculates his nose or eyes, which then initiates the pattern of viral replication on the epithelial surface. Cold symptoms usually appear 2 to 4 days later. Infection is acute and spreads locally on respiratory epithelium. Shedding and symptoms abate when nasal epithelium regenerates, usually in 3 to 4 days for rhinoviruses, although they may last longer than 10 days. Chilling, wet feet, and drafts play no role in "catching a cold."

CLINICAL PRESENTATION

All causative viruses produce a similar symptomatology, although influenza and respiratory syncytial (RS) viruses typically cause more serious illness than rhinoviruses and coronaviruses. No distinctive clinical characteristics are unique to any of the viruses. Nasal involvement is usually the first sign of infection and must always be present for the diagnosis. Mild nasal congestion may precede a watery rhinorrhea. Sneezing and a sore throat are usually present, and the child may also have fever, conjunctivitis, headache, and myalgias. Symptoms in infants tend to be more variable, as does a febrile response. Low-grade fevers are most common, but fevers of between 103°F and 104°F are not rare. After about the second day of illness, the nasal discharge typically becomes mucopurulent and less copious. Symptoms usually persist for at least 2 more days and the rhinorrhea often becomes more purulent. A nocturnal cough attributable to a post-nasal drip is often present. The rhinitis and cough may linger occasionally for weeks. Although colds are self-limited, complications or spread of the disease frequently occur. The most common bacterial complication is an acute suppurative otitis media. Other pyogenic and nonpyogenic complications include sinusitis, adenitis, pneumonia, croup, and bronchitis.

DIFFERENTIAL DIAGNOSIS

Colds should be distinguished from other upper respiratory tract illnesses, such as pharyngitis, sinusitis, and obstructive airway disease. A cold-like illness may be the prodrome for other diseases such as measles and pertussis. A streptococcal infection in infancy may be clinically indistinguishable from the common cold.

Allergic rhinitis is probably the most common and difficult entity to differentiate from the common cold, particularly when symptoms first occur. A strong family history of atopia and seasonal recurrence incriminate allergies. Violaceous, edematous nasal mucosa, itching eyes, and other allergic facies (e.g., nasal crease, allergic shiners, and the allergic salute) strongly indicate an allergic etiology. Vasomotor rhinitis, although more commonly seen in adults, should also be considered in the differential diagnosis.

A thick (i.e., purulent) nasal discharge usually indicates a resolving cold, but it may be due to a bacterial primary or superinfection. Other relatively common causes of purulent rhinitis include allergy (although a thin nasal discharge is more common), sinusitis, adenoiditis, nasal polyps, septal deviations, and systemic illness such as cystic fibrosis. A unilateral, thick, foul-smelling, or bloody discharge strongly suggests a foreign body.

Rhinitis secondary to chronic medication use such as topical decongestants, drug abuse (e.g., cocaine), and leakage of cerebrospinal fluid is thin. The use of a bulb syringe for longer than 5 days may result in mechanical trauma to the nasal turbinates, causing mucopurulent rhinitis.

WORK-UP

History

The physician should ask if there is a history of seasonal or perennial rhinitis. Children with allergies obviously get colds, but an abrupt onset of nasal symptoms suggests an infectious etiology. Is the child otherwise healthy and thriving? If the child has been symptomatic for several days, the physician should find out whether the rhinorrhea is becoming less copious and thicker; whether the discharge is bilateral; and whether there are other likely causes for rhinitis (e.g., forced hot air heating without humidification or prolonged use of a bulb syringe). Since the initial onset of chronic rhinitis in the adolescent may be caused by the use of cocaine, the physician should be alert to this possibility.

Physical Examination

A child with rhinitis warrants a complete examination of at least the respiratory tract, including the ears. Although bilateral purulent rhinitis is more likely caused by bacterial infection than is mucopurulent or thin rhinorrhea, bacterial primary and secondary infections are uncommon. It is, therefore, of little clinical significance to place importance on the color and thickness of the nasal discharge. As already mentioned, a foul-smelling or unilateral discharge suggests the presence of a foreign body and pale blue and swollen turbinates suggest an allergic etiology.

Laboratory Tests

No laboratory test ought to be considered routine and no single test "rules in" or "rules out" a cold. Throat cultures are neither helpful nor indicated. Flora from a nasopharyngeal (NP) culture, even if a pure growth is recovered, is difficult to interpret because it may reflect colonization rather than infection. NP cultures should be obtained only selectively, such as if pertussis is suspected. Wright or Hansel staining of nasal secretions is useful to look for eosinophils. Large numbers of eosinophils suggest an allergy and large numbers of neutrophils suggest an infection. Since the peripheral white blood cell count is usually normal, but may be elevated, it should not be routinely ordered. Sinus roentgenograms may help diagnose sinusitis, but the radiation exposure, the age of the child (the younger the child, the more difficult it is to interpret), and the duration of symptoms must be considered prior to ordering sinus films (see Chap. 85).

TREATMENT AND MANAGEMENT

Hundreds of cold preparations are marketed for the treatment of the common cold. To reduce their unnecessary use, parents should be told that none are curative and that all may have side effects potentially worse than the cold symptoms themselves.

Most preparations contain a decongestant. Topical decongestants are vasoconstrictors and probably provide as great or greater symptomatic relief than other classes of medications. Although they generally have fewer side effects, they must be used cautiously because systemic absorption may cause the same troublesome side effects as the oral decongestants. A rebound effect may result in obstructive apnea in young infants. If used for longer than 4 days, rebound congestion may develop, which may then lead to *rhinitis medicamentosa*. The most widely used topical decongestants are phenylephrine (*e.g.*, Neosynephrine) and oxymetazoline (*e.g.*, Afrin). Oral decongestants do not cause a rebound, but they have more side effects. Most oral cold preparations have an antihistamine, which may be useful to counter the stimulatory side effects of the decongestants, to control an allergic component (if suspected), or for sedation (*e.g.*, at bedtime). Manufacturers claim, though have not proven, that the anticholinergic effects of antihistamines reduce nasal secretions. Although the efficacy of medications for treatment of the common cold is controversial, one study found chlorpheniramine effective in reducing cold symptoms.

Beneficial nonpharmacologic approaches include isotonic saline followed by bulb syringe suctioning for rhinorrhea or congestion. Suctioning should be gentle to avoid rebound swelling, and should be discontinued after 4 consecutive days. Suctioning may resume in 1 to 2 days if rhinitis persists. Hydration is as effective as any medication to relieve a dry or scratchy throat. Candy, gum drops, or lozenges can also relieve an irritated throat. Since dry air can mimic or exacerbate cold symptoms, humidification (either central or bedside) may be helpful.

Antibiotics should be used only for presumed bacterial complications and never for the treatment of the common cold or to prevent complications. The weight of current evidence is against vitamin C in preventing colds or shortening their clinical course. Acetaminophen may be used for malaise or high fevers. Aspirin should be avoided because it increases viral shedding and may cause Reye's syndrome.

COMPLICATIONS AND REFERRALS

Major complications from the common cold are unusual, and children rarely require hospitalization. A referral to an allergist for the initial evaluation of chronic rhinitis is common, although frequently unnecessary if the primary physician takes a thorough history and performs a baseline workup. A referral, however, is warranted if the rhinitis does not respond to environmental control and appropriate medications.

ANNOTATED BIBLIOGRAPHY

Cherry JD: The common cold. In Feign RD, Cherry JD: Textbook of Pediatric Infectious Diseases, pp 97–103. Philadelphia, WB Saunders, 1981. (Complete and authoritative discussion with an exhaustive bibliography.)

Douglas RM, Moore BW, Miles HB et al: Prophylactic efficacy of intranasal alpha 2-interferon against rhinovirus infections in the family setting. N Engl J Med 314:65–70, 1986 (This report and a confirmatory following report in *New England Journal of Medicine* show that intranasal interferon reduces both the number of colds and duration of symptoms, especially from rhinoviruses. Probably the best potential for preventive and therapeutic application.)

Howard JC, Kantner TR, Lilienfield LS et al: Effectiveness of antihistamines in the symptomatic management of the common cold. JAMA 242:2414–2417, 1979 (One of the few controlled trials. When compared to placebo, benefit from chlorpheniramine was statistically significant.)

Marcy SM: Prevention of respiratory infection. Pediatr Infect Dis 4:442–446, 1985. (Good overview of the limited ways in which viral and bacterial infections of the respiratory tract can be prevented.)

Pruitt AW: Rational use of cold and cough preparations. Pediatr Ann 14:289–291, 1985. (Succinct and current rundown.)

Simons FER: Chronic rhinitis. Pediatr Clin North Am 31:801–819, 1984 (Excellent presentation of this elusive entity.)

A persistent cough in children causes much parental concern. A cough is not an illness but a sign for which a cause should be sought. The term *persistent cough* is synonymous with a *chronic cough*, because it is often difficult to differentiate between the two types. Some authorities use it interchangeably with the *chronic bronchitis complex in children*. *Persistent* is usually defined as lasting from 2 to 4 weeks. Coughing is largely a host defense mechanism to expectorate foreign matter from the respiratory tract and to clear secretions that are already there; thus, the presence of a cough does not necessarily (indeed frequently) require suppression.

Cough receptors located throughout the pharynx to the bronchioles comprise the afferent limb of the cough reflex. Once stimulated, impulses travel along the vagus nerve to the brain stem. Efferent fibers then travel to the larynx, intercostal muscles, diaphragm, and muscles of the abdomen and pelvis, and they trigger a cough. There is, however, some voluntary control over coughing.

CLINICAL PRESENTATION AND DIFFERENTIAL DIAGNOSIS

The history and physical examination often suggest the etiology. The cause of a persistent cough is sometimes obvious, but not uncommonly, a proven etiology will be elusive, even after an extensive work-up. The two most common causes of a persistent cough are recurrent viral bronchitis and asthma. It is sometimes difficult to differentiate initially between these two conditions because they share many features.

In reactive airway disease (most often asthma), wheezing is not often present. However, a history of wheezing, a good therapeutic response to bronchodilators, a nocturnal cough or a cough after exercise suggests asthma. Upper respiratory tract infections (URI) may trigger asthmatic attacks but may also lead to persistent infectious bronchitis. Viral etiologies of bronchitis are much more common than bacterial superinfections. Some children are prone to recurrent bouts of bronchitis, a tendency that lessens by 8 to 9 years of age.

Major Causes of Persistent Cough

1. Bronchitis
   A. Infectious
      1. Viral
      2. Bacterial
   B. Reactive
      1. Asthma
      2. Allergic
   C. Chemical
      1. Pollution (*e.g.*, tobacco smoke)
      2. GE reflux
2. Chronic upper airway disease (with or without postnasal drip)
3. Suppurative lung disease
   A. Cystic fibrosis
   B. Bronchiectasis
4. Postinfectious (*e.g.*, pneumonia, bronchiolitis)
5. Focal lesion
   A. Foreign body
   B. Mediastinal or pulmonary tumors, cysts, or nodes
   C. Laryngeal and tracheal stenosis, cysts, or hemangiomas
6. Psychogenic

(Adapted from Cooper D: Chronic cough. In Kelley V [ed]: Practice of Pediatrics. Vol 2, Chap 43, p 3. Hagerstown, Harper & Row, 1985)

It is useful to consider the age of onset when formulating differential diagnoses (see the box, Major Causes of Persistent Cough).

Infancy

A young infant with a chronic cough has an increased likelihood of congenital malformations such as tracheoesophageal fistula, cysts, and vascular rings. A perinatal infection must also be considered if the cough started within the first few weeks of life. Chlamydial pneumonia with its characteristic staccato cough occurs in the young infant. Bronchiolitis is another disease of infancy and pertussis is more common in young children. In both, as with any infection of the lower respiratory tract, coughing may persist for weeks after the infectious process has resolved. Pulmonary manifestations of cystic fibrosis may occur in this age group. Recurrent coughing is a well known manifestation of symptomatic gastroesophageal (GE) reflux, and, when symptomatic, it is more likely to be diagnosed in infancy.

Preschool Age

Toddlers are at greatest risk of foreign body aspiration. Since a history of choking is not always elicited, the diagnosis may require a high index of suspicion. Breath sounds may be asymmetric. Hyperinflation or air-trapping on inspiratory-expiratory chest roentgenograms strongly suggests aspiration. Bronchoscopy is indicated when the diagnosis remains doubtful.

Most children with persistent coughs appear healthy. The preschooler with cystic fibrosis may look frail, and he may have associated gastrointestinal (GI) problems such as steatorrhea and increased appetite. Cystic fibrosis (CF) and bronchiectasis must always be considered in a child with a chronic, suppurative cough.

A chronic upper airway disease such as sinusitis often has an associated bronchitic component. Although it is debatable whether a postnasal drip causes a chronic cough by itself, it is common practice to attribute it to a postnasal drip in a child who coughs only when in a supine position. Children with a GE reflux may also cough when in a supine position.

School Age

Mycoplasma pneumoniae infections peak in school-aged children and coughing may persist from 1 to 3 months after other symptoms resolve. A psychogenic cough is more common in older children. The cough disappears during sleep and is exacerbated during times of stress. Cigarette smoking may also cause a persistent cough.

Other conditions without an age predilection include chronic atelectasis secondary to suppurative lung disease, passive smoking, air pollution, and smoke inhalation (*e.g.*, from wood-burning fireplaces).

WORK-UP

History

The physician should discover if the child ever had a persistent cough and also if medications were used during the previous episodes. The medications should be noted with their response. Asthma is suggested if the cough is nocturnal; precipitated by exercise; improved by bronchodilators; exacerbated during the spring or summer; or if there is a strong family history of asthma. GE reflux is suggested in the infant with a chronic cough, but without the above mentioned symptoms. A chronic cough during winter suggests a recurrent or persistent viral bronchitis, although asthma and irritation (*e.g.*, from fireplaces and dry air) may be causative.

The physician should determine the nature of the sputum. The sputum in asthma and chronic infectious bronchitis, if productive, is clear, mucoid, or tenacious. A dry hacking cough is characteristic of tracheal irritation. Purulent sputum suggests CF and bronchiectasis, and if advanced, hemoptysis may be present. Since a progressive cough that becomes productive and often blood-streaked is also consistent with tuberculosis (TB), the physician should inquire about exposure to TB. A history of aspiration is difficult to elicit in young children. The physician should also determine if the cough was preceded by a choking episode; if there is (or was) drooling; and if the child sounds hoarse.

Paroxysms of coughing suggest pertussis, a pertussis-like syndrome, CF, and a chlamydial infection. The cough that disappears at night may be psychogenic.

Physical Examination

The complete physical examination should concentrate on the following:

General. Does the child appear robust or wasted? Are the height and weight age-appropriate and the growth parameters being maintained? CF, bronchiectasis, and immunodeficiency disorders must be considered in children who fail to thrive.

Chest. An increased chest circumference suggests CF or other causes of chronic air trapping secondary to pulmonary disease. Generalized wheezing, crackles (rales), or prolonged expirations suggest asthma, whereas focal crackles, if coarse and low pitched, suggest bronchiectasis. If associated with decreased aeration, the presence of a foreign body is suggested. Viral or mycoplasma pneumonia is the likely diagnosis if only fine inspiratory crackles are heard, and, less commonly, a fibrotic process. The auscultatory examination is usually normal in children with bronchitis, but rhonchi may be heard. A chronic cough with stridor suggests an anatomic lesion in the larynx, subglottic region, or upper trachea.

Other. Finger clubbing suggests CF and purulent rhinitis may be a sign of sinusitis. The physician should also look for other evidence of atopia such as the allergic salute and allergic rhinitis.

Laboratory Tests

With few exceptions, a TB skin test, chest roentgenogram, and sweat chloride test should be part of the initial evaluation in all children who have unexplained persistent coughs. A barium swallow is often helpful if structural lesions (either congenital or acquired masses), GE reflux, or foreign body aspiration is suspected. A complete blood count (CBC) looking for eosinophilia (indicating asthma), neutrophilia (suggesting a bacterial infection), and lymphocytosis (suggesting pertussis or a viral infection) is also a reasonable screening test. Eosinophilia may be seen in chlamydial infections. If the cough is productive, Wright and Gram stain the sputum. Eosinophils suggest asthma whereas bacteria and pus cells indicate infection.

Spirometry is a simple office test to detect airway obstruction. Asthma may be diagnosed if bronchodilators reverse the airway narrowing. Other tests ordered selectively include toxoplasma, rubella, cytomegalovirus, herpesvirus (TORCH) titers if the cough began in early infancy, serologic testing for Mycoplasma, and α_1-antitrypsin levels.

TREATMENT

Treatment is based on the diagnosis or diagnostic probabilities revealed by the work-up. Simple recommendations such as home air humidification, keeping the throat moist, or stopping cigarette smoking at home often eliminate the cough.

A chronic, dry irritative cough (especially if it keeps the child or family awake at night) exhausts the child or is socially disruptive (*e.g.*, at school). The cough may be suppressed by either codeine or dextromethorphan. Both are centrally acting antitussives. Codeine is more effective, but the drawbacks include its addiction potential and respiratory depression. It should never be given to young infants. The dose is 0.6 to 1 mg/kg/day in three to four divided doses and should not exceed 60 mg/day. Dextromethorphan is much safer, and the dose is the same or slightly higher than for codeine. A purulent cough should never be suppressed. Other productive coughs constitute relative contraindications for prescribing antitussive medications.

A diagnostic (and therapeutic) trial of a bronchodilator is appropriate before prescribing antitussives if airway hyperreactivity is suspected, but a poor clinical response does not necessarily rule out that diagnosis. It may be used in the absence of atopia. Beta-adrenergic medications such as metaproterenol and albuterol are less toxic than theophylline. Cromolyn sodium may be administered by a metered dose inhaler. In the latter instance, it may be given in conjunction with a β agonist. The child who has failed a trial of bronchodilators should be given a 10- to 14-day course of erythromycin for presumptive bacterial bronchitis. It is, however, reasonable to use erythromycin initially if infectious bronchitis is the more likely diagnosis. The dose of theophylline must be reduced by ~25% if given with erythromycin since the half-life of theophylline is prolonged by erythromycin.

Expectorants and mucolytic agents such as guaifenesin (glyceryl guaiacolate) are usually ineffective. Antihistamines may be prescribed if a postnasal drip is thought to cause or contribute to the cough. Diphenhydramine has been used as an antitussive, but it is not as effective as codeine or dextromethorphan.

It is axiomatic that the child should be well hydrated, but overhydration should be avoided because it may compromise a pulmonary function. Sinusitis should be treated with cefaclor or amox-

---

Consultants and When to Refer

1. Cystic fibrosis center if the child is diagnosed as having CF
2. Allergist—Allergy skin testing may be helpful in differentiating allergic from other etiologies.
3. Pulmonologist—Formal and definitive provocative testing for airway hyperreactivity using histamine or methanocholine. Also, refer if the work-up has been negative.
4. Bronchoscopist (*e.g.*, surgeon, ENT, or pulmonologist)—Referral should be to whomever has the greatest experience and the most appropriate instrument. Bronchoscopy is indicated if a foreign body aspiration or anatomic lesion is suspected. Without a specific clinical suspicion, its yield is low.
5. Surgeon—GE reflux must be corrected if medical therapy fails to prevent recurrent pneumonia. Consult a pediatric pulmonary or general pediatric surgeon for conditions such as anatomic lesions and chronic bronchiectasis. A radiologist may then need to perform bronchography.
6. Immunologist—For children with immunodeficiencies

icillin (see Chap. 85), and erythromycin should be prescribed for mycoplasma and chlamydial infections. Chest physical therapy and postural drainage are usually unnecessary unless there is a suppurative pulmonary infection or secondary atelectasis.

INDICATIONS FOR REFERRAL OR ADMISSION

Most children with persistent coughs who are worked up systematically by their primary care physician do not need to be referred to a specialist. Outside consultation may be indicated if the etiology of the cough remains unclear; if the clinical response to therapy is unsatisfactory; if the disease is rare or complex; or if the parents or primary physician want "a second opinion." Many disciplines may be involved in the care of these children. These specialists and also indications for hospitalization, are listed in the box, Consultants and When to Refer.

ANNOTATED BIBLIOGRAPHY

Agents used to treat cough. In AMA Drug Evaluations, 4th ed, pp 467–475. New York, John Wiley, 1980 (Comprehensive review of cough medications.)

Eigen H: The clinical evaluation of chronic cough. Pediatr Clin North Am 29:67–78, 1982 (Excellent, in-depth review.)

Morgan WJ, Taussig LM: The chronic bronchitis complex in children. Pediatr Clin North Am 31:851–864, 1984 (Defines the CB complex; relates it to the child with a persistent cough; and emphasizes the importance of the hyperactive airway as its major cause. Also presents a staged, practical protocol on the management of children with the CB complex.)

Over-the-counter cough remedies. Med Lett 21:103–104, 1979 (Quick overview on the efficacy of therapeutic options.)

161
Stridor

ELLEN M. FRIEDMAN

Stridor is a nonspecific term that means noisy breathing. Stridor, in itself, is not pathognomonic or diagnostic of any disease process. Stridor may not even be related to otolaryngologic abnormalities. An initial consideration of stridor in the neonate should include congenital cardiac malformations, neurologic disorders, or general toxicity. If these etiologies are ruled out, the physician should look to the airway as the most likely source of difficulty.

PATHOPHYSIOLOGY

Stridor is caused by an increase in turbulence when air passes through a narrow inlet. Due to the small size of the infant and the pediatric airway, a small amount of airway narrowing may result in a significant obstruction. The prolonged and tubular curved omega shape of the infant epiglottis and the redundant aryepiglottic folds may further compromise the airway. The elastic cartilage of the pediatric larynx is flexible and, therefore, may partially obstruct the airway with the dynamic changes associated with respiration. By determining if the stridor is present on inspiration, expiration, or both, the physician should be able to approximate the anatomic location of the obstruction.

Stridor will occur on inspiration if a narrowed area is in the nasopharynx, pharynx, or supraglottis. This is the result of the increased negative pressure on inspiration that causes the supraglottic structures to collapse into the airway. Expiration will force these structures open and allow unobstructed air flow; therefore, there will be no audible sound on expiration with supraglottic obstruction. The subglottic space is encompassed by the circumferential cricoid ring, which is inflexible; therefore, changes in the phase of respiration will not alter the stridor. An obstruction in this region will result in noisy breathing present on expiration and inspiration, or biphasic stridor. Stridor, associated with pathology of the lower trachea, will be present on expiration only. The relative positive pressure associated with expiration will further infringe on the already narrowed tracheal lumen, resulting in a low-pitched expiratory wheeze. Inspiration will be unobstructed.

Table 161-1.   Signs and Symptoms
Associated With Lesions

	SUPRAGLOTTIC	SUBGLOTTIC	TRACHEAL
Stridor	Inspiratory	Biphasic	Expiratory
Dysphagia	Present	Absent	Absent
Cry/voice	Muffled	Normal	Normal
Retractions	Mild	Present	Present

Table 161-2.   Supraglottic Stridor

CONGENITAL	INFLAMMATORY	NEOPLASMS	TRAUMA
Choanal atresia	Adenotonsillar	Benign	Postoperative
Nasal septal deviation	hypertrophy/infection	Dermoid	Caustic ingestion
Epiglottic cyst	Retropharyngeal	Cystic hygroma	
Laryngomalacia	abscess	Malignant	
	Supra(epi)glottitis	Lymphoma	
		Rhabdomyosarcoma	

CLINICAL PRESENTATION AND EVALUATION

Stridor may or may not be associated with respiratory distress. Frequently, loud inspiratory stridor may occur in a very pink, happy child without a significant obstruction. If air hunger and significant obstruction are present, however, it is essential for the physician to proceed promptly and aggressively to alleviate the obstruction. The degree of respiratory distress can be estimated by assessing certain parameters: color, retractions, respiration rate, air entry, and state of consciousness. When actual respiratory distress is absent, stridor may be evaluated with leisure. Questions regarding birth history, mode and age of onset, and the presence of associated symptoms will be most helpful. Associated symptoms, such as feeding difficulties, quality of cry/voice, and the presence or absence of retractions may complete the clinical picture and will help elucidate the final diagnosis. A summary of the signs and symptoms associated with lesions in the different anatomic areas is listed in Table 161-1.

Most cases of stridor ($\sim 60\%$) are secondary to problems at the level of the larynx. *Laryngomalacia* is a frequent diagnosis that causes low-pitched, fluttering inspiratory stridor. This diagnosis is a benign, self-correcting condition and is thought to represent immaturity of the laryngeal cartilages. The stridor gradually improves as the soft cartilage matures. This condition usually resolves without any intervention between the ages of 12 to 18 months. A partial list of specific lesions in specific locations is given in Tables 161-2, 161-3, and 161-4.

TREATMENT

Overzealous handling or investigations of the child with respiratory distress may exacerbate the situation. The ensuing work-up, therefore, should be determined by the degree of toxicity and respiratory distress of each patient. Observation of the patient in various positions and during feeding is helpful. Radiographic studies, including fluoroscopy of the airway and barium swallow, are helpful in order to determine dynamic changes associated

Table 161-3.   Subglottic Stridor

CONGENITAL	INFLAMMATORY	NEOPLASM
Web	Croup	Benign
Stenosis	Angioneurotic	Papillomatosis
Vocal cord	edema	Hemangioma
paralysis		Malignant
		Rhabdomyosarcoma

Table 161-4.   Tracheal Stridor

CONGENITAL	INFLAMMATORY	NEOPLASM	TRAUMA
Tracheoesophageal fistula	Bacterial tracheitis	Benign Papillomatosis Adenoma	Foreign body
Tracheomalacia		Malignant Chondrosarcoma	Stenosis

with respiration and the possibility of an extratracheal cause for obstruction, such as a vascular ring.

In general, no further blood tests or laboratory studies are routinely indicated. However, in specific cases special tests (*e.g.*, C-reactive protein or pulmonary functions tests) may be required. The diagnosis is established most commonly by laryngoscopy and bronchoscopy. The airway of the neonate and premature infant can be evaluated with the use of the magnifying telescope. The rigid ventilating bronchoscope allows for a relatively leisurely inspection of the entire length of the larynx, trachea, and upper bronchi. A controversy arises concerning the role of diagnostic flexible bronchoscopy because of both its advantages and disadvantages.

Although flexible laryngoscopy and bronchoscopy can be performed without anesthesia, there are significant limitations. Without the benefit of an endotracheal tube, the airway control is not assured, which limits the duration of a safe examination. Many of the more complex situations are difficult to assess with only a brief visualization. The small size of the pediatric flexible endoscopes allows limited capability for suctioning and secre-

tion removal, and no possibility of foreign body removal or obtaining a biopsy. The significant advantage of flexible endoscopy is the ability to view the larynx and trachea in the dynamic state of spontaneous respirations without an obstructed view due to an endotracheal tube.

A referral to an otolaryngologist should be based on the degree of stridor and associated airway obstruction. An unusual history or progressive clinical course should alert the physician that a consultation is needed. Laryngoscopy and bronchoscopy should be performed by an experienced pediatric endoscopist with the aid of an experienced pediatric anesthesiologist.

ANNOTATED BIBLIOGRAPHY

Cotton R, Reilly JS: Stridor and airway obstruction. In Bluestone CD, Stool SE (eds): Pediatric Otolaryngology. Philadelphia, WB Saunders, 1983

Holinger LD: Etiology of stridor in the neonate, infant and child. Ann Otol 89:397, 1980

Holinger PH, Brown WT: Congenital webs, cysts, laryngoceles and other anomalies of the larynx. Ann Otol Rhinol Laryngol 76:744, 1976 (Good overview of the various congenital anomalies.)

162
Foreign Body Aspiration
VICTOR C. BAUM

Accidental aspiration of foreign matter into the airway is a major cause of childhood morbidity and mortality and results in several hundred deaths each year in children in the United States. Approximately 10% of children with foreign body aspiration are less than 1 year of age; 50% to 75% are 1 to 3 years of age; and 15% to 30% are over 3 years of age. The most commonly aspirated material is food, with nutmeats accounting for 50% of all aspirations (with peanuts being the most common). About half of the children who ultimately present to a physician do so within the first 48 hours of aspiration;

up to 20% may not develop symptoms, or may have their symptoms overlooked for over 1 month.

PATHOPHYSIOLOGY

Foreign objects in the airway can do damage either by partial or complete occlusion of a portion of the tracheobronchial tree or by direct trauma to the mucosa. Although it is said that aspirated material is typically aspirated into the right lung, a review of several large series reveals this predeliction does not occur often enough to be clinically useful.

Indeed, in one series, a preponderance of foreign bodies was located in the left main-stem bronchus. The final resting place is determined by the size of the aspirated material in relation to the size of the airways. The main-stem bronchi are the site of impaction in 75% to 80% of cases; the trachea (typically the distal trachea) in about 10%; and the larynx in ~4% of cases. The onset of symptoms, the nature of symptoms, and the radiologic findings depend on three factors: (1) Type of object: sharp or irritating objects may result primarily in hemoptysis and blood-tinged sputum, unlike organic or other objects that cause damage primarily by airway obstruction. (2) Location of the object: resulting in upper (extrathoracic) or lower (intrathoracic) airway obstruction. (3) Complete or partial obstruction: because airway diameters vary with changes in airway pressure during the respiratory cycle, aspirated objects may either completely obstruct airways to produce atelectasis or may allow air entry during inspiration, but obstruct during exhalation, resulting in localized air trapping.

CLINICAL PRESENTATION

Over 90% of children present with some respiratory distress, usually dyspnea and cough. As mentioned, the clinical presentation is determined by the type of foreign object, the location of the object, and whether aspiration has resulted in a partial or complete obstruction of that portion of the airway. Obstruction of the larynx by a large object results in immediate cessation of effective ventilation and progresses rapidly to cyanosis and syncope (*cafe coronary*). Impaction in the upper, extrathoracic airway results primarily in difficulty during inspiration with retractions and inspiratory stridor. Intrathoracic partial obstruction results in a cough and primarily in difficulty during exhalation with expiratory wheezing. Smaller aspirated particles may not produce symptoms for several weeks at which time an afebrile chronic cough or a lower respiratory tract infection becomes apparent. Only a few, however, present with a chronic infection or bronchiectasis. Few patients present with hemoptysis from excoriation of the airway mucosa by a sharp or rough object.

DIFFERENTIAL DIAGNOSIS

The differential diagnosis of foreign body aspiration includes all causes of upper and lower airway obstruction. Congenital abnormalities causing airway obstruction typically present with chronic obstruction, however, these may develop acute exacerbations mimicking foreign body aspiration. Since foreign body aspiration can present with a chronic, indolent course, causes of chronic pulmonary infiltrates, such as pulmonary sequestration, should be considered.

A partial list of causes of acute airway obstruction includes asthma, massive tonsillar enlargement, peritonsillar or retropharyngeal abscess, croup (laryngotracheal bronchitis), epiglottitis, bacterial tracheitis, diphtheria, subglottic stenosis, laryngomalacia and tracheomalacia, anaphylaxis, craniofacial anomalies with macroglossia or mandibular hypoplasia, subglottic hemangioma, laryngeal papillomatosis, vascular anomalies such as vascular rings and pulmonary artery sling.

WORK-UP

History

A history of foreign body aspiration is usually elicited. Various series, however, report a positive history in only 50% to 90% of cases, leaving a sizeable minority in whom clinical suspicion is a major factor in instituting further evaluation. With a positive history and appropriate symptoms, a foreign body can be found on bronchoscopy in 90% of cases.

Physical Examination

The physical findings depend on the location of the object and the degree of airway obstruction. A partial obstruction of the upper, extrathoracic airway results primarily in inspiratory difficulty with inspiratory stridor. Lower, intrathoracic airway obstruction results primarily in expiratory difficulty. The location in lobar or segmental bronchi produces unilateral findings of asymmetric breath sounds, focal wheezing, or localized decreased air entry. Aspiration of a foreign body may also result in the findings of a chronic infiltrate with a chronic cough, crackles, and fever.

Laboratory Tests

Though most aspirated foreign bodies are radiolucent, radiologic imaging procedures are the most effective diagnostic tests. Fluoroscopy of the chest can demonstrate evidence of an aspirated foreign body in 90% of bronchial foreign bodies and 30% of laryngotracheal foreign bodies. Most laryngeal foreign bodies, however, will be missed. Laryngeal obstruction from any cause can produce a dilated hypopharynx. Signs on fluoroscopy include an inspiratory shift of the mediastinum, mediastinal widening on inspiration, and air trapping with reduced expiratory diaphragmatic excursion on the affected side. Plain chest radiographs can produce evidence for foreign body aspiration in ~75% of cases. The most common findings are unilateral hyperaeration, infiltrates, and atelectasis. Less common findings (less than 10%) are a radiopaque foreign body, a narrowed tracheal lumen, bronchiectasis or lung abscess, pneumomediastinum, or pneumothorax. A film obtained at end-exhalation will make unilateral hyperexpansion more apparent. If the child cannot cooperate, obtaining bilateral decubitus films or pushing up on the epigastrium with a gloved hand will also demonstrate unequal lung volumes. The subglottic tracheal lumen should be evaluated for evidence of croup (*pencil point* or *church steeple* sign). A lateral neck film should be evaluated for an enlarged epiglottis if that diagnosis is a consideration and the child's clinical status allows it (see Chap. 163).

THERAPY

The current consensus for life threatening airway obstruction in children older than 12 months and adults is to deliver 6 to 10 abdominal thrusts (*Heimlich maneuver*) until the foreign body is expelled. If unsuccessful, four sharp blows should be delivered to the victim's back between the shoulder blades, and if still necessary, the Heimlich maneuver should be repeated.

The current recommendation for the choking infant younger than 1 year is to support the prone infant on one arm of the rescuer with the head lower than the trunk and to deliver four back blows. If unsuccessful, the infant is turned to the supine position, supported between two hands, and four chest thrusts are delivered. These thrusts are identical to external cardiac compressions and they are delivered to the chest rather than to the abdomen because of the relatively large size of the liver in infants. If the infant is unconscious and the airway cannot be opened with the aforementioned maneuvers, an attempt should be made to ventilate mouth-to-mouth following correct positioning of the neck and jaw and removal of any foreign body visualized in the oropharynx.

Bronchoscopy is indicated for any known foreign body aspiration; the urgency is determined by the location and degree of respiratory distress. This should be done, if at all possible, by a bronchoscopist/anesthesiologist/operating room team experienced in pediatric endoscopy. A rigid bronchoscope is preferred and these objects can be removed by various instruments and manipulations. The removal of one foreign body does not exclude the presence of another. In one series 15% of patients required a second examination due to a second foreign body not noted during the first procedure or incompletely removed. A thoracotomy is only rarely required (less than 1%). Postbronchoscopy complications include laryngeal edema that responds to racemic epinephrine and steroids. Most patients are rapidly discharged from the hospital. One series reported 88% of their patients were discharged within 24 hours of admission and 36% were discharged home directly from the recovery room.

Postural drainage alone is not indicated as a primary therapy. It may not be successful and may relocate a foreign body from one bronchus to the other, resulting in a foreign body in one bronchus and an edematous airway on the other side. The foreign body may also be dislodged producing laryngeal obstruction. Postural drainage may be indicated if bronchoscopy does not identify a foreign body, suggesting small fragments.

INDICATIONS FOR REFERRAL

Any history of foreign body aspiration deserves further evaluation and a documented foreign body in the airway requires referral to a skilled endoscopy team. A history of unexplained cough, wheeze, or decreased air entry also provides a reason for referral as does unexplained hemoptysis and a chronic localized infiltrate.

PATIENT EDUCATION

Appropriate foods for age should be part of routine well-child discussions with parents because most aspirated material is food matter.

ANNOTATED BIBLIOGRAPHY

Blazer S, Naveh Y, Friedman A: Foreign body in the airway. Am J Dis Child 134:68, 1980 (Series of 200 cases of foreign body aspiration in children.)

Cohen SR, Herbert WI, Lewis GB, Geller KA: Foreign body in the airway. Ann Otol 89:437, 1980 (Retrospective review that concentrates on perioperative management.)

Cotton E, Yasuda K: Foreign body aspiration. Pediatr Clin North Am 4:937, 1984 (General review of foreign body aspiration.)

Kosloske AM: Bronchoscopic extraction of aspirated foreign bodies in children. Am J Dis Child 136:924, 1982 (Well-illustrated discussion of various bronchoscopic extraction maneuvers.)

163

Inflammatory Illnesses of the Pediatric Airway

ELLEN M. FRIEDMAN

As discussed in Chapter 161, due to the anatomy of the pediatric airway, a small amount of edema may lead to significant airway obstruction. Inflammatory conditions are second only to congenital anomalies as the most common cause for airway obstruction. The three most common inflammatory illnesses of the pediatric airway are supraglottitis (epiglottitis), croup, and bacterial tracheitis. Each of these entities has a fairly distinctive clinical presentation and requires specific intervention. Since these illnesses can progress rapidly to complete respiratory obstruction, it is imperative that the physician is familiar with the proper method to diagnose and treat each disease.

SUPRAGLOTTITIS

Supraglottitis is a true pediatric emergency. The clinical progression from partial to complete airway obstruction is rapid and requires prompt intervention. The morbidity and mortality associated with supraglottitis has decreased over the past 30 to 40 years with the use of antibiotics and endotracheal intubation.

Pathophysiology

Supraglottitis is a bacterial infection that is most commonly secondary to *Hemophilus influenzae* type b. The bacterial invasion causes inflammation of the lingual surface of the epiglottis, the aryepiglottic folds, ventricular bands, and paraglottic space. The involvement of all of these structures has supported supraglottitis as the preferred name for the entity previously known as epiglottitis. Due to the massive supraglottic edema, inspiratory stridor is a predominant clinical feature. Swelling in the area of the esophageal inlet results in difficulty with secretions and subsequent drooling.

Children with supraglottitis are usually between 3 and 5 years old and in previous good health. A consistent male predilection is demonstrated with this disease, as in many airway ailments. The clinical picture rapidly evolves from a mild sore throat

to severe respiratory distress, with inspiratory stridor and drooling. The child becomes increasingly toxic within hours, and has a high fever and a rapidly increasing respiratory rate. The frightened child will sit upright, with head extended, jaw thrust forward, and mouth open in an attempt to maintain a patent airway. The child will become limp and will relinquish this posture only when he is completely exhausted and is hypoxic. Such a change in position indicates collapse and impending respiratory arrest.

Due to the fragile nature of the compromised airway in supraglottitis, a physical examination of the child should be minimized. Overzealous handling of a child in this condition can be disastrous. Although some physicians feel that direct visualization of the epiglottis with a tongue depressor in the emergency room will confirm or rule out the diagnosis, the serious possibility of inducing laryngospasm and subsequent respiratory arrest does not warrant such an examination. The patient should remain with the parent and must not be alarmed or disturbed. Blood tests should not be performed and intravenous lines should not be established. All attempts should be directed at the prompt establishment of a secure artificial airway.

Supraglottitis is a clinical diagnosis and does not require a confirmatory radiogram. The possibility of a sudden complete respiratory obstruction in the radiology suite is real. Although there is a diagnostic radiographic appearance of supraglottitis, it does not warrant delay in the establishment of a secure airway. In cases where the possibility of supraglottitis is raised but considered unlikely, a radiogram may be useful in ruling out the diagnosis. In this setting, the patient must be sent for a radiogram accompanied by resuscitation equipment and experienced staff if intubation becomes necessary.

In general, hospitals with a well-defined protocol for the management of supraglottitis have lower morbidity and mortality rates. The team approach has proven most successful. Team members include a pediatrician, an otolaryngologist, an anesthesiologist, or an intensive care unit staff member. It is important for each member to be familiar with the procedure in order to minimize confusion and to smoothly organize the management of the patient.

Supraglottitis used to be treated either by intubation, tracheotomy, or close observation in the intensive care unit. The option of monitored observation should be highly discouraged. The progression of this illness is rapid and may be unpredictable. There is a 6% mortality rate in patients who are closely monitored without airway support, but this rate decreases to less than 1% mortality with the establishment of an artificial airway. Such data reemphasize the need to establish an artificial airway and highlight the fact that observation is an unacceptable practice.

The decision to intubate rather than to establish a tracheotomy depends on the clinical facilities available. Certain hospital personnel are more comfortable with the postoperative care and management of the tracheotomized patient. The complication rate associated with pediatric tracheotomies has been reported between 10% and 19%. Complications include hemorrhage, pneumothorax, and subglottic stenosis. A general preference for nasotracheal intubation in this illness has emerged because it is highly effective and has fewer inherent risks. When nasotracheal intubation is selected, it is important to use an endotracheal tube that is ~1 mm smaller than the normal tube size. Due to the smaller tube size, attentive nursing care and frequent suctioning will alleviate the possibility of mucous plug obstruction. Meticulous taping of the tube will avoid an accidental extubation. The nasotracheal tube is able to be removed immediately when the supraglottic edema has resolved. Since there is no need to await tracheotomy decannulation, shorter hospitalization has been the rule.

Since supraglottitis is usually due to *H. influenzae* type b, intravenous antibiotic therapy directed against this organism should be started immediately.

CROUP

Croup is a term that is used interchangeably to describe various respiratory illnesses. Three specific entities comprise the croup syndromes: spasmodic croup, laryngotracheitis, and laryngotracheobronchitis. Characteristics common to each of the diseases are a varying degree of respiratory obstruction, barking cough, and toxicity. Each entity is discussed separately, although in practice they may not always be distinguishable.

Spasmodic Croup

Spasmodic croup usually begins with difficulty in breathing at night and the sudden onset of a barking cough. It occurs throughout the ages of childhood and may recur. The children are usually afebrile and nontoxic. A mild upper respiratory infection may precede the development of a spasmodic croup.

The etiology is undetermined, but spasmodic croup is currently felt to reflect an allergic phenomenon or a low-grade viral infection. Symptoms resolve quickly when treated with humidity (*i.e.*, running the shower or going out in the night air) and reassurance. Other medications that have been used with varying responses include corticosteroids, syrup of ipecac, diphenhydramine elixir, and subcutaneous epinephrine. Airway intervention in the form of intubation or tracheotomy is rarely necessary.

Laryngotracheitis

Laryngotracheitis is a viral infection in which submucosal edema is present in the subglottic space. Due to the inflammation and swelling, there is destruction of the ciliated epithelium with poor mucous transport without increased humidification. The fibrinous exudate will dry out and become hardened crusts, which will further compromise the airway.

Laryngotracheobronchitis

Laryngotracheobronchitis refers to an infection that extends further and involves the entire respiratory tract. The most common viruses are parainfluenza and respiratory syncytial viruses. When the respiratory tract is extensively involved, a bacterial suprainfection may occur. When there is a bacterial component, it is usually secondary to streptococcus, staphylococcus, or *Hemophilus influenzae*.

The children involved are usually less than 3 years of age. They appear ill but not toxic. They have the characteristic croupy cough and biphasic stridor. Laryngotracheitis and laryngotracheobronchitis are most common during the winter. Significant yearly variations are determined by the virulence of the specific viruses.

The history is fairly straightforward. A mild preceding upper respiratory infection usually occurs. The symptoms may intensify at night and then wane during daytime. Most commonly, croup will resolve within 3 to 7 days. Prolonged or recurrent episodes of croup should alert the physician to the possibility of underlying congenital malformation (*e.g.*, congenital subglottic stenosis), the presence of a foreign body, or a bacterial infection.

A PA radiogram of the airway will reveal the characteristic narrowing of the subglottic space: This is referred to as the *steeple sign* or the *pencil point sign*. No other studies are useful in the work-up.

Most patients with any of the croup syndromes do not require hospitalization. Humidification is crucial and is effective in reducing the airway obstruction and may be implemented at home. It is helpful to use a croup score or another established criterion to evaluate the child who has croup. A suggested croup scoring symptom includes the following parameters: (1) stridor; (2) retraction; (3) air entry, (4) color; (5) level of consciousness.

Children who do not respond to humidification and oxygen administration will require racemic epinephrine. The response to racemic epinephrine should be dramatic; however, do not assume that this response will be long-lived. After one administration of racemic epinephrine in the emergency room or in one's office, the patient should be admitted to the hospital for observation. A deterioration of the clinical status or actual pharmacologic rebound may occur following even one dose of racemic epinephrine.

Airway support should be considered in those few patients with an increasing croup score, a decreasing response to epinephrine, or the need for more frequent epinephrine injections. Controversy surrounds the decision to intubate children who have an inflamed, narrowed subglottis. The fear is that the foreign body response to an endotracheal tube will heighten the subglottic irritation and will result in an acquired stenosis. Tracheotomy has been suggested as an alternative.

The role of steroids is also controversial in the management of croup. Reports in the literature are difficult to analyze, since frequently in the various papers the specific croup syndrome is not defined and there are significant differences in dosages and dosage schedules. It appears that a significant dose (*i.e.*, 1.5 mg/kg, up to 20 mg) of Decadron may decrease the amount and the duration of subglottic inflammation.

Most children who have croup can be managed at home with humidification and reassurance. In cases where the clinical symptoms of airway obstruction are progressing, the child should be evaluated in an emergency room. Signs of increasing obstruction are patient fatigue, increasing stridor, retractions and cyanosis. A referral should be made to a pediatric otolaryngologist for an endoscopy if croup recurs more than three times a year; if it is prolonged beyond reasonable expectation; or if it does not clear between recurrences.

BACTERIAL TRACHEITIS

Bacterial tracheitis is an acute infectious disease of the airway in infants and children and has features common to both croup and epiglottitis. It is felt that bacterial tracheitis represents a true infection of the trachea and not merely a suprainfection of viral croup.

Pathophysiology

Bacterial tracheitis is characterized by subglottic edema and copious mucopurulence in the trachea. The bacterial infection impedes mucociliary flow and there is stasis of the secretions. Bronchoscopy on these patients reveals thick mucus with a disruption and sloughing of the tracheal mucosa.

The most common causative organism is *Staphylococcus aureus*, although *Hemophilus influenzae* type b and streptococcus have also been isolated. The blood cultures are uniformly negative, although the blood count will show an elevated white blood cell count with a shift to the left.

Clinical Presentation

The age of children who have bacterial tracheitis may be from several months old to early adolescence. A preceding mild upper respiratory infection usually occurs with an 8- to 10-hour deterioration of clinical status. During this period, there is a progressive hoarseness, brassy cough, and inspiratory or biphasic stridor. Cardiopulmonary arrest has been reported with increasing obstruction.

On physical examination, the patient with bacterial tracheitis will appear to have a varying degree of respiratory distress. Stridor, cough, retractions, and cyanosis are also present. The patients are frequently febrile and may have a concomitant pneumonia. A lateral neck x-ray shows cloudiness of the tracheal air column, with an irregularity or scalloping of the tracheal wall. The sloughed tracheal mucosa sometimes gives the radiographic impression of a foreign body and has been misread as such.

Many centers recommend positioning an artificial airway in patients with bacterial tracheitis. Most series, even with intubation or tracheostomy, report a significant number of cardiac arrests and death. These occurrences have been related to mucous plug formation and obstruction of the artificial airway or the bronchi. Thus, meticulous suctioning of the airway is the key to the successful management of these patients. Bronchoscopy will not only be diagnostic but will also be therapeutic in that it will allow for direct visualization as well as a complete removal of debris. Further management involves humidity, appropriate intravenous antimicrobial therapy, and close monitoring in the intensive care setting. Intubation or tracheotomy is reserved for those patients in whom adequate ventilation is impossible without such intervention.

ANNOTATED BIBLIOGRAPHY

Davis HW, Gartner JC, Galvis AG et al: Acute upper airway obstruction, croup and epiglottitis. Pediatr Clin North Am 4(28), 1981

Fried MP: Controversies in the management of supraglottitis and croup. Pediatr Clin North Am 4(26):931–942, 1979

Jones R, Santos JI, Overall JC, Jr: Bacterial tracheitis. JAMA 242:721–276, 1979 (The three references listed here provide good overviews of the topics indicated by their respective titles.)

164
Bronchiolitis

HENRY L. DORKIN

Bronchiolitis is one of the more prevalent respiratory illnesses encountered by pediatricians who treat young infants. Usually the result of a viral infection, the more common causative agents in this age group are respiratory syncytial virus (RSV), parainfluenza type III, adenovirus, and, occasionally enteroviruses.

PATHOPHYSIOLOGY

The exact immunologic nature of the host–virus interaction is not fully understood, but the resultant pathophysiology is well described. A necrotizing desquamation occurs along the epithelium of the bronchioles. This results in deposition of luminal debris which both increases airway resistance and leads to air trapping in alveoli behind the partially obstructed airway lumina. Because of the air trapping and hyperinflation, much more negative pressure must be generated by the muscles of inspiration in order to move the same tidal volume of air more easily inhaled at a healthy functional residual capacity. Such large negative pressures in the pulmonary interstitium upset the hydrostatic forces that keep interstitial fluid content low. The increased interstitial fluid that results adds to the work of breathing not only by increasing airflow obstruction, but also by further decreasing pulmonary compliance. The respiratory rate increases to minimize this work of breathing and maintain respiratory function.

CLINICAL PRESENTATION

Bronchiolitis usually begins as a mild upper respiratory tract infection with rhinitis or cough. There is usually little or no fever, although a high fever has been reported. After 1 or 2 days, there is onset of a wheeze and tachypnea. The child is somewhat irritable and often has less interest in feeding. The child's color may be normal or slightly cyanotic. The nares are often flared and the child may be using accessory muscles of respiration. The chest is, to some degree, hyperinflated with intercostal or subcostal retractions. Abdominal organs are often easily palpated below the costal margins. Wheezes are prominent on auscultation, but crackles and rhonchi may also be heard diffusely throughout the lung fields.

DIFFERENTIAL DIAGNOSIS

In a child under 2 years of age, bronchiolitis is one of the most common causes for episodic airflow obstruction. Asthma can be difficult to differentiate from bronchiolitis; in fact, some physicians will not try to separate borderline cases, referring to them only as *wheezing associated respiratory illness* (WARI). In clearcut cases with strong family history of asthma, marked response to bronchodilators, and clinical symptoms in the absence of a predisposing viral respiratory tract infection, the physician can feel slightly better about diagnosing asthma in an infant. Cystic fibrosis often presents in a child as repetitive episodes of bronchiolitis. A recurrent presentation outside of the epidemic time frame or the presence of other complicating cystic fibrosis symptoms (*e.g.*, diarrhea, failure to thrive, meconium ileus) suggests that the child be sent to a cystic fibrosis center for a sweat test (see Chap. 205). Anatomic abnormalities such as vascular rings or tracheomalacia do not remit during the standard bronchiolitis time course. Chest fluoroscopy with barium swallow may reveal the etiology. Gastroesophageal reflux is often a confounding factor in the differential diagnosis of bronchiolitis. All infants reflux to some degree, and this may be enhanced secondarily as a result of the hyperinflation of bronchiolitis. Nevertheless, the presence of recurrent symptoms associated with emesis, acid reflux on a *p*H probe or esophagitis on biopsy all suggest that there may be a contribution of reflux to the recurrent wheeze. This is important in the differential diagnosis because many of the drugs that are used for bronchodilation will decrease lower esophageal sphincter tone and hence exacerbate the reflux (see Chap. 103). Aspiration of a foreign body has to be considered in a child who wheezes for the first time, especially if otherwise well. The wheezing, however, is usually paroxysmal in onset and can often be related to a choking episode with feeding or play (see Chap. 162). Numerous other diagnoses, including immunodeficiency, dysmotile cilia syndrome and α_1-antitrypsin deficiency, can occur but are less likely in the absence of a positive family history. In addition, congestive heart failure in a child with congenital heart disease may present with wheezing and respiratory distress.

WORK-UP

History

Several features of the history are important. The physician should discover if the baby has been active, playful, or is merely lying in the crib or stroller interacting little with his environment. He should determine if the child has been fed relatively normally or with great difficulty and if the child is breathing so quickly that he can only nurse for a few moments before coughing and choking. Both the intake over the previous 24 hours and whether the baby has been urinating as frequently as usual should be noted. The child's temperature should be taken and the physician should observe how prolonged the temperature elevation has been. The mother's experience in dealing with illness of small children should also be determined.

Physical Examination

The physical examination can confirm or refute some of the information from the history. It is important to unclothe the child so that only a diaper remains. A complete assessment of respiratory function cannot be performed adequately in a dressed infant. The child's color in particular should be noted. The presence of pallor or cyanosis should be taken as an indication of hypoxemia. A child who has any degree of nasal flaring, cervical accessory respiratory muscle use, intercostal or subcostal retractions has the potential for respiratory failure. The inferior liver margin should be palpated and the upper border percussed. It is important to ascertain whether the liver edge is depressed secondary to lung hyperinflation, or the liver is enlarged possibly due to congestive heart failure. In any event, careful measurements are useful in following the course of the child's illness. The physician should pay particular attention to chest wall and abdominal motion. As the diaphragm tires, the abdomen no longer moves outward with inspiration, but rather inward and towards the thorax. Such breathing is an ominous sign.

Laboratory Tests

There is little in the standard office laboratory that will help the physician discern the severity of the illness. If urine can be collected, a urine specific gravity can be useful in determining hydration status. In children old enough to concentrate their urine, dilute urine (specific gravities below ~1.008) suggests that the child is adequately hydrated. Concentrated urine (specific gravities greater than ~1.015) suggests that the child is being forced to preserve his intravascular status. Other laboratory data helpful in assessing the child may be available at the local hospital.

Historically, the arterial blood gas has been the standard method for determining the level of hypoxemia and hypercarbia. This information, if carefully gathered, is invaluable, but the physician must be aware that the agitation of arterial puncture may produce spurious results. (The physician can sometimes administer local Xylocaine, allow the child to fuss briefly, and then obtain the arterial sample through the anesthetized region when the child has calmed down.) A specimen obtained by venipuncture can be used if the *p*H and Pco_2 are corrected.

Usually, venous pH is 0.04 pH units lower and venous P_{CO_2} is 6 Torr higher than the corresponding arterial values. Syringes with dry heparin should be used because liquid heparin will dilute the sample. Although this will have little effect on the pH, it can severely effect the P_{CO_2} results, falsely suggesting that the problem is predominantly one of acidemia secondary to metabolic acidosis and not carbon dioxide retention. Alternative methods may be used such as a determination of hemoglobin saturation through pulse oxymetry. Information from poorly obtained blood gases and improperly attached oxymeters can lead to incorrect therapeutic decisions, reminding us that bad data are worse than no data.

MANAGEMENT

Management of patients with a severe or mild disease is relatively straightforward. Oxygen, critical monitoring of vital signs and oxygen/carbon dioxide levels, ventilatory support, intravenous nutrition, antiviral agents where appropriate, antibacterial agents where superinfection has been proven, and bronchodilators where a response has been established, are the standard approach in hospital for the severely ill child. Reassurance, nasal suctioning, judicious feedings, and appropriate use of antipyretics suffice for the limited illness in most children. The remaining group, those that are borderline between outpatient care and hospitalization, tax the physician's medical acumen and skill most of all.

Close observation and family contact are important in outpatient management. A follow-up phone call in a few hours or even a return office visit allows the physician to develop a perspective on the child's illness and the progression or resolution of incipient respiratory failure. It must be remembered that there is little warning when children with bronchiolitis begin to tire out. Retractions will lessen and the child may appear not to work as hard as earlier in the illness. This is an ominous sign when coupled with lack of playfulness, decreased interest in feeding, and persistent tachypnea.

The usefulness of bronchodilators and methylxanthines is controversial. Smooth muscle bronchospasm, theoretically, does not play a large role in the pathogenesis of bronchiolitis. These drugs also have little effect on luminal debris and mucus plugging. Moreover, despite relative airway specificity, even the most selective β-2 agonist may have some cardiac chronotropic effect. The situa-tion is less clear in children with chronic lung disease. Airway reactivity has been demonstrated in children with bronchopulmonary dysplasia and, for some investigators, bronchodilators appear to produce a desired response. The clinical data on methylxanthines are also unclear. Retrospective studies and clinical impressions are somewhat at variance. In recent years, there has been at least theoretical support for the use of this drug because of its properties as a diaphragmatic inotrope. The drug, nevertheless, has not been satisfactorily studied; likewise, no conclusive data support the use of corticosteroids in this illness.

It is reasonable to try a β agonist or methylxanthine in the treatment of these children. Clinical observation, however, is important. Failure to document a clinical response to a medication trial would argue for the cessation of such therapy before problems developed from drug side effects. It is also important not to develop a false sense of security because a wheezing child has been placed on bronchodilators.

Chest physiotherapy and large particle mist are often considered adjunct care. With regard to chest physiotherapy, the benefits of helping expectoration of luminal debris must be balanced against the agitation and possible oxyhemoglobin desaturation that may result. If begun, the child should have adequate time to rest between sessions. Large particle mist has little chance of getting to the lower respiratory tract and may theoretically increase airway resistance. Careful suctioning of the nasopharynx, with saline nose drops just prior to suctioning, may be much more useful. Mist tents hide the child from caretakers and make it more difficult to perceive deterioration.

Future trends in control of infection and management of disease can be extrapolated from current knowledge. Simple hand washing by family members and caretakers, as well as preventing cohorts with respiratory infection from attending daycare centers, may decrease the incidence of the disease. Previous attempts at immunization were unsuccessful, but newer vaccines or temperature sensitive viral mutants may play a future role in prevention. Although the use of aerosolized antiviral agents such as ribovirin is currently limited to hospital administration for proven viral infection in the compromised host (chronic lung disease, congenital heart disease, immunoincompetent patient), further investigation could lead to some form of outpatient administration for the general population at risk. At present, however, the physician's best weapon in caring for the infected child is to understand the pathophysiology and to anticipate the individual patient's course so that intervention can prevent respiratory failure.

ANNOTATED BIBLIOGRAPHY

Denny FW, Collier AM, Henderson FW et al: The epidemiology of bronchiolitis. Pediatr Res 11:234–236, 1977

Hall CB: The shedding and spreading of respiratory syncytial virus. Pediatr Res 11:236–239, 1977 (This and the above reference detail the natural history of RSV infection.)

Hall CB, McBride JT, Walsh EE et al: Aerosolized ribovirin treatment of infants with respiratory syncytial virus infection. N Engl J Med 308:1443–1447, 1983 (Proof that an aerosolized antiviral agent can be useful.)

Outwater KM, Crone RK: Management of respiratory failure in infants with acute viral bronchiolitis. Am J Dis Child 138 (11):1071–1075, 1984 (Logical approach to progressive respiratory failure in infants. Certain therapies such as the use of theophylline are suggested although supporting data are predominantly by clinical impression.)

Webb MS, Martin JA, Cartlidge PH et al: Chest physiotherapy in acute bronchiolitis. Arch Dis Child 60(11):1078–1079, 1985 and

Wohl ME: Bronchiolitis. In Kendig, Chernick (eds): Disorders of the Respiratory Tract in Children, pp 283–293. Philadelphia, WB Saunders, 1983 (Extensive reviews of the subject with good discussions of the pathophysiology of postulated immunologic interaction.)

165
Pneumonia
KENNETH M. BOYER

Pneumonia is a potentially serious respiratory infection often encountered by the pediatrician practicing in an ambulatory setting. Incidence ranges from 40:1000 children/year at ages less than five to 7:1000 children/year at ages 12 to 15. Although pneumonia at present generally has an excellent prognosis with treatment, the pediatrician should remember that this diagnosis may engender fear on the part of parents because of its frequent fatal outcome in the preantibiotic era.

PATHOPHYSIOLOGY

The usual first step in the pathogenesis of pneumonia is damage to the mucociliary clearance mechanism induced by viral respiratory infection. This damage may be more severe in patients with pre-existing clearance abnormalities such as bronchopulmonary dysplasia or cystic fibrosis. Particularly in the young infant, involvement of terminal airways leads to bronchiolitis, air trapping, and segmental atelectasis. Extension into the adjacent interstitial tissues leads to interstitial pneumonia. Alveolar inflammation (lobar pneumonia) usually represents a superimposition of bacterial infection on previously damaged terminal airways as the result of minor aspiration.

Complications of nonbacterial pneumonia include atelectasis, bronchospasm, apneic spells, and respiratory failure. Complications of bacterial pneumonia include septicemia, pleural extension (effusion or empyema), and lung abscess.

CLINICAL PRESENTATION

The clinical presentation of pneumonia varies with age and with infecting agent. A young baby with pneumonia generally has minimal systemic signs but obvious respiratory distress. On general inspection, tachypnea, retractions, and nasal flaring are usually apparent. A cough may or may not be present. The older child or adolescent generally has more obvious signs of systemic illness, including fever and prostration. Rather than respiratory distress, pulmonary involvement is usually manifested by cough, chest pain, or sputum production. All of these manifestations may be present in the older infant or toddler with pneumonia.

Nonbacterial pneumonia generally has a gradual onset that correlates with the gradual progression of disease from the upper to the lower airways and interstitial tissues. Bacterial pneumonia often presents as a sudden change in a previously mild respiratory illness, usually with a recrudescence of fever or chills. Common nonbacterial and bacterial causes of pediatric pneumonia are summarized in Table 165-1, with clinical clues that may suggest specific etiologies in an individual patient.

Table 165-1. Nonbacterial and Bacterial Agents Causing Pediatric Pneumonia, According to Age*

AGE GROUP, INFECTING AGENT	CLINICAL CLUES	AGE GROUP, INFECTING AGENT	CLINICAL CLUES
YOUNG INFANT (≤3 MONTHS)		Human immunodeficiency virus	Blood transfusion, maternal IV drug abuse
Nonbacterial agents			
Chlamydia trachomatis	Afebrile, "staccato cough," conjunctivitis	*Mycoplasma pneumoniae*	Cold agglutinins, no coryza
RS virus†	Low-grade fever, wheeze, apnea, winter season	Bacteria	
		Streptococcus pneumoniae	Lobar consolidation, antigenuria
Cytomegalovirus†	"Blueberry muffin," transfused premie	*Hemophilus influenzae*	Lobar consolidation, pleural effusion, antigenuria, penicillin Rx failure
Parainfluenza viruses†	Sibling or parental URIs or LTB, Fall or Spring season		
Influenza viruses†	Parental or sibling "flu" illness, winter season, community epidemics	*Staphylococcus aureus*†	Pneumatoceles, empyema
		Bordetella pertussis	Immunization history, lymphocytosis, pertussoid cough
Bacteria			
Group B streptococcus†	Amniotic fluid infection, antigenuria	Group A streptococci†	Empyema, scarlatiniform rash
Staphylococcus aureus†	Skin pustules, empyema, pneumatoceles	Oral anaerobes†	Aspiration secondary to neuromuscular or anatomic abnormality
Klebsiella pneumoniae†	Nosocomial pneumonia in a premie		
Oral anaerobes†	Aspiration secondary to neuromuscular or anatomic abnormality	**OLDER CHILD/ADOLESCENT (6–16 YEARS)**	
		Nonbacterial agents	
OLDER INFANT/TODDLER/YOUNGER CHILD (4 MONTHS–5 YEARS)		*Mycoplasma pneumoniae*	Cold agglutinins, no coryza
Nonbacterial agents		Influenza viruses	Parental or sibling "flu" illnesses, winter season, community epidemics
RS virus	Wheeze, winter season	Adenoviruses	Exudative pharyngitis
Parainfluenza viruses	Sibling or parental URIs or LTB, Fall or Spring season	Measles virus	Rash, immunization history
Influenza viruses	Sibling or parental "flu" illness, winter season, community epidemics	Bacteria	
		Streptococcus pneumoniae	Lobar consolidation, antigenuria
Adenoviruses†	Severe, may involve liver, CNS, skin	*Staphylococcus aureus*†	Pneumatoceles, empyema
Measles virus	Rash, immunization history	Group A streptococci†	Empyema, scarlatiniform rash

* Agents in each category are listed in approximate order of frequency. Clinical clues may suggest a specific etiology, but are not definitive.
† Inpatient management mandatory.

DIFFERENTIAL DIAGNOSIS

The major categories of disease that need to be differentiated in patients with pneumonia are (1) bacterial etiologies that require specific antimicrobial therapy, (2) nonbacterial etiologies that may require antiviral or broad spectrum antimicrobial therapy, (3) noninfectious conditions that may simulate pneumonia but for which other forms of therapy may be essential, and (4) unusual or "exotic" infections. Additional considerations that enter into differential diagnosis include the status of the host, whether compromised or normal, the age of the patient, the exposure history, and the season of the year.

Pneumonias caused by bacteria characteristically are lobar in distribution and exhibit consolidation on x-ray. Atelectasis, on the other hand, is common in nonbacterial pneumonia and must be distinguished from a true consolidation. Pleural effusions, circular infiltrates, consolidations with convex margins, and pneumatoceles all favor a bacterial etiology. Because of the association of bacteremia with high fever and significant leukocytosis in the young child, these clinical features also favor bacterial etiology. Positive cultures of blood, pleural fluid, or lung aspirates establish etiology in bacterial pneumonia.

In certain settings, the diagnosis of nonbacterial pneumonia may be made with relative certainty based on the clinical presentation, season, and age. Viral pneumonias characteristically appear as bronchopneumonia on chest roentgenogram, with hyperinflation, segmental atelectasis, or interstitial infiltrates. Despite recent advances in techniques for rapid viral diagnosis, however, in most instances this category of pulmonary infection remains a diagnosis of exclusion. Mycoplasma pneumonia is usually lobar in distribution, but not densely consolidated. Serologic tests usually permit diagnosis in the acute phase.

The list of noninfectious conditions that may simulate pneumonia should be kept in mind and is

---

Noninfectious Conditions That May Simulate or Underlie Acute Pneumonia in Children

PHYSIOLOGIC

Prominent thymus
Breast shadows
Underpenetrated chest radiograph

CHRONIC PULMONARY DISEASE

Asthma
Cystic fibrosis
Bronchiectasis
Bronchiolitis obliterans
Pulmonary sequestration
Congenital lobar emphysema
Pulmonary hemosiderosis
Desquamative interstitial pneumonitis

RECURRENT ASPIRATION

Gastroesophageal reflux
Tracheoesophageal fistula
Cleft palate
Neuromuscular disorders
Familial dysautonomia

ATELECTASIS

Mucous plug
Foreign body

ALLERGIC ALVEOLITIS

Dusts (farmer's lung)
Molds (allergic aspergillosis)
Excreta (pigeon breeder's lung)

DAMAGE BY PHYSICAL AGENTS

Bronchopulmonary dysplasia
Lipoid pneumonia
Kerosene pneumonia
Near drowning
Smoke inhalation

IATROGENIC PULMONARY DAMAGE

Drugs (nitrofurantoin, bleomycin)
Radiation pneumonitis
Graft-vs-host disease

PULMONARY INFARCTION

Sickle vaso-occlusive crisis
Fat embolism

MISCELLANEOUS

Congestive heart failure
Adult respiratory distress syndrome
Systemic lupus erythematosis
Sarcoidosis
Neoplasms (lymphoma, teratoma, neuroblastoma)
Pleural effusion or reaction
Bronchogenic cyst
Vascular ring
Histiocytosis X

provided in the box, Noninfectious Conditions That May Stimulate or Underlie Acute Pneumonia in Children. The line of demarcation between infectious and noninfectious conditions is not always sharp. In the child with sickle cell anemia, for example, a pulmonary vascular occlusive crisis presents with fever, leukocytosis, and patchy pulmonary infiltrates. Differentiation from pneumococcal, hemophilus, or mycoplasmal pneumonia, to which the child with sickle cell anemia has increased susceptibility, may be difficult or impossible. Early recognition of noninfectious conditions either mimicking or underlying pneumonia may prevent a recurrence or improve prognosis. Asthma, for example, is the most frequent cause of recurrent pneumonia. Treatment with bronchodilators may prevent recurrences. Similarly, early recognition and treatment of cystic fibrosis as an underlying condition has a clear beneficial effect in slowing irreversible pulmonary damage.

Other infectious conditions that may present as acute pediatric pneumonia include mycobacterial, fungal, or parasitic infections. Patients who have tuberculosis are frequently considered to have acute pneumonia when first examined. Thus, tuberculin testing is an important consideration in the initial evaluation of a patient with pneumonia and is especially important for children residing in urban areas, recent immigrants, and native American Indians. Fungal pneumonia, particularly coccidioidomycosis and histoplasmosis, should be considered in children residing in or visiting endemic areas. A suggestive exposure history may often be elicited such as backyard swimming pool excavations, clean up chores in old barns or sheds, or exposure to dust storms. Other fungal pneumonias, such as aspergillosis and cryptococcosis, occur almost exclusively in the setting of immunosuppression. Pneumocystis pneumonia implies a major defect in cell-mediated immunity and may be the presenting problem in congenital immunodeficiency or pediatric AIDS.

WORK-UP

History

Key elements in the history of a child with pneumonia are the family history, the past medical history, and a history of unusual exposures. Family history may uncover relatives with genetic diseases that may affect the lungs (*e.g.*, cystic fibrosis) or an atopic tendency (*e.g.*, asthma, eczema, or hayfever). A factor that is frequently overlooked but is perhaps more important than these is a history of recent infectious illnesses in the family such as flu-like illnesses, upper respiratory infections, or croup. Such a history makes an infectious process, usually viral, more likely than a noninfectious condition. In the past medical history, a low-birth-weight premature infant may have a higher probability of having nosocomial pathogens or a greater predisposition to apnea (and hence a stronger indication for hospitalization) during pneumonia. Gaps in immunization may indicate a susceptibility to measles, pertussis, or *Hemophilus influenzae* type b infection. Previous hospitalizations for pneumonia should alert the physician to the possibility of an underlying anatomic or immunologic disease. Patients known to have chronic diseases, such as cystic fibrosis, bronchopulmonary dysplasia, asthma, sickle cell disease, or congenital heart disease may have unusual pathogens or an unusual severity of illness. A recent history of "choking" should suggest the possibility of foreign body aspiration. Recent travel, exposure to pets, or unusual activities may increase the possibility of fungal disease, psittacosis, Q fever, or unusual bacterial pathogens.

Physical Examination

A physical examination is usually sufficient to indicate a strong probability of pneumonia (and thus the need for laboratory confirmation). More importantly, it identifies the child with respiratory decompensation (which may require hospitalization for oxygen therapy or mechanical ventilation) or dehydration (which may require other forms of supportive therapy most appropriate in a hospital setting). General appearance is the most important aspect of the physical examination, particularly in the infant or young child. By inspection of the child at rest, the physician can best estimate the severity of respiratory involvement and the presence of tachypnea, grunting, flaring, or retractions. (The experienced clinician often recognizes pneumonia on the basis of these findings alone.) Findings on auscultation may vary and may range from a normal examination to localized diminished breath sounds to the more classic findings of rales, tubular breath sounds, or egophony.

Laboratory Tests

The essentials in laboratory work-up of pediatric pneumonia include a PA and lateral chest radiograph, a white blood cell count and differential, a tuberculin test, and cold agglutinins. The Gram stain and culture of sputum, standard in the adult work-up, are generally not practical in pediatrics. Blood culture, although a "low-yield" test, is an appropriate one for the highly febrile child less than 2 years of age with a markedly elevated white count. Ten to twenty percent of these children are bacteremic. Establishing a specific etiology in those that have positive blood cultures is worth the expenditure. Tests for bacterial polysaccharide antigens in urine may help in diagnosing bacterial pneumonia, but unfortunately they are not sufficiently sensitive to permit a bacterial process to be completely ruled out in an individual patient. The reagents for these tests are best for *Hemophilus influenzae* type b and group B streptococcus. Viral cultures, previously considered to be an academic exercise, are becoming increasingly important in the hospital management of young infants with pneumonia due to the recent availability of the antiviral drug ribavirin. The diagnosis of infection by respiratory syncytial virus by means of immunofluorescense microscopy or enzyme-linked-immunosorbent assay now makes it possible to identify patients who would benefit from this inhalational drug therapy. Such tests are particularly appropriate for the young baby with underlying cardiopulmonary disease who is at high risk for serious consequences of RSV pneumonia. With the exceptions of tests for mycoplasmal or chlamydial infection, serologic tests are a futile exercise.

In the patient with significant respiratory compromise, blood gas determinations or ear oximetry are indicated. The latter, using simple noninvasive instruments, is a real advance in the hospital management of the sick infant with pneumonia. Finally, for immunocompromised hosts, whose range of possible pathogens is wide and who are particularly susceptible to a progressive disease, invasive diagnostic procedures such as bronchoalveolar lavage or open lung biopsy are usually indicated.

TREATMENT

Although most textbooks conveniently describe the most appropriate therapeutic regimens for specific etiologic agents of pneumonia, the reality of clinical practice is that most children with acute pneumonia must be treated as *pneumonias of unknown cause*. The patient's age, radiographic findings, and white count may be guides to probable etiologies. However, the goal of diagnostic efforts should be to replace empiric by specific treatment.

In the baby within the first 5 days of life, major considerations for treatment are early-onset infections due to perinatally acquired bacteria. An appropriate combination therapy for such babies is ampicillin and gentamicin. The premature infant who has had a prolonged hospitalization is susceptible to nosocomial pneumonia with hospital pathogens. Under these circumstances, the parenteral combinations of nafcillin/gentamicin or nafcillin/ceftriaxone are reasonable empiric treatments. Normal babies who develop pneumonia in the first 3 months of life are most likely to have either chlamydial or respiratory syncytial viral infections. Erythromycin is a reasonable oral regimen for such babies.

In the older baby and young child between 4 months and 5 years of age, about two thirds of pneumonias are due to viruses and one third is due to bacterial etiologies. For the child who can be treated as an outpatient in whom a bacterial etiology appears likely, or cannot be excluded, treatment with oral amoxicillin or amoxicillin/clavulanic acid is reasonable. The use of inhalational ribavirin is now recommended for the child with pre-existing cardiopulmonary disease and an apparent viral pneumonia. In the child who requires hospitalization for an apparent bacterial pneumonia, parenteral antibiotic regimens with broad activity against the most likely pathogens (*e.g.*, pneumococci, *Hemophilus*, and *Staphylococcus aureus*) are indicated. Cefuroxime or the combinations of nafcillin and chloramphenicol or nafcillin and ceftriaxone are good initial empiric regimens. The child older than 6 years of age with pneumonia is most likely to have mycoplasma or pneumococcal pneumonia. In that setting, erythromycin should be considered the preferred oral drug, with cefuroxime or erythromycin and cefuroxime for hospitalized patients.

Most children with mild to moderate disease can be managed satisfactorily with oral antimicrobial agents outside the hospital. Commonly used oral agents are summarized in Table 165-2, with their "coverage" and recommended dosages. (Initial therapy with these agents would be inappropriate for some pathogens, such as *S. aureus*, but they may be used judiciously during convalesence.) The child managed as an outpatient should be seen within 72 hours of initiation of therapy to document improvement; parents should be instructed to return with the child earlier if there are any signs of a progression of disease. Children who require hospitalization are those with severe disease at onset or who appear to be deteriorating on outpatient management, children with underlying pulmonary or cardiac problems, and those whose families lack

Table 165-2.   Oral Antimicrobial Agents for Outpatient Treatment of Pediatric Pneumonia

DRUG	EFFECTIVE AGAINST	DOSAGE (MG/KG/24 HOURS)
Amoxicillin	S. pneumo, group A strep* Some H. flu	40 ÷ Q8H
Amoxicillin/Clavulanic acid	S. pneumo, all H. flu, group A strep, S. aureus,* oral anaerobes*	40 ÷ Q8H
Cefaclor	S. pneumo, all H. flu, group A strep*	40 ÷ Q8H
Chloramphenicol	All H. flu, S. pneumo, oral anaerobes*	50–75 ÷ Q6H
Clindamycin	S. aureus*, oral anaerobes*, group A strep*	20–30 ÷ Q8H
Dicloxacillin	S. aureus*, S. pneumo, Group A strep*	25–50 ÷ Q6H
Erythromycin	S. pneumo, M. pneumo, B. pertussis, C. trachomatis	40 ÷ Q6H
Erythromycin/sulfisoxazole	S. pneumo M. pneumo, B. pertussis, C. trachomatis	40 ÷ Q6H (erythromycin component)
Penicillin	S. pneumo, group A strep*	25–50 ÷ Q6H
Trimethaprim/sulfamethoxazole	All H. flu, S. pneumo, P. carinii*	10–20 ÷ Q12H (trimethaprim component)

* Initial therapy should be parenteral (inpatient).

the ability to reliably provide therapy and supportive care. Special concern is needed for infants under 1 year of age whose signs of respiratory disease may be subtle, who may progress rapidly, and who are experiencing their first major infectious illness and are of unproven immunologic competence.

Durations of treatment vary with etiology. A 10-day course is recommended for outpatient antimicrobial therapy of most pneumonia cases. For viral disease being treated in hospital with ribavirin, a brief duration of 3 to 5 days is generally considered adequate. For the complicated case, for example a child with S. aureus pneumonia, empyema, and prolonged chest tube drainage, 3 to 6 weeks of treatment (parenteral followed by oral) may be necessary. Follow-up chest roentgenograms are not mandatory but are a reasonable way to document the resolution of a disease at 6 to 8 weeks after onset. They should always be performed on hospitalized children and selectively in children managed as outpatients who have a persistent cough or who fail to return to normal activities or weight gain.

INDICATIONS FOR REFERRAL

Indications for outpatient referral are primarily a failure to clear the first episode of pneumonia or recurrent disease. Indications for inpatient consultation or transfer include a failure to respond to parenteral regimens (in terms of fever and toxicity) within 48 to 72 hours of admission, respiratory failure necessitating intensive respiratory therapy or mechanical ventilation, development of empyema, or suspicion of a foreign body indicating the need for bronchoscopy.

ANNOTATED BIBLIOGRAPHY

Beem MO, Saxon E: Respiratory-tract colonization and a distinctive pneumonia syndrome in infants infected with Chlamydia trachomatis. N Engl J Med 296:306, 1977 (Exemplary study of the afebrile pneumonitis syndrome of infancy that established C. trachomatis as a common etiologic agent.)

Dennehy PH, McIntosh K: Viral pneumonia in childhood. In Weinstein L, Fields BN (eds): Seminars in Infectious Disease, p 173. Vol 5: Pneumonias. New York, Thieme–Stratton, 1983 (Scholarly review of the pathogens and clinical features of pneumonias caused by viral agents in children.)

Denny FW, Clyde WA, Jr: Acute lower respiratory tract infections in nonhospitalized children. J Pediatr 108:635, 1986 (Most recent in an outstanding series of studies of respiratory infection in a Chapel Hill, NC, group practice that have defined patterns of illness associated with common respiratory viral pathogens.)

Griscom NT, Wohl MEB, Kirkpatrick JA, Jr: Lower respiratory infections: How infants differ from adults. Radiol Clin North Am 16:367, 1978 (Well-illustrated article demonstrating the most common features—air trapping and segmental atelectasis—seen in pediatric viral pneumonia.)

Grossman LK, Wald ER, Nair P et al: Roentgenographic follow-up of acute pneumonia in children. Pediatrics 63:30, 1979 (Prospective study of 129 children with acute pneumonia demonstrating that follow-up chest x-rays may be done selectively based on persistent respiratory symptoms or failure to thrive.)

Hall CB, McBride JT, Gala CL et al: Ribavirin treatment of respiratory syncytial viral infection in infants with underlying cardiopulmonary disease. JAMA 254:3047, 1985 (Comparative trial of ribavirin aerosol treatment vs placebo in 53 infants with respiratory syncytial virus infection and underlying bronchopulmonary dysplasia or congenital heart disease. Treated infants did significantly better, establishing a role for ribavirin treatment in this high-risk patient group.)

Long SS: Treatment of acute pneumonia in infants and children. Pediatr Clin North Am 30:247, 1983 (Comprehensive review of pediatric pneumonias, with the emphasis on epidemiologic, clinical, and laboratory features that aid in diagnosis, and a rational approach to antimicrobial and supportive therapy.)

Ramsey BW, Marcuse EK, Foy HM et al: Use of bacterial antigen detection in the diagnosis of pediatric lower respiratory tract infections. Pediatrics 78:1, 1986 (Etiologic study of 162 children with acute lower respiratory infections. Antigenuria was found in 24% of the children, suggesting that bacterial etiology may be more common in pediatric pneumonia than is generally believed and that empiric antibiotic treatment is reasonable in most cases.)

Seto DSY, Heller RM: Acute respiratory infections. Pediatr Clin N Am 21:683, 1974 (Review of classic pneumonia syndromes in pediatrics, according to specific etiology, with representative radiographs.)

166
Tuberculosis: Screening and Prophylaxis
L. GERARD NIEDERMAN

The screening of asymptomatic children for tuberculous infection, a traditional part of pediatric office care, is based on three premises: (1) tuberculous disease (*i.e.*, the presence of symptoms or clinical signs consistent with tuberculosis) is curable; (2) tuberculous disease progresses from tuberculous infection (*i.e.*, the presence of a positive tuberculin skin test in the absence of symptoms and clinical findings suggesting tuberculosis); and (3) the progression from infection to disease is preventable with chemoprophylaxis. Recent recommendations for screening have advised concentrating efforts in high risk groups. In an era when the morbidity and mortality from tuberculosis are decreasing, control is directed towards finding and treating active disease in order to eliminate transmission.

In 1985, 22,201 cases of active tuberculosis were reported in the United States. 1261 cases were children less than 15 years old, of whom 789 were less than 5 years old. The occurrence in children is clear evidence of the ongoing transmission of tuberculosis and emphasizes the need for vigorous continued, comprehensive control programs.

WHO SHOULD BE SCREENED?

All children should be screened by taking a careful history for risk factors, particularly children with clinical signs and symptoms suggestive of tuberculous disease. However, in most areas of the United States the prevalence of tuberculous infection in children is well below 1% (often between 0.1% and 0.5%), making mass screening of the general population with tuberculin skin tests an inefficient method of finding infection and disease. In this situation, most positive tuberculin reactions are false positives, particularly in areas where atypical mycobacteria exposure is likely. Screening, however, is indicated for groups in which the prevalence is not low or where the risk of infection poses a higher risk of subsequent disease with its attendant morbidity or mortality.

Groups with a high risk of infection include immigrants from Asia, Africa, the Caribbean, Latin America, and the Middle East; some groups of American Indians and Eskimos; and children who are contacts of proven or suspected cases of tuberculosis. Children who have signs or symptoms that suggest tuberculous disease and children who have findings on chest radiographs compatible with past tuberculosis should be evaluated for tuberculous infection or disease. Children living in inner city, low socioeconomic environments are generally *not* at high risk of infection. Local public health departments, however, can provide risk estimates for particular communities.

HOW TO SCREEN—SKIN TESTING AND INTERPRETATION

Usually within a period of 2 to 10 weeks after infection with *Mycobacterium tuberculosis*, delayed (cellular) hypersensitivity develops, which may be manifested by a positive tuberculin skin test. The Mantoux test is the preferred method of testing. One tenth (0.1) ml of PPD containing 5 tuberculin units (TU) is injected intracutaneously on the volar aspect of the forearm with a short-bevel, 26- or 27-gauge needle. With proper administration, a discrete 6-mm to 10-mm wheal is produced. The Mantoux test should be read on the second or third day after injection, which is the time when induration is usually most evident. Significant induration, however, may persist for 5 to 7 days. The margins of induration (not erythema) should be determined by palpation or by using a ball-point pen, measured in millimeters transversely to the long axis of the forearm and recorded.

Though not recommended for screening, various multipuncture tests are currently in widespread use. Concentrated tuberculin (OT or PPD) is introduced into the skin with an applicator coated with dried tuberculin or by a puncture through a film of liquid tuberculin. The dose introduced often exceeds 5 TU, because it cannot be administered precisely; thus, these tests are not meant for diagnostic use but rather for screening asymptomatic persons. After 48 to 72 hours, induration of the largest single papule or induration of coalescence of papular reactions should be measured and recorded. The test is interpreted as positive if vesiculation is present. Reactions of 2 mm or more of induration are doubtful and need verification by the standard Mantoux test. Induration of less than 2 mm is considered a negative reaction.

Induration measuring 10 mm or more is frequently considered the definition of a positive Mantoux test. Interpretation of tuberculin skin tests, however, should be done in the clinical context of why the test was performed. Induration measuring 15 mm or greater is almost always due to *M. tuberculosis* infection or disease, and reactions less than 5 mm usually exclude tuberculosis. Reactions between 5-mm and 15-mm induration are more difficult to interpret.

False-positive tuberculin tests are most often due to reactions caused by nontuberculin mycobacteria. In the southeastern United States as well as other areas of the world where infection with nontuberculous mycobacteria is common, cross-reactions may outnumber true reactions to *M. tuberculosis*. This is particularly true when there is no history of tuberculous exposure and the population has a low prevalence of tuberculosis. In such areas, preventive treatment might be reserved for children with reactions greater than 15-mm induration. On the other hand, reactions between 5 mm and 10 mm should be considered due to *M. tuberculosis* when there is a history of contact with an infectious case of tuberculosis, or when there is radiographic evidence of present or past tuberculosis.

The interpretation of tuberculin skin tests in children purportedly vaccinated with bacillus Calmette–Guerin (BCG) may be confusing. The intensity and duration of positive tuberculin skin reactions following BCG vaccination is variable, and there is no completely reliable way to distinguish reactions due to *M. tuberculosis* from those due to BCG. The child with a positive skin test reaction and a history of vaccination with BCG should be managed based on the clinical risk of tuberculous infection and disease. Prophylactic therapy with isoniazid is reasonable if there is a history of tuberculous exposure and the chance of transmission to the child is significant, particularly since BCG vaccination is not completely protective.

False-negative skin tests occur and reasons for their occurrence are presented in the box, Causes for False-Negative Tuberculin Reactions.

PREVENTIVE MANAGEMENT OF TUBERCULOUS INFECTION AND CONTACT

Preventive treatment with isoniazid (INH) is indicated for children with positive tuberculin skin tests who have no evidence of clinical disease and also for children with significant exposure to an infectious (or presumed infectious) case of tuberculosis. The highest risk of developing disease occurs in the first 2 years after infection, and the risk of

Causes for False-Negative Tuberculin Reactions

FACTORS RELATED TO THE PERSON BEING TESTED

Infections that cause temporary anergy
Live virus vaccinations (*e.g.,* measles, mumps, polio)
Metabolic and nutritional derangements
Diseases affecting lymphoid organs
Corticosteroid and immunosuppressive drugs
Age (newborns, elderly patients with "waned" sensitivity)
Recent infection with *M. tuberculosis*

FACTORS RELATED TO THE TUBERCULIN USED

Improper storage and dilution
Chemical denaturation and adsorption
Contamination

FACTORS RELATED TO THE ADMINISTRATION AND INTERPRETATION

Injection errors (*e.g.,* too little antigen, subcutaneous)
Inexperienced or biased reader
Error in recording

(Adapted from American Thoracic Society: The tuberculin skin test. Am Rev Respir Dis 124:356–363, 1981)

disease and its complications increases with decreasing age. Other risk factors for developing tuberculous disease include diabetes, particularly poorly controlled insulin-dependent diabetes, corticosteroid or immunosuppressive therapy, malnutrition either primary or secondary to other illnesses, acquired or congenital immunodeficiency diseases, and children with malignancies of lymphoid tissue.

A child or adolescent with a positive tuberculin skin test should be evaluated with a chest roentgenogram. If it is normal, and no previous antituberculous treatment has been received, preventive therapy with isoniazid should be initiated. Household contacts and other close contacts with a proven or potentially infectious case of tuberculosis should also receive preventive therapy. When the index case is identified, all family members should have a tuberculin skin test performed. If it is positive (5 mm or more induration in this clinical situation), or if there is clinical suspicion of tuberculosis, a chest radiograph should be done. If the tuberculin test is positive and there is no evidence of tuberculous disease, preventive therapy for 1 year should be given. If the tuberculin test is negative, treatment for 10 to 15 weeks should be given, particularly for infants and children. The tuberculin test should be repeated at the end of this treatment period, and, if it is positive, treatment should be continued for 1 year. If, after 3 months, the skin test is negative and the risk of transmission has been eliminated, INH can be discontinued. In the newborn infant born to a mother with active, contagious tuberculosis, the mother and child should be separated until the mother has been treated and is noncontagious. Preventive treatment is usually continued for 6 months in such a high-risk situation. If compliance with isoniazid prophylaxis is questionable or is contraindicated, and exposure to infectious tuberculosis cannot be avoided, BCG vaccination may be considered.

Currently, INH is given in a single daily dose of 10 mg/kg/day, not to exceed 300 mg/day. Twelve months of treatment is recommended, although there is evidence to suggest that 6 months of treatment may be almost as effective. Future recommendations may be for a shorter duration of treatment. Alternatively, if compliance with daily administration of INH cannot be assured, INH can be administered in a dose of 20 to 40 mg/kg/day (not to exceed 900 mg) twice a week. Prophylaxis with rifampin (10 mg/kg/day, up to 600 mg) should be given for 12 months if there is proof that infection has occurred with an isoniazid-resistant organism. Combined INH and rifampin treatment may be given pending sensitivity results if resistance is suspected.

Hepatotoxic reactions to INH are rare in children and adolescents, and routine monitoring of liver enzymes is not indicated. Monthly personal or telephone contact should be made with parents or patients receiving INH, and they should be instructed to report symptoms suggesting hepatitis (*e.g.,* fever, anorexia, nausea, vomiting, malaise, jaundice, dark urine, or right upper quadrant abdominal pain). Peripheral neuritis may occur, particularly in malnourished children receiving INH, and may be prevented by concurrent administration of daily pyridoxine (1 mg per 10 mg of INH).

ANNOTATED BIBLIOGRAPHY

American Thoracic Society: The tuberculin skin test. Am Rev Respir Dis 124:356–363, 1981 (This and the following two references provide current, comprehensive guidelines for the office management of tuberculosis [and much more!])

American Thoracic Society, CDC: Control of tuberculosis. Am Rev Respir Dis 128:336–342, 1983

American Thoracic Society, CDC: Treatment of tuberculosis infection in adults and children. Am Rev Respir Dis 134:355–363, 1986

Donaldson JC, Elliott RC: A study of co-positivity of three multipuncture techniques with intradermal PPD tuberculin. Am Rev Respir Dis 118:843–846, 1978 (If you use a multipunture tuberculin skin test, use the Mono-Vacc.)

Ferebee SH: Controlled chemoprophylaxis trials in tuberculosis: A general review. Adv Tuberc Res 17:29, 1969 (Treatment for 1 year with INH is effective in reducing pulmonary and systemic complications of tuberculosis.)

Snider DE: Bacille Calmette–Guerin vaccinations and tuberculin skin tests. JAMA 253:3438–3439, 1985 (Sound practical advice on this confusing clinical problem.)

167

Pulmonary Function Tests

ROBERT G. ZWERDLING

Morbidity due to respiratory illness in childhood results in more loss of time at school than from any other cause. The physician who cares for children must, therefore, have the proper tools to evaluate the functional status of the respiratory tract in an objective and quantitative fashion.

An overview of techniques available for such evaluations is provided in this chapter. In most cases such assessments can be accomplished in a noninvasive and cost-effective manner, and they are well suited to the ambulatory setting. The reader is directed to more extensive sources for a detailed discussion of pulmonary physiology (West, 1985) and pulmonary function testing (Ruppel, 1979).

INDICATIONS FOR PULMONARY FUNCTION TESTS

Pulmonary function tests (PFT) are used to assess the degree and type of physiologic derangement, the responses to pharmacologic intervention, and the progress of various diseases. They are indicated for the evaluation of children having or suspected of having lung disease when the physician needs to have physiologic (functional) information regarding the patient. Children presenting with recurrent or chronic cough or dyspnea ("can't keep up," "won't keep up") are easily evaluated using such tests. On the other hand, chest radiographs are used to visualize anatomic defects but are relatively insensitive and difficult to quantitate physiologic abnormalities.

TECHNIQUES FOR MEASURING PULMONARY PHYSIOLOGY

Respiratory Rates

The respiratory rate, although generally felt to be part of the physical examination, is a reprodu-

Table 167-1. Respiratory Rates by Age and Sex

AGE (Years)	BOYS (Mean ± SD)	GIRLS (Mean ± SD)
0–1	31 ± 8	30 ± 6
1–2	26 ± 4	27 ± 4
2–3	25 ± 4	25 ± 3
3–4	24 ± 3	24 ± 3
4–5	23 ± 2	22 ± 2
5–6	22 ± 2	21 ± 2
6–7	21 ± 3	21 ± 3
. . .	. . .	. . .
17 – 18	16 ± 3	17 ± 3

Active children have rates that are considerably higher. (Iliff A, Lee VA: Pulse rate, respiratory rate, and body temperature of children between two months and eighteen years of age. Child Dev 23:237, 1952)

cible measure of pulmonary function. It is affected by virtually all severe derangements of pulmonary physiology. However, one must appreciate that it varies with age, activity, and state of consciousness (Table 167-1). It is often useful to have parents keep a log of sleeping respiratory rates at home. Respiratory rates and assessment of oxygenation often constitute the only readily available measures currently obtainable for the young or uncooperative infant and child.

Arterial Blood Gases

Arterial blood gases (ABG) reflect gas exchange and, with various transcutaneous measurements, are often one of a few measurements for use in infants and young children. To properly evaluate the results, the physician must know the concentration of inspired oxygen; that the sample is solely composed of arterial blood; and that excess heparin is not used (because it will falsely depress the P_{CO_2}).

Table 167-2.   Causes of Abnormal Arterial Blood Gases

| | Po₂ | | |
	RA	100%	Pco₂
V/Q mismatch	↓	↑	↓
Diffusion def	↓	↑	↓
Hypoventilation	↓	↑	↕
R to L shunt	↓	↓	↓

RA = room air; V/Q = ventilation/perfusion; R = right; L = left.

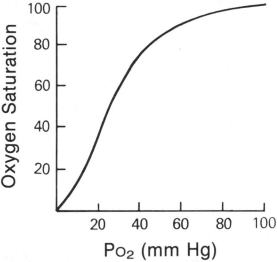

Figure 167-1.   The oxygen saturation curve relates the percent saturation of oxygen with the partial pressure of oxygen.

Diseases that involve the lung in a diffuse manner virtually always result in hypoxemia if the patient is breathing room air. This becomes more pronounced with exercise. In addition, there may be a derangement of acid-base status most often caused by hyperventilation.

The pattern of blood gas abnormalities varies in a characteristic way depending on the type and severity of the problem (Table 167-2). Diffuse pulmonary disease such as bronchiolitis, cystic fibrosis, and pneumonia result in a mismatch of ventilation to perfusion(V/Q). Characteristically, the ABG seen in such a situation is that of hypoxemia and hypocapnia with the hypoxemia being correctable by oxygen supplementation. Right to left shunts are produced by intracardiac or intrapulmonary shunting. These shunts also produce hypoxemia and hypocapnia. In this case, however, oxygen supplementation only minimally corrects the resultant hypoxemia. Hypoventilation, most often a manifestation of neuromuscular disease, drug overdose, or obstruction of the upper airway, produces hypoxemia correctable with oxygen supplementation as well as hypercapnia.

hemoglobins. Keeping these factors in mind, oximetry is simple, rapid, and easier than transcutaneous oxygen measurements. The increasing numbers of children on home oxygen due to cystic fibrosis, bronchopulmonary dysplasia, and other less common respiratory diseases makes this measurement particularly attractive.

Lung Volumes

Lung volumes refer to the amount of gas in the lungs at varying degrees of inspiration (Fig. 167-2). Total lung capacity (TLC) is the amount of gas con-

Pulse Oximetry

Pulse oximetry is now becoming a widely available method for the measurement of oxygen saturation. It is noninvasive, accurate, and suitable for office and even home measurements. The reading is of oxygen saturation rather than the more familiar partial pressure of oxygen (Po₂). The relationship between oxygen saturation and Po₂ is shown in Fig. 167-1. For example, a oxygen saturation of 90% corresponds to a Po₂ of 60 mm Hg. It must be noted that the curve is shifted to the left by alkalosis, hypothermia, fetal as well as other unusual types of hemoglobin and to the right by acidosis, hyperthermia, hypercapnia, and certain other abnormal

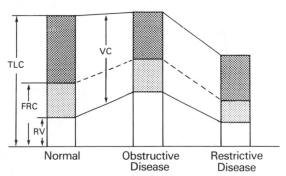

Figure 167-2.   The expected changes in lung volumes with obstructive and restrictive defects are demonstrated.

tained at a full inspiration; residual volume (RV) is the amount of gas left in the lung after the patient expires completely. The vital capacity (VC) is the amount of gas that the patient can expel and is the most widely measured value. The office-based pediatrician will most commonly measure VC either as part of a complete pulmonary function evaluation or when following a child with neuromuscular weakness, such a Guillain–Barré syndrome. The measurement of VC requires the cooperation of the child and is, therefore, rarely accurate for a child under 5 years of age.

Flow Rates

Flow rates are the most widely used and useful measurement of pulmonary function in the ambulatory setting (Fig. 167-3). This is because of the high prevalence of asthma and other airway diseases in childhood. These are generally measured as volume *vs* time or flow *vs* volume as demonstrated in Figure 167-3. Flow rates can also be measured before and after bronchodilators, exercise, cold air, and occasionally antigen challenge to evaluate the degree and nature of airway reactivity (see the section on challenge testing). These tests also require cooperation on the part of the child. Simple measurements of peak expiratory flow can often be performed at 3 years of age, although more extensive testing usually requires that the child be over 5 years of age.

Peak Expiratory Flow Rates

The peak expiratory flow rate (PEFR) is a simple, inexpensive, and reproducible gauge of obstruction. It is a measurement of the highest expiratory flow rate achieved and is generally reported in liters/min. The child blows into a mechanical device and the reading is taken directly off of a meter. Since this study is effort dependent, one must be sure that the effort is maximal. This may be confirmed if the patient's readings are within 5 to 10 l/min on a least two occasions. With practice, children 3 years of age and older are readily tested.

Interpretation is based on comparing the patient's reading with normal values which, in childhood, are generally based on height (Hsu). It is also useful to compare the patient's own previous values with those of the current study. In addition, if there is an indication that the patient has an obstructive defect, the child should be retested after receiving a bronchodilator (see challenge testing). Although the PEFR is one of the least sensitive of the PFTs, it is significantly more sensitive than the physician using a stethoscope. The PEFR will drop to 50% to 60% of predicted before the physician or patient detects obstruction. It is, therefore, an excellent early warning system for airway obstruction, allowing for the early institution or modification of therapy.

The use of PEFRs in the home allows the patient and family to determine when to institute additional

Flow Volume Loop

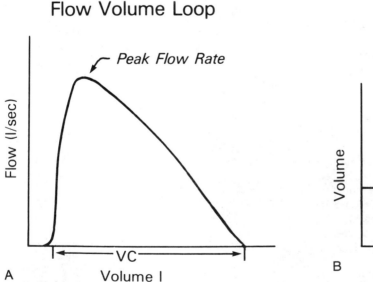

Spirogram

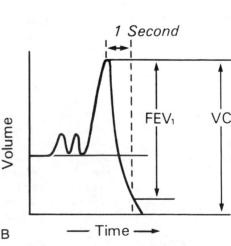

Figure 167-3. (*A*) An expiratory flow volume curve (flow *vs* volume) is illustrated. (*B*) An example of spirometry (volume *vs* time) is given.

therapy, to call the physician, or to visit the emergency room. The result is a significant decrease in anxiety for all concerned.

GUIDELINES FOR THE PERFORMANCE AND ANALYSIS OF PULMONARY FUNCTION TESTS

Standards for the performance of PFTs in childhood have been established (Taussig, 1980). It is the responsibility of the primary care physician to be sure that the laboratory to whom these patients are referred adheres to these standards.

Pulmonary function tests report the patient's observed value, predicted value (variously based on height, sex, age, and race), and the percent of the predicted value. The latter is the observed divided by the predicted value. In addition, an interpretation is usually provided by the pulmonologist directing the laboratory. That individual also evaluates the technical aspects of the test as part of the interpretation.

Outside of a formal pulmonary function laboratory, the primary care physician is most successful using a simple measure of obstruction such as the PEFR in a consistent way rather than becoming involved with complete testing. Pressure from the vendors of pulmonary function equipment who paint rosy clinical and economic pictures should be resisted.

PATTERNS OF PULMONARY FUNCTION ABNORMALITIES

Three patterns of pulmonary function abnormalities are seen: These consist of restrictive, obstructive, and mixed obstructive and restrictive defects.

Restrictive patterns result in a decrease in most lung volumes while preserving the ability to empty gas from the lung rapidly (Table 167-3). Thus, the percent of the vital capacity that is emptied in the first second (FEV_1/VC) is normal or elevated. Space occupying lesions such as tumors, pleural effusions, interstitial fluid as well as neuromuscular weakness are common causes for such findings.

Obstructive patterns (Table 167-3) result in decreased air flow, an elevation of residual volume, functional residual capacity, and an elevation of total lung capacity. The amount of the vital capacity emptied in the first second (FEV_1/VC) is decreased. Common diseases such as asthma, chronic obstructive lung disease, and cystic fibrosis usually produce such findings.

Mixed patterns are seen in situations such as a patient who has an airway obstruction with mucous plugging and atelectasis.

INHALATION CHALLENGE TESTING

Any measure of lung volume or flow rate can be determined after being given a challenge of bronchodilator, methacholine, histamine, cold air, exercise, or antigen. As a result, the dynamic properties of the lung are readily assessed. For practical purposes, one usually needs only to measure the FEV_1 and perhaps vital capacity after a particular challenge. Patients who are obstructed should receive an inhaled bronchodilator and have a repeat FEV_1. An increase of 15% to 20% or greater indicates bronchodilator responsiveness. Patients who have normal flow rates are often retested after exercise, breathing cold air, or inhalation of progressive concentrations of methacholine. This enables the physician to determine the degree of airway reactivity which is helpful in the analysis of complaints of chronic cough, dyspnea, and unexplained recurrent pneumonia. Such studies should only be performed in laboratories directed by physicians experienced in such testing. This is important because there is a small but real danger of significant airway obstruction associated with these studies. I strongly urge that the guidelines for inhalation challenge testing provided by the American Thoracic Society (Cropp) be followed.

BIBLIOGRAPHY

Cropp GJA, Bernstein IL, Boushey HA et al: Guidelines for bronchial inhalation: Challenge with pharmacologic and antigenic agents. ATS News Spring, 1980

Hess D, Kochansky M, Hassett L et al: An evaluation of the Nellcor N - 10 Portable Pulse Oximeter. Respiratory Care 31:796, 1986

Hsu KHK, Jenkins DE, Hsi BP et al: Ventilatory functions of normal children and young adults—Mexican-American, white, and black. I: Spirometry. J Pediatr 95:14, 1979

Table 167-3. Patterns of Lung Function Abnormalities

	OBSTRUCTIVE	RESTRICTIVE
VC	↓	↓
FEV_1	↓	↓
FEV_1/VC	↓	↑

VC = vital capacity; FEV_1 = forced expiratory in 1 second.

Iliff A, Lee VA: Pulse rate, respiratory rate, and body temperature of children between two months and eighteen years of age. Child Dev 23:237, 1952

Ruppel G: Manual of Pulmonary Function Testing. St. Louis, CV Mosby, 1979

Taussig LM, Chernick V, Wood R et al: Standardization of lung function testing in children. J Pediatr 97:668, 1980

West J: Respiratory Physiology. Baltimore, Williams & Wilkins, 1985

20

Toxicologic Problems

MICHAEL A. MCGUIGAN,
Section Editor

168
Therapeutic Drug Monitoring in Pediatric Practice

DANIEL A. GOLDSTEIN

Therapeutic drug monitoring (TDM) is now recognized as essential to the provision of standard medical care. This chapter focuses on the principles of pharmacology and therapeutic monitoring necessary for the practice of ambulatory pediatrics. Exact prediction of drug levels over time is rarely necessary and frequently impractical in general practice. Therefore, a nonmathematical approach with emphasis on practical dosage adjustments for orally administered drugs is presented. Following a discussion of principles, individual attention is given to theophylline, the anticonvulsants, digoxin, and aspirin. The aminoglycosides are mentioned briefly because of the frequency with which these drugs are used even by office-based pediatricians. The adjustment of dosage in renal or hepatic failure and the existence of important drug interactions are outlined when appropriate. Illustrative examples are provided at the end of the chapter. The general pediatrician should be aware that TDM has important applications in the use of anti-infective, psychotropic, antineoplastic, and antiarrhythmic drugs whose infrequent use does not warrant inclusion in this chapter.

INDICATIONS FOR THERAPEUTIC DRUG MONITORING

Before deciding to use therapeutic monitoring in a particular clinical situation, consideration must be given to the nature of the drug and to the use of the derived information. An adequate assay must be available, and there must be a clinically meaningful relationship between the response to the drug (therapeutic or toxic) and the serum level. The drug should have a narrow therapeutic index (i.e., therapeutic and toxic ranges are close or overlapping). Finally, the absorption or elimination of the drug must vary substantially among patients so that a simple dosing scheme will not ensure therapeutic levels.

The indications for using TDM are as follows:

1. Therapeutic failure—TDM can be helpful in establishing whether or not the patient has achieved a therapeutic level. If the levels are appropriate, the drug may be ineffective for the condition being treated. A low level may mean noncompliance, but may also mean that the patient is absorbing the drug poorly or excreting it rapidly. In this situation it may be helpful to measure levels following a witnessed dose in order to characterize absorption and excretion.
2. Suspected toxicity or overdosage—Drug levels are helpful in establishing the diagnosis of drug intoxication, particularly if the drug response of the patient is already known. Because patients vary widely in their ability to tolerate any particular drug level, other causes of "toxic" symptoms should be sought in patients whose dose–response is not well known.
3. "Routine" monitoring—This is recommended

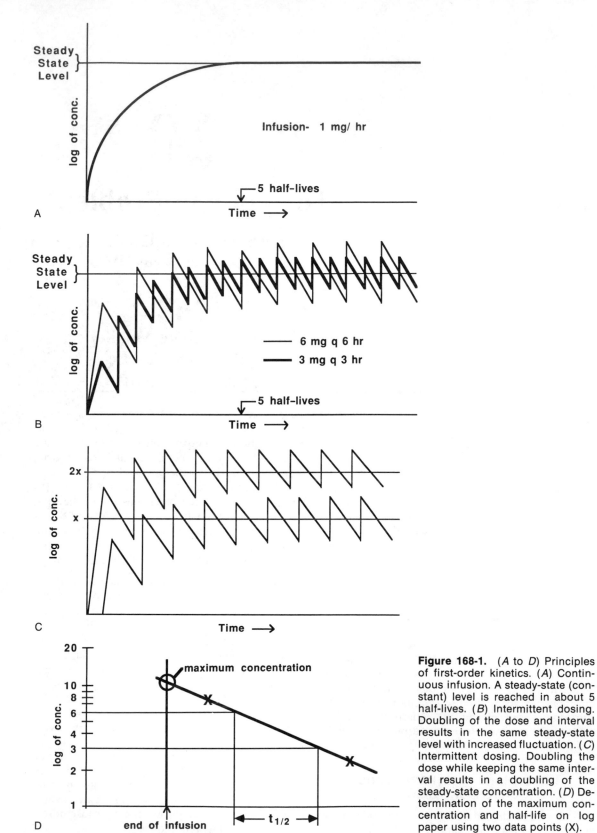

Figure 168-1. (*A* to *D*) Principles of first-order kinetics. (*A*) Continuous infusion. A steady-state (constant) level is reached in about 5 half-lives. (*B*) Intermittent dosing. Doubling of the dose and interval results in the same steady-state level with increased fluctuation. (*C*) Intermittent dosing. Doubling the dose while keeping the same interval results in a doubling of the steady-state concentration. (*D*) Determination of the maximum concentration and half-life on log paper using two data points (X).

only for drugs whose side effects tend to be unpredictable but serious, and for which a clinical assessment does not indicate impending toxicity. Digoxin and aspirin (in antirheumatic doses) are excellent examples.

4. Predictable drug interactions—TDM can be used to assure therapeutic levels in the face of predictable interactions between drugs or between a drug and other environmental factors.
5. Disease states—Many disease states affect drug absorption and excretion. TDM is particularly useful when patients have renal or hepatic disorders.

When interpreting drug levels for all of these applications, it is important to recall that some patients will be able to tolerate levels well into the purported "toxic" range, whereas others will be unable to tolerate even marginally "therapeutic" levels. Using the laboratory ranges as a guide, the physician must always seek the patient's own optimal therapeutic range. Finally, when the patient has had the desired clinical response without developing unacceptable toxicity, the physician should not feel obligated to perform TDM simply to document "therapeutic" levels.

PRINCIPLES OF PHARMACOKINETICS

An understanding of basic pharmacokinetics is essential in order to interpret and apply the results of therapeutic monitoring. This section will attempt to impart a nonmathematical understanding of pharmacokinetic terminology and principles and to make useful generalizations about different types of drug kinetics.

Linear (First-Order) Kinetics

Linear kinetics adequately describes the disposition of most drugs when levels are in the usual therapeutic range. Exceptions include aspirin, phenytoin, and sometimes theophylline. The term *linear kinetics* implies only that a constant *fraction* of the drug is removed per unit of time (*e.g.*, one third of the drug in the body is removed each hour), regardless of the actual amount of drug in the body. In effect, the rate of excretion increases exactly in proportion to rising serum levels. For convenience, the rate of removal is usually expressed as the time needed to remove half of the drug from the body— the *half-life*. A drug is usually assumed to dissolve into a hypothetical volume of body fluid, the *volume of distribution*, expressed in liters/kg of body weight.

Several important generalizations can be made about first order kinetics:

1. A continuous infusion will give a constant level (Fig. 168-1*A*). The level is determined *only* by the half-life of the drug and the dose given. This level is directly proportional to the dose in a particular patient (*i.e.*, doubling the dose doubles the level).
2. If an infusion is started with no drug in the body, it will take 5 half-lives to reach this constant level, which is known as the *steady state level*.
3. Intermittent IV or oral doses will give the same *average* level as a continuous infusion of the same dose over the same interval. As doses are given further apart, the size of the dose must increase to obtain the same average level, and the amount of fluctuation in the levels increases (Fig. 168-1*B*).
4. With intermittent dosing, the serum levels at any time remain proportional to the dose (*i.e.*, if 1 mg given every 6 hours gives a certain level 2 hours after the dose, then 2 mg every 6 hours will give twice that level at the same time after dosing) (Fig. 168-1*C*).
5. Whenever a drug dose or infusion is changed, it again takes 5 half-lives (not 5 doses) to reach a new steady state.
6. After a dose, the highest level is called the *peak* and the lowest level (just prior to the next dose) is called the *trough*. The peak (mg/L) after any dose can be estimated by dividing the dose (mg) by the volume of distribution (L) and adding the previous trough level (mg/L). This can also be done by extrapolating (on semi-log paper) the level *vs* time line back to the time of drug administration (Fig. 168-1*D*).
7. Slow-release drugs do not have a longer half-life. Like a continuous infusion, they slowly release the drug into the body, giving less fluctuation of levels between doses. Five half-lives (not five doses) are still required to reach steady state. The timing of "peaks" and "troughs" is erratic with these preparations and a half-life cannot be calculated using levels obtained between doses.

Nonlinear (Zero-Order) Kinetics

This type of kinetics is used to describe the behavior of aspirin and phenytoin. Theophylline also behaves in this way when serum levels are high. Zero-order kinetics is much more complex than linear kinetics, and a direct prediction of serum levels over time becomes difficult.

With nonlinear kinetics, the body is not able to increase the amount of drug eliminated in proportion to serum levels. This results in an apparent slowing of elimination as blood levels increase. It is important to remember that the amount excreted per unit of time is not actually diminished at high levels, but simply approaches a plateau at which it is impossible for the body to further increase elimination (*saturation*). As a result, the fraction of the total drug in the body excreted per unit time becomes smaller as serum levels rise. It is often stated that nonlinearly excreted drugs have a longer half-life at higher serum levels. Although this is conceptually useful, it is not mathematically correct, because *half-life* is a derived term applicable only to linear kinetics.

Important generalizations about nonlinear kinetics are as follows:

1. A constant infusion produces a constant steady state level.
2. The volume of distribution of a nonlinear drug is still useful for calculating initial concentrations (using level = dose/volume of distribution) after a loading dose.
3. It may take a long time (weeks) to reach equilibrium following a change in dosing regimen.
4. Changes in blood levels are disproportionately large compared to changes in dose or infusion rate. Small changes in the dosage of a drug may result in a dramatic change in levels.

Drug Dosage in Renal and Hepatic Failure

The excretion of almost all drugs is affected to some degree by alterations in hepatic or renal function. In cases of altered drug excretion, it is important to remember that the initial or *loading dose* needed to achieve a therapeutic level generally remains the same because the volume of distribution for the drug *is not usually altered*. Rather, it is the dosage used to maintain a therapeutic level that must be reduced in the face of organ dysfunction.

Many renally excreted drugs are eliminated in direct proportion to the glomerular filtration rate (GFR) (*e.g.*, aminoglycosides), and hence can be easily adjusted once the GFR has been estimated. Nomograms or formulas for conversion of serum creatinine to GFR are readily available. For hepatically excreted drugs and for drugs with substantial tubular resorption or excretion, no simple method is available for dosage prediction.

Theophylline

Theophylline is one of the most frequently monitored drugs. There are a variety of preparations, including several slow-release formulations that are designed to provide more stable serum levels. In general, the absorption from all of these preparations is complete and, in the standard preparations, rapid. In certain individuals the absorption of slow-release preparations may be poor, irregular, or both. Despite this, the convenience, improved compliance, and more stable blood levels seen in most patients using slow-release preparations generally outweigh this unpredictability.

Theophylline has a volume of distribution of about 0.5 l/kg. The drug is eliminated by hepatic metabolism with a variable half-life. In children, half-lives range from 2 to 10 hours. Half-lives tend to prolong throughout childhood, particularly at puberty, and to approach the adult mean of 8.7 hours. Therapeutic levels are 10 μg/ml to 20 μg/ml.

When serum levels exceed 20 μg/ml, the ability of the patient to eliminate theophylline may be limited. Caution should be used in adjusting dosages upward when the serum level is at or near 20 μg/ml, since larger than expected changes in blood levels may occur.

Age-specific dosage recommendations with adjustment for smoking habits in older patients are widely available and should be used for the initiation of therapy when no other patient data are available. With rapid release forms, dosage adjustment can be made based on peak and trough levels obtained after 5 half-lives (~24 hours in a typical child). Peak levels should be obtained 2 hours after dosing to allow for complete absorption. With slow-release (SR) dosage forms, a single predose level in the midtherapeutic range is often all that is necessary to assure that the patient is within the therapeutic range. If a patient is responding poorly to SR therapy or shows signs of toxicity, it may be worth obtaining one or more levels 2 to 10 hours after dosing in order to document the patient's absorption profile. The "peak" level may occur at any time following SR dosing, although 4 to 6 hours is typical.

No adjustment of theophylline dosage is required in renal failure. The drug should be used cautiously in hepatic disease. A large number of drugs interfere with theophylline metabolism, particularly erythromycin and cimetidine. Viral illness may also significantly impede elimination in some subjects.

Phenobarbital and Primidone

Phenobarbital (PB) has a distribution volume of 0.8 l/kg. 80% to 90% of an ingested dose is absorbed. It is eliminated primarily by hepatic metabolism with a half-life of 40 to 70 hours in children. This long half-life allows once a day dosing with minimal fluctuation in serum levels. Once the patient has reached a steady state, which may take 8 to 14 days, a single blood level obtained at any time is adequate to allow dose adjustment. The generally accepted therapeutic range is 40 μg/ml to 80 μg/ml.

Primidone is converted into two active metabolites—PB and phenylethylmalonamide. The latter is not usually measured, but primidone and PB levels should both be measured whenever primidone is used. Primidone has a distribution volume of 0.6 l/kg body weight and a half-life of 24 to 40 hours. Therapeutic primidone levels are 5 μg/ml to 12 μg/ml. Plasma PB:primidone ratios are ~1:1, but there is wide variation depending on the rates of PB production and elimination. PB may have to be given along with primidone to achieve therapeutic levels of both drugs. When evaluating levels, sufficient time should be given for both drugs to come to steady state. Since PB generally has the longer half-life, this will require 8 to 14 days. Poor compliance with primidone can create a confusing picture in which the patient has a substantial PB level at a time when there is little primidone present.

PB and primidone levels can be easily adjusted using first order kinetics because the serum levels are directly proportional to the dose. When adjusting primidone dosage to achieve therapeutic levels, the physician should remember that PB levels will also change.

PB enhances the metabolism of many drugs, including other anticonvulsants. In hepatic disease the elimination of both drugs is diminished to a variable extent.

Carbamazepine

Carbamazepine (CBZ) is rapidly becoming the preferred drug for many seizure disorders in the pediatric age group because of its effectiveness and lack of unacceptable cosmetic and behavioral side effects. The behavior of the drug can be reasonably approximated by assuming 100% absorption with a distribution of volume of 1 l/kg body weight. Actual absorption is probably variable and incomplete, with peak levels occurring 3 or more hours following a dose. The half-life is generally in the 5 to 12 hour range. The monitoring of carbamazepine is complicated by two considerations. First, the drug appears to induce its own metabolism (*i.e.*, the drug causes an increase in enzymatic activity that increases the elimination of the drug). Current dosage recommendations reflect this phenomenon in the fact that CBZ is begun at a low dosage and gradually increased at biweekly intervals. Second, a portion of the activity of CBZ is due to the presence of a metabolite. Fortunately, the levels of the metabolite, which are not generally measured, are proportional to the levels of the parent compound.

The simple first order rules for dosage adjustment apply to CBZ if one recalls that a true steady state level can only be measured after enzymatic induction is complete, usually 1 to 2 weeks after a change in dose. Increases in blood level may be less than predicted after an increase in dosage because of enzyme induction. Conversely, when dosage is diminished, enzymatic induction will also decrease, so that levels may not fall as far as predicted. Finally, slow absorption makes it difficult to obtain a peak level or to estimate half-life. A single predose level can be used to determine whether the patient is within the therapeutic range. In the child with rapid metabolism, it may be helpful to obtain two or more levels between doses in order to define a plasma concentration curve.

The addition of CBZ will generally accelerate the metabolism of other anticonvulsants. Similarly, the addition of anticonvulsants other than valproic acid will accelerate the metabolism of CBZ. The use of CBZ is not recommended in patients who have liver disease. Use in renal disease has not been extensively studied, but dosage probably requires adjustment only in the severely uremic patient.

Valproic Acid

Valproic acid (VPA) is a unique anticonvulsant whose pharmacology differs significantly from the other anticonvulsants. The drug is well absorbed in all dosage forms and by all routes, including rectal administration. The enteric coated tablets are completely absorbed, but delays of up to 6 hours may occur before peak levels are reached. Food may significantly delay the absorption of standard preparations. The kinetics of VPA vary widely among individuals, as indicated by the wide dosing range of 10 to 60 mg/kg/day. Determination of half-life following initial dosing has been shown to be advantageous in achieving therapeutic levels rapidly. It may be helpful to establish a dosing regimen using a nonenteric dosage form and then change to an enteric coated form if the patient develops gastric intolerance.

The volume of distribution of VPA is only 0.2 l/kg and half-lives in children range from 4 to 17 hours. Dosing intervals may range from 6 to 24 hours. Therapeutic levels are 50 μg/ml to 100 μg/ml. VPA is highly protein bound, but the protein binding is saturated at high levels. Because the unbound drug is metabolized, saturation results in less than predicted changes in levels when dosage is adjusted. This is not usually clinically significant.

Samples for half-life determination should ideally be taken 2 to 8 hours after an oral dose of non-enteric VPA, either at steady state or after a single dose. Dosage can then be predicted as in Example 2. Because absorption is slowed with food or enteric coating, monitoring of a predose level will be most helpful in the uncontrolled clinical situation.

The metabolism of VPA is enhanced by other anticonvulsants. VPA generally slows the metabolism of other anticonvulsants (and many other hepatically excreted drugs). VPA displaces phenytoin from protein-binding sites, which may lead to acute phenytoin intoxication.

Because of hepatotoxicity, VPA is contraindicated in liver disease. In renal disease the protein binding of VPA is significantly reduced, leading to more pronounced drug effects at any given serum level.

Ethosuximide

Ethosuximide (ESX) is less commonly used and less well studied than the other anticonvulsants. Absorption is excellent. ESX follows first order kinetics, with a volume of distribution of 0.7 l/kg and a half-life of 14 to 72 hours in children. The therapeutic range is 40 µg/ml to 100 µg/ml. In general, a single daily dose is satisfactory and random levels will reflect steady state values, because daily fluctuation will be fairly small. The occasional rapid metabolizer may require twice daily dosing. Peak and trough levels may be obtained in these patients, but the control of absence events appears to be good in many patients despite fluctuating serum levels.

The kinetics of ESX in hepatic and renal failure is inadequately studied, and caution is needed when ESX is combined with other anticonvulsant drugs. Interactions have been reported anecdotally, but have not been studied systematically.

Phenytoin

Phenytoin (diphenylhydantoin [DPH]) is a commonly used anticonvulsant, and therapeutic problems are frequently encountered because of nonlinear kinetics and substantial protein binding. The drug is about 80% absorbed, with a substantial variation among individuals. Nasogastric feedings can nearly abolish absorption. The volume of distribution is 0.7 (0.5 to 1.2) l/kg. The half-life in children is 4 to 12 hours. During puberty the half-life prolongs toward the adult range of 20 to 40 hours. This change can be anticipated, and may be an indication for periodic monitoring. Therapeutic levels are 10 µg/ml to 20 µg/ml. It is not infrequent for children to require up to twice the maximal recommended starting dosage for phenytoin.

In childhood, monitoring of peak and trough levels is often useful. In adolescents, where the half-life is long, serum levels fluctuate minimally and a single random determination is adequate. The measurement of fluctuation may aid in determining dosing interval, which may range from every 6 hours in toddlers to once daily for adults. Many weeks may be required to achieve a steady state. For this reason a loading dose may be needed to establish therapeutic levels. Serum levels can be repeated at intervals of several weeks in order to determine a steady state level. Dosage adjustment is largely empirical, but it should certainly be more conservative than estimates based on linear kinetics. Nomograms have been developed for dosage adjustment.

DPH variably affects other anticonvulsants. Valproic acid displaces DPH from protein-binding sites and may cause acute phenytoin toxicity. Dosage adjustments are required for both hepatic and renal dysfunction.

Digoxin

The therapeutic monitoring of digoxin is plagued by several problems. The drug suffers from erratic absorption, with a bioavailability of about 60% to 80%. Medications, dietary changes, and changes in bowel flora all alter absorption. Following absorption there is a prolonged equilibration phase of 6 to 12 hours during which digoxin slowly enters the body tissues. The apparent volume of distribution is about 10 liters/kg, reflecting concentration in body tissues. Because of the prolonged distribution phase, peak levels of digoxin are meaningless and a half-life cannot be determined from peak and trough values. Finally, the presence of an "endogenous digoxin-like substance," particularly in the newborn or fluid overloaded patient, places the value of current digoxin assay systems in question.

Practical monitoring of digoxin is restricted to the measurement of trough levels, which should be in the 0.9 to 2 ng/ml range. It can generally be assumed that trough levels will be proportional to daily dosage, and adjustment can be made accordingly. The half-life of digoxin in children ranges from 16 to 40 hours, so that steady state levels may not be achieved for 1 week or more. For newly digitalized or unstable patients, it may be necessary to check levels prior to steady state in order to ensure that excessive accumulation is not occurring. Dosage adjustment is required in both hepatic and renal failure as well as for many disease states and drug interactions.

Aminoglycosides

The therapeutic monitoring of aminoglycosides has become a matter of routine practice. After intravenous administration, the aminoglycosides have an apparent volume of distribution of 0.5 l/kg and a half-life of about 2 hours. Effective mathematical methods for dose adjustment are available. Detailed examples of gentamicin dosage adjustment are given at the end of this chapter and can be applied to the other aminoglycosides. It is important to modify the dosing interval as well as the dose when adjusting aminoglycoside dosages for rapid or slow excretion. Therapeutic levels of gentamicin and tobramycin are peaks of 6 μg/ml to 10 μg/ml and troughs less than 2 μg/ml Amikacin and kanamycin have recommended peaks of 20 μg/ml to 25 μg/ml and troughs of 1 μg/ml to 4 μg/ml.

The aminoglycosides are excreted exclusively by glomerular filtration and maintenance dosage adjustment based on serum creatinine or creatinine clerance is required in renal failure. No adjustment is required in hepatic failure. The major interaction with aminoglycosides is increased nephro- and oto-toxicity when combined with furosemide and possibly vancomycin.

Salicylates

The monitoring of salicylate (ASA) levels is only necessary when the drug is used in antirheumatic doses. Monitoring is critically important because the control of pain is not considered an adequate index of anti-inflammatory activity and because the therapeutic levels are close to toxic levels. Any patient beginning antirheumatic therapy should be observed for signs of salicylism.

The absorption of ASA is rapid and complete. The volume of distribution is roughly 0.16 l/kg. Elimination is largely by hepatic metabolism with urinary excretion of metabolites. A steady state level is usually established within 2 weeks. Typical initial doses are 60 to 80 mg/kg/day, divided into four doses. The goal of therapy is to establish trough levels of 200 μg/ml to 300 μg/ml (20 to 30 mg/dl) by gradually increasing the dosage. Because of the marked nonlinearity of salicylates, increases should be limited to increments of 10 to 20 mg/kg/day. Doses in excess of 130 mg/kg/day are rarely required. Once levels are established, salicylates are often continued for months to years and periodic monitoring is recommended.

Caution is required in the presence of hepatic or renal failure.

EXAMPLES

Example 1. Phenobarbital

Q. A 4-year-old patient has been chronically on 6 mg/kg/day of PB. Following an isolated seizure, you check a random level and obtain a value of 40 μg/ml. How would you get his level to 60 μg/ml?

A. Since levels of PB are proportional to dose (first order kinetics), you increase the dose to 60/40 or 1.5 times the original dose. The patient does well on 9 mg/kg/day.

Example 2. Valproic acid (approach could apply equally well to theophylline)

Q. Your patient has not responded well to a dose of 30 mg/kg/day of VPA. You suspect noncompliance, thus you obtain levels 2 and 8 hours after a witnessed dose. The 2-hour level is 80 and the 8-hour level is only 25. The patient has a brief seizure in your office. How do you interpret the results? What do you do to improve therapy?

A. You plot these levels on log-linear paper and discover a half-life of only 4 hours. His extrapolated level at 12 hours is about 10. His volume of distribution is 0.2 l/kg (15 mg/kg/dose divided by a change in level (peak-trough) of 70), which is typical. You conclude that the patient is compliant, but is a rapid metabolizer and thus requires a dose increase and (more importantly) a q6 hour dosing schedule. He responds well to 40 mg/kg/day divided every 6 hours.

Example 3. Gentamicin

Q. Your patient is on standard doses of gentamicin—2.5 mg/kg every 8 hours. Pre- and postdose levels are obtained at 1 and 7 hours after a dose. Assuming that the patient is at steady state, what would you do with the following levels (μg/ml):
  a. pre = 3.0, post = 15.0
  b. pre = <1 (lower limit of detection)
     post = 13
  c. pre = 3.5, post = 10.0

A. a. Both pre and post levels are about 1.5

times too high and the half-life is typical of gentamicin. You cut the dose proportionately to two thirds of 2.5 mg/kg, or 1.6 mg q 8 hours.

b. Pre-levels are fine, but peaks are too high. The half-life is short. (If you assume that the pre-level was 1, the half-life would plot out to 1.8 hours.) The best solution is to shorten the dosing interval to q 6 hours, keeping the same daily dose. Since each dose will be three quarters as large as before, peaks will be roughly two thirds of 13, or about 10. The trough will, of course, still be less than 1.

c. The half-life obtained from these data is prolonged—about 4 hours. You elect to increase the interval to q 12 hr without changing the size of the dose. This gives two thirds of the previous daily dose, thus peaks will be roughly two thirds of 10; (*i.e.*, about 7). Twelve hours (three half-lives) later the trough should be $\frac{1}{2} \times \frac{1}{2} \times \frac{1}{2} \times 7$, which is less than 1.

Example 4. Aspirin

Q. You start a patient on ASA for rheumatoid arthritis, beginning with a dose of 80 mg/kg/day. One week later a predose level is 150 µg/ml. What do you do?

A. If ASA had linear kinetics, you would increase the dose by 25/15 or 1.6 times to 130 mg/kg/day. This initial calculation is helpful because it places an upper limit on the size of dose adjustment needed. You know, however, that ASA has nonlinear kinetics. You opt for the maximum recommended dose increase of 20 mg/kg/day (to 100 mg/kg/day), since this is still only 40% of the calculated correction with linear kinetics.

Example 5. Phenytoin

Q. A colleague asks you what to do with a 5-year-old patient who "can't get a level above 3.5" on the maximum recommended dose of DPH. What do you suggest?

A. If phenytoin had linear kinetics, you would have to triple the dose just to get into the low therapeutic range. Since you know that kinetics is nonlinear, you suggest doubling the dose and checking levels biweekly for 6 weeks in order to determine the new equilibrium level. You point out that toddlers often require large doses of phenytoin.

ANNOTATED BIBLIOGRAPHY

Bauer LA: Interference of oral phenytoin absorption by continuous nasogastric feedings. Neurology 32:570–572, 1982

Benet LZ, Sheiner LB: General principles. In Gilman AG, Goodman LS, Rall TW, Murad F (eds): The Pharmacological Basis of Therapeutics. New York, Macmillan, 1985 (Good general coverage of basic principles and specific drug information.)

Chiba K, Takashi I, Miura H, Michaelis–Menton KM: Kinetics of diphenylhydantoin and application in the pediatric age group. Pediatrics 96:479–484, 1980 (Normogram for phenytoin dosage adjustment; slightly complex, but useful.)

Dettli L: Drug dosage in renal disease. In Gibaldi M, Prescott L: Handbook of Clinical Pharmacokinetics, pp 261–276. New York, ADIS Health Sciences Press, 1983 (Practical approach to dosage adjustment in renal disease.)

Eadie MJ, Tyrer JH: Anticonvulsant Therapy. Pharmacological Basis and Practice. New York, Churchill Livingstone, 1980 (Practical text covering anticonvulsant use, interactions, kinetics, and monitoring.)

Evans WE, Schentag JJ, Jusko WJ (eds): Applied Pharmacokinetics. San Francisco, Applied Therapeutics, 1980 (Comprehensive textbook devoted to phenytoin, digoxin, theophylline, aminoglycosides, and drugs not covered here.)

Hendeles L, Weinberger M: Theophylline—a state of the art review. Pharmacotherapy 3:2–44, 1983 (Up to date review of all aspects of theophylline therapy.)

Taylor WJ, Finn AL (eds): Individualizing Drug Therapy. New York, Gross, Townsend, Frank, 1981 (This comprehensive, concise, and well-referenced series, with pocket handbook, is available to physicians free of charge through Syva or Syntex representatives; omits salicylates.)

Prescription and over-the-counter cough and cold preparations are common in households with young children. Children are not only encouraged to take them, but the medications are also designed specifically to be attractive in color and flavor. It is no wonder that cough and cold preparations are involved commonly in accidental ingestions.

Cough and cold medications form a heterogenous group of pharmacologic agents. Medications used to treat nasal congestion include sympathomimetics (decongestants) and antihistamines. Those agents used for the treatment of coughing include suppressants (opiates and opiate derivatives, including dextromethorphan) and expectorants (usually guiafenesin). Many commercially available preparations also include aspirin or acetaminophen or both.

This chapter will discuss the clinical toxicology of the three main classes of cough and cold medications: antihistamines, decongestants (phenylpropanolamine), and cough suppressants (opiate derivatives).

ANTIHISTAMINES

Pathophysiology

Literally dozens of chemically different antihistamines are currently available. Although there are subtle differences in the effects produced by each of these antihistamines, for practical purposes, it is reasonable to consider them as a single group.

Antihistamines, in general, are absorbed rapidly from the gastrointestinal tract and are distributed widely throughout the body. These compounds are excreted by way of the hepatic metabolism with an elimination half-life following an overdose of up to 8 hours. The exact mechanism of toxic effect is uncertain, but is believed to be related to peripheral antihistamine antagonism and direct central nervous system effects.

Clinical Presentation

Children who ingest excessive amounts of one of the standard formulations of antihistamines will demonstrate signs of toxicity within 4 hours. Clinical effects may not begin for 6 to 8 hours if a slow-release preparation has been ingested. Evidence of central nervous system stimulation was noted in nearly 85% of the reported cases of overdoses involving antihistamines. Common excitation manifestations include insomnia, restlessness, nystagmus, ataxia, tremor, hyperreflexia, myoclonic jerks, and hallucinations. Convulsions occurred more commonly with large ingestions; seizures were reported in ~70% of pediatric antihistamine overdoses in the literature. Central nervous system depression may also occur (38% of reported cases) and is manifest as drowsiness or lethargy, or coma. Anticholinergic (or atropine-like) effects occur but their frequency has not been documented. Findings may include dilated pupils, xerostomia, tachycardia, low-grade fever, and flushed dry skin. Multifocal premature ventricular contractions are an uncommon complication of a severe antihistamine overdose.

Differential Diagnosis

The differential diagnosis of a child who overdoses on an antihistamine that was being used to treat his upper respiratory infection includes Reye's syndrome and encephalitis or meningitis. Other toxins that may produce a clinical picture similar to that caused by an antihistamine overdose include chronic salicylate intoxication and the acute ingestion of phenothiazines, lithium, tricyclic antidepressants, sympathomimetics (e.g., cocaine, phenylpropanolamine, amphetamines), and plants containing belladonna alkaloids (e.g., deadly nightshade). Thryotoxicosis (either endogenous or from ingestion of thyroid hormone) and hypoglycemia should also be considered in the differential diagnosis.

Work-Up

The correct identification of the product is essential. Each active ingredient and its concentration should be identified and the maximum quantity ingested should be estimated. In products in which several different antihistamines are combined, it is reasonable to add all antihistamines together in calculating a single ingested dose. The toxic dose of antihistamines is not well established but ingestions of more than 10 mg/kg are likely to result in unwanted effects. Not only must the product and the dose be accurately identified, but the time of ingestion must be estimated in order to determine whether or not therapeutic intervention would be reasonable. If symptoms are present, they should be detailed with regard to the time and sequence of onset.

A careful physical examination may reveal the anticholinergic signs as well as evidence of drowsiness, central nervous system excitation, or hallucinations. Laboratory investigations are not useful in antihistamine overdoses except in eliminating other causes of similar syndromes. Documentation of antihistamines in the blood or urine is confirmatory but not beneficial in managing the acute overdose. Many liquid antihistamine preparations contain ethanol; thus, measurement of blood ethanol and blood sugar levels are important considerations.

Treatment

Treatment should consist of the administration of ipecac to an asymptomatic child at home within 2 hours of an overdose. Activated charcoal will bind unabsorbed antihistamine within the gastrointestinal tract and its use is recommended. Symptomatic supportive care should be used to treat most of the clinical effects. Intravenous diazepam, phenytoin, or barbiturates may be used to control convulsive activity. Hallucinatory activity often responds to nonpharmacologic treatment: quiet reassurance in a normally lit room. If the hallucinations do not respond to such therapy and are becoming disruptive, a small dose of a short-acting benzodiazepine (*e.g.*, lorazepam) may be beneficial.

Physostigmine has been used to treat serious complications of antihistamine overdose but because physostigmine itself is potentially toxic and its duration of action is short, it should not be used unless the effects of the antihistamine overdose are potentially life threatening. If it appears that physostigmine is necessary, a discussion with a regional poison center is recommended.

Indications for Admission or Referral

A medical evaluation is recommended for any child who has ingested an unknown or potentially toxic amount (more than 10 mg/kg) of an antihistamine. Admission to hospital is recommended for any patient who is symptomatic within 4 hours of an overdose.

DECONGESTANTS

Available oral sympathomimetics include drugs such as ephedrine, orciprenaline, pseudoephedrine, phenylephrine, and phenylpropanolamine (PPA). Toxicity resulting from ingestion of any of these drugs is rare, except for PPA.

Pathophysiology

PPA is readily absorbed through the stomach and exerts its toxic effects both by direct stimulation of α-adrenergic receptors and by causing the release of stored epinephrine. If PPA is ingested in conjunction with the antihistamine chlorpheniramine, the duration of toxicity may be prolonged because the antihistamine inhibits the re-uptake of catecholamines by the nerve endings.

Clinical Presentation

Ingestion of excessive amounts of PPA results most commonly in headache, hypertension, and bradycardia. Other less commonly reported symptoms of PPA overdose include dizziness, nausea, sweating, agitation, and various cardiac arrhythmias.

Differential Diagnosis

The differential diagnosis of PPA overdose should include previously unrecognized causes of hypertension (*e.g.*, renal, vascular, and adrenal) or the ingestion of other sympathomimetic drugs such as amphetamines or cocaine, or hallucinogenic drugs such as phencyclidine. Certain combinations of symptoms and signs may suggest hypoglycemia or the effects of nicotine or insecticides.

Work-Up

In any case of PPA overdose, not only must the quantity of PPA be estimated but efforts must also be made to identify other ingested drugs that may interact adversely (*e.g.*, chlorpheniramine or caffeine). Acute doses of PPA in excess of 10 mg/kg may result in toxicity. A physical examination should be directed primarily at the central nervous system and cardiovascular system. No specific laboratory tests are available to confirm a PPA overdose or to help evaluate its severity. Routine laboratory tests may be used to help eliminate renal disease and hypoglycemia.

Treatment

The early induction of vomiting may be useful but the administration of ipecac should be considered in light of the rapidity with which PPA is absorbed from the stomach and the vomiting-induced delay in the administration of activated charcoal. In any event, treatment should include the administration of activated charcoal to patients who have ingested toxic doses of PPA. The use of activated charcoal is especially important because many preparations are mixtures of different drugs. Dividing the amount of PPA ingested by the patient's weight can be used to estimate the expected toxicity. Physical examination should include a careful look for narcotic symptoms and signs as well as an evaluation of the respiratory function (at rest).

No specific guidelines are available for the treatment of hypertension associated with PPA ingestion. Recommendations include treatment of blood pressure in excess of 180/100 or at lower levels if the patient has a headache, signs of encephalopathy, or a blood pressure that rises over 30 minutes of observation. Patients who have a congenital heart disease which may be adversely affected by hypertension should receive antihypertension therapy at lower levels of hypertension. The initial treatment of PPA-induced hypertension consists of placing the patient in a head-elevated position because PPA-induced hypertension appears to be more severe in the supine position. If this does not reduce the blood pressure, the preferred pharmacologic agent is nitroprusside.

Acidification of the urine will increase the renal clearance of PPA but this therapy should be reserved only for severely affected patients. Convulsions secondary to PPA should be treated with rapidly acting intravenous anticonvulsant drugs, such as diazepam.

INDICATIONS FOR ADMISSION OR REFERRAL

Patients with ingestions of PPA alone in quantities exceeding the minimum toxic dose (10 mg/kg) should be observed for 4 to 8 hours for symptoms of sympathetic stimulation. Patients who are objectively toxic need to be admitted to hospital for observation and care.

OPIATE DERIVATIVES

Pathophysiology

Codeine, hydrocodone, hydromorphone, and dextromethorphan are the opioid drugs most commonly used as cough suppressants. In overdose, they all exert similar affects: miosis, and central nervous system and respiratory depression to a variable degree. Dextromethorphan overdose has been associated with convulsions in rare instances.

Clinical Presentation

The triad of central nervous system depression, miosis, and respiratory depression is characteristic of opioid drugs. Head trauma secondary to a fall may result when an ingestion of a depressant results in neuromuscular unsteadiness.

Differential Diagnosis

A similar clinical picture may result with a pontine hemorrhage (a rare occurrence) or from the ingestion of large quantities of ethanol, barbiturates, phenothiazines, or clonidine. An overdose of benzodiazepines may produce central nervous system depression and miosis without respiratory depression.

Work-Up

A work-up must include identification of the drug ingested and its formulation (liquid vs tablet, regular vs sustained-release) as well as any other ingested drugs. The timing is important; thus, establishing when the ingestion occurred is critical. The milligram quantity of the drug ingested divided by the patient's weight can be used to estimate the expected toxicity (see the section on admission). A physical examination should include vital signs as part of a careful look for narcotic symptoms and signs as well as an evaluation of the respiratory function (at rest). No definitive laboratory procedures are useful in diagnosing or assessing the degree of toxicity. When a patient requires hospitalization, a qualitative identification of the drug in question should be done for purposes of documentation. Liquid preparations of cough suppressants may contain ethanol; thus, measurements of blood sugar and blood ethanol concentrations may be warranted.

Treatment

Activated charcoal effectively binds the opioid drugs and should be used. Patients with clinical toxicity to the point of respiratory compromise (as documented by cyanosis or abnormal blood gas values) should be treated with ventilatory support and perhaps endotracheal intubation. Naloxone (0.03 mg/kg intravenously) may be used to reverse the signs of a narcotic overdose. It may be repeated at 2- to 3-minute intervals. If a dramatic response in the level of consciousness and respiratory effort does not occur following a naloxone dose of 0.1 mg/kg, the diagnosis of opiate overdose should be reconsidered.

Indications for Admission or Referral

Medical evaluation is indicated for children who, by history, ingest toxic doses of the common opioid cough suppressants: dextromethorphan > 10 mg/kg; codeine > 2 mg/kg; hydrocodone > 0.6 mg/kg; and hydromorphone > 0.2 mg/kg. Admission to hospital is recommended for any child who demonstrates symptoms and signs compatible with opioid overdose within 6 hours of ingestion. If respiratory support or naloxone therapy is required, the child should be cared for in a hospital that is capable of providing pediatric intensive care.

ANNOTATED BIBLIOGRAPHY

Bernstein E, Diskant BM: Phenylpropanolamine: A potentially hazardous drug. Ann Emerg Med 11:311–315, 1982 (Pathophysiology and clinical presentation of PPA overdose.)

Committee on Drugs: Use of codeine and dextromethorphan-containing cough syrups in pediatrics. Pediatrics 62:118–122, 1978 (Excellent review of both the therapeutic and toxic sides of the subject.)

Hooper RG, Conner CS, Rumack BH: Acute poisoning from over-the-counter sleep preparations. JACEP 8:98–100, 1979 (Good presentation of a large series of patients; useful frequency data.)

Howrie DL, Wolfson JH: Phenylpropanolamine-induced hypertensive seizures. J Pediatr 102:143–145, 1983 (Interesting report that implies possible interaction with the caffeine.)

Krenzelok EP, Anderson GM, Mirick M: Massive diphenhydramine overdose resulting in death. Ann Emerg Med 11:212–213, 1982 (Case presentation with a good discussion of pathophysiology.)

Shaul WL, Wandell M. Robertson WO: Dextromethorphan toxicity: Reversed by naloxone. Pediatrics 59:117–119, 1977 (One of the few cases of serious toxicity from dextromethorphan.)

vonMuhlendahl KE, Scherf–Rahne B, Krienke EG et al: Codeine intoxication in childhood. Lancet 2:303–305, 1976 (Good discussion of the likelihood and timing of symptoms following acute codeine overdose.)

170
Salicylate and Acetaminophen Poisoning

L. GERARD NIEDERMAN

Preparations containing salicylates or acetaminophen are widely used for children and adolescents as analgesics and antipyretics. Aspirin (acetylsalicylic acid) and acetaminophen, both nonprescription drugs, are present in numerous over-the-counter preparations, as well as in many combination prescription medications. Other salicylates may be found in analgesic ointments and liniments (methyl salicylate), sunscreens (homomenthyl salicylate), and keratolytic agents (salicylic acid). Toxicity from both acetaminophen and salicylates may follow accidental or intentional ingestion. Accidental ingestion usually occurs in younger children whereas intentional ingestion is more common in adolescents. Chronic salicylate poisoning occurs in all ages though more commonly in young children, and most common in infants.

SALICYLATE POISONING

Pathophysiology

When salicylates are taken in therapeutic doses, they are rapidly absorbed in the stomach and small intestine. However, when large doses are ingested, absorption may be prolonged by delayed tablet dissolution and by delayed gastric emptying. Enteric-coated tablets are even more erratically absorbed in overdosage. Aspirin is rapidly hydrolyzed to salicylic acid, which at low serum concentrations is largely bound to plasma proteins, primarily albumin. Salicylate, with a pKa of 3.5, is present primarily in the ionized fraction, which penetrates biologic membranes poorly and remains largely in the blood. As blood concentrations increase, albumen binding is saturated and, if acidemia occurs, there will be an increase in the nonionized fraction of salicylate. Both these factors facilitate passive diffusion of salicylate across cell membranes, increasing tissue drug levels and toxicity. Alkalemia, on the other hand, increases the proportion of ionized salicylic acid, thus impeding tissue penetration.

The symptoms of salicylism are related to the direct stimulating effect on the central nervous system, particularly the respiratory center of the brain; the uncoupling of oxidative phosphorylation with increased oxygen consumption, carbon dioxide accumulation, and heat production; the alteration of Krebs' cycle enzymes with resultant accumulation of organic acids; and, in severe poisoning, to central nervous system depression.

One of the complex manifestations of salicylism is a derangement of acid-base balance. Early in its course, direct respiratory center stimulation results in hyperventilation and respiratory alkalosis which, if present for any duration, will be compensated by renal bicarbonate excretion. This may be the only alteration in acid-base balance or, with more severe toxicity, metabolic acidosis may occur. The acidosis is not the result of accumulated salicylic acid, but rather is due to the accumulation of organic acids (lactate and pyruvate) secondary to salicylate-induced derangements of Krebs' cycle function. Underlying caloric deprivation and dehydration as well as stimulation of lipid metabolism also result in the production of ketoacids. Further adding to the acidosis is the accumulation of CO_2 and depletion of O_2 resulting from the uncoupling of oxidative phosphorylation.

Significant alteration in fluid and electrolyte balance often accompanies the acid-base derangements described above. Increased heat production from uncoupled oxidative phosphorylation, hyperpnea, and hyperventilation all increase insensible water loss and result in some salt loss through perspiration. Early renal compensation for respiratory alkalosis results in sodium and potassium loss, as hydrogen ion is initially conserved. Later, renal excretion of organic acids in acidemic patients results in further water and salt depletion. Vomiting and poor oral intake also aggravate the fluid balance in the young child. The sum of these effects may be considerable water, sodium, and potassium depletion, particularly with chronic salicylism.

Rarely, inappropriate ADH has been reported, which is probably due to the direct effect of salicylate on the hypothalmus.

Either hypoglycemia or hyperglycemia may be present with salicylism. Even though blood glucose measurements may be normal or high, central nervous system hypoglycemia may occur and cause mental status changes. Bleeding phenomena rarely occur with salicylate poisoning, although platelet function is altered and prothrombin time is prolonged.

At relatively low blood concentrations, salicylate is conjugated in the liver, but at toxic concentrations these enzymes are saturated and salicylic acid accumulates. The half-life for salicylate at low blood levels is ~ 2 to 3 hours whereas at toxic levels the half-life may be as long as 30 hours. Salicylate and its conjugates are primarily excreted in the urine, and urinary alkalosis enhances salicylate excretion several fold.

Clinical Presentation

The early clinical symptoms include nausea and vomiting, tinnitus (described only by older children), confusion, hyperpyrexia, and most commonly, hyperpnea and hyperventilation. Lethargy, convulsions, and coma may occur with increased toxicity. For reasons not entirely clear, children and particularly infants are more likely to develop serious acidemia. Chronic intoxication, rather than a single dose ingestion, is also more likely to result in acidemia.

Differential Diagnosis

The differential diagnosis of salicylism can be organized around the central nervous symptoms (confusion and lethargy); the respiratory symptoms (hyperpnea and hyperventilation); and the metabolic acidemia. Head trauma, Reye's syndrome, CNS infections, and other intoxicants such as alcohol may present with changes in mental status similar to those seen with salicylate toxicity. Children with head trauma may also manifest central neurogenic hyperventilation, though usually history and other physical signs make confusion with salicylism unlikely. Anxiety attacks with hyperventilation and respiratory illness such as asthma may also be initially confused with salicylism. Metabolic acidosis is seen in diabetes mellitus, gastroenteritis with dehydration, hypoperfusion, severe renal disease, ethylene glycol and methanol intoxication, as well as the other less common metabolic diseases. A careful history will provide recognition of the child with gastroenteritis or diabetes who may have concomitantly been given aspirin for fever or analgesia.

Evaluation and Treatment of the Child with Salicylism

Salicylate intoxication can usually be suspected by a history of acute ingestion, a history of repeated therapeutic overdosage, or recognition of the characteristic symptoms. Salicylism should also be suspected in any child with an unexplained metabolic acidosis or nonfocal neurologic signs. Single dose ingestions of greater than 150 mg/kg of salicylate may result in toxic symptoms. Chronic salicylism may occur even at therapeutic dosages (80 to 100 mg/kg/day), though it more commonly occurs with higher daily intakes.

Urine ferric chloride testing is a simple bedside test that can confirm the presence of salicylic acid in the urine, though it has no quantitative value. A few drops of 10% ferric chloride solution is added to about 5 ml urine, and a stable purple color, persisting after heating the urine to boiling (which removes ketones), indicates a positive test for salicylic acid. Another bedside test that has some

semiquantitative value is to test plasma or serum with a Phenistix. A tan reaction indicates an approximate serum salicylate value of less than 40 mg/dl; a deeper brown to purple color indicates a level of 40 to 90 mg/dl; and a pure purple color indicates a level of greater than 90 mg/dl. Although these tests are helpful, if salicylate intoxication is suspected a serum salicylate level will confirm this diagnosis. The Done nomogram is useful in prognosticating the severity of intoxication for an acute single-dose exposure (Fig. 170-1). It is not useful, however, when managing the child with chronic salicylism, where the severity of intoxication correlates less with the serum salicylate level and more with the tissue distribution of salicylic acid. Serial salicylate determinations are necessary to determine when peak levels occur and also to follow the effects of therapeutic intervention.

A careful laboratory evaluation of the acid-base and fluid and electrolyte manifestations of salicylism requires serial determinations of arterial blood gases and serum electrolytes. A clinical pitfall that should be avoided is the use of only an arterial or venous pH to try to gauge the significance of these disturbances. Not infrequently, the pH may be normal or almost normal in a child with mixed respiratory alkalosis and metabolic acidosis. Other ap-

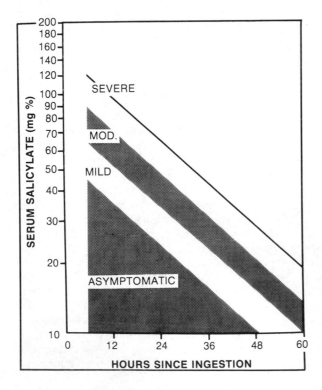

Figure 170-1. This nomogram relates serum salicylate concentration and expected severity of intoxication at varying intervals following the ingestion of a single dose of salicylate. (Done AK: Salicylate intoxication: Significance of measurements of salicylate in blood in cases of acute ingestion. Pediatrics 26:800, 1960. Reproduced by permission of Pediatrics, 1960)

propriate studies, especially in the child requiring hospitalization, include measurements of glucose, prothrombin time, and hepatic enzymes.

The initial treatment of salicylate poisoning includes ipecac-induced emesis, or gastric lavage in the unresponsive patient, followed by the administration of activated charcoal in a dose of 1 to 2 g/kg. Both these attempts to prevent absorption are most effective if performed within 4 hours of ingestion. Osmotic cathartics (*e.g.*, magnesium citrate or sorbitol) may also prevent absorption, particularly with enteric-coated aspirin preparations.

Rapid and careful correction of water, electrolyte, and glucose deficits are crucial particularly with chronic salicylism. Hypoglycemia should be treated aggressively. Seizures should be treated with anticonvulsants, and if unresponsive a trial of intravenous glucose should be considered.

The brain is the most vulnerable organ in salicylate poisoning and therapy is aimed at reducing the amount of salicylate that enters the central nervous system. Systemic alkalinization both prevents tissue penetration of salicylate and enhances the urinary excretion of unbound plasma salicylic acid.

Alkalinization can usually be achieved by adding bicarbonate to intravenous fluids. The goal of therapy is to maintain a normal or slightly alkalotic serum *p*H (7.35 to 7.45) while producing an alkaline urine. Care must be taken to provide adequate potassium, because sudden shifts in the *p*H from acidemic to alkalemic may precipitate arrhythmias in the child with intracellular potassium depletion. In the face of potassium depletion, a paradoxical aciduria may also occur despite adequate systemic alkalinization.

Hemodialysis has been shown to remove salicylate more rapidly than alkaline diuresis and should be considered in the child with severe acidemia or salicylate levels over 80 mg/dl, and in the child showing clinical deterioration despite adequate bicarbonate therapy.

ACETAMINOPHEN POISONING

Pathophysiology

Acetaminophen, when ingested, is rapidly absorbed in the upper gastrointestinal tract. Peak serum levels are achieved in ½ to 2 hours after ingestion depending on the formulation taken, although with toxic ingestions, peak levels may be delayed.

Hepatotoxicity is the major, clinically important condition resulting from acetaminophen (N-acetyl-

para-aminophenol) poisoning. In therapeutic doses, acetaminophen is metabolized by the liver primarily into conjugates of glucuronic and sulfuric acid, with smaller amounts being oxidized by the mixed function oxidases. With increasing dosages, the capacity to conjugate acetaminophen is exceeded, resulting in the oxidation of larger amounts of acetaminophen. A reactive intermediate metabolite of acetaminophen oxidation is, under normal conditions, conjugated with glutathione to acetaminophen–mercapturate which is excreted in the urine. Following larger doses of acetaminophen or under conditions where the mixed function oxidases are induced, glutathione becomes depleted, resulting in the direct covalent binding of this intermediate reactive metabolite to intracellular proteins, with resultant centrilobular hepatic necrosis.

Clinical Presentation

Children tolerate larger overdosages without hepatotoxicity than do adolescents and adults, although severe toxicity may occur in children. Ingestion of toxic amounts of acetaminophen usually causes mild symptoms during the first 24 hours. Nausea, vomiting, abdominal pain, anorexia, and malaise may occur several hours after ingestion. Diaphoresis may be seen in adolescents and adults, though rarely in children. These symptoms cease within 24 hours of ingestion and the child appears well for the next 24 to 48 hours. During this silent period, however, laboratory evidence of hepatic necrosis and dysfunction is present in the untreated patient. Transaminase levels (SGOT, SGPT) and bilirubin begin to rise and prothrombin time (PT) is prolonged. Evidence of hepatic injury becomes clinically apparent between 2 to 4 days postingestion. Jaundice, malaise, nausea, vomiting, and in severe cases symptoms consistent with fulminant hepatic necrosis and hepatic encephalopathy may occur. Fortunately, such severe cases have been described only rarely in children less than 6 years old. The recovery of hepatic function usually occurs in 6 to 8 days after ingestion and does not result in cirrhosis.

Differential Diagnosis

Acetaminophen toxicity may be confused with various forms of hepatitis particularly when there is not a clear history of ingestion. Infectious causes include hepatitis A, hepatitis B, non-A, non-B hepatitis, cytomegalovirus, Epstein–Barr, herpes simplex, Coxsackie and ECHO viruses, as well as hepatitis due to toxoplasmosis. Toxic hepatitis may occur from trichloroethylene, carbon tetrachloride, yellow phosphorus, the mushroom *Amanita phalloides*, as well as from medications such as halothane, isoniazid, aspirin, valproic acid, furosemide, and methyldopa. Reye's syndrome should be distinguished from acetaminophen intoxication by its different clinical presentation and by the characteristic fatty infiltration without significant inflammation seen on histologic appearance of the liver in Reye's syndrome.

Evaluation and Treatment

When faced with the situation where a child may have ingested acetaminophen, it is important to obtain an accurate history of the timing of the ingestion and the amount of acetaminophen that was ingested. With an intentional overdosage, it is important to assess whether additional drugs may have been taken. A single acute ingestion of 140 mg/kg of acetaminophen is a potentially toxic dose and requires a careful assessment including a plasma acetaminophen level. The Rumack–Matthew nomogram is useful for prognosticating the severity of a single, acute ingestion of acetaminophen (Fig. 170-2). It is important that the plasma acetaminophen level be obtained at least 4 hours post-

ingestion. A level of 200 µg/ml at 4 hours after ingestion indicates that the child is at risk for hepatic injury and should be treated. Multiple acetaminophen levels obtained to calculate the plasma half-life rarely add helpful information to the assessment or management of the child.

The successful treatment of a significant acetaminophen ingestion requires the removal of unabsorbed acetaminophen from the stomach and treatment with oral N-acetylcysteine (NAC). Syrup of ipecac or gastric lavage should be used within 4 hours of ingestion to remove unabsorbed acetaminophen. Activated charcoal is effective in binding acetaminophen but may also bind NAC and inhibit its absorption. Activated charcoal is not currently recommended in situations where acetaminophen is the sole toxin, but it may be used if other substances have been ingested concomitantly. If used, one should lavage the stomach to remove charcoal before initiating treatment with NAC.

Oral N-acetylcysteine is, in the United States, the current preferred treatment for potentially hepatotoxic acetaminophen poisoning. The treatment should be initiated as soon as possible after ingestion. NAC should be started within 12 hours of ingestion to be maximally efficacious. If unsure of the time of ingestion, the initial loading dose of

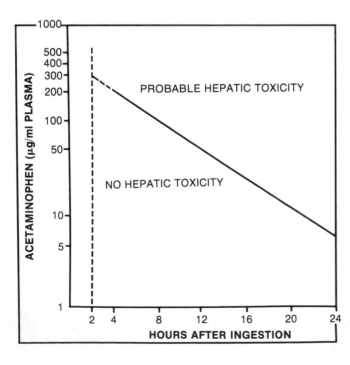

Figure 170-2. Semilogarithmic plot of plasma acetaminophen levels versus time. (Rumack BH, Matthew H: Acetaminophen poisoning and toxicity. Pediatrics 55:871, 1975. Reproduced by permission of Pediatrics, 1975)

NAC can be given while awaiting further history and laboratory confirmation of ingestion. Treatment initiated more than 24 hours after ingestion probably does not prevent hepatotoxicity. The initial loading dose of NAC is 140 mg/kg and the treatment is continued with 70 mg/kg given every 4 hours for 17 additional doses. NAC can be diluted in water, juices, or sodas to increase palatability. If not tolerated orally, NAC can be administered through a gastric or duodenal tube.

Tests to evaluate hepatocellular necrosis (SGPT, SGOT) and hepatic function (PT, bilirubin) should be performed daily. Hepatic coma and encephalopathy should be anticipated with severe ingestions, and appropriate supportive care should be initiated.

ANNOTATED BIBLIOGRAPHY

Done AK: Salicylate intoxication: Significance of measurements of salicylate in blood in cases of acute ingestion. Pediatrics 26:800, 1960 (Clinical study in which the Done nomogram was developed.)

Done AK, Temple AR: Treatment on salicylate poisoning. Mod Treat 8:528, 1971 (Still an excellent clinical review.)

Hill JB: Salicylate intoxication. N Engl J Med 288:1110, 1973 (Provocative animal research supporting bicarbonate therapy and extracorporeal removal of salicylate in severe poisoning.)

Mitchell JR, Jollow DJ, Potter WZ et al: Acetaminophen induced hepatic necrosis. I. Role of drug metabolism. J Pharmacol Exp Ther 187:185, 1973 (First of a series of four consecutive papers in the same issue providing experimental evidence for the pharmacopathology of acetaminophen induced hepatic injury and its treatment.)

Rumack BH, Peterson RC, Koch GG, Amara IA: Acetaminophen overdose: 662 cases with evaluation of oral acetylcysteine treatment. Arch Intern Med 141:380, 1981 (Clinical study from which standards for treating with oral N-acetylcysteine were developed.)

171
Iron Overdose
PIERRE GAUDREAULT

Iron is present in a large number of over-the-counter medications. The accidental ingestion of these products is relatively common in childhood. In 1984, 4329 cases of iron poisoning were reported in United States, and more than 90% of these cases involved children less than 6 years old. Although rarely fatal (only three deaths were reported), the ingestion of a substantial amount of iron may lead to serious sequellae. Iron preparations are usually dispensed as ferrous sulfate, fumarate, or gluconate. The amount of elemental iron ingested determines the severity of the intoxication. The percentage of elemental iron varies with each salt. It ranges from 33% for the fumarate salt to 20% and 12% for the sulfate and gluconate salt respectively. Most iron poisonings result from the ingestions of multivitamin preparations or prenatal vitamins containing iron.

PATHOPHYSIOLOGY

The pathophysiology of iron intoxication has not been clearly elucidated. The morbidity and mortality result from the toxic effect of the iron on several systems including gastrointestinal irritation with hemorrhage, cardiovascular depression with hypotension, hepatic injuries, and metabolic changes such as acidosis and coagulation defects. Ferrous iron is absorbed primarily by the duodenum and jejunum, oxidized to its ferric state, and bound to ferritin, which is an iron-storage protein. The ferric iron is then released into the plasma where it is bound to transferrin. Transferrin becomes attached to sites in the bone marrow and releases the iron necessary for erythropoiesis. The iron content of the body is mainly regulated by absorptive mechanisms. Indeed, there are no specific excretory mechanisms. Approximately 1 mg iron is lost each day from the intestine, skin, or urinary tract. This phenomenon explains the accumulation of iron that occurs following an overdose. With an overdose, tranferrin's binding capacity is exceeded and the remainder of the iron circulates in the free form. It is the unbound iron that causes systemic toxicity.

Gastrointestinal symptoms such as vomiting, hematemesis, and bloody diarrhea result from a direct toxic effect of iron on the mucosa. The mucosa, submucosa, and basement membrane cytoplasm and nuclear tissue show heavy iron staining. Hemorrhages and necrotic lesions to the stomach and the proximal small bowel may result and segmental infarctions characterized by marked mucosal congestion and submucosal venous thrombosis in the distal small bowel have also been described. The large intestine is usually not affected. Although the loss of blood and fluids from the damaged structures is usually not sufficient to result in death, these losses contribute to the severity of the shock.

Shock appears rapidly in animals given lethal doses of iron. The exact mechanism of action has not been clearly elucidated. The circulatory failure may be induced by a direct action of iron on blood vessels. The circulating free iron damages the vessels, inducing an increase in the capillary permeability and a postarteriolar vasodilation. These changes result in a decrease of the effective circulatory blood volume as well as the total blood volume that leads to a decrease in the cardiac output.

It has also been noted in animals that plasma concentrations of ferritin, serotonin, and histamine are elevated following an iron overdose. These substances are well known vasodilators that may play a role in the generation of hypotension. The fluid loss in the gastrointestinal tract also contributes to the hypotension.

The liver damage results from the uptake of iron by hepatic cells once plasma transferrin has been saturated. Iron is localized primarily in the area of the mitochondria, which cause alterations in several hepatic cell oxidative processes. Hepatic necrosis may result and is usually limited to the periportal parenchymal cells. In humans, hepatocellular damages have not been incriminated as a causative factor in death.

The release of hydrogen ions from the conversion of ferrous iron to its ferric form is the main factor responsible for the metabolic acidosis. The accumulation of organic acids such as lactic and citric acid from anaerobic metabolism may also contribute to the acidosis. The inhibition of enzymatic processes in the Krebs' cycle aerobic metabolism may be secondary to a direct action of iron or to cardiovascular insufficiency.

The coagulation defects are secondary to a direct action of iron on the various proteins involved in blood coagulation. Animals poisoned with high doses of iron (700 mg/kg) developed prolongation in clotting time, thrombocytopenia, hypoprothrombinemia, and qualitative changes in fibrinogen. Coagulation defects, however, are not a major factor in the lethality of iron overdose.

CLINICAL PRESENTATION

The severity of an acute iron intoxication is proportional to the amount of elemental iron ingested. Although the oral lethal dose is generally accepted to be ~200 to 250 mg/kg of elemental iron, doses in excess of 20 mg/kg may lead to toxicity. The clinical presentation usually evolves through phases.

First Phase

Following an acute oral overdose, signs and symptoms appear ½ to 6 hours after the ingestion. Nausea, vomiting, hematemesis, abdominal pain, melena, and bloody diarrhea may be seen. In severe cases, the decrease of effective circulatory as well as total blood volume results in hypotension with reflex tachycardia.

Central nervous system manifestations range from lethargy and hypotonia to seizures and coma secondary to decreased cerebral perfusion or a direct effect of iron on the central nervous system. Laboratory findings may include metabolic acidosis, hyperglycemia, and leukocytosis. Shock or coma during this period usually indicates a grave prognosis.

Second Phase

The patient may experience a period of relative stability following the first phase. The appearance and duration of this period is probably related to the severity of the intoxication. Since the patient's status may deteriorate, it is imperative to pursue adequate treatment during this phase. Following this period of quiescence, the patient may develop shock, coma, seizures, and he may die. Elevated levels of hepatic enzymes and hypoglycemia may be seen.

Late Phase

Pyloric or antral strictures may develop 2 to 5 weeks after the ingestion. Diffuse fibrosis of the liver with fatty degeneration has been reported.

WORK-UP

History

The physician should determine the type of iron preparation and the maximal amount of elemental iron that has been ingested. Ingestion of multivitamins with iron (~4 mg to 5 mg elemental iron/pill) rarely causes serious morbidity.

In contrast, iron preparations (60 mg to 65 mg elemental iron/pill) used as supplemental intake during pregnancy are responsible for most serious intoxications.

Physical Examination

The physical examination should be directed toward the evaluation of the clinical signs expected with this intoxication.

Laboratory Tests

The severity of an iron intoxication correlates with serum iron concentrations as long as the blood sample is obtained within a few hours after the ingestion. Indeed, the rapid clearance of iron from the plasma may be responsible for deceptively low serum iron concentrations within a few hours of a substantial ingestion. Normal serum iron concentrations range from 100 μg/dl to 125/μg/dl. Concentrations less than 300 μg/dl are usually associated with no or mild symptoms such as nausea, vomiting, or melena. Abdominal cramps, bloody diarrhea, and lethargy may occur with concentrations between 300 μg/dl to 500 μg/dl. Patients who have concentrations above 500 μg/dl may develop mild hypotension as well as the gastrointestinal manifestations. Concentrations of more than 750 μg/dl to 1000 μg/dl may be associated with hypotension, shock, metabolic acidosis, coma, and death.

If an iron determination cannot be obtained rapidly, a white blood count and a blood sugar level should be performed because elevated results (leukocytosis greater than 15,000 mm^3 and blood glucose levels above 150 mg/dl) correlate with high serum iron concentrations. Hematocrit, hemoglobin level, serum electrolytes, and acid-base status should be monitored.

A flat plate of the abdomen done early in the course of the intoxication may reveal the presence of ingested iron tablets. It can usually detect prenatal iron preparations but not multivitamin preparations with iron. A film can also document the success or failure of the gastrointestinal decontamination.

Treatment

Since the severity of the intoxication is proportional to the amount of iron absorbed, measures to prevent its gastrointestinal absorption should be undertaken. The removal of iron from the stomach is accomplished best by emesis induced with ipecac syrup. However, if the patient is obtunded, gastric lavage should be performed with the largest bore tube possible. If evidence of iron (radiopaque material) persists in the stomach, these procedures should be repeated. Iron pills will rarely form a mass of concretions requiring surgical removal. After the completion of these procedures, the instillation of 50 ml to 100 ml of 1% solution of bicarbonate should be performed in patients having ingested a large amount of iron (>50 mg elemental iron/kg) presenting with signs or symptoms other than mild gastrointestinal upset. Phosphate containing preparations have been associated with complications and are not recommended. Activated charcoal does not adsorb heavy metals and therefore should not be administered. Cathartics should not be given because their efficacy has never been demonstrated and they could aggravate the diarrhea induced by the iron.

Once iron has been absorbed, measures should be taken to reduce the free toxic fraction. Deferoxamine is a chelating agent that binds the free iron and competes for the iron with transferrin and ferritin. It removes only a small amount of the iron from transferrin and does not bind the iron in the cytochrome system or hemoglobin. Deferoxamine may be given intramuscularly (IM) or intravenously (IV) to chelate the absorbed iron.

A deferoxamine provocative chelation challenge (dose of 50 mg/kg with a maximum of 1 g IM or IV) should be given to patients with a history of a large ingestion (>50 mg elemental iron /kg), signs or symptoms of more than mild gastrointestinal upset, a serum iron concentration above 300 μg/dl, a leukocytosis greater than 15,000/mm^3 or a blood glucose above 150 mg/dl.

If the patient passes a vin rosé colored urine within 2 hours of the administration of deferoxamine, it signifies that free iron was chelated to deferoxamine and that therapy should be continued. The patient should be given 50 mg/kg (maximum 1g) every 4 hours IM or as a constant IV infusion until signs of toxicity have subsided, serum iron concentrations are less than the total iron-binding capacity and the vin rosé colored urine has stopped for 4 to 6 hours.

The IV infusion rate should usually not exceed 15 mg/kg/hr to avoid the risk of inducing hypotension. The IV route should be used in patients with hypotension, metabolic acidosis, or those who have a severe ingestion.

Patients remaining asymptomatic 6 hours after the ingestion, without vin rosé urine and an abdominal roentgenogram demonstrating no residual iron tablets can be safely sent home.

There are no efficacious procedures to increase the elimination of free iron. Dialysis and exchange transfusion do not remove the free fraction and remove only a small portion of the iron-chelate complex. Dialysis should be used in patients with renal failure.

Finally, adequate supportive care should be instituted to correct fluid losses, hypotension, and metabolic acidosis.

ANNOTED BIBLIOGRAPHY

Lacouture PG, Wason S, Temple AC et al: Emergency assessment of severity in iron overdose by clinical and laboratory methods. J Pediatr 99:89,1981 (Use of laboratory tests [leukocytosis and blood sugar] as predictors of serum iron concentrations.)

Robotham JL, Lietman PS: Acute iron poisoning. A review. Am J Dis Child 134:875,1980 (Very good review of the pathophysiology and the treatment of iron overdose.)

Westlin WF: Deferoxamine as a chelating agent. Clin Toxicol 4:597,1971 (Good review of deferoxamine.)

Whitten CF, Brough AJ: The pathophysiology of acute iron poisoning. Clin Toxicol 4:585,1971 (Pathophysiology of iron poisoning is reviewed.)

Whitten CF, Gibson GW, Good MH et al: Studies in acute iron poisoning. 1: Deferoxamine in the treatment of acute iron poisoning: Clinical observations, experimental studies, and theoretical considerations. Pediatrics 36:322, 1965 (Among the first articles evaluating the efficacy of deferoxamine.)

172
Plants

MICHAEL A. MCGUIGAN

Plants, as a group, account for one of the most common ingestions in childhood. Potentially dangerous plants are available to children nearly every day of their lives. Poisonous plants grow wild, but are often cultivated and even brought into the home as ornamental plants. Although every plant contains toxic chemicals, the concentration of these toxins is generally so low as to render most plants nontoxic (see the box, Nontoxic Plants). Certain plants do contain quantities of chemicals that may pose a toxic hazard. An important factor is that the concentrations of the toxic elements in any plant will vary with the season, climate, age of the plant, and degree of cultivation, among other variables. Some plants have small amounts of toxins that have a high "scare potential," such as cyanide or cardiac glycosides. This chapter will discuss the clinical toxicology of plants containing oxalates, gastrointestinal irritants, cyanogenic glycosides, and cardiac glycosides.

The prevention of plant poisoning can be accomplished by taking the following simple precautions:

1. All plants in and around the home should be identified.
2. Plants and related parts (*e.g.*, seeds, fruit, bulbs) should be kept away from young children.
3. Children should not drink out of flowers or use leaves, seeds, or berries to make "tea."

Nontoxic Plants	
African violet	Prayer plant
Begonias	Rubber plant
Coleus	Schefflera
Dracena	Spider plant
Ferns	Swedish ivy
Jade plant	

4. Do not make children's playthings from unknown plants or trees.

OXALATE

Pathophysiology

Crystals of calcium oxalate are found in all parts of house plants such as dieffenbachia, dumbcane, elephant's ear, and philodendron as well as in the leaves of outdoor plants such as rhubarb, jack-in-the-pulpit, wild cala, and skunk cabbage. Although the exact mechanism of the toxicity of these plants is uncertain, it is generally stated that by chewing the part of the plant that contains the oxalate crystals, they will be released, resulting in irritation of the mucous membranes. Proteolytic enzymes have also been found in the sap of the dieffenbachia plant.

Clinical Presentation

Topical symptoms and signs develop within minutes of chewing or sucking on these plants. Typical symptoms include a burning sensation and irritation of the mucous membranes, edema, and inflammation of the lips and tongue, and excessive drooling. Dysphagia is common. Rarely, mucous membrane bullae may develop. Facial edema may occur in areas that have come in contact with the sap. Systemic symptoms do not occur. Acute symptoms generally last only a few hours, although necrotic areas resulting from severe irritation may take longer to heal.

Differential Diagnosis

The differential diagnosis should include the causes of urticarial reactions, viral or bacterial stomatitis/pharyngitis, and the ingestion of caustic or corrosive products. The inflammation of the oral mucous membranes and excessive drooling may mimic epiglottitis although coughing and fever are usually absent in oxalate-induced inflammation.

Work-Up

The evaluation of the child who ingested a plant containing oxalate should include a proper identification of the plant. If the care-giver does not know the name of the plant, a nursery, florist, or local botany department may be able to identify it based on a telephone description. The main thrust of the physical examination is to evaluate the possibility of the inflammation obstructing the airway. Laboratory investigations are not helpful in the diagnosis or assessment of severity. Hypocalcemia and oxalate crystaluria have not been demonstrated. The use of soft-tissue x-ray examinations of the neck has not been reported.

Treatment

Plant debris in the mouth should be removed immediately. Administration of cool soothing substances such as water, milk, popsicles, or ice cream may bring symptomatic relief. The use of ipecac syrup or activated charcoal is not recommended. Prophylactic intubation should be considered if airway obstruction is a possibility.

Indications for Admission or Referral

Most cases may be managed at home or in an ambulatory setting. Hospitalization may be necessary if the oral lesions are severe, if the child is unable to tolerate fluids, or if there are symptoms or signs of airway compromise.

GASTROINTESTINAL IRRITANTS

Pathophysiology

Many plants contain substances that cause gastrointestinal irritation. The gastroenteritis may be due to any of a variety of substances such as saponins (e.g., horse chestnuts, amaryllis, wisteria), resins (e.g., iris), or irritant oils (e.g., buttercup). The exact mechanism of action of these substances is uncertain although the effect is believed to occur at the gastrointestinal level with, perhaps, some stimulation of the vomiting center in the brain.

Clinical Presentation

The time interval between ingestion and the onset of gastrointestinal effects is highly variable, ranging from a few minutes to several hours. The severity of the presenting symptoms or signs may also vary considerably, ranging from minor abdominal discomfort to severe vomiting, abdominal cramps, and explosive diarrhea. Oral irritation may also occur as a sole finding.

Differential Diagnosis

The differential diagnosis should include viral or bacterial gastroenteritis and ingestion of other toxins that cause gastroenteritis such as iron or arsenic. Staphylococcal food poisoning should be considered. Oral lesions must be differentiated from viral or bacterial stomatitis or ingestion of caustic substances (e.g., lyes or acids).

Work-Up

A work-up should include a thorough history of events preceding the onset of the symptoms, especially identifying where the child was playing and what potential toxins might have been available. A physical examination may reveal signs of irritation of the oral mucous membranes or findings compatible with dehydration secondary to severe diarrhea. No specific diagnostic or laboratory tests are available for this type of poisoning. Laboratory investigations, therefore, should be aimed at assessing the severity of the effects rather than trying to identify the cause. Renal and hepatic function tests may be indicated in patients who are severely symptomatic.

Treatment

The "toxic dose" of any of these plants is unknown, so that if a child has ingested one of these plants but no symptoms have occurred, a "wait and watch" approach is recommended.

The efficacy of gastrointestinal decontamination procedures has not been investigated. Emesis or lavage is not indicated. Although activated charcoal theoretically *may* be beneficial, its use in practice is difficult. Prophylactic use is not recommended and toxin-induced vomiting may preclude its administration. Cathartics should not be used in the face of existing diarrhea. Fluid and electrolyte replacement may be required to prevent or correct imbalances and shock. The use of antiemetics and antidiarrheal agents is not indicated.

Indications for Admission or Referral

The indications for admission depend on the severity of the symptoms, the presence of dehydration, and the ability of the child to take adequate oral fluids.

CYANOGENIC GLYCOSIDES

Pathophysiology

Cyanogenic glycosides are contained in a number of fruit pits or seeds such as apple, wild cherry, elderberry, and peach and apricot kernels. The products of cultivated apricot plants may contain as little as one twentyfifth the concentration of cyanogenic glycosides found in the wild plants. Following ingestion, the glycosides are hydrolized within the gut to liberate cyanide which is absorbed into the body. Cyanide, once absorbed, distributes to the cells where it binds to and inhibits cytochrome oxidase activity, thus blocking cellular respiration.

Clinical Presentation

Patients who ingest large quantities of the appropriate fruit material may present ½ to 2 hours later with symptoms and signs of cyanide poisoning: malaise, vomiting, weakness, unsteadiness, confusion, tachypnea, and coma.

Differential Diagnosis

The differential diagnosis of acute collapse may include central nervous system hemorrhage, convulsions, or exposure to toxic gases such as hydrogen sulfide or carbon monoxide.

Work-Up

A historical evaluation may identify the suspected fruit and the circumstances. The toxic dose of each fruit pit or seed is difficult to establish. However, it has been estimated that for cultivated peaches, the toxic dose of peach pit kernels is ~ one kernel/kg. A physical examination will reveal an unconscious or deteriorating child with hypotension and bradycardia but not cyanosis. The bitter almond smell of cyanide may be noted. Laboratory investigations may document elevated cyanide levels as well as metabolic (lactic) acidosis.

Treatment

If a large quantity of seeds or pits has been ingested, it is reasonable to use ipecac syrup followed by activated charcoal. Ipecac may be used within 2 hours of the ingestion. Unless the diagnosis is certain, treatment should be symptomatic and supportive. Ventilatory assistance with supplemental oxygen is indicated and also support of circulation using volume expanders and pressor agents. Acidosis should be corrected with sodium bicarbonate. Once the diagnosis of cyanide poisoning has been made, standard therapy consists of the intravenous administration of sodium nitrite followed by sodium thiosulfate.

Indications for Admission or Referral

Indications for admission include any child with a positive history and compatible symptoms.

CARDIAC GLYCOSIDES

Pathophysiology

Many attractive plants contain cardiac glycosides. Lily-of-the-valley, foxglove, and oleander are all popular flowering plants that contain variable quantities of cardiac glycosides. Following ingestion of these plants, the digitalis-like glycoside is absorbed and exerts an effect on the myocardium similar to that produced by digoxin.

Clinical Presentation

Symptoms usually become evident within 2 hours of ingestion. Vomiting is the most common presenting complaint. Topical or oral irritation may be present and also salivation, abdominal pain, and diarrhea. Cardiac symptoms may begin 1 to 6 hours after the ingestion and consist of bradycardia, hypotension, and cyanosis.

Differential Diagnosis

The differential diagnosis includes acquired cardiac disease of other causes as well as an ingestion of pharmaceutical digitalis preparations.

Work-Up

A history of exposure or availability of these plants is important, but the reliable "toxic dose" of these plants has not been established. No documented cases of lily of the valley poisoning have been reported in children. A physical examination may document oral irritation and an atrioventricular block. An electrocardiogram may demonstrate conduction defects compatible with digitalis cardiotoxicity: exaggerated sinus arrhythmia, sinus bradycardia, and second- or third-degree block. Hyperkalemia may occur.

Treatment

Treatment is not necessary for accidental ingestion of lily-of-the-valley. Ingestion of wild oleander or foxglove should be treated with ipecac syrup or gastric lavage, followed by activated charcoal.

Atropine has been useful in the treatment of oleander-induced bradyarrhythmias. Other therapy should follow the guidelines established for the treatment of digoxin overdose (*e.g.*, electrical pacing for atropine-resistant heart block). Fab antibody fragments have not been used for the treatment of this type of cardiac glycoside poisoning.

Indications for Admission or Referral

Patients who ingest lily-of-the-valley do not need to be admitted to hospital. For patients who have ingested wild oleander or foxglove, admission is recommended if any symptoms or signs occur within 6 hours of ingestion. Patients with cardiac abnormalities should be hospitalized in a center capable of monitoring and treating them.

ANNOTATED BIBLIOGRAPHY

Ansford AJ, Morris H: Fatal oleander poisoning. Med J Aust 1:360–361, 1981 (Case history and clinical presentation.)

Arditt J, Rodriguez E: Dieffenbachia: Uses, abuses and toxic constituents: A review. J Ethonopharmacol 5:293–302, 1982 (Scientific more than clinical review.)

Haynes BE, Bessen HA, Wightman WD: Oleander tea: Herbal draught of death. Ann Emerg Med 14:350–353, 1985 (Case history and clinical presentation.)

Lasch EE, El Shawa R: Multiple cases of cyanide poisoning by apricot kernels in children from Gaza. Pediatrics 68:5–7, 1981 (Clinical case presentations.)

Rubino MJ, Davidoff F: Cyanide poisoning from apricot seeds. (letter) JAMA 241:359, 1979 (Clinical case presentations.)

Shaw D, Pearn J: Oleander poisoning. Med J Aust 2:267–269, 1979 (Case history and clinical presentation.)

173
Hydrocarbon Ingestion
MICHAEL A. MCGUIGAN

Accidental exposure to a hydrocarbon product occurs commonly in children. More than 10,000 cases were reported in 1983 by Poison Centers in the United States. Hydrocarbons have been classified or divided in many ways: aromatic *vs* aliphatic, petroleum distillate *vs* nonpetroleum distillate, high viscosity (thick) *vs* low viscosity (thin), halogenated *vs* nonhalogenated, and, finally, hydrocarbons with toxic additives *vs* those without additives.

Aromatic hydrocarbons are aromatic ring structures and they include such compounds as benzene, toluene, turpentine, and xylene. The aromatic ring is important because it appears that the aromatic hydrocarbons are absorbed from the gastrointestinal tract in quantities sufficient to cause systemic toxicity. Aliphatic hydrocarbons are formed from the distillation of crude petroleum.

Viscosity is important only with respect to the risk of developing widespread aspiration pneumonitis. Most hydrocarbons are of low viscosity and, therefore, pose a risk of aspiration pneumonitis. High-viscosity hydrocarbons such as greases, petroleum jelly, or tar are hazardous only as a foreign body and have no toxic effects.

Halogenated hydrocarbons (*e.g.*, carbon tetrachloride, trichloroethane) and hydrocarbons with toxic additives (*e.g.*, pesticides) are unique entities and are not discussed. It is important to remember, however, that the therapeutic approach to the patient who ingested one of these products may depend on the *additive* and not on the hydrocarbon.

This chapter discusses only the low viscosity nonhalogenated additive-free aliphatic petroleum distillate hydrocarbons: gasoline, kerosene, lighter fluid, lubricating oils, furniture polish (mineral seal oil), mineral spirits, and naphthas. These compounds are dealt with as a group and are referred to as petroleum distillate hydrocarbons (PDH).

PATHOPHYSIOLOGY

Drinking a PDH results in mild irritation of the mucous membranes of the mouth. These substances are not significantly absorbed through the gastrointestinal tract and, therefore, will produce no pulmonary or nonpulmonary (systemic) disease as a result of an uncomplicated ingestion. Chemical pneumonitis arises only as a result of pulmonary aspiration of the hydrocarbon liquid. Following aspiration of significant quantities of PDH, central nervous system (CNS) depression may develop secondarily to hypoxemia or from the CNS effects of PDH absorbed through the lung.

CLINICAL PRESENTATION

Most patients present shortly after the exposure has been discovered. The commonest symptom resulting from the ingestion of PDH is vomiting, which occurs in 50% of ingestions. Coughing occurs in 40% of children, but ~20% of the children present with no respiratory complaints. Drowsiness is an unusual presenting complaint, occurring in 10% of cases. Dyspnea (6%) and abdominal pain or diarrhea (3%) are rare complaints. The smell of hydrocarbon in the child's mouth may be noticeable. Because children often spill while drinking from ungainly containers, their skin and clothes may smell of hydrocarbons.

DIFFERENTIAL DIAGNOSIS

The correct diagnosis is usually not difficult to make because PDHs have a distinct petroleum smell and an accurate history is volunteered. Poisoning with insecticides (*e.g.*, organophosphates or carbamates) that inhibit the enzyme cholinesterase will produce a clinical picture similar to that caused by PDH ingestion and aspiration: vomiting, excess salivation, tachypnea, drowsiness, and chest findings. Other diagnoses to consider in a child who presents with an acute onset of vomiting and abdominal pain are infectious gastroenteritis (bacterial or viral) and ingestion of other substances such as acetaminophen, salicylates, caffeine, iron, digitalis products, theophylline, and tobacco. The differential diagnosis of an acute consolidation on a chest roentgenogram includes viral or bacterial infections and foreign body aspiration.

WORK-UP

History

The most important questions to answer are "What was the product?" and "Did the child aspirate?" The correct identification of the product as a pure PDH is essential; estimates of the volume missing are less important. In assessing whether or not the child aspirated, the presence or absence of respiratory *symptoms* can be a useful guide. If the episode was observed by a reliable witness and there is no history of coughing, choking, gagging, vomiting, or burping, then the likelihood that the child aspirated is negligible.

Physical Examination

If the child exhibits any symptoms or signs that suggest the trachea was endangered, then the child may have aspirated and may need a careful examination. A low-grade fever may be noted. During the physical examination the physician should attempt to detect the smell of PDH in the child's mouth and to look for irritated oral mucous membranes. Procedures that might induce gagging or choking, such as the depression of the tongue with a tongue-blade, should be avoided. The respiratory rate and depth should be documented, although tachypnea has been noted infrequently. The chest should be examined carefully. Although rhonchi and crepitations may be found, the physician should remember that an examination within a short time after aspiration may give false-negative results. The examination should thus be repeated several times over a period of 6 hours after the ingestion before the results may be considered reliable.

Central nervous system depression, if present, is usually mild. More severe findings (*e.g.*, stupor or convulsions) are rare (1% of reported cases) on presentation.

Finally, the skin around the mouth and on the neck, chest, abdomen, and groin should be examined for evidence of irritation.

Laboratory Tests

If the child is not severely ill, a chest roentgenogram should be delayed until 4 to 6 hours after the aspiration. In patients who eventually develop pneumonitis, a chest roentgenogram is positive in only 60% by 1 hour after the aspiration. Therefore, a negative chest roentgenogram 1 hour after aspiration may have to be repeated after several hours. The chest roentgenogram, when positive, demonstrates a unilobar infiltrate in 83% of patients and a perihilar pattern in only 9%. The white blood cell count may be elevated as high as 16,000 cells/mm^2 in patients with pneumonitis.

TREATMENT

Neither induced vomiting nor gastric lavage should be used to treat patients with PDH ingestion because PDHs are not absorbed to a significant degree through the gastrointestinal tract. Activated charcoal binds the PDH, but its use is impractical because such large quantities are required. The administration of mineral or paraffin oil, or saline cathartics is not recommended. For children with no or mild symptoms, the best therapy consists of careful observation. The child may be discharged when enough time has passed to allow for emptying of the PDH from the stomach through the pylorus.

If the clothes or skin are contaminated, clothing should be removed and the skin gently washed with lukewarm water and a mild soap.

When aspiration pneumonitis has been documented, treatment should consist of chest physical therapy and humidified air or supplemental oxygen (if needed). Ventilatory assistance using endotracheal intubation and mechanical ventilation may be necessary if normal arterial blood gases cannot otherwise be maintained. Corticosteroids have no place in either the prophylaxis or the treatment of hydrocarbon pneumonitis. The use of systemic antibiotics is indicated if secondary bacterial infections is suspected or documented.

INDICATIONS FOR ADMISSION OR REFERRAL

Patients who have severe pneumonitis should be admitted immediately to a hospital capable of providing adequate respiratory care. Patients presenting with symptomatology of a moderate degree should be admitted and observed for a progression of symptoms and signs. Patients with minor presenting complaints should be observed for 6 hours before deciding whether or not to admit the patient. The patient may be sent home at the end of the 6-hour period, if both the patient's physical examination *and* chest roentgenogram are normal. If, on the other hand, either the patient's physical examination *or* chest roentgenogram is abnormal, the patient should be admitted to hospital for observation. Patients who have been entirely asymptomatic following ingestion can be observed at home and their progress can be re-evaluated in 2 to 4 hours by telephone.

The clinical course of aspiration pneumonitis is usually fairly benign unless the aspiration is severe. Fever, tachycardia, and tachypnea may last for less than 2 days. The mean duration of hospitalization in one study was 4 days. Severe cases of aspiration pneumonitis may require intubation and ventilation to maintain adequate arterial blood gas values. There have been no common clinically significant residual pulmonary effects from routine PDH aspiration.

ANNOTATED BIBLIOGRAPHY

Baldachin BJ, Melmed RN: Clinical and therapeutic aspects of kerosene poisoning: A series of 200 cases. Br Med J 2:28–30, 1964 (Excellent brief presentation of children with clinical toxicity.)

Dice WH, Ward G, Kelly J et al: Pulmonary toxicity following gastrointestinal ingestion of kerosene. Ann Emerg Med 11:138–142, 1982 (Most recent experimental evaluation of the question of gastrointestinal absorption.)

Majeed HA, Bassyouni H, Kalaawy M et al: Kerosene poisoning in children: A clinico-radiological study of 205 cases. Ann Trop Paediatr 1:123–130, 1981 (One of the largest studies; a great deal of useful information is presented.)

Marks MI, Chicoine L, Legere G et al: Adrenocorticosteroid treatment of hydrocarbon pneumonia in children—a cooperative study. J Pediatr 81:366–369, 1972 (Excellent review, with duration of symptoms and hospitalization information.)

Wolfsdorf J: Kerosene intoxication: An experimental approach to the etiology of CNS manifestations in primates. J Pediatr 88:1037–1040, 1976 (Good presentation of the role of gastrointestinal absorption *vs* aspiration in the production of CNS findings.)

174
Caustic Ingestions
PIERRE GAUDREAULT

The ingestion of caustic substances is a significant problem. Although rarely fatal, such ingestion carries serious immediate and long-term morbidity. The morbidity is greater in adolescents and adults who ingest these products in an attempt to commit suicide. The morbidity related to liquid or solid caustic substances results from perforation or stenosis secondary to severe esophageal or gastric injuries.

In 1984, 7007 cases of caustic ingestion were reported in the United States. Most of these cases (72%) involved children less than 6 years old. Three deaths were related to such ingestions.

Lye was previously the alkali agent most frequently ingested. With the introduction of drain cleaners, sodium or potassium hydroxide has become more prevalent. Other alkali products encountered are laundry and dishwasher detergents (*e.g.*, carbonate, phosphate), denture cleaners (*e.g.*, bicarbonate, phosphate), and Clinitest tablets (sodium hydroxide).

The acidic compounds encountered most frequently are toilet-bowl cleaners (*e.g.*, hydrochloric, phosphoric, and sulfuric acids), antirust compounds (*e.g.*, hydrochloric, phosphoric, and sulfuric acids), automobile battery fluids (sulfuric acid), and slate cleaners (hydrofluoric acid).

Household bleach products (containing less than 8% of sodium hypochlorite) usually cause only a mild irritation to the esophagus; they rarely cause tissue necrosis and virtually never cause strictures. Most authors, therefore, do not treat bleach ingestions as a caustic ingestion.

PATHOPHYSIOLOGY

Alkali products destroy tissues by partially dissolving tissue proteins, a process which is referred to as *liquefaction necrosis*. This destruction permits deep penetration into tissues. In contrast to alkali agents, acids are potent dessicants and coagulate tissues. This coagulation necrosis limits acid penetration and frequently results in damage only to the mucosa.

Factors that influence the severity of the tissue destruction and the development of complications include the pH, the concentration and the quantity of the product ingested, the length of contact with the mucosa, and the relative tonicity of the pyloric sphincter. Alkali products with a pH greater than 12 are more likely to produce severe esophageal injuries.

Alkali and acid burns usually evolve through three stages. The acute phase is characterized by a marked inflammatory response with edema. This inflammation may extend through the muscle layer with severe burns, and perforation may occur.

Vascular thrombosis and hemorrhages can be seen. Cell death and necrotic tissue accumulation end 4 to 7 days after the insult. The necrotic tissue is sloughed; edema decreases; neovascularization begins; and granulation takes place. This second phase occurs between the second and third week postingestion. The last phase begins with the proliferation of fibroblasts and the formation of connective tissue. This cicatrization phase begins at the end of the third week. During this period, if the burn is deep, adhesions may form and narrowing or obliteration of the esophageal lumen may occur. Reepithelization occurs between the third and sixth week postingestion.

CLINICAL PRESENTATION

The ingestion of caustic substances primarily induces burns to the gastrointestinal tract, particularly to the oropharynx, esophagus, and stomach. The severity of these burns and associated symptoms depends on several factors such as the type of product (acid *vs* alkali), the nature of the product (solid *vs* liquid), the amount ingested, the concentration, and the pH of the substance.

The ingestion of solid products usually causes severe burns to the mouth, pharynx, or upper portion of the esophagus. Solid products may adhere to the mucosa causing deeper burns. In contrast, since liquid substances are easier to swallow, they often cause less injury in the mouth but extensive damage to the esophagus or stomach. The extent of the burns ranges from slight erythema and edema to severe ulcerations with grayish pseudomembranes.

Alkali agents have traditionally been considered to damage mainly the esophagus whereas acid products affect primarily the stomach. However, in a review of 378 cases of caustic ingestions treated in our hospital, we found that the incidence of esophageal lesions was similar with acid or alkali agents.

Injuries to the oral or esophageal mucosa may be accompanied by excessive salivation, drooling, dysphagia, painful swallowing, and retrosternal pain. Nausea, vomiting, hematemesis, epigastric or abdominal pain, or tenderness may be experienced. Substernal or back pain, and abdominal pain with rigidity may also indicate mediastinitis or peritonitis. The presence of hoarseness, aphonia, stridor, or dyspnea suggest laryngeal, tracheal, or pulmonary involvement secondary to aspiration.

The major clinical questions with caustic ingestion are to determine the location of the burn (if it occurred in the esophagus or the stomach) and the extent and the depth of the injury. Several studies have demonstrated that the presence of clinical manifestations cannot predict the presence or severity of esophageal lesions. However, patients who present with unprovoked vomiting, drooling, or stridor are more likely to have severe esophageal lesions.

The acute manifestations last 1 to 3 days, depending on the severity of the intoxication. The patient is at the highest risk for perforation during the first 72 hours following the ingestion. This period is followed by a latent phase that lasts for several weeks. Delayed complications such as stricture formation may occur toward the end of this phase. Progressive dysphagia secondary to stricture formation may be noted 3 to 4 weeks after the ingestion but may take months to appear, again depending on the severity of the mucosal burn.

Several classifications of esophageal injury have been proposed. These classifications are based on the depth of burn. The absence of an esophageal lesion is termed grade 0. Burns that are limited to the mucosa and are characterized by the presence of edema or erythema are classified as grade 1. Grade 2 burns penetrate beyond the mucosa and are characterized by the presence of ulcerations or whitish membranes. Finally, the presence of perforation is classified as grade 3. Burns that are circular or penetrate in the muscle layer carry the greatest risk of inducing a stricture formation.

WORK-UP

History and Physical Examination

The clinician should determine the type of product involved and, as much as possible, the quantity ingested. Particular attention should be given to detect the appearance of respiratory distress or signs of perforation, as well as to the determination of the presence of certain signs or symptoms (*e.g.*, vomiting, stridor, drooling) that suggest an increased risk of serious esophageal involvement.

Laboratory Tests

Esophagoscopy is the most accurate way to evaluate the involvement of the esophagus and stomach following the ingestion of caustic substances. Therefore, an esophagoscopy is recommended for all patients who have ingested a caustic substance regardless of the presence or absence of clinical signs or symptoms. The esophagoscope should not be advanced beyond the first area of ulceration to avoid the risk of perforation. This procedure carries a low risk of morbidity when performed by an experienced endoscopist using a flexible endoscope.

Children who have a questionable history of ingestion without oropharyngeal burns, dysphagia, stridor, drooling, or vomiting should be observed for 3 to 4 hours. They may be discharged without an esophagoscopy if they remain asymptomatic. Other laboratory tests should be performed as dictated by the clinical status of the patient.

An esophagram (barium swallow) is not as accurate as an esophagoscopy in determining esophageal involvement in the acute phase. Indeed, because there is no clear correlation between esophagraphic findings during the acute stage and the final outcome, such a procedure should be reserved for the documentation of a perforation or to observe the progress of a stricture.

TREATMENT

The initial treatment should consist of immediate washing with water to remove the caustic substance from the esophagus, unless the patient demonstrates signs of airway swelling, obstruction, or evidence of gastrointestinal perforation. The use of neutralizing agents such as vinegar to neutralize alkali agents or sodium bicarbonate to neutralize acid agents is not useful and may increase the esophageal injury by producing an exothermic reaction.

Emesis induced with Ipecac syrup is contraindicated because it would subject the esophagus to repeated exposure to the caustic agent. Gastric lavage is also contraindicated because the blind passage of a nasogastric tube may cause an iatrogenic esophageal perforation. If a nasogastric tube is necessary for nutritional support, it should be positioned under direct visualization during an esophagoscopy.

Results from an esophagoscopy enable the clinician to rapidly discharge patients without esophageal involvement and to start the appropriate treatment in other patients. The esophagoscopy should be performed within 48 hours of the ingestion, when the risk of perforation is low.

The role and efficacy of steroids in the prevention of stricture formation following a caustic ingestion remain unclear. Studies in animals have shown that the early administration of steroids delays the formation of connective tissue and reduces the incidence and severity of esophageal strictures following lye ingestion. Randomized controlled studies that evaluate the efficacy of steroids in humans do not exist. Some authors have reported beneficial effects of steroids in reducing the incidence of stricture formation following alkali ingestions whereas others did not find any beneficial effects.

Furthermore, there are no data evaluating the best dosage. Until such data are available, a dose of 1 to 2 mg/kg/day of prednisone (maximum 60 mg/day) or its equivalent should be sufficient. This dose should be tapered after 21 days, a time period adequate to reduce the inflammatory response during the acute injury and early reparative phases. Treatment should be started as soon as possible in patients with grade-2 esophageal burns in order to benefit from the antifibroblast action of steroids. If an esophagoscopy cannot be performed soon after an alkali ingestion, steroids should be started immediately and their necessity re-evaluated after the esophagoscopy. Patients with grade-0 or grade-1 lesions do not require treatment. Patients with grade-3 lesions need surgical intervention and do not benefit from steroids.

The use of prophylactic antibiotics in patients treated with steroids is controversial. Their use was based on animals studies demonstrating an increased mortality rate in animals treated with steroids but without antibiotics. These data are not supported by human data. In our experience with more than 100 children treated with steroids but without antibiotics, none developed any measurable deleterious effects. Prophylactic antibiotics, therefore, should not be used. Antibiotics should be reserved for patients who develop signs of secondary infection or who experience esophageal or gastric perforation.

Adequate nutrition is essential because inadequate calorie intake inhibits appropriate healing and increases susceptibility to infection. Parenteral nutrition should be started early in patients with severe esophageal lesions. Furthermore, if oral intake is delayed for a long time, a gastrostomy for the placement of a gastrojejunal feeding tube may be indicated.

After 3 to 4 weeks, the status of esophageal injuries should be reassessed. An esophagram or an esophagoscopy should be performed. A contrast esophagram will depict the functioning of the esophagus while the esophagoscopy will give the physician a visual image of the healing process.

If stricture formation has begun, dilation and bougienage should be started. The success of these techniques relates in part to the severity of the stricture and the presence of any esophageal lumen. Some physicians recommend the insertion of a nasogastric tube in order to maintain a lumen that can be dilated later. The efficacy and safety of this procedure remains unclear and is not recommended. Patients who develop stricture with lye may have an increased risk of developing esophageal carcinoma. Patients who do not respond to dilation or who develop a complete obliteration of their esophageal lumen may need a colon interposition.

PREVENTION

Prevention of caustic ingestions remains the best way to avoid serious sequellae in children. Corrosive materials should be kept out of the reach of children in locked cabinets and in their original containers with child-resistant closures. Furthermore, physicians should provide parents with adequate anticipatory guidance so that they may provide a safe environment for their children.

ANNOTATED BIBLIOGRAPHY

Appelqvist P, Salmo M: Lye corrosion carcinoma of the esophagus. A review of 63 cases. Cancer 45:2655, 1980 (Good study evaluating the risk of developing an esophageal carcinoma following a lye stricture.)

Crain EF, Gershel JC, Mezey AP: Caustic ingestions. Symptoms as predictors of esophageal injury. Am J Dis Child 138:863, 1984 (Good study evaluating symptoms as predictors of esophageal lesions.)

Friedman EM, Lovejoy FH Jr: The emergency management of caustic ingestions. Emerg Med Clin North Am 2(1):77, 1984 (Good review of the subject.)

Gaudreault P, Parent M, McGuigan MA et al: Predictability of esophageal injury from signs and symptoms. A study of caustic ingestion in 378 children. Pediatrics 71:767, 1983 (Study on signs or symptoms as predictors of esophageal injuries.)

Hawking DB, Demeter MJ, Barnett TE: Caustic ingestion: Controversies in management. Laryngoscope 90:98, 1980 (Very good article on the treatment of caustic ingestions.)

Wasserman RL, Ginsburg CM: Caustic substance injuries. J Pediatr 107:169, 1985 (Very good review of the subject.)

175
Food Poisoning
MILTON TENENBEIN

The patient or his caretaker often wonders if it was something that the patient ate recently that was responsible for an acute onset of illness. Indeed, the recognition of food as a vector of illness and disease is a basic requirement for human survival. Safe foods and preparation practices have been learned through the process of trial and error. These include sanitation and food preservation through the processes of heating, freezing, fermentation, and treatment with chemical additives.

Food poisoning can be considered as an acute onset of illness caused by the consumption of a particular food. This concept of food-induced illness, however, is too broad because it includes the abdominal pain and diarrhea following the consumption of a glass of milk by an individual with lactase deficiency. It is better to think of *foodborne disease*, recognizing that the food is a vector for the agent responsible for the symptoms and that the presence of the agent (the poison) is unexpected. This excludes naturally toxic "foods" such as poisonous plants, mushrooms, fish, and shellfish.

It is generally agreed that foodborne disease is common but underreported. The agent may be biologic (*e.g.*, bacteria, viruses) or chemical (*e.g.*, heavy metals, pesticides). One epidemiologic survey reported that 24% of outbreaks of foodborne disease are caused by chemical agents. The food may become toxic prior to, during, or after its processing. Most cases (70% in one series), however, are caused by errors in food-handling practices, either in restaurants or in homes. In the same series, only 3% of the total outbreaks were accounted for by commercial food processing establishments. An overview of the clinical features of food poisonings from multiple organisms is presented in Table 175-1. For food poisoning due to chemical agents, the clinical features are dependent on the toxin that has contaminated the food.

CLINICAL PRESENTATION

The patient with a foodborne illness usually presents with an acute onset of gastrointestinal illness. The most common symptoms are abdominal pain, nausea, vomiting, and diarrhea. Fever may be present if there is an infectious etiology. Depending on the responsible agent, alternative presentations may include neurologic symptoms such as headache, paresthesias, weakness, and paralysis.

DIFFERENTIAL DIAGNOSIS

The most common clinical presentation of food poisoning is an acute onset of gastrointestinal symptoms including abdominal pain, nausea, vomiting, and diarrhea. The differential diagnosis of this presentation is reviewed in Chapter 104. Whether or not these symptoms are a result of foodborne disease, they are usually due to a microbiologic agent. Although the management of the patient with gastrointestinal illness is usually the same regardless of whether the etiology is due to a primary gastrointestinal infection or an infection acquired from food, there are specific preventive and public health concerns that make this distinction important.

WORK-UP

History

If the patient or the caretaker is concerned that the illness is associated with food, it is important to inquire regarding the presence of symptoms in others who have eaten the same foods. If it is the physician who is considering food poisoning as the cause of an illness, he should inquire if any unusual, esoteric, or tainted foods have recently been eaten. He should also determine if the patient has recently broken his normal routine and eaten a meal, for

Table 175-1. Food Poisoning: Differential Diagnosis of Gastrointestinal Presentation

ORGANISM	PATHOGENESIS	INCUBATION PERIOD	SYMPTOMS	FOODS
Staphylococci	Ingestion of enterotoxin	1–6 hours	Nausea, vomiting, diarrhea, abdominal cramps; no fever; several hours' duration	Cream-filled desserts, cold meats, salads
Clostridium perfringens	Formation of enterotoxin in vivo	8–12 hours	Watery diarrhea and abdominal cramps; fever and vomiting are uncommon; several hours' duration	Cooked meats
Bacillus cereus I	Ingestion of enterotoxin	1–6 hours	Nausea, vomiting, diarrhea, and abdominal cramps; no fever; less than 24 hours' duration	Rice, starches, vegetables, meats
Bacillus cereus II	Formation of enterotoxin in vivo	8–12 hours	Watery diarrhea and abdominal cramps; no fever; less than 24 hours' duration	Rice, starches, vegetables, meats
Shigellae	Bacterial invasion of colonic mucosa	24–96 hours	Diarrhea (often bloody), abdominal pain, and fever; dehydration, meningismus, and seizures can develop	Water supply
Salmonellae	Bacterial invasion of intestinal mucosa	12–48 hours	Diarrhea (may be bloody); nausea, vomiting, and abdominal pain less common; fever; up to 5 days' duration	Poultry, egg products, water
Vibrio	Uncertain	12–24 hours	Explosive diarrhea; occasionally cramps, nausea, and vomiting; ~3 days' duration	Seafood
Campylobacter	Bacterial invasion of intestinal mucosa	48–120 hours	Diarrhea (may be bloody), abdominal pain, and fever; vomiting uncommon; several days' duration	Water supply

example, at a school picnic or on a camping trip. Preparation of food in advance, improper storage and inadequate cooking, cooling, and reheating are the most common factors contributing to food poisoning. The interval between food consumption and onset of symptoms is important. Rapid onset (within a few hours) supports the ingestion of a bacterial toxin or chemical food poisoning. Later onset (many hours to a few days) is consistent with an enteric infection.

Physical Examination

The patient with a gastrointestinal presentation should be assessed for dehydration. The remainder of the physical examination usually contributes little except in the patient with botulism.

Laboratory Tests

A complete blood count, serum electrolytes, creatinine, and BUN may be necessary depending on the clinical severity. Samples of vomitus and stool for culturing and toxin analysis should be taken. This often requires the involvement of the local public health agency. Any suspected food should be submitted for testing.

MANAGEMENT

Clinical management of foodborne illness is dependent on its etiology, which can be divided into bacterial and chemical agents.

Bacterial Food Poisoning

Food poisoning caused by bacteria is due to an infection by the agent or to the effects of a toxin elaborated by the agent. The clinical features of the various bacterial food poisonings presenting with gastrointestinal symptoms are described in Table 175-1. Botulism, a neurologic disease, is discussed separately.

Staphylococci, C. perfringens, and *Salmonellae* are the most common causes of food poisonings. The gastrointestinal food poisoning syndromes due to toxins (*Staphylococci, C. perfringens*, and *B. cereus*) usually do not last a long time and thus require no specific therapy. Dehydration is uncommon, as is the need for hospitalization. Those syndromes due to direct invasion of gastrointestinal mucosa (*Shigellae, Salmonellae*, and *Campylobacter*) have longer courses and symptoms can be more severe. Dehydration may result, especially in in-

fants. Hospitalization, therefore, may be required for intravenous therapy. Those with moderate to severe illness due to *Shigellae* or *Campylobacter* should also receive antibiotics (either ampicillin or trimethoprim–sulfamethoxazole for the former and erythromycin for the latter).

Botulism

The toxin of *Clostridium botulinum* is the most toxic substance known to man. It is elaborated under anaerobic conditions at a pH greater than 4.5. Ingestion of the preformed toxin produces botulism (except for infant botulism). This consists of anticholinergic symptoms since the toxin irreversibly binds to the peripheral neuromuscular junction blocking transmission by preventing acetylcholine release. Initially there may be some gastrointestinal symptoms such as nausea, vomiting, and abdominal pain. Neurologic symptoms and signs develop within several hours to a few days. Cranial nerve involvement appears early. Thus, patients may present with dry mouth, diplopia, dysarthria, dysphagia, and third- and sixth-nerve palsies. The severity of ocular symptoms may be of prognostic value. Systemic skeletal muscle paralysis follows cranial nerve involvement with death being due to respiratory failure.

The differential diagnosis is large and may include myasthenia gravis, Guillain–Barré syndrome, tick paralysis, poisonings (*e.g.*, carbon monoxide, atropine, organophosphate insecticides, and soluble barium salts), and trichinosis. Most cases of botulism are caused by foods canned at home.

Botulism should be suspected in any patient with a recent onset of cranial nerve palsies and a history of eating home-canned foods. Confirmation of the diagnosis requires a demonstration of the organism or toxin in the food, vomitus, or stool. Serum can be tested for toxin. All of these tests take time and a specific therapy should be instituted if there are reasonable clinical grounds to suspect the diagnosis. This involves the administration of specific trivalent antitoxin. Mechanical ventilation may be required if respiratory failure develops. Penicillin therapy is not indicated because botulism is an intoxication and not an infection. Guanidine therapy is controversial.

Infant botulism differs from classical botulism in that the toxin is elaborated from organisms growing within the gastrointestinal tract. This entity is limited to infants from 3 to 26 weeks of age. They present with constipation followed by lethargy, weakness, and poor feeding. Generalized weakness and hypotonia ensue, which can be followed by respiratory failure. Diagnosis can be confirmed by a demonstration of organisms or toxin in the stool. Serum is negative for the toxin. The treatment consists of meticulous respiratory and nutritional support. The roles for antitoxin, penicillin, and guanidine are unclear. Honey is implicated as a source of *C. botulinum* organisms and it should not be fed to infants less than 1 year of age.

Chemical Food Poisoning

There are many reports of foodborne illness due to chemicals. Examples include insecticide poisoning from cucumbers, tin poisoning from tomato juice, solanine poisoning from potatoes, and methemoglobinemia from meats. Food poisoning due to chemicals is characterized by the rapid onset of symptoms (within 1 to 2 hours) and multiple victims. Cases of food poisoning involving a single victim are usually not recognized as such. The chemical may contaminate the food during the production, processing, distribution, or preparation. The management of cases depends on the specific toxin and the degree of illness.

PUBLIC HEALTH CONCERNS

When faced with a single case of acute gastrointestinal illness, food poisoning is difficult to confirm. When the history identifies multiple victims, the pediatrician should ensure that implicated foods are saved and he should initiate specimen collection (vomitus, stool). The local public health authority should be notified in order that these samples and specimens can be tested. They will investigate the

situation with the goal of prevention of additional cases and the correction of improper food-handling practices.

ANNOTATED BIBLIOGRAPHY

Brown LW: Commentary: Infant botulism and the honey connection. J Pediatr 94:337–338, 1979 (Honey as a risk factor for infant botulism and a recommendation not to feed it to infants.)

Donadio JA, Gangarosa EJ, Faich GA: Diagnosis and treatment of botulism. J Infect Dis 124:108–112, 1971 (Review of classical botulism with a good discussion on its differential diagnosis.)

Grady GF, Keusch GT: Pathogenesis of bacterial diarrheas. N Engl J Med 285:831–841; 891–900, 1971 (Good general review of the clinical features of bacterial diarrheas.)

Hughes JM, Merson MH: Fish and shellfish poisoning. N Engl J Med 295:1117–1120, 1976 (Good general review of poisoning due to toxic fish and shellfish.)

Johnson RO, Clay SA, Arnon SS: Diagnosis and management of infant botulism. Am J Dis Child 133:586–593, 1979 (General review of infant botulism and its management.)

Roberts D: Factors contributing to outbreaks of food poisoning in England and Wales 1970–1979. J Hyg Camb 89:491–498, 1982 (Analysis of those factors contributing to food poisoning.)

Sours HE, Smith DG: Outbreaks of foodborne disease in the United States, 1972–1978. J Infect Dis 142:122–125, 1980 (Review of the epidemiology of food poisoning.)

Terranova W, Palumbo JN, Breman JC: Ocular findings in botulism type B. JAMA 241:475–477, 1979 (Relates the ocular findings in classic botulism to the patient's prognosis.)

176
Alcohol Intoxication
STEVEN M. MARCUS

Calls to poison centers across the United States for exposure to alcohol represent ~ 5% of the total call volume. The source of the ingested alcohol varies widely and includes alcoholic beverages, mouth washes, cosmetics, solvents, breath deodorants, record cleaners, windshield-wiper fluid, and even innocent-appearing "glo-sticks." Most of the accidental ingestions produce few, if any, symptoms. The potential, however, for serious toxicity from

alcohol-containing products varies greatly and depends on the nature of the offending alcohol and the dose ingested. The dose ingested is, in turn, related to the mixture involved, the taste, and the age of the patient.

Patients ingesting alcohol-containing products range in age from infancy up. The cause of the ingestion ranges from accidental ingestion in a child to intentional suicidal ingestion in the adolescent age group. In intentional or suicidal ingestions, alcohol is frequently the second or third substance ingested rather than the primary one.

All alcohols depress the central nervous system (CNS) function; they all cause stupor, coma, and, in excessive quantities, even death. Death may occur from respiratory depression or the direct toxic effect on the neuron. Many of the effects of alcohol occur outside the CNS and can produce serious morbidity and mortality.

Alcohol is absorbed rapidly from the gastrointestinal tract. Absorption begins in the mouth and may be delayed by food present in the stomach or by high concentrations of consumed alcohol. Peak blood levels after ingestion are achieved within 20 minutes on an empty stomach. Alcohols diffuse rapidly throughout the body and, because of their solubility in water, they distribute throughout total body water.

The CNS effects of alcohol frequently appear more rapidly than elevations in venous blood alcohol determinations. Arterial concentrations of alcohol rise more rapidly than venous concentrations and, hence, result in the rapid onset of lightheadedness and stupor after the ingestion of alcohol. Alcohols are metabolized in the liver by alcohol dehydrogenase. The elimination of ethanol by the kidneys, lungs, and sweat glands represents only 2% to 5% of the total ingested dose. The rate of alcohol oxidation by alcohol dehydrogenase is relatively constant at 100 mg/kg/hr of the index alcohol. This represents a mean of 16 mg/dl/hr when expressed as a decline in blood alcohol concentrations.

Since all alcohols are osmotically active, significant overdoses may predispose to a hyperosmolar state. This fact can also be used to approximate blood alcohol concentrations if levels are unavailable. A blood ethanol concentration of 100 mg/dl increases the serum osmolality by ~ 22 mosmol/L. Alcohol intoxication is unlikely if osmolality is only slightly increased or normal.

ETHANOL

Ethanol is the index alcohol for discussion. Ethanol, which is contained in beverages, mouthwashes, cosmetics, pharmaceuticals, elixirs, solvents, in some brands of medicinal rubbing alcohol, and in cooking products such as vanilla extract, is found in almost every household in the United States.

Experimental data suggest that most individuals with blood ethanol levels over 100 mg/dl will show signs of inebriation. As a "rule of thumb," 1 ml/kg of *absolute* ethanol results in blood alcohol levels above this value. Many individuals, however, particularly small children, will begin to show signs of insobriety, particularly stupor and even coma, at considerably lower levels.

The most common source of alcohol exposure is alcoholic beverages. Concentrations of ethanol in alcoholic beverages are reported in *proof*, which expresses approximately double the alcohol concentration in percent *volume*. Thus, a beverage that contains 80 proof contains 40% alcohol by volume. Since ethanol is less dense than water, the quantity of alcohol in weight is slightly less than the volume.

Pathophysiology

Reports of hypoglycemia leading to convulsions, brain damage, and death have been reported as serious complications of acute ethanol ingestions in small children. The hypoglycemic effect of ethanol appears to be related to the impairment of gluconeogenesis related to an increased NADH/NAD ratio.

Some patients with ethanol overdose have a mild to moderate metabolic acidosis, which appears to be a true lactic acidemia secondary to the metabolism of the ethanol, the enhanced release of free fatty acids, and the accumulation of acetone and β-hydroxybuterate. Vasodilatation and depression of the cardiovascular centers of the brain may lead to pooling of blood in the periphery and an increased heat loss with subsequent hypothermia.

Ethanol is a competitor of antidiuretic hormone (ADH). Acute intoxications have produced a diabetes insipidus-like syndrome with excessive fluid losses. The metabolism of ethanol also requires 7 molecules of water for every molecule of ethanol metabolized. These fluid losses, when combined, can represent substantial fluid shifts and can produce serious dehydration (Table 176-1). Aside from symptomatic treatment, especially of hypoglycemia, no specific therapy is available. The recommendations for the severely intoxicated patient are

1. Protect the patient's airway. If the patient is not breathing, tracheal intubation should be provided to facilitate respiratory support.
2. Provide intravenous fluids to counteract any dehydration and give sufficient fluids to prevent dehydration.
3. Administer dextrose intravenously if the patient is hypoglycemic.
4. Treat by aggressive use of fluid and bicarbonate if metabolic acidosis is present.

Table 176-1. Ethanol Intoxication

BLOOD ETHANOL LEVEL	CLINICAL SYNDROME
40–50 mg/dl	Inebriation, excessive laughter, hyperactivity or lethargy, slurred speech, blurred sensory input, relaxed inhibitors
100 mg/dl	Considered as presumptive evidence of impairment in most states
200 mg/dl	Marked muscular incoordination, blurred vision, stupor
300 mg/dl	Profound lethargy or stupor, hypoglycemia common, hypothermia not uncommon
500 mg/dl	Coma, depressed vital signs— potentially fatal

5. Induction of emesis is rarely indicated. Absorption of alcohol is generally completed by the time the patient is seen.
6. Activated charcoal fails to bind significant amounts of ethanol and, therefore, is of little use.
7. Consider hemodialysis with potentially lethal concentrations of ethanol.

METHANOL

Methyl alcohol, wood alcohol, acetone alcohol, or Manhattan spirit is a well-known substance that is used frequently as an industrial solvent, antifreeze, and fuel. Common sources of methanol exposure in children are windshield-wiper fluid and phonographic record-cleaning fluid.

Methanol intoxication can present with significant CNS effects similar to ethanol. The more serious effects of methanol, however, are extraneurologic.

Oxidation, like that of ethanol, proceeds in the liver by way of the enzyme alcohol dehydrogenase. In the case of methanol, the metabolite formic acid is considerably more toxic than the metabolite of ethanol, acetaldehyde. Symptoms of methanol poisoning may be delayed for a long time due to the delay in metabolic production of the toxic product. Once the latent period is over, characteristic findings include a significant metabolic acidosis with swelling, edema, and redness of the retina and optic disc.

The early period of insobriety or inebriation is followed characteristically by an asymptomatic latent period. The characteristic symptoms and signs may appear between 6 and 30 hours after the ingestion. These signs consist of vertigo, vomiting, abdominal pain, diarrhea, back pain, shortness of breath, motor restlessness, blurring of vision, and hyperemia of the optic disc. The visual disturbance may proceed to optic atrophy, and pupillary light reflexes may be diminished or absent.

Data suggest that the prognosis in methanol overdose is more closely related to the delay in onset of therapy and to the presence of acidosis than to the concentration of methanol. The treatment of methanol intoxication depends on the preferential metabolism of ethanol by alcohol dehydrogenase. The administration of ethanol depresses the rate of oxidation of methanol and, hence, delays or prevents its metabolism to formic acid, blocking its biochemical and clinical effects.

Methanol is excreted only to a small extent by the lung, the sweat glands, and the kidneys. Treatment with hemodialysis is recommended if evidence of toxicity from methanol exists, or with significant elevations in methanol concentration. The following protocol is suggested:

1. If a significant methanol ingestion is suspected, a blood determination of methanol concentration, electrolytes, and blood gases should be obtained. A measurement of serum osmolality and comparison with a calculated osmolality can be used to estimate the concentration of methanol in the blood if a blood methanol level cannot be obtained.
2. Attention to the airway and to the circulatory volume is essential. Correction of any acidosis with bicarbonate is imperative.
3. Administration of ethanol in all cases of significant methanol intoxication to achieve and maintain a blood ethanol concentration of 100 mg/dl. Once the concentration of methanol is available, a decision can be made regarding whether it is reasonable to remove the methanol by hemodialysis. It is generally accepted that when blood methanol levels are greater than 50 mg/dl, hemodialysis should be considered.

ISOPROPYL ALCOHOL

Isopropyl alcohol is found widely in the home and in industry, both as a solvent and as *rubbing alcohol* or as a sterilizing agent.

In the home, isopropyl alcohol is found in small quantities in various skin lotions, hair tonic, some aftershave lotions, window-cleaning solutions, and household detergents. Isopropyl alcohol is most commonly encountered in 70% solution, intended for use as rubbing alcohol. Not all solutions labeled as rubbing alcohol will contain isopropyl alcohol, because some will contain *denatured* ethanol rather than isopropyl alcohol. Most of the preparations of rubbing alcohol are packaged in pint containers without child-resistant packaging or child-resistant caps.

Isopropyl alcohol appears to be more toxic than ethyl alcohol, but significantly less toxic than methanol. On a molar basis, it is about twice as potent as ethanol in producing insobriety. Isopropyl alcohol is absorbed rapidly and completely. In addition to rapid absorption through the gastrointestinal tract, it is absorbed rapidly by inhalation. Isopropyl alcohol appears to be metabolized at a slower rate than ethanol.

The use of isopropyl alcohol in water to lower fever in children has been reported to cause stupor and even coma secondary to the absorption of isopropyl alcohol both from inhalation and transdermal absorption. It is thought, however, that the inhalation route is the more important route of absorption. The metabolism of isopropyl alcohol produces relatively large quantities of acetone without the production of appreciable quantities of acetoacetate, acetoacetic acid, or β-hydroxybutyric acid and, thus, the diagnosis of isopropyl alcohol ingestion is made frequently on the basis of the presence of nonacidotic ketosis.

The ingestion of isopropyl alcohol frequently produces gastritis with vomiting and occasional hematemesis. Most emesis occurs early and is thought to be a local reaction. Systemic symptoms, such as stupor and insobriety, frequently occur within 30 minutes of ingestion.

Treatment

As with most ingested alcohol, absorption occurs so rapidly that gastric lavage or gastric emptying may not be efficacious. However, since isopropyl alcohol is frequently ingested in concentrated form and since high concentrations of alcohol lower the rate of absorption of alcohol, gastric emptying may remove significant quantities of isopropyl alcohol.

BENZYL ALCOHOL

The presence of benzyl alcohol as a preservative in many intravenous (IV) fluids leads to a syndrome of *gasping* in neonates. This appears to occur from the metabolism of benzyl alcohol by way of oxidation to benzoic acid and hippuric acid. In prematures with relatively low renal clearances, this leads to an accumulation of these compounds in the serum. Following the reports of illness in several infants in whom solutions of benzyl alcohol were used, a warning was released by the Food and Drug Administration alerting clinicians to the dangers from exposure in infancy. Careful attention must be paid to the possibility that IV medications and heparin may contain benzyl alcohol if used in small infants or in patients with inadequate renal function.

ETHYLENE GLYCOL

Ethylene glycol is commonly found in permanent antifreeze and is available in many homes. In addition to its widespread use, it is frequently packaged as an attractive, colorful but odorless liquid. The liquid has a pleasant, warm, sweet taste; thus, ingestions are frequently in substantial quantities. Although it has a low toxicity, ethylene glycol is metabolized by alcohol dehydrogenase to oxalic acid and this metabolite may cause cardiac and renal toxicity as well as significant and sometimes profound acidosis.

On presentation, the patient may appear to be inebriated as with all alcohols, although in this ingestion the absence of an alcoholic breath is characteristic. As in methanol overdose, there may be a time lag of several hours between the ingestion and the onset of toxicity due to the formation of a toxic metabolite. Many patients experience nausea, vomiting, and hematemesis; however, the major effects are those in the CNS, with the patient frequently presenting in coma. As with methanol, there may be a latent period when the patient appears to be getting better followed by progressive acidosis, flank pain, and oliguric acute renal failure.

Ethylene glycol poisoning must be suspected in patients who appear inebriated but who have no smell of alcohol on their breath. With a history of ingestion of some form of antifreeze, ethylene glycol should be the primary consideration. The presence of oxalate crystals in the urine supports the diagnosis of ethylene glycol intoxication. The finding of an elevated measured serum osmolality lends further support to the diagnosis of ethylene glycol intoxication.

Once the presumptive diagnosis of ethylene glycol intoxication is made, the further conversion of ethylene glycol must be blocked through the administration of ethyl alcohol. Hemodialysis or hemoperfusion may be necessary to remove the un-metabolized ethylene glycol.

ANNOTATED BIBLIOGRAPHY

Gershanik J, Boecler B, Ensley H et al: The gasping syndrome and benzyl alcohol poisoning. N Engl J Med 307:1384–1388, 1982 (Describes the experience with 10 neonates and discusses the metabolism of benzyl alcohol.)

McCoy HG, Cipolle RJ, Ehlers SM et al: Severe methanol poisoning: Application of a pharmacokinetic model for ethanol therapy and hemodialysis. Am J Med 67:804–807, 1979 (Two case reports, with a general discussion and literature review.)

Moss MH: Alcohol-induced hypoglycemia in coma caused by alcohol sponging. Pediatrics 4:445–446, 1970 (Report of alcohol intoxication secondary to the absorption of inhaled ethyl or isopropyl alcohol vapor during sponge bathing.)

Ricci L, Hoffman S: Ethanol induced hypoglycemic coma in a child. Ann Emerg Med 11:202–204, 1982 (Case report of ethanol-induced hypoglycemic coma in a small child after an accidental ingestion of ethanol with a nice review.)

Smithline N, Gardner KD: Gaps—anionic and osmolal. JAMA 236:1594–1597, 1976 (Discussion of anionic and osmolar gaps with clinical implications.)

Stokes JB, Aueron F: Prevention of organ damage in massive ethylene glycol ingestion. JAMA 243:2065–2066, 1980 (Case report of massive ethylene glycol poisoning and brief discussion of therapy.)

177
Street Drugs

MICHAEL A. MCGUIGAN

Street drugs are defined as those psychoactive chemicals that can be purchased without medical authorization from a nonlicensed dispenser for the purpose of sensory alteration. Street drugs, therefore, may be legal as well as illicit drugs or chemicals. Drugs that are commonly used illicitly include cannabis (marijuana, hashish), hallucinogens (LSD, PCP, peyote, mescaline), depressants (barbiturates, benzodiazepines, and other hypnotic-sedative medications), stimulants (amphetamines, cocaine, phenylpropanolamine), opiates (*e.g.*, heroin), and inhalants (gasoline, glues, trichlorethane, and other solvents). Legal drugs that are widely used by young people are ethanol and tobacco.

Many studies have established the use, prevalence, and demographics of young drug users. Because the drug-use epidemic may well be a series of overlapping miniepidemics, one can anticipate that both the drugs and their popularity will vary with geography, time, and the age of the population studied.

Although recent surveys have documented an apparent stabilization or even decrease in drug-use prevalence among children, there is still cause for concern. Ethanol is still widely consumed (41% of adolescents had five or more drinks in the 2 weeks prior to a 1983 survey) and more than one third of nonproblem adolescent drinkers became problem drinkers in adulthood. Thus, not only is drug use a contemporary concern, but the pediatrician has also a responsibility for practicing preventative medicine.

The discussion in this chapter has two goals. The first is to provide guidelines to help the practicing pediatrician identify and treat children with drug-related problems. The second is to provide an overview of the syndromes of acute overdose with cannabis products and with cocaine.

Pathophysiology

The child, adolescent, or teenager begins to use legal drugs (ethanol or tobacco) in an experimental or recreational way. Street drugs may be encountered as early as the late elementary school grades. Peer pressure and a desire to be accepted may be contributing causal factors in the initiation of drug use. One of the strongest influences on a child's decision to use marijuana is that he has a friend who uses it. Other factors that influence young (adolescent) children to try marijuana include prior unapproved use of ethanol or cigarettes. Parental influence appears to be important for the initiation of ethanol use and the use of illicit drugs other than marijuana. It must be stressed, however, that the use of "legal drugs" (ethanol, tobacco) does *not* mean that the child *will* progress to the use of illicit drugs. The converse is also true: a certain number of teenagers will initiate marijuana use without prior use of either ethanol or tobacco.

The pleasure and excitement derived from "recreational'' use may reinforce further use of the drug. A progression in drug use and a predisposition to dependence is recognized when the frequency of use increases, when the use of drugs interferes with normal daily activities, or when the drug is used for the purpose of dealing with stress.

As drug dependence becomes established, school, social, and family situations deteriorate. Depression and suicidal thoughts may be manifest. Full dependency on drugs occurs when the adolescent no longer uses drugs for their pleasurable effects but uses them to maintain a feeling of normalcy. By this stage, the victim's social environment has deteriorated and the physical health of the individual may be declining.

Clinical Presentation

The adolescent drug user may present to the pediatrician in several ways. The child may come forward spontaneously or on questioning with an admission of drug use. Indirect clues to the diagnosis of drug use may include a deterioration in family life or functional or behavioral problems in a younger sibling. Social problems consistent with, but by no means diagnostic of, drug use include deteriorating school or athletic performance, truancy, and law breaking. The difficulty in coping that many of these children have may lead to suicide gestures. Adolescents who have drug problems may also present to the hospital emergency room with trauma or overdose.

Not infrequently, the pediatrician may examine young drug users for drug-use-related ''functional'' complaints such as fatigue, sore throat, cough, chest or abdominal pain, or headache. In any adolescent or teenager with these complaints, a contributing diagnosis of drug use should be considered.

The complications of chronic drug abuse are more commonly seen in adult populations but may also be found in older teenagers. Some of these problems are hepatitis, streptococcal arthritis, anorexia, weight loss, bacterial endocarditis, osteomyelitis, fever, convulsions, and renal disorders.

Differential Diagnosis

None of the clinical presentations are pathognomonic for drug use. Because drug-related medical problems have protean manifestations, it should be considered in the differential diagnosis of each specific complaint or presenting symptom or sign.

Work-Up

Once it has been established that an adolescent is using drugs, the pediatrician must identify the drug(s) and assess the extent of use. An inquiry into the adolescent's drug history may follow general questions about drug use at school or social functions. Areas to explore are the settings in which the drugs are used and the amount of disruption in social, academic, athletic, or work-related life that can be attributed to the drugs. It is also important to try to identify the perceived benefits from using drugs. During this assessment phase, it is necessary to establish certain drug-related facts, such as which drugs, how much of each drug, and how often the drugs are used.

If the answers to direct questions appear misleading or the patient is uncooperative, the extent or degree of drug involvement may need to be established indirectly from the history of behavior. The pediatrician may have to seek information from the parents and the school representatives to obtain a history about an uncooperative child. Parents may be able to give a history of cigarette smoking, argumentative behavior, refusal to accept responsibility, irritability, and mood swings. Asking the parents about their child's friends may elicit negative feelings. The parents themselves may be feeling stress at their child's drug use and this stress may be manifested as insomnia, short-temper, or altered sexual performance. Interviews with school representatives may reveal a deteriorating school performance such as declining grades, truancy, drowsiness in class, poor memory, lack of motivation, or the need for special classes. A review of the patient's past medical history is important and may reveal numerous functional complaints, involvement with a child psychiatrist or psychologist, or that the child has been and still is developmentally immature.

A physical examination is less likely to be revealing. There may be a recent weight loss or other evidence of the complications of drug abuse.

Laboratory identification of the drug(s) in question in blood or urine is likely to be unrewarding. A sophisticated analytical laboratory is required and, even then, the chemical assays are not reliable for some of the substances in question. Furthermore, many of the drugs used are eliminated rapidly from the body so that the analysis may be negative even in the face of regular use. Cannabis is relatively unique in that tetrahydrocannabinol, the active ingredient, is stored in the body for long periods of time, and metabolites may be detected in the urine for 1 to 2 weeks after use.

Treatment

Prevention may be the most important aspect of treatment. Although the use of any street drug should not be condoned, there is evidence that the younger the child is at the age of initiation, the greater the risk of progression in use and the subsequent development of serious drug problems. It may be sufficient only to postpone the initial illicit drug exposure until late adolescence to prevent significant drug dependency.

Once street drug use is identified, the pediatrician has the obligation to intervene therapeutically. Even for a cooperative child, clear-cut, detailed, and successful therapeutic approaches have not been established for the management of adolescent drug users, although certain general guidelines can be formulated. The therapeutic approach chosen will depend on the perceived severity of the drug use and the availability of resources.

In the early stages, before dependency and deterioration have occurred, physician-guided parental intervention may be successful. Lacking capable parents, a surrogate (social worker, counsellor, teacher, athletic coach, or physician) may be effective. The emphasis at this stage is on educating the child and the parents regarding the adverse, and perhaps unappreciated, aspects of drug use. It is also necessary to help the parents and child build the child's self-image and to teach social and communication skills. These aspects may help the child to resist the pressure to use drugs that come from his social environment. The clear relationship between drug use and automobile accidents must also be discussed.

Other approaches to the therapy of adolescent drug users include keeping daily records, self-assessment of leisure activity, and routine drug screening. Daily records should include the number, the time, and the activity associated with drug cravings, drug refusals, and drug uses. It is important that the patient learn to identify the triggers or stimuli for his drug use. Special emphasis may be put on the methods that the patient used to refuse drug use at any time. The adolescent who uses drugs generally has a problem in using free or leisure time constructively. Time needs to be spent in evaluating how unstructured time is spent, the degree to which drugs are used during these periods, and how and to what extent drug use is acting as a barrier to doing what he wants. Daily urine samples should be collected. The treatment period must be drug-free. Although spontaneous confessions of drug use should be encouraged, the requirement of a daily urine sample for drug analysis will help the adolescent achieve and maintain a drug-free state. Of course, not every sample needs to be analysed.

More severely affected children may require more aggressive therapy and the pediatrician should be aware of the local facilities available for treatment purposes. Outpatient or ambulatory care services such as social services, peer counseling groups, psychiatry, or adolescent medicine may be useful. In-patient drug treatment facilities for adolescents may be unavailable. The adolescent who requires hospitalization for drug use will usually end up in a general pediatric ward or in an adolescent medicine or psychiatric unit. The ultimate goals of therapy are to change or dampen the stimuli for drug use, to establish alternate methods for achieving the rewards that drugs provided, and to change the adolescent's peer group.

Because there is no clearly successful approach to treating adolescent drug abusers, the pediatrician must constantly monitor the effectiveness of whatever treatment program is started. Relapses are common. Treatment must be individualized and the physician must consider both the child and his family.

Indications for Admission or Referral

In-patient therapy or referral to a tertiary care specialty center may be necessary if ambulatory care is unsuccessful or cannot be followed. Adult treatment centers usually do not accept adolescents and young teenagers and would not be appropriate for these patients. Unfortunately, many pediatric medical centers are not equipped for treating such patients.

CANNABIS

Cannabis generally refers to the active substances (primarily $\triangle$-9-tetrahydrocannabinol or THC) that come from the plant *Cannabis sativa*. Marijuana refers to the flowering tops and leaves of the *Cannabis sativa* plant and is 1% to 3% THC. Sensimilla is the seedless unpollenated flowering tops of the female plant and has a higher concentration of THC (3% to 5%). Hashish, the crude resin from the plant may range in THC content from 2% to 15%. Hash oil is a dark viscous liquid extracted from the flowering tops of the plant; it contains up to 22% THC.

Pathophysiology

The mechanism of action of THC is unknown. The psychotomimetic and physiologic effects are related to the amount of drug absorbed and the experience of the user. The potentially lethal dose of THC is in the range of 30 mg/kg.

Clinical Presentation

Patients who suffer from an acute overdose of THC demonstrate a nonspecific syndrome. Conjunctival hyperemia is common. Tachycardia and mild hypertension or postural hypotension may be noted. Skeletal muscle jerking and a fine tremor may occur but convulsions are a risk only in individuals who have a pre-existing convulsive disorder. Occasionally, a patient will demonstrate a panic reaction or rapid extreme swings in mood. The most common features of acute overdose are euphoria and central nervous system depression, poor coordination, ataxia, slurred speech, lethargy, and stupor. Frank coma and respiratory depression do not occur unless other drugs have also been ingested. Significant symptoms and signs usually last for no longer than 6 to 12 hours.

Treatment

Most serious acute overdoses are due to the ingestion of THC, thus the administration of activated charcoal orally or by nasogastric tube is recommended. Most patients will do well with just quiet observation in a normally lighted room. Panic reactions that do not respond to nonpharmacologic care may be treated with small doses of a short-acting benzodiazepine.

Indications for Admission or Referral

Significantly symptomatic patients may need short-term observation in hospital. Infants or small children who inadvertently ingest THC should be hospitalized if any symptoms or signs develop within 2 hours. It is unlikely that a patient with an acute overdose of THC will require a transfer to a referral center.

COCAINE

Cocaine is a white, crystalline, water-soluble powder obtained from the leaves of the plant *Erythroxylan coca*; as yet, there is no "synthetic" cocaine. A major concern about illicit cocaine is its purity. Most street samples contain other chemicals including, but not limited to, sugars, local anesthetics, caffeine, amphetamines, and phenylpropanolamine.

Pathophysiology

Cocaine is absorbed from all routes. Peak blood levels occur 30 to 60 minutes after intranasal application. The half-life of the drug in the plasma is in the range of 20 to 90 minutes. The pertinent pharmacologic effects are on the central nervous system where cocaine interferes with the neurotransmitters, producing first stimulation and then depression of function. Peripherally, cocaine stimulates the sympathetic nervous system.

Clinical Presentation

The development of symptoms of cocaine intoxication is rapid. Symptoms and signs begin within 5 to 10 minutes. They reach a maximum within 30 minutes, and they may last for another 30 minutes. In a case of extreme overdose, the time between the onset of symptoms and the development of coma may be only a few minutes. Central nervous system abnormalities include excitement, euphoria, confusion, and apprehension. Mydriasis, hyperpyrexia, nausea, and vomiting may occur. Hyperreflexia and convulsions may give way to muscular paralysis, areflexia, and coma. Cardiovascular effects include tachycardia and hypertension. The respiratory rate and depth may be increased. Death has been reported from cardiovascular collapse, convulsions, or respiratory insufficiency.

Differential Diagnosis

The syndrome produced by acute cocaine overdose is similar to bacterial or viral meningitis/encephalitis, or poisoning with salicylates, antihistamines, amphetamines, or phenylpropanolamine.

Work-Up

The minimum toxic dose of cocaine has not been established. Even if it were, an accurate application to the impure cocaine bought illicitly would be impossible. Exposure to any amount should be considered as potentially serious. Because cocaine is absorbed from any mucous membrane, the route of administration must be established. The time of administration is also important. The duration of existing symptoms should be established. In a physical examination, the physician should try to document objective signs of cocaine intoxication, especially the vital signs (T, P, R, BP) and the degree of central nervous system excitation in order to be able to appreciate future changes. Routine laboratory evaluations are not helpful in the diagnosis or management of cocaine intoxication.

Treatment

Because cocaine is absorbed rapidly, gastric decontamination procedures such as ipecac-induced emesis or gastric lavage are not warranted. If an ingestion has occurred within 1 hour, the administration of activated charcoal may be beneficial. If the overdose has occurred through the nose, the nasal mucosa should be irrigated to remove unabsorbed drug. Supportive care should include frequent determinations of vital signs, a cardiac monitor, and the establishment of a secure intravenous (IV) line. Significant hypertension should be treated with rapidly acting hypotensive agents such as nitroprusside or diazoxide. The treatment of cocaine-induced cardiovascular abnormalities has included the administration of propranolol or chlorpromazine. However, the usefulness of either drug has not been demonstrated satisfactorily in the clinical setting. Convulsions should be treated vigorously with IV diazepam or phenytoin. If the convulsions fail to respond to these drugs within 30 minutes, thiopental anesthesia should be considered.

Indications for Admission or Referral

Any patient with a history of exposure to cocaine should be examined by a physician for an evaluation. All symptomatic patients should be admitted to a hospital for observation and care. The rapidity of the clinical course may preclude the transfer of the patient to a distant medical center.

ANNOTATED BIBLIOGRAPHY

AAP Committee on Adolescence: The role of the pediatrician in substance abuse counselling. Pediatrics 72:251–252, 1983 (Good review and approach to the subject.)

AAP Committee on Drugs: Effects of marijuana on man. Pediatrics 56:134–143, 1975 (Very good, though a little old, review of the pharmacology/toxicology of marijuana.)

AAP Committee on Drugs: Marijuana. Pediatrics 65:652–656, 1980 (Nice coverage of the basic concerns regarding marijuana use.)

Anonymous: Adverse effects of cocaine abuse. Med Lett Drugs Ther 26:51–52, 1984 (Brief run-down of adverse effects of cocaine use.)

Gay GR, Inaba DS, Sheppard CW et al: Cocaine: history, epidemiology, human pharmacology, and treatment. A perspective on a new debut for an old girl. Clin Toxicol 8:149–178, 1975 (Enjoyable reading concerning many aspects of cocaine use and abuse.)

Kandel DB et al: Patterns of drug use from adolescence to young children. Vols I to III. Am J Public Health 74:660–681, 1984 (Excellent, though somewhat technical, epidemiologic study covering three aspects: periods of risk for initiation, continued use, and discontinuation; sequences of progression; predictors of progression.)

MacDonald DI: Drugs, drinking and adolescents. Am J Dis Child 138:117–125, 1984 (Insights, advice, and an approach from an experienced individual.)

Robins LN: Editorial: The natural history of adolescent drug use. Am J Public Health 74:656–657, 1984 (Summarizes and comments on DB Kandel's three-part study.)

Schwartz RH: Marijuana: A crude drug with a spectrum of underappreciated toxicity. Pediatrics 73:455–458, 1984 (Discussion of some of the lesser appreciated effects of marijuana.)

Weinberg D, Lande A, Hilton N et al: Intoxication from accidental marijuana ingestion. Pediatrics 71:848–850, 1983 (Case reports and brief discussion of common management problems.)

21

Signs, Symptoms, and Systemic Problems

178
Identification of a Sick Child
PAUL L. MCCARTHY

Children in the first 2 years of life have approximately four to six acute infectious episodes/year. The number of episodes each year lessens as the child grows older. Thus, the young child with an acute infectious illness is a common problem for pediatricians. This review concentrates primarily on the differentiation of the child with an acute illness who has a minor or trivial illness from the child with an acute illness that is serious.

DIFFERENTIAL DIAGNOSIS

Of the 1169 consecutive children with fever of all ages coming to the Yale pediatric emergency room, ~30% had otitis media, 50% had diagnoses of *viral syndrome, viral URI, viral gastroenteritis,* or *flu-like* illness. Approximately 18% had diagnoses of the more common serious illnesses that the physician sees in pediatric patients with acute infectious illnesses: pneumonia (12%), bacteremia (4%), urinary tract infections (1%). One patient in 300 had bacterial meningitis. Other diagnoses, such as varicella and DPT reaction, made up the remainder.

In another study, 330 consecutive children less than 24 months of age with a fever ≥104°F, were evaluated extensively in the same emergency room and were followed carefully until they became well. The diagnoses in these children are shown in Table 178-1. Bacteremia, bacterial meningitis, and pneumonia were seen slightly more often than in the first series of 1169 unselected patients.

Table 178-1. Diagnosis in 330 Children <24 Months with Temperature ≥104°F

DIAGNOSIS	NUMBER*
Recognizable bacterial infection:	
Bacterial meningitis	4
Bacteremia	20
Urinary tract infection	2
Cellulitis	3
Shigellosis—other	2
Pneumonia	51
Otitis media	122
Recognizable viral illness:	
Exanthem—enanthem	19
Croup	5
Gastroenteritis	6
Aseptic meningitis	12
Nonspecific illness	84

* Children with two positive laboratory tests are classified under only one final diagnosis.

CLINICAL PRESENTATION

Do these common serious illnesses in febrile children represent a diagnostic challenge? In a study of 330 children with high fever, the examining physician was asked to list a diagnosis based on the history and physical examination and before laboratory data were obtained. Ninety-five percent of 20 instances of bacteremia without meningitis, over 50% of 52 episodes of pneumonia, and all 3 instances of urinary tract infection were not diagnosed by the initial history and physical examination. All 4 instances of bacterial meningitis were diagnosed by the initial history and physical examination. The 49 episodes of unrecognized serious illnesses occurred when the impression after the history and physical examination was either otitis media (7 patients with pneumonia and 9 patients with bacteremia) or a nonspecific febrile illness (20 instances of pneumonia, 10 of bacteremia, and 3 of urinary tract infection).

It is not surprising that these common serious illnesses may be clinically silent in the febrile child of <24 months. An optimal chest examination in the young child is difficult because of noncooperation and a respiratory rate more rapid than the adult. Bacteremia, especially that caused by *Streptococcus pneumoniae*, most frequently presents in the febrile child as a minor illness such as a URI, a fever without an apparent source, or otitis media. Most patients with a urinary tract infection (UTI) may present with nonspecific findings such as fever, irritability, decreased feeding, or mild gastrointestinal symptoms. Bacterial meningitis may be an occult infection in a child. Samson found that 11 of 152 patients with bacterial meningitis did not have nuchal rigidity, Brudzinski sign, bulging fontanelle, or depressed sensorium. All of these children were less than 16 months of age and had had a febrile seizure. Meningeal signs may, therefore, not be reliably present in the age group at greatest risk for meningitis. Serious illnesses are special diagnostic challenges in children less than 3 months of age. In this group, there is a higher occurrence of sepsis and meningitis and the organisms causing these infections are often *group B streptococcus* or gram-negative organisms. Pneumonia may be caused by *Staphylococcus aureus* or gram-negative bacteria. Finally, there is a higher occurrence of bacteremic UTIs in these patients.

WORK-UP

Information that the pediatrician has available for the diagnosis of the child with an acute infectious illness comes from several sources:

1. Observing the child
2. Taking a history
3. Performing a physical examination
4. Assessing age and temperature risk factors
5. Utilizing laboratory tests

Observing a febrile child before the history and the physical examination is a key part of the diagnostic process. These observation data supplement the history and physical examination. The his-

tory has some limitations in evaluating febrile children because the child often cannot tell us what "hurts." For example, costovertebral angle pain in a child with pyelonephritis might present in the history only as the mother's perception of fever, crying, and decreased appetite. The two most frequently used observation variables to judge the degree of illness concern the use of the child's eyes (looking at the observer and looking around the room). Eye function or appearance can be described in many ways; for example, shiny, bright, looks at observer, glassy, stares vacantly into space. These descriptions probably reflect what pediatricians mean by the term *alertness*.

Other observation data that are also frequently used include the child's sitting, moving arms and legs on table or lap, lays limply on table, and no movement in mother's arms. These phrases describe and define what is often referred to as *motor ability*.

Several of the most commonly used observation variables including vocalizing spontaneously, playing with objects, reaching for objects, smiling, and crying with noxious stimuli are descriptions of data that are referred to as *playfulness* and severe impairment termed *irritability*.

Another commonly used observation variable is the response of a crying child to being held by the parent. A normal response is that the child stops crying when held by the parent. Severe impairment can be indicated, for example, by a continual cry despite being held and comforted. These data probably represent a more precise description of what is termed *consolability*. Most observation variables correspond to the child's response to stimuli rather than to "organic" variables such as petechiae and nasal flaring. In variables relating to eye appearance or function, for example, stimulus–response data about the eyes (*e.g.*, looks at pen being offered) are noted much more often than "organic" data about the eyes (*e.g.*, sunken, red, glassy). More experienced pediatricians rely more heavily on stimulus–response data than less experienced physicians. Thus, the judgment of the degree of illness by observation is based largely on the assessment of the interaction between the child and his environment. The extent of the interaction is often immediately apparent. The child smiles at the observer and reaches for the proffered pen. At other times, the child cries and clings to the mother. The experienced examiner orchestrates the stimuli in an attempt to make the child act normally. To accomplish this, the pediatrician must be a developmentalist and must know what is an appropriate stimulus for children of various ages and what is a developmentally appropriate response. Thus, observation of febrile children is a complex process including both development skills and clinical skills. Pediatricians must assess the child's responses to multiple stimuli and must also be alert to clinical clues such as sunken eyes or cyanosis.

Observation data have been further examined to identify those criteria that are the key predictors of serious illness in febrile children. Six items have been identified and each has a three-point scale: 1 = normal, 3 = moderate impairment, and 5 = severe impairment. The items and their scales are termed the Yale Observation Scales (Table 178-2). Note that 4 of 6 items concern the child's response to stimuli. When these six items and their scales are used in practice, the best possible score is 6 × 1 = 6: the worst possible score is 6 × 5 or 30. Nearly 2 of 3 children with acute illnesses have been found to have scale scores ≤10 (*i.e.,* appear well) and less than 3% of these children have serious illnesses. On the other hand, severely ill-appearing children with a scale score ≥16 are relatively uncommon; but if such a child is seen, the chance of serious illness is high (92% in one study). Approximately one in four children appear moderately ill (scale score 11 to 15) and, even here, the chance of a serious illness is high (26% in the same study). The occurrence of serious illness in mod-

erately or severely ill-appearing febrile children as defined by a scale score >10 is 13 times greater than the occurrence in well-appearing children (scale score ≤10).

What is the relation between data gathered by observation and the results of the history and physical examination? In one study, 36 of 350 children with acute infectious illness had a serious illness. Ill appearance, abnormal history, or abnormal physical examination were equally important in detecting serious illnesses. The history and physical examination together detected ~78% (28 of 36) of children with serious illnesses. However, it was a combination of observation, history, and physical examination that had the highest sensitivity for serious illnesses and detected 86% (31 of 36) of children with such illnesses.

The abnormalities found on a history and a physical examination have also been analyzed. Findings relating to the pulmonary or central nervous systems represent most abnormalities; in addition, abnormalities of the pulmonary and central nervous systems have the strongest correlation with serious illnesses. This is not surprising because diseases of these systems represent 60% to 65% of serious illnesses in children with acute infectious illnesses.

Children with acute infectious illnesses can also be assessed for age or temperature risk factors. Se-

Table 178-2. Six Observation Items and Their Scales

OBSERVATION ITEM	1 NORMAL	3 MODERATE IMPAIRMENT	5 SEVERE IMPAIRMENT
Quality of cry	Strong with normal tone OR content and not crying	Whimpering OR sobbing	Weak OR moaning OR high pitched
Reaction to parental stimulation	Cries briefly then stops OR content and not crying	Cries off and on	Continual cry OR hardly responds
State variation	If awake → stays awake OR If asleep and stimulated → wakes up quickly	Eyes close briefly → awake Awakes with prolonged stimulation	Falls to sleep OR will not rouse
Color	Pink	Pale extremities OR acrocyanosis	Pale OR cyanotic OR mottled or ashen
Hydration	Skin normal, eyes normal AND mucous membranes moist	Skin and eyes are normal, AND mouth is slightly dry.	Skin doughy OR tented AND dry mucous membranes OR sunken eyes
Response (talk, smile) to social overtures	Smiles OR alerts (≤2 mo)	Brief smile OR alerts briefly (≤2 mo)	No smile Face anxious, dull, expressionless OR no alerting (≤2 mo)

lected serious illnesses occur in febrile children <3 months (see Chap. 191). There is also an association between height of temperature and serious illnesses. As the degree of fever increases, so does the occurrence of bacteremia. The occurrence of bacteremia in young children is ~7% when the temperature is ≥104°F, 13% when the temperature is 105°F to 105.9°F, and increases to 26% when the temperature is ≥106°F. In addition, there is a 50% occurrence of bacterial meningitis when the fever is ≥106°F (see Chap. 192).

Laboratory Tests

Screening laboratory studies may be helpful in identifying the child at increased risk for many of the common serious illnesses discussed. For example, a WBC ≥15,000 per cu mm or ESR ≥30 mm/hr in children ≤24 months with a fever ≥104°F places those children at five times the risk of bacteremia (15% *vs* 3%) compared to children in whom the WBC is <15,000 and the ESR <30. A similar efficacy of combinations of WBC ≥15,000 per cu mm, PMN count ≥10,000 per cu mm and band count ≥500 per cu mm in detecting bacteremia has been found. The risk of *any* serious illness in febrile children is approximately twice as great if the WBC was ≥15,000 per cu mm or the ESR ≥30 mm/hr than if neither of these elevations is present. Thus, screening laboratory tests, though far from perfect in detecting serious illnesses in febrile children, can point towards an increased risk of these illnesses.

The foregoing considerations in this chapter have implications for ordering laboratory tests in children with acute infectious illnesses. Children at greatest risk for serious illnesses are those who either have an ill appearance, abnormal history findings, or abnormal physical examination findings. Such patients comprise 20% to 30% of febrile children. The specific findings from observation, history, and physical examination dictate the laboratory evaluation. For example, if abnormal physical examination findings suggest pneumonia, a chest roentgenogram is indicated. An ill appearance, with or without other abnormal findings, warrants a laboratory evaluation. The studies ordered can be based on other associated findings. For example, an ill-appearing febrile child with rhinorrhea is a better candidate for blood culture, lumbar puncture, and chest roentgenogram than for a urine or stool culture. The history information may provide clues to the diagnosis; for example, the child with a history of bloody diarrhea with a nonspecific

physical examination should have a stool culture performed. The interpretation of an ill appearance, abnormal history, or physical examination and the subsequent ordering of laboratory tests can be aided by a consideration of age and temperature risk factors. Ill appearance with a nonspecific physical examination in a <3-month-old child warrants, at least, an evaluation for sepsis and meningitis. Fever ≥104°F in an ill-appearing febrile child, with or without abnormal history or physical examination findings, suggests a bacterial blood stream invasion, and a blood culture should be part of the laboratory evaluation.

A child with an acute infectious illness may, on the other hand, appear well and may demonstrate no abnormal history or physical examination findings suggestive of a serious illness. That is, the illness seems nonspecific or otitis media may be present. Laboratory studies are not indicated if no age or temperature risk factors are present. The child may be followed expectantly or the otitis media may be treated. The largest proportion of febrile children, perhaps 60% to 65%, meet these criteria. The risk for serious illness is low, and it is reasonable to forego a laboratory evaluation.

In well-appearing children with acute illness, without an abnormal history or physical examination, the implications of age <3 months or temperature ≥104°F for ordering laboratory tests are less clear. Some would argue that these risk factors alone are indications for a further work-up; others would argue that no work-up is indicated. Until data prove otherwise, it is prudent and reasonable to perform sepsis work-ups on febrile children <3 months and to admit these patients to the hospital for observation. The use of expectant antibiotics once the infant is hospitalized and while awaiting cultures is a matter of judgment, but it is probably wise in children <6 weeks of age. If high fever (≥104°F) is detected in a child between 3 and 24 months, a blood culture is indicated; a screening WBC or WBC/ESR may aid in the decision to obtain a blood culture.

MANAGEMENT/ADMISSION

The decision to admit a child with an acute infectious illness to the hospital or to follow the child as an outpatient is based on several considerations:

1. *Age*—The management and treatment of febrile infant <3 months was discussed above.
2. *Appearance*—The child who appears ill, even in

the absence of a specific diagnosis after the initial clinical and laboratory evaluation, should be admitted to the hospital. Antibiotics can be started once bacterial cultures have been obtained.

3. *Diagnosis*—Certain diagnoses, such as bacterial meningitis, warrant admission and intravenous antibiotics. Other diagnoses, such as pneumonia, do not necessarily warrant admission. Factors such as the degree of distress, the extent of organ involvement (in this case, the extent of the pneumonia), the ability of the parents to observe and care for the child and keep follow-up appointments are critical in decisions regarding admission.

If the decision is made to follow the child on an outpatient basis, then the follow-up evaluation can serve many purposes. The physician can ascertain if symptoms are resolving. If a significant illness, such as pneumonia, has been diagnosed, one can ascertain if the child is responding to therapy. Outpatient follow-up can become part of the diagnostic process when the diagnosis was not apparent at the initial visit. The follow-up visit can also serve as an opportunity to support and educate the parents.

ANNOTATED BIBLIOGRAPHY

Baron MA, Fink HD: Bacteremia in private pediatric practice. Pediatrics 66:171–175, 1980 (Discusses the use of screening laboratory tests in private pediatric practice to detect serious illness, such as bacteremia, in febrile children.)

McCarthy PL (ed): The Evaluation and Management of Febrile Children. Norwalk, CT, Appleton–Century–Crofts, 1985 (Concentrates on the use of clinical judgment in detecting the common serious illnesses in children with acute infections: meningitis, pneumonia, bacteremia, bacterial diarrhea, urinary tract infection.)

McCarthy PL, Jekel JF, Dolan TF: Temperature greater than or equal to 40°C in children less than 24 months of age: A prospective study. Pediatrics 59:663–668, 1977 (Large series of children ≤24 months with high fever which discusses differential diagnosis and the value of screening laboratory tests.)

McCarthy PL, Jekel JF, Stashwick CA et al: Further definition of history and observation variables in assessing febrile children. Pediatrics 67:687–693, 1981 (Definition of the observation data on which pediatricians rely to make a judgment of toxicity.)

McCarthy PL, Sharpe MR, Spiesel SZ et al: Observation scales to identify serious illness in febrile children. Pediatrics 70:802–809, 1982 (Scales that can be used to judge, in a systematic way, the appearance of a child with an acute infectious illness.)

Samson JH: Febrile seizures and purulent meningitis. JAMA 210:1918–1920, 1969 (Discusses the problem of a lack of selected clinical findings in children with bacterial meningitis.)

Wright PF, Thompson J, McKee KT et al: Patterns of illness in the highly febrile young child: Epidemiologic, clinical and laboratory correlates. Pediatrics 67:694–700, 1981 (Describes the value of a pediatrician's impression of toxicity in detecting febrile children with serious illnesses.)

179
Fever
ROBERT A. DERSHEWITZ

Fever in children arouses much parental, and occasionally provider, concern. Its presence is one of the most common reasons for parents to seek medical care.

Because of circadian variations and the influence of multiple factors, such as activity on the body's temperature, the healthy child's temperature fluctuates within a *normal* range. If the temperature exceeds 38°C (100.4°F) rectally, 37.8°C (100°F) orally, or 37.2°C (99°F) axillary, the temperature is said to be *elevated*, and hence, the child has a fever.

Most fevers in children result from infection. In response to invasion from any type of organism, it is believed that endogenous pyrogen is released from neutrophils, monocytes, and Kupffer cells. The pyrogens, in turn, interact with prostaglandins to act on the *central thermostat* believed to be located in the anterior hypothalamus.

DETERMINATION OF FEVER

Although the touch cannot yield a precise measurement of temperature, one can usually tell by touch when the child's temperature is high (*i.e.*, above 103°F). A glass mercury thermometer has been the traditional instrument for measuring temperature, but for reasons of sanitation and speed, electronic thermometers are becoming more popular. Many pediatricians fear using oral thermometers in children under 4 to 5 years of age. The accuracy of axillary measurements is controversial. In clinical practice, it is usually used in newborn nurseries (to avoid risk of cross-contamination and rectal perforation), the infant or toddler with diarrhea, the uncooperative child, and in any child when simply knowledge of the presence, rather than an exact temperature, is desired.

Regardless of which method is chosen, all children must remain still when their temperatures are taken. A lubricated rectal thermometer is gently inserted about 1 inch and left inside for 2 minutes with the buttocks squeezed together. An oral thermometer should be placed on either side of the posterior sublingual pocket and left in place for 3 minutes. Parents should be cautioned not to give the child hot or cold food just before taking the temperature. An axillary temperature should have a thermometer left in a dry axilla for 4 minutes.

Liquid crystal forehead strips have become popular for reasons of ease, convenience, and safety. Unfortunately, they are not as accurate as glass or electronic thermometers.

TO TREAT OR NOT TO TREAT

By itself, the presence of fever is not necessarily the marker of a child sicker than one who has the same symptoms but who is without fever. In fact, hypothermia is usually much more ominous than hyperthermia. Although most febrile children have trivial illnesses, fever should provoke high anxiety in certain conditions. These include neonates (especially under 5 weeks of age), fever above 105°F (greater incidence of bacteremia), and in the febrile child with associated immunodeficiency, lethargy, and inconsolability. The febrile child with disorientation, meningismus, petechiae, or purpura constitutes a medical emergency (see Chap. 178 for the relationship of fever to illness, a work-up for fever, and indications for hospitalization).

Clearly, all children with fevers do not need antipyretic medication. Most children are not made ill or uncomfortable solely by a temperature elevation. Children who appear to be uncomfortable by the fever, regardless of its height, should receive medication. Although brain damage does not occur with a fever below 107°F (41.7°C), most clinicians recommend antipyretics in children whose fevers are 105°F (40.5°C) or greater to prevent temperatures from reaching dangerous levels (a rare event) and to prevent febrile seizures. Children with a history of febrile seizure, and those in whom the side effects of a fever may be harmful (e.g., borderline dehydration, compensated cardiac disease) should have aggressive fever management.

The argument against treating febrile children derives from a growing body of data (and opinion) that show that fever helps in the host-defense mechanisms against infection. At least experimentally, fever increases T cell production, leukocyte mobility, and the effectiveness of interferon. Other reasons include the avoidance of overdose and untoward effects of the antipyretic and obscuring the fever pattern in a child with a prolonged fever (see Chap. 180).

DIFFERENTIAL DIAGNOSIS

Most fevers in children are of viral etiology. Typically, the fever does not exceed 104°F and resolves within 3 days, although it may last as long as 14 days. Infections from bacteria and mycoplasma result in the only other common causes of fever in children. Malignancy, collagen–vascular disease, CNS lesions, and hyperthyroidism usually cause signs and symptoms other than pyrexia to suggest the diagnosis. Fever in a child with gastroenteritis may be due to hypernatremia or dehydration. In a previously well child with a fulminant onset of hyperthermia, environmental causes (e.g., sitting in a car parked in the sun with windows rolled up) and heat stroke should be considered. Other causes of acute onset of fever include insect bites (e.g., tics, spider, snake) and ingestions (e.g., salicylates and anticholinergics).

TREATMENT

The mainstay of treatment is acetaminophen and salicylate. Acetaminophen is being increasingly favored because of the association of salicylate with Reye's syndrome and because aspirin is not available as a liquid preparation. Both medications are equally effective antipyretics and both have the same dose (i.e., 10 to 15 mg/kg/dose, given every 4 hours as needed). It is not recommended to give them together because they have similar mechanisms of action (interferes with prostaglandin synthesis) and of the lack of data demonstrating efficacy. Another common practice with probably little benefit is alternating aspirin and acetaminophen every 2 hours.

If the temperature is high or if aggressive fever management is indicated, children may be sponged, but only after the antipyretic medication is given. This is to lower the hypothalamic set-point (which sponging does not), thereby avoiding shivering after the sponging which may, in itself, raise the body temperature. The water should be luke-warm, and the water temperature should be raised if the child shivers. The greater the exposure of skin to the water, the more rapid will the body temperature fall. Iced water enemas and sponging with alcohol should be avoided. Do not use ice blankets or baths except in the case of malignant hyperthermia, heat stroke, and environmental causes. Regardless of the etiology, the febrile child should not be bundled or overdressed. Recent data have shown that there is no relationship between the fever response (either to the antipyretic alone or in combination with sponging) to the infectious etiology. Thus, a high fever unresponsive to an antipyretic or sponging is not a clue to a bacterial infection.

PARENTAL EDUCATION

Much of a pediatrician's illness management is devoted to mitigating or dispelling fever phobia. Parents should be taught that fever is a sign, not a disease, and that it is more important to note how the child is acting, rather than how high is the fever. Many parents, however, will want more firm guidelines on when and how to treat their child's fever. Open lines of communication (including telephone) between the physician and the parent should always be fostered. Parents should be told to call immediately if their neonate has a fever, if their child's fever is over 105°F, or if the child is twitching, lethargic, inconsolable, has a stiff neck or a purplish rash. The physician should also be contacted immediately when high-risk children (*e.g.*, with sickle cell disease, immunodeficiency) develop fevers. Less urgent indications for calling include a child whose fever persisted for more than 3 days; if the child acts ill; or if the parents want reassurance. If the child has had a febrile convulsion, prompt and aggressive fever management should be instituted for that and future episodes. Parents should be told that although febrile convulsions should be avoided, they do not result in neurologic damage.

ANNOTATED BIBLIOGRAPHY

Casey R, McMahon BA, McCormick MC et al: Fever therapy: An educational intervention for parents. Pediatrics 73:600–605, 1984 (Demonstrates that parents can be taught appropriate fever management.)

Fruthaler GJ: Fever in children: Phobia vs facts. Hosp Practice pp 49–53, 1985 (Good review; strong on differential diagnosis and treatment.)

Kresch MJ: Axillary temperature as a screening test for fever in children. 104:596–599, 1984 (Concludes that because of its poor sensitivity, axillary temperatures should not be used.)

Norris J: Taking temperatures: The changing state of the art. Contemp Pediatr pp 22–39, 1985 (Current discussion on the various ways of taking a temperature.)

Schmitt B: Fever in childhood. Pediatrics (Suppl) 74:929–936, 1984 (Good overall discussion, with excellent section on parent education.)

180
Fever of Unknown Origin
PAUL L. MCCARTHY

Fever of unknown origin (FUO) tests the diagnostic acumen of pediatricians. The array of laboratory tests that can be ordered is great; the clinician's goal should be to minimize the cost and trauma of studies while maintaining diagnostic accuracy.

DEFINITION AND PATHOPHYSIOLOGY

The differential diagnosis of fever of unknown origin encompasses many disease entities. The pathophysiology of FUO is related to its etiology. For example, the cause of a fever from an infection *vs* an autoimmune disorder is different. The duration of fever qualifies an illness to be termed *FUO*. Unfortunately, the definition of *duration* varies from one study to another. Pizzo and associates define FUO as fever $\geq 38.5°C$ on more than four occasions for at least a 2-week period. McClung's criteria are that the fever should last for 3 weeks and that the cause should remain undiagnosed despite an active outpatient evaluation or for longer than 1 week despite inpatient diagnostic efforts. Fevers associated with most uncomplicated viral infections rarely last beyond 5 days. When a child has been febrile for 10 days or more and no cause is apparent, it is reasonable for the pediatrician to undertake the thorough evaluation mandated by the term *FUO*.

DIFFERENTIAL DIAGNOSIS

In their classical work of FUO, Petersdorf and Beeson reported on 100 adult patients and outlined an evaluative approach. However, recent work by Pizzo and associates and McClung raise many questions regarding the applicability of the adult experience with FUO (especially the differential diagnoses of FUO in adults) to children.

The occurrence of diagnostic categories in adults and children is compared in Table 180-1. The occurrence of infectious illnesses in adults and children is similar except for children less than 6 years of ago who, in Pizzo's series, had a higher incidence of infectious illnesses (65%). Infections in the adult series were unusual and included 11 patients with tuberculosis, 7 patients with hepatobiliary infections, and 4 patients with abdominal abscesses. Children, on the other hand, had other infections. In Pizzo's series, 34 of 100 children had bacterial infections and 18 children had viral illnesses. Of note, 22 of the 34 bacterial infections were those commonly seen in the pediatric age group: UTI (4), pneumonia (4), tonsillitis (4), sinusitis (3), meningitis (3), septicemia (2), and streptococcosis (2). In McClung's series of 99 patients, 28 had bacterial infections and only one had a viral infection. Again, most bacterial illnesses (17 of 28) were not unusual infections: UTI (4), pneumonia (4), septicemia (3), tonsillitis (2), sinusitis (2), and meningitis (2).

Neoplastic disease is more common in adults: 19% *vs* 6% (Pizzo) and 8% (McClung). The types of tumors also differed. In adults, one half of tumors were solid tumors or disseminated carcinomas. In children, most were leukemias and lymphomas.

Collagen inflammatory diseases, most commonly systemic lupus erythematosus and acute rheumatic fever, were diagnosed in 13% of Petersdorf's patients. Collagen inflammatory diseases represented 20% of Pizzo's patients and only 11% of McClung's patients, with juvenile rheumatoid arthritis causing approximately one half of the illnesses in both series. In Pizzo's series, 33% of children 6 years of age or older had juvenile rheumatoid arthritis (JRA). In Pizzo's series, 10% of children had miscellaneous diagnoses such as "CNS fever" (2%), dehydration (1%), Behcet's disease (1%), hepatitis (1%), ruptured appendix (1%), and other (4%). McClung had six patients in a miscellaneous category that included regional enteritis (3), thyroiditis (1), salicylate toxicity (1), and *erythroblastopenia* (1).

Twelve children remained undiagnosed in Pizzo's series; at least three continued to have symptoms for which an etiologic diagnosis was not established. In McClung's series, a total of 11 patients remained undiagnosed and continued to have symptoms such as arthralgias, abdominal pain, and fever.

WORK-UP

History

The most critical diagnostic maneuver in arriving at a diagnosis of a child with FUO is a carefully performed history and physical examination. In Pizzo's series, the history and physical examination could have diagnosed 62 of 100 patients. In McClung's series, the history and physical examination suggested the diagnosis in 87 of 99 patients.

It is necessary first to establish that the child does, in fact, have a fever. Dinarello and Wolff re-

Table 180-1.   Causes of FUO in Adults and Children

| | ADULT PATIENTS (N = 100)* | CHILDREN (N = 100)† | | | CHILDREN (N = 99)‡ |
		<6 Yr	≥6 Yr	Total	
Infection	36%	65%	38%	52%	29%
Neoplastic	19%	8%	4%	6%	8%
Collagen	13%	8%	33%	20%	11%
Miscellaneous	25%	14%	6%	10%	10%
No diagnosis	7%	5%	19%	12%	11%
					30% (normal or resolving illness)

* Petersdorf RG, Beeson PB: Fever of unexplained origin: Report on 100 cases. Medicine 40:1, 1961
† Pizzo PA, Lovejoy FH Jr, Smith DH: Prolonged fever in children: Review of 100 cases. Pediatrics 55:468, 1975
‡ McClung HJ: Prolonged fever of unknown origin in children. Am J Dis Child 124:544, 1972

ported on over 400 patients who were said to have FUO and found that 18% actually did *not* have a fever. Most commonly, the fever was factitious (in 6%) or the technique of temperature taking or interpretation of temperatures was erroneous (12%).

Physical Examination

Pizzo found the following signs and symptoms most useful:

- *Skin findings:* These include rash, pruritus, edema, or infection. Of the 24 patients with such findings, 6 patients had a malignancy and 8 patients had a fatal outcome.
- *Joint pain:* 14 patients had arthralgia including 9 patients with a collagen-inflammatory disorder.
- *Joint findings:* Of the 9 patients with these findings, 6 had a collagen-inflammatory disorder.
- *Significant heart murmurs:* 4 of the 8 patients with a significant heart murmur had subacute bacterial endocarditis.
- *Chest pain, cyanosis, dyspnea:* 6 of 7 patients with these findings had a fatal outcome.
- *Hepatosplenomegaly:* This sometimes pointed toward malignancy.

Although Pizzo noted that fever patterns, anorexia, fatigue, chills, sweats, weight loss, abdominal pain, and adenopathy were unrelated to diagnosis or prognosis, the experiences of others are different. For example, the once daily elevation of fever at the same time each day, often in association with abdominal and joint pain, may suggest juvenile rheumatoid arthritis (see Chap. 132). Weight loss and abdominal pain may indicate occult inflammatory bowel disease, whereas significant adenopathy may point toward malignancy or juvenile rheumatoid arthritis. The physician should, therefore, carefully seek those signs and symptoms associated with the most common etiologies of FUOs in children. He should search carefully in particular for clues in a patient's history or physical examination that indicate bacterial infections, which may present as FUOs (*e.g.*, pneumonia, meningitis, UTI, sinusitis, tonsillitis, subacute bacterial endocarditis, and bacteremia-sepsis).

Laboratory Tests

A WBC, differential, platelet count, and erythrocyte sedimentation rate should always be obtained. In McClung's series, 4 to 5 children with leukemia had abnormalities of the white blood count, differential, or platelet count. Pizzo found that anemia and elevated ESR indicated an active process; on the other hand, of 20 children with ESR <10 mm/hr, 18 had a fever secondary to a nonserious or viral illness. A shift to the left on the WBC suggests collagen-inflammatory disorders and bacterial infections.

The urinalysis is mandatory. In Pizzo's series, it helped establish the diagnosis in 4 patients with urinary tract infections, 3 with subacute bacterial endocarditis, and 5 with collagen-inflammatory disorders.

All children in Pizzo's series had chest roentgenograms performed and 13 of these studies were abnormal.

Appropriate bacterial cultures of urine, blood, throat, cerebrospinal fluid, and stool are important for diagnosing common serious bacterial infections that can cause an FUO.

Since the occurrence of collagen-inflammatory disorders is high in children with FUO, investigating this possibility should be part of the initial laboratory evaluation and should include antinuclear antibodies, rheumatoid factor, quantitative immunoglobulins, and a serum complement profile.

A PPD along with Candida, mumps, and Trichophyton controls should also be applied.

Consideration should be given to a bone marrow examination if the aforementioned studies do not result in a diagnosis. In Pizzo's series, 6 of the 14 bone marrow examinations were diagnostic: leukemia (4), lymphosarcoma (1), and agranulocytosis (1). An additional 6 of the 14 bone marrow examinations suggested either a collagen-inflammatory disease (with a plasma cell predominance) or an infectious process (with a *shifted-cell line*).

Other, more invasive biopsy, surgical, or radiologic procedures should be done only if the child continues to be symptomatic and no diagnosis has been established. These procedures may include an IVP, GI series, barium enema, laparotomy, and biopsies (*e.g.*, lymph node, liver). The yield from a liver biopsy and laparotomy in pediatric patients is far less than in adult patients. A Gallium scan is useful if the physician is concerned about an occult infectious focus that has not been identified by the bacterial cultures discussed previously. Thus, this test should be reserved for more perplexing patients with persisting symptoms that remain undiagnosed.

ADMISSION/TREATMENT

The decision to hospitalize a child should be based on several considerations. If the child does not appear severely ill and has no findings that suggest a serious illness, an outpatient work-up may be initiated. The technique of temperature taking should be reviewed with the parents and a fever diary may be kept. If, on the other hand, the child appears more severely ill, or has findings suggestive of a serious illness (*e.g.*, hepatosplenomegaly), then inpatient care is warranted. Admission to the inpatient service may also be needed to document that the child has a fever. The temporal characteristics of the illness can also be appreciated better while the child is an inpatient. For example, the child with systemic juvenile rheumatoid arthritis may have a fleeting *salmon* rash only once a day when the fever peak occurs and these findings may be associated with severe joint achiness.

The therapy of FUO depends on the etiology. If it is established that the child has a fever, treatment with an antipyretic such as acetaminophen is reasonable. If the disease is a collagen-inflammatory process, an initial therapeutic trial of salicylates is warranted. In other circumstances, no antipyresis is warranted. These may include, but are not limited to, the following:

- Situations in which the fever has not been sufficiently documented or in which a purpose of the inpatient evaluation is to define the temperature pattern

- Situations in which acute rheumatic fever is suspected and the physician wishes to establish whether the pattern of joint complaints is migratory. It may be wise to withhold salicylates because joint complaints in this disease often respond dramatically to aspirin.

Contraindications to using antipyretics include salicylates in a child with thrombocytopenia or acetaminophen in a child with liver disease.

ANNOTATED BIBLIOGRAPHY

Dinarello CA, Wolff SM: Pathogenesis of fever in man. N Engl J Med 298:607–612, 1978 (Discussion of mechanisms of fever with some comments on the NIH experience with FUO.)

McClung HJ: Prolonged fever of unknown origin in children. Am J Dis Child 124:544–550, 1972 (Value of the history and physical examination is clearly shown in this study.)

Petersdorf RG, Beeson PB: Fever of unexplained origin: Report on 100 cases. Medicine 40:1–30, 1961 (Classic article on FUO in adults.)

Pizzo PA, Lovejoy FH Jr, Smith DH: Prolonged fever in children: Review of 100 cases. Pediatrics 55:468–473, 1975 (Experience with FUO at a large children's hospital.)

181
Child with Recurrent Infections
RAOUL L. WOLF

Recurrent infections are frequent in childhood, mainly as a consequence of exposure in nursery schools and other reservoirs of infection. The difficulty lies in determining when this problem indicates an underlying disorder, such as an immune defect. A careful history, noting the pattern of infections and a planned clinical investigation, can generally resolve this dilemma.

PATHOPHYSIOLOGY

Most recurrent infections occur within tubular structures, which are usually the middle ear, the lung, the nose and paranasal sinuses, and the kidney. The problem can be considered as a result either of resistance of the organism to therapy or a defect in the host. Organisms, such as staphylococci, frequently become resistant to antibiotics. The choice of antibiotic may be incorrect or may lack specificity for the organism. Resistance to antibiotics or an inappropriate choice of antibiotic is the most common cause for persistent infection. The host defects may be local or systemic. Local etiologic factors result in an obstruction to the lumen, causing stasis of air or fluid. Pathogenic organisms then persist in the lumen and become invasive. The infection responds to therapy, only to recur weeks or months later when stasis provides a medium for a pathogenic organism to proliferate.

A wide range of systemic disorders actually cause recurrent infections by producing an immunologic dysfunction. Diabetes mellitus and sickle cell disease are examples of this. In diabetes there is a reduction in lymphocyte function and a loss of tissue barriers. Patients with sickle cell disease suffer from a lack of opsonins in plasma and poor to absent splenic function. Immune defects can generally be considered as primary (congenital) or secondary. The primary defects involve either antibody production (humoral) or the interaction and function of lymphocytes and monocytes (cell mediated). These two processes are intimately linked. The lymphocytes are divided into two main groups: T cells and B cells. The T cells orchestrate the immune response, receiving signals from macrophages and other adherent cells. Macrophages process antigens and react to their presence, activating T cells during this sequence. The T cells pass information to and stimulate B cells, which proliferate, giving rise to plasma cells that secrete specific antibody binding. The antibody binds to the stimulating antigen, activating the complement pathway. This attracts polymorphonuclear cells to the site where they ingest and destroy the complex. This intricate system can break down at many points.

The production of antibody may be defective, resulting in repeated otitis media, rhinosinusitis, and pneumonia, with rarer episodes of meningitis or sepsis. T cell abnormalities result in severe infections or infections with unusual organisms such as *Pneumocystis carinii* or mycoplasma. Growth retardation is prominent and these children usually die at an early age. Associated anomalies are common. Defects in killing by polymorphonuclear cells result in an unusual condition called the *cold* abscess. This is the formation of an abscess without an inflammatory response that may involve the skin and viscera. Its presence is diagnostic of a functional defect in polymorphonuclear cells. The patient with recurrent *Neisseria* infectious organisms should be suspected of having a deficiency of the sixth or eighth component of serum complement.

CLINICAL PRESENTATION

Recurrent upper respiratory infections are common in childhood. Most of these are of viral etiology; recurrent bacterial infections are more likely to be associated with an immune defect. Several physical signs (*e.g.*, high fever, rigors, purulent discharge, and sputum production) indicate bacterial infection. There are few physical signs that might indicate the need to work-up a patient for an immune defect. The occurrence of 3 or more separate, presumed bacterial otitis media episodes within a 6-month period has been used as a guide by some centers. In such a patient, the absence or paucity of lymphoid tissue, especially tonsillar tissue, strongly suggests a B cell deficiency. Arthritis involving large joints is often associated with immunodeficiency. Other features associated with

immune defects may occur, such as thrombocytopenia, eczema, and cardiac defects; however, these occur in rare syndromes and are usually associated with severe infections.

A common problem (frequently frustrating to both patient and physician) is the question of recurrent boils and furuncles: These are rarely caused by an underlying immunologic or chronic systemic disease. Poor hygiene is more likely to be the reason for this type of persistent infection. The patient who has a deep abscess formation without an inflammatory response (cold abscess) is an exception. This is associated with an inability of polymorphonuclear cells to kill and is peculiar to this problem.

Recurrent urinary tract infections are usually based on an underlying mechanical problem and are rarely associated with systemic diseases and immune defects.

DIFFERENTIAL DIAGNOSIS

There are two major differential considerations: the cause for recurrent infections lies with the organism or with the host.

Organisms

The infectious agent may be resistant to antibiotics or the antibiotic may be incorrect or in a low concentration. The organism may become sequestered in an inaccessible area (*e.g.*, renal parenchyma). The infection may be caused by an unusual or unexpected organism such as atypical mycobacteria. Another example could be a salmonella species causing osteomyelitis.

Host Factors

Since most recurrent infections occur in hollow viscera, the causes can be considered in mechanical terms. These may lie in the lumen, in the wall, or outside the wall.

In the Lumen. Here one must consider the presence of a foreign body. This is one of the most common causes of recurrent infection in childhood. It may be a pea in a nostril or a peanut in a bronchus. A "check-valve" effect results in intermittent obstruction and also intermittent stasis. This cycle leads to clearing of infection followed by a recurrence of symptoms. Other causes in this category include deformities of the lumen such as congenital webs and strictures. Cystic fibrosis causes thickened mucus. Conditions in which there is a reservoir of infection are a related group of conditions. Bronchiectasis and chronic sinusitis are examples where seeding of infection to the lung is frequent. The infections are self-perpetuating because of an obstruction.

In the Wall. Distortions of the wall from tumors, benign or malignant, belong in this group. These masses may be carcinomata or hemangiomas. Inflammatory conditions can cause chronic thickening of the bronchial wall with an obstruction leading to poor drainage of secretions and repeated secondary infections. Granulomas, which occur in sarcoidosis, can obstruct drainage. Muscle dysfunction causes poor peristalsis. This often occurs in the ureter, with stasis then leading to a recurrent urinary tract infection.

Outside the Wall. Vascular anomalies often compress a bronchial lumen. Tumors may cause an obstruction to ureters, bronchi, and sinuses. For example, granulomatous conditions, such as Wegener's granulomatosis, often present with repeated infections, particularly of the sinuses.

Several local conditions result from a combination of these three groups. Dysfunctional cilia syndrome is an unusual condition in which the cilia are abnormal and do not clear secretions. It results in recurrent sinusitis, bronchitis, pneumonia, and bronchiectasis. When a pneumonia recurs in the same lobe, usually the left lower lobe, the physician should consider a sequestration of that lobe or lobule. This is a congenital malformation in which the bronchi of the sequestered lobe do not communicate with the main bronchi. There is also no connection with the pulmonary vasculature. The blood supply is derived from the aorta by way of the bronchial vessels. Because of the poor communication with the rest of the lung, air stasis results in repeated infections and seeding to other parts of the lung.

SYSTEMIC CONDITIONS

Immunodeficiency

This group of diseases results from defects in humoral or cellular immunity; humoral defects are more frequent. These humoral disorders can be considered in two groups: selective defects and total or pan-hypogammaglobulinemia.

Humoral-Selective Deficiency. IgA deficiency is a selective defect and is the most common of the immune defects. It occurs with a frequency of 1:600. Patients present with sinopulmonary infections and diarrhea.

Subclass IgG deficiency is a defect of IgG_2. There are 4 subclasses of IgG and IgG_2 is concerned with the control of encapsulated organisms, such as *H. influenzae* and *S. pneumoniae*. These patients also develop sinopulmonary infections.

Humoral-Total Deficiency. Pan-hypogammaglobulinemia is best described by an X-linked disorder, known as *Bruton's agammaglobulinemia*. In this disorder, there is an absence of mature B cells and antibody levels are low. Recurrent sinopulmonary infections are common and meningitis occurs occasionally.

Another category of conditions is classified together as a *common variable immunodeficiency*. This group encompasses a variety of underlying problems, such as the inability to synthesize an antibody or to release it from cells.

Cellular Defects. Defects of cell-regulated immunity are much rarer. These patients develop severe systemic infections often with opportunistic organisms such as *Pneumocystis carinii* and *Mycoplasma pneumoniae*. Many patients have associated abnormalities that may draw attention to the immunologic problem. Failure to thrive is common. Viremia and septicemia often cause an early demise. There is a wide range of underlying defects in this condition. The thymus may be absent, stem cells may not mature into T cells, or an arrest may occur in development of T cells.

There are subclasses of T cells, predominantly helper and suppressor. Several conditions cause disturbances in the normal cell ratio of 2 helper : 1 suppressor. The most striking example of this problem is the acquired immunodeficiency disease syndrome (AIDS). This disease is caused by a virus, HIV, that destroys helper T cells. This results in excessive suppression, leading to overwhelming infection by cytomegalovirus, hepatitis B virus, and Epstein–Barr virus. Malignancy is common. The condition occurs in children, usually associated with hemophilia and blood transfusions, or transmission of the virus by an infected mother (see also Chap. 206). Epstein–Barr virus may also cause severe immunologic disturbances.

Polymorphonuclear Cell Defects. Defects in the ability of polymorphonuclear cells to kill organisms causes recurrent abscess formation when the defect is in the ability of these cells to kill. The cold abscess is typical of this deficit and the lung is often involved. Neutropenia, on the other hand, is associated with septicemia rather than with localization to an abscess.

Chronic Diseases

Diabetes mellitus is associated with recurrent infections, especially of the skin, but all organs may be involved. This is due to a loss of the barrier function of the skin as well as reduced T cell function.

Cardiac disease is another chronic problem that can cause recurrent pneumonia because of persistent pulmonary edema.

Chronic renal disease is associated with systemic infections and pneumonia. In this condition there is an accumulation of toxic peptides that block T cell function.

WORK-UP

History

A careful history is essential in the evaluation of patients with recurrent infections. The physician should ask the following questions:

- Has the child been well between infections? This will distinguish a persistent infection from repeated separate infections.
- Are the episodes associated with high fever? This implies a bacterial origin.
- Is the same organ involved (*e.g.*, are the infections confined to the respiratory tract)? In this circumstance a structural anomaly may be present or an obstruction, such as a foreign body.
- Do the infections occur in the same site, for example one lobe of the lung? This may indicate an anomaly such as sequestration.
- Has the child been in any unusual areas or in rural areas or farm lands? Unusual organisms are possible, such as animal-borne diseases.
- Has any other family member had a similar problem? This question will expose a possible hereditary or familial disorder.
- Have any siblings, cousins, or other relatives had repeated infections or died from overwhelming infections? This expands on genetic problems and immune defects.
- Are there symptoms that suggest an acute illness or are the infections silent? Silent infections imply that the usual immune response with polymorphonuclear cell activation is not present.

Physical Examination

This is specific for the site of infection. In accessible areas, such as the nose, one should look for a foreign body if unilateral purulent rhinitis is present. Evidence of unequal respiration or breath sounds, or unilateral wheezing, may suggest a foreign body within the lung. The most notable sign in patients with recurrent upper respiratory tract infections is a lack of tonsillar tissue. This often indicates an underlying immune defect because tonsillar tissue has a high content of B lymphocytes and one would expect the tonsils to be enlarged under these circumstances.

Laboratory Tests

The specific nature of the tests performed depends on the site and the type of infection. A complete blood count will indicate deficiencies of neutrophils, lymphocytes, or platelets. A left shift would indicate that the infection is possibly bacterial. Cultures should be taken of sputum, nasal secretions, blood, and obviously infected tissues to determine the type of infection and the degree of sensitivity to antibiotics.

X-ray studies will be determined by specific needs. Persistent purulent rhinitis is an indication for sinus roentgenograms. Chest roentgenograms taken at different times in the patient with recurrent pneumonia should be compared for the site of infection and evidence suggesting an obstructed bronchus. Infection occurring in one site is indicative of a sequestered lobe or an obstructive lesion.

A suspicion of an immune defect can be addressed by a two-step approach. The first includes a blood count and differential count to exclude numerical deficiencies in lymphocytes or polymorphonuclear cells. Serum quantitative immunoglobulins must be compared to age-appropriate controls because levels are low in the first few years of life. Isohemagglutinins (anti-blood group A or B substances) provide an easy measurement of endogenous antibody production. This can also be measured by specific antitetanus or antidiphtheria antibodies; and, if the child has had a booster shot, a rise in the titer can be expected. A low immunoglobulin level or a lack of response to tetanus or diptheria is an indication of an immune defect. Skin testing for cell-mediated responses can be done using intradermal injections of candida albicans antigen, mumps, streptokinase/streptodornase from streptococcal antigens. These are read at 72 hours. A measurement of serum complement is rarely indicated, because deficiencies are unusual. Complement defects are suggested by recurrent Neisseria infections and rheumatoid disease with recurrent infections. If the preliminary series of tests outlined is normal, one can assume that an immune defect is unlikely and observe the patient over several months. However, if there is an abnormality, the patient should have a full immunologic work-up included in the second step. The basic procedures are an enumeration of T cells and B cells and the evaluation of their function *in vitro*. This type of testing can be done at a high level of sophistication, and it is often possible to precisely delineate a defect.

TREATMENT AND MANAGEMENT

Acute episodes of infection should be treated with the appropriate antibiotic, and resistant organisms should be detected by cultures. In cases of persistent infection, unusual organisms can be considered and treated if found.

Structural defects can be treated where appropriate. A sequestered pulmonary lobe may be resected surgically; a foreign body can be removed from a bronchus or other obstructed site.

An underlying defect, such as an immune deficiency, requires an avoidance of risk situations. These children should avoid nursery schools and other known risk areas. Live vaccines should never be given because of the risk of disseminated viral infection. In patients with immunodeficiency, tetanus toxoid and diphtheria toxoid will not induce a response and should not be given. Whole blood must be avoided in patients with immune defects because of the risk of graft *vs* host disease. In this condition, the recipient who cannot develop an immune response is rejected by viable T cells that are infused with the whole blood. If blood must be given, only packed, washed red cells should be used.

Patients with panimmunoglobulin defects can be well controlled with replacement gamma globulin, given monthly at 100 mg/kg either by the intramuscular or intravenous route. Care must be taken even with new IV preparations, and blood pressure must be monitored since there is a risk of shock if the infusion is too rapid. IV infusion is best administered in a specialized clinical hospital setting. With cellular immune deficiencies, transplantation of bone marrow or thymus may offer a cure, but these circumstances are rare.

Prophylactic antibiotics are used for patients with immune defects where replacement gamma globulin therapy is insufficient or in other diseases that cause recurrent infections such as cystic fibrosis. It is best to rotate the drugs on a 4-month cycle. Trimethoprim–sulfamethoxazole is efficacious, especially in patients with hypogammaglobulinemia.

INDICATIONS FOR REFERRAL

When a physician suspects an underlying structural defect, an immunologic or other underlying disease such as cystic fibrosis, a referral to a specialist is appropriate.

ANNOTATED BIBLIOGRAPHY

Aytag A, Yurdakul Y, Ikizler C et al: Inhalation of foreign body in children. Report of 500 cases. J Thorac Cardiovasc Surg 76:145–151, 1977 (Good discussion of the spectrum of foreign body in the airway.)

Blazer S, Naveh Y, Friedman A: Foreign body in the airway: A review of 200 cases. Am J Dis Child 134:68–71, 1980 (Good discussion of the spectrum of foreign body in the airway.)

Buckley RH: Immunodeficiency. J Allerg Clin Immunol 72:627–644, 1983 (Well-referenced review.)

Fraser RG, Paré JAP: Pulmonary abnormalities of developmental origin. In Fraser RG, Paré JAP (eds): Diagnosis of Diseases of the Chest, pp 602–628. Philadelphia, WB Saunders, 1977 (Excellent review of sequestration and lung abnormalities.)

Gallin JI, Wright DG, Malech HL et al: Disorders of phagocyte chemotaxis. Am Intern Med 92:520–538, 1980 (Difficult reading, but a good discussion of the topic.)

Gotoff SP: The secondary immunodeficiencies. In Stiehm ER, Fulginiti VA (eds): Immunologic Diseases in Infants and Children, 2nd ed., pp 399–430. Philadelphia, WB Saunders, 1980 (Detailed review of diseases that cause infection by altering the immune function.)

Ross SC, Densen P: Complement deficiency states and infection: Epidemiology, pathogenesis and consequences of Neisserial and other infections in an immune deficiency. Medicine 63:243–273, 1986 (Review of recurrent Neisserial infections—good coverage of a difficult topic.)

Wilson CB: Immunologic basis for increased susceptibility of the neonate to infection. J Pediatr 108:1–12, 1986 (Discussion focused on group B streptococcus, herpes virus, and nonviral intracellular pathogens.)

182
Pain
RUSSELL S. ASNES

Among the first questions asked when eliciting the medical history of a sick or injured child is "Where does it hurt?" Pain is one of the most subjective symptoms. It is considered an important indication of the presence of tissue injury, which may be due to trauma, inflammation, or obstruction. Although most children experience pain as a manifestation of an acute illness, a significant number of children have chronic pain syndromes. By the time children enter early adolescence, 20% complain of frequent headaches, 10% to 15% complain of recurrent abdominal pain, and 15% experience intermittent limb pain.

Most physicians have the wish or the expectation that their patients will be able to define their pain in terms of its location, quality, intensity, periodicity, and duration. Furthermore, these physicians would like their patients to relate those factors that precipitate, intensify, and relieve their pain. The evaluation of the pediatric patient with pain presents the unique challenge that the symptom must be elicited and assessed within the context of a developmental framework. Children, particularly young children, lack the ability to describe pain in adult terms and thus the symptom is often difficult to assess. There have been various attempts to standardize the evaluation of pain in children and these have led to the development of instruments such as The Pediatric Pain Questionnaire, The Visual Analogue Scale or Pain Thermometer, and the Observational Distress Scale for Infants and Young Children.

It has been shown that a child's level of cognitive development directly influences or defines his perception of pain. The fetus will respond to noxious stimuli by withdrawal, and the newborn will exhibit several behavioral and physiologic responses when subjected to pain or discomfort. The pain reaction in infants between 3 and 12 months of age begins to become more localized, and by 1 year of age children can localize pain and have memories of painful experiences. However, the presence of irritability, restlessness, poor feeding, a particular cry, tachycardia, excessive sweating, and sleep disturbances may be the only indication that the infant or preverbal child is in pain. Preschool children are unable to relate their pain to their injury or illness and are incapable of understanding the reasons for their discomfort. When experiencing pain, particularly repetitive pain, they may become withdrawn, quiet, and clingy and they may exhibit other evidence of regressive behavior. Children may view pain in terms of punishment. (The word *pain* is derived from the Greek word *poine*, which means punishment.) It has been suggested that many children may suffer in silence because they believe that their pain is a result of having been bad. With the development of the ability to recall painful experiences, there is the evolving ability to anticipate painful experiences. This accounts for the resistance of many children between 1 and 3 years of age in coming to the physician's office. The child between 4 and 7 years of age will frequently respond to pain with increased anxiety and aggressive behavior. The school-aged child may be fearful of bodily injury and may tend to exaggerate minor bruises and injuries. By 7 years of age, an age that corresponds to Piaget's concept of the origin of concrete thinking, children are capable of a more logical and relative understanding that their pain is the consequence of injury or illness. For children between 10 and 12 years of age, a major component of their concept of pain may be their anxiety and fear of the loss of control.

There are several critical biologic, social, and psychologic variables that must be considered in the evaluation of a pediatric patient with pain. These variables include the child's age, sex, developmental stage, temperament, personality style, affective state, cultural background, past experiences with pain, and coexisting intrafamilial stresses. Most studies suggest that pain-prone families are more likely to have pain-prone children and that there is a clear relationship between maternal anxiety and the degree of distress experienced by children. Children tend to follow the family style of expressing and coping with pain. Thus, in some families, the children are encouraged to express pain and are provided with a "pain language" to express their symptoms. In other families, the expression of pain is considered a sign of weakness and the children are chided to "grin and bear it."

Studies have demonstrated that children experiencing painful illnesses, injuries, or procedures are less likely to receive attention to and treatment for their symptoms of pain than are adults in similar situations. Children receive fewer analgesics, at longer intervals and for shorter periods of time, than do adults. In addition, children who are unable or unwilling to communicate the extent of their discomfort are least likely to receive relief. Many medical personnel continue to believe that children do not experience pain with the same intensity as do adults, that children quickly forget painful experiences, that children recover more quickly and do not need pain control, and that narcotic analgesics should be avoided in children because they become addicted more easily than adults. These concepts have all been disproven.

Physicians and nurses need to have a high index of suspicion to determine if their pediatric patients are in pain and they need to be aware of the physiologic alterations that accompany pain, such as increased heart rate, respiratory rate, blood pressure, and sweating. They should not rely solely on children's complaints. A guiding principle in the prevention and relief of pain in children is that any procedure, injury, or illness that is painful for an adult will be painful for a child. It has been reported that the younger the child, the lower the pain threshold and the greater the sensitivity to pain.

NONPHARMACOLOGIC PAIN RELIEF

Children who have been provided with clear and realistic explanations about their illness and treatment have been shown to experience less pain and less anxiety. Most painful experiences that result from illness, injuries, and diagnostic studies can be anticipated. There are many excellent children's books available that describe common illnesses, what the child can expect in a visit to the doctor's office and hospitalization procedures. In addition, permitting parents to be present during medical procedures may contribute to pain relief or make the pain more tolerable.

The application of local measures to relieve and control pain is a component of the care repertoire of most parents. The use of a cold compress immediately after an injury and the subsequent application of warm soaks will usually provide temporary relief. Apley has suggested that the kiss and caress, among the oldest approaches to the treatment of pain, may help not only by providing compassion and security, but may also stimulate large afferent nerves and thereby modify pain transmission.

A variety of cognitive-psychological measures has been reported to lessen the fear and anxiety associated with expected and actual pain and thus help the child cope with the pain. Pain relief has been achieved through the use of transcutaneous nerve stimulation, biofeedback, and hypnotherapy.

Hypnosis is a specific behavioral method that has been used to reduce pain and anxiety experienced by children and adolescents during various medical procedures (*e.g.*, dressing changes in burn patients, bone marrow aspirations, and recurrent injections). Hypnotherapy has also been successfully used in patients with sickle-cell disease and asthma. Patients are taught how to narrow their attention, to limit awareness of peripheral stimuli, and to become so focused, concentrated, and relaxed that they are able to exclude specific stimuli. When a person is able to achieve this level of altered awareness, he is said to be in a hypnotic or trance state. In a trance state, the patient has no loss of consciousness and he is not asleep. He is in full control and can leave or come out of the trance state at will.

Approximately 60% to 70% of the general population can be successfully hypnotized and children have been shown to be more hypnotizable than adults. Children as young as 4 years of age can be taught the technique of self-hypnosis whereby they can learn to modify or ignore painful stimuli. Several excellent books and courses are available for those clinicians who wish to learn how to use hypnotic techniques in their practices.

PHARMACOLOGIC PAIN RELIEF

The usual prescribing practice of ordering analgesics *pro re nata* (prn) is both ineffective and impractical. Who is to determine when pain relief is needed? Children may lack the language facility to communicate that they are experiencing pain and to indicate the intensity of their pain. They may be unaware that relief is available or may be afraid that pain relief can only be provided by a "shot." Angell has suggested that pain dosing regimens be flexible, whereby the patient is asked at fixed intervals whether relief from pain is needed and is given the choice between a small or a large dose of medication. Analgesics are more effective when given when the pain is slight, rather than severe. This approach provides patients with some control over their treatment, which may have positive psychological benefits.

Aspirin

Aspirin, which has both analgesic and anti-inflammatory properties, remains one of the most effective medications for the treatment of mild to moderate pain. It exerts its action by repressing the synthesis of prostaglandins. Prostaglandins are released in tissue as the result of injury or inflammation and sensitize those nerve endings that relay pain signals. Aspirin reaches a peak level 2 hours after oral administration and has a half-life of 3 hours. The usual therapeutic dose is 10 to 15 mg/kg/dose and the therapeutic blood level is between 15 mg/dl to 30 mg/dl. Aspirin is available as tablets, chewable tablets, enteric-coated tablets, and suppositories. Suppositories, although widely used by parents, are less effective due to their unpredictable absorption. Until recently, aspirin was the analgesic most commonly used by parents for the treatment of pain. With the recent warnings and publicity suggesting an association between the use of aspirin in children with influenza and chickenpox and the development of Reye's syndrome, many parents have been reluctant or have refused to use aspirin under any circumstances or condition.

Acetaminophen

Acetaminophen is presently the most popular analgesic used for children. Although it is as effective as aspirin with regard to its analgesic properties, it has no anti-inflammatory activity and is thus less useful in the treatment of pain associated with inflammatory conditions. Acetaminophen does not have the gastrointestinal side effects commonly encountered with aspirin; it is rapidly absorbed; peak levels are achieved within 30 to 60 minutes; and it has a half-life of 2 to 5 hours. Acetaminophen is available in the form of drops, elixir, tablets, chewable tablets, and suppositories.

Codeine

Codeine is the preferred drug for the treatment of moderate pain that is not relieved by aspirin or acetaminophen. Codeine is available in both liquid and tablet dosage form and as a parenteral preparation for subcutaneous injection. When codeine is used in combination with aspirin or acetaminophen, its analgesic effect is potentiated. Codeine is well absorbed. Peak levels are reached 1 to 1½ hours after oral administration, and it has a duration of action of 4 to 6 hours. The dosage for analgesia is 3 mg/kg/day in 3 to 4 divided doses. Commonly encountered side effects are drowsiness, lethargy, apathy, nausea, vomiting, and constipation. Prolonged usage may produce physical dependence. Unfortunately, many physicians undertreat children with narcotic analgesics because they are afraid of overmedicating them.

Morphine

Morphine is the most effective analgesic for the treatment of severe pain. At therapeutic doses, it produces selective analgesia without altering the other senses. Peak levels are attained within 30 minutes following subcutaneous (SQ) or intramuscular (IM) administration and the half-life is 2 to 3 hours. The therapeutic dose is 0.1 to 0.2 mg/kg/dose administered every 4 hours. Paregoric, which is tincture of morphine, contains 0.4 mg morphine/ml and can be administered orally to infants and young children. Morphine should be used when control of severe pain is needed, but it should be used cautiously. Respiratory depression is a serious and potentially fatal side effect of overdosage in patients with compromised pulmonary function. The duration of treatment with morphine must be carefully monitored since tolerance and physical dependency are commonly encountered.

Meperidine

Meperidine (Demerol) is an effective analgesic, although it is not as potent as morphine. It has the advantage of oral or parenteral administration. The dosage is 1 to 1½ mg/kg/dose. Peak levels are reached within ½ to 1 hour after administration and its duration of action is 2 to 4 hours. Side effects are similar to those of morphine, although additional caution is needed with the use of meperidine in patients with sickle cell disease and renal failure, because it may induce seizures.

Nonsteroidal Anti-inflammatory Agents

Several nonsteroidal anti-inflammatory drugs have been demonstrated to have beneficial analgesic effects. However, these agents have no advantage over aspirin or acetaminophen and they are not approved for use as simple analgesics.

INDICATIONS FOR REFERRAL OR ADMISSION

It is difficult to offer specific guidelines regarding when or to whom a child with persistent, recurrent, or chronic pain should be referred or hospitalized. However, among the most important considerations in this decision making process are (1) the degree to which the clinician is confident with his understanding or diagnosis of the etiology of the patient's pain, and (2) the degree of dysfunction that the child or his family is experiencing from his symptoms. If the findings from the history, physical examination, or initial laboratory screening suggest a specific diagnosis, referral to a "specialist" might be appropriate. For example, if the child with recurrent abdominal pain has a history of intermittent diarrhea and weight loss, and he is found to have an elevated erythrocyte sedimentation rate, referral to a pediatric gastroenterologist for a further evaluation would be appropriate. Although many general pediatricians may feel confident and may have the knowledge and experience to manage their patient's specific condition, parents may request, or insist, on obtaining the advice of a specialist.

If there is a significant history of psychosocial problems that could be presenting as a somatic pain syndrome, referral to a psychiatric social worker, psychologist, or child psychiatrist could be of assistance to both the pediatrician and the patient.

If the history is confusing, the physical findings inconsistent, and the results of laboratory studies inconclusive, a brief period of hospitalization for the purpose of observation might be helpful. We can frequently learn a great deal by following Gellis' dictum: "Don't just do something, stand there . . . and observe and think."

ANNOTATED BIBLIOGRAPHY

Asnes RS: Pain in childhood. Pediatr Consult 4:1–8, 1985 (Helpful discussion of chronic pain syndromes and the assessment of the child in pain.)

Beyer JE, Knapp TR: Methodological issues in the measurement of children's pain. Children's Health Care 14:233–241, 1986 (Review of methods for measuring painful experiences by children. The validity of various instruments is described.)

Beyer JE, Beyer ML: Knowledge of pediatric pain: The state of the art. Children's Health Care 13:150–159, 1985 (Excellent review of pain as it relates to children's developmental stages and various approaches to pain management.)

Gardner GG, Olness K: Hypnosis and Hypnotherapy with Children. New York, Grune and Stratton, 1981 (Comprehensive review of the application of hypnotherapeutic technique to children.)

Jerrett MD: Children and their pain experience. Children's Health Care 14:83–89, 1985

Schechter NL: Pain and pain control in children. Curr Probl Pediatr Vol XV, No 5, May 1985 (Superb review of pain, including a discussion of the neurophysiology, assessment, psychosocial factors, clinical implications, and treatment of pain in children.)

183

The Overweight Child

EVAN CHARNEY

In a society obsessed with fitness and a sleek body image, the overweight infant, child, or adolescent may be presented for medical scrutiny and "therapy." Equally often, during child health supervisory visits the clinician may perceive medical or psychological problems related to the child's weight status that the family may have not considered to be a problem. In either case, the physician caring for children who are overweight has an important role to play. The first task is to identify those few children who have medical conditions associated with obesity and who need to be brought under therapy. For most of the remaining cases, the clinician needs to determine whether a problem exists, who the patient is, and how best to influence the body fat depot, the whole child, and the whole family.

PATHOPHYSIOLOGY

Obesity implies an excess of body fat rather than just increased body weight, which also reflects lean body mass. Ideally, the definition of what is excessive fat ought to be related to some pathologic condition that becomes manifest when the fat depot attains a certain mass. We could then comfortably identify which patient has the "disease" and proceed accordingly. In reality, there is no such point in overweight children short of morbid obesity, which may cause respiratory embarrassment. We are left with a statistical definition—those children at some arbitrary percentile or weight-for-height status are declared overweight or obese. Although there are many other biologic conditions that have a range of intermediate values bridging normality and disease (*e.g.*, hemoglobin concentration, blood pressure), the condition of overweight is a good example of labeling by statistics. Children with greater-than-average body weight have no significant morbidity in childhood. Their "disease" is based on two factors: they deviate from a socially defined ideal weight, and their condition has a well-defined risk of tracking into adulthood, where the hazards of overweight appear to be real.

The underlying pathophysiology of obesity is not well defined at present. Genetic factors are clearly important; for example, recent studies suggest that adult weight status of adopted children correlates more strongly with their biologic parents than with their adoptive parents. Twin studies show double the concordance rate for overweight among monozygotic compared to dizygotic twins. The physiologic mechanism by which this genetic tendency becomes manifest is less evident. A host of studies have failed to clarify whether obese children eat more and exercise less than their normal weight peers, although the preponderance of data suggest both to be the case to some degree. Once an individual becomes obese, little additional caloric intake is required to maintain that status, since the fat depot is not metabolically active. Can some aberration in metabolism account for obesity over and above a simple imbalance between calories ingested and energy expended? Differences between obese and lean individuals (and animals) in carbohydrate metabolism and energy storage have been described but may be evidence of a consequence rather than a cause of obesity. We are not yet at a point where metabolic or biochemical differences between those destined to be obese can be identified, much less subject to alteration.

CLINICAL PRESENTATION AND DIFFERENTIAL DIAGNOSIS

"If he looks fat, he is fat" may be a workable definition of adult obesity but it does not apply to children. Since the normal amount of subcutaneous fat and body muscle mass varies with age, the child who is at the 50th percentile for both height and weight looks quite different at different points in childhood. Thus, the premature infant appears thin

(the bulk of body weight is gained in the third trimester, most rapid linear growth in the second). The 6- to 12-month-old child has more subcutaneous fat than at any point before puberty, and therefore the "Buddha" appearance of late infancy is normal. Toddlers appear progressively thinner as linear growth rates stabilize at 2″ to 3″/yr while the rate of gain in weight progressively slows and the thickness of the subcutaneous fat layer actually diminishes. Children appear most lean at about 6 years of age and the chubby-appearing child at that age is usually markedly overweight. From age 5 or 6 years to the time of the adolescent growth spurt, both muscle mass and subcutaneous fat increase rapidly, and the preadolescent boy or girl normally has a chubbier or at least a stockier build. Both the family and clinician should distinguish these physiologic variations in the child's appearance from true deviations from normal.

There is no universally accepted definition of overweight or obesity in childhood because, as indicated, there is no identified weight status or body fat distribution pattern that correlates with a clear disease state. Weight-for-length percentiles (or merely a weight percentile greatly in excess of length percentile) are simplest to use. Some experts suggest the use of skinfold calipers, because triceps and subscapular skinfold thicknesses correlate reasonably well with total body fat measured by more precise means such as densitometry, K40 analysis, or prompt gamma ray emission methods. However, *fatfold thickness* is difficult to measure reliably by caliper in infancy or early childhood and may add more apparent than real scientific precision to what is a clinical estimate. For practical purposes, *overweight* can be defined as a weight 110% to 120% above the comparable weight for the child's height percentile, and *obesity* can be defined as a weight in excess of 120% of that figure.

Plotting the child's weight and height on the National Center for Health Statistics Growth Chart (published in 1976) is the first step. These most current growth standards can be applied in all American children if racial and genetic variations are taken into account. The rate of the child's weight gain and linear growth should track regardless of genetic factors between 2 years and adolescence.

If the child is of at least normal height for age and has had a normal growth velocity, endocrinologic abnormalities such as acquired hypothyroidism and Cushing syndrome are excluded, and thyroid studies and serum electrolyte values do not need to be obtained. In fact, most obese children have a somewhat accelerated linear growth that parallels their weight gain. If the child is of short stature and is hypertensive, then Cushing's syndrome should be ruled out. If the child is both short and mentally slow, the Prader–Willi or Laurence–Moon–Biedl syndromes should be considered.

WORK-UP

History

It is important to determine who the patient is. The physician should determine who wishes the child to lose weight (*e.g.*, one or both parents; the grandparents; or the child himself). Since family weight status is a strong predictor of the child's ultimate weight status, it is important to assess both parents' current weight and height and, if they are obese, when that condition developed. A family history of hypertension, noninsulin dependent (type II) diabetes, and cardiovascular disease should be obtained. The family's social class and educational level are worth noting because those factors correlate strongly with the child's ultimate weight status. Beginning just prior to adolescence in girls, there is a dramatic sorting out process: the prevalence of obesity increases among girls in the lower social class and diminishes among girls in the upper social class. That trend is both less marked and in the opposite direction for boys; richer boys (and their fathers) tend to be heavier; poorer boys (and their fathers) tend to be leaner. How are these data useful to the clinician? In the low income family, if the overweight mother or adolescent girl who is rapidly gaining weight are not concerned about weight status or even consider heaviness a desirable social trait, the clinician will have little influence. Intervention strategies are thus unlikely to succeed. Conversely, the thin affluent parents of the newly chubby preadolescent girl can be reassured that she will probably lose weight during or after adolescence, without any externally imposed diet. In fact, emphasizing her "overweight" status may only encourage a tendency toward anorexia or bulimia, which may pose more important health risks for her than obesity. The clinician should be alert to the preadolescent whose weight is "socially dissonant"; that is, the fat child in an affluent family of thin adults or the thin girl in a family of poor obese women. The obese child in a thin, upper income family will need support from the physician in the future to temper the alternating enthusiasm and despair associated with a series of dietary manipulations of varying degrees of rationality. Conversely, the slender girl in a low income family with many

obese adults may also need guidance and support regarding the normality of her body weight.

Physical Examination

A complete and careful examination is particularly important where weight and, by implication, health status are concerned. Both the parent and the child need to be reassured that all is well independent of weight, if that is the case. Blood pressure measurement and height and weight plotted on growth charts are essential. Further assessment of the obese child, who is less than 50% for height or who is developmentally slow, is indicated.

Laboratory Tests

Serum cholesterol and triglyceride levels should be obtained in children whose families have a strong history of cardiovascular disease. No other screening laboratory tests are necessary without a specific indication.

TREATMENT

"There is no known safe, effective, long-term treatment for obesity" is the summary of the 1981 Statement by the Committee on Nutrition of the Academy of Pediatrics. In 1985, the Committee concluded that "the long-term success rate for treatment of obesity is poor, and it remains to be seen whether efforts at prevention will be effective." No therapeutic modalities have been developed since then to alter the validity of those conclusions. Studies using behavioral techniques, particularly group programs involving the family, report encouraging weight reductions in children lasting 1 to 2 years; a longer follow-up on any large series is not yet available. There are no medications that will result in sustained weight loss in children (or adults). The use of thyroid hormone is both ineffective and potentially hazardous. Surgical techniques such as a gastric bypass or a jaw-wiring carry serious risks and are contraindicated in all but the morbidly obese patient; even in those cases, hazards are likely to outweigh benefits.

The physician who is confronted with a family concerned about the child's weight status is in a difficult position. We would like our overweight patients to lose weight, and if we had safe and effective therapy we would be overjoyed to prescribe it. The reality, however, is that current intervention strategies are not efficacious in perhaps 80% of cases. At best, these strategies may "help" 20%

and probably leave some patients more obese than before our intervention. In what other area of medicine do we recommend therapy for a clinical condition with unclear morbidity, where our intervention is usually ineffective and often leaves the child with the same problem but less self-esteem than he had prior to seeking our advice? Given this current reality, what help can we offer? The clinician can be an important resource in helping the child and his family cope with, if not "cure," the problem.

PRIMARY PREVENTION

Birth weight is not correlated with weight status in childhood or adulthood. Although the risk of early adult obesity is doubled if the infant exceeds the 90th percentile for weight in the first year of life, two thirds of heavy infants will be normal-weight adults. Since genetic factors are such a strong influence, the physician should consider offering anticipatory guidance when one or both parents are significantly overweight. Recommending breast-feeding, delaying the introduction of solids until 4 to 6 months of age, and, in bottle-fed infants, counseling the family against using the bottle as a pacifier seems reasonable advice, but it must be acknowledged that there is no good evidence that these strategies work. Skim milk formulas are contraindicated before 1 year of age, but a reduced fat milk thereafter is prudent for those at high familial risk of obesity. Counseling the family to offer the infant and toddler a balanced diet, with limited high caloric snack foods, may help establish appropriate eating habits while the child's intake is under the family's control. If, however, the parents are serious about limiting the risk of evolving obesity, a change in the entire family's eating habits may then be necessary. They will need to consider essentially excluding high-calorie snack foods from the home and setting the habit of eating only at the dinner table and only at meal times. Eating while watching television is another "high risk" habit that should be avoided, because long hours of television viewing have been associated with obesity in older children, probably from a combination of inactivity and increased snack food intake. Establishing patterns of regular family exercise (*e.g.*, bicycle riding, swimming, walking, and hiking) may be particularly worth cultivating in the child who is at a high risk of becoming obese. We must, however, be cautious in giving this advice to families because no clinical trials demonstrate the efficacy of these interventions (logical though they appear to be) and because excessive zeal may alienate the family and child

who will need our ongoing support. It would seem prudent to titrate the forcefulness of our primary prevention advice against the perceived risks. The family in which one or both parents are obese, particularly where early cardiovascular disease or type II diabetes is present, merits an attempt at intervention. Less advice is necessary or indicated when these conditions are not present. A cautionary note about excessive fear of obesity is in order: Some lean parents become concerned lest their normally growing child develops obesity, and they may interpret the appropriate chubby appearance of the 5- to 12-month-old child as pathologic. They need reassurance that their child is well.

SECONDARY PREVENTION

The age at which the child is obese is predictive of adult weight status. Perhaps one third of overweight infants are at risk (compared to 10% to 15% of all infants); ~40% of obese 7-year-olds and ~70% of obese adolescents will be obese adults, with the powerful influence of family factors increasing or decreasing that risk. Mild to moderately obese children should have no dietary limitations beyond a reduction of dietary fat (*e.g.*, use of low-fat or skim milk and a reduced intake of fried foods, gravies, salad dressings) and a restriction of high-calorie snacks. Family exercise patterns should be encouraged. At present, the physician must be cautious about casually prescribing more severe dietary interventions. They have not been successful, and the risk of beginning a life-time habit of alternating diet and normal eating with weight swings is of little value and may perhaps be harmful. The early adolescent who has just become overweight, particularly in a normal weight family, has the best prognosis, and no intervention is necessary. If more severe calorie-limiting diets are invoked, abundant daily protein intake (1 to 1.5 g/kg ideal body weight) is essential to limit the effect that all such diets have on linear growth. Family and group-based programs and those involving behavior modification measures are more likely to demonstrate short-term results (eat only at designated times, in designated places, and eat slowly). Weight control programs in middle school and high school have been attempted in some communities, involving dietary advice and exercise groups. The physician should be alert to the possibility that such programs may add to the social labeling (and further lowering of self-esteem) that is already the plight of the overweight child. Vigorous aerobic exercise programs in schools, unless part of a family pattern, are inappropriate, and no long-term benefits have been documented. For most obese children, a reasonable goal is the maintenance of weight status and the avoidance of a super-obese state, which is even more refractory to intervention.

The clinician's role with the obese child and family therefore transcends diet and exercise advice. As outlined, a complete history and physical examination are sufficient to rule out an underlying medical disease or to suggest that specific diagnoses be pursued. If the child is over 6 years of age and is not motivated to lose weight, individual dietary advice is inappropriate and alterations in the family's caloric intake and energy output are more appropriate subjects for discussion. Is the family using the obese child as a scapegoat for parental conflict? If this is the case, that conflict should be addressed. Perhaps we can be of most help by resisting the scenario in which the overweight (but otherwise low risk) child is labeled by the doctor as in need of treatment. Diet and exercise are prescribed and the child is told to return periodically for *checkups*. The high rate of failure of this approach means that the physician becomes one more authority figure, along with parents, friends, and gym teachers, who conclude that the child is abnormal. Moreover, when the child fails to lose weight or to sustain any weight loss, his inadequacy is further confirmed and a potentially supportive relationship with the physician is compromised. It may be more important to examine the child carefully, to reassure him of his basic normality and personal worth, and to offer to be available for guidance and advice over the years while he copes with the blizzard of advice on cures for his affliction. At present, the advice to "first do no harm" remains the most appropriate one in dealing with the overweight child.

ANNOTATED BIBLIOGRAPHY

American Academy of Pediatrics, Committee on Nutrition: Nutritional aspects of obesity in infancy and childhood. Pediatrics 68:880–883, 1981 (Balanced, authoritative, if gloomy, statement. See also American Academy of Pediatrics: Pediatric Nutrition Handbook, 2nd ed., pp 247–254, 1985)

Dietz W: Childhood obesity: Susceptibility, cause and management. J Pediatr 103:676–686, 1983 (Concise, clearly written review with dietary guidelines. See also the article by W Dietz and S Gortmaker on the fattening influence of television viewing. Pediatrics 75:807–812, 1985)

Freedman D, Burke G, Harsha D et al: Relationship of changes in obesity to serum lipid and lipoprotein changes in childhood and adolescence. JAMA 254:515–520, 1985 (As part of the Bogalusa Heart Study, an analysis of 1598 5- to 12-year-olds suggests that an increase in obesity over this time is accompanied by an increasingly atherogenic lipoprotein profile.)

Garn S: Continuities and changes in fatness from infancy through adulthood. Curr Prob Pediatr XV:4–47, 1985 (Thorough discussion of the epidemiology of overweight by an authority and scholar of the field.)

Malick M: Health hazards of obesity and weight control in children: A review of the literature. Am J Publ Health 73:78–82, 1983 (Critical and skeptical review concludes that further research is necessary before enlightened clinical practice is possible.)

Stunkard A, Sorensen T, Hanis C et al: An adoption study of human obesity. N Engl J Med 314:193–198, 1986 (Study of 540 Danish adoptees found that genetic factors are far more important than familial environment. See also article by Stunkard A et al: JAMA 256:51–54, 1986)

Weil W: Obesity in children. Pediatr Rev 3:180–189, 1981 (Well-outlined approach to appraisal and management, with guidelines on distinguishing simple obesity and endocrine disorders.)

184
Failure to Thrive
DONALD M. BERWICK

Failure to grow or to gain weight can be a consequence of the majority of major physical and psychological problems of infancy and childhood. When it is the presenting problem, therefore, failure to thrive (FTT) is a formidable diagnostic challenge for the pediatrician. An evaluation and management are further complicated by the strong feelings that can easily come to surround the child who is growing poorly: guilt and a sense of failure in the parents, anxiety and accusatory impulses in the professional caregivers, and, often, irritability or emotional unavailability of the child. The long-term consequences of severe growth failure are disturbing, and the diagnostic evaluation can easily be infused with a sense of urgency that poor growth is laying the seeds of more general future impairment.

An effective diagnosis and management of FTT depend on restrained, structured investigation, and strict attention to maintaining an alliance with the child's parents. The pediatrician must also remember that FTT rarely has a single cause in a particular patient, but rather results from many factors working together against adequate caloric intake and use. Approaching FTT with a search for a unitary cause will almost always lead to oversimplification and continued frustration.

PATHOPHYSIOLOGY

Failure to gain weight in children is usually due to problems in caloric balance: either failure to ingest calories, or failure to use calories, or excessive caloric loss. The exceptions include failure to grow due to genetic short stature, achondroplastic dwarfism, and prenatal insults, such as congenital rubella syndrome and fetal alcohol syndrome. These disorders affect skeletal growth and are associated with a failure in both weight gain and linear growth. On the whole, however, the forms of poor weight gain commonly encountered in the general pediatric practice involve excessive loss or inadequate intake of calories. Emotional deprivation syndromes, long known to be associated with FTT, impair physical growth both through decreased nutrition and through secondary disorders of endocrine function.

Caloric intake may seem adequate or even excessive in certain states involving hypercatabolism, malabsorption, or occult loss of nutrients. In these conditions, the diagnosis rests on discovering the source of an abnormally high calorie requirement or nutrient loss, such as chronic diarrhea or vomiting, celiac disease, or congenital heart disease.

Once the cycle of poor growth begins, secondary abnormalities may develop which aggravate the problem and may even confuse the diagnosis. Pituitary insufficiency, depressed levels of growth hormone, abnormal glucose tolerance, elevated liver function tests, retardation of skeletal development, and anemia may appear as secondary conditions in children with FTT, even when the growth failure has primarily psychosocial origins.

CLINICAL PRESENTATION

Despite its importance, FTT has no universally accepted clinical definition. Commonly, the label is applied to children below the third percentile of weight for age or with weights less than 80% of ideal for age. Some authors focus concern on children whose weights are "crossing percentiles"; thus, a child who has moved from the 50th to the 15th percentile of weight for age may be said to be *failing* to thrive. The use of growth chart criteria for FTT may be misleading for ethnic groups of characteristically short stature and thin build. In the end, the pediatrician's judgment must determine when to become concerned about a particular child, at least until clearer physical criteria emerge from future research.

Among hospitalized children with growth failure of any cause, FTT is a secondary consequence of a prior known disease in 70% to 90% of cases. Cardiac, neurologic, and gastrointestinal diseases, along with cystic fibrosis, lead the list of the underlying causes, and in these severe cases, the underlying disease is rarely subtle. With modern improvements in supportive technologies, the number of chronically ill children with special needs is increasing, and skill in managing nutrition, feeding strategies, and parental support and education are essential to good outcomes for these children.

Other case series report on children with FTT for whom no underlying disease is at first apparent and who are admitted to hospital for evaluation, sometimes after an extensive outpatient investigation. Such children tend ultimately to be placed in one of three diagnostic groups: (a) FTT on the basis of organic disease, (b) FTT on the basis of environmental deprivation, and (c) FTT without explanation. When a major physical disease is not the obvious cause of FTT, the clinical presentations of these three groups may be remarkably similar. Among children admitted specifically to find a cause for FTT, only about one third ultimately receive a specific organic diagnosis. No matter what the cause of the FTT, by the time FTT is severe enough to warrant hospitalization, many parents may have developed feelings of guilt or anger toward the child. These feelings may be reactions to the child's rejecting behaviors, a response to the common sense of helplessness, or signs of deficient emotional or physical resources for parenting. Physicians are unwise if they draw conclusions about the etiology of FTT from casual initial observations of parent–child interactions. No matter what the cause of FTT, the parent–child dyad may be dysfunctional by the time that a detailed evaluation begins.

DIFFERENTIAL DIAGNOSIS

The differential diagnosis of FTT is virtually the same as the list of all serious diseases of infancy and childhood. The underlying disease is readily apparent for most organic causes. Even for the child with an obvious major physical illness, however, such as a large ventricular septal defect, cerebral palsy, or multiple congenital anomalies, the diagnostic dilemma does not end with the labeling. The pediatrician should seek secondary causes contributing to growth failure, especially when the growth curve indicates a discontinuity in a child's usual growth pattern. When the trajectory of growth shows such an abrupt change, issues worth considering include superimposed metabolic burdens such as infection, gaps in parents' skills such as feeding techniques and selection of foods, superimposed social and emotional stresses in the family, and difficult developmental issues arising in the child around separation and individuation.

When the physical cause of FTT is not evident, occult and nonorganic causes must be considered, including primary breakdowns in environmental support for the child.The list of potential causes is long, but, in younger children if an organic disease exists, it is most likely to be one of a rather small set of possibilities. These include primarily gastrointestinal disorders, such as chronic diarrhea, chronic gastroesophageal reflux, malabsorption (primarily celiac disease), and, possibly, occult infection (primarily of the urinary tract). Occult cardiac, neurologic, renal, and endocrine diseases occur, but they are much less common. In inpatient series of children admitted specifically to evaluate FTT, generally about one third eventually receive an organic diagnosis, and over three fourths of these are gastrointestinal disorders.

Approximately 40% to 50% of children admitted to hospital specifically for an evaluation of FTT are assumed eventually to have primarily environmentally induced growth failure. Although formerly a diagnosis of exclusion, *nonorganic FTT* is now a diagnosis that the modern pediatrician should pursue actively in parallel with a search for organic disease. A sound classification scheme for failures of the child's environment is not yet available, but at least three general categories of disability in the parent–child dyads appear to lead to FTT. First, some children with nonorganic FTT have mothers with recent losses and acute, reactive depressions. Growth in these children is likely to be restored as the mother's depression resolves. Second, some children with FTT reside in homes characterized by some combination of chronic loss, social isolation, and poverty. Here, parental depression is more chronic and resistant to therapy and grieving processes, but parents remain emotionally concerned and positively disposed toward their children. The third group of children, for whom the prognosis may be worst, have parents with chronic problems in interpersonal relationships, not necessarily grounded in physical impoverishment, and who tend to see their children as "bad," "uncooperative," or otherwise causing their own growth failure. The boundary between FTT and issues of neglect and abuse is blurred for this minority of FTT families.

In inpatient series, nearly one fourth of children with FTT remain inscrutable even after an extensive evaluation. Many children within this group have genetic short stature; they are on their own genetic program; and they are really not failing to thrive. No cause of FTT whatsoever is identified for a substantial portion of the remainder.

Cross-sectional and longitudinal community-based studies of children with growth failure show a spectrum of final diagnosis quite different from that in hospital series. Children below the third percentile in a rural community, for example, who lacked an obvious organic disease, almost never received significant organic diagnoses later on which could have explained their poor growth. Controlled community-based studies are few, but it is likely that the office-based pediatrician will discover an occult organic disease in children with FTT far less frequently than is reported in a hospital-based series. In the primary care setting, skill in pursuing possible environmental issues actively is especially important. It is an error to seek environmental problems only after all possible organic diseases have been ruled out.

WORK-UP

History

An evaluation of a child with FTT is best guided by specific clues from a history or a physical examination, not by extensive laboratory screening. A careful history should seek prenatal and perinatal injuries, as well as signs of developmental delay. A family history may reveal a pattern of short stature, which can be highly reassuring in cases of equivocal severity. Efforts should be made to determine the stresses on the mother and family that may impede social interactions with the infant, and a detailed nutritional history may occasionally reveal aberrant feeding habits, which explain the growth failure directly. If the infant is exclusively breast-fed, a careful and supportive assessment of the nursing pattern is important, since, in a few instances, supplemental bottle feeding can provide a dramatic improvement in growth.

Physical Examination

A physical examination must begin with the careful measurement of length, weight, and head circumference. Children with genetic short stature will generally have concordant length and weight. A global judgment of the child's appearance is also sensible; a robust-looking small infant does not generally require a detailed investigation. Other specific clues to diagnosis can include a murmur or cyanosis suggestive of cardiac disease, cataracts suggesting congenital infection, a protuberant abdomen (classically associated with celiac disease, malabsorption, or cystic fibrosis), or signs of chronic respiratory disease. A neurologic examination may suggest previously undiagnosed cerebral palsy or other central nervous system problems.

One general principle in the examination of the child with FTT is that, despite anecdotes to the contrary, most organic disease severe enough to cause FTT will yield clues in a careful physical examination. FTT may be due to a truly hidden organic illness, but usually this is not the case. If an organic disease is present, it is likely to betray itself in a history or a physical examination.

Laboratory Tests

When the cause of FTT is not apparent, the diagnostic evaluation should be guided by the history and the physical examination. Laboratory fishing expeditions are unlikely to reveal problems that are not suggested by the history and the physical examination, and they will almost certainly lead the pediatrician down costly and uncomfortable blind alleys. The hazard is compounded by the many secondary biochemical and hematologic abnormalities that may derive from FTT. Mild elevations of liver enzymes, for example, are common, and work-ups usually lead nowhere.

Some basic laboratory studies are probably worthwhile in most cases and include hematocrit, urinalysis, urine culture, blood urea nitrogen or creatinine, serum calcium, and serum electrolytes. In high-risk populations, a tuberculin test should be performed, and, in older children, some experts suggest a thyroid function test. The remainder of the laboratory investigation should be guided strictly by specific clues from the history, epidemiologic circumstances, and physical examination.

In a carefully reported series of hospitalized children, organic disease is almost never discovered on the basis of laboratory testing alone, without prior clues on a history or a physical examination.

MANAGEMENT

Four important philosophies should guide the management of the child with FTT, and they apply equally well to FTT of organic and nonorganic origin:

1. Involve the parents in the process of diagnosis and treatment. The maintenance of this alliance is important whenever possible. Feelings of guilt in the parent and moral judgments by clinicians confound effective understanding and treatment. The pediatrician may need to spend effort helping other professionals to deal with their own countertransference reactions and impulses to judge apparently neglectful parents harshly.
2. Involve other disciplines. The demands of the child with FTT often go beyond the skills of the pediatrician to manage, and consultation with nutritionists, developmental specialists, mental health workers, and others may be important.
3. Take the long view. FTT is a chronic problem and is rarely simply "cured." In follow-up studies, about one third of infants with FTT are physically small as much as a decade later. In addition, half of the children in hospital follow-up series have behavioral or psychoeducational difficulties during latency and afterward.
4. Assume multiple causes. Growth failure involves self-sustaining cycles of cause and effect. Even for the child with an apparent singular cause of FTT, issues commonly arise in the emotional relationship between the parents and the child, in skills needed for appropriate feeding, in the effect of stress on the physical and emotional resources of the family, and in the ability of the family to use appropriate community supports. When growth fails, more than one cause is likely to exist.

One problem in managing infants with FTT arises in the exclusively breast-fed baby whose growth fails despite an adequate attempt at nursing with appropriate instructions to the mother. In such infants, supplemental feeding may be required in addition to breast-feeding. When this is necessary, the pediatrician must be particularly sensitive to the feelings of guilt and failure that can arise for the mother.

INDICATIONS FOR REFERRAL
OR ADMISSION

The use of hospitalization to assist in diagnosing FTT is controversial. Hospitalization is indicated usually only if the safety of the child is in question, or if special combinations of disciplines are required and can be assembled only inside the hospital. One theory suggests that organic FTT can be differentiated from nonorganic FTT by observing growth in the hospital; the child with an environmental deprivation will grow (according to the theory), while the child with an organic disease will not. Empirical evidence for the diagnostic value of in-hospital growth is sparse, and the in-hospital "trial period" should be used cautiously. When weight gain does occur in the hospital, it frequently does not begin until the second or third week of hospitalization, presumably when the child has become somewhat adjusted to the new surroundings. Observations of the child's behavior and of the parent–child dyad in the hospital can also be misleading. In some hospitals, special units exist to permit such observations to occur under circumstances that are especially comfortable for the parents and child, but the ambience of the average hospital is hardly designed to show parent–child interactions at their best.

On occasion, placement of a child with FTT outside of the home may be the only safe choice, especially when parents are clearly neglectful and unable to see themselves or their child as troubled, or when the child's physical condition poses parents with emotional and logistic problems beyond their capacities even with outside support. The decision is, of course, difficult and is best undertaken only with the deep involvement of appropriate social service agencies.

ANNOTATED BIBLIOGRAPHY

Berwick DM: Non-organic failure to thrive. Pediatr in Rev 1:265–270, 1980 (General review article, stressing the need for a systematic, targeted evaluation of children with FTT, instead of a dragnet of laboratory investigation.)

Berwick DM, Levy JC, Kleinerman R: Failure to thrive: Diagnostic yield of hospitalization. Arch Dis Child 57:347–351, 1982 (In a case series of 122 infants aged 1 to 25 months, admitted to a teaching hospital to evaluate FTT of obscure origin, 34% had no diagnosis even after evaluation, 32% received a social or environmental diagnosis, and 31% had a specific organic diagnosis. Organic disease usually offered a clue on history or physical examination.)

Kotelchuck M, Newberger EH: Failure to thrive: A controlled study of family characteristics. J Am Acad Child Psychiatr 22:322–328, 1983 (Compared with control families matched for SES, mothers of children with FTT perceived their infants as sickly and tended to perceive less positive support from friends and neighbors.)

Mitchell WG, Gorrell RW, Greenberg RA: Failure-to-thrive: A study in a primary care setting, epidemiology, and follow-up. Pediatrics 65:971–977, 1980 (One of the few studies of slow growth in a rural, primary care population. The problem seems less ominous and the outcomes more favorable than in the usual reports from referral hospitals.)

Oates RK, Peacock A, Forrest D: Long-term effects of nonorganic failure to thrive. Pediatrics 75:36–40, 1985 (Long-term follow-up of 14 children with FTT showed significant behavioral and intellectual problems 12 years later. This paper also contains an excellent review of the FTT follow-up literature.)

Pollitt E, Eicher A: Behavioral disturbances among failure to thrive children. Am J Dis Child 130:24–29, 1976 (Classic discussion of the possible causes and effect of disturbances of normal nurturance in infants with FTT.)

Rosenn DW, Loeb LS, Jura MB: Differentiation of organic from nonorganic failure to thrive syndrome in infancy. Pediatrics 66:698–704, 1980 (Effort to define the behavioral characteristics of infants with FTT of environmental causes, as distinguished from those with organic disease. The former preferred distant social encounters or inanimate objects; the latter responded more positively to close, personal interactions.)

Sills RH: Failure to thrive: The role of laboratory evaluation. Am J Dis Child 132:967–969, 1978 (One of the largest [185 subjects] and clearest published case series of children hospitalized to diagnose the reason for their FTT. Fifty-five percent received a nonorganic diagnosis, and 26% remained unexplained after evaluation.)

Dehydration is a relatively common clinical problem in pediatric practice resulting usually as a complication of gastroenteritis. Infants and young children are at particular risk for dehydration because of their small size and lack of free access to replacement fluids. The spectrum of dehydration ranges from mild dehydration, marked only by increased thirst and easily corrected with simple oral rehydration, to profound dehydration resulting in hypovolemic shock or major electrolyte abnormalities. In this latter state, there is a high risk of mortality or major morbidity either from the disease or from inappropriate management.

Over the past several decades the general approach to moderate or severe dehydration in children has been hospitalization and intravenous therapy. However, using extensive experience developed in Third World nations, oral rehydration with carefully formulated oral rehydration solutions is becoming more accepted in current American practice.

PATHOPHYSIOLOGY

Dehydration is characterized by an excessive loss of fluid from the body. The pathophysiologic processes and clinical presentation depend on the net composition of the abnormal losses (*i.e.*, the relative net loss of water and of solute [most importantly Na^+]). The net loss of these will result from the type of fluid lost (*e.g.*, diarrhea, gastric, third space) and by the type of oral fluids that have been given (balanced salt solutions, inappropriately hypertonic solutions, or hypotonic fluids). Other factors, such as small body size, an abnormal thirst mechanism, a lack of appropriate renal water reabsorption, tachypnea, a hot dry atmosphere, or limited water access may contribute to excessive losses of water over solute. Abnormal sweat electrolytes or endocrinopathies involving the mineralocorticoids may cause excessive solute loss. With dehydration the kidney attempts to reabsorb water by producing a concentrated urine, followed by oliguria as dehydration results in decreased renal perfusion.

Dehydration is commonly classified as hypo-natremic when the serum Na^+ is less than 125 mEq/L, isonatremic, when losses of salt and water are balanced, and hypernatremic when the loss of water is greater than the loss of Na^+ and the resultant serum Na^+ is >150 mEq/L. The terms *hyponatremic, isonatremic*, and *hypernatremic* dehydration are often used interchangeably with the terms hypotonic, isotonic, and hypertonic dehydration respectively. In actuality, if abnormal amounts of osmotically active agents, such as glucose or urea, or abnormal osmotic agents such as mannitol are not present, these terms may be roughly interchangeable, since Na^+ is the predominant osmotic agent in the extracellular fluid.

Isonatremic Dehydration

Isonatremic dehydration results in a loss of Na^+ and water in concentrations similar to that of the extracellular fluid. Thus, the fluid left behind will not be significantly altered in composition, although the total body Na^+ and water will be depleted.

Hyponatremic Dehydration

Hyponatremic dehydration results primarily in a depletion of the extracellular fluid. Water, which can freely pass through the cell membranes, moves from the now diluted extracellular fluid to the intracellular fluid. Thus, an early compromise of circulating blood volume occurs.

Hypernatremic Dehydration

Hypernatremic dehydration produces relative sparing of the extracellular fluid at the expense of intracellular fluid. With increased osmolality of the plasma and extracellular fluid, water moves out of the cells and into the extracellular fluid in order to try to equilibrate the differences in osmolality. With significant hypernatremia, cells generate *idiogenic osmols* that are thought to be primarily products of protein breakdown. These small molecules increase osmolality within the cells to help balance the osmolality differential and draw back the extracellular fluid.

Hypernatremic dehydration has a higher mortality rate and central nervous system morbidity (*e.g.*, seizures, hemorrhage, thrombosis) than hyponatremic or isonatremic dehydration. This may be due to a decreased brain volume and a rupture of blood vessels. In addition, if water is given too rapidly during attempted rehydration, water passes readily into brain cells that now have a higher osmotic load because of idiogenic osmol production. This results in swelling of these cells and cerebral edema. Pulmonary edema may also occur with rapid rehydration.

CLINICAL PRESENTATION

The best method of judging acute fluid losses is by serial weights or by a comparison to a recent weight. Since these data are often unavailable, estimates of the extent of dehydration can be made based on the physical examination. For any degree of dehydration, the physical examination may be altered in the presence of hypernatremia or hyponatremia. It is important to understand that 1% = 1 ml fluid/100 g body weight. Therefore, 1% dehydration indicates that the individual has lost 10 ml fluid/kg. An individual who is 5% dehydrated has lost 50 ml/kg.

Traditionally, dehydration is estimated and expressed as follows:

- <5% loss in body weight: slightly increased thirst, no change in physical examination
- 5% to 10%: moderate thirst, decreased urine production, irritability, dry mucous membranes, decreased tearing (normally newborn infants do not cry with tears). There is also tenting of the skin. Skin turgor is determined by pinching up on anterior abdominal wall skin. Normally, this skin rapidly retracts to its normal position. In dehydrated states it remains pinched up. Chronically malnourished children may have tenting in the absence of dehydration and older children may not have tenting when dehydrated. The anterior fontanel may be depressed.
- 10% to 15%: intense thirst, irritability or lethargy, absent tears, sunken anterior fontanel, decreased blood pressure, poor peripheral perfusion, pallor
- >15%: inability to maintain blood pressure

Because most of these physical findings result from decreased extracellular fluid, physical findings are greatest in hyponatremic dehydration for any degree of fluid loss. These patients may also have central nervous system symptoms with lethargy and seizures, but typically these do not occur until the serum Na^+ is <120 mEq/L.

Hypernatremic dehydration is primarily a loss of intracellular fluid; therefore, physical findings may not be as marked for any degree of loss of body weight. Because of the relative maintenance of circulating blood volume, they may not be as oliguric as infants with isonatremic or hyponatremic dehydration and shock is a late finding. These infants may be lethargic but when stimulated they become irritable with a shrill cry. They are hyperreflexic with increased muscle tone and may have seizures. The skin does not tent, but rather has a thick "doughy" feel. An intense thirst is usually present. Approximately one half have hyperglycemia and 10% are hypocalcemic, but only rarely are these clinically significant. As with any small, stressed infant with decreased glycogen reserves, infants with dehydration may also present with hypoglycemia.

DIFFERENTIAL DIAGNOSIS

It must first be determined that the child is dehydrated. Hypernatremia without dehydration, for example, can be caused by salt poisoning (*e.g.*, by incorrect preparation of powdered or concentrated formula or the feeding of inappropriately hypertonic fluids such as boiled skim milk). Water overload (pathologic water drinking or inappropriately dilute oral feedings) or excessive antidiuretic hormone (SIADH), a sequela of various pathologic processes, can cause hyponatremia without dehydration.

Once it is determined that the child has had adequate access to appropriate oral fluids, the cause of excessive fluid loss must be determined. Gastroenteritis with diarrhea and vomiting is the most common cause of excessive enteric losses. However, there may be other causes of excessive gastrointestinal losses such as structural gastrointestinal abnormalities. Examples include hypertrophic pyloric stenosis in young infants, malrotation, and intusussception.

A renal concentrating defect in which the kidneys cannot reabsorb water appropriately is another potential etiology of excessive water loss. Examples are central or nephrogenic diabetes insipidus and renal tubular acidosis.

The most common endocrinologic disease that can present with dehydration is diabetic ketoacidosis. The various salt-losing endocrinopathies such as congenital adrenal hyperplasia, Bartter's syndrome, and Addison's disease produce hyponatremia. Hyponatremia can also occur in cystic fibrosis with excessive Na^+ losses in sweat, and in renal diseases with salt wasting such as chronic renal insufficiency, and with chronic diuretic use.

WORK-UP

History

An accurate history is essential and should stress: (1) urinary frequency and volume (*e.g.*, do the diapers need to be changed as frequently as usual and when they are changed are they as heavy as usual? Frequent diarrhea may make urine production difficult to evaluate, however.), (2) urinary concentration (*e.g.*, does the urine smell stronger than usual?), (3) an estimate of stooling or emesis in terms of volume and frequency, (4) the child's mental status, and (5) most important, what the most recent weight has been. In addition, the physician should determine what fluids the child has been offered and how much he has taken.

Physical Examination

All dehydrated children should be weighed both to objectively assess the dehydration and to establish a baseline should their clinical status worsen. Vital signs must be obtained in all patients. Hyperpnea and tachypnea suggest that decreased tissue perfusion has resulted in metabolic acidosis. Decreased circulating blood volume causes tachycardia, which can exceed 200 beats/min in infants. It is not uncommon for small, stressed infants to become hypothermic after lying unwrapped on an examination table. Blood pressures should be obtained in all children considered dehydrated with an appropriate-sized cuff. If an automatic or auscultatory blood pressure is not obtainable, a systolic blood pressure should be determined by palpation. The inability to obtain a blood pressure reading may suggest hypotension or poor peripheral circulation. The extent of dehydration (*e.g.*, mental status, skin turgor, mucous membranes, anterior fontanel, peripheral perfusion, and peripheral pulses) should be evaluated. A careful examination of the abdomen should be performed to exclude signs of surgical disease, such as bowel obstruction and pyloric stenosis.

Laboratory Tests

The extent of laboratory investigation is largely dependent on the degree of dehydration. A urinalysis should be obtained. The specific gravity in the absence of glycosuria and proteinuria will indicate the severity of dehydration. Mild proteinuria may be present with significant dehydration. An alkaline urine with moderate to severe dehydration suggests renal tubular acidosis. Ketonuria and glycosuria are seen with diabetic ketoacidosis. Mild degrees of ketonuria are commonly seen in ill children who may not have been eating regularly. On microscopic examination there may be some cellular debris, but excessive cellular elements suggest the presence of renal disease. With moderate to severe dehydration, the physician should obtain blood for a laboratory evaluation. Electrolytes, BUN, and creatinine should be determined to aid in evaluating the degree of dehydration (hemoconcentration will result in elevated BUN). Blood glucose can be evaluated initially by a semiquantitative indicator strip rather than waiting for an official result from a laboratory. In infants with severe dehydration, an arterial blood gas should be obtained to determine if acidosis is present. If a renal concentrating defect is considered, serum osmolality can be measured and compared to urine osmolality.

THERAPY

The approach to the management of dehydration is changing from the use of intravenous fluids in hospitals to an approach that encourages oral rehydration. As more experience is gained with the latter method by American physicians, the oral approach will likely be increasingly used.

The first, and most critical step in managing a patient with dehydration is to assure an adequate circulating blood volume. The evaluation is based on a history and a physical examination. Inadequate circulating blood volume requires urgent intervention with intravenous fluids. If there is adequate peripheral circulation, therapy can be either by the oral or by the intravenous route (these will be discussed separately). It should be stressed that no matter which route is taken, clinical estimates of fluid and electrolyte requirements are only approximate and that with adequate renal function a general approximation of the degree of dehydration is sufficiently accurate.

Oral Rehydration

There has been a long and successful experience with oral rehydration solutions in Third World nations. Current recommendations are that these contain ~60 to 90 mEq/L Na^+, 20 mEq/L K^+, 30 mEq/L bicarbonate, and 80 mEq/L chloride. Citrate is often substituted for bicarbonate. Since sodium and glucose are transported on an equimolar basis, the optimal solution contains ~111 mMol/L glucose (equivalent to 2½% glucose); the final osmolality is 331 mOsm/L. It should be noted that this differs significantly from earlier oral electrolyte solutions available in the United States such as Pedialyte and Lytren, which had too much glucose, too little Na^+, and no bicarbonate and which were relatively hyperosmotic. These solutions have been reformulated to more closely approximate current recommendations. Commercially available flavored electrolyte solutions that are advertised for adults as sources of fluids and electrolytes are inadequate for oral rehydration in infants, having excessive glucose and inadequate sodium, potassium, and alkali (see also Chap. 106).

Intravenous Therapy

The specific requirements of intravenous fluid therapy depend on the degree and the type of dehydration. However, the emergency therapy of all three types is similar. The ongoing intravenous hydration of hospitalized patients is not discussed.

Emergency Considerations

An adequate circulating blood volume should be assured. Although the exact composition of the rehydration solution depends on the serum Na^+, isotonic fluids (normal saline or Ringer's lactate) can be given to any child with dehydration without worsening electrolyte imbalance. Thus, the initiation of therapy should not await the return of blood tests from the laboratory. Although adults often become hyperglycemic with stress, young children more commonly become hypoglycemic; thus, it is recommended that the first unit of fluid be D_5 normal saline or D_5 Ringer's lactate. Boluses of 10 ml/kg over 10 to 15 minutes can be given and repeated for a total of 20 to 30 ml/kg, depending on mental status, blood pressure, heart rate, and perfusion. As a rule, colloids (*e.g.*, albumin, plasma, dextran, hetastarch) are not necessary in the absence of hypoalbuminemia.

Although acidosis will resolve spontaneously with adequate fluid repletion, profound metabolic acidosis ($pH < 7.0$) should be treated with small amounts of bicarbonate (1 mEq/kg). Seizures may occur with hypernatremia or hyponatremia. Unlike hypernatremia, which needs to be corrected slowly, hyponatremia with seizures should be corrected

rapidly with 3% saline (513 mEq Na^+/L). Approximately 5 mEq/kg/hr can be given to rapidly bring the serum sodium to safe (but still low) levels. The Na^+ deficit (correcting to 125 mEq/L) in mEq is calculated as follows: (125 − patient's serum Na^+) × 0.6 × patient's weight in kg. 0.6 is the apparent volume of distribution of sodium. In treating hypernatremic dehydration, care must be given to avoid too rapid declines in serum Na^+. As discussed earlier, rapid infusion of dilute solutions can result in cerebral edema. Normal saline or Ringer's lactate is also used for acute repletion of intravascular volume. However, with hypernatremia, Ringer's lactate may be a better choice because it provides a lower chloride load. A serum sodium Na^+ of >180 mEq/L has a high incidence of central nervous system sequelae and emergency peritoneal dialysis should be considered.

INDICATIONS FOR ADMISSION

The development of specific oral rehydration fluids has allowed for the oral therapy of many children with mild to moderate dehydration who previously would have been admitted to a hospital for intravenous therapy. It is anticipated that an increasing acceptance of oral rehydration by the medical community and the increasingly cost-effective approach by third-party payers will encourage oral, outpatient therapy. There will always remain, however, a group of children in whom hospitalization will be indicated.

Hospitalization with intravenous therapy is indicated in the presence of shock, profound metabolic acidosis, and symptomatic hypernatremia and hyponatremia. Although oral rehydration has been used with adequate results for hypernatremic dehydration, until a further evaluation is available, intravenous therapy is probably indicated for moderate or severe hypernatremic dehydration. Serum Na^+ at high levels requires dialysis. Hospitalization may also be indicated if oral fluids cannot be tolerated either due to emesis or exhaustion. Finally, the physician must be comfortable that the infant's caretakers are capable of caring for and rehydrating the infant.

ANNOTATED BIBLIOGRAPHY

Feig PU, McCurdy DK: The hypertonic state. N Engl J Med 297:1444, 1977 (Excellent discussion of the physiology of the hypernatremic state.)

Hirschhorn N: The treatment of acute diarrhea in children. An historical and physiologic perspective. Am J Clin Nutr 33:637, 1980 (Review of the historical and physiologic rationales for oral rehydration.)

Segar WE: Parenteral fluid therapy. Curr Probl Pediatr 3:1, 1972 (Thorough discussion of intravenous fluid

therapy. Particularly good for its explanation of maintenance fluid therapy.)

Tamer AM, Friedman LB, Maxwell SRW et al: Oral rehydration of infants in a large urban U.S. medical center. J Pediatr 107:14, 1985 (American, urban experience with oral rehydration.)

186
Pallor
PAUL G. DYMENT

"Doctor, my child always looks so pale" is a refrain heard almost daily in a busy pediatric practice. Although frequently accompanied by other nonspecific complaints such as fatigue and listlessness, pallor may be the symptom of most concern to the parent because it is often considered synonymous with anemia and may indicate leukemia.

PATHOPHYSIOLOGY

A child may appear pale for many reasons. The manifestation of pallor can be affected by the state of vasoconstriction of the cutaneous blood vessels, by the presence of edema, and by anemia (*i.e.*, an insufficient amount of circulating hemoglobin in the blood). Children frequently appear pale if they are tired; if they have an acute respiratory or gastrointestinal infection; if they have minimal exposure to sunlight; and if they have a chronic infectious or inflammatory disease, even in the absence of anemia. Acute causes of pallor are usually obvious and patients generally have signs other than pallor that dominate the clinical picture.

CLINICAL PRESENTATION AND DIFFERENTIAL DIAGNOSIS

Probably the most common cause of pallor in pediatric practice is the presence of a fair complexion, which is frequently a familial trait. However, at least one pediatrician believes that food allergy ("the Great Masquerader") is the most common cause of a group of symptoms including pallor, fatigue, and nervousness. Crook reports his findings after having examined more than 4000 children in his practice in whom non-IgE mediated food allergy was the principal cause of this symptom complex (Crook, 1975). The actual prevalence of this

entity has been the subject of great controversy because many consider that it is overdiagnosed and infrequently encountered. What is accepted, however, is that atopic individuals often appear pale.

Anemia is the most frequent serious cause of pallor. Classical symptoms of anemia in children and adolescents include headache, palpitations, light-headedness, fatigue, and irritability. However, since profound anemia can occur even without these symptoms, a hemoglobin or a hematocrit should be obtained in children who could be anemic.

Many other diseases can cause pallor. Among the more common ones are chronic inflammatory diseases (*e.g.*, rheumatoid arthritis and inflammatory bowel disease), and chronic infectious diseases (*e.g.*, chronic pyelonephritis, cystic fibrosis, nephrosis, malnutrition, juvenile diabetes mellitus, uremia, and hypothyroidism).

The causes of pallor of acute onset are varied. Pallor from closed head trauma with any degree of severity and significant acute infectious processes such as acute pyelonephritis and bacteremia are commonly encountered in a busy pediatric practice. An acute blood loss or sudden hemolytic process even without shock causes pallor. Paroxysmal disorders such as seizures, breath-holding spells, and migraine often lead to or have associated pallor. Another common cause in an otherwise healthy child is a reaction to a DPT or DT immunization. This can be associated (but not necessarily) with screaming, fever, or hypotonia. In one British study of 10,000 children who received either of these immunization combinations, 10 children demonstrated an episode of acute pallor within 24 hours and from which they recovered quickly (Pollock, 1984). Syncope, hypoglycemia, and intussusception are less common, though not rare causes of pallor.

WORK-UP

The history should determine whether the pallor is acute or chronic; if the child is sick or well; and if the child has any of the aforementioned conditions associated with pallor. A complete physical examination should always be performed with careful attention paid to the complexion and general appearance of the child. For an initial physical assessment of anemia, the physician may compare the lividity of his palm to the patient's palm to see if pallor is truly present and to carefully look at the degree of pallor of the inferior palpebral conjunctiva. A clue to the diagnosis of food allergy or other atopic conditions is the presence of dark circles under the eyes (*allergic shiners*).

If the child has always appeared pale; if he is healthy and growing well; and if the complete physical examination is normal (the usual scenario), then a basic hemoglobin or hematocrit to rule out anemia is all that is indicated. A history suggestive of, or positive for, nonconstitutional factors (*e.g.*, failure to thrive) or positive physical findings (*e.g.*, edema, jaundice, chronic cough, arthritis, lymphadenopathy, splenomegaly) or a laboratory diagnosis of anemia, necessitates a further work-up that should be directed by the suspected diagnosis.

TREATMENT AND INDICATIONS FOR REFERRAL

A child who is pale on the basis of constitutional make-up needs only parental reassurance. As a general health recommendation and not expressly for the treatment of pallor, the child who stays indoors a great deal should be encouraged to spend more time outdoors. The diagnosis of milk allergy should be confirmed by the response of the symptoms to an elimination diet. If anemia is present, the specific cause of anemia should be treated. The urgency and extent of the work-up and management is largely determined by the severity of the anemia. Similarly, other conditions previously listed, if not of a transient nature, should be treated. Pallor immediately following minor closed head trauma and breath-holding spells may simply require reassurance, whereas other conditions may need to be treated as emergencies (*e.g.*, neurologic signs or symptoms resulting from head trauma, severe blood loss, shock, and serious infectious disease). These children will likely require immediate hospitalization, and the primary care physician may elect to consult with the appropriate subspecialist. It is advisable to have a subspecialist participate in the management of children with more complex chronic conditions such as uremia, cystic fibrosis, and nephrosis. A surgeon should be consulted if a potentially surgical condition, such as intussusception, is suspected.

ANNOTATED BIBLIOGRAPHY

Crook WG: Food allergy: The great masquerader. Pediatr Clin North Am 22:227–238, 1975 (Written by a general pediatrician with many years of office-practice experience. The points he raises are reasonable, and perhaps most physicians do underdiagnose food allergy.)

Pollock TM, Miller E, Mortimer JY et al: Symptoms after immunizations with DPT and with DT vaccine. Lancet 2:146–149, 1984 (This large prospective study of 10,000 children who received either of these vaccines showed no difference in the rate of acute reactions.)

Tunnessen WW Jr: Signs and Symptoms in Pediatrics, pp 60–62. Philadelphia, JB Lippincott, 1983 (Excellent outline of the acute and chronic causes of pallor.)

187
Syncope
PETER T. HEYDEMANN

Syncope is a common, potentially serious symptom that occurs in all age groups and has been estimated to occur in more than one quarter of adolescents. The term *syncope* is used to describe a rapid loss of consciousness and postural tone due to a sudden diminution in the brain's blood (or oxygen) supply. In addition to symptomatic treatment, the physician's major issues in evaluating a rapid loss of consciousness are determining whether the episode was due to a cause other than syncope (*e.g.*, epilepsy, hypoglycemia, or behavior and, if not, what specific factor predisposes the patient to syncope.

CLINICAL PRESENTATION AND PATHOPHYSIOLOGY

Since syncope is an intermittent phenomenon, the patient is usually without symptoms or signs in

Factors Predisposing to Syncope

VASCULAR—DECREASED VENOUS RETURN

Pregnancy
Anemia
Dehydration
Hypovolemia
Obstructive venous disease
Poor autonomic reflexes (*e.g.*, dysautonomia, neuropathy)
Spinal cord disease
Medications (*e.g.*, diuretics, phenothiazines)

VASODEPRESSOR SYNCOPE

Pain
Emotional shock

OTHER REFLEX SYNCOPES

Breath-holding spells (see Chap. 203)
Cough syncope
Micturition syncope
Defecation syncope
Carotid sinus stimulation

VASCULAR—ARTERIAL DISEASE

Subclavian steal syndrome

CARDIAC DISEASE—OBSTRUCTIVE

Hypertrophic aortic stenosis
Mitral stenosis
Cardiac tamponade
Tetralogy of Fallot

CARDIAC DISEASE—ARRHYTHMIC

Tachyarrhythmias
    Paroxysmal atrial tachycardia
    Prolonged QT syndrome
    Recurrent ventricular tachycardia
Bradyarrhythmias
    A-V conduction block (Stokes–Adams)

the doctor's office. Predisposing conditions may be apparent: heart disease, dehydration, anemia, or pregnancy (see the box, Factors Predisposing to Syncope). Orthostasis is a common element of many kinds of syncope.

There are four phases of syncope: a preceding event, the early symptoms, a loss of consciousness and postural tone, and the recovery period. Syncope is commonly preceded by an event or activity that causes destabilization of autonomic function or cardiac output. Such factors include sudden standing, an overheated environment, hyperventilation, pain, and emotional shock. Often more than one of

the preceding events will occur in combination. The early symptoms last a few seconds to several minutes. When they are brief, only a sense of lightheadedness and dimmed vision is noted along with pallor. If the early symptoms last longer, there is a sense of apprehensiveness accompanied by clammy perspiration and epigastric discomfort similar to nausea (but often distinct). Pallor is prominent, due to peripheral vasoconstriction, and is associated with an initial tachycardia and pupillary dilation (similar to the fight or flight reaction). An urge to urinate or defecate is often noted. The patient may feel the need to lower his head to aid cerebral blood flow. Visual blurring and clouded consciousness occur as the tachycardia gives way to a slowing of the heart rate. If the attack is not interrupted, a loss of postural tone and consciousness ensue. The unconsciousness commonly lasts only 10 seconds and ends when the blood pressure and cerebral blood flow are re-established. Awakening is accompanied by pallor, mild confusion, and unsteadiness, which lasts seconds to minutes. This should be distinguished from the more prolonged postictal state following a generalized seizure.

If cerebral blood flow is not re-established quickly, then convulsive syncope may occur. A loss of postural tone is protective in syncope because the patient falls, which lowers the head and allows the low systemic blood pressure to reach the cerebrum more easily. Thus convulsive syncope is more likely to occur when the patient is prevented from falling because he is seated in a chair, standing in a phone booth, or being held upright by a parent or bystander. The convulsion has all the typical characteristics of a grand mal seizure and may be associated with incontinence of the bowel or the bladder and a more prolonged postictal state.

As indicated, the pathophysiology of syncope relates directly to the effects of decreased arterial blood flow on the cerebrum. There are 3 major mechanisms of diminished blood flow: (1) cardiac disease including arrhythmias and outflow obstruction; (2) vascular disorders generally resulting in inadequate venous return to the heart; and (3) reflex syncopes, most commonly vasodepressor syncope. With cardiac syncope, a decreased rate or stroke volume results in syncope when effective circulation to the brain cannot be maintained. Exercise is frequently the stimulus that brings on cardiac syncope.

Vascular disorders causing syncope are predominantly arteriolar and venous, but may rarely involve the great arteries. When there is ineffective venous return to the heart, due either to hypovolemia or overexpansion of the peripheral vascular bed, syncope may result from the consequent diminished cardiac output. The act of rising to a standing position is frequently the final event that aggravates the already diminished venous return and results in orthostatic syncope. Hypovolemia should never be overlooked because it is common and easily treated. An unusual arterial vascular disease is known as *subclavian steal syndrome*. It is due to proximal obstruction of the subclavian artery and consequent shunting of blood from the brain to the arm by way of the ipsilateral vertebral artery, especially during arm exercise.

Vasodepressor or vasovagal syncope is the most common of the reflex syncopes. The actual reflex arc is complex. An emotional shock or surprise is interpreted rapidly by the limbic system and results in a vasomotor outpouring that causes marked peripheral vasodilation, particularly in the mesenteric and skeletal muscle beds. Thus, total systemic peripheral resistance suddenly drops. Cerebral perfusion cannot be maintained because cardiac output does not increase appropriately to compensate. Although increased vagal input to the heart may be the reason that a compensatory tachycardia does not occur, atropine does not abolish vasodepressor syncope. Like all other syncopes, it is aggravated by the upright posture. Other reflex syncopes, with varying mechanisms, include cough, micturition, and defecation syncopes, in addition to pallid breath-holding spells of infancy.

DIFFERENTIAL DIAGNOSIS

When a patient faints, syncope is only one of several diagnostic alternatives. Epilepsy, hypoglycemia, basilar artery migraine, hyperventilation spells, and hysteria are the primary alternatives. In addition, vertigo may be confused with presyncopal lightheadedness.

Akinetic seizures and complex partial seizures may produce a sudden loss of postural tone and a clouding or loss of consciousness. These spells are not consistently related to activity or postural changes. Like syncope, akinetic seizures (or drop seizures) may have a minimal postictal state; however, akinetic spells seldom have premonitory symptoms such as lightheadedness. Complex partial (psychomotor) seizures may include such premonitory symptoms (though rarely the whole group of "early symptoms"), but sudden loss of postural tone is a rare occurrence. In addition, primary grand mal seizures must be differentiated from seizures secondary to syncope. In one series, more

than 50% of original diagnoses of primary epilepsy were later changed to syncope (see also Chap. 146).

Just as syncope results from an inadequate supply of the substrate oxygen, hypoglycemic attacks result from inadequate supply of the substrate glucose. Hypoglycemic attacks share certain characteristics with syncope: pallor, perspiration, abdominal discomfort, lightheadedness, confusion, unconsciousness, and seizures may occur in both. Hypoglycemic attacks are more gradual in onset and recovery (unless glucose is administered, in which case recovery is more rapid); they do not occur during or soon after meals; and the presyncopal symptoms do not improve with supine or Trendelenberg posture.

Basilar artery migraine, a variety of classic migraine, may occur with abdominal discomfort, dizziness, visual symptoms including "blackout," and a loss of postural tone. The nonsyncopal symptoms of tinnitus, scotomata, vomiting, and true vertigo may occur during the early attack. Postural changes do not affect symptoms. After the early symptoms, a headache is prominent (though not necessarily in each individual attack), and most patients prefer to sleep. A family history of migraine is common (see also Chap. 145).

Hyperventilation spells are a variety of syncope because intense cerebral vasoconstriction is part of the pathophysiologic process. The typical spell consists of a feeling of apprehensiveness with deep sighing respirations that are often unnoticed by the patient. Such spells are similar to slow onset syncopal attacks in that patients may note abdominal discomfort, palpitations, lightheadedness, and (rarely) loss of consciousness. The same emotional situations that sometimes produce syncope may also result in hyperventilation spells. Supine posture may improve symptoms in hyperventilation attacks primarily because lying down helps a patient to relax and reverse the anxiety–hyperventilation cycle.

Episodic behavior simulating fainting may occur as a conscious act or as a subconscious conversion symptom (hysteria). The pace of onset of symptoms varies, but is often faster than typical syncope and without the usual premonitory findings. Pallor and hypotension are not part of the attack. Since most presyncopal symptoms are subjective, a sophisticated teenager may give an accurate syncopal history; however, the history is often accompanied by an indifferent affect. The spells generally last longer than brief syncopal spells, and there may be unusually good recall of events during the period of "unconsciousness." These spells occur typically in an emotionally charged setting; they do not relate consistently to postural changes; and they are rare before 10 years of age. Diagnosis is often difficult and may require hospitalization with electrophysiologic and video monitoring.

Vertigo and the presyncopal symptom of lightheadedness are often confused. A postural change may bring on either of these symptoms, and pallor, unsteadiness, and nausea-like symptoms may accompany both. Vertigo consists of a sensation of the room moving around the patient; in addition, any movement may aggravate the vertiginous feeling, not simply movement to an upright posture as is common in lightheadedness. Children are often unable to make such a distinction, and the diagnosis of vertigo in preschool children is difficult.

WORK-UP

History

An accurate and detailed history surrounding the syncopal event is the key to a proper diagnosis. Crowds, overheated environments, emotionally loaded settings, prolonged prior bed rest, and the physical activity and posture of the patient are critical points. Most syncope occurs either with prolonged immotile upright posture or a change to an upright posture. If the spells occur during vigorous exercise, a cardiac origin of the syncope should be thoroughly evaluated. The patient's sequential sensations at the onset of the spell should be elucidated with special reference to dizziness, lightheadedness, confusion, awareness of surroundings, tingling, palpitations, involuntary movements, abdominal discomfort, perspiration, and aberrations of the special senses (auditory, visual, and olfactory). With regard to the period of apparent unconsciousness, questions should focus on the length of the spell, awareness of surroundings and ongoing events, posture, skin color, body movements, incontinence, and self-injury such as biting. After the period of unconsciousness, the nature and time course of the recovery period should be evaluated. It is often important, in fact critical with small children, to speak to the most reliable person who observed the spell, such as a school teacher. This may necessitate making several telephone calls to get the most accurate history.

Physical Examination

In the majority of syncopes, the physical examination is normal. Nevertheless, a careful search must be made for abnormalities to help define a specific cause. An evaluation for cardiac disorders is particularly important because of the possibility of sudden death. It is essential to examine the pulse rate and rhythm as well as blood pressure for orthostatic changes. Orthostasis is evaluated supine and again after standing for 15 seconds and 120 seconds. A drop of more than 15 points in systolic pressure is abnormal, especially if there is a failure to increase heart rate in compensation. Observation of the general body habitus is important in looking for the asthenia of adrenal insufficiency, along with the associated increased palmar pigmentation. Mucous membranes and skin turgor must be checked for hydration status. Pallor of the lips or palpebral conjunctivae indicates anemia. The examination for cardiac disease is important. Conditions that decrease stroke volume such as aortic stenosis, pulmonary stenosis, carditis, and pericardial effusion should be carefully evaluated. Weakness of peripheral pulses may indicate focal obstructive vascular disease, such as seen with a unilaterally decreased radial pulse in the subclavian steal syndrome. The physician should pay particular attention to the possibility of pregnancy, a common predisposing condition for syncope. Evidence of neuropathy, spinal cord disease, bulbar disease, or movement disorder must be sought by an observation of gait and movements and an examination of cranial nerves and deep tendon reflexes. Thus, muscle wasting, hyporeflexia, hyperreflexia, and gait or postural abnormalities may indicate an underlying neurologic disease.

Laboratory Tests

The laboratory work-up may range from minimal to extensive. In the case of an otherwise healthy teenager who faints immediately after getting an emotional shock, an ECG may be the sole laboratory evaluation if the physical examination suggests no clues to an underlying disorder. When an otherwise healthy teenager, who is mildly dehydrated, faints when standing, it is reasonable to perform no laboratory evaluation and simply suggest rest and oral rehydration. At the other extreme, if the teenager has fainted many times during exercise, an exhaustive laboratory search for cardiac disease must be made. When the spells are repetitive and their nature is unclear, it may be necessary to perform detailed testing to differentiate syncope from the alternative causes of brief spells listed above. A detailed first visit laboratory work-up *might* include: ECG, chest roentgenogram, electrolytes, fasting blood sugar, hemoglobin, and

EEG. A subsequent work-up becomes more detailed and directed toward particular suspicions. Along with a cardiac consultation, Holter monitoring, exercise testing, cardiac echogram, and cardiac catheterization (for His-bundle study or angiogram) may become necessary. In the differential diagnosis of epilepsy, 24-hour ambulatory EEG may be helpful if a spell can be elicited; prolonged simultaneous video-EEG-ECG monitoring is even better. A neurologic consultation will be helpful. A further neurologic work-up may include a CT scan of the brain and, less commonly, spine roentgenograms, nerve conduction study, electromyogram, magnetic resonance imaging of the spine, myelogram, and measurement of blood catechols.

MANAGEMENT

The treatment for simple vasovagal syncope is patient education and reassurance. The patient must avoid obvious predisposing circumstances, such as prolonged standing in an overheated environment or rising rapidly from a warm bathtub. While keeping in mind that exercise syncope may suggest cardiac disease, susceptible athletes and others prone to dehydration should focus on preventive fluid intake. When the early presyncopal symptoms are noted, it is essential not to ignore them as the self-conscious teenager is likely to do. The head must be lowered by lying down or flexing the head and body forward in an effort to increase cerebral blood flow. The patient with a history of syncope during venipuncture should always have the procedure performed supine. Tensing one's muscles provides further protection against syncope by increasing the vascular resistance in the skeletal muscle bed.

Other treatment depends on individual circumstances, and *correctable primary disorders must be addressed*. For instance, anemia, dehydration, and cardiac arrhythmia have specific treatments. Predisposing medications may be withdrawn or substituted. Cough syncope may be controlled by addressing the causes of a chronic cough, such as asthma.

In frequently recurring pallid breath-holding spells, atropinic agents may be used. The patient who faints due to hyperventilation must be taught consciously to slow the respiratory pattern, to relax, and to use a paper bag for rebreathing. Propranolol has been used effectively for hyperventilation when simple measures were ineffective.

When syncopal episodes persist with no obvious cause despite these simple measures, then symptomatic management to increase venous return to the heart is indicated. Elastic stockings aid venous return from the legs. In addition, fluorinated mineralocorticoids are used to expand plasma volume.

ANNOTATED BIBLIOGRAPHY

Beder SD, Cohen MH, Riemenschneider TA: Occult arrhythmias as the etiology of unexplained syncope in children with structurally normal hearts. Am Heart J 109:309, 1985 (Emphasis on the diagnosis of arrhythmias as a cause of syncope.)

Boudoulas H, Weissler A, Lewis R, Warren J: The clinical diagnosis of syncope. Curr Probl Cardiol October 1982 (Thorough discussion of syncopal mechanisms with emphasis on cardiovascular mechanisms.)

Gastaut H: Syncopes: Generalized anoxic cerebral seizures. In Vinken and Bruyn (eds): Handbook of Clinical Neurology, Vol 15, pp 815–835. Amsterdam, North–Holland, 1974 (Discussion of syncope with focus on neurologic aspects and pathophysiology.)

Joorabchi B: Expressions of hyperventilation syndrome in children. Clin Pediatr 16:1110, 1977 (Interesting discussion of the findings in hyperventilation syndromes and the use of propranolol in refractory cases.)

Katz RM: Cough syncope in children with asthma. J Pediatr 77:48, 1970

Ormerod AD: Syncope. Br Med J 288:1219, 1984 (Presents an interesting algorithm to the approach of syncope.)

Sapire D, Shah J, Black I: Prolonged atrioventricular conduction in children and adolescents—the role of increased vagal tone. South African Med J 55:669, 1979 (Prolonged A-V conduction is often normal, and vagal tone plays an important role in prolonged A-V conduction.)

Sledge W: Psychological factors in the onset of vasovagal syncope. Psychosom Med 40:568, 1978 (Discusses psychological circumstances in individuals who have recurrent vasovagal syncope.)

188
Edema

JODY R. MURPH AND
JEROLD C. WOODHEAD

Edema, which may be generalized or localized to one region of the body, represents an abnormal accumulation of fluid within the interstitial space. Its presence may be indicative of several disease states.

PATHOPHYSIOLOGY

Fluid volumes within the intravascular and interstitial compartments maintain equilibrium only when capillary membrane permeability is intact and a balance exists between plasma oncotic pressure and intravascular hydrostatic pressure. Interstitial fluid accumulates when oncotic pressure decreases or when capillary membrane permeability or hydrostatic pressure increases. Edema forms as fluid escapes from the intravascular space to the interstitial space within the capillary bed. In healthy children, colloid oncotic pressure, produced by plasma proteins, is exceeded by hydrostatic pressure at the arterial end of the capillary bed and causes movement of fluid into the interstitium. The reverse occurs at the venous end of the capillary bed where hydrostatic pressure is less than oncotic pressure and fluid is reabsorbed. Fluid movement is normally balanced and there is no net change in fluid volumes. A shift in this equilibrium causes localized or generalized interstitial fluid accumulation; edema develops.

Increased hydrostatic pressure accompanies several disease states including congestive heart failure, constrictive pericarditis, and portal hypertension. In these situations edema forms because the force driving fluid out of the vascular compartment is greater than the oncotic force that promotes fluid reabsorption. Decreased oncotic pressure occurs in illnesses characterized by protein loss such as nephrotic syndrome or protein-losing enteropathy.

Increased capillary permeability may play a role in the formation of edema, which occurs as a result of allergic reactions, hereditary angioneurotic edema, chemical or thermal injury, and certain infections such as Rocky Mountain spotted fever. Localized edema may occur more commonly in disease states associated with altered capillary permeability than with altered hydrostatic or oncotic pressures.

Renal handling of sodium and water also plays a role in the development of edema. Approximately two thirds of the glomerular filtrate undergoes obligatory reabsorption in the proximal tubule. Excretion or reabsorption of the remainder of the filtrate is regulated by the action of aldosterone and antidiuretic hormone in the distal tubule. Excretion of these hormones is altered in certain disease states such as congestive heart failure, cirrhosis, and the nephrotic syndrome, thereby contributing to edema formation.

DIFFERENTIAL DIAGNOSIS

Localized edema may result from discrete areas of altered capillary permeability (e.g., an insect bite) or may be one of the first manifestations of a systemic illness that produces a generalized edema (e.g., nephrotic syndrome). The periorbital area is particularly predisposed to edema formation because of the low tissue tension that allows the ready accumulation of interstitial fluid. Acute glomerulonephritis, nephrotic syndrome, Rocky Mountain spotted fever, angioneurotic edema, serum sickness, congestive heart failure, and hypothyroidism may all cause periorbital or more generalized edema. Periorbital edema, as a localized reaction, may also occur with sinusitis, scarlet fever, infectious mononucleosis, roseola, conjunctivitis, orbital or periorbital cellulitis, conjunctival foreign body, insect sting or bite, and local allergic reaction. Other forms of localized edema include mumps-related edema of the anterior chest wall, pretibial edema of hypothyroidism, edema of the hands and feet in newborns with Turner syndrome or Milroy disease, and in older children with sickle cell anemia (hand–foot syndrome) or Kawasaki disease, and edema of the forehead or scrotum in Henoch–Schönlein (anaphylactoid) purpura.

Generalized edema or anasarca (edema plus ascites) may occur at any age and may result from disease processes in several organ systems. Cardiovascular causes of generalized edema include congestive heart failure, pericardial effusion, or constrictive pericarditis. Gastrointestinal disorders may produce edema by protein malabsorption (*e.g.*, cystic fibrosis) or protein loss (*e.g.*, protein-losing enteropathy, celiac disease, ulcerative colitis, regional enteritis, and chronic infection or infestation, such as Giardiasis, with severe or chronic diarrhea). Hepatic causes include biliary atresia, Chiari syndrome, cirrhosis, hepatitis, hepatic failure, and portal hypertension. Nutritional deficiencies of protein (kwashiorkor), vitamin C (scurvy), and vitamin B_1 (beriberi) produce generalized edema. The infant with severe anemia may develop edema, and edema is the primary clinical feature of the newborn with hydrops fetalis. Collagen vascular diseases and systemic allergic reactions may also produce generalized edema, as may drugs such as oral contraceptives and other steroids.

Renal protein loss causes the most commonly seen form of edema in childhood. The combination of massive proteinuria plus edema, hypoalbuminemia, and hypercholesterolemia constitutes the nephrotic syndrome and represents the end result of various different pathologic processes within the kidney. Minimal change nephrotic syndrome (also called idiopathic nephrotic syndrome) is the most common form of nephrotic syndrome in children. Features that distinguish minimal change nephrotic syndrome include (1) age of onset between 1 and 9 years (most commonly between 3 and 6 years), (2) normal serum complement, (3) absence of persistent hematuria, hypertension, or reduced renal function, and (4) response to prednisone therapy. Other causes of nephrotic syndrome in children include acute gomerulonephritis, focal glomerulosclerosis, membranoproliferative glomerulonephritis, the nephritis of lupus erythematosis, and numerous other types of nephritis.

WORK-UP

Children present most commonly with localized edema associated with minor trauma, infection, or allergic reactions. Generalized edema, although more uncommon, may represent a serious systemic disease, often cardiovascular or renal in origin. The extent of edema, its duration and associated signs and symptoms direct the physician's approach to the edematous patient.

History

Parents may not remember the onset of edema unless the physician focuses attention on rapid changes in clothing size, such as shoes that have become suddenly tight or belts or pants that have become too small. Complaints of puffiness of the eyes, protuberant abdomen, or swollen labia or scrotum may lead to the diagnosis of generalized edema.

Localized edema should prompt the physician to identify the etiology such as trauma, insect bite, burn, foreign body, and infection. Generalized edema demands a more comprehensive history. Diarrhea or other alteration in stool quantity or quality may suggest a gastrointestinal disease. A change in urine volume or color may suggest a renal etiology. Rapid heart or respiratory rate, decreased exercise tolerance (often noted by parents as fatigue or inability to keep up with peers), shortness of breath, or a persistent cough may indicate congestive heart failure. In infancy, however, irritability, tiring during feeding, and restlessness while supine or prone may be the presenting feature of congestive heart failure, long before edema is evident. A history of a rash may suggest infectious or collagen vascular etiology. Drug ingestion, either prescribed or illicit, may be associated with edema because of idiosyncratic, allergic, or toxic causes. Cyclical edema may occur in adolescent girls because of premenstrual fluid retention; or edema may relate to oral contraceptive use. Pregnant adolescents may complain of dependent edema in the second and third trimester.

The child with generalized, persistent edema has an increased risk of infectious complications. Immunoglobulin loss in addition to altered cellular host-defense mechanisms caused by increased interstitial fluid and ascites predisposes to soft tissue or intraperitoneal infection.

Physical Examination

Although localized edema would appear to result from a truly local phenomenon, the physician should be alert for findings that suggest a more generalized process such as periorbital edema without obvious local irritation. Bilateral involvement of extremities also suggests a more generalized process. Generalized edema, especially anasarca, is easily detected. An evaluation of a child with this degree of edema must include careful attention to weight and vital signs including pulse and respiratory rates, temperature, and blood pressure. A weight change gives the best indication of fluid retention. Orthostatic changes in blood pressure suggest serious depletion of intravascular volume and potential for shock. Hypertension may occur in some edematous states in response to the disease process or as a response to contracted intravascular volume. The presence of a pulsus paradoxus of more than 12 mm mercury suggests pericardial tamponade or constriction. A fever must prompt a thorough search for infection, and likewise for local areas of tenderness and erythema. Tachypnea and respiratory distress, rales, wheezes, and areas of diminished breath sounds may indicate pneumonia or pulmonary edema. Abdominal fluid is obvious when a fluid wave can be produced in a distended abdomen. Lesser degrees of ascites present as dullness to percussion. Abdominal tenderness suggests peritonitis, but rebound tenderness may be absent, difficult to elicit, or delayed in appearance when ascites is present. Scrotal and labial edema may cause marked enlargement and discomfort. In the presence of edema, cyanosis, jugular venous distention, hepatomegaly, and petechiae or purpura may be ominous signs.

Laboratory Tests

A history and a physical examination allow the formulation of a differential diagnosis which, in turn, determines the laboratory evaluation. Suspicion of a cardiac etiology should prompt a chest roentgenogram that may demonstrate an enlarged heart, pulmonary edema, the "bag of water" silhouette associated with hemodynamically significant pericardial effusion, or calcifications in the cardiac shadow suggestive of constrictive pericarditis. The electrocardiogram may reveal arrhythmias or may support the diagnosis of pericardial effusion with low-voltage QRS complexes. Echocardiography has become the preferred diagnostic tool for the detection of pericardial effusion and many other cardiac disorders.

Since renal disease is the leading cause of generalized edema in children, a urinalysis is mandatory. Proteinuria greater than $1+$ (30 mg/dl) on a dipstick evaluation of a random urine specimen should prompt a repeated urinalysis. With persistent proteinuria on random urine specimens, a timed 12- to 24-hour urine sample should be collected for protein quantification. More than 150 mg protein in 24 hours is generally considered abnormal, although some growing adolescents may spill up to 300 mg protein in 24 hours during their rapid growth spurt. Children with edema caused by renal protein loss typically have proteinuria >50 mg/kg/24 hours (usually more than 2 g total in 24 hours). Because protein loss decreases oncotic pressure, intravascular fluid depletion may occur and reduced circulating volume may cause diminished renal per-

fusion. Renal function may consequently decline. Endogenous creatinine clearance should be determined whenever 24-hour urine collections are made so that renal function may be assessed (see Chap. 116 for a complete discussion of proteinuria). Hematuria, when associated with proteinuria and edema, is indicative of active inflammation within the kidney and suggests causes other than minimal change nephrotic syndrome. Serum total protein and albumin, electrolytes, creatinine, urea nitrogen, cholesterol, and complete blood count should be performed. All children with generalized edema should also be screened for collagen vascular and immune complex mediated diseases with antinuclear antibody, C_3 and C_4 complement components, and antistreptolysin O titer (or similar streptococcal antibody screen) determinations. Sickle cell screening, intravenous pyelogram, and renal biopsy may be selectively indicated.

Other laboratory tests such as liver enzymes, cultures of blood, urine, stool, wounds, and pharynx, and tests of gastrointestinal function are reserved for specific clinical settings.

MANAGEMENT

The therapy for edema should, if possible, be directed towards a resolution of the underlying disease state. Edema caused by localized processes may respond to topical measures such as the application of ice, heat, or steroid cream, or the elevation of an edematous extremity. Antihistamines, aspirin, nonsteroidal anti-inflammatory agents, or antibiotics may be indicated in specific instances. When localized edema results from systemic illness, therapy aimed at the illness may reduce the edema.

The management of generalized edema must be directed at its cause, but some generalizations apply. Fluid restriction is unnecessary in most instances and is difficult to enforce outside of the hospital. When fluid *must* be restricted, water intake should be reduced to a volume equal to the child's daily insensible water loss plus urine output. Insensible water loss is age dependent, ~30 ml/kg/24 hours in the 1- to 3-year-old child, 20 ml/kg/24 hours in the 3- to 10-year-old child, and 15 ml/kg/24 hours in the child over 10 years. Fever and elevated respiratory rate increase insensible water loss.

Salt restriction greatly aids in the control of edema. Severe restriction leads to poor dietary compliance and promotes "cheating." The best compliance is associated with a no added salt diet. Parents should be instructed to cook family meals without added salt, to remove salt shakers from the table, and to avoid foods high in salt, such as processed meats, pickles, certain cheeses, and snack foods including salted potato chips, pretzels, and nuts.

Diuretics may provide some relief of generalized edema but cannot be considered a definitive therapy. Diuretics may actually be detrimental when edema results from decreased plasma oncotic pressure because interstitial fluid accumulates at the expense of intravascular volume. The diuretic action may not produce the desired diuresis when the intravascular volume is depleted, thus prompting an increase in subsequent doses. Continued high-dose diuretic therapy in this situation may result eventually in a severe depletion of intravascular fluid, and shock may ensue. Cautious use of diuretics requires a prior assessment of serum proteins and an estimation of intravascular depletion. In general, when serum albumin is below 2.5 g/dl, and when anasarca is present, the intravascular fluid volume will be depleted and the use of potent diuretics will be dangerous unless accompanied by intravenous colloid. In situations such as nephrotic syndrome refractory to steroid therapy, the combination of furosemide plus intravenous salt-poor albumin produces effective diuresis and temporary reduction of edema. Such therapy requires hospitalization and close supervision.

Since minimal change nephrotic syndrome represents one of the most common causes of generalized edema seen in an office-based practice, the subsequent discussion of the management of edema is directed toward this entity. The details of management for other causes of generalized edema are beyond the scope of this text because most require referral to specialists or hospitalization.

Corticosteroids are the mainstay of therapy for minimal change nephrotic syndrome. Children who meet the clinical criteria discussed in the section on differential diagnosis may be started on corticosteroid therapy without a prior renal biopsy and without a referral to a pediatric nephrologist. For this form of nephrotic syndrome, the management of the disease process is synonymous with the management of edema.

Minimal change nephrotic syndrome typically responds to prednisone therapy within 4 weeks. Diuresis, cessation of proteinuria, and resolution of edema occur in 95% of children treated with steroids. The initial treatment is usually with prednisone, 60 mg/m^2/day (or 2 mg/kg/day) with a maximum daily dose of 60 to 80 mg. Prednisone is divided into 2 equal doses daily and is continued for 4 weeks. At the end of 4 weeks, if the nephrotic syndrome has resolved, prednisone should be switched to an every-other-day schedule with 60 mg/m^2/day of prednisone (maximum 60 to 80 mg/day) given as a single, morning dose, on alternate days, for an additional 4 weeks. Finally, prednisone should be tapered over a 3-week period at a maximum rate of 20 mg/week.

A relapse occurs in ~80% of cases and is often associated with a mild, intercurrent infection. A relapse is defined as proteinuria >2+ (100 mg/dl) on dipstick of random urine specimens for 3 consecutive days and is accompanied usually by the recurrence of edema.

To treat a relapse, prednisone (60 mg/m^2/day, maximum 60 to 80 mg/day) should be given, in divided doses until edema has resolved and urine is protein-free (or has at most trace protein on dipstick) for 7 *consecutive days*. Alternate day prednisone as a single dose is then given for 1 week, followed by a slow tapering at a rate of 10 mg/week.

Infection may be difficult to detect and may have a serious outcome in children with anasarca. Signs of the inflammatory process may be blunted and may delay the identification of an infection. A history of fever in an edematous child should prompt an evaluation for potentially serious infection. Abdominal pain and erythema or increasing pain or discomfort at sites of minor trauma may also indicate infection. Peritonitis caused by many different types of bacteria, including *Escherichia coli* and *Streptococcus pneumoniae*, occurs with increased frequency in patients with anasarca. This is a serious complication that requires the identification of the infecting organism by abdominal paracentesis with a culture and a Gram's stain. A child with anasarca and peritonitis should be hospitalized in a center with pediatric intensive care facilities where intravenous antibiotics can be administered and the patient carefully monitored for evidence of overwhelming sepsis.

INDICATIONS FOR REFERRAL

Indications for referral to a pediatric nephrologist include (1) failure to respond to initial or relapse treatment after 1 month of high-dose daily prednisone, (2) frequent relapses (defined as 3 or more relapses/year), (3) inability to maintain a remission without steroid therapy, (4) signs of steroid toxicity (*e.g.*, growth failure, cataracts, hypertension, marked Cushingoid changes), (5) children for whom the cause of edema is not obvious or whose clinical presentation is complicated. Such patients may require renal biopsy or treatment with cytotoxic medications such as cyclophosphamide. In addition, children with serious infectious complications of nephrotic syndrome, such as peritonitis, may require a referral to a center with pediatric intensive care facilities.

ANNOTATED BIBLIOGRAPHY

Boyer JL, Lewy JE: Pathogenesis and treatment of edema in infancy and childhood. In Moss AJ (ed): Pediatrics Update: Reviews for Physicians, 1984 ed, pp 281–292. (Review of pathophysiology of edema and mechanism of action of commonly used diuretics.)

Holzgreve W, Holzgreve B, Curry CJR: Nonimmune hydrops fetalis: Diagnosis and management. Semin Perinatol 9:52–67, 1985 (Review of the etiology, diagnosis, and management of nonimmune hydrops fetalis.)

International Study of Kidney Disease in Children: The primary nephrotic syndrome in children. Identification of patients with minimal change nephrotic syndrome from initial response to prednisone. J Pediatr 98:561–564, 1981 (Presents guidelines for diagnosing MCNS.)

Lewey JE: The pathogenesis of edema in renal disease and other disorders affecting the kidney. In Edelmann C (ed): Pediatric Kidney Disease, pp 315–324. Boston, Little Brown, 1978 (Excellent general reference. See also pp 452–457 for management.)

McEnery PT, Strife CF: Nephrotic syndrome in childhood: Management and treatment in patients with minimal change disease, mesangial proliferation, or focal glomerulosclerosis. Pediatr Clin North Am 89:875–893, 1982 (Pathogenesis, evaluation, and management of nephrotic syndrome with extensive references.)

Oliver WJ, Kelsch RC: Nephrotic syndrome due to primary nephropathies. Pediatr in Rev 2:311–317, 1981 (Excellent overall review of the nephrotic syndrome.)

Paller MS, Schrier RW: Pathogenesis of sodium and water retention in edematous disorders. Am J Kidney Dis 2:241–254, 1982 (Extensive review of edematous disorders.)

Sugel W, Goldberg B, Krassner LS, Hayslett JP: Long-term follow-up of children with steroid-responsive nephrotic syndrome. J Pediatr 81:251–258, 1972 (Discussion of steroid therapy modifying the natural history of minimal change disease.)

189
Cyanosis
VICTOR C. BAUM

Cyanosis, derived from the Greek *kyanos* or blue substance, results from an excess of desaturated hemoglobin. Cyanosis depends on the presence of a critical absolute amount (not percent) of desaturated hemoglobin. This is often said to be 5 g/dl desaturated hemoglobin. However, with careful observation, cyanosis can be detected in the presence of only 3 g/dl desaturated hemoglobin. Cyanosis is usually categorized as *central* or *acrocyanosis*. With central cyanosis, there is excessive desaturated hemoglobin in arterial blood in all areas of blood flow that can be observed (*e.g.*, skin, lips, tongue, and oral mucosa). Acrocyanosis is the result of an excessive removal of oxygen from localized distal areas of the circulation (*e.g.*, hands, feet, and perioral area).

PATHOPHYSIOLOGY

The hemoglobin level and the oxygen–hemoglobin dissociation curve may affect whether cyanosis is present at any particular arterial Po_2.

Hemoglobin Level. A lower blood hemoglobin requires a higher percent desaturation in order to result in a total of 5 g/dl desaturated hemoglobin. A higher blood hemoglobin level can have 5 g/dl desaturated hemoglobin with a higher percent saturation. For example, a profoundly anemic individual with a total blood hemoglobin of 5 g/dl (hematocrit about 15%) might never be visibly cyanotic, no matter how desaturated the blood became. On the other hand, a polycythemic individual with a hemoglobin of 20 g/dl (hematocrit about 60%) could have an oxygen saturation of 75% to 85% (15% to 25% desaturation) and be cyanotic.

Oxygen–hemoglobin Dissociation Curve. This curve relates oxygen saturation of hemoglobin (in percent) on the y-axis to Po_2 on the x-axis and results in the well-known sigmoid-shaped curve. A left-shifted curve results in a higher hemoglobin saturation for any given Po_2. Thus, cyanosis will only become apparent at a lower Po_2. Factors that shift this curve to the left include *decreased* Pco_2, *decreased* temperature, *decreased* levels of, or affinity for, 2,3-DPG, and fetal hemoglobin. Neonates will become cyanotic at lower Po_2 levels than older individuals with predominantly hemoglobin A.

Although decreased oxygen saturation of arterial blood can be the result of a variety of factors, cyanosis results from one of the following five pathophysiologic mechanisms:

1. Alveolar hypoventilation: While decreased ventilation of the lungs can result in hypoxemia, the primary effect of alveolar hypoventilation is an increase in arterial carbon dioxide content (hypercarbia).

2. Right to left shunt: In right to left shunting, systemic venous blood bypasses ventilated alveoli and returns to the left side of the heart or the aorta without being oxygenated. The site of shunting can be intracardiac (*e.g.*, tetralogy of Fallot), at the great vessel level (*e.g.*, pulmonary hypertension with shunting through a patent ductus arteriosus), or intrapulmonary with perfusion of nonventilated areas of the lung. The individual responds to hypoxemia with hyperventilation in an attempt to maintain arterial P_{O_2}. The arterial P_{CO_2} is usually lower than normal.

3. Ventilation/perfusion (V/Q) mismatch: Normally, within the lung, areas of decreased ventilation are matched with decreased blood flow. Abnormal oxygen saturation can result if this relationship is altered.

4. Impairment of diffusion: Before hemoglobin can be oxygenated, oxygen molecules must diffuse from the alveoli into the pulmonary capillaries. Anything that interferes with this diffusion will affect oxygenation of hemoglobin.

5. Decreased affinity of hemoglobin for oxygen: Since cyanosis depends on the presence of desaturated hemoglobin, the presence of an abnormal hemoglobin with decreased affinity for oxygen at any given P_{O_2} can result in cyanosis. Oxygenation of hemoglobin can occur only when the iron atom is in its ferrous (Fe^{2+}) state. There is normally a small production of hemoglobin with iron in the ferric (Fe^{3+}) state that is unable to bind with oxygen and is termed *methemoglobin*. This is reduced back to the ferrous state by the enzyme methemoglobin reductase. An excessive production of methemoglobin results in cyanosis and may be produced by exposure to various agents including nitrobenzene, aniline dyes, acetanilid, chloral hydrate, amyl nitrite, and even "exposure" to carrot juice and other sources of dietary nitrites. A functionally abnormal methemoglobin reductase can be inherited as an autosomal recessive trait. Certain abnormal hemoglobins, referred to as the *hemoglobins M*, in which a specific amino acid substitution in either the α or β globin chain prevents the return from the ferric to the ferrous state, result in methemoglobinemia. In addition, several other rare hemoglobins have decreased oxygen affinity. Since infants normally have a low level of methemoglobin reductase, they are particularly prone to the induction of methemoglobinemia when exposed to potentially toxic agents.

Acrocyanosis is typically due to pooling of blood in the extremities resulting in increased local extraction of oxygen from hemoglobin. Thus, it can be the result of any factor that slows blood flow through the affected tissues such as poor cardiac output, vasoconstriction, or peripheral vascular disease. Increased venous pressure can also result in decreased local blood flow with venous suffusion and cyanosis.

CLINICAL PRESENTATION

The presence of central cyanosis is always pathologic. Acrocyanosis may be a normal finding. Newborn infants typically have cyanotic hands and feet during the first day of life. Infants may have cyanosis of the hands and feet when cold and may have a bluish color in the perioral moustache and goatee areas with crying.

Dark skin or lip color can sometimes make a diagnosis of cyanosis difficult at marginal levels of desaturated hemoglobin. The tongue and oral mucosa should always be examined in children with heavily pigmented skin.

The clinical presentation depends on whether cyanosis is acute or chronic. The age at onset depends on the underlying lesion. Children with acute cyanosis may present with tachypnea and metabolic acidosis from decreased oxygen delivery. They have normal hematocrits. Children with chronic cyanosis are often well compensated and stable. They become polycythemic as a response to the decreased oxygen saturation of their hemoglobin. Children with chronic cyanosis typically develop clubbing (hypertrophic osteoarthropathy) of the fingers and toes after 1 to 2 years of age. Clubbing can, however, be due to noncyanotic causes and can be familial. Children with chronic cyanosis can grow and develop surprisingly well, particularly if they are not in congestive heart failure. However, right to left shunting predisposes to two potentially catastrophic complications: cerebral thrombosis (stroke) and brain abscess. Cerebral thrombosis occurs most often in children less than 2 years of age. The viscosity of blood increases markedly above a hematocrit of ~65%, resulting in the sludging of blood in small vessels. This hyperviscosity is exacerbated by anything that makes red blood cells stiffer, such as iron deficiency. Brain abscesses occur in ~2% of children over 18 months of age with cyanotic congenital heart disease. Although children with chronic cyanosis are frequently thrombocytopenic, this is rarely severe enough to result in nonsurgical hemorrhagic complications.

Many children with cyanotic congenital heart defects present in the newborn nursery with cyanosis. Others present with a later onset of cyanosis. There may be adequate shunting through a patent ductus arteriosus to prevent visible cyanosis until the ductus arteriosus closes at about 7 to 14 days of age, at which time they become profoundly cyanotic. Other cyanotic congenital heart defects, such as tetralogy of Fallot or the Eisenmenger syndrome, may not develop enough right to left shunting to result in cyanosis until several years of age.

Because of their relative frequency, the cyanotic spells associated with tetralogy of Fallot deserve special mention. These "tet spells," in which children frequently squat down, can be the first symptom in a child with tetralogy of Fallot who has not previously been cyanotic. They often first occur in the early morning after awakening. These children develop anxiety, hyperpnea, cyanosis, and a softening of their murmur. If allowed to progress, irritability, lethargy, loss of consciousness, and even death can ensue. When the episode resolves, the child returns to his previous state without any changes in cardiac or mental status.

DIFFERENTIAL DIAGNOSIS

Although cyanosis is usually a consequence of cardiac or pulmonary disease, disorders in other organ systems must be considered in the differential diagnosis. Numerous specific pulmonary diseases and cardiac malformations can result in cyanosis (see Chap. 54 for a more complete discussion on cardiac causes).

The various diagnoses that should be considered derive from the pathophysiologic mechanisms discussed earlier:

1. Alveolar hypoventilation: Airway obstruction, either congenital or acquired (e.g., aspiration of a large foreign body), space-occupying thoracic lesions (e.g., pneumothorax or diaphragmatic hernia), decreased lung volume (e.g., congenitally hypoplastic lungs), decreased pulmonary compliance (e.g., pulmonary edema), neuromuscular disease resulting in weakness of the respiratory muscles, central nervous system abnormalities affecting control of respiration (e.g., seizure activity, infection, trauma, depressant drugs, breath-holding spells)

2. Right to left shunt: Congenital heart disease, pulmonary hypertension with a ductal shunt (e.g., persistent fetal circulation also termed persistent pulmonary hypertension), pulmonary disease with atelectasis, pulmonary arteriovenous fistula

3. Ventilation/perfusion mismatch: Respiratory distress syndrome, asthma, pulmonary aspiration, drugs that abolish pulmonary hypoxic vasoconstriction (e.g., isoproterenol, dopamine, inhalational anesthetics)

4. Impairment of diffusion: Pulmonary edema, certain uncommon pulmonary alveolar diseases, central nervous system diseases resulting in neurogenic pulmonary edema

5. Decreased affinity of hemoglobin for oxygen: Exposure to toxic substance as described under pathophysiology, absent or functionally abnormal methemoglobin reductase, presence of an abnormal hemoglobin

The age of development of cyanosis with the hemoglobinopathies depends on the specific defect. Abnormalities of the α-globin chain present with cyanosis at birth. Infants with β-globin defects may not develop cyanosis until the β-chain becomes predominant over the fetal γ-chain during the first year of life. Methemoglobinemia results in a more grayish-blue or slate-gray color than does typical cyanosis.

A useful mnemonic to remember the major cyanotic lesions is the five Ts: Tetralogy, Transposition of the great vessels, Truncus arteriosus, Total anomalous pulmonary venous return, and Tricuspid atresia. With the addition of pulmonary atresia, with or without ventricular septal defect, most of the cyanotic lesions are represented.

Sepsis, polycythemia, hypoglycemia, and hypocalcemia must also be considered in the cyanotic newborn.

The differential diagnosis of acrocyanosis includes any cause of decreased cardiac output as well as cold and polycythemia. Acrocyanosis is typical on the first day of life.

Although cyanosis is almost always due to organic illness, breath-holding spells in young children can result in cyanosis. These children have violent crying followed by apnea, cyanosis, and hypotonia. There is a prompt resolution without sequelae and these episodes are rare after 3 years of age.

WORK-UP

History

It should be determined whether the cyanosis is of chronic or recent onset. A full prenatal and neonatal history should be obtained. A congenital heart defect that results in a murmur in the neonatal period may be responsible for the development of cyanosis many months later. A history of squatting or early morning cyanosis suggests the possibility of tetralogy of Fallot. Evidence of a pulmonary infection should be investigated. The possibility of drug ingestion or foreign body aspiration should be considered. A family history is also important. A family history of congenital heart disease raises the likelihood of congenital heart disease as an etiology and a family history of chronic cyanosis may suggest a hemoglobinopathy.

Physical Examination

Acrocyanosis and central cyanosis should be differentiated by evaluating the extremities and oral mucosa. In acrocyanosis the blood that immediately refills a compressed extremity will not be cyanotic. Children with borderline contents of desaturated hemoglobin have a plethoric look before frank cyanosis develops. The physician should consider a shunt at the level of the ductus arteriosus if there is differential cyanosis in the young infant (upper *vs* lower extremities), which may be made more obvious by breathing supplemental oxygen. Methemoglobinemia results in a more slate-gray color rather than the typical blue of cyanosis. Evidence of respiratory distress (*e.g.*, nasal flaring, grunting, retractions, crackles, wheezing, or stridor) suggests airway or pulmonary disease whereas tachypnea without dyspnea suggests a cardiac or metabolic etiology. The presence of a murmur may be helpful, but serious cyanotic congenital heart disease may not be associated with a murmur, and children may develop very loud functional murmurs when stressed (Fig. 189-1).

Laboratory Tests

Any child in whom a diagnosis of congenital heart disease is considered should have an electrocardiogram and a chest roentgenogram. However, the electrocardiogram may be normal for age in newborns with certain congenital heart defects. The chest roentgenogram should be evaluated for cardiac size and shape, the presence of increased or decreased pulmonary blood flow, and evidence of abnormal situs (dextrocardia or abnormal shape or position of the liver or stomach). The lung fields should be examined for evidence of space-occupying lesions, pneumothorax, infiltrates, and foreign body aspiration. Since lateral chest roentgenograms are only rarely helpful in newborn infants, an anteroposterior view alone is usually adequate.

Arterial blood gases will document hypoxemia. Crying infants, however, may spuriously lower oxygen saturation compared to samples obtained at rest. Elevated Pco_2 suggests lung disease. Pco_2 will typically be normal or low in the presence of right to left shunting. A hyperoxia test in which an infant breathes 100% oxygen is often used in neonates to differentiate cyanosis due to pulmonary disease from cyanosis due to cardiac disease. Since blood that has not been shunted is normally fully saturated, arterial Po_2 will increase minimally in the presence of a right to left shunt (*i.e.*, cyanotic congenital heart disease). While breathing 100% oxygen, an arterial Po_2 of less than 150 torr strongly suggests a cardiac etiology. Three points, however, need to be remembered: (1) the physiology of cyanotic heart lesions may be complicated by associated pulmonary disease (*e.g.*, total anomalous pulmonary venous return with obstruction to pulmonary venous flow and pulmonary edema); (2) cyanotic lesions associated with a markedly elevated pulmonary blood flow may have a significant increase in arterial Po_2 when breathing oxygen; (3) severe pulmonary disease can also result in hypoxemia while breathing oxygen-enriched gas. Pulmonary disease of this severity is, however, readily apparent on a chest roentgenogram. Capillary Po_2 is often measured in neonates but it is not as reliable beyond the neonatal period. It is also unreliable in the presence of poor cardiac output. Venous Po_2 does not correlate with arterial Po_2. The blood of patients with methemoglobinemia and the other cyanotic hemoglobinopathies will have an appropriate Po_2 but an inappropriately low hemoglobin saturation because the problem is one of oxygen binding to hemoglobin. Hemoglobin saturation must be measured, however, and must not be derived from the Po_2 level. Blood containing methemoglobin becomes brownish after standing in room air.

MANAGEMENT

Cyanosis is most commonly treated in the hospital by various subspecialists, most often cardiologists. Although the specific therapy of cyanosis depends on the specific etiology, several general principles apply. Cyanosis of acute onset at any age

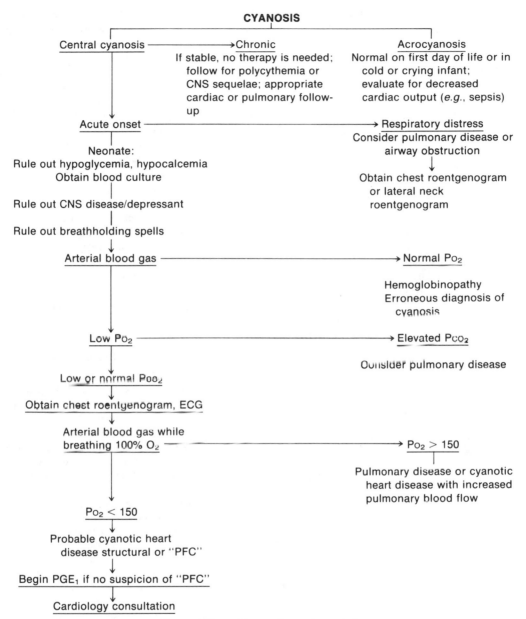

Figure 189-1. The work-up of cyanosis.

is an absolute indication for hospitalization. If there is not an obvious pulmonary etiology, a referral to a pediatric cardiologist is indicated. Pulmonary disease producing cyanosis is an absolute indication for referral to a skilled bronchoscopist (for airway obstruction) or to a pediatric critical care unit for therapy of severe pulmonary disease. Dehydration increases the risk of thrombosis in polycythemic patients and should be avoided. Due to the large red blood cell production in polycythemic patients, an adequate iron and folate intake should be assured, particularly because an iron deficiency may be partially masked by the elevated hematocrit and iron-deficient blood is more viscous than normal blood. Scrupulous care must be taken to assure that no air is introduced into intravenous lines in the presence of right to left shunting because of the potential of air emboli traveling to the systemic arterial circulation.

An acute reduction in the hematocrit in polycythemic patients who have hematocrits greater than 65% should be done by an isovolemic exchange transfusion rather than by phlebotomy in order to avoid hypovolemia. This is best done by exchanging aliquots of blood with 5% albumin in saline (5 g albumin/100 ml saline). The total amount exchanged equals:

$$\frac{\text{Initial hematocrit—desired hematocrit}}{\text{Initial hematocrit}}$$
$$\times \text{ body weight (kg)} \times \text{blood volume}$$

Blood volume varies from 85 ml/kg in newborns to 60 ml/kg in adults. In severe cyanotic conditions the hematocrit should be kept at ~55% to 65% if possible. Persistently higher hematocrits are an indication for surgical correction or palliation of the cardiac defect.

In the immediate newborn period, cyanosis usually precedes a specific cardiac diagnosis. Since this can be life-threatening, therapy should not be delayed until a complete diagnosis is made. As discussed above, supplemental oxygen typically does not raise the arterial Po_2 very much. However, some additional oxygen is useful because even a small increase in arterial oxygenation is helpful. The maintenance of ductal patency is crucial because many cyanotic lesions depend on blood shunting across the patent ductus arteriosus to bring deoxygenated blood to the lungs or oxygenated blood to the aorta. This is accomplished by a continuous infusion of prostaglandin E_1 (PGE_1) in the neonate, which is diluted and infused at a constant rate of 0.05 μg/kg/min. This can be given through any vascular access. If the infant is later shown not to have a ductal-dependent defect, the prostaglandin can be stopped without having caused problems.

The "tet spells" of tetralogy of Fallot can be treated by various therapies. Initial approaches include oxygen (which will not have a major impact),

flexing the legs at the hips and knees to simulate the knee–chest position of squatting, and giving the child morphine 0.2 mg/kg IM (or morphine 0.15 mg/kg IV). Other therapies include propranolol 0.1 mg/kg IV, an α sympathomimetic such as methoxamine (0.1 mg/kg IV) or phenylephrine (Neo-synephrine, 0.02 mg/kg IV), and the calcium channel blockers, all of which decrease right to left shunting. Bicarbonate can be given if acidosis is severe, and transfusions should be given for a hemoglobin less than 15 g/dl. Emergency surgery (a palliative shunt or complete correction) should be performed if all of these methods fail.

Acquired methemoglobinemia is treated with methylene blue, 1% solution, 1 to 2 mg/kg IV followed by daily oral doses of 2 mg/kg. The cyanotic hemoglobinopathies do not respond to methylene blue therapy.

Chronic cyanosis is well tolerated. These children, if stable, are readily followed as outpatients with referral only as required for diagnosis or management.

ANNOTATED BIBLIOGRAPHY

Feig SA: Methemoglobinemia. In Nathan DG, Oski FA (eds): Hematology of Infancy and Childhood, 2nd ed. Philadelphia, WB Saunders, 1981 (More detailed discussion of methemoglobinemia.)

Kendig EL, Chernick V (eds): Disorders of the Respiratory Tract in Children, 4th ed. Philadelphia, WB Saunders, 1983 (General pediatric pulmonology text that discusses the numerous pulmonary causes of cyanosis in more detail.)

Lees MH: Cyanosis of the newborn infant. Recognition and clinical evaluation. J Pediatr 77:484, 1970 (Discussion of the diagnosis and pathophysiology of cyanosis, specifically in the newborn.)

Lombroso CT, Lerman P: Breathholding spells (cyanotic and pallid infantile syncope). Pediatrics 39:563, 1967 (Discussion in detail of cyanotic breath-holding spells.)

Rudolph AM: Congenital Diseases of the Heart. Chicago, Year Book, 1974 (Prime source for more reading on the pathophysiologic processes underlying the structural congenital heart diseases.)

190
Jaundice
COLETTE DESLANDRES–LEDUC AND
RONALD E. KLEINMAN

An overview of bilirubin metabolism is important in understanding the pathophysiology and differential diagnosis of jaundice in the pediatric population. Bilirubin is the principal degradation product of heme in humans. The major source of heme (80%) is hemoglobin from senescent erythroid cells which is degraded in the reticuloendothelial system of the spleen, liver, and bone marrow. The other sources of bilirubin (10% to 20%) derive from nonerythroid sources, such as hepatic cytochrome P. 450. Once heme is dissociated from the globin, it is converted to biliverdin, which is then reduced to bilirubin. This free (unbound to plasma protein) unconjugated bilirubin is a potential toxin. After binding to albumin in the systemic circulation, bilirubin is transported to the hepatocyte where it is released from albumin and taken up by the hepatocyte. In the hepatocyte, the unconjugated (indirect) bilirubin is conjugated to glucuronide, a polar molecule, by the action of UDP-glucuronyltransferase. The conjugated (direct) bilirubin is not toxic and is secreted in the bile. More than 97% of the bilirubin arriving in the gastrointestinal (GI) tract is in this form.

In the GI tract, direct bilirubin is reduced by bacterial action to mesobilirubin, stercobilinogen, and urobilinogen. The latter two are colorless and are oxidized to the colored pigments urobilin and stercobilin. These oxidized compounds may contribute part of the brown color to normal feces. Fuscins, probably originating from early labeled hemes, are responsible for most of the color of stools. About 75% of the urobilinogen and stercobilinogen are reabsorbed in the ileum by way of the portal circulation and are excreted in the urine.

The differential diagnosis of hyperbilirubinemia (jaundice) can be related to the pathways of bilirubin metabolism. Excessive degradation of red blood cells, displacement of indirect bilirubin from albumin by drugs, abnormal uptake of indirect bilirubin by the hepatocyte, and abnormalities of conjugation by a lack or deficiency of UPD-glucuronyltransferase lead to unconjugated or indirect hyperbilirubinemia (Table 190-1). Abnormalities after the conjugation step will lead to a direct hyperbilirubinemia, which is also called *cholestasis*.

CLINICAL PRESENTATION

Jaundice may present with a constellation of symptoms depending on its cause. A neonate may appear ill, vomit, and fail to thrive as with galactosemia, tyrosinemia, or sepsis, or may be healthy in the first month of life as with breast milk jaundice or extrahepatic biliary atresia. Viral hepatitis may be accompanied by fatigue, fever, anorexia, and vomiting along with jaundice. Pallor, right upper quadrant pain, poor weight gain, pruritus, arthritis, clay-colored stools, and dark urine are commonly associated with jaundice in a variety of different disorders.

DIFFERENTIAL DIAGNOSIS

The age of the patient and the type of hyperbilirubinemia (direct *vs* indirect) are major considerations in an evaluation of a child with jaundice.

Birth to 14 Days of Age

In this age group, indirect hyperbilirubinemia is the most frequent cause of jaundice and physiologic jaundice is the leading diagnosis in this category. In the term infant, the peak rise in bilirubin is noticed at 3 days of age and rarely exceeds 15 mg/dl. The preterm infant tends to have earlier and higher peaks and the duration of jaundice is longer. Numerous hypotheses exist to explain the causes of physiologic jaundice. These hypotheses include immaturity of uptake and conjugating pathways, excessive heme from red cells and muscle, and shunting around the liver by a persistently patent ductus venosus.

Hemolytic diseases such as ABO incompatibility are the second most common cause of indirect hyperbilirubinemia in the first week of life. In this case, the quantity of indirect bilirubin overwhelms the hepatocyte's capacity to conjugate. Rh incom-

Table 190-1. Differential Diagnosis of Jaundice in Infancy

AGE	INDIRECT HYPERBILIRUBINEMIA	AGE	DIRECT AND MIXED HYPERBILIRUBINEMIA
1–14 days	Physiologic jaundice* Rh and ABO incompatibility Breast milk jaundice Lucey–Driscoll syndrome Crigler–Najjar types I and II	1 day–3 months	Infections: 　E. coli sepsis 　Urinary tract infection 　TORCH 　Neonatal hepatitis*
2 weeks–3 months	Breast milk jaundice* Lucey–Driscoll syndrome Crigler–Najjar types I and II Congenital hypothyroidism Pyloric stenosis		Anatomic: 　Choledochal cyst 　Extrahepatic biliary atresia 　Inspissated bile syndrome 　Alagille syndrome Metabolic: 　Galactosemia 　Fructosemia 　Tyrosinemia 　α_1-antitrypsin deficiency
Postneonatal period	Hemolytic diseases: 　G6PD deficiency 　Congenital spherocytosis 　Autoimmune 　Gilbert disease*	Postneonatal period	Viral hepatitis* Wilson disease Rotor syndrome Dubin–Johnson syndrome

* Most frequent cause in the specific age group.

patibility is less frequent but more dramatic. A failure to control high peaks of indirect bilirubin in the neonatal period may lead to kernicterus. The hemolytic diseases usually present in the first 36 hours of life.

Toward the end of the first and the beginning of the second week of life, breast milk jaundice should be considered in a breast-fed infant with indirect hyperbilirubinemia. This benign condition often recurs in siblings. Theoretically, a substance(s) contained in breast milk inhibits UDP-glucuronyltransferase. The Lucey–Driscoll syndrome is a dramatic situation seen rarely in breast-fed infants in which kernicterus may be a serious complication of high indirect serum bilirubin levels occurring during the first few days of life.

Rarer causes of indirect hyperbilirubinemia in the first 2 weeks of life are the Crigler–Najjar types I and II syndromes where UDP-glucuronyltransferase is respectively lacking or deficient and peaks of indirect bilirubin may be high. Congenital hypothyroidism should also be considered in a neonate with prolonged indirect hyperbilirubinemia. Finally, an abdominal obstruction and pyloric stenosis may be responsible for indirect hyperbilirubinemia.

Between 2 Weeks and 3 Months of Age

Jaundice is usually cholestatic after 2 weeks of age and a differentiation between *hepatocellular* and *extrahepatic* causes is mandatory. Among the

hepatocellular causes, metabolic, anatomic, infectious, and toxic possibilities must be excluded. In most neonates with hepatocellular cholestasis, no cause is found (see Chap. 110). Infectious disorders are the second largest category. Toxoplasmosis, rubella, cytomegalovirus, herpes, enteroviruses, syphilis, hepatitis B, hepatitis A, *Listeria monocytogenes*, group B streptococcus, and *Escherichia coli* are the most common offending agents.

Toxic etiologies include parenteral nutrition, particularly in premature infants who received only this form of nutrition for a prolonged time. Metabolic causes are much rarer and include galactosemia, fructosemia, α_1-antitrypsin deficiency, and tyrosinemia. Anatomic causes include inspissated bile syndrome, which follows severe hemolysis and which is characterized by plugs of bile in the hepatic canaliculi. Furthermore, intrahepatic bile ducts may be hypoplastic as part of Alagille syndrome (syndromic paucity of interlobular bile ducts) or as an isolated finding. Finally, cystic fibrosis may also be a cause for cholestasis in a neonate.

Extrahepatic obstructive causes of cholestasis must be recognized quickly because they may have a surgical cure. Extrahepatic biliary atresia is a rare disorder occurring in 1:8000 to 1:14,000 live births. Early intervention (before 2 months of age) with a portoenterostomy gives some hope for survival. A choledocal cyst may also be responsible for an obstruction of the biliary tree and may require early surgical intervention.

Postneonatal Period

After the first 3 months of age, the appearance of jaundice in a previously well child is most frequently secondary to a viral hepatitis: HAV, HBV, nonA–nonB hepatitis, cytomegalovirus (CMV), and Epstein–Barr virus (EBV) should all be considered as possible causal agents. Hemolytic diseases such as glucose-6 phosphate dehydrogenase (G6PD) deficiency may manifest when a susceptible toddler is given an oxidizing agent. Severe anemia and indirect hyperbilirubinemia may develop. Although the following disorders may be encountered in other age groups, they are more frequent in late childhood and adolescence. Gilbert's disease occurs in up to 5% of white people and it is the most frequent cause of indirect hyperbilirubinemia in this age group. This disease is a benign condition and presents as mild, intermittent, indirect hyperbilirubinemia. Jaundice is exacerbated with fasting or intercurrent illness. Gallstones may obstruct the biliary tree and produce jaundice (direct type) with severe right upper quadrant pain, nausea, and vomiting. In this age group, specific attention should be given to a hemolytic disease such as congenital spherocytosis and sickle cell disease as the cause of the gallstones. Autoimmune hemolytic diseases are seen in systemic lupus erythematous (SLE) disease, Mycoplasma infection, drug ingestion (e.g., α-methyldopa) or they may be idiopathic. Anemia and jaundice may be acute and impressive. Wilson's disease may also present as an acute hemolytic anemia with acute hepatitis and jaundice (mixed hyperbilirubinemia). Rotor's syndrome and Dubin–Johnson syndrome rarely present in the pediatric population. They are benign syndromes and present with cholestasis secondary to abnormalities in conjugated bilirubin excretion pathways from the hepatocyte.

WORK-UP

History

In the neonatal period, special attention should be given to the age in the days when jaundice was first noticed; the history during pregnancy to determine the role of intrauterine infection, pre-eclampsia, diabetes, or hypothyroidism; complications at delivery; and the weight at birth. Important antecedents *post natum* include the type of feeding, blood group incompatibility between mother and child, intolerance to feedings, failure to thrive, age of first stool, and color of stools and urine.

After the neonatal period, special attention should be given to the mode of onset and the duration of jaundice. A history of contact with viral hepatitis, day care attendance, blood transfusions, IV drug abuse, travel in foreign countries, and drug or shellfish ingestion should be sought. A family history of hepatic or hemolytic disease, and a history of early onset of cholelithiasis in siblings may also be important clues.

Physical Examination

The initial appearance of the patient including congenital malformations and dysmorphism (Alagille syndrome) should be noted. The skin color may be yellow, greenish, or pale. The skin examination may reveal xanthomas, spider angiomas, palmar erythema, or hematomas.

Upon examination of the eyes, chorioretinitis, seen in toxoplasmosis or cytomegalovirus infections or the typical Kayser–Fleischer ring of Wilson disease, may immediately indicate the cause of jaundice. Conjunctivae will become icteric at a bilirubin over 2.5 mg/dl.

The physical examination of the liver should include an appreciation of the size, firmness, and texture of the surface. An acutely enlarging liver is often painful. The gallbladder will be palpable only if it is inflamed or if the outflow of bile is obstructed. Ascites and collateral circulation over the abdomen may also be noted. Splenomegaly may be an important sign in hemolytic disease.

Among other important findings, the auscultation of the heart may reveal the murmur of pulmonary artery hypoplasia that accompanies paucity of intrahepatic bile ducts. Clubbing of the extremities indicates an intrapulmonary right-to-left shunting, which is often seen with cirrhosis.

Laboratory Tests

The first step in evaluating jaundice is to differentiate between direct and indirect hyperbilirubinemia by obtaining a total and direct serum bilirubin (by the Van den Bergh reaction). SGOT, SGPT, alkaline phosphatase, and 5'nucleotidase are useful indicators of hepatocellular or bile ductular disease. A general classification of appropriate laboratory tests according to the type of hyperbilirubinemia is presented in Table 190-2.

Imaging Techniques. Ultrasonography of the gallbladder and the portal structures will detect a choledocal cyst. The presence of a gallbladder *does not* exclude extrahepatic biliary atresia. Hepatobiliary scintigraphy is a safe and important tool in

Table 190-2.   Laboratory Work-up of Hyperbilirubinemia*

INDIRECT HYPERBILIRUBINEMIA	DIRECT (CHOLESTATIC) HYPERBILIRUBINEMIA	
	Neonatal Period	
CBC	5'nucleotidase	Serum α_1-antitrypsin
Reticulocyte count	Serum cholesterol	Pi typing of α_1-antitrypsin
Red blood cell smear	Blood, urine culture	Galactose-1-uridyl transferase
Platelet count	VDRL test	activity in RBC
Direct and indirect Coombs'	TORCH antibody titers	Amino acid screen of urine
test	HB$_s$Ag in mother and child	and blood
Serum haptoglobin	Reducing substances in urine*	Sweat test
Cold agglutinins	*Postneonatal Period*	
Antinuclear antibodies (ANA)		
G6PD activity in RBC	5'nucleotidase	CMV antibody titers
Thyroid function tests	Serum cholesterol	Serum ceruloplasmin
Urine culture	HB$_s$Ag + IgM antiHB$_c$Ag	24-hr collection of urine for
	IgM anti-HAV	copper
	Monotest	Serum α_1-antitrypsin level

* Serum bilirubin (total and direct), SGOT, SGPT, alkaline phosphatase should be the initial studies.
† Galactose and fructose are both reducing substances in the urine: They are Clinitest $(+)$ and Clinistix $(-)$. They may not be detected in urine if not ingested in sufficient quantities.

the evaluation of neonatal cholestasis. It is done with iminodiacetic acid (IDA) derivatives labeled with technetium 99m. A 5- to 7-day treatment with phenobarbital is recommended before the scintigraphy.

TREATMENT

Jaundice may be part of a disorder that is curable through medical or surgical means. Frequently, however, palliative measures may be all that can be offered to alleviate the complications of the primary disease.

Diet

Special dietary manipulation may be useful in the treatment of metabolic disorders such as galactosemia or fructosemia. In prolonged cholestasis, medium-chain triglycerides (MCT) should be the major source of lipids because they are less dependent on bile salts for absorption. In a neonate with cholestasis, formulas such as Portagen, which contains 87% MCT, can be used. Fat-soluble vitamins, especially vitamin E, must be supplied in adequate amounts to compensate for losses. Adequate protein of either animal or vegetable origin must be supplied to maximize the growth potential without causing hyperammonemia. Micronutrient repletion, including calcium, phosphorous, and magnesium, is also essential for growth.

Drugs

Phenobarbital has been used to promote bile secretion and alleviate pruritus, thereby improving the quality of life. Bile acid binding resins such as cholestyramine may accomplish the same purpose. Both of these agents may have adverse metabolic effects. Pruritus has been treated with a wide range of antihistamines, although severe cases are often refractory to standard therapies.

Phototherapy

Indirect bilirubin in the skin absorbs light energy and is transformed into nontoxic products excreted by the liver and kidney. The spectrum of light at which phototherapy is most effective corresponds to the maximum absorption peak of bilirubin:420 nM to 460 nM, which is in the blue light range. The management of hyperbilirubinemia depends on the age (in days) of the patient and the levels of serum indirect bilirubin.

Exchange Transfusion

An exchange transfusion is performed when phototherapy is ineffective in lowering the rapidly rising levels of indirect bilirubin that occur with brisk hemolysis.

Surgery

Surgical intervention is indicated to relieve an obstruction to the bile flow as with obstructive gallstones and a choledocal cyst. A portoenterostomy (Kasai procedure) is usually the preferred surgery for extrahepatic biliary atresia and an early intervention (before 2 months of age) is associated with a better outcome.

INDICATIONS FOR REFERRAL

When a neonate presents with persistent cholestasis, and no hepatocellular causes have been found, he should be referred to a tertiary center for an abdominal ultrasound and hepatobiliary scintigraphy. A liver biopsy (percutaneous or during a laparotomy) is mandatory if these tests are inconclusive. Since the Kasai procedure is more successful in a neonate below 2 months of age, there should be *no delay* in referral. Unexplainable jaundice in older pediatric patients is an indication for referral to a pediatric gastroenterologist.

ANNOTATED BIBLIOGRAPHY

Alter MJ: Hepatitis surveillance, 1982–1983. MMWR 34:1SS, 1SS–10SS (Review of the incidence of HAV, HBV, nonA–nonB hepatitis.)

Altman RP: The portoenterostomy procedure for biliary atresia: A five year experience. Ann Surg 188:351–362, 1978 (Outcome of 43 patients with extrahepatic biliary atresia who underwent a Kasai procedure.)

Butler DA, MacMillan JP: Relationship of breast feeding and weight loss to jaundice in the newborn period: Review of the literature and results of a study. Cleve Clin Q 50:263–268, 1983 (Review of the literature on breast milk jaundice and report on a study of 588 newborns.)

Cashore WJ, Stern L: The management of hyperbilirubinemia. Clin Perinatol 11:2, 339–357, 1984 (Review of the management of hyperbilirubinemia in the neonate.)

Gollan JL, Schmid R: Bilirubin update: Formation, transport, and metabolism. Prog Liver Dis VII-261–283, 1982 (Update on bilirubin metabolism.)

Kirks DR, Coleman RE, Filston HC, Rosenberg ER, Merten DF: An imaging approach to persistent neonatal jaundice. Am J Radiol 142:461–465, 1984 (Sonography and radionuclide scintigraphy studies in 15 patients with persistent neonatal jaundice: A diagnostic approach.)

Odell GB: "Physiologic" hyperbilirubinemia in the neonatal period. N Engl J Med 277:193–194, 1967 (Review of the various mechanisms incriminated in the development of *physiologic jaundice*.)

Reichen J: Familial unconjugated hyperbilirubinemia syndromes. Semin Liver Dis 3:24–35, 1983 (Review on Gilbert's disease and the Crigler–Najjar syndrome.)

22

Other Common Infections

191
Neonatal Infections
SAMUEL P. GOTOFF

Congenital and neonatal infections include all infections acquired during gestation, the perinatal period, and the first month of life. Most of these infections will be inapparent, some will be symptomatic during the neonatal period, and others will produce clinical manifestations later in childhood. Infections in the first months of life may be localized or systemic. Systemic infections, such as meningococcemia, occur at any age, but systemic infections with less invasive organisms, such as gram-negative enterics, are more likely to occur in the very young infant. The premature infant, whose defense mechanisms are even less well developed, is more likely to be at risk for septicemia. A disruption of normal barriers to infection and an introduction of foreign bodies (central lines or ventriculoperitoneal shunts) increase the risk of infection at any age.

The localization of infection by clinical and laboratory examinations permits a more restricted consideration of etiologic agents than in the situation where one encounters a sick infant with a suspected systemic infection. Selected localized and systemic infections are discussed in this chapter because they may differ significantly in etiology and management when compared to older children. However, it is important to remember that most of the infections seen in older children may occur in the young infant, depending on exposure and the status of transplacental immunity.

PATHOGENESIS

The transplacental passage of infectious agents may occur at any time during gestation. An intrauterine infection may result in abortion, stillbirth, prematurity, symptomatic neonatal infection, delayed manifestations, or inapparent infection depending on the etiologic agent, timing of infection during gestation, dosage, and host factors. In each case of congenital infection, there is maternal bacteremia, viremia, or parasitemia, and the placental barrier fails to prevent fetal infection. Early in gestation, infection may affect organogenesis with resulting congenital malformations. Later in gestation, inflammatory responses lead to pathologic manifestations at birth or later in life. The spectrum of signs resulting from congenital syphilis illustrates this problem. Only a single organ may be involved leading to deafness, ocular manifestations, cerebral damage, or hepatitis. In other cases, multiple organ systems may be involved.

Late in pregnancy the ascending amniotic infection syndrome is the principal route of infection. Usually with ruptured membranes, but occasionally with presumably intact membranes, organisms inhabiting the birth canal invade the amniotic fluid and are aspirated or ingested prior to or during delivery. Perinatal infection may be signalled by fetal distress or symptoms may be delayed until after birth. The duration of ruptured membranes correlates with the risk of amnionitis and neonatal infection. If maternal fever, attributed to endometritis, is present, the risk of infection in the newborn is greatly increased. In the nursery, the newborn may be exposed to pathogenic microbial flora from other infants, hospital personnel, and fomites. The mother, other members of the family, and community contacts are also sources of postnatally acquired infection.

OPHTHALMIA NEONATORUM

Mild chemical conjunctivitis is commonly seen within 6 to 24 hours after the installation of 1% silver nitrate. Gonococcal ophthalmia appears typically 2 to 5 days after birth, but it has been reported at birth or weeks later due to postnatal acquisition. *Neisseria gonorrhoeae* usually produces an acute purulent conjunctivitis but the spectrum of infection ranges from asymptomatic cases to panophthalmitis. Perinatally acquired herpes simplex ophthalmia is usually seen within a few days after birth but postnatally acquired HSV infection may present later in the neonatal period. Fluorescein staining of the cornea is a helpful screening test; diagnosis is made by culture. Several other bacteria have been associated with conjunctivitis in the newborn: These include *Staphylococcus aureus, Streptococcus pneumoniae*, enterococci, and *Hemophilus* species. The most common cause of neonatal conjunctivitis is *Chlamydia trachomatis*. The inflammatory response, which typically involves the tarsal conjunctivae, may be mild or severe, unilateral or bilateral, and may persist for weeks. Symptoms usually appear between 5 and 14 days of age although the range of reported cases extends from 2 days to weeks after birth. The perinatal infection may be prevented by erythromycin or tetracycline topically at birth in place of silver nitrate. Chlamydial conjunctivitis should be treated with erythromycin po (see Chap. 94 for a complete discussion).

RESPIRATORY INFECTIONS

Otitis media, ethmoid and maxillary sinusitis, and pneumonia are the major respiratory tract infections in the newborn infant. Infections that present in the first few days are due to bacterial pathogens acquired from the birth canal. Group B streptococcus is currently the most common organism producing perinatal pneumonia. Postnatal infections with *Staphylococcus aureus, H. influ-*

enzae, and *Streptococcus pneumoniae* also contribute to late onset respiratory tract infections. Postnatal pneumonias may also be due to respiratory viruses (respiratory syncytial virus), and the most common agent is *Chlamydia trachomatis*.

Chlamydial pneumonia may appear as early as 2 weeks of age but occurs typically between 4 and 11 weeks. The infant is usually afebrile with tachypnea and a paroxysmal staccato cough. Other respiratory tract signs, such as conjunctivitis, nasal obstruction, and abnormal tympanic membranes are common. X-rays show bilateral interstitial infiltrates and air trapping. A diagnosis is made by culturing chlamydia from the respiratory tract or demonstrating a serologic response, rising titers, or IgM antibody to *C. trachomatis*. Topical administration of antibiotics does not prevent chlamydial pneumonia. One study indicates that erythromycin treatment of colonized women can prevent chlamydial infections in infancy. Erythromycin in a dose of 40 mg/kg/day po for 2 weeks should be used for the treatment of chlamydial infections (see also Chap. 165).

GASTROENTERITIS

Gastroenteritis in the newborn infant, presenting as diarrheal disease, is caused by the same agents that produce symptoms in older children. The etiologic agents may be divided into those that produce inflammation, characterized by fecal leukocytes, and those that do not. Inflammatory diarrhea is caused by *Salmonella, Shigella, Campylobacter*, invasive *E. coli, Vibrio parahemolyticus, Yersinia enterocolitica, E. histolytica*, and others. Noninflammatory diarrhea is usually caused by rotaviruses, enterotoxigenic *E. coli*, and, less commonly, enteroviruses and other agents. A bacteriologic culture and tests for rotavirus antigen will usually define the problem. Several noninfectious causes of neonatal diarrhea must also be considered (see also Chap. 106).

URINARY TRACT INFECTIONS

The estimated incidence of urinary tract infection (UTI) in newborn infants ranges from 0.1% to 1%. UTIs are commonly asymptomatic and are detected in screening programs. A UTI may occur as a result of hematogenous spread from a systemic infection or through the ascending route. When they occur in conjunction with a generalized infection, the infection is less likely to originate in the urinary tract than to spread from some other focus, but a determination of the initial focus may be difficult. The diagnosis of UTI is made by an examination and a culture of the urine. The urine sediment may or may not contain leukocytes. Abnormal urines should be cultured, but many infants with UTIs do not have pyuria. Gram-stained organisms in urine correlate well with positive cultures ($\geq 10^5$ colonies/ml). A major problem in the diagnosis of UTI in young infants is in obtaining an uncontaminated urine sample for culture. A negative bag specimen is useful in excluding a UTI, but a positive urine culture must be confirmed by a clean-voided urine specimen or one obtained by suprapubic bladder aspiration.

Clinical signs of UTI may be nonspecific, ranging from low-grade fever and failure to thrive to more acute signs of sepsis. If jaundice is a manifestation of UTI, it is usually associated with bacteremia. Focal signs of UTI include balanitis, urethritis, orchitis, and prostatitis.

The etiologic agents of neonatal UTI are usually *E. coli* and other enteric bacteria. Antimicrobial agents are selected with the same guidelines as in the treatment of neonatal septicemia (see also Chap. 114).

CUTANEOUS INFECTIONS

Skin and subcutaneous infections may be localized or they may occur as manifestations of systemic infections. They may result from a hematogenous spread of bacteria, viruses, and candida or from injury to the skin due to circumcision, birth trauma, and fetal monitoring. The umbilical cord is a common focus for local or systemic bacterial infection. The source of a local skin infection is frequently not determined.

The type of skin lesion may suggest the etiology. Characteristic skin lesions include the staphylococcal scalded skin syndrome and ecthyma gangrenosum due to *Pseudomonas aeruginosa*. More often, the cutaneous manifestation suggests a limited number of possibilities that must be confirmed by Gram stain, culture, or histologic examination. *Staphylococcus aureus* is the most frequent cause of skin infections in the newborn infant, presenting as impetigo, pustules, bullae, and abscesses. A large number of bacteria, viruses and, less commonly, fungi may produce skin lesions early in infancy. Skin lesions, such as petechiae or *Herpes simplex* vesicles, may be the initial manifestation of a systemic infection (see also Chaps. 64 and 67).

EARLY ONSET AND LATE ONSET INVASIVE DISEASE IN THE NEWBORN

Systemic neonatal infections may be classified by the age at onset into early and late onset disease. The precise cutoff for early onset infection varies from 2 days to 1 week, but the implication is that early onset disease has a perinatal pathogenesis. Infection may be acquired *in utero*, with signs present in the delivery room, or during parturition, with a latent period before the development of disease. Obstetric risk factors for neonatal early onset disease such as premature delivery, prolonged rupture of maternal membranes, amnionitis, and twinning have been identified. The most common agent, the group B streptococcus, has been studied extensively. The attack rate is 2 to 3:1000 live births; but it becomes considerably higher in infants with risk factors.

Invasive bacterial infections must be considered in the differential diagnosis of any infant who becomes ill in the nursery. The clinical signs are often vague. Poor feeding, vomiting, abdominal distention, lethargy, temperature changes, respiratory distress, jaundice, hepatomegaly, seizure activity, and petechiae are significant clues that should lead to a diagnostic evaluation and presumptive therapy. Most infants with early onset disease have a respiratory tract focus and are bacteremic. Some will have meningitis, involvement of other organs (*e.g.*, liver, kidneys, musculoskeletal system), or be overwhelmingly ill due to high level bacteremia (septicemia) manifested by septic shock (apnea, hypotension, and disseminated intravascular coagulation).

Late onset infections may present with the same spectrum as early onset disease, but are more often localized to the lungs, meninges, bones, or joints. Fever, without localizing signs, may be the initial presentation.

When an invasive bacterial infection is suspected in the newborn, blood, cerebrospinal fluid, and urine should be obtained for culture, and the CSF and urine examined. Group B streptococci, *E. coli*, and *Listeria monocytogenes* are the most common etiologic agents but a large number of bacterial species may produce disease. Several viruses, fungi, and protozoa may also lead to systemic infections in the newborn. A laboratory diagnosis is essential.

If the physician makes a presumptive diagnosis of systemic bacterial infection or even considers this possibility, then antibiotics should be begun immediately. If there are no clues to the etiologic agent from an examination of biologic fluids (CSF, urine, joint aspiration, pus), broad spectrum treatment is begun with a penicillin and an aminoglycoside. If a staphylococcal infection is suspected, a penicillinase-resistant penicillin should be included. Certain third generation cephalosporins may be employed for the treatment of gram-negative bacillary meningitis. When bacteriologic cultures are negative in infants with a syndrome consistent with septicemia, the physician should consider other nonbacterial etiologies such as HSV, enteroviruses, rubella, CMV, and toxoplasmosis, and he should obtain appropriate specimens for diagnosis. The management of these serious infections frequently requires consultation with an expert in infectious diseases.

SPECIFIC AGENTS

Cytomegalovirus

Cytomegalovirus (CMV) is a common infection. From 3% to 12% of pregnant women have viuria, and ~10% of the infants born to infected women will also excrete CMV. While 90% to 95% of infected infants are asymptomatic in the neonatal period, 10% to 20% of apparently normal newborns excreting CMV may ultimately have sensorineural or intellectual defects. The clinical manifestations of congenital CMV infection include microcephaly, periventricular calcifications, optic atrophy, cataracts, chorioretinitis, microphthalmia, coloboma, jaundice, hepatosplenomegaly, pneumonia, meningoencephalitis, and thrombocytopenic purpura as isolated problems or in combination.

Neonatal infections are transmitted vertically by way of the transplacental route and, more commonly, through cervical secretions at the time of parturition. CMV may also be transmitted by blood transfusion, breast milk, and horizontally in the nursery. Clinical infection is more likely to result from the hematogenous route. The diagnosis is made by isolation of virus from urine or other biologic fluids in the first few days of life. Isolation of virus later in life does not differentiate between congenital and natal or postnatal acquisition. Cytomegalic inclusion bodies may be observed in urine by light microscopy, a test that is more rapid but much less sensitive. IgM antibody in the infant's serum is also evidence for infection. Serologic tests that measure IgG reflect maternal antibody and must be interpreted accordingly. A stable or rising titer would indicate congenital infection.

Currently, there is no therapy for CMV infection. Both vaccines and antiviral chemotherapy are under investigation. Since subclinical infection is not uncommon in the newborn nursery, good handwashing techniques should be observed routinely. Screening high-risk pregnant women for CMV excretion is not recommended as a cost-effective approach to the prevention of congenital CMV. Only CMV antibody-negative blood should be used for transfusions in newborn infants.

Rubella

Rubella is a mild febrile exanthem that has major consequences during pregnancy. Rubella-associated abortions, miscarriages, stillbirths, fetal anomalies, and the congenital rubella syndrome have been significantly diminished by the rubella immunization program. In the 1980s, less than 20 cases of congenital rubella syndrome were reported annually in the United States.

The range of disease manifestations is extensive. Cardiac, ophthalmologic, auditory, and neurologic anomalies are well described. In addition, newborn infants may have growth retardation, hepatosplenomegaly, interstitial pneumonia, thrombocytopenia purpura, and radiolucent bone disease. Although major abnormalities are easily recognized in the neonatal period, mild cases with cardiac disease, deafness, developmental problems, and endocrinopathies may not be detectable for months or years. So-called "silent" rubella infections in young infants are more common than those that are symptomatic. The most common sequellae are auditory and are often associated with problems in language development.

If infected infants born to women with first trimester rubella are monitored for at least 2 years, up to 80% will be affected. The congenital rubella syndrome occurs in 20% to 25% of infants born to women who acquire rubella during the first trimester. Subclinical rubella infection, detected by IgM RIA, occurred in over 50% of infants following maternal rubella between 12 and 16 weeks of gestation. Although fetal infection can occur at any stage of pregnancy, defects rarely occur after infection beyond the 20th week.

Congenital rubella infection is best diagnosed by culturing the virus from pharyngeal or conjunctival secretions, cerebrospinal fluid, or urine. A serologic diagnosis is made by a demonstration of rubella-specific IgM antibodies or the persistence of rubella antibodies for more than 3 months at a level beyond that expected from passive transfer or maternal antibodies. The hemagglutination inhibition

(HI) test is now being replaced by a number of more sensitive antibody assays.

The diagnosis and management of rubella during pregnancy are not discussed here. There is no established treatment for congenital infection. Active immunization affords a method to prevent congenital rubella infection and is clearly attainable.

Herpes Simplex Virus (HSV)

The estimated number of annual cases of neonatal herpes in the United States is between 300 and 1500. While the frequency of genital HSV infection in pregnant women is 5 to 10:1000, not all of these infections are active at the time of delivery. Most infants with neonatal herpes are born to women who are asymptomatic for genital herpes and without a history of genital herpes or a sexual partner with a vesicular rash (see also Chaps. 67 and 195).

A neonatal infection is most frequently acquired at birth. In utero acquisition is rare. Postnatal transmission may occur, usually from contact with saliva from individuals with oral herpes or with virus on the hands of parents, relatives, or hospital personnel.

In contrast to CMV, neonatal HSV is almost always symptomatic and is frequently associated with significant morbidity and mortality. The disease may be limited to the portal of entry (eye, mouth, skin) or may progress to the CNS or widespread dissemination. Congenital lesions may be noted at birth, but most natal infections present at the end of the first week. Postnatally acquired infections may appear even later. Vesicles are typical and frequently cluster, but the lesions become pustular and scab with evolution and may be mistaken for impetigo. Skin lesions typically recur. Occasionally, neonates with apparently only skin lesions may ultimately develop ocular or CNS sequelae. Eye findings include keratoconjunctivitis and chorioretinitis, which may appear later. The disseminated disease frequently resembles septicemia with temperature alterations, lethargy, and involvement of the liver, lungs, and adrenal glands. The brain is involved in ~70% of HSV infections; about one third of children have localized CNS infections. The mortality rate is about 80% in untreated disseminated disease and 50% in localized CNS disease.

When skin, conjunctival, or oral lesions are present, a presumptive diagnosis may be established by a cytologic examination and may be confirmed by cell culture. Intranuclear inclusions and multinucleated giant cells are typical of HSV and varicella-zoster virus (VZV) infection. The sensitivity of cytology is only about 60%, thus virology is preferred. Other sites for virus culture include the nose, throat, conjunctivae, urine, CSF, and stool. Serology is generally not helpful, except to document maternal seroconversion.

Treatment should be instituted with an effective antiviral agent. Vidarabine and acyclovir have been shown to decrease morbidity and mortality, but residual neurologic abnormalities remain a problem. Acyclovir is currently the recommended treatment.

It is generally accepted that pregnant women with active genital herpes should be delivered by cesarean section. Thus, genital cultures should be obtained in women with a history of genital herpes beginning at 34 to 36 weeks. The management of infants delivered vaginally to women with active genital herpes remains controversial. There are no data to resolve the question, and there are a number of considerations. First, although vidarabine treatment of clinically infected infants has not eliminated death and neurologic residua from neonatal herpes, earlier therapy may further improve the outcome. Second, the risk of transmission of infection to infants is about 40% in mothers with primary infection whereas only 3% in the case of recurrent genital herpes. Thus, prophylactic or very early treatment may be beneficial in the infant whose mother has a primary infection; however, a large study would be necessary to demonstrate efficacy. Some experts now recommend cultures of infants delivered vaginally to mothers with active genital herpes between 24 and 48 hours after delivery. Positive cultures would reflect the proliferation of virus in the infant, an indication for antiviral therapy prior to clinical signs.

Women with active herpes need not be isolated from their infants if careful handwashing is performed. Breast-feeding is contraindicated if breast lesions are present. Individuals with herpes labialis should wear masks.

Toxoplasmosis

The incidence of congenital infections with *Toxoplasma gondii* is ~1:1000 live births in the United States. Most of the infections are asymptomatic at birth with sequelae manifested after the neonatal period. Congenital toxoplasmosis refers to the disease. The classical findings in congenital toxoplasmosis are hydrocephalus, chorioretinitis, and intracranial calcifications. Neurologic signs such as seizures, increased intracranial pressure, and nystagmus are common. Approximately one third show signs of systemic infection including fever, jaundice, hepatomegaly, splenomegaly, lymphadenopathy, anemia, and abnormal spinal fluid. Pneumonitis, abnormal bleeding, and eosinophilia are less common.

The common sequellae of congenital infections are chorioretinitis, which may not become apparent until adolescence, retardation, seizures, and other neurologic abnormalities.

A diagnosis is established easily by the demonstration of organisms or antigens in tissues or body fluids. The placenta should be examined, if it is available. The interpretation of serologic tests may be more difficult. Nonspecific laboratory clues to diagnosis are eosinophilia and high spinal fluid protein values.

Several serologic tests for the diagnosis of toxoplasma infection are available. These include the Sabin–Feldman dye test, complement fixation, ELISAs, indirect fluorescent antibody, and indirect hemagglutination. An interpretation of the results of these tests is often difficult in practice.

The diagnosis of acquired toxoplasmosis in the mother can be established by the demonstration of a significant increase in antibody titers. Since high titers may persist for years following infection, a single high titer is not diagnostic. A screening dye test during pregnancy will establish whether the woman is susceptible (negative test). A positive dye test and a negative IgM antibody test (IFA or ELISA) indicates prior infection. The duration of IgM antibody is variable, depending on the assay, thus a negative IgM antibody test late in pregnancy may not exclude infection in the first trimester.

Serologic diagnosis in the newborn is even more complicated. The antibody in cord blood or neonatal sera may reflect IgG passed transplacentally from the mother. While the presence of IgM antibodies to toxoplasma is diagnostic of congenital infection, the IgM IFA test is negative in 75% and the IgM ELISA is negative in 20% of neonates with congenital toxoplasmosis. Subsequent testing will show the decline of maternally derived antibody in uninfected infants; however, antibody synthesis in some infected infants is delayed until 3 or 4 months of age.

Unfortunately, there is a considerable variation in antigen preparations, relative contributions of IgG and IgM antibodies to titers, and the assays used in different laboratories. In questionable cases, it is best to consult a reference laboratory.

Treatment is recommended for all cases of congenital toxoplasmosis because of the late manifestations. Although an evaluation of therapy is difficult, the morbidity and mortality are serious enough to warrant treatment. Several chemotherapeutic agents have been used for therapy, but the experience is limited. Spiramycin appears to be most promising but is not presently available in the United States. In this country, the combination of pyrimethamine and sulfadiazine is recommended for a 3-week course. With evidence of inflammation (meningitis, chorioretinitis), prednisone is added. Folinic acid is recommended during pyrimethamine therapy.

Hepatitis

The newborn infant may be exposed to a mother with hepatitis A or B. Although transplacental transmission may occur, neonatal infection usually takes place at the time of delivery or postnatally. With the prolonged incubation period of these viruses, there are usually no early clinical manifestations. Newborn infants of women with hepatitis B are at risk for acute or chronic active hepatitis and hepatocellular carcinoma many years later. Asymptomatic hepatitis B antigenemia is more frequent in certain high risk groups. Screening during pregnancy is recommended for women of Asian, Pacific Island, or Alaskan Eskimo descent; women born in Haiti or Sub-Saharan Africa; women who have histories of liver disease, contact with hemodialysis or institutionalized mentally retarded patients; frequent exposure to blood; multiple episodes of venereal disease; or percutaneous use of illicit drugs.

Effective prophylaxis is now available for hepatitis B. HBIG (0.5 ml) and hepatitis B vaccine (0.5 ml) should be given IM at separate sites, preferably within 12 hours of birth. The vaccine may be delayed as much as 7 days and should be repeated at ages 1 and 6 months. Immune serum globulin should be administered to infants of women with hepatitis A.

While HB$_s$Ag is found in breast milk, breast-feeding is not contraindicated if infants are given HBIG prophylaxis. In the absence of prophylaxis, the risks and benefits of breast-feeding must be weighed on an individual basis (see also Chap. 110 for a complete discussion).

Varicella

Early intrauterine infection may result in cicatricial skin lesions, hypoplastic limbs, cortical atrophy, and ocular abnormalities. Neonatal varicella usually presents with a limited vesicular rash, but can involve multiple organs and the central nervous system. The severe form of the disease may be complicated by disseminated intravascular coagulation, and fatality rates up to 30% have been reported.

A diagnosis is apparent when typical skin lesions are noted in the mother and infant. A presumptive diagnosis of a herpes virus (VZV or HSV) infection is made by an examination of Tzanck preparations of vesicles. Varicella antigen in fluid or culture of virus from the vesicle provides diagnostic confirmation. Infection may also be documented by a fourfold or greater rise in V-Z antibody or specific IgM antibody in a single specimen.

Although there are no published studies, a serious infection in the newborn should be treated with acyclovir, 30 mg/kg/day for 7 to 10 days. Congenital varicella may be prevented or modified in neonates born to mothers with the onset of chickenpox less than 5 days before delivery by administration of VZIG or ZIG in a dose of 1.25 ml IM. No deaths have been reported in infants whose mothers had rash 5 or more days prior to birth, as transplacental antibody appears at this time. Newborn infants whose mothers have chickenpox postnatally are susceptible and may have a severe infection. They should probably be given VZIG although supportive data are lacking (see also Chap. 197).

Syphilis

The incidence of congenital syphilis is less than 1:10,000 live births. A diagnosis may be difficult because of the timing of the infection and interpretation of serologic tests, and management of the infant with a reactive test for syphilis on a cord blood specimen is a repetitive problem for the pediatrician.

The fetus is infected transplacentally. The placenta is large due to inflammation and *T. pallidum* are usually demonstrable. Systemic spread may involve liver, spleen, lung, kidney, gastrointestinal tract, nervous system, and bones.

At birth, infants with congenital infection are usually asymptomatic. Late manifestations of infection may be delayed for a few months to years. Signs of early congenital syphilis include various mucocutaneous lesions, with persistent rhinitis (snuffles), generalized lymphadenopathy, hepatosplenomegaly, jaundice, Coombs' negative hemolytic anemia, hydrops fetalis, various ocular and central nervous system abnormalities, nephrotic syndrome, osseous lesions that are usually asymptomatic but may result in pseudoparalysis, pneu-

monitis, and changes in peripheral blood (thrombocytopenia, anemia, leukemoid reaction).

The signs of late congenital syphilis include Hutchinson's triad (abnormal permanent central incisors, interstitial keratitis, and eighth nerve deafness), mulberry molars, saddle nose, rhagades, and residual central nervous system and skeletal abnormalities.

The diagnosis of congenital syphilis is made by darkfield or histologic examination, or by a combination of epidemiologic, clinical, roentgenologic, and serologic criteria.

The Venereal Disease Research Laboratory (VDRL) and rapid plasma reagin (RPR) tests measure antibody to cardiolipin. These tests are usually used for screening and reactivity depends on the duration and status of infection. The test may be positive in nonsyphilitic conditions and may be negative in maternal and cord blood if infection occurred late in gestation.

Several tests have been developed to detect specific antibodies to *T. pallidum*. The fluorescent treponema antibody absorbed with nonpallidum treponemes (FTA–ABS) test is usually available in health department laboratories. FTA-IgM and FTA-IgG tests have been developed to differentiate fetal and maternal antibody in cord blood and neonatal sera. Unfortunately, not all infants with congenital syphilis make IgM antibody and a positive FTA-IgM test may be due to an IgM anti-IgG antibody to *T. pallidum* analogous to a rheumatoid factor.

The management of a newborn infant with suspected syphilis depends on several variables. If maternal syphilis is treated correctly with penicillin during pregnancy, the risk to the infant is minimal. The infant should be monitored clinically and serologically, with a demonstration of falling titers, to assure the effectiveness of maternal therapy on fetal infection. If maternal treatment is inadequate or if an alternative treatment such as erythromycin is employed or if the infant cannot be properly monitored, then the infant should be treated with penicillin.

Current recommendations for treatment differentiate between infants with and without neurosyphilis. A 10-day course of either aqueous crystalline or procaine penicillin G is recommended for the former with a single dose of benzathine penicillin G for the latter. Neurosyphilis may be difficult to ascertain since most infants have no neurologic abnormalities. A diagnosis of neurosyphilis rests usually on cerebrospinal fluid abnormalities. A positive VDRL on CSF indicates neurosyphilis but a negative test does not exclude it. Elevated CSF protein and pleocytosis are compatible with neurosyphilis but are not diagnostic. The interpretation of CSF results (including FTA tests) remains controversial. The most conservative approach is to examine the CSF in all infants when treatment for congenital syphilis is indicated and to treat for 10 days if the CSF is abnormal without an alternative explanation (see also Chap. 195).

ANNOTATED BIBLIOGRAPHY

Texts

Feigin RD, Cherry JD (eds): Textbook of Pediatric Infectious Diseases. Philadelphia, WB Saunders, 1981 (Detailed reference.)

Remington JS, Klein JO (eds): Infectious Diseases of the Fetus and Newborn Infant. Philadelphia, WB Saunders, 1983 (Detailed reference.)

Articles

Centers for Disease Control: Postexposure prophylaxis of hepatitis B: Recommendation of the Immunization Practices Advisory Committee (ACIP). MMWR 33:285, 1984

Leland D, French MLV, Kleiman MB, Schreiner RL: The use of TORCH titers. Pediatrics 72:41, 1983 (Emphasizes limitations of TORCH titers.)

Nankervis GA: Cytomegaloviral infections: Epidemiology, therapy, and prevention. Pediatr Rev 7:169, 1985 (Recent review.)

Pickering LK: Diagnosis and therapy of patients with congenital and primary syphilis. Pediatr Infect Dis 4:602, 1985 (Recent review.)

Schachter J, Sweet RL, Grossman M et al: Experience with the routine use of erythromycin for chlamydial infections in pregnancy. N Engl J Med 314:276, 1986 (Effective method of prophylaxis of neonatal chlamydial infections.)

Whitley RJ, Hutto C: Neonatal herpes simplex virus infections. Pediatr Rev 7:119, 1985 (Recent review.)

192
Bacteremia
ROBERT A. DERSHEWITZ

Children may have bacteria in their blood at any age. Bacteremia may be primary (often used interchangeably with *occult* and *unsuspected*) or secondary to a focal infection (*e.g.*, pneumonia). Although definitions, risk factors, and management strategies are somewhat controversial, this chapter offers a reasonable clinical approach to this problem.

Children between 3 and 24 months of age are at greatest risk for unsuspected bacteremia. It is uncommon in children older than 36 months. Neonates represent a special category. Most recommendations require any febrile newborn under 2 months old and any "septic-looking" or "toxic" child to be hospitalized, to have a full sepsis work-up, and to be started on parenteral antibiotics. Children between 2 and 3 months of age do not have as great a risk as neonates and hence they may be managed less conservatively if no risk factors other than fever are present. Indeed, recent trends are to admit less infants who are at risk because of the great expense, the risk of nosocomial infections, the complications such as drug toxicity, stress to the family, and most importantly, no demonstrable improved outcome.

In addition to age (3 to 24 months), elevations in fever and white blood cells (WBC) comprise the classic triad of risk factors for occult bacteremia. In one representative study, only 0.9% of children less than 24 months of age, who had fevers less than 38.9°C, were bacteremic. 4.1% were bacteremic if the fever was between 38.9°C and 39.4°C, and the incidence rose to 8.0% when it was greater than or equal to 40°C. There is a fivefold increased risk of bacteremia if the WBC is greater than 15,000. The presence of both temperature elevation and leukocytosis, or the greater degree of either, increases the likelihood for bacteremia. Race, socioeconomic status, and sex are not risk factors.

Septicemia is a different entity compared with bacteremia and a septic (*i.e.*, toxic) child represents a more serious problem. These children require immediate hospitalization with aggressive management. In most instances, however, the highly febrile infant does not appear toxic, and management decisions should be individualized based on various factors, such as clinical judgment. Clinical judgment, however, is not highly accurate. Pediatric residents, attending physicians in emergency rooms, and private practitioners are usually incorrect when they are asked to predict if the febrile infant whom they examined has bacteremia. On the other hand, physicians are more accurate in predicting specificity (*i.e.*, identifying children who are not bacteremic). The ultimate goal is clearly not to diagnose bacteremia, but to prevent its complications such as sepsis and meningitis.

PATHOPHYSIOLOGY

Bacteremia from any organism may resolve spontaneously; it may respond to antibiotic therapy; or it may result in fulminant disease, despite appropriate antibiotics. *Streptococcus pneumoniae* is the most common cause of bacteremia (65%). *Hemophilus influenzae* type b accounts for 20% to 25% of the cases, and *Neisseria meningitidis, Escherichia coli, Salmonella* species, *Enterobacter–Klebsiella* species, and group A β-hemolytic streptococci are other pathogens. Possible contaminants include *Staphylococcus aureus, Streptococcus viridans*, Moraxella, Candida, and mixed organisms. A determination of the pathogenicity, however, must be based on the clinical context. *Staphylococcus epidermidis*, α streptococci, diphtheroids, and bacillus species are probable contaminants.

S. pneumoniae is the least aggressive of the common pathogens; most resolve spontaneously or promptly with or without antibiotic therapy. In contrast, *H. influenzae* type b is usually associated with soft tissue invasion. Common "metastatic" spread includes pneumonia, meningitis, epiglottitis, cellulitis, and otitis media. *N. meningitidis* bacteremia results in the worst outcome. In one series (Dashefsky et al, 1983), 4:12 cases of unsuspected bacteremia resulted in meningitis or death, compared to 7% from *H. influenzae* type b and 4% from *S. pneumoniae*.

Children with congenital or functional asplenia are at considerably increased risk of overwhelming sepsis from bacteremia, especially from *S. pneumoniae*. Children with sickle cell disease have a tenfold increase of pneumococcal septicemia and meningitis. Immunocompromised children are also at an increased risk of septicemia, most commonly from gram-negative bacilli and staphylococci. Close contacts (siblings and day care) of children with serious invasive *H. influenzae* type b and meningococcal disease are also at increased risk.

CLINICAL PRESENTATION

In one study (Dershewitz et al, 1983), 25 of 699 nonhospitalized children between 3 and 24 months with temperatures of 39.5°C or higher had occult bacteremia. Twelve children presented with otitis media, 2 had URIs, 2 had pneumonia, 1 had a UTI, 1 had purulent rhinitis, and 7 has no focus of infection. The most common organism was *S. pneumoniae*, which presents typically as a relatively minor illness in the febrile child. At any point in the illness, even while seeming to recover, the child may develop complications such as meningitis. It should be reemphasized that the moribund child, the *toxic* child, or one with a primary diagnosis such as osteomyelitis, septic arthritis, or meningitis in which secondary bacteremia is common presents an entirely different clinical situation. These children, regardless of whether or not risk factors for bacteremia are present, must be hospitalized, worked-up completely, and treated aggressively.

WORK-UP

The work-up should help the clinician decide which children will be started on expectant antibiotic therapy.

History

Determine how sick is the infant. Has the child been less playful, alert, or active or is he inconsolable? Has there been a recent or concurrent exposure or predisposing illness to bacteremia, such as pneumonia? Does the child have medical conditions, such as malignancy, splenectomy, shunt, or in-dwelling catheters that would increase the likelihood of bacteremia?

Physical Examination

Optimal observation is important. The observer must avoid haste. The physician should ensure that the child is comfortable. If necessary, he should reassess the child repeatedly, especially after the fever is lowered. He should take note if the child is looking about, consolable, or playful. McCarthy and associates have stressed the importance of observation variables such as cry, reaction to parents, state variation, color, state of hydration, and response to social overtures (see Chap. 178 for a detailed discussion of identifying sick from non-toxic appearing children). The physician should perform a complete physical examination to look for focal infection. He should test carefully for meningismus. Certain findings on physical examination are clues to etiology: pustules suggest *S. aureus*, ecthyma gangrenosum indicates a pseudomonas infection and petechiae or purpura, although not pathognomonic, are characteristic of meningococcemia. Purpura, however, may occur in as many as one third of cases of invasive *H. influenzae* infection.

Laboratory Tests

No laboratory test should be considered routine, but should be based on the clinical situation. The clinician must decide why a test is ordered. Is it part of a sepsis work-up or to help decide which children should receive expectant antibiotic therapy for occult bacteremia? If the child appears well, and particularly if he is to receive antibiotics for a focal infection such as otitis media, no laboratory studies are necessary. A WBC is recommended for highly febrile infants who look neither well nor toxic; who are without focal illness; or for whom a careful follow-up is questionable. The clinician should do a blood culture if the WBC is greater than 16,000 but should also realize that bacteremia may be present when the WBC is below this level. Many clinicians order a complete blood cell count because of the evidence that the more abnormalities on the CBC (*e.g.*, elevation in total WBC, bands, polys, erythrocyte sedimentation rate [ESR]), the increased likelihood of bacteremia. Although data are inconsistent, the ESR is probably as sensitive as any combination of tests. Other acute phase reactants such as C-reactive protein are probably not more sensitive. Slide agglutination tests and counterimmunoelectrophoresis (CIEP) have not been proven efficacious in screening for occult bacteremia. Vacuolization and toxic granulation in polymorphonuclear neutrophils, and acridine orange stains of buffy coat smears are sensitive, but not practical for office screening. A lumbar puncture (LP), chest roentgenogram, and urine culture are more appropriate as part of a sepsis work-up than to rule out bacteremia.

Infants who appear ill or toxic should be hospitalized and should have a full sepsis work-up, including an LP. Although an association in children under 1 year of age with an LP and later development of bacterial meningitis has been reported (but subsequently refuted), an LP should be performed if the procedure *is indicated*.

TREATMENT

Although there is no consensus of approach, data and current opinion favor expectant antibiotic therapy in children at high risk for bacteremia. Retrospective studies also show that children treated initially with antibiotics improve faster and suffer less complications.

Any child who does not look well; who is less than 24 months; or who has a temperature of at least 39.5°C and a WBC of greater than 16,000 is a candidate for expectant therapy. Antibiotics should also be started more readily in patients who are perceived as less compliant; who have poorer access to medical care; and whose parents are unlikely to observe subtle changes in the condition. Traditionally, this has been targeted to, but is obviously not limited to, an inner-city clinic population. It is obvious that the presence of a focal infection such as otitis media or pneumonia usually eliminates the decision of whether or not to initiate antibiotic therapy. Amoxicillin, 50 mg/kg/day for 10 days, is the preferred antibiotic for outpatient therapy because it covers all major pathogens. However, resistance, especially from *H. influenzae* type b is a major concern, and Augmentin is a reasonable alternative. If the child is allergic to penicillin, either cefaclor or trimethoprim–sulfamethoxazole should be used.

Most physicians would agree that blood cultures should be drawn prior to the initiation of therapy and may be discontinued if the blood cultures are negative, providing that there is no concomitant focal infection. Perhaps most important, and regardless of whether or not expectant therapy is begun, the child should have a close and careful follow-up. While expectant antibiotic therapy greatly reduces the possibility of a metastatic spread of infection, it does not eliminate this risk. Patients must be told to notify their physician if their status worsens because it may indicate complications such as meningitis, septicemia, septic arthritis, epiglottitis, endocarditis, pneumonia, cellulitis, and otitis media.

HOSPITALIZATION

Any toxic-appearing child, regardless of whether or not "risk" factors for bacteremia are present, should be hospitalized. Any child whose condition worsens while on expectant antibiotic therapy should also be hospitalized. The child should have a sepsis work-up and should receive intravenous antibiotics. A dilemma may arise when blood cultures are positive in children who are NOT receiving antibiotic therapy. All children should be re-examined and treated for 10 days, even if they are clinically well. The organism and condition of the child determine the need for hospitalization. Because of their high complication rate, infants with *H. influenzae* type b and meningococcal bacter-

Table 192-1. Summary of Management of the Highly Febrile Infant

CLINICAL SITUATION	MANAGEMENT
Serious infection or looks toxic	Hospitalize; sepsis work-up; treat
Nonwell, but "nontoxic" appearing without focal illness	Obtain WBC and, if elevated, send for a blood culture. Treat for presumptive bacteremia. Careful follow-up mandatory. If questionable, hospitalize.
Nonwell, but "nontoxic" appearing with focal illness	WBC and B/C unnecessary. If compliance is questionable, do a B/C only if WBC is elevated. Careful F/U is mandatory.
Well-appearing without focal illness	Careful F/U mandatory. WBC is optional, but if drawn and elevated (or close F/U questionable), send B/C and start expectant treatment.
Well-appearing with focal illness	No laboratory studies are necessary.

B/C = blood culture; F/U = follow-up;
WBC = white blood cell count.

emia, unless they are *completely* well or greatly improved, should be hospitalized. They should have a full sepsis work-up, including an LP to rule out meningitis, and they should receive parenteral antibiotics. With pneumococcal bacteremia, no laboratory studies other than repeating the blood culture are necessary if the child is well. The child should be hospitalized if his condition remains unchanged, and a full sepsis work-up should be done. If the child is still sick, though improved, an LP should be performed. If negative, the patient may either be treated in the hospital or followed carefully as an outpatient. In the latter case, if no improvement is made in 18 to 24 hours, the child should be hospitalized for intravenous therapy (Table 192-1).

Combination therapy, such as penicillin G (200 mg/kg/day divided q 4 to 6 hrs) and chloramphenicol (100 mg/kg/day divided q 6 hr), has been the standard treatment of sepsis; however, this treatment is rapidly being replaced by third-generation cephalosporins such as ceftriaxone or cefuroxime as a single medication. Intravenous antibiotics should be given initially and, when improvement occurs, they should be switched to oral therapy for the remaining 10 days.

PREVENTION

The contacts of patients who have a serious invasive disease such as bacteremia must seek medical attention at the first sign of illness. Specific prophylactic measures are available to reduce the risk of secondary spread of *N. meningitidis* and *H. influenzae* type b infections. All household, day care, nursery, and classroom contacts of patients with meningococcemia should receive rifampin chemoprophylaxis, 10 mg/kg/dose every 12 hours for 4 doses with a maximum dose of 600 mg. All household contacts of children less than 4 years old with *H. influenzae* type b bacteremia should receive rifampin, 20 mg/kg/dose, once a day for 4 days, with a maximum dose of 600 mg. The treatment of day care and classroom contacts of serious *H. influenzae* type b disease is somewhat controversial. Whereas some recommendations call for chemoprophylaxis to all contacts, most experts recommend rifampin only with outbreaks of at least two cases in the setting within a 60-day period. Since index cases may still harbor either organism in their nasopharynx and then reintroduce it into their households, they should also receive rifampin prophylaxis prior to discharge from hospital.

ANNOTATED BIBLIOGRAPHY

Carroll WL, Farrell M, Singer JI et al: Treatment of occult bacteremia: A prospective randomized clinical trial. Pediatrics 72:608–612, 1983 (Data to support treating the high-risk infant with expectant antibiotic therapy for presumptive occult bacteremia.)

Dashefsky B, Teele DW, Klein JO: Unsuspected meningococcemia. J Pediatr 102:69–72, 1983 (Outcome data showing that *N. meningitides* is the worst bacteria to have in the blood.)

Dershewitz RA, Wigder HN, Wigder CM et al: A comparative study of the prevalence, outcome and prediction of bacteremia in children. J Pediatr 103:352–358, 1983 (Major conclusions: (1) race and SES are not risk factors for bacteremia; (2) the limitation of clinical judgment in the prediction of bacteremia; (3) since highly febrile infants treated for focal illness do well, most do not need laboratory studies.)

Feigin RD: Prevention of infection with *Neisseria meningitidis* and *Haemophilus influenzae* type b. Pediatr in Rev 7:88–94, 1985 (Comprehensive discussion, including indications for active immunizations.)

McCarthy PL: Controversies in pediatrics: What tests are indicated for the child under 2 with fever. Pediatr in Rev 1:51–56, 1979 (Most of the controversies and uncertainties persist.)

McCarthy PL, Lembo RM, Baron MA et al: Predictive value of abnormal physical examination findings in ill-appearing and well-appearing febrile children. Pediatrics 76:167–171, 1985 (The Yale Observation Scale is useful in teaching, screening, and predicting which febrile infants are at greatest risk of serious illness.)

Roberts KB: Blood cultures in pediatric practice. Am J Dis Child 133:996–998, 1979 (This classic editorial is as timely now as it was in 1979.)

Roberts KB: Management of young, febrile infants. Am J

Dis Child 137:1143–1144, 1983 (Succinct, practical approach to managing the febrile neonate.)

Teele DW, Marshall R, Klein JO: Unsuspected bacteremia in young children. Pediatr Clin North Am 26:773–784, 1979 (Detailed description of risk factors for occult bacteremia, and the influence of the organism on outcome.)

193
Infections in Day Care Centers
MARGARET HIGHAM

The past decade has witnessed a steady trend toward the care of young children outside of the home. Over 11 million children now receive part- or full-time day care, primarily in day care centers or smaller day care homes. The increase in child day care has been accompanied by the recognition that these settings can act as foci for the development and spread of communicable diseases.

The common causes of infections in day care centers (DCC) are identified in this chapter. The epidemiology of these infections is discussed and the management of outbreaks is outlined. A DCC is defined as a facility outside the home that provides regular care to 2 or more unrelated children; this definition includes small day care homes as well as larger centers.

PATHOPHYSIOLOGY

The close proximity of young children, who often have poor personal hygiene, facilitates the spread of infections in DCC. Two modes of transmission are responsible for the dissemination of most DCC-associated infections: fecal–oral spread and respiratory spread.

Fecal–oral spread gives rise to diarrheal diseases and hepatitis A. Fecal contamination occurs widely in DCC environments occupied by young children in diapers, particularly on the hands of children and caretakers, and in diaper changing areas. Many enteric pathogens survive for a long time on environmental surfaces. DCCs often suffer from understaffing and poor training in hygienic standards. These factors lead to the ready spread of enteric organisms. Unsatisfactory physical facilities with inadequate handwashing and diaper changing areas contribute further to the problem.

Respiratory spread accounts for the transmission of acute upper respiratory tract infections and also the transmission of invasive pathogens such as *Hemophilus influenzae* type b and *Neisseria meningitidis*. Direct person-to-person spread by infected droplets and spread by fomites contribute to respiratory transmission.

The size and structure of a DCC are factors that influence the incidence and spread of disease. Day care centers that allow a mixture of children from different age groups promote the spread of diarrheal outbreaks throughout the facility. Outbreaks are more likely to be contained when groups are separated. Children in larger DCCs have higher rates of diarrheal disease than children cared for in smaller day care homes. This is thought to reflect the greater chance for the introduction of a pathogen prevalent in the community into the larger group with subsequent spread within the group. The return of children to their families each day then allows disease to be spread back to their households.

CLINICAL PRESENTATION

Diseases Transmitted by Fecal–Oral Spread

Hepatitis A. Outbreaks of hepatitis A in DCCs constitute a health problem not only for young children, but also for the community. Up to 40% of hepatitis A cases in the community can be traced to DCC contact. In most cases, children less than 4 years of age are either asymptomatic or develop only mild nonspecific symptoms; infection is anicteric in 80% of cases. In contrast, 75% of infected adults develop clinical illness. Thus, outbreaks are recognized usually by illness in employees and household contacts. Infected but asymptomatic young children excrete virus and may transmit infection to adult contacts within the DCC and at home.

The enrollment of children less than 2 years of age in the DCC is the most important determinant of the incidence and spread of hepatitis A. Employees and household members who have regular contact with toddlers less than 2 years old are at greatest risk for acquiring a symptomatic disease. Outbreaks of hepatitis A occur in >50% of DCCs enrolling infants and toddlers less than 2 years old. In contrast, <10% of DCCs enrolling children over 2 years of age have significant outbreaks.

Rotavirus. Rotavirus is a leading cause of DCC-associated diarrhea. Whether children in DCCs are more likely than children cared for at home to contract rotavirus infection is unknown. The epidemiology of rotavirus in DCCs is similar to that observed in the general population. Outbreaks occur primarily during cooler weather and infants have the highest attack rates. Up to 70% of infants in affected groups have developed disease during outbreaks. Asymptomatic excretion of rotavirus has been found in over 10% of children less than 2 years old attending DCC. Thus, a large reservoir of this organism exists in the DCC setting.

Giardia. *Giardia lamblia* is a parasite that has been identified with increasing frequency in children attending DCCs. Children 1 to 3 years old are most likely to acquire giardiasis. Children in this age group are still in diapers and fecal–oral transmission occurs readily. The infective innoculum for *Giardia* is low, facilitating person-to-person transmission.

Children who attend a DCC are significantly more likely to excrete *Giardia* cysts in their stools than are children who do not attend a DCC. *Giardia* prevalence ranging from 17% to 70% has been reported in DCCs from different areas of the country with a prevalence in age-matched controls of 2% to 5%. Family contacts of children in day care have higher attack rates than families who do not use child day care. Asymptomatic excretion appears to be common; it has been identified in up to 25% of children attending DCCs. A wide spectrum of disease is associated with giardiasis (see Chap. 201). Diarrhea, often lasting greater than 5 days, is accompanied in some cases by abdominal pain, bloating, anorexia, or weight loss.

Bacterial Gastroenteritis. Various bacterial enteric pathogens have been identified as causes of DCC-related diarrheal outbreaks, including *Shigella, Salmonella*, and *Campylobacter*. A stool culture is necessary to identify the specific pathogen.

Outbreaks of diarrhea due to *Shigella* have been well described. Symptomatic disease can be initiated by an innoculating dose as small as ten organisms, a characteristic that facilitates person-to-person spread in the DCC setting. Although children of all ages may be affected, attack rates are often highest in the younger groups. The spread of disease to household contacts is common.

Campylobacter jejuni has been identified occasionally as a pathogen among DCC attendees with diarrhea. *Salmonella* has only rarely been described as the cause of gastroenteritis in DCCs. It is not known if children attending DCCs are more likely to contract salmonellosis or *Campylobacter* enteritis than children cared for at home.

Despite careful research, an etiologic organism is not identified in most cases of gastroenteritis occurring in DCCs. A diagnosis is more likely to be made during outbreaks than for sporadic cases of diarrhea. When more data accumulate, other agents responsible for diarrhea in this setting may be described. *Clostridium difficile* and *Cryptosporidium* have recently been implicated.

Diseases Transmitted by Respiratory Spread

Upper Respiratory Tract Infection. Upper respiratory tract infections are the most commonly diagnosed illnesses among young children. Children in day care average eight respiratory infections each year; the frequency is highest in infants less than 1 year of age and decreases with each succeeding year. Only one study has compared the incidence of respiratory infections in children attending DCCs with that of children cared for at home; it demonstrated a higher number of febrile episodes in children less than 2 years old attending DCCs compared with those at home. Afebrile respiratory infections were not monitored. The viruses responsible for respiratory infections have been recovered both from acutely symptomatic children and from about 10% of asymptomatic children in day care.

Hemophilus Influenzae Type b. *Hemophilus influenzae* type b (Hib) is the leading cause of bacterial meningitis in the United States. Other systemic forms of Hib disease also occur frequently. The contagious nature of this organism, particularly among young children, has only been recognized in the last decade.

Two studies have identified DCC attendance as a significant risk factor for primary Hib infection. Overall, they found children who attended a DCC were approximately twice as likely to develop Hib disease. The relative risk varied with age in both studies. In one study, only children over 1 year of age had a significantly increased risk, and risk increased further in direct proportion to DCC size. In the other study, DCC attendees under 1 year of age had the greatest relative risk for Hib infection. Thus, children in day care do seem to be at greater risk for contracting primary Hib disease than children cared for at home. Further study will be required to delineate more clearly the relative contributions of age and DCC size to this increased risk.

The risk of secondary Hib disease among children exposed to a primary case in a day care is currently unclear because different studies have come to differing conclusions. Two large prospective studies have not demonstrated any increased risk of secondary disease among classroom contacts in a DCC. Two other studies, however, have found a substantial risk of secondary disease in DCC contacts. This risk was age-dependent, with children under 2 years of age having the greatest risk of developing Hib disease following a classmate's infection. Secondary disease also appeared to be related to the number of hours spent in day care. Those children attending for more hours per week were more likely to transmit or acquire infection. The risk of secondary disease appeared to be similar whether the index case had meningitis or another invasive form of the disease. The disparities in the magnitude of risk for DCC associated secondary Hib disease among these studies remains unexplained and will require further research for clarification.

Neisseria Meningitidis. Outbreaks of meningococcemia and meningococcal meningitis have been described in DCCs. The epidemiology is assumed to be similar to Hib infection, except that teachers are also at risk for acquiring disease. One study from Belgium found significantly increased secondary attack rates for DCC attendees; children 2 years of age and under were at greater risk than older preschool children.

Cytomegalovirus. The precise mechanisms of cytomegalovirus (CMV) transmission in the community are not completely understood. Infected children shed virus in saliva and urine for long periods of time. It has been suggested that repeated close contact with secretions and excretions of infected children either directly or indirectly from toys is a major mode of CMV transmission.

Cytomegalovirus excretion occurs frequently among DCC attendees. A comparison of CMV infection among children of similar socioeconomic backgrounds and ages show rates of viral infection that are 2 to 3 times greater in children attending DCCs than among children cared for at home. The prevalence of viral excretion among children in DCC varies with age. CMV infection appears to be uncommon during the first year of life but most toddlers in a DCC will acquire CMV. The dramatic increase in incidence of infection among toddlers is probably related to the development of their ambulatory abilities, which results in frequent close contact and ready transmission of oral secretions and urine.

Most CMV infections in children and adults are asymptomatic. However, a primary CMV infection among pregnant women may result in a symptomatic congenital infection of the newborn. Thus, the major concern is that infected children may in turn infect susceptible pregnant women, particularly their own mothers and DCC providers.

The magnitude of risk for a seronegative mother or child care worker is unknown. An infected child can clearly transmit a virus to a susceptible mother. Day care workers may be at less risk of acquiring CMV from their infected charges. Many questions about the potential risks of DCC-related CMV infection remain unanswered.

WORK-UP

Pediatricians need to be aware of the diseases that are associated with day care facilities. They must keep in mind the child care arrangements of the children whom they evaluate for diarrheal and systemic illness. Early identification of significant pathogens and appropriate management can help to curtail further spread of disease. Day care center directors need to keep the parents of attendees informed of the occurrence of disease. This epidemiologic information can assist pediatricians in the early diagnosis of ill contacts.

Details of the work-up for each of the diseases discussed are not presented here. The reader should refer to the appropriate chapters elsewhere in the text. A diagnosis in most cases depends on appropriate culture results or body fluid examination.

MANAGEMENT

Diseases Spread by Fecal–Oral Transmission

Procedures designed to minimize fecal–oral spread may reduce the amount of enteric infection experienced at a DCC and may help curtail ongoing epidemics. Handwashing is the most important factor in reducing the spread of enteric infection and, if performed conscientiously, handwashing has been demonstrated to decrease the amount of diarrheal disease in DCCs. Fecal contamination of the child, child handler, and environment occurs most often during diaper changing. Since enteric pathogens may be shed asymptomatically or for a long time after recovery from acute infections, attention to good hygienic practices should become a matter of habit during the diaper changing of all children. Diaper changing areas should be designed to facilitate cleaning and handwashing after each use. When possible, staff who prepare food should not be involved in diaper changing.

Single children who are acutely ill with diarrhea should probably be excluded from the DCC until symptoms subside. The management of an outbreak of diarrheal disease involving several children is more difficult. Various strategies have been used including exclusion, cohorting of sick children in the DCC, and the development of alternative care resources. There are advantages and disadvantages to each alternative and consultation with public health officials is recommended.

Hepatitis A. Gamma globulin prophylaxis can help terminate hepatitis A outbreaks and reduce the incidence of hepatitis A in the general community. Current recommendations for the use of gamma globulin depend on the ages of children in the affected DCC and on the distribution and number of identified cases. Since the spread of hepatitis A is limited in centers enrolling only older children, the use of gamma globulin can also be limited. When a single case of hepatitis A occurs in an employee or child attending a DCC accepting only children over 2 years, gamma globulin (0.02 ml/kg IM) should be administered to all center employees and to children in the same classroom as the index case. Hepatitis A tends to spread widely in DCCs accepting children who are still in diapers, and gamma globulin prophylaxis should be more extensive. If a single case of hepatitis A occurs in an employee or child in a DCC accepting children in diapers, or if cases occur among household contacts of 2 children within 3 weeks of one another, a gamma globulin injection should be given to all staff and children at the DCC, including all new enrollees for up to 6 weeks after the last case is identified. If more than 3 weeks has elapsed from the initial case to the recognition of the outbreak, or if 3 or more families report disease, prophylaxis should also be considered for household contacts of all children under 3 years of age who are enrolled in the DCC.

Giardia Lamblia. The management of giardiasis in children attending DCC is controversial. Treatment is clearly indicated for all symptomatic cases with an appropriate antiparasitic agent. Three drugs are available in the United States: furazolidone (6 to 8 mg/kg/day divided qid for 10 days, maximum dose 400 mg/day); quinacrine (6 mg/kg/day divided tid for 7 days, maximum dose 300 mg/day); and metronidazole (15 mg/kg/day divided tid-qid for 10 days, maximum 750 mg/day). Metronidazole is not approved for the treatment of giardiasis by the Food and Drug Administration.

The management of infected but asymptomatic children attending DCC is less clear. The drugs used for the treatment of giardiasis are not without toxicity. They can cause unpleasant side effects and they are only effective in 85% to 95% of cases. A longitudinal study of these children has shown that *Giardia* excretion is well tolerated. The public health effects of untreated cyst excretors and their role in perpetuating the spread of disease is unknown.

Bacterial Gastroenteritis. When *Shigella* enteritis is diagnosed in a child who attends day care, a stool culture should be obtained from all symptomatic staff and attendees. Infected children and adults should receive antibiotic therapy with either ampicillin (not amoxicillin) or trimethoprim–sulfamethoxazole. Because of the low innoculum needed to cause disease, infected individuals should not have contact with uninfected children in the DCC until three negative stool cultures are documented; this may involve excluding children or cohorting if several children are affected.

A stool culture should be obtained for all DCC contacts of an individual with salmonellosis. It is currently recommended that ill children should be excluded from the DCC until three negative stool cultures have been obtained, but this recommendation is difficult to carry out as some children may excrete salmonella for weeks to months. In this case, a return to the DCC with strict observation of hand washing policies may prove more practical.

The treatment of *Campylobacter* enteritis with erythromycin may not shorten the course of the disease but it will eliminate stool excretion in most cases. Children may return to day care once cultures are negative.

Diseases Spread by Respiratory Transmission

Procedures designed to minimize the spread of respiratory secretions may help to control respiratory disease in the DCC setting. Strict attention to handwashing and hygiene are essential. The proper disposal of tissues saturated with respiratory secretions and handwashing after contact with such secretions should be emphasized. Children should be taught to cover their mouths when they sneeze or cough.

Upper Respiratory Tract Infection. Children who have afebrile upper respiratory infections should not be excluded from the DCC. There is no conclusive evidence that the elimination of such children lessens the incidence of serious infection, and viral spread will probably have already occurred before the onset of symptoms.

Hemophilus Influenzae Type b. The prevention of invasive Hib disease is available with the use of a vaccine. Unfortunately, the current vaccine is immunogenic only in children over 18 months of age, which leaves a large proportion of susceptible children unprotected. Until a more immunogenic vaccine is available, the focus must be on an early diagnosis of Hib disease and on strategies for the prevention of secondary spread within the DCC.

Rifampin is effective in eliminating nasopharyngeal carriage of Hib, unlike other commonly used antibiotics that only temporarily suppress Hib nasopharyngeal colonization without eradicating the organism. The CDC currently recommends that when a case of systemic Hib occurs in a DCC classroom in which one or more children under 2 years of age have been exposed, strong consideration should be given to administering rifampin prophylaxis to all children and staff in the classroom. The dose of rifampin is 20 mg/kg once daily for 4 days (maximum 600 mg/day); for infants less than 1 month of age 10 mg/kg is given once daily for 4 days. The ill child should also receive rifampin before he returns to the DCC. Physicians diagnosing Hib disease in a DCC attendee should notify public health officials, who will help communicate to parents the possibility of the risk of disease for their children. In some states public health officials will also help with the coordination and implementation of chemoprophylaxis. Chemoprophylaxis is unlikely to be effective if less than 75% of contacts receive rifampin.

Not all infectious disease specialists agree with the CDC recommendations; they would withhold prophylaxis unless two or more cases of invasive Hib disease occur in a DCC.

Neisseria Meningitidis. When a physician diagnoses meningococcal disease in a DCC attendee, he should immediately notify public health officials.

Chemoprophylaxis with rifampin is recommended for all children and staff in the same classroom. The dose of rifampin recommended for prophylaxis of meningococcal disease is 10 mg/kg twice a day for 2 days (maximum dose 1200 mg/day). The index patient should also receive rifampin before returning to the DCC. For a further discussion on prophylaxis against *Hemophilus influenzae* type b and *Neisseria meningitidis*, see Chapter 194.

Vaccine Preventable Diseases

Routine childhood immunizations are particularly important for children attending a DCC. Strict adherence to recommended schedules for polio, DPT, and MMR vaccine administration should be maintained.

INDICATIONS FOR REFERRAL

The heterogeneity of day care facilities and the range of pathogens that cause disease can pose dilemmas in management. Local public health departments can be helpful in providing guidelines for the management of specific situations. When a significant pathogen is identified in a child attending day care, public health authorities can assist in the implementation of infection control recommendations and in the identification of related cases.

PATIENT EDUCATION

Pediatricians are able to advise parents about their arrangements for child day care and to provide anticipatory guidance. Parents should be aware of the potential for disease transmission within the day care setting. They should understand the need for good hygienic practices and they should work to implement them. The importance of handwashing in particular, which is a simple but often neglected procedure, should be stressed both at the DCC and at home.

ANNOTATED BIBLIOGRAPHY

Bartlett AV, Moore M, Gary GW et al: Diarrheal illness among infants and toddlers in day care centers. I: Epidemiology and pathogens. II: Comparison with day care homes and households. J Pediatr 107:503, 1985 (Prospective study of causes, patterns, and incidence of diarrhea in children in DCC and a comparison with children cared for at home.)

Child Day Care Infectious Disease Study Group: Public health considerations of infectious diseases in child day care centers. J Pediatr 105:683, 1984 (Excellent review of current information and policies on day care associated infections; extensive bibliography.)

Dashefsky B, Wald E, Li K: Management of contacts of children in day care with invasive *Hemophilus influenzae* type b disease. Pediatr 78:939, 1986 (Well reasoned commentary on the issues involved in using rifampin prophylaxis to reduce secondary Hib disease, and practical recommendations.)

Fleming DW, Leibenhaut MH, Albanes D et al: Secondary *Haemophilus influenzae* type b in day-care facilities. JAMA 254:509, 1985 (Demonstrates increased risk of secondary Hib disease in children in DCC.)

Istre GR, Conner JS, Broome CV et al: Risk factors for primary invasive *Haemophilus influenzae* disease: Increased risk from day care attendance and school-aged household members. J Pediatr 106:190, 1985

Murphy TV, Clements JF, Breedlove JA et al: Risk of subsequent disease among day-care contacts of patients with systemic *Hemophilus influenzae* type b disease. N Engl J Med 316:5, 1987 (Prospective study in Texas demonstrating no increased risk of secondary Hib disease among DCC contacts.)

Osterholm MT, Pierson LM, White KE et al; The risk of subsequent transmission of *Hemophilus influenzae* type b disease among children in day care. N Engl J Med 316:1, 1987 (A second prospective study in Minnesota also showing increased risk for secondary Hib disease in DCCs.)

Redmond SR, Pichicher ME: *Hemophilus influenzae* type b disease. JAMA 252:2581, 1984 (Describes increased relative risk for primary Hib infection in children in day care.)

194
Antimicrobial Prophylaxis
ELLEN R. WALD

The purpose of this review is to provide the pediatric practitioner with access to the rationale, indications, and recommendations for prophylactic antimicrobials to prevent bacterial and parasitic infections in office practice. Prophylaxis for surgical procedures or for the immunosuppressed patient is not discussed.

ESTABLISHED INDICATIONS FOR ANTIMICROBIAL PROPHYLAXIS

There are eight established indications for antimicrobial prophylaxis in pediatric patients that are accepted and noncontroversial. These indications include antimicrobial prophylaxis to prevent endocarditis in patients with structural cardiac disease who undergo procedures likely to be associated with bacteremia; penicillin prophylaxis to prevent rheumatic fever recurrences; ophthalmic antimicrobials to prevent neonatal conjunctivitis caused by *Neisseria gonorrhoeae* or *Chlamydia trachomatis*; prophylaxis after exposure to a sexual contact with gonorrhea or syphilis; prophylaxis to prevent recurrent urinary tract infections; isoniazid prophylaxis for household contacts of individuals with tuberculosis; and malarial prophylaxis for travelers to an endemic area. The preferred drugs and route of administration are shown in Table 194-1.

Endocarditis

Prophylaxis for endocarditis is indicated in patients with congenital heart disease (except uncomplicated secundum atrial septal defect), rheumatic fever or other acquired valvular heart disease, idiopathic hypertrophic subaortic stenosis, and mitral valve prolapse syndrome. Patients with rheumatic fever who have been on penicillin prophylaxis to prevent a recurrent infection due to group A streptococci may harbor viridans streptococci that are resistant to penicillin. Accordingly, for these patients and for those who are penicillin allergic, erythromycin is preferred to penicillin for prophylaxis against infectious endocarditis.

Rheumatic Fever

After diagnosing rheumatic fever, the patient is started on prophylactic penicillin, the thrust of which is to prevent recurrent group A streptococcal pharyngitis that might lead to recurrent rheumatic fever (particularly rheumatic fever with carditis). Although recurrent episodes of rheumatic fever tend to mimic the initial episode with regard to the major manifestation, a cross-over may occur (*i.e.*, patients initially presenting with arthritis or chorea may develop carditis during recurrences). The most serious outcome is that children who initially

Table 194-1.   Established Indications for Prophylaxis

INDICATION	ANTIMICROBIAL AGENT	ROUTE OF ADMINISTRATION	DOSE AND DURATION
1. Endocarditis	Penicillin V	Oral	> 60 lb: 2 g 1 hr before procedure and 1 g 6 hr later. < 60 lb: ½ of the above dose
	Erythromycin	Oral	20 mg/kg (max 1.0 g) 1½ to 2 hr prior to procedure, then 10 mg/kg (max 500 mg) q6h for 8 doses
2. Rheumatic fever	a. BenzathinePenicillinG	Intramuscular	1.2 million units
	b. Penicillin V,G	Oral	250 mg bid
	c. Sulfisoxazole	Oral	1.0 g/day
	d. Erythromycin	Oral	250 mg/day
3. Ophthalmia neonatorum a. Gonococcal	a. Silver nitrate	Topically	Once at delivery
	b. Erythromycin 0.5%	Topically	Once at delivery
	c. Tetracycline 1.0%	Topically	Once at delivery
b. Chlamydia	Erythromycin 0.5%	Topically	Once
4. Gonorrhea exposure	a. Procaine penicillin G plus probenecid	Intramuscular Oral	4.8 million units or 100,000 units/kg 1.0 g or 25 mg/kg
	b. Tetracycline	Oral	0.5 g four times daily for 5 days
	c. Amoxicillin plus probenecid	Oral Oral	3.5 g or 50 mg/kg 1.0 g or 25 mg/kg
5. Syphilis exposure	Regimens that treat gonorrhea are effective for incubating syphilis.		
6. Urinary tract	SMX–TMP	Oral	10 and 2 mg/kg respectively hs
	Nitrofurantoin	Oral	2 mg/kg hs
7. Mycobacterium tuberculosis	Isoniazid	Oral	10 mg/kg/day
8. Malaria	Chloroquine base	Oral	5 mg/kg once weekly starting 1 week before and for 6 weeks after leaving endemic area

present with carditis will develop recurrent carditis with severe sequelae including early mortality. It is important to recognize that the twice daily penicillin prophylaxis does not protect patients with rheumatic fever from endocarditis. Although the recommendations regarding prophylaxis against endocarditis have not been subjected to critical clinical evaluation, their use represents the current standard of care.

The duration of twice daily penicillin prophylaxis to prevent streptococcal infections in individuals with rheumatic fever is controversial. The decision must be based on the likelihood of the index case having contact with others who may be infected with group A streptococci. Since these infections are endemic in the age group 5 to 15 years, an evaluation of the degree of contact with school-aged youngsters is critical. Accordingly, continued prophylaxis is indicated for parents of school-aged children or teachers of primary and secondary grade schools who continue to be vulnerable. If one elects to use benzathine penicillin G in younger children, these injections should be spaced ~3 weeks apart.

Ophthalmia Neonatorum

This syndrome is usually due to infection with either *C. trachomatis* or *N. gonorrhoeae*. Topical therapy with an erythromycin ophthalmic preparation is effective in preventing both and is accordingly the preferred drug for this indication.

Exposure to Gonorrhea or Syphilis

The victim of sexual abuse or a known sexual contact of an individual infected with *N. gonorrhoeae* or *Treponema pallidum* should be provided with prophylaxis for these infections. The regimens shown in Table 194-1 are all effective for gonorrhea and likewise for incubating syphilis. If a nontreponemal test for syphilis shows reactivity, then an alternate treatment will be required for established or primary infection with *T. pallidum* (see Chap. 195).

Recurrent Urinary Tract Infection

The two categories of patients that are best managed with chemoprophylaxis include children with demonstrable vesicoureteral reflux and those without anatomic problems who are subject to closely spaced recurrent acute urinary tract infections. In the former category, the intention of prophylaxis is to prevent renal damage by maintaining the sterility of the refluxing urine. In the latter, the aim of prophylaxis is simply to reduce the morbidity associated with frequent infections. The efficacy of nitrofurantoin, sulfamethoxazole–trimethoprim (SMX–TMP), and methanamine mandelate as prophylactic agents in urinary tract infections is well established. The first two are most commonly used in childhood. The third requires acidification of the urine, which is often accomplished by the coadministration of ascorbic acid. An acid *p*H allows the disassociation of mandelamine to formic acid, thereby providing an antiseptic intravesicular environment. Both nitrofurantoin and SMX–TMP are well absorbed from the gastrointestinal tract. Accordingly, little active drug reaches the colon to be exposed to coliforms (a population of microorganisms that is likely to ultimately colonize the periurethral area and to be introduced into the bladder urine). On the other hand, antimicrobial agents such as amoxicillin, sulfisoxazole, or cephalexin are only moderately well absorbed orally. Consequently, sufficient drug reaches the colon thereby providing an opportunity for secondarily resistant coliforms to become predominant and to emerge ultimately as the infectious pathogen.

One concern regarding urinary tract prophylaxis is the safety of the recommended antimicrobial agents. Nitrofurantoin has been shown to be a cause of pneumonitis and hepatitis and thereby requires monitoring during chronic usage. SMX–TMP may cause bone marrow suppression and Stevens–Johnson syndrome. A half dose of either at bedtime is usually sufficient to maintain sterile urine. When prescribed for reflux, the prophylactic agent should be used until the reflux resolves. An assessment of the persistence of reflex should be undertaken every 6 to 12 months with a radionuclide voiding cystourethrogram. When the indication for prophylaxis is frequent acute infections, a 6-month trial of prophylaxis is appropriate. Repeated courses may be required if frequent infections recur after the prophylaxis has been discontinued (see also Chap. 114).

Mycobacterium Tuberculosis

Prophylaxis for *M. tuberculosis* is indicated for skin-test-negative household contacts of active cases of pulmonary tuberculosis. The skin test is repeated after 3 months of treatment; no further medication is necessary if the skin test is still negative.

Another isoniazid treatment group is asymptomatic, tuberculin skin-test-positive patients. Although asymptomatic, these patients have an infection and therefore the isoniazid is not a prophylaxis but rather an appropriate treatment (see Chap. 166).

Malaria

Travelers to malaria endemic areas are at risk of acquiring an infection. In areas of chloroquine-resistant *Plasmodium falciparum*, additional measures beyond those mentioned in Table 194-1 may be required. The former recommendation was once weekly pyremethamine–sulfadoxine (Fansidar); however, since several deaths have been reported after use of Fansidar, risk–benefit considerations are essential in the final individual recommendations.

CONTROVERSIAL INDICATIONS FOR PROPHYLACTIC ANTIMICROBIALS

There are seven controversial areas involving prophylactic therapy that are common clinical situations for the practitioner and they deserve a more detailed discussion. These areas include prophylaxis for *Neisseria meningitidis* and *Hemophilus influenzae* type b, otitis media, animal bites and lacerations, pertussis, asplenia, and early-onset group B streptococcal sepsis.

Neisseria Meningitidis and Hemophilus Influenzae Type B

Intimate contacts of a patient with infection caused by either *Neisseria meningitidis* or *Hemophilus influenzae* type b are at an increased risk of developing invasive disease caused by these two bacterial species. The risk for both infections is highest for children between the ages of 3 months and 4 years, a time when many children lack the protective antibody that is directed against the polysaccharide capsule of the organism (anticapsular antibody). The risk for secondary meningococcal infection extends into adulthood with a second peak in the 15 to 24 year age group, when crowding due to dormitory style housing (military barracks or college campus) facilitates the transmission of the organism. In contrast, the risk of secondary illness due to *H. influenzae* type b is decreased dramatically beyond the fourth birthday and is virtually nil in adults.

Pharyngeal colonization with *N. meningitidis* or *H. influenzae* type b is not rare. Under circumstances in which there has been no exposure to an individual with invasive disease caused by *N. meningitidis* or *H. influenzae*, the pharyngeal colonization rate with these two bacterial species is ~ 10% and 2%, respectively. When there has been a case of invasive disease due to either of these pathogens, the pharyngeal colonization rate amongst contacts is usually dramatically increased—in the range of 30% to 70%. The individuals who are at highest risk of developing illness after an exposure to a patient with invasive disease are those who are not colonized and are antibody-negative. (There is a suggestion that those individuals who are carriers are actually at low risk of invasive disease, probably because many already possess anticapsular antibody). When a susceptible (antibody-negative) noncolonized individual is exposed to the invasive pathogen, one of two outcomes can be anticipated: either the individual will become a healthy carrier of the organism or invasion and subsequent disease will evolve. Factors favoring the latter outcome have not been delineated but may include the development of, or exposure to, viral agents that cause an upper respiratory infection. Thus, to protect antibody-negative, noncolonized individuals from acquiring colonization with these pathogens, we try to create a Neisseria or Hemophilus-free environment. This can be accomplished with rifampin, an antimicrobial capable of eradicating these pathogens from the throats of those who are colonized. Most secondary cases in the household environment occur within a few days of the primary case. Since conventional throat cultures for the identification of *N. meningitidis* and *H. influenzae* are time consuming and insensitive, the strategy employed to protect the unidentified individual who is at highest risk is the use of rifampin for all contacts who may be colonized without obtaining prior throat cultures. This will create (at least temporarily) a pathogen-free environment, consequently protecting against acquisition of the bacterial species by a potentially susceptible individual.

Other important information in guiding decisions regarding prophylaxis are: (1) index cases have persistent pharyngeal colonization even after parenteral therapy for their primary infection, (2) individuals less than 2 years of age may fail to develop protective antibody even after invasive infections. Thus, the following procedure is recommended:

a. All household and intimate contacts of children with invasive illness due to meningococcal disease should receive rifampin at a dose of 10 mg/kg twice daily for 2 days (not to exceed 600 mg twice daily). A household contact may be defined as someone who lives with the index case or is a nonresident who spends considerable time with the index case. Day care contacts or close neighborhood friends may be included by this definition. The index case should also receive rifampin at the end of treatment for the primary infection.

b. All household and intimate contacts of children less than 2 years of age with invasive disease caused by *H. influenzae* type b should receive rifampin at a dose of 20 mg/kg/day (not to exceed 600 mg) as a single daily dose for 4 days.

c. If the index case with disease caused by *H. influenzae* type b is older than 2 years, the requirement to provide prophylaxis is contingent on there being an additional age-susceptible child in the household. If there are no other children less than 4 years of age, then prophylaxis for household members is not recommended. If there are children less than 4 years, the procedure is as in (b) (see also Chap. 193 for a further discussion of prophylaxis in a day care setting).

Otitis Media

Antimicrobial prophylaxis has been recommended for children with recurrent episodes of acute otitis media. The objective of prophylaxis is to reduce the morbidity—otalgia and hearing loss—associated with these episodes. Although several studies have addressed this issue, they are imperfect in their design and do not provide conclusive evidence of the benefits of prophylaxis. Nonetheless, the consensus is that antimicrobial prophylaxis with an appropriate agent will prevent symptomatic episodes of acute otitis media. The suggested indications for initiating prophylaxis are three episodes of acute otitis media in 6 months or four episodes in a year. The best studied regimen is sulfisoxazole at 75 mg/kg in two divided doses; others recommend amoxicillin at 20 mg/kg/day as a single nighttime dose. Although symptomatic episodes of otitis media may be prevented by these regimens, their impact on the persistence of middle ear effusion has been less thoroughly evaluated. Consequently, it is recommended that patients on antimicrobial prophylaxis be examined at regular intervals (at least once monthly) to evaluate the possibility of persistent effusion. Persistence of middle ear fluid beyond the 3-month mark—particularly if associated with significant hearing loss—may require an alternative management strategy. The duration of prophylactic antimicrobial therapy depends on the length of the remaining respiratory infection season. For example, if a patient experiences three episodes of acute otitis media by November, it will probably be necessary to treat prophylactically for 6 months, or until the respiratory season is over. Alternatively, if prophylaxis is not initiated until March or April, it may only be necessary to treat for 1 to 2 months (see also Chap. 80).

Animal Bites and Lacerations

The role of prophylactic antibiotics in dog bites has not been settled. However, there is consensus that antibiotic prophylaxis is not indicated for non-facial or hand dog-bite-inflicted wounds that are adequately cleaned, irrigated, and debrided. In contrast, a small study (11 patients) of prophylactic therapy with oxacillin for cat bites showed a significant decrease in the infection rate in the treated group (see also Chap. 141).

Pertussis

Primary prevention of pertussis is accomplished with the use of a whole killed bacterial vaccine. The exposure of an unimmunized host to active illness is likely to cause disease. The exposure of partially immunized individuals also provides some risk of infection.

Limited data suggest that erythromycin is an effective agent with which to provide prophylaxis for pertussis if the exposure is recognized early in the incubation period. Erythromycin prophylaxis was provided for one immunized and 12 unimmunized children who were exposed to an active case of pertussis within the family; only three children developed mild respiratory symptoms. In a hospital outbreak of pertussis in Cincinnati, only one of six infected staff who received erythromycin prophylaxis developed the disease. Within a nursery setting, administration of erythromycin to seven infants exposed to a 6-week-old child with pertussis appeared to prevent the appearance of clinical disease. In contrast to these reports, there is ample documentation that once the paroxysmal stage of illness has evolved, antimicrobial agents are not effective in modifying the course of illness.

Although no prospective randomized controlled trials have systematically evaluated erythromycin prophylaxis for pertussis, the Committee of Infectious Diseases of the American Academy of Pediatrics recommends that infants who are exposed to pertussis should receive erythromycin prophylaxis as soon as possible at a dose of 40 mg/kg/day in four divided doses for 7 days.

Asplenia

The role of oral penicillin prophylaxis in preventing pneumococcal infection in patients with sickle cell disease or asplenia has been evaluated in a randomized, double-blind, multicenter trial. The risk of septicemia from *S. pneumoniae* was decreased by 84% and no deaths occurred in the group that received penicillin. Although compliance with the oral regimen could not be adequately monitored, oral penicillin prophylaxis is an effective strategy when combined with neonatal screening for sickle cell disease, pneumococcal vaccine, and comprehensive health care. The dose of phenoxymethyl penicillin was 25 mg/kg/day in two divided doses.

Early Onset Group B Streptococcal Sepsis

Pregnant women with heavy vaginal colonization with group B streptococci may transmit this organism to their neonates. If other high-risk factors are present such as prematurity, prolonged rupture of membranes, or maternal perinatal fever, the infant may develop early onset sepsis with group B streptococci. Studies show that intrapartum antimicrobial therapy with ampicillin can effectively prevent colonization of and disease in the neonate. The strategic problem that has evolved is identifying the mother with heavy colonization in a timely fashion so as to selectively identify the mother–infant pair at risk and to minimize the use of intrapartum antimicrobials in those who do not require them.

ANNOTATED BIBLIOGRAPHY

General

Feder HM: Chemoprophylaxis in ambulatory patients. Pediatr Infect Dis 2:251, 1983 (Nice review of eight indications for prophylaxis.)

Scheifele DW: Prophylactic antibiotics in children. Pediatr Infect Dis 1:420–424, 1982 (Attempts to identify key elements of successful chemoprophylaxis.)

Endocarditis

American Heart Association Committee report: Prevention of Bacterial Endocarditis Circulation. 56:139A–143A, 1977 (Standard recommendations for prophylaxis in patients with structural heart defects.)

Urinary Tract Infections

Hellerstein S: Recurrent urinary tract infections in children. Pediatr Infect Dis 1:271–182, 1981 (Provides useful guidelines for the evaluation and management of children with urinary tract infections.)

Holmberg L, Boman G, Bottiger LE et al: Adverse reactions to nitrofurantoin: Analysis of 921 reports. Am J Med 69:733–788, 1980 (Detailed account of toxicity related to nitrofurantoin use.)

Malaria

Adverse reactions to Fansidar and updated recommendations for its use in the prevention of malaria. Morb Mortal Week Rep 33:713–714, 1985

Otitis Media

Paradise JL: Antimicrobial prophylaxis for recurrent acute otitis media. Oto Rhinol Laryngol 905:53–57, 1981 (Analysis of studies concerning prophylaxis for otitis media reported before 1981. More recent studies suffer from similar methodologic flaws but purport the same result—apparent efficacy of sulfisoxazole in preventing symptomatic episodes of acute otitis media.)

Pertussis

Altemeier WA, Ayoub EM: Erythromycin prophylaxis for pertussis. Pediatr 59:623–625, 1977 (Limited experience with erythromycin as a prophylactic drug for pertussis.)

Animal Bites and Hand Lacerations

Boenning DA, Fleisher GR, Campos JM: Dog bites in children: Epidemiology, microbiology, and penicillin prophylactic therapy. Am J Emerg Med 1:17–21, 1983 (Routine use of prophylactic penicillin is not required for simple nonfacial and non-hand dog bites in children.)

Rosen RA: The use of antibiotics in the initial management of recent dog-bite wounds. Am J Emerg Med 3:19–23, 1985 (Antibiotics are not indicated in the initial management of dog bite wounds. However, most guidelines state that prophylaxis is indicated for bites to the hand and face and those at high risk for infection [see Chap. 141].)

Sexually Transmitted Diseases

STD treatment guidelines. MMWR 34:75–1085, 1985

Prophylaxis for H. Influenzae and N. Meningitidis

Shapiro E: Prophylaxis for contacts of patients with meningococcal or *haemophilus influenzae* type b disease. Pediatr Infect Dis 1: 132–138, 1982 (Comprehensive review of presumed epidemiology and pathogenesis of secondary or associated cases of illness.)

Asplenia

Gaston MH, Varter JI, Woods G et al: Prophylaxis with oral penicillin in children with sickle cell anemia. N Engl J Med 314:1593–1599, 1986 (Reports an 84% reduction in episodes of sepsis in penicillin treated patients compared to controls.)

Group B Streptococcal Sepsis

Boyer KM, Gotoff SP: Prevention of early-onset neonatal group B streptococcal disease with selective intrapartum chemoprophylaxis. N Engl J Med 314:1665–1669, 1986 (Presents an effective and practical strategy for reducing GBS sepsis; women at high risk received intrapartum ampicillin.)

195
Sexually Transmitted Diseases

BARRY DASHEFSKY

The primary care pediatrician encounters sexually transmitted diseases (STD) in newborn, prepubertal, pubertal, and postpubertal patients. Each practitioner must decide *a priori* whether his office practice will be inclined and equipped to provide appropriate questioning, physical examination (including pelvic examination), laboratory studies, and confidential management for STD or be prepared to refer patients elsewhere for these services. Although consideration is usually given to STD when symptomatology is overt and obvious (*e.g.*, when the patient presents with urethral or vaginal discharge or genital lesions), anticipation and vigilance are required to facilitate their diagnosis when the presentation is vague, subtle, or frankly asymptomatic or when the patient is unable or unwilling to direct our attention.

Despite the fact that only traditional venereal diseases (*i.e.*, gonorrhea, syphilis, chancroid, granuloma inguinale, and lymphogranuloma venereum) are mandatorily reported to public health authorities and, even these conditions are grossly underreported, epidemiologic data indicate that the incidence of nearly all STD and their complications have burgeoned to epidemic proportions in industrialized countries during the past 30 years, especially among women, adolescents, and homosexuals.

Most adolescents with STD, like adults, are unwitting victims of voluntary (although perhaps unacknowledged) sexual contact. The clinical manifestations and consequences of these infections are identical to those in adults. The changing physiology of the maturing female genitourinary tract may explain a greater predilection of adolescents to endocervical infection due to *Neisseria gonorrhoeae* and *Chlamydia trachomatis*.

Although nonvenereal transmission by fomites or close nonsexual contact with infected adults is a tenable, albeit rare, explanation of an STD infection in a prepubertal child, involuntary sexual contact (*i.e.*, sexual abuse) must always be suspected and explored as the most likely cause.

Neonates and infants may present with protean features of STD infection incurred *in utero* (either by hematogenous transplacental transmission or by retrograde extension from the maternal genital tract), during parturition (by direct contact with an infected birth canal), or postnatally.

This chapter is not intended to provide a comprehensive listing of all STD agents and their most common clinical manifestations in children and adolescents. Rather, selected aspects of the clinical presentation, diagnosis, and management of four of the most common STD (gonorrhea, chlamydia, herpes simplex virus, and syphilis) are presented. The reader is referred to the following chapters in this volume where information regarding many of the STD is presented according to the presenting clinical syndrome: Chapters 66 (Warts and Molluscum Contagiosum), 93 (Conjunctivitis), 110 (Hepatitis), 114 (Urinary Tract Infections), 115 (Dysuria and Frequency), 119 (Genital Pain), 120 (Vulvovaginitis), 122 (Pelvic Inflammatory Disease), 165 (Pneumonia), 191 (Neonatal Infections). Additionally, the reader is referred to related topics in chapters 14 (Sexuality Education), 20 (Child Abuse), 42 (Contraception), and 44 (Teenage Pregnancy). (For a more detailed discussion of STD, see the references by Holmes, 1984 and Bell, 1983, which are listed in the bibliography.)

A few general statements regarding the evaluation and management of STD are germane: (1) Multiple STD often coexist. Suspicion or diagnosis of one infectious agent should generally result in (laboratory) assessment for additional candidate pathogens. (2) Sexual partners should be identified and (often presumptively, on the basis of a history of contact) treated for infection due to the agent(s) identified in the index case. (3) Follow-up tests for proof of cure should be routinely obtained; sexual activity should be strongly discouraged pending results of follow-up tests. (4) The value of barrier contraception, especially condoms, in lowering, but not eliminating the risk of contracting and transmitting STD should be stressed in patient education.

GONORRHEA

Background

Infection due to *Neisseria gonorrhoeae* is the most common reportable infectious disease in the United States. Approximately one million cases are reported each year with an estimated additional one to two million cases unreported annually. Age-specific rates indicate that teenagers and young adults are at highest risk for acquiring gonorrhea. Although the highest overall rate of disease occurs in the 20- to 24-year-old age bracket, more than one quarter of all cases occur among pediatric patients less than 19 years old of whom girls, between the ages of 15 and 19 years, have the highest rate of infection (~900/100,000). Although gonorrhea is usually a mild disease, 10% to 20% of infected females develop salpingitis of whom a significant proportion become involuntarily infertile (at least 13% after one episode of salpingitis, 36% after two episodes, and 75% after three or more episodes). At least 1% of infected individuals develops disseminated gonococcal infection.

Clinical Presentation

Pubertal and Postpubertal Adolescents. The clinical manifestations of gonorrhea in children who have undergone puberty are similar to those in adults. Most females and a significant proportion of males are asymptomatic.

Males. Although gonococcal urethritis is uncommon among prepubertal males, it is the most common form of gonococcal infection in males after puberty. Following an incubation period of 1 to 14 (average 2 to 7) days, disease presents with the sudden onset of dysuria, urgency, frequency, and a purulent, often thick and yellow discharge. Edema and erythema of the penile meatus may occur. If left untreated, the majority will resolve spontaneously within weeks; persistent, asymptomatic urethral carriage is considered rare.

Females. Urogenital disease is the most common manifestation of gonococcal disease in pubertal and postpubertal females. In that age group, under the effect of estrogen, the vagina develops cornified epithelium and an acidic milieu that render it relatively resistant to gonococcal infection (in contrast to the prepubertal vagina). The primary site of infection is the endocervical canal; the urethra is also often colonized simultaneously. Although most women with gonococcal cervicitis are asymptomatic, within 10 days of infection, those females who do develop symptomatic disease manifest mucopurulent vaginal discharge, dysuria, urgency, frequency, menstrual irregularities, and lower abdominal pain. A physical examination reveals mucopus emanating from the cervical os. The cervix may be inflamed, erythematous, friable, and tender on manipulation. There may also be an expressible urethral or periurethral gland exudate.

Pelvic inflammatory disease (PID), which is an infection of the endometrium, fallopian tubes, and possibly the ovaries and peritoneum may develop in 10% to 20% of women with cervical infection due to *N. gonorrhoeae* following the ascent of infecting organisms through the uterine cavity to the endosalpinx. Tubo-ovarian abscess, peritonitis, and perihepatitis (Fitz–Hugh–Curtis syndrome) are possible complications. PID often occurs at or within a few days of the onset of menses. A vaginal discharge is present in ~60% of cases of PID, but its absence does not preclude the diagnosis. In addition to vaginal discharge, the onset of PID may be heralded by fever, chills, nausea, and vomiting. The major findings on physical examination are cervicitis, marked pain on cervical manipulation, and adnexal tenderness or masses. The specific microbiologic etiology of a particular episode of PID is difficult to determine. In addition to *N. gonorrhoeae*, suspect organisms include one or more of the aerobic and anaerobic genital flora, *Chlamydia trachomatis*, and *Mycoplasma hominis*. Endocervical, even culdocentesis cultures do not clearly identify the cause of PID and accordingly, empiric antimicrobial therapy must be broader than regimens only adequate to treat gonorrhea (see Chap. 122).

Pharyngeal gonorrhea is associated with orogenital sexual activity and is found in 10% to 20% of heterosexual women, 10% to 25% of homosexual men, and 3% to 7% of heterosexual men with gonococcal infection. It is usually asymptomatic but may produce pharyngitis and cervical adenitis. It is often difficult to treat effectively.

Anorectal gonorrhea is common in women with cervical infection (40%) and homosexual males. It seldom produces symptomatic infection (less than 10%), but when it does, it presents as proctitis with pruritus, tenesmus, purulent and often hemorrhagic rectal discharge.

Disseminated gonococcal infection (DGI) with gonococcal bacteremia occurs in 1% to 3% of infected patients. It is the leading cause of septic arthritis in sexually active populations and uncommonly causes endocarditis, meningitis, pneumonia, or osteomyelitis. DGI occurs mostly in females and presents usually during the first menses (7 to 30 days) after the onset of an asymptomatic genitourinary tract or other local infection. The illness varies in its severity. A typical course is manifested by migratory polyarthralgias involving large joints and a rash of varying description usually involving extremities and sparing the face and trunk (most often pustules on an erythematous base but sometimes papules, petechiae, or hemorrhagic bullae) during the first week of symptoms. Twenty-five percent of patients will have tenosynovitis. Blood cultures are frequently positive during the first week of illness. Subsequently, a portion of patients will develop septic arthritis in one or two joints (usually with positive synovial fluid cultures) with variable degrees of fever and toxicity.

Prepubertal Child. Beyond infancy, involuntary sexual contact is the most likely mode of gonococcal acquisition in prepubertal children aged 1 to 9 years. Rarely, it occurs through fomites or nonsexual transmission from infected close contacts. The infection is most often acquired within the household during the mother's absence. Accordingly, gonococcal infection in this age group necessitates an assiduous evaluation for neglect or abuse. In children aged 10 to 14 years, both voluntary and involuntary sexual activity figure significantly in the pathogenesis of gonococcal infection.

Most (up to 85%) prepubertal gonococcal infections occur among girls and they present most often as vaginitis. Most cases of vaginitis in the prepubertal age, however, are not attributable to a specific etiology. This is because of the physiology of the prepubertal vagina which, unlike the mature vagina, is characterized by unestrogenized, nonglycogen filled, uncornified atrophic epithelium and has a relatively alkaline *p*H, factors that make it susceptible to gonococcal colonization and disease. Because the endocervix is not patent in the prepubertal girl, it is uncommon for an infection to produce endocervical infection or PID. Gonococcal vaginitis presents with variable amounts of vaginal discharge, itching, and occasionally dysuria, usually in the absence of features of systemic illness. Abdominal pain and fever may occasionally be present in the rare instance of associated salpingitis or peritonitis. Asymptomatic vaginal colonization may occur and should be sought when sexual abuse is suspected.

Neonates. Neonatal gonococcal infection is acquired from a symptomatically or an asymptomat-

ically infected mother *in utero* (secondary to amnionitis), during delivery through an infected birth canal, or following intimate exposure postnatally. Ophthalmia neonatorum is the most common manifestation among newborns, usually appearing by the end of the first week of life (from 1 to 12 days). Formerly a highly virulent infection, the severity of gonococcal ophthalmia is purportedly more variable at present. It presents clinically as an intense, bilateral inflammation with a profuse exudate. If left untreated, the infection may progress from a superficial infection of the conjunctiva to an invasion and necrosis of the cornea. Gonococcal ophthalmia was one of the most common causes of blindness prior to widespread practice of prenatal screening and ophthalmic prophylaxis (see Chap. 94).

DGI occurs rarely in neonates. When it does occur, it presents most often at 1 to 2 weeks of age with constitutional features of illness (fever and irritability) and septic arthritis, often involving multiple joints.

Work-Up

The diagnosis of gonococcal infection depends usually on the isolation of *N. gonorrhoeae* from the site of infection (*e.g.*, blood, cerebrospinal fluid, synovial fluid, vagina, endocervix, urethra, conjunctiva), which is often suggested by a Gram stain and is confirmed by a culture. Identification by use of immunofluorescent antibody tests is available through specialized facilities. Most practitioners will transport specimens to laboratories for culture diagnosis although Gram stains can be assessed in the office.

Because of the fastidious growth requirements of *N. gonorrhoeae*, specimens for culture must be obtained and processed carefully. Warm water rather than a petroleum product should be used to lubricate instruments that come in contact with the specimen. Calcium alginate rather than cotton swabs should be used to sample urethral specimens. Culture and transport media should be warmed to room temperature before inoculation. Urethral specimens can be obtained by the insertion of the swab 2 cm to 4 cm into the urethra or collecting the first 10 ml to 20 ml of a voided urine specimen.

Specimens from normally sterile sites (*e.g.*, blood, cerebrospinal fluid, synovial fluid, peritoneal fluid, petechial scrapings) can be cultured on nonselective chocolate agar. Cultures from sites that are normally colonized by various flora (*e.g.*, conjunctiva, cervix, vagina, rectum, pharynx) require selective culture media such as Thayer–Martin, Martin–Lewis, or New York City agar which consist of chocolate agar containing antibiotics which inhibit normal flora including most nonpathogenic Neisseria species. Specimens must be plated immediately and must be incubated at 35°C in 5% to 10% carbon dioxide or transported in an appropriate commercially prepared holding medium such as Transgrow (which contains modified Thayer–Martin agar in a carbon dioxide atmosphere).

Gram-stained smears of exudates from symptomatic individuals, which show typical intracellular organisms within polymorphonuclear leukocytes, are highly suggestive of gonococcal infection. For males with symptomatic urethritis, such a finding is 90% to 95% sensitive and 95% to 100% specific compared with culture results and is considered adequately diagnostic. Confirmatory cultures are required in almost all other circumstances. In postpubertal females, the finding of intracellular organisms on Gram stain of endocervical smears is only 50% to 70% sensitive, although 95% to 100% specific in expert hands.

Appropriate specimens for culturing are dictated usually by the presenting symptomatology. Rectal and pharyngeal cultures, however, should be processed routinely in addition to genitourinary specimens when evaluating homosexuals, sexually abused patients, patients with oral or anal exposure to *N. gonorrhoeae*, and patients who are assessed for DGI.

Treatment and Management

Recommended antimicrobial regimens for the several clinical syndromes associated with *N. gonorrhoeae* are outlined in Table 195-1 (For the treatment of Pelvic Inflammatory Disease, see Chap. 122). Other management issues are briefly considered below:

1. Hospitalization and parenteral therapy of patients with acute PID (of whatever etiology) should be strongly considered if (1) the diagnosis is uncertain, (2) an abscess is suspected, (3) tolerance of or compliance with oral regimens is suspect (4) the patient is pregnant, or (5) a trial of outpatient therapy has failed. Because of the frequency of poor compliance and the substantial long-term morbidity associated with PID, the threshold for hospitalizing adolescents with PID should be low and patients with PID treated as outpatients should be reevaluated within 48 to 72 hours.

   DGI, as well as septic arthritis, endocarditis, meningitis, and ophthalmia neonatorum due to *N. gonorrhoeae* likewise require hospitalization and parenteral therapy.

2. Because of the frequent polymicrobial etiology of PID (difficult to document with specificity in a particular case), antimicrobial regimens should be empirically selected to be sufficiently broad to be effective against *C. trachomatis*, anaerobes, gram-negative enteric organisms, and *M. hominis*, as well as *N. gonorrhoeae*.

   Because of the frequent coincidence of other STD in genitourinary gonorrhea (in addition to PID), especially *C. trachomatis* (present in up to 45% of patients with gonorrhea), preferred antimicrobial regimens are often selected to be inclusive of both *N. gonorrhoeae* and *C. trachomatis*.

3. Follow-up cultures should be obtained as a test of cure ~4 to 7 days after the completion of therapy and to detect reinfection 4 to 6 weeks later. All women with genitourinary gonorrhea should have rectal cultures obtained at a follow-up examination.

4. All cases of gonorrhea should be reported to public health authorities to facilitate contact tracing.

5. Sexual contacts should be identified and evaluated for gonorrhea. The presumptive treatment of sexual contacts of persons with gonorrhea should be implemented. Child victims of sexual abuse are thought to be at low but uncertain risk of contracting STD and, therefore, need not be prophylactically treated unless the assailant is known to be infected.

6. All isolates of *N. gonorrhoeae*, especially those isolated from treatment failures, should be evaluated for sensitivity to penicillin (to identify resistant strains including penicillinase-producing *N. gonorrhoeae* [PPNG]). Patients with such isolates or other treatment failures should be treated with one of the alternative regimens listed in Table 195-1 (often ceftriaxone or spectinomycin).

7. A serologic test for syphilis (STS) should be obtained for all infected patients to look for coexisting infection at the time of first evaluation and again in 6 weeks to exclude the possibility of incubating syphilis.

8. The major adverse reaction to treatment for gonorrhea is the rare reaction to procaine (when procaine penicillin G is administered parenterally), which can cause agitation, hallucination, convulsion, or hypertension which can be managed by reassurance, sedatives, or restraint. Anaphy-

Table 195-1. Treatment of Gonorrhea

TYPE OR STAGE	PREFERRED DRUGS	DOSAGE	ALTERNATIVES
Gonorrhea Urethritis or cervicitis	Amoxicillin *plus* probenecid OR ceftriaxone	3 g oral once 1 g oral once 125–250 mg IM once	Penicillin G procaine 4.8 million U IM once *plus* probenecid 1 g oral once Spectinomycin 2 g IM once Cefoxitin 2 g IM once *plus* probenecid 1 g oral once
Anal Women	As for urethritis or cervicitis		
Men	Ceftriaxone	As for urethritis	Penicillin G procaine 4.8 million U IM once *plus* probenecid 1 g oral once Spectinomycin 2 g IM once
Pharyngeal	Ceftriaxone	As for urethritis	Penicillin G procaine 4.8 million U IM once *plus* probenecid 1 g oral once Trimethoprim–sulfamethoxazole 9 tablets daily × 5 days
Ophthalmia (adults)	Penicillin G *plus* saline irrigation	10 million U IV daily × 5 days	Cefoxitin 1 g or cefotaxime 500 mg IV qid or ceftriaxone 1 g IM daily × 5 days *plus* saline irrigation
Bacteremia and arthritis	Penicillin G *followed by* amoxicillin	10 million U IV daily × 3 days 500 mg oral qid × 4 days	Ceftriaxone 1 g IV daily × 7 days Cefotaxime 500 mg or cefoxitin 1 g IV qid × 7 days Tetracycline 500 mg oral qid × 7 days
Meningitis	Penicillin G	At least 10 million U IV daily for at least 10 days	Cefotaxime 2 g IV q4h for at least 10 days Ceftriaxone 2 g IV daily for at least 10 days Chloramphenicol 4 to 6 g/day for at least 10 days
Endocarditis	Penicillin G	At least 10 million U IV daily for at least 3 to 4 weeks	
Neonatal Ophthalmia	Penicillin G *plus* saline irrigation	100,000 U/kg/day IV in 4 doses × 7 days	Cefotaxime 25 mg/kg q8–12h × 7 days
Arthritis and septicemia	Penicillin G	75,000 to 100,000 U/kg/day IV in 4 doses × 7 days	Cefotaxime 25–50 mg/kg q8–12h × 10–14 days
Meningitis	Penicillin G	100,000 U/kg/day IV in 3 or 4 doses for at least 10 days	Cefotaxime 50 mg/kg q8–12h × 10–14 days

Table 195-1. Treatment of Gonorrhea (*continued*)

TYPE OR STAGE	PREFERRED DRUGS	DOSAGE	ALTERNATIVES
Children (under 45 kg) Urogenital, anal, and pharyngeal	Amoxicillin *plus* probenecid OR ceftriaxone	50 mg/kg oral once 25 mg/kg (max. 1 g) once 125 mg IM once	Penicillin G procaine 100,000 U/kg IM once *plus* probenecid 25 mg/kg (max. 1 g) once Spectinomycin 40 mg/kg IM once
Arthritis	Penicillin G	150,000 U/kg/day IV × 7 days	Cefoxitin 100 mg/kg/day or cefotaxime 50 mg/kg/day IV in divided doses × 7 days Ceftriaxone 50 mg/kg/day (max. 2 g) IV × 7 days Tetracycline (over 8 years old) 10 mg/kg oral qid × 7 days
Meningitis	Penicillin G	250,000 U/kg/day IV in 6 divided doses for at least 10 days	Ceftriaxone 100 mg/kg/day (max. 2 g) IV × 7 days Cefotaxime 200 mg/kg/day IV for at least 10 days Chloramphenicol 100 mg/kg/day IV for at least 10 days

(Abramowicz M [ed]: Treatment of sexually transmitted diseases. Medical Letter 28:23–28, 1986)

lactic reactions to either penicillin or procaine are rare and require appropriate cardiorespiratory supportive measures.

CHLAMYDIA

Background

Chlamydia trachomatis is the most common STD in the United States. Although not an officially reportable condition, it causes an estimated three to four million infections each year. The high and increasing prevalence of such infections is most striking among young and poor single women and it has been reported to be as high as 37% among pregnant inner-city adolescents. Young males are also affected more often than older males. The risk of disease varies with the number of sex partners. In many of its clinical presentations, disease produced by *C. trachomatis* resembles that produced by *N. gonorrhoeae* and the two infections frequently coexist. Both of them usually produce superficial mucosal genital infections, but they are also capable of producing more invasive diseases.

This discussion does not include the disease pro-

duced by serotypes of *C. trachomatis* responsible for trachoma or lymphogranuloma venereum, which are uncommon problems in the United States.

Clinical Presentation

As with many STD the asymptomatic or mildly symptomatic infection due to *C. trachomatis* must be suspected and sought to be diagnosed. Most women with chlamydial cervicitis; most homosexuals with chlamydial proctitis (4% to 8% of homosexual males seen in STD clinics); and up to 30% of heterosexual males with chlamydial urethritis are asymptomatic or mildly symptomatic.

Pubertal and Postpubertal Males. *C. trachomatis* is the major cause of nongonococcal urethritis (NGU) and acute epididymitis in males 35 years of age or younger in the United States and is responsible for ~50% of cases of each. *C. trachomatis* can be cultured from up to 11% of asymptomatic sexually active males. In ~15% to 30% of heterosexual and 5% of homosexual males with gonococcal urethritis, *C. trachomatis* can be concomitantly isolated. Treatment of the gonococcal urethritis may result in persistent, relapsing, or (due to its longer incubation period) belatedly manifest NGU due to *C. trachomatis*.

NGU due to *C. trachomatis* usually produces less dysuria and less purulent (clear to white) urethral discharge than urethritis due to *N. gonorrhoeae*, but the differentiation cannot be made securely on clinical grounds. Presenting symptoms include urethral discharge, itching, or dysuria after an incubation period of 7 to 21 days. A physical examination may further reveal meatal irritation. The diagnosis of NGU is based on a demonstration of urethritis and exclusion of gonorrhea by Gram stain and culture. The objective diagnosis of urethritis requires a demonstration of at least four polymorphonuclear leukocytes for each oil-immersion field on a gram-stained smear of a urethral exudate or at least 10 to 15 polymorphonuclear leukocytes for each high-power field in the sediment of the first 10 ml to 15 ml of a voided urine specimen.

Epididymitis or epididymo-orchitis presents with unilateral scrotal pain, swelling, tenderness and fever, usually with accompanying NGU. In addition to *C. trachomatis*, the differential diagnosis includes epididymitis due to *N. gonorrhoeae*, uropathogens such as Enterobacteriaceae, and testicular torsion.

Proctitis due to *C. trachomatis* should be considered in homosexual males presenting with mild to moderate rectal discharge, anorectal pain, tenesmus, or constipation. *C. trachomatis* is possibly implicated etiologically in some cases of prostatitis and Reiter's syndrome.

Pubertal and Postpubertal Females. Like gonorrhea, chlamydial infection in females is frequently asymptomatic. Mucopurulent cervicitis is the most common symptomatic form of infection and *C. trachomatis* is isolated from 30% to 50% of women who have mucopurulent endocervical discharge; it is isolated coincidentally in 25% to 50% of cases of gonococcal infection. A physical examination often reveals a creamy endocervical discharge. Ectopy is the normal physiologic state of the cervix of the child and variably of the adolescent until, with full maturity, it converts to squamous epithelium. Ectopy is felt to predispose to chlamydial and gonococcal infection because it tends to persist in women who use oral contraceptives. The use of oral contraceptive and nonbarrier forms of contraception are thought to represent risk factors for cervical infection due to *C. trachomatis*. In addition, chlamydial cervicitis is associated with an increased risk of cytologic atypia and dysplasia. The objective diagnosis of mucopurulent cervicitis is based on a demonstration of ten or more polymorphonuclear leukocytes for each oil immersion field in a smear of exudate.

C. trachomatis is a frequent cause of PID being implicated in 25% to 50% of the one million cases seen annually in the United States. As previously discussed in the section on *N. gonorrhoeae*, PID is frequently of polymicrobial etiology; causative agents cannot be reliably distinguished from each other on clinical grounds. *C. trachomatis* purportedly presents with milder signs and symptoms but this tendency may be deceiving because the consequences of chlamydial PID may be as severe as those of *N. gonorrhoeae*. The complications include peritonitis and perihepatitis (Fitz–Hugh–Curtis syndrome). Long-term sequelae include ectopic pregnancies and infertility (see Chap. 122).

C. trachomatis is also responsible for urethritis in women (producing the dysuria–pyuria syndrome); up to two thirds of women with pyuria and sterile bladder urine have evidence of chlamydial infection (see Chap. 115).

Prepubertal Females. Rarely, *C. trachomatis* is isolated from vaginal specimens of asymptomatic girls. More often, it is isolated in the context of symptomatic nongonococcal vaginitis and indicates sexual abuse.

Neonates and Young Infants. *C. trachomatis* is the most common cause of neonatal conjunctivitis and one of the most common causes of interstitial pneumonitis in the first 3 to 6 months of life. The frequency of neonatal chlamydial infection is a function of the rate of colonization among pregnant women. The rates vary from 2% to 37% with most studies reporting rates of 8% to 12% in the United States. Although most colonized pregnant women are asymptomatic, 28% to 66% of their vaginally delivered offspring will become colonized, of whom 50% to 75% will develop conjunctivitis and 11% to 29%, afebrile pneumonia due to *C. trachomatis*.

Chlamydial conjunctivitis is the most commonly documented cause of ophthalmia neonatorum (13% to 74%; mean, 29%) in the developed western countries where the frequency of gonococcal ophthalmia has declined because of effective prophylaxis and prenatal maternal screening. Eighteen to 50% of infants born to infected mothers will have conjunctivitis between 1 and 3 weeks (usually 5 to 12 days) of age. Infection usually presents with a unilateral mucoid discharge associated with eyelid edema, bulbar and palpebral conjunctival inflammation and bilaterality within 1 week of onset. Severity is variable. Other causes cannot be distinguished clinically. Smears of ocular discharge reveal both polymorphonuclear and mononuclear leukocytes. Intracytoplasmic inclusions are noted on giemsa-stained smears of epithelial cells. The conjunctivitis usually resolves spontaneously within weeks to months without visual sequelae (see Chap. 93).

Chlamydial pneumonia is one of the most common causes of pneumonia in the first 6 months of life. It develops in 3% to 18% of infants born to infected mothers. It usually presents between 3 and 11 weeks of age with tachypnea and a characteristic staccato cough in an afebrile child with a prior 1- to 2-week history of mucoid rhinorrhea. Fine rales, usually without wheezes, are noted on auscultation. Approximately 50% of infants have prior or concurrent conjunctivitis. A chest roentgenogram shows hyperinflated lungs with diffuse interstitial or alveolar infiltrates. The leukocyte count is usually normal, but a moderate degree of eosinophilia is noted in 50% to 65% of cases. In most instances, the course of disease is mild and the infant improves gradually over 5 to 7 weeks without the benefit of therapy. Hospitalization is usually not clinically indicated. The risks of long-term sequelae including asthma, chronic cough, and abnormal pulmonary function tests are incompletely elucidated (see Chap. 191).

A role for *C. trachomatis* in producing otitis media, gastroenteritis, or apnea in infancy is uncertain.

Work-Up

Tissue culture coupled with fluorescent antibody identification of intracellular inclusions constitute the "gold standard" for the diagnosis of infection due to *C. trachomatis*. Antigen detection using either a fluorescent antibody technique (FA) applied directly to a smear (available commercially as Microtrak, manufactured by Syva Diagnostics) or enzyme-linked immunoabsorbent assay (ELISA, available commercially as Chlamydiazyme, manufactured by Abbott Diagnostics) offer alternative, more rapid, though somewhat less sensitive methods for detecting the presence of *C. trachomatis* from conjunctival or genital specimens. Designated transport media must be used for culture and ELISA studies. Prior to inoculation into cell culture, specimens may be stored at 4°C for up to 12 to 24 hours, but thereafter, must be frozen at −70°C.

Cytologic identification of intracytoplasmic inclusions on giemsa-stained smears of epithelial cell scrapings is a diagnostic method that the clinician can use in the office. However, it is only in detection of neonatal chlamydial conjunctivitis that this method is sufficiently sensitive (95%) for routine use. Serologic diagnosis of chlamydia is not useful in routine practice.

Treatment

Chlamydial urethritis and cervicitis are treated with either tetracycline or erythromycin 500 mg po qid for 7 days. Both neonatal ophthalmia and pneumonia are treated with erythromycin 12.5 mg/kg po or IV qid for 14 days. Other issues pertinent to management follow:

1. Patients with symptoms compatible with the following chlamydia-associated syndromes (even without diagnostic confirmation), as well as their identified sexual contacts of the prior 30 days should receive presumptive antimicrobial therapy adequate for chlamydial infection: (1) nongonococcal urethritis, (2) mucopurulent cervicitis, (3) pelvic inflammatory disease, and (4) epididymitis in men who are 35 years of age or younger.

2. Mothers and sex partners of mothers of infants with neonatal conjunctivitis or pneumonitis confirmed to be due to *C. trachomatis* should be treated for presumed genital chlamydial infection.

3. Neonatal ophthalmic prophylaxis, using either topical erythromycin (0.5%) or tetracycline (1%) ointments, but not silver nitrate, instilled within 1 hour of birth, is effective in preventing chlamydial (and gonococcal) conjunctivitis in the newborn. Neither regimen, however, will prevent nasopharyngeal colonization by chlamydia, which is considered a requisite precondition for the development of chlamydial pneumonia.

4. Two weeks of systemic erythromycin therapy for chlamydial conjunctivitis without concomitant topical therapy is effective in both treating the ocular infection and in reducing nasopharyngeal colonization. Although based on uncontrolled observations, 2 weeks of systemic erythromycin therapy is also recommended to decrease shedding and effect clinical improvement in established chlamydial pneumonia.

5. Post-treatment cultures are advised in pediatric populations. No tetracycline-resistant chlamydia have been reported, although persistence of symptoms may be due to tetracycline-resistant

Ureaplasma urealyticum infection. Positive post-treatment cultures usually reflect noncompliance or reinfection from an untreated infected sex partner and repeat treatment should be initiated.

6. Patients should be advised to abstain from sexual activity or, at least, use condoms or other barrier methods of contraception, pending the completion of therapy and a follow-up assessment.

HERPES SIMPLEX VIRUS— GENITAL INFECTION

Background

There are two serotypes of herpes simplex virus (HSV): HSV-1 and HSV-2. HSV-1 usually produces primary herpetic gingivostomatitis, pharyngitis, or conjunctivitis, typically in young children during the first 5 years of life. HSV-2 is responsible for most (70% to 95%) of sexually transmitted herpetic genital lesions. Genital herpes is classified as (1) primary genital infection (disease due to the first experience with either HSV-1 or HSV-2), (2) nonprimary first infection (the first clinically apparent genital infection in a person with prior experience with either HSV-1 or HSV-2), and (3) recurrent infection (repeat genital infection(s) in an individual with prior manifest genital infection). Although not a reportable condition, genital herpetic infections are estimated to have increased tenfold between 1966 and 1981. This epidemic increase in frequency, coupled with both their propensity for recurrence from latent status (60% to 70%) and their frequently asymptomatic status (50% to 70%) help explain the significance of genital herpes infections.

Clinical Presentation

HSV, mostly HSV-2, is responsible for 40% to 60% of all ulcerative genital lesions. Herpetic genital lesions are most commonly found among adolescents and young adults 2 to 7 days after exposure. Sometimes herpetic genital infection (due to either HSV-1 or HSV-2) may be transmitted by nonvenereal means, such as by contaminated hands (including autoinoculation from oral lesions) or fomites. Most often, however, it is sexually transmitted, and its diagnosis in nonvoluntarily sexually active individuals must raise concern for sexual abuse.

The characteristic genital herpetic lesion consists of a vesicle on an erythematous base which,

in males, is found on either the penile glans or shaft and, in women, on the vulva, perineum, buttocks, cervix, or vagina. The exanthem typically begins with nonspecific papules and evolves through the characteristic vesicular stage, becoming sequentially pustular, ulcerated, and finally scabbed.

Primary herpetic genital infections tend to have both systemic and local clinical features that are more severe and more prolonged than other nonprimary first infections or recurrent genital infections. Women tend to be more symptomatic and tend to suffer more complications than men. First genital infections that are not true primary herpetic infections (*i.e.*, the patient previously had a nongenital herpetic infection) tend to be milder than true primary genital infections.

Systemic features of primary genital herpetic infection include fever, headache, malaise, and myalgias and they occur in 40% of infected males and in 70% of females. These symptoms peak in the first 3 to 4 days and resolve by the end of the first week. Local symptoms include pain, itching, dysuria, and vaginal or urethral discharge. Painful genital lesions occur in 95% of males and in 99% of females and they have a mean duration of 10 to 12 days.

The ulcerative stage of lesions may persist for 4 to 15 days until crusting occurs. New lesions occur in more than 75% of cases during the fourth to tenth days of infection. The mean duration of viral shedding from lesions is 12 days and shedding remains a concern until the completion of scabbing. Cervical lesions occur in 90% of women with genital lesions due to primary HSV-2 infection and 70% of women with genital lesions due to primary HSV-1 or initial but nonprimary HSV-2 genital disease (but in only 12% to 20% of women with recurrent external genital herpetic lesions). Cervical involvement can be asymptomatic. If symptomatic, herpetic cervicitis is usually associated with mucopurulent discharge with or without a friable, red, and ulcerated exocervix (in contrast to the endocervical site of gonococcal and chlamydial infections). The differential diagnosis of the genital lesion includes chancroid, syphilis, excoriation, erythema multiforme, candidiasis, and Behçet's disease.

Dysuria occurs in 44% of males and 83% of females. Urethral discharge tends to be clear or mucoid. Local pain tends to increase in severity during the first week of symptomatic disease and tends to peak and recede by the end of the second week. Tender inguinal lymphadenopathy occurs during the second and third weeks of the disease and then resolves slowly.

Other sites of primary herpetic infection include the pharynx, which occurs coincidentally in 11% of primary HSV-2 genital infections, or rectum, especially among homosexuals.

Secondary or recurrent genital herpetic lesions occur in 80% of those who suffer primary HSV-2 genital disease. The characteristic lesions are identical to those suffered in primary disease but there are usually few, if any, systemic features and a particular episode tends to be less severe and shorter than in primary infection. Approximately 50% of patients suffer prodromal symptoms of local tenderness, burning, or tingling sensations hours before the presentation of genital lesions. Lesions are on the penis in males and most often on the labia minora and majora and perineum in females with only 15% to 30% of women suffering concomitant cervicitis. Dysuria occurs in only ~27% of females. Lesions are frequently unilateral; they involve only approximately one tenth the area of the primary attack; they are associated with viral shedding for ~4 days; and they heal over the course of 6 to 10 days.

Complications of primary herpetic disease include extragenital infections, aseptic meningitis, encephalitis (which is most often due to HSV-1), transverse myelitis, autonomic nervous system dysfunction, disseminated disease, and bacterial or fungal superinfection. Neonatal infection due to the retrograde extension of genital herpes infections or the passage of the neonate through an infected genital tract (more often but not exclusively in primary disease) occurs in one in 3000 to one in 30,000 live births. HSV-2 genital infection is a risk factor for the development of cervical carcinoma.

Work-Up

Viral tissue culture of vesicular fluid or specimens obtained from other infected sites is the preferred diagnostic method and clearly requires the use of a specialized laboratory equipped to perform such tests. Typical cytopathic effects appear quickly (usually within 4 days). Specimens must be planted promptly or transported in an appropriate holding medium; they may be held at 4°C to 9°C for up to 4 hours or at −70°C if a longer delay is incurred. A rapid presumptive diagnosis may be made with a Tzank smear of scrapings of skin or mucosa from suspect lesions that are smeared, air-dried, fixed (with ethanol or methanol), and stained with Giemsa or Wright's stain. The presence of ballooned and multinucleated giant cells indicates the lesion is due to one of the Herpetoviridae, but this is an insensitive detection method. A Papanicolaou smear of cervical or vaginal secretions may demonstrate suggestive intranuclear inclusions.

Treatment and Management

The efficacy of acyclovir in the treatment of genital herpes lesions has been studied only in adults. Since it has not been explicitly approved for use in pediatric patients, it should be used selectively in this population.

In adults with primary genital infection, oral acyclovir reduces the duration of systemic and local signs, symptoms, and viral shedding by ~3 to 5 days if initiated within 6 days of the onset of symptoms. It has no effect on the rate or severity of recurrences. The recommended dosage is 200 mg orally five times each day for 7 to 10 days. This regimen should be considered in pediatric patients only if they have no prior history of herpes infection, including oral lesions (i.e., if they have a true primary genital infection). Topical acyclovir produces a slight but inferior benefit in the reduction of clinical features and viral shedding. Intravenous acyclovir is reserved for severely infected or complicated hospitalized patients. Acyclovir is not recommended for use during pregnancy. Routine treatment of sex partners is not recommended.

Oral acyclovir offers a marginal benefit in the treatment of recurrent genital infections and, when given continuously to adults with frequent recurrences, has resulted in fewer recurrences during the period of therapy. It is not recommended for use in pediatric patients for either recurrent genital disease or suppressive therapy.

Patients are to be urged to abstain from sexual activity while symptomatic lesions are present, even if they are receiving acyclovir. The use of barrier methods of contraception (e.g., condoms) is recommended to reduce the risk of transmission and, because the risk of transmission in the asymptomatically infected individual is unknown, they should be considered for routine contraceptive use in patients with a history of genital herpes.

Women with genital herpes should have yearly Papanicolaou smears and, when pregnant, should inform their obstetricians of their history.

SYPHILIS

Background

Syphilis is the third most commonly reported communicable disease in the United States, ranking after gonorrhea and varicella. In 1983, 32,698 cases of primary and secondary syphilis were reported, representing a rate of 14.1:100,000 population. In 1985, 268 cases of congenital syphilis were reported, representing a decline of 98% since 17,600 cases were reported in 1941; however, the frequency of cases is increasing since the nadir of 108 cases reported in 1978.

Syphilis is a disease of protean clinical expression caused by the spirochete *Treponema pallidum*. Its natural course is divided into four stages: (1) primary syphilis, which is manifested by a nonpainful chancre (usually genital) and regional (usually inguinal) adenopathy after a mean incubation period of ~3 weeks; (2) secondary syphilis, which is manifested by mucocutaneous or visceral lesions with lymphadenopathy following hematogenous dissemination; (3) latent syphilis, which is a period of subclinical infection; and (4) late or tertiary syphilis, which is manifested by ascending aortitis and involvement of the central nervous and other organ systems including skin, bone, liver, and spleen.

Syphilis is most often transmitted sexually, but may also be acquired through saliva, blood transfusion, direct inoculation from moist mucocutaneous lesions, or transplacentally. Most cases occur in patients between the ages of 15 and 30 years; one third of cases occur in homosexuals. Although it is uncommonly diagnosed in pediatric populations, it serves as an easily diagnosed useful marker of sexually transmitted diseases and should be considered and sought whenever another STD is diagnosed or suspected.

Clinical Presentation

Primary syphilis begins at the site of inoculation as a single, painless papule that evolves into a chancre (a nontender, eroded ulcer with a smooth, clean base and raised, firm margins). Multiple chancres may occur. The usual sites of chancres include the external genitalia, cervix, anal canal, perianal region, and oral cavity. Regional lymphadenopathy is usually moderately large, firm, nonsuppurative, and painless. Irrespective of treatment, chancres typically resolve in 2 to 6 weeks whereas the lymphadenopathy persists longer. The differential diagnosis of genital chancres and inguinal adenopathy includes herpes simplex (typically clustered vesicles), chancroid (typically painful, exudative, indurated ulcers with suppurative adenopathy), traumatic genital lesions, early venereal warts, granuloma inguinale, lymphogranuloma venereum, tuberculosis, atypical mycobacteria, tularemia, sporotrichosis, anthrax, and rat-bite fever.

Secondary syphilis develops in the untreated patient, 2 to 8 weeks after the onset of the primary chancre. Following hematogenous dissemination, highly contagious mucocutaneous lesions may develop. Skin lesions may be macular, maculopapular, papular, or pustular and typically involve the trunk and extremities including the palms and soles. Painless, moist, gray-white to erythematous plaques called *condylomata lata* may occur in intertriginous regions. Mucous patches consisting of silvery-gray superficial erosions with erythematous margins may also occur. In addition, any of the following systemic or local features may develop: fever; malaise; pharyngitis; laryngitis; anorexia; weight loss; arthralgia; generalized, painless lymphadenopathy (including epitrochlear nodes); aseptic meningitis (which is only symptomatic in 1% to 2% of cases); immune-complex-mediated glomerulonephritis; hepatitis; splenomegaly; uveitis; synovitis; osteitis; or periostitis. Mucocutaneous lesions of secondary syphilis usually resolve within 2 to 12 weeks irrespective of therapy but patients are subject to relapses, most of which occur within the first 2 years. The differential diagnosis of skin lesions of secondary syphilis includes pityriasis rosea, measles, infectious mononucleosis, erythema multiforme, leukemia, lymphoma, tinea, sarcoid, granuloma annulare, and lichen planus.

Latent syphilis is defined as the stage in which there are no clinical manifestations of infection. A diagnosis requires serologic testing. During early latency (defined as the first 4 years) relapses, mostly mucocutaneous, may occur, but 90% occur within the first year.

During late latency or tertiary syphilis, untreated patients may manifest the slowly progressive inflammatory disease of neurosyphilis, cardiovascular, or gummatous syphilis. This stage is not encountered in pediatric-aged patients.

For a discussion of congenital syphilis, see Chapter 191.

Work-Up

The practitioner must utilize specialized, widely available laboratory facilities to make the diagnosis of syphilis.

In primary, secondary, and early congenital syphilis, a definitive diagnosis is made by a dark-field examination of serous transudate obtained from moist lesions such as chancres, condylomata lata, or mucous patches. Serologic tests for syphilis (STS) are the only means of diagnosing syphilis during the latent stage and often provide corroborative evidence for the diagnosis of primary, secondary, or congenital syphilis. STS include nontreponemal reaginic tests (*e.g.*, rapid plasma reagin [RPR], Venereal Disease Research Laboratory [VDRL]) and specific Treponemal tests (*e.g.*, fluorescent treponemal antibody absorption [FTA–ABS], micro-hemagglutination assay for *Treponema pallidum* [MHA–TP], *Treponema pallidum* immobilization [TPI]).

Nontreponemal STS are 70% to 80% and 99% sensitive in detecting primary and secondary syphilis, respectively. These tests are not specific for *T. pallidum* and a positive test requires a confirmation by a specific Treponemal test. Nontreponemal STS have the virtue of being quantifiable and, therefore, can be repeated serially to gauge the response to therapy and to detect relapses or reinfections. False-positive tests can occur in the context of acute bacterial or viral infection, immunization, drug addiction, collagen-vascular disease, hyper-gammaglobulinemic states, and pregnancy.

As the name implies, specific Treponemal STS measure antibodies specific for infection due to *T. pallidum*, and they are used for serologic confirmation of the diagnosis of syphilis. They are 50% to 80% and 97% to 100% sensitive in detecting primary and secondary syphilis, respectively. These tests are not readily quantifiable and a positive test does not revert to negative; therefore, they are not helpful for monitoring the response to therapy. False-positive tests are uncommon but they can occur.

IgM specific for *T. pallidum* is not a practicable serologic diagnostic tool.

Treatment

The reader is referred to Table 195-2 for antimicrobial therapy for syphilis. Additional issues involving management are included in the following list:

1. Adequate treatment of primary, secondary, or early latent syphilis requires sustained blood levels of penicillin (of ≥ 0.3 μl/ml) for at least 7 days; this is afforded by intramuscular (IM) benzathine penicillin G at a dose of 50,000 U/kg. Early incubating syphilis would be eradicated by standard treatment for gonorrhea (4.8 million units of IM aqueous procaine penicillin G and 1 g oral probenecid) but this treatment would not be adequate for the treatment of an established syphilis infection. Single large doses of ampicillin or amoxicillin orally or 7-day courses of tetracycline or doxycycline orally probably eradicate incubating syphilis; spectinomycin and trimethoprim–sulfamethoxazole do not. Erythromycin's capacity to do so is undetermined.

2. Repeat quantitative nontreponemal STS should be performed in congenital, primary, secondary, and early latent syphilis at 3, 6, and 12 months after treatment. They should be repeated again at 24 months for syphilis of more than 1 year's duration prior to therapy. Repeat treatment should be given if there is failure of the titer to decrease fourfold within 1 year.

3. The self-limited Jarisch–Herxheimer reaction of fever and generalized malaise within a few hours of beginning therapy for syphilis requires only an anticipatory warning to penicillin recipients

Table 195-2. Treatment of Syphilis

TYPE OR STAGE	PREFERRED DRUG	DOSAGE	ALTERNATIVES
Early (Primary, secondary, or latent less than 1 year)	Penicillin G benzathine	2.4 million U IM once	Tetracycline 500 mg oral qid × 15 days Erythromycin 500 mg oral qid × 15 days
Late (more than 1 year's duration, cardiovascular)	Penicillin G benzathine	2.4 million U IM weekly × 3 weeks	Tetracycline 500 mg oral qid × 30 days Erythromycin 500 mg oral qid × 30 days
Congenital CSF normal CSF abnormal	Penicillin G benzathine Penicillin G OR Penicillin G procaine	50,000 U/kg IM once 25,000 U/kg IM or IV bid for at least 10 days 50,000 U/kg IM daily for at least 10 days	

(Abramowicz M [ed]: Treatment of sexually transmitted diseases. Medical Letter 28:23–28, 1986)

and expectant observation of those who experience it.

4. Because the moist mucocutaneous lesions of primary and secondary syphilis are highly contagious, drainage and secretion precautions are necessary. Infants with proven or suspected congenital syphilis likewise require drainage, secretion, and blood precautions until therapy has been administered for at least 24 hours.

5. STS are recommended for all pregnant women in early and late pregnancy. They are also recommended for high-risk populations (especially prostitutes and homosexuals) and patients with other documented or suspected STD and their contacts.

6. Recent sexual contacts (within the preceding 3 months) of individuals with acquired syphilis should be evaluated and presumptively treated for early syphilis.

ANNOTATED BIBLIOGRAPHY

Abramowicz M (ed): Treatment of sexually transmitted diseases. Medical Letter 28:23–28, 1986 (Succinct and authoritative tabular presentation of preferred antimicrobial therapies for common STD agents.)

Bell TA: Major sexually transmitted diseases of children and adolescents. Pediatr Infect Dis 2:153–161, 1983 (Brief but useful discussion of STD in the pediatric age group; both an overview of the topic and a review of specific clinical syndromes, their differential diagnosis, and management.)

Corey L: The diagnosis and treatment of genital herpes. JAMA 248:1041–1049, 1982 (Clinically oriented presentation of the elements of diagnosis and therapy for genital herpes.)

Emans SJ: Vulvovaginitis in children and adolescents. Pediatr Rev 2:319–326, 1981

Emans SJ: Vulvovaginitis in the child and adolescents. Pediatr Rev 8:12–19, 1986 (These two articles by Emans provide a practical approach to the evaluation, differential diagnosis, microbiologic considerations, and management of dysuria and vaginal discharge in children and adolescents.)

Hart G: Syphilis tests in diagnostic and therapeutic decision making. Ann Intern Med 104:368–376, 1986 (Review of guidelines for diagnosing syphilis and the diagnostic capabilities of the various STS.)

Holmes KK, Mårdh PA, Sparling PF, Wiesner PJ (eds): Sexually Transmitted Diseases. New York, McGraw–Hill, 1984 (Definitive comprehensive text including discussions of the general subject of STD as well as current, well-referenced chapters on each of the specific agents.)

Hook EW, Holmes KK: Gonococcal infection. Ann Intern Med 102:229–243, 1985 (Recent review of the topic including current material on epidemiology, microbiology and pathogenesis, clinical manifestations, diagnosis, therapy [including issues of antimicrobial resistance], and prospects for prevention.)

Murphy DM: Office laboratory diagnosis of sexually transmitted diseases. Pediatr Infect Dis 2:146–152, 1983 (Review of the capabilities and limitations of the office laboratory in making at least preliminary diagnosis of such STD as Candida, Trichomonas, Gardnerella, and *N. gonorrhoeae*.)

Rettig PJ: Chlamydial infections in pediatrics: Diagnostic and therapeutic considerations. Pediatr Infect Dis 5:158–162, 1986 (Review of the diagnostic and therapeutic aspects of chlamydial infections in pediatric patients.)

Rettig PJ: Infections due to *Chlamydia trachomatis* from infancy to adolescence. Pediatr Infect Dis 5:449–457, 1986 (Review of the epidemiologic and clinical features of chlamydial infections of neonates, children, and adolescents.)

Straus SE (moderator): NIH conference: Herpes simplex virus infection: Biology, treatment, and prevention. Ann Intern Med 103:404–419, 1985 (Current review of epidemiology, biology, diagnosis, treatment, and prospects for prevention of herpes simplex virus infection.)

US Department of Health and Human Services/Public Health Service: 1985 STD treatment guidelines. MMWR (Suppl) 34(4S):75S–108S, 1985 (Authoritative and specific management guidelines from CDC for each STD agent, including advice concerning counseling, follow-up, and special considerations.)

196
Pertussis
STEPHEN I. PELTON

In 1982 and 1983, 4358 cases of pertussis were reported by *Morbidity and Mortality Weekly Report* (MMWR). Outbreaks were reported in selected religious groups that generally do not advocate immunizations, as well as statewide in Oklahoma.

More than 50% of cases occurred in children less than 1 year of age, with the majority in children less than 6 months of age. Fifteen children died, and 13 of these deaths occurred in children less than 6 months of age.

Most reported cases of pertussis occur among children who have not received appropriate immunizations. Complications of the disease, as well as severity, are also greatest in inadequately immunized children. Although the benefits of immunization are generally accepted, rare but serious complications have resulted in concern among consumers, in legal action against manufacturers, and in re-evaluation of the risk–benefit ratio of pertussis vaccine.

Pertussis remains an important cause of morbidity in young children. Recognition of the disease in its early stage is important to reduce its spread within the community. Supportive therapy is necessary to reduce morbidity. Vaccination of appropriate children is critical to maintain immunity within the population and to prevent local or widespread epidemics such as those observed in Japan and England when vaccine use declined because of adverse publicity.

PATHOPHYSIOLOGY

Pertussis represents infection with the bacterium *Bordetella pertussis* in most cases. On rare occasions, *Bordetella parapertussis* and *Bordetella bronchiseptica* have been isolated from children with clinical whooping cough. However, these members of the *Bordetella* genus play a minor role. In one series, 188 of 190 bacteriologically confirmed cases were due to *B. pertussis*, whereas the other members of this genus were each isolated only once.

A viral etiology in this clinical illness was hypothesized after the isolation of adenovirus from several children with clinical whooping cough. The clinical syndrome was typical, but repeated attempts to isolate *Bordetella* or demonstrate an antibody response were unsuccessful. Although some cases of whooping cough may be due to adenovirus, more recent investigations have isolated adenovirus in a small percentage of patients in association with positive bacterial cultures, and most authorities do not consider it an important etiologic agent.

B. pertussis is spread by way of droplet to susceptible contacts. It is a highly contagious illness with an attack rate of ~90% in people who are susceptible. The incubation period is 3 to 15 days. The bacteria reside in the respiratory tract, attached to ciliated mucosal cells. At this point, the patient has mild respiratory symptoms, and *B. pertussis* is easily isolated from respiratory secretions.

As the disease progresses, and the frequency of positive bacterial cultures declines, the child's paroxysmal cough becomes predominant. Biologically active toxins have been proposed as clinically important. The most likely candidate is pertussis toxin, which can be associated *in vitro* with lymphocytosis promoting activity, histamine sensitization, and islet cell activation.

CLINICAL PRESENTATION

The manifestations of pertussis are dependent on the age and immunization status of the patient as well as the development of complications such as pneumonia and encephalopathy. Its classical description, paroxysmal staccato cough occurring during expiration followed by an inspiratory "whoop" is easily recognized by the clinician. The disease, however, is usually in its second week before such paroxysms begin, and they are often absent in young infants, immunized patients, and adolescents, making the diagnosis more difficult in these patients.

The disease begins as an upper respiratory infection. This stage, catarrhal or initial, is associated with cough, coryza, and sneezing. Fever is variable and rarely remarkable. During the second week, the cough becomes spasmodic and the classical respiratory whoop is observed. The children are seriously ill and may become cyanotic during attacks, which may last 60 seconds. Profuse mucus covers the face, and epistaxis and subconjunctival hemorrhage may be observed. The whoop heralds the end of the paroxysm; however, inspiration occurs only with great effort. Several paroxysms may occur back to back, profuse sweating is observed, and finally the child vomits mucus and appears exhausted.

An improvement begins weeks after the paroxysms have begun. Coughing paroxysms become less severe and less frequent. Recovery requires several additional weeks.

When the illness progresses from catarrhal to paroxysmal to convalescent, it is easily recognized. A paroxysmal cough was reported in 85% of cases in 1960, while recent reports from the MMWR suggest that such episodes may be less common. A whoop has been described in 50% to 61% of patients and apnea has been reported in 40% of patients under 1 year of age.

Other atypical cases are reported in adolescents and partly immunized children in whom a persistent cough may be the presenting sign and bronchitis the clinical diagnosis. Such cases cause special concern, since numerous contacts may be exposed before the correct diagnosis is made.

COMPLICATIONS

Complications are most frequent in children less than 6 months of age. 49% of cases require hospitalization, with a higher rate of hospitalization in children less than 6 months of age. The three most serious complications are pneumonia, seizures, and encephalopathy. All three are most common in children less than 1 year of age and in children who have not been immunized.

Confirmed pneumonia occurred in 16% of patients reported in 1982 to 1983 to the MMWR. It may be due to *Bordetella pertussis* or associated with bacterial superinfection. Peribronchial roentgenogram changes, which may persist throughout the clinical course, are most often due to *B. pertussis* alone. Secondary bacterial pneumonias occur rarely. Death is more frequent in children with pneumonia than in uncomplicated cases.

Seizures and encephalopathy occurred in 1.9% and 0.3% of children with pertussis, respectively. It appears that the etiology of CNS disease is related to various pathophysiologies. Anoxia, petechial or subarachnoid hemorrhage, edema, and possible postinfectious encephalitis have been incriminated.

The long-term prognosis of children with per-

tussis is favorable if the child survives the acute illness. Although bronchiectasis has been reported in the past, current studies do not reveal chronic pulmonary disease in patients who have had pertussis. The neurologic prognosis for children without encephalopathy also appears comparable to controls. The prognosis for those with clinical encephalopathy, however, is less favorable, with persistent sequelae in as many as 50% of survivors.

WORK-UP

History

The most important history is that of exposure. Any child who presents with a history of paroxysmal cough for more than 1 week associated with vomiting, whoop, or cyanosis should prompt a clinical suspicion of pertussis. If the child is incompletely immunized against pertussis, a further evaluation is warranted. Although 3% to 8% of cases of pertussis occur in children who are fully immunized, a reliable history of complete immunization makes whooping cough unlikely.

Identification of a potential contact requires the physician to ask about mild illness, possibly in adults or older adolescents. The presence of a persistent paroxysmal cough and mucous production may be the clues to diagnosis. Asymptomatic patients, usually older and partially or completely vaccinated, who are culture or fluorescent antibody positive have been identified. These may be the source of infection for patients for whom no symptomatic contact can be identified.

Physical Examination

In the earliest stage, the physical examination reveals URI symptoms. Only when the cough becomes paroxysmal or the inspiratory whoop appears is it possible to make a clinical diagnosis of pertussis.

Laboratory Tests

The preferred culture is the nasopharyngeal swab (Calgi swab, Colab Laboratory, Chicago Heights, IL). The swab is passed through the naris about 2 in. into the nasopharynx and kept in place while the child coughs. It is then streaked directly onto fresh Bordet–Gengou medium, a specially prepared medium that contains 20% fresh horse, sheep, or rabbit blood and penicillin (0.2 units/ml) or methicillin (4 μg/ml). In many states, this medium is available from the state laboratory upon request.

A fluorescent antibody (FA) test is also available. The clinician smears the nasopharyngeal swab onto a glass slide. The slide can be sent to the laboratory where antisera, antibodies to *B. pertussis* conjugated with a material that fluoresces under ultraviolet light, is added. The slide is washed to remove antibody-conjugate complexes not specifically attached to *B. pertussis*. The slides are examined by experienced technicians with a fluorescent microscope.

Controversy over the relative sensitivity of FA *vs* culture are evident in the literature. False-negative and false-positive FA tests have been reported by some investigators when compared to culture. However, FA appears to be the more readily available test.

Prior antimicrobial therapy and the timing of the culture affect the frequency of isolation of *B. pertussis* from nasopharyngeal cultures. Cultures taken during the catarrhal stage are more often positive than those performed during the paroxysmal stage. In addition, isolation of *B. pertussis* is less likely from patients who have been treated with erythromycin or tetracycline prior to culture. Prior treatment with penicillin or ampicillin appears to have no effect on isolation rates for *B. pertussis*. The white blood cell count can be helpful when the characteristic leukocytosis (WBC > 15,000) and lymphocytosis (70%) are present. These parameters are much less valuable in children younger than 6 months of age. Leukemoid reactions (WBC > 50,000/mm^3) are infrequently seen but may be associated with severe disease.

DIFFERENTIAL DIAGNOSIS

Infection due to *B. pertussis, B. parapertussis*, and *B. bronchisepticum* produce clinical syndromes that are indistinguishable.

Other illnesses that are associated with a spasmodic cough may initially require consideration. In young infants, disease due to *Chlamydia trachomatis* and respiratory syncytial virus may present with spasmodic cough, apnea, and respiratory distress. Roentgenographic findings may be helpful in distinguishing disease due to *Chlamydia*. Specific microbiologic testing, however, will be most useful.

In the older infant and child, tuberculosis, cystic fibrosis, bacterial pneumonia, foreign body aspiration, and sinusitis need to be considered in the child with persistent paroxysmal coughing. Again, the history of a contact, inspiratory whoop, and

specific microbiology will be most useful in confirming the diagnosis of pertussis.

TREATMENT

Specific therapy to reduce the severity of illness is unavailable. The effect of erythromycin on the eradication of *B. pertussis* from the nasopharynx is well established, with a reduction in mean duration of nasopharyngeal carriage from more than 12 days in untreated patients to 3.6 days. However, no effect on the duration of hospitalization was observed following erythromycin, suggesting that antibiotics are not effective once the child reaches the paroxysmal stage. Some controversy continues concerning the possible benefit of erythromycin given during the catarrhal stage. The British Medical Research Council reported that cases treated "early" demonstrated fewer paroxysms than controls, and fewer children progressed to severe disease. Realistically, the debate is academic, because erythromycin is used to eradicate nasopharyngeal carriage and communicability.

Supportive therapy is most important for the child with pertussis. It is for this reason that most patients with pertussis less than 1 year of age, and children over 1 year with moderate or severe illness, require hospitalization. Suctioning to reduce thick mucus, nutrition, oxygen to prevent anoxia, calming, and comfort are all employed to prevent malnutrition, wasting, and exhaustion. Suctioning will clear copious secretions, but may stimulate paroxysms. Experienced clinicians suggest that suctioning should be performed immediately after a paroxysm when the child is less likely to begin coughing again. Nutrition is important, and gavage or intravenous feeding may be necessary to prevent weight loss. Finally, humidified air and oxygen should be utilized as necessary. Many infants will require as much as 50% FiO$_2$ during some part of the course. Cough suppressants are ineffective and sedatives are rarely, if ever, appropriate.

Recent studies have evaluated corticosteroids or solbutamol in patients with pertussis. In two studies, corticosteroids reduced the number and severity of paroxysms when compared with untreated controls. These preliminary studies suggest that such therapy may be beneficial and might be appropriate in a young infant with severe disease. Several studies have demonstrated that solbutamol at 0.3 to 0.5 mg/kg/day reduces the number of paroxysms, the duration of paroxysms, and the patients' distress. Not all studies of solbutamol have demonstrated a beneficial effect.

Bacterial pneumonia or otitis media may be complications of infection with *B. pertussis* and require appropriate therapy. In one series, 3 of 190 children developed secondary bacterial pneumonia—one due to *Pseudomonas* and two due to *S. aureus*.

PREVENTION

The controversy over the use of pertussis vaccine was precipitated by adverse publicity concerning serious reactions to the vaccine and the question of vaccine efficacy. Over the last decade, studies of secondary attack rates have clearly established the efficacy of the vaccine in the prevention of disease among close contacts. There is a 91.4% efficacy after three or more doses among household contacts aged 6 months to 9 years compared to unvaccinated household contacts. Immunization has also been associated with milder disease in children who have not been completely protected as well as a reduced incidence of pneumonia and hospitalization in partially immunized children compared to children who have not been immunized.

Unfortunately, the current vaccine is associated with a large number of side effects. Although most of these reactions are mild, some are severe. 35% to 40% of patients have local redness or swelling; more than 50% report pain or fretfulness, and 20% of patients demonstrate fever or drowsiness. More serious reactions include prolonged screaming, convulsions, hypotonic–hyporesponsive episodes, and frank encephalitis. The screaming is usually high pitched, beginning 3 to 6 hours after immunization and lasting for several hours. Convulsions occur within the first day following immunization and are usually brief and associated with fever, although multiple seizures occasionally are reported. The reactions of pallor, hypotonia, and unresponsiveness lasting minutes or hours is unique to pertussis vaccine and usually only occur in children between 2 and 18 months of age.

Frank encephalitis is the most serious vaccine complication and may be associated with permanent neurologic disability. The rate of each of these serious reactions is variable. High-pitched crying reportedly occurs in 1:1000 doses; convulsions occur between 1:1750 and 1:800,000 doses; and hypotensive-hyporesponsive episodes vary from 5 episodes in 969 injections in Belfast to 1 in 73,000 immunized children in South Holland.

Permanent neurologic disability following seizure or hypotonic–hypotensive episodes are un-

likely. However, estimates of the frequency of encephalopathy vary greatly; estimates for United States licensed products are 1 in ~300,000 doses.

This problem reflects the current vaccine which is preparedfrom whole killed *B. pertussis*. In this country, the preparation is alum precipitated. The schedule of dosing is 2, 4, 6, and 18 months for the primary series. The dose is 0.5 ml or 4 units. The current approach to reducing side effects has been twofold: first, not immunizing children at high risk for serious complications, and second, development of a less toxic vaccine.

The American Academy of Pediatrics has recommended that pertussis immunization is contraindicated in patients who have had the following reactions after administration of vaccine: (1) severe neurologic reactions, (2) persistent screaming for 3 hours or more, (3) a hyporesponsive, hypotensive episode, (4) temperature of 105°F or higher, (5) convulsion within 48 hours following immunization, or (6) allergic reaction. The Committee on Infectious Diseases has recommended delaying immunization of children who have a history of convulsions, children with neurologic conditions such as tuberous sclerosis or metabolic defects that predispose to convulsions, and children with neurologic syndromes that are evolving in character. These children should be reassessed frequently and considered for immunization if circumstances change (*e.g.*, enrollment in a day care center, planned travel to endemic areas).

Reduced dosage schedules have been suggested as another approach to reducing the incidence of serious reactions. Although it is clearly established that reduced vaccine doses are associated with a reduction in local reaction rates, data regarding protective efficacy are incomplete. The current data pertaining to reduced dosage schedules fail to provide sufficient evidence of either effectiveness or reduced incidence of severe side effects. Reduced dosage schedules remain controversial, and they are not advocated by the Committee on Infectious Diseases of the American Academy of Pediatrics.

The most promising development in this controversy is that of an acellular vaccine that is being developed and evaluated in Japan. Early experience shows that this vaccine is effective and is associated with a lower febrile reaction rate than whole cell vaccines. Efficacy studies in household contacts in Japan show a 79% reduction in vaccinated compared with unimmunized children. A further evaluation of the experience in Japan is necessary to document that the rare but serious side effects associated with whole cell preparations do not occur with increased use of this product. Field trials are being conducted in the United States to evaluate safety and immunogenicity.

BIBLIOGRAPHY

Altemeier WA III: Pertussis and parapertussis. In Kelley VC (ed): Practice of Pediatrics. Philadelphia, Harper & Row, 1986

Baraff LJ, Wilkins J, Wehrle P: The role of antibiotics, immunizations, and adenoviruses in pertussis. Pediatrics 61:224, 1978

Baraff LJ, Cody CL, Cherry JD: DTP-associated reactions: An analysis by injection site, manufacturer, prior reactions, and dose. Pediatrics 73:31, 1984

Barkin RM, Samuelson JS, Gotlin LP: DTP reactions and serologic response with a reduced dose schedule. J Pediatrics 105:189, 1984

Bass JW: Pertussis: Current status of prevention and treatment. Pediatr Infect Dis 4:614, 1985

Brooksaler F, Nelson JD: Pertussis: A reappraisal and report of 190 confirmed cases. Am J Dis Child 114:389, 1967

Cody CL, Baraff LJ, Cherry JD et al: Nature and rates of adverse reactions associated with DTP and DT immunizations in infants and children. Pediatrics 68:650, 1981

Committee on Infectious Diseases: Pertussis vaccine. Pediatrics 74:303, 1984

197
Chickenpox
JANET L. SCHWANER

Chickenpox or varicella is a common, usually mild childhood disease caused by the varicella-zoster virus. The disease is highly contagious and infection confers lifetime immunity; more than 90% of adults are immune. Adults and immunocompromised patients who develop chickenpox are more likely than normal children to develop severe disease or complications. After the disease subsides the virus may remain dormant for decades and may then reappear as herpes zoster, a unilateral varicella-like eruption in the distribution of one to three sensory nerves of dorsal root ganglia or cranial nerve extramedullary ganglia.

CLINICAL PRESENTATION

The incubation period ranges from 10 to 21 days; most cases occur 14 to 17 days after exposure. The contagious period extends from 1 day before the rash erupts until all of the lesions have crusted. Chickenpox is spread person-to-person by direct contact or by the respiratory route. The prodrome, which may be mild or absent in young children but tends to be more severe in adolescents and adults, consists of 1 to 2 days of fever, headache, malaise, and anorexia.

The rash, often pruritic, begins as a macule and progresses rapidly through the stages of papule, vesicle, and crusted lesion. The spots first appear on the face or trunk and, at the height of the illness, are more numerous centrally than distally. The lesions erupt in crops for 3 to 4 days, and it is char-

acteristic of the rash that lesions in different stages of development may be found in one area.

The vesicle is a 2-mm to 3-mm oval filled with clear fluid surrounded by an erythematous base. The fluid clouds and a crust forms within 1 day. Lesions occurring on the mucous membranes do not crust but form a shallow ulcer. Scars are unusual except at the site of secondary infections and where scabs have been pulled off rather than allowed to fall off. Inflamed skin such as the diaper area may have more lesions than other areas, and these lesions are more likely to be in the same stage of development.

The *congenital varicella syndrome* may develop in babies whose mothers have clinical varicella before 29 weeks' gestation. The percentage of such women who deliver affected babies is unknown. This rare and devastating syndrome includes hypotrophic limbs, cicatricial skin scarring, eye abnormalities, and severe psychomotor and growth retardation.

Maternal varicella 4 days or less before delivery may result in severe disseminated or fatal chickenpox in the newborn. Twenty percent of babies in these circumstances will develop varicella; death occurs in up to 30% to 35% of affected newborns. The development of neonatal chickenpox is probably related to the presence or absence of maternal antibody. Varicella–zoster immune globulin (VZIG) may modify the course of newborns whose mothers develop chickenpox during the critical period. Infected newborns should be treated with acyclovir, 30 mg/kg/day for 7 to 10 days (see also Chap. 191).

COMPLICATIONS

Secondary bacterial infection of lesions, most often with staphylococci or β hemolytic group A streptococci, is the most common complication. Systemic antibiotics may be necessary for infections, such as cellulitis, that do not respond to local care. Bullous varicella, which occurs usually in children under 2 years of age, is caused by phage group II toxigenic *S. aureus* and is self-limited. Primary varicella pneumonia is uncommon in healthy children but affects immunocompromised patients and up to 35% of normal adults. The disease varies from mild to severe and may be fatal.

Encephalitis follows varicella in less than 1:1000 cases. The involvement of the cerebellum alone has an excellent prognosis, whereas cerebral involvement manifested as change in sensorium, convulsions, stupor, coma, or paralysis may result in permanent brain damage or death. Less common neurologic complications are Guillain–Barré syndrome, transverse myelitis, optic neuritis, and facial nerve palsy.

Along with influenza, chickenpox is one of the most common antecedents of Reye's syndrome. The relationship between salicylate use in varicella and the development of Reye's syndrome is being investigated.

Idiopathic thrombocytopenic purpura, purpura fulminans, nephritis, appendicitis, gastritis, gangrene, myocarditis, and arthritis are rare complications.

DIFFERENTIAL DIAGNOSIS

Formerly, it was important to distinguish chickenpox from smallpox. The differentiation is unnecessary since the eradication of smallpox in the 1970s. Early impetigo is vesicular and may be pruritic, but the rash is not widespread and has a predilection for the nasolabial area. Insect bites are papular and itchy but do not occur in crops; they are not vesicular; and they have no systemic symptoms. Scabies is often accompanied by burrows between the fingers or toes. Urticarial lesions are usually large and short-lived, and they do not develop vesicles. Patients who have eczema herpeticum have a history of eczema. The distribution of lesions is similar to that of the eczema, and the patients often appear toxic.

WORK-UP

Chickenpox is usually easy to diagnose, and laboratory tests are rarely needed. A mild leukocytosis may occur. Vesicle scrapings contain multinucleated giant cells, and vesicular fluid contains virus in the first several days of illness. The scabs do not contain virus. Virus grows in a number of human tissue culture cell lines. Acute and convalescent complement fixation titers confirm varicella–zoster virus infection.

TREATMENT AND MANAGEMENT

In most cases, only symptomatic treatment is necessary. Calamine lotion or a skin moisturizer containing menthol (*e.g.*, Sarna) is helpful for pruritus, as also are baths of pulverized oatmeal. More severe pruritus may respond to oral antihistamines such as diphenhydramine and hydroxyzine. The patient's fingernails should be cut short and the skin kept clean to prevent secondary infection from scratching. Acetaminophen is the preferred drug for fever control. Aspirin should *not* be used in children and adolescents because of mounting evidence linking its use in chickenpox and influenza to the development of Reye's syndrome.

Because of their potential seriousness, varicella infections in immunocompromised patients require more vigorous treatment. VZIG given as prophylaxis within 72 hours of exposure can attenuate the disease. Acyclovir (750 mg/sq/m/day for 7 days in patients under 12 years of age; 15 mg/kg/day in older patients) is the preferred drug for high-risk patients who develop varicella rash. Interferon and vidarabine are also effective but more toxic. Antiviral therapy is not required for high-risk patients who have received active or passive immunization and subsequently develop the disease unless they are severely affected. VZIG is recommended for newborns whose mothers develop chickenpox between 5 days before and 2 days after delivery. The dose is 1.25 ml/10 kg body weight; the minimum dose is 1.25 ml and the maximum dose 6.25 ml.

A live attenuated varicella vaccine has been developed and is undergoing clinical trials. It has been useful in preventing chickenpox in immunocompromised patients. Its use in normal children will be controversial.

INDICATIONS FOR REFERRAL OR ADMISSION

Health care professionals can usually help the child's caretakers manage chickenpox with telephone contact alone. The patient should be evaluated in the office if he develops signs of bacterial infection, respiratory symptoms, central nervous system changes, severe vomiting, or if he is immunocompromised. Patients requiring hospital referral include those with bacterial infections unresponsive to oral antibiotics, severe respiratory disease, central nervous system signs, and Reye's syndrome.

If there is eye involvement, it is prudent to have an ophthalmologic consultation within 24 to 36 hours to rule out infection of the cornea. A child with suspected keratitis (*e.g.*, photophobia, tearing, or decreased vision), should be referred promptly. Herpetic corneal ulcerations constitute an emergency and usually require hospitalization.

ANNOTATED BIBLIOGRAPHY

Brunell P: Varicella-zoster infections. In Feigin R, Cherry J: Textbook of Pediatric Infectious Diseases, p 1206. Philadelphia, WB Saunders, 1981 (Concise but thorough.)

Fleisher G, Henry W, McSorley M et al: Life-threatening complications of varicella. Am J Dis Child 135:896, 1981 (5 years' experience in a large children's hospital.)

Gershon A: Live attenuated varicella vaccine. J Infect Dis 152:859, 1985 (Especially useful is its presentation of the current status and future use of the vaccine.)

Gordon J: Chickenpox: An epidemiological review. Am J Med Sci 224:362, 1962 (The classic work; includes a section on history beginning with the 9th century A.D.)

Hermann KL: Congenital and perinatal varicella. Clin Obstet Gynecol 25:605, 1982 (Clear presentation of a complicated topic.)

Hurwitz E et al: Public health service study on Reye's syndrome and medications: Report of the pilot phase. N Engl J Med 313:849, 1985 (Well-designed and clinically important preliminary study; the main study involving 50 pediatric centers is underway.)

Varicella–zoster infections. In Krugman S, Katz S, Gershon A, Wilfert C (eds): Infectious Diseases of Children. St. Louis, CV Mosby, 33:433, 1985 (Complete; good diagrams and pictures.)

198
Mumps
THOMAS G. DEWITT

Mumps is a highly contagious viral illness primarily affecting children and young adults. Parotitis is the principal presentation of this illness. The annual incidence of this disease in the United States has diminished from over 200,000 cases to less than 4,000 cases since the introduction of a live-attenuated virus vaccine in 1967, though sporadic outbreaks still occur.

PATHOPHYSIOLOGY

The infectious agent in mumps is an RNA virus, *myxovirus parotiditis*. It belongs to a group of viruses that cause influenza, parainfluenza, and Newcastle disease. The mumps virus is pathogenic only in humans.

The virus is transmitted primarily through saliva though it has been found in blood, urine, stool, and breast milk. Acquired through the respiratory tract, the virus proliferates locally and in regional lymph nodes. A viremia then occurs after an incubation period of 18 days (range of 14 to 25 days). During this viremia, the virus may be disseminated widely to an array of tissues including salivary, pancreas, testes, ovaries, thyroid, breast, and meninges. The shedding of the virus in saliva tends to occur 2 to 3 days before, and persists for up to a week after the onset of symptoms. After infection, antibodies develop to both the nucleoprotein core (soluble [S] antigen and a hemagglutinin surface (viral [V]) antigen. An immunity to the disease correlates with the acquisition of antibody to the surface antigen and not to the core antigen. Both parainfluenza and Newcastle disease viruses can elicit antibodies that cross-react with the mumps virus.

CLINICAL PRESENTATION

General malaise, anorexia, and myalgia with a low-grade fever are the nonspecific prodromal symptoms of a mumps infection followed, most commonly, by a high fever and parotitis. Other manifestations may include pancreatitis, oophoritis, orchitis, mastitis, myocarditis, meningoencephalitis, and cranial nerve involvement. These symptoms can occur singly, sequentially, or concurrently. One third of patients infected with a mumps virus show no clinical symptoms.

The parotitis often presents initially as an earache with no tympanic membrane abnormalities.

Parotid edema begins with erythema and tenderness above the angle of the mandible within 1 or 2 days from the onset of the earache. Edema increases over several days and then persists for ~1 week. It may progress to above the eye, to the mastoid area, or to the chin and anterior neck. Typically, the edema obliterates the angle of the mandible making palpation of it difficult and may also cause an upturning of the earlobe. An examination of the buccal mucosa often reveals erythematous and edematous orifices of Wharton's and Stensen's ducts. In approximately three quarters of the patients, the parotid edema is bilateral, with the involvement of one gland tending to precede that of the contralateral gland by 1 to 5 days. Concurrent with the increasing parotid involvement is an increase in fever, which may be as high as 40°C. The temperature subsides with the reduction in size of the glands.

When parotitis is the initial presentation of mumps, the other focal manifestations tend to occur 1 week or more after the onset of parotid edema. Although rare in prepubertal males, orchitis may occur in as many as 30% of postpubertal males. In 25% of these affected males, the orchitis is bilateral. Symptoms include testicular edema and tenderness, nausea, vomiting, and temperature. The testicle may increase to four times the normal size. Although the extreme pain tends to subside in a few days, the edema and tenderness may last for weeks. Mild atrophy of one testes may develop in many cases, but sterility is uncommon.

As with orchitis, oophoritis is also found primarily in postpubertal patients. The incidence, however, is ~5% and the clinical presentation often mimics that of an acute abdomen. Although mastitis is rare in prepubertal females, it has been described in as many as one third of postpubertal females.

One of the more significant manifestations of mumps is meningoencephalitis. The presence of white blood cells in the spinal fluid has been reported in over half of the patients infected with mumps. Most patients, however, have subclinical involvement. Unlike many of the other manifestations of mumps, the meningoencephalitis commonly presents (25% to 50%) without an associated parotitis. Males are affected more commonly than females by 3:1. If the principal manifestation is meningitis, the patient presents with the symptoms of fever, headache, nausea, vomiting, and nuchal rigidity. In mumps encephalitis, the patient may present with convulsions, focal neurologic signs, movement disorders, or marked changes in sensorium. One may occasionally find symptoms of muscular weakness and a loss of reflexes, reflecting myelin involvement.

A small percent of people with mumps may develop unilateral deafness. The onset may be sudden or gradual, and the hearing loss tends to be complete and permanent.

Mumps may affect other organs and glandular tissue. Pancreatitis may be a manifestation, presenting with upper abdominal pain and tenderness in the epigastrium. The incidence of subclinical pancreatitis may be as high as 5%. Myocarditis and pericarditis occur primarily in adults, presenting with ECG changes of a prolonged AV conduction time. Joint, thyroid, renal, and prostate involvement may also occur.

DIFFERENTIAL DIAGNOSIS

Since most patients presenting with mumps have parotitis, the differential diagnosis must focus principally on other causes of parotid swelling. However, as the mumps virus may infect many glandular tissues, the general considerations that follow may also be generalized to other glandular involvement.

The most common other causes of parotid swelling are infections. The viral agents, parainfluenza types I and III, Coxsackie A, EBV, CMV, and ECHO viruses may all cause parotitis. More important, suppurative parotitis, most often caused by staphylococcus, pneumococcus, or gram-negative bacilli, should be strongly considered when the patient presents with systemic toxicity. The expression of purulent material from Stensen's duct may help delineate this condition.

Noninfectious causes of parotid enlargement include obstruction, tumors (particularly lymphocytic), congenital or acquired cysts, and drugs such as iodides and phenothiazines. Malnutrition, or rapid refeeding after malnutrition, can be associated with enlarged parotid glands. Pneumoparotitis may occur in a child blowing up balloons or learning to play the trumpet.

Several systemic diseases can cause parotid enlargement, including diabetes mellitus, obesity, and cystic fibrosis. Parotid involvement, however, is an uncommon presentation in all of these.

Other conditions in the area of the angle of the mandible may, on superficial examination, resemble parotitis. The most common problem in children is cervical lymphadenitis. Typical and atypical mycobacteria, as well as cat-scratch fever may affect preauricular nodes. Dental abscesses and severe otitis externa should also be considered. In the small child, infantile cortical hyperostosis (Caffey's disease) and a branchial cleft cyst may resemble parotitis.

WORK-UP

History

The most important history to obtain in a child who has parotid swelling or encephalitis is that of prior exposure to, or previous vaccination for, mumps. With an average incubation period of 18 days, exposure to a person with symptoms suggestive of mumps 2 to 3 weeks prior to the onset of the patient's symptoms may also be helpful. It is important to remember that although parotitis is the most common presenting symptom of mumps, other manifestations, such as pancreatitis, encephalitis, and orchitis, can occur without parotid involvement. Since the live-attenuated virus vaccine is about 95% effective, a history of previous mumps' vaccination would mitigate against the mumps virus as an etiology. A small percentage of patients can obviously have mumps despite previous vaccination, and illnesses suggestive of recurrent mumps have been reported.

Physical Examination

In the child with suspected mumps, the physical examination should determine whether the child actually has parotitis; whether he has other tissue involvement; or whether he has any abnormal neurologic signs.

The area of the parotid gland should be palpated to determine if the edema includes the angle of the mandible. An examination of Stensen's and Wharton's ducts for inflammation may help to confirm the diagnosis of parotitis. Palpation of the neck for thyroid enlargement and tenderness, and the abdomen for epigastric tenderness should follow the parotid examination. In women, particularly postpubertal, the breasts and lower abdomen should be examined for evidence of mastitis and oophoritis. Likewise in postpubertal males, the testes should be examined. Remember, however, that involvement of these and other glands may occur 1 week or more after parotid involvement. Patients should be assessed neurologically for signs of meningeal irritation, sensory changes, or weakness.

Laboratory Tests

Since mumps is primarily a clinical diagnosis, laboratory tests are usually not helpful. Serum amylase may aid in differentiating between parotitis and other diseases that mimic it, but will not confirm a diagnosis of mumps. Most laboratories are also not equipped to differentiate between parotid and pancreatic amylase. The presence of antibodies to the nucleoprotein core (S) antigen indicates a current, or recent, mumps infection whereas antibodies to the hemagglutinin surface (V) antigen indicates a past history of mumps infection. These antibody assays are not readily available and are probably not indicated unless there are compelling epidemiologic or diagnostic reasons. A lumbar puncture is necessary in a patient with "hard" neurologic findings. The presence of only headache or photophobia makes the need for a lumbar puncture more of a clinical judgment. Other laboratory tests are indicated only as they may rule in, or out, other diseases listed in the differential diagnosis. In particular, an elevated white blood count with a left shift may be helpful in identifying suppurative parotitis.

TREATMENT AND MANAGEMENT

The optimal treatment is prevention, which is accomplished by the use of a live-attenuated virus vaccine. Given intramuscularly to children older than 12 months of age, it provides an adequate immune response in over 95% of patients. Children younger than 1 year who receive the vaccine may have a poorer response due to the presence of maternal antibodies.

Since no antimumps viral agent is available, the treatment of patients with mumps is symptomatic. Analgesics and antipyretics are helpful. Steroids and antibiotics have not been shown to be efficacious.

In cases of meningitis or meningoencephalitis, supportive therapy is again indicated, with particular attention to the complications of cerebral edema and seizures. The use of steroids does not seem to alter the course of these conditions, including the development of deafness.

INDICATIONS FOR REFERRAL OR ADMISSION

In the patient with mumps, the principal indications for referral or admission are significant neurologic involvement or metabolic derangements due primarily to nausea and vomiting. Most patients with mumps, regardless of the site of involvement, have a self-limited disease that with good supportive care and close follow-up resolves spontaneously without a need for hospitalization.

In the child or adolescent who has had mumps, the physician should be aware of some potential long-term effects. Deafness has been described in patients with mumps and may occur without meningitis or encephalitis. A follow-up hearing screen should be done on patients who have had mumps. In addition, although the association has not been clearly defined, there is some suggestion that diabetes mellitus may be associated with a previous mumps infection.

ANNOTATED BIBLIOGRAPHY

Azimi PH, Gramblett HG, Haynes RE: Mumps meningoencephalitis in children. JAMA 207:509, 1969 (Relates the spectrum of clinical presentation of mumps meningoencephalitis.)

Centers for Disease Control: Mumps Surveillance, January 1977–December 1982. United States Department of Health and Human Services; September, 1984 (Good epidemiologic information with a focus on mumps vaccine and immunization.)

Feldman HA: Mumps. In Feigin RD, Cherry JD: Textbook of Pediatric Infectious Disease, pp 419–440. Philadelphia, WB Saunders, 1981 (Comprehensive review of mumps with an extensive [152] list of references.)

Jones GF, Ray CG, Fulginiti VA: Perinatal mumps infection. J Pediatr 96:912, 1980 (Good brief review of perinatal mumps.)

Marcy SM, Kibrick S: Mumps. In Hoeprich PD: Infectious Diseases, pp 621–627. New York, Harper & Row, 1977 (Excellent listing of differential diagnoses.)

199
Influenza
KENNETH M. BOYER

Influenza is an acute respiratory infection caused by strains of the orthomyxoviruses. The first of the human respiratory viruses to be isolated and characterized, influenza viruses have also been studied the most extensively. Yet, despite great sophistication in our understanding of it as a disease, influenza continues to elude preventive measures. The pediatrician whose busy practice has been overwhelmed during an influenza epidemic is only too aware of this.

Influenza infections are seldom definitively proven by virus isolation in outpatient practice. Characteristic "influenza-like" illnesses with abrupt onset, fever, headache, myalgia, and respiratory symptoms are easily recognized, however. Influenza viruses are the most likely cause of such illnesses, although parainfluenza viruses, enteroviruses, and adenoviruses may also cause the syndrome.

MICROBIOLOGY AND PATHOPHYSIOLOGY

Influenza viruses are negative strand RNA viruses of three major antigenic types—A, B, and C—and multiple antigenic subtypes. All have the property of hemagglutination and possess the enzyme neuraminidase. The World Health Organization system of nomenclature for influenza virus strains specifies type, host (for strains of animal origin), geographic source, strain number, and year of isolation, to which code designations of hemagglutinin and neuraminidase subtypes are appended. Thus, the original "Shope strain" of swine influenza virus is designated A/swine/Iowa/15/30 ($H_{sw}N1$); the recent *Taiwan* influenza A strain is designated A/Taiwan/1/86 (H1N1).

The biologic and antigenic diversity of influenza viruses is attributable partly to their unique, segmented RNA genome. A variation in hemagglutinin and neuraminidase specificity is the basis for antigenic *drift* and *shift* in prevalent viruses. Drift implies a minor change in either antigen, without a change in subtype; shift implies a major change in either or both antigens, with a change in subtype.

To establish infection, influenza viruses must penetrate the mucous blanket lining the respiratory tract and escape inactivation by nonspecific inhibitors as well as specific local antibodies. The major site of infection is the ciliated columnar epithelial cell. Influenza pneumonia may occur as a result of primary viral infection, bacterial superinfection, or combined bacterial-viral infection. In recent years, the pathologic entity of diffuse encephalopathy and fatty degeneration of the liver (Reye's syndrome) has been established as a potential complication of influenza, particularly type B, in children. It is becoming increasingly clear that the use of aspirin during the acute infection is a major cofactor in pathogenesis of this syndrome.

Immunity against influenza results from a complex interplay of humoral, secretory, and cell-mediated mechanisms. Because of the brief incubation period of the disease, anamnestic stimulation of antibody affords little protection. Thus, some degree of pre-existing antibody appears to be essential to prevent infection. The sequential antigenic changes that occur in the virus in the course of antigenic drift afford each new variant a selective advantage in establishing infection; the major antigenic changes that accompany antigenic shifts render larger populations susceptible and account for pandemic spread.

EPIDEMIOLOGY

Outbreaks of influenza may be localized, nationwide, or global; sporadic cases rarely occur. On the whole, other agents (*e.g.*, respiratory syncytial virus, parainfluenza viruses, and *Mycoplasma pneumoniae*) account for most serious respiratory illnesses in childhood. During periods of epidemic or pandemic spread, however, respiratory infections by influenza viruses may exceed all other etiologies. In the peak month of a composite of 11 consecutive influenza A virus outbreaks observed in Washington, DC, influenza A virus was isolated from 68% of croup patients and 36% of all hospitalized children with respiratory disease.

Influenza infections have marked seasonality. In temperate climates, epidemics occur almost exclusively in winter months. Off-season infections are documented infrequently. Droplet spread, with inhalation of large airborne particles produced by coughing and sneezing, is generally accepted as the most common mode of natural influenza transmission. Once infection is established, peak virus shedding coincides with clinical symptoms. Virus may be recovered for 1 day prior to the onset of symptoms and for a variable period, usually less than 6 days, afterward. The incubation period of influenza ranges from 1 to 7 days but is commonly 2 to 3 days. This brief incubation period, coupled with the large amount of infectious virus in secretions and the relatively small amounts necessary for infection of susceptibles, accounts for the sharpness of influenza outbreaks.

CLINICAL PRESENTATION

Disease due to epidemic influenza A virus is unique in that persons of all ages in a population become ill with febrile respiratory complaints. In contrast, whereas other noninfluenzal respiratory viral agents may also cause community epidemics that involve both children and adults, the illness is different in both age groups. Young children with primary viral infections with noninfluenzal agents have febrile illnesses. Older children and adults with similar infections most commonly have common colds and other upper respiratory involvement with no or minimal fever.

The symptoms and signs of "classic" influenza in older children and adolescents include abrupt onset, with fever and associated flushed face, chills, headache, myalgia, and malaise. The temperature range is between 39°C and 41°C (102°F to 106°F) with a general inverse correlation with age. Systemic symptoms are generally more severe in the older patient. Although a dry cough and coryza are also early manifestations of influenza, these symptoms may go unobserved by the patients because of the severity of the systemic manifestations. A sore throat occurs in over half the cases and is usually associated with nonexudative pharyngitis. Ocular symptoms include tearing, photophobia, burning, and pain with eye movement (ophthalmodynia).

In uncomplicated illness, the fever usually persists for 2 to 3 days but may last up to 5 days. A biphasic temperature pattern may occur even without apparent secondary bacterial complications. By the second to the fourth days, respiratory symptoms become more prominent, and the systemic complaints begin to subside. The cough is dry and hacking and usually persists for 4 to 7 days; occasionally a cough, in association with some degree of general malaise, will persist for 1 to 2 weeks or longer after the rest of the illness has subsided.

In younger children, the manifestations of influenza viral infections are frequently similar to those resulting from other respiratory viruses. Laryngotracheitis, bronchitis, bronchiolitis, pneumonia, and the common cold all occur. Primary infection with influenza A in these age categories is typically seen as an undifferentiated febrile upper respiratory illness. Fever tends to be high and will exceed 39.5°C in most patients. Affected children appear moderately toxic, with clear nasal discharge, cough, and irritability as almost constant findings. Pharyngitis is usually present, with diffuse erythema and boggy, enlarged tonsillar tissue. Between 5% and 10% of those infected will have some degree of pulmonary involvement; in hospitalized children, this percentage may be as high as 50%. Gastrointestinal symptoms have been noted in several studies of influenza infection in young children. Febrile convulsions, precipitated by fever of abrupt onset, have also been cited as common presenting complaints in several studies. Acute laryngotracheitis (croup) has been noted as a prominent feature of influenza A. Illness tends to be more severe than is the rule for the croup syndrome induced by parainfluenza viruses. An increased severity of influenza should be anticipated in children with pre-existing cardiac, pulmonary, and neuromuscular disease.

DIFFERENTIAL DIAGNOSIS

The differential diagnosis of influenza includes an extensive list of febrile conditions, most commonly caused by other respiratory viruses and *S. pyogenes*. In common pediatric practice, influenza and other common respiratory viral illnesses are often grouped casually as viral URI. A definitive diagnosis of influenza in even a few children greatly increases the likelihood that other pediatric respiratory illnesses are caused by the same agent and may be useful in forecasting the development of serious influenzal infections in high-risk patients within a practice or community.

WORK-UP

Routine laboratory studies provide little help in the differentiation of influenza from other viral respiratory diseases. Hematologic manifestations are variable, with marked leukocytosis frequently observed in infants. Chest radiographs are useful primarily to determine the presence of complicating interstitial or lobar pneumonia.

A definite diagnosis of influenza depends on either virus isolation from respiratory secretions or a significant rise in serum antibody during convalescence. In contrast to shedding of adenoviruses or herpes simplex from the respiratory tract, asymptomatic carriage of influenza viruses is rare. Thus, virus isolation alone is considered conclusive evidence for an etiologic role in an illness. Serologic diagnosis may be accomplished using either complement–fixation or hemagglutination–inhibition techniques, but it is not useful unless sera are paired.

TREATMENT

Symptomatic treatment is the cornerstone of management. Bed rest, adequate hydration with oral fluids, control of fever and myalgia with acetaminophen, and maintenance of comfortable breathing by means of nasal decongestants and humidified air suffice in most cases. Prophylactic administration of antibiotics should be discouraged. A persistent irritative cough during convalescence can often be relieved with dextromethorphan or codeine.

Complicated illnesses demand the physician's clinical judgment in the use of other therapeutic modalities. Bacterial infections, suggested by a prolonged febrile course or recrudescence of fever during early convalescence, should be identified with regard to site, and appropriate cultures should be obtained. Antibiotic therapy is then indicated and should be guided and modified by the results of cultures.

Inhalation therapy is an integral part of the management of illnesses complicated by airway compromise (croup), apneic spells, or diffuse pneumonia. Such patients should be hospitalized and monitored carefully. Humidified air alone is an important element in the management of croup, but nasotracheal intubation or tracheostomy is required in a high percentage of patients with croup due to influenza. The provision of supplemental oxygen and, as indicated by oximetry or arterial blood gas analysis, mechanical ventilation may be required in patients with apnea or respiratory failure due to pneumonia.

The antiviral agent amantadine hydrochloride is active *in vitro* against influenza A viruses and has been shown to provide prophylactic and therapeutic benefit in adults. Amantadine lacks activity against influenza B viruses. During a documented community epidemic of influenza A, however, amantadine may be used to treat infants and children who present with fever and croup, bronchiolitis, or pneumonia. The drug may also be used in unvaccinated patients in high-risk categories either prophylactically or at the onset of a febrile upper respiratory illness under similar epidemic circumstances. The dosage is 4 to 6 mg/kg/day orally in two divided doses for 5 days. Dosage should not exceed 150 mg/day in young children. Children older than 10 years can take a 100-mg tablet twice a day.

PREVENTION

Immunization is the best method for the prevention of influenza. A prediction of the nature of new influenza virus variants and their potential for epidemic spread is the major difficulty. Vaccines must contain antigens identical or similar to those of the potential infecting agent in order to be effective. In years when a new variant arises and causes widespread outbreaks, the available vaccine may contain a previous variant with only modest heterologous immunizing potential. Conversely, in years in which new variants do not arise, vaccines may be formulated ideally, but the epidemic potential of virus strains that already have circulated may be minimal. Thus, by virtue of changes in either virus antigens or prevalences of natural immunity, the prevention of epidemics through the widespread use of vaccine has been difficult.

Only inactivated (formalin-treated) influenza vaccines are licensed for use in the United States. Several improvements have been made in these vaccines since their introduction in the late 1930s. These innovations have included enhanced vaccine production using recombinant virus strains that grow rapidly in eggs, exclusion of host antigens and other toxic impurities by zonal ultracentrifugation (current *whole virus* vaccines), and disruption of viral particles with ether or detergents (current *split-product* vaccines). Split-product vaccines, by virtue of their minimal reactogenicity, are preferred for the vaccination of children. Reactions, when they occur, include mild fever, "flu-like" symptoms of malaise and myalgia, and local tenderness at the site of inoculation.

The emphasis of current influenza vaccination strategy continues to be on the prevention of complicated illness in population groups at highest risk. Such rates are highest in children with (1) cardiovascular disorders such as rheumatic, congenital, or hypertensive heart disease; (2) chronic bronchopulmonary disease such as bronchopulmonary dysplasia, cystic fibrosis, and asthma; (3) chronic metabolic diseases such as diabetes mellitus; (4) chronic glomerulonephritis and nephrosis; and (5) chronic neurologic disorders, especially those associated with weak or paralyzed respiratory muscles. It is clear from recent experience that use of inactivated vaccines in children of all ages can produce acceptable levels of antibody with minimal side effects. Current and future influenza vaccines deserve wider use in pediatric patients.

ANNOTATED BIBLIOGRAPHY

Bryson YJ: The use of amantadine in children for prophylaxis and treatment of influenza A infections. Pediatr Infect Dis 1:44, 1982 (Clear summary of the available data on prophylactic and therapeutic use of amantadine, with prescribing guidelines for pediatricians.)

Centers for Disease Control: Prevention and control of influenza. Morbid Mortal Weekly Rep 36:373, 1987 (Most recent of the recommendations concerning influenza vaccination developed by the CDC Advisory Committee on Immunization Practices. These recommendations [updated annually] are the definitive reference for American physicians using influenza vaccination.)

Couch RB, Kasel JA, Glezen WP et al: Influenza: Its control in persons and populations. J Infect Dis 153:431, 1986 (Review of the extensive surveillance studies of influenza infections and immunization conducted during the past decade by the Influenza Research Center in Houston.)

Hurwitz ES, Barrett MJ, Brogman D et al: Public Health Service Study on Reye's syndrome and medications. Report of the pilot phase. N Engl J Med 313:849, 1985 (Case-control study that provides the strongest evidence for the association of Reye's syndrome and aspirin use.)

Jordan WS, Denny FS, Badger GF et al: A study of illness in a group of Cleveland families. XVII. The occurrence of Asian influenza. Am J Hyg 68:190, 1958 (Classic clinical and epidemiologic study of influenza A infections in the "Cleveland family study." This paper clearly delineates the clinical spectrum of influenza A infections in children and adults.)

Wright PF, Ross KB, Thompson J et al: Influenza A infections in young children. Primary natural infection and protective efficacy of live-vaccine-induced or naturally acquired immunity. N Engl J Med 296:829, 1977 (Delineates the clinical features of influenza A in a large prospectively studied group of young children aged 6 weeks to 3 years of age.)

200
Cat-Scratch Disease
HUGH A. CARITHERS

Cat-scratch disease is an infection that has been recognized world-wide. It is associated with direct cat contact and it has a benign course with a good prognosis in most patients. After obvious cutaneous infections and infections of the nose and throat, it is probably the next most common cause of unilateral regional adenitis in childhood. Complications and unusual manifestations sometimes make the diagnosis imperative, such as when a malignancy of the lymph nodes is considered.

PATHOPHYSIOLOGY

The probable cause of cat-scratch disease (CSD) is a pleomorphic, small, gram-negative bacillus. The organism causing CSD is thought to be transmitted directly or indirectly only by the domestic cat. In those few patients in whom cat contact is strongly denied, an inoculation by an object in which the cat was in contact may have resulted in an infection. The organism causing the disease enters the body through a break in the skin, which rarely may be a bite or other injury caused by another animal.

Cats that transmit the disease are usually immature and not ill, and they have no distinctive features. The length of time in which they are capable of transmitting the disease is unknown. An older child or adult who denies cat contact may have had a brief encounter as long as 1 month prior to the recognition of lymphadenopathy.

Pathologists usually report findings as "compatible with" or "suggestive of" CSD because lymph node changes are not diagnostic. The basic pathology is the formulation of a granuloma. There are three stages of change in lymph nodes: an enlargement with hypertrophy of the germinal centers and a thickening of the cortex; the formation of granulomas with invasion of lymphocytes and epithelial cells; and the fusion of the granulomas with central necrosis and infiltration with neutrophils. All may be present simultaneously but regression occurs usually before pus formation. Pus may be loculated.

CLINICAL PRESENTATION

About 3 to 5 days after an intimate exposure to a cat, usually immature, an inoculation site appears and progresses through stages similar to chickenpox lesions. First, a pink or red macule becomes papular and later forms a vesicle filled with sterile, opaque liquid. On breaking, a brief crust phase may be observed, which is much shorter than that of chickenpox. These changes, which usually last 1 to 3 days, often pass unnoticed but the remaining papule, a few millimeters to 1 cm in diameter, may be present for weeks. A remaining macule may be observed for as long as 2 to 3 months.

In most patients, the illness is mild with generalized aching, malaise, anorexia, and rarely nausea and abdominal pain. About 40% of patients are afebrile. Only about 10% have temperatures above 102°F.

Although virtually all patients have lymphadenopathy, the extent of the involvement and clinical course are highly variable. It may be concurrent with recognition of the papule, but due to the location or size of the lymph node, it may be undetected for 1 month or more. It may increase in size for several weeks and then regress over a period of 2 or more months. In approximately 12% of the cases, the involved lymph node proceeds to suppuration.

Lymphadenopathy in CSD is usually single. When regional, usually only two nodes are enlarged; three nodes are occasionally enlarged, and four or more are rarely enlarged. The location of involved lymph nodes among my 1200 patients with CSD is shown in Table 200-1.

Generalized lymphadenopathy has been reported. In a disease which almost always involves single or regional lymph nodes, such manifestation appears unlikely unless an immune deficiency is present.

An accurate measurement is essential at the initial examination to detect the progression or regression of lymphadenopathy. Since enlarged lymph nodes are sometimes ovoid rather than round, two planes, horizontal and vertical, should be measured. A convenient way to assure accuracy is by using calipers. Those used in electrocardiographic interpretation are readily available.

By a great majority, the most unusual manifestation of CSD is the oculoglandular form (of Parinaud) that is manifested by a granuloma of the conjunctiva, preauricular lymphadenopathy, no purulent discharge from the eye, and a surprising

Table 200-1. Location of Lymphadenopathy Among 1200 Patients with Cat-Scratch Disease

LOCATION	NUMBER	PERCENT
Total upper extremity	610	46.1
Axillary	586	
Epitrochlear	24	
Total neck and jaw	340	26.1
Cervical	191	
Submandibular	149	
Total groin	228	17.5
Inguinal	143	
Femoral	85	
Preauricular	87	6.6
Postauricular	2	
Clavicular	31	2.3
Chest	4	

Note: The number of patients totals 1302; some had more than one location.

Diagnosis of Cat-Scratch Disease: *The Rule of Five*

Lymphadenopathy, single (mostly) or regional (sometimes)	1.0
Intimate exposure to a cat (usually immature)	2.0
Inoculation site	2.0
Positive skin test	2.0

Note: Five points strongly suggest cat-scratch disease; seven points indicate a definite diagnosis.

lack of local discomfort. The prognosis is excellent. Other rarely encountered manifestations include erythema nodosum, thrombocytopenia, erythema marginatum, and an osteolytic lesion, which has been reported in only five patients. Encephalopathy accompanying CSD is abrupt and severe in onset; convulsions are often the first sign. This form of encephalopathy has a better prognosis than most other types or encephalitis.

DIFFERENTIAL DIAGNOSIS

A helpful aid in the diagnosis of CSD is the *Rule of Five* as shown in the box, Diagnosis of Cat-Scratch Disease: *The Rule of Five*.

Some authorities believe that other causes of lymphadenopathy should be eliminated before making a diagnosis of CSD. The differential diagnosis, however, is usually apparent. For example, infectious mononucleosis may begin as a single enlarged lymph node, almost always in the neck, but acute tonsillopharyngitis distinguishes it from CSD. The Kawasaki syndrome is characterized by lymphadenopathy, but confusion with CSD is highly unlikely because of the scattering of enlarged nodes and other features.

A mycobacterial infection has caused more difficulty in differential diagnosis. Lymphadenopathy caused by *Mycobacterium tuberculosis*, which is usually regarded as a bilateral infection of the lymph nodes of the neck, can be diagnosed readily in most patients. On the other hand, with atypical mycobacteria, single node lymphadenopathy in the neck is characteristic.

A malignant disease involving the lymph nodes may present as a single node or regional lymphadenitis. In children, especially, other nodes usually become involved quickly.

WORK-UP

The diagnosis of CSD presents little difficulty in most patients. All have lymphadenopathy, usu-

ally single, sometimes regional and rarely bilateral; therefore, the diagnosis primarily depends on determining the cause of lymph node enlargement or excluding other causes of lymphadenopathy.

A history of handling a cat, usually an immature one that is not ill, is almost essential in the diagnosis. Finding the inoculation site may clinch the diagnosis. Locating the entry site of the organism that causes CSD is the most neglected feature in the study of patients. When it is not apparent, a history from the patient and his family will often reveal a lesion remembered as a "bump" or pimple at the time or just before the recognition of lymphadenopathy.

Laboratory work is not helpful, although there may be an elevation of the white blood cell count and occasionally an eosinophilia. The sedimentation rate may be elevated, but not consistently.

Skin Test

The skin test need not be performed in most patients; however, it can be invaluable in complicated cases. When the physician is unwilling to observe a patient with lymphadenopathy, rather than embark on a complicated diagnostic evaluation and treatment such as lymph node removal, the test can be the means of avoiding unnecessary surgery and use of antibiotics. It may thus be argued that the skin test, in preventing anguish among patients and their families with regard to the cause of undiagnosed lymphadenopathy, far outweighs its vague danger, as yet undiscovered or even defined.

The test uses a crude substance made from pus aspirated from a fluctuant node of a patient with the disease. If the test is applied more than 1 week after the enlargement of the involved node, all patients should have a positive result. There may be an occasional false-positive reaction, but I believe that many such patients have had an inapparent infection in childhood.

A reaction to the test in the form of a wheel may be immediate in a few patients. An anaphylactic reaction has not been reported.

TREATMENT

Treatment is usually symptomatic and is aimed at the protection of the involved lymph node. Isolation of the patient is not indicated. Antibiotics do not appear to shorten the duration of the disease or to prevent a progression to suppuration of involved lymph nodes.

A limitation of activity is advised to prevent trauma to enlarged lymph nodes. Analgesics and bed rest are indicated for the minority of patients who have a fever. Normal activity may be continued by most patients during the weeks to a few months required for the complete regression of lymphadenopathy.

Aspiration is indicated in patients who have suppuration of lymph nodes. This should be done with a 16- or 18-gauge needle after ethyl chloride has been sprayed over the puncture site. The skin is usually too thin to permit the injection of a local anesthetic. Unless there is considerable pain, a delay of aspiration until suppuration is marked may prevent repeated aspiration.

Surgical removal of involved lymph nodes is not justified except rarely when diagnosis is in doubt and a delay might hinder the treatment of a malignancy. Moreover, an incision of suppurant lymph nodes is not recommended because aspiration is nearly always successful and is less likely to result in chronic drainage.

The patient and his family are almost always interested in the care of the involved cat. Since these animals are not ill and the length of time during which they may transmit disease is unknown, I do not recommend the removal of the cat.

ANNOTATED BIBLIOGRAPHY

Carithers HA: Cat scratch disease: An overview based on a study of 1,200 patients. Am J Dis Child 139:1124–1133, 1985 (Extended study.)

Carithers HA: Cat scratch disease: Notes on its history. Am J Dis Child 119:200–203, 1970 (Tells of discovery and Franco-American connections.)

Carithers HA: Oculoglandular disease of parinaud, manifestations of cat scratch disease. Am J Dis Child 132:1195–1200, 1978. (Describes this most common unusual manifestation.)

Carithers HA: Cat scratch disease associated with an osteolytic lesion. Am J Dis Child 137:968–970, 1983 (Describes in detail this unusual manifestation.)

Lyon LW: Neurologic manifestations of cat scratch disease. Arch Neurol 25:23–27, 1971 (The only survey of neurologic manifestations.)

Margileth AM: Cat scratch disease: Non-bacterial regional lymphadenitis. Pediatrics 42:803–818, 1968 (Excellent reference.)

Margileth AM, Wear DJ, Hadfield TL et al: Cat scratch disease: Bacteria in skin at primary inoculation site. JAMA 252:928–931, 1984 (Important advance in understanding the disease.)

Wear DJ, Margileth AM, Hadfield TL et al: Cat scratch disease: Bacterial infection. Science 221:1403–1405, 1983 (First description of the probable cause of the disease.)

201
Common Intestinal Parasites
MARGARET HIGHAM

Intestinal parasitic infections are often considered uncommon and esoteric by primary care practitioners. There are, however, several intestinal parasites that pediatricians are likely to be required to recognize and treat. The ubiquitous *Enterobius vermicularis* or pinworm is well known to pediatricians. *Giardia lamblia* is the most frequently identified parasite in stool samples. The association of *Giardia* with day care centers indicates that it will become an increasingly important pediatric pathogen. *Ascaris lumbricoides* and *Trichuris trichiura* are particularly prevalent in the southeastern part of the country. The recognition and management of these four most commonly encountered intestinal parasites in the United States are reviewed in this chapter.

PATHOPHYSIOLOGY

Enterobius Vermicularis

Adult pinworms are thread-like worms about 1 cm long that live in the human cecum. Gravid females migrate to the perianal area at night, where they cause pruritus and lay their eggs. The eggs become widely disseminated in the environment and can remain infective for up to 20 days. When eggs are ingested, they hatch in the duodenum and the larvae pass to the large intestine where maturation occurs.

Pinworms are the most common intestinal parasite in the United States. The highest prevalence occurs among 5- to 9-year-olds. Disease transmission usually occurs by hand-to-mouth spread following perianal scratching or following handling of contaminated fomites such as bedding or clothing. Inhalation of eggs in dust can also initiate infection. Reinfection is common. Crowded household and institutional settings seem to promote infection.

Giardia Lamblia

Infection with *Giardia* begins with ingestion of the infectious stage of the organism, the cyst. Once ingested, the noninfectious trophozoite emerges in the upper small intestine where it adheres to the microvillus epithelium. When trophozoites are swept away in the fecal stream, they change back to cysts and are passed in the feces. Cysts are relatively hardy and can remain in the environment for days to weeks. When diarrhea and rapid intestinal transit time are present, trophozoites may be found in stool specimens.

Water-borne and person-to-person transmission are the most common modes of disease spread. Person-to-person spread in day care centers appears to be particularly important in the United States. Factors that contribute to the prevalence of giardiasis in day care centers include the low innoculum needed to initiate infection, poor personal hygiene among young children, and the widespread fecal contamination occurring in environments occupied by diapered toddlers.

Giardia prevalence ranging from 17% to 70% has been reported in day care centers. Children 1 to 3 years old are most likely to acquire giardiasis. Once infected, children can then return home and spread the disease to siblings and parents. *Giardia* infection has been found in as many as 25% of household contacts exposed to an infected child in day care.

Ascaris Lumbricoides

Adult *Ascaris* are distinguished by their large size, reaching 10 cm to 35 cm in length. The usual habitat of these worms is the small intestine. Female worms produce an average of 200,000 eggs/day. The eggs are resistant to changes in the external environment. After being swallowed, the infective egg hatches in the small intestine and follows a circuitous path through the body before returning to the small intestine. Newly hatched larvae penetrate the intestinal wall and migrate to the lungs by way of lymphatics and venules, where they break out of pulmonary capillaries into alveoli. Once in the alveoli, they migrate up the tracheobronchial tree to the glottis where they are swal-

lowed and pass back to the small intestine. The process of migration and maturation takes about 2 months.

Ascariasis is most prevalent in warm climates where sanitation is poor, particularly the rural South and Puerto Rico. Transmission is primarily fecal–oral following contact with contaminated soil or ingestion of fecally contaminated fruits and vegetables. The spread of infection is facilitated by the enormous egg output of the worms and the hardiness of the eggs. Infection rates and intensity of infection are greatest in children.

Trichuris Trichiura

The whipworm is a thin worm 3 cm to 4 cm long. Its usual habitat is the large bowel; it inserts its tip into intestinal tissue from which minute amounts of blood are sucked. Eggs are passed in feces and they develop outside the host. Infective eggs are ingested, hatch, mature, and make their way to the large intestine.

The epidemiology of whipworm is similar to *Ascaris*; geographic distribution and modes of spread are similar and indeed dual infection with *Ascaris* and *Trichuris* often exists. The intensity of infection is greatest in children 2 to 3 years old.

CLINICAL PRESENTATION

Enterobius Vermicularis

Most pinworm infections are asymptomatic. When symptoms do occur, perianal and perineal pruritus are most common. Sleep disturbance, irritability, teeth grinding, abdominal pain, enuresis, and vaginitis have been reported in conjunction with pinworm infection. None of these associations has been substantiated in carefully controlled studies. Any association between urinary tract infections and pinworms also remains unproven.

Giardia Lamblia

The clinical manifestations of giardiasis can be variable. Asymptomatic excretion appears to be common both in children attending day care centers and in adult contacts of children with giardiasis. Symptomatic patients are most likely to present with watery diarrhea of greater than 5 days' duration. Various other gastrointestinal complaints may be present including intermittent constipation and diarrhea, abdominal distention and cramps, anorexia and weight loss. In some patients, gastrointestinal symptomatology can be subtle, and diarrhea may be minimal or absent. More rarely, failure to thrive or chronic diarrhea may develop. Giardiasis should be considered in any patient who has an unexplained weight loss or chronic gastrointestinal signs and symptoms.

Ascaris Lumbricoides

Ascariasis appears to be asymptomatic in most cases. Symptomatology is probably related to worm burden, which is greatest among children; even so, heavy infection is uncommon.

Because *Ascaris* worms absorb nutrients ingested by the host, there has been concern over possible impairment of nutritional status, particularly among children with large parasite loads and poor dietary intake. A carefully controlled evaluation of American children with moderate to heavy worm burdens has not revealed any differences in nutritional status compared to uninfected controls.

During the worm's migratory phase, pulmonary manifestations may occur, such as pneumonitis or wheezing. The most serious consequence of ascariasis is intestinal obstruction. This occurs primarily in children less than 5 years old with heavy infections. An obstruction occurs at the level of the small bowel; it is manifested by vomiting, abdominal distention, and pain. Adult worms may be found in the vomitus. Other acute gastrointestinal manifestations include biliary obstruction, volvulus, and intussusception.

Trichuris Trichiura

Trichuriasis is asymptomatic in all but a small proportion of infected individuals. When symptoms do present, they seem to be related to worm burden. The amount of blood lost from whipworm infection is so small that mild anemia develops only in massively infected young children. Rectal prolapse has been reported in heavily infected children.

DIFFERENTIAL DIAGNOSIS

The signs and symptoms of intestinal parasites are frequently nonspecific. Intestinal manifestations may be protean, particularly in giardiasis, and they may mimic any gastrointestinal disease including viral or bacterial gastroenteritis, lactase deficiency, ulcer disease, hiatal hernia, pancreatitis, colitis, occult malignancy, malabsorption syndromes, spastic colon, or functional abdominal

pain. The pulmonary manifestations of ascariasis may mimic asthma or pneumonia.

WORK-UP

History

A parental report of tiny worms in the rectal area suggests pinworm infection, but care should be exercised in accepting the diagnosis without confirmatory evidence as a thread or piece of lint may be mistaken for a worm.

Epidemiologic associations are most important in suggesting the possibility of a parasitic infection. Factors that should prompt investigation for giardiasis in a patient with gastrointestinal tract symptoms include day care center attendance, contact with a day care center attendee, contact with an individual with giardiasis, recent travel to an endemic area, or exposure to water that might be contaminated. Even without a suggestive epidemiologic history, *Giardia* infection should be considered in anyone with persistent gastrointestinal symptoms, failure to thrive, or unexplained weight loss.

Residence in a geographic region endemic for *Ascaris* and *Trichuria*, or recent travel to such an area, may suggest infection with these worms. A history of contact with soil, pica, or ingestion of unwashed fruits or vegetables should be sought. Wheezing or pneumonia in patients with the appropriate geographic exposure should suggest ascariasis if eosinophilia is present.

Physical Examination

The physical examination is usually noncontributory unless a worm found in vomitus, stool, or the perianal area is brought for inspection.

Laboratory Tests

Enterobius vermicularis is best identified by an examination of the perianal area for eggs. A piece of scotch tape or one of the commercially available *pinworm paddles* is applied repeatedly to the perianal skin in the morning just before washing. The freshly laid eggs will adhere to the tape or paddle and can then be recognized by their characteristic shape under $\times 100$ magnification. Since worm migration and egg laying may be variable from one night to another, repeated tests are sometimes necessary to detect infection. Three tests will detect

90% of infections; 5 tests will detect 99%. Pinworm eggs are only rarely found in stool examination.

Giardiasis can be diagnosed by an examination of several types of specimens from the gastrointestinal tract. Stool samples are most readily obtained and can be examined for trophozoites and cysts. Trophozoites are labile outside the gastrointestinal tract, thus liquid stools should be examined within 1 hour of passage or be preserved. Fresh stool examination is usually impractical in the ambulatory setting. Ova and parasite collection kits are commercially available that allow convenient preservation of stool specimens until a laboratory examination can be performed. Since cyst excretion is intermittent, stool specimens collected over several days are needed for optimum results. In patients in whom the diagnosis is strongly suspected but stool samples are negative, a duodenal fluid examination should be performed either by duodenal intubation and aspiration or through the use of the string test. String inside the Entero-Test capsule is swallowed until it reaches the duodenum. When the string is withdrawn, jejuenal fluid is squeezed from the distal end and examined for trophozoites. A biopsy of the duodenal mucosa may be needed if other methods have failed. In experienced hands, duodenal fluid examination and biopsy are more sensitive than stool examination.

Due to the tremendous numbers of eggs passed each day, *Ascaris* infection is readily diagnosed by stool examination. Eosinophilia does develop in patients with ascariasis and may prompt stool examination. Trichuriasis is easily identified by a stool examination. Eosinophilia does not occur.

TREATMENT

Enterobius Vermicularis

Mebendazole is a wide spectrum antihelmintic that is the preferred drug for most roundworm infections. A single dose of 100 mg has a 96% cure rate in enterobiasis. Because mebendazole is active only against worms and has no effect on eggs, the Center for Disease Control recommends a repeat dose 2 weeks after the initial dose to eradicate newly hatched worms. Toxicity of mebendazole is infrequent; rarely, local gastrointestinal disturbances may occur. Pyrantel pamoate is an acceptable alternative in the treatment of pinworms. A single dose of 11 mg/kg (maximum dose 1 g) has a 90% cure rate and, like mebendazole, should be repeated in 2 weeks.

Because of the contagious nature of pinworms and the frequency of infection and reinfection among household members, simultaneous treatment of the entire family is sometimes recommended. Hygienic measures should not be overly stressed since even stringent housecleaning and personal sanitation have not helped to prevent reinfection.

Giardia Lamblia

When a case of giardiasis is diagnosed, family members and symptomatic day care contacts should be examined for *Giardia*. Testing of all asymptomatic day care contacts is not routinely recommended although a controversy exists around this issue.

Individuals with symptomatic giardiasis should be treated with one of the three available effective agents: quinacrine, metronidazole, or furazolidone. Quinacrine (6 mg/kg/day divided tid for 7 days, maximum 300 mg/day) is the least expensive and has a >90% cure rate. However, it has a bitter taste and causes frequent gastrointestinal upsets, particularly in children under 5 years of age. Metronidazole (15 mg/kg/day divided tid–qid for 10 days, maximum 750 mg/day) is as effective as quinacrine, but is not approved for use in giardiasis by the Food and Drug Administration because of its carcinogenic effect on animals. Furazolidone (6 to 8 mg/kg/day divided qid for 10 days, maximum 400 mg/day) is the only drug available in a liquid preparation. It has lower cure rates but gastrointestinal upset is less common. Because no drug is completely effective, treatment failures are not uncommon in giardiasis. These can be managed by retreatment with the same agent for a similar or longer course or by switching to one of the alternative agents.

Treatment of children with asymptomatic *Giardia* infection is controversial. Because of evidence that asymptomatic infection is common among children in day care centers, and generally well tolerated, overly vigorous treatment with potentially toxic drugs cannot be routinely recommended. The role of asymptomatic cyst excretion in perpetuating the spread of disease in the day care center or community is not well delineated.

General hygienic measures are clearly important in controlling the spread of giardiasis. Careful handwashing, proper diaper changing technique, and good environmental sanitation, especially in diaper changing areas, are all important in preventing the spread of infection.

Treatment efficacy should be determined following therapy by an examination of stool samples. Since nonviable cysts may be excreted for up to 1 week after treatment, repeat stool samples should be collected more than 1 week after the completion of therapy.

Ascaris Lumbricoides

Mebendazole in a dose of 100 mg twice a day for 3 days is 99% effective in the treatment of ascariasis. Alternative regimens include pyrantel pamoate 11 mg/kg (maximum 1 g) in a single dose and piperazine citrate 75 mg/kg daily (maximum 3.5 g/day) for 2 days. Piperazine citrate paralyzes the worms and is particularly effective for the treatment of intestinal obstruction because it may relax a matted bolus of worms.

There is no specific treatment for the pulmonary manifestations of ascariasis, which are self-limited and usually last 2 to 3 weeks. Symptomatic measures are helpful when indicated. Intestinal antihelmintic therapy can be provided later, when the worms have developed to maturity in the small intestine. An intestinal obstruction should be treated conservatively with nasogastric suction, intravenous hydration, and piperazine citrate. Surgical intervention can be avoided in most cases.

Trichuris Trichiura

The treatment of trichuriasis is mebendazole 100 mg twice daily for 3 days. A cure rate of 70% to 96% can be expected.

INDICATIONS FOR REFERRAL

Infection with pinworms, Ascaris, Trichuria, and most cases of giardiasis can be readily handled by the pediatrician. In cases where Giardia is strongly suspected but stool samples are unrevealing, a referral to a gastroenterologist is indicated.

ANNOTATED BIBLIOGRAPHY

Craft JC: Giardia and giardiasis in childhood. Pediatr Infect Dis 1:196, 1982 (Comprehensive review.)

Davidson RA: Issues in clinical parasitology: The treatment of giardiasis. Am J Gastroenterol 79:256, 1984 (Reviews treatment options for giardiasis with a good discussion of the comparative efficacy and toxicity.)

Pickering LK: Problems in diagnosing and managing giardiasis. Pediatr Infect Dis (Suppl) 4:6, 1985 (Concise clinically oriented review.)

Pickering LK, Woodward WE, Dupont HL et al: Occurrence of Giardia lamblia in children in day care centers. J Pediatr 104:522, 1984 (Prevalence survey of giardiasis in day care centers and long-term surveillance of a small group of children.)

Warren KS, Mahmoud AAF: Algorithms in the diagnosis and management of exotic diseases; Enterobiasis. J Infect Dis 132:229, 1975 (Excellent review of all facets of pinworm infection.)

Warren KS, Mahmoud AAF: Algorithms in the diagnosis and management of exotic diseases; Trichuriasis. J Infect Dis 133:240, 1976 (Excellent review of current knowledge about trichuriasis.)

Warren KS, Mahmoud AAF: Algorithms in the diagnosis and management of exotic diseases; Ascariasis and Toxocariasis. J Infect Dis 135:868, 1977 (Excellent review of Ascaris infection.)

Weller TH, Sorenson CW: Enterobiasis: Its incidence and symptomatology in a group of 505 children. N Engl J Med 224:143, 1941 (Established that subclinical enterobiasis is common and that gastrointestinal symptoms are no more common in infected than uninfected children.)

23
Miscellaneous Conditions

202
Apnea of Infancy
DOROTHY H. KELLY

The sudden unexpected and unexplained death of infants has been reported since biblical times. In recent years, many researchers have investigated numerous hypotheses of the causes of such deaths. As a result of these investigations, it seems probable that the sudden infant death syndrome (SIDS) is due to *multiple causes*. *One* the factors that can result in the sudden death of infants is an abnormal control of ventilation. This was first documented in 1972 by a report of the sudden death in two infants in one family who were SIDS siblings and who had prolonged apnea. Since that time others have reported sudden and unexpected deaths in some infants with idiopathic apnea of infancy. It is a clinical challenge for the primary care physician to evaluate and manage infants with apnea.

PATHOPHYSIOLOGY

Numerous physiologic studies of infants with apnea have documented abnormalities in the control of ventilation in some of these infants including a decreased ventilatory response to breathing carbon dioxide, mild hypoventilation in quiet sleep, absent arousal response to hypoxia and hypercarbia, prolonged sleep apnea, excessive short apnea, periodic breathing, and obstructive sleep apnea. Others have failed to document such abnormalities. Many of these abnormalities have been present in infants with apnea of infancy who subsequently died. However, the cause(s) of these abnormalities remain(s) unknown. Only two autopsy studies on infants with apnea of infancy (AOI) have been reported. In the first study, increased muscularity of the pulmonary vasculature was reported in five infants and in the second gliosis in the brainstem was described in one infant. Both findings can be associated with chronic hypoxia either as a cause or as an effect.

In summary, many abnormalities in control of ventilation have been found in infants with AOI, some of whom have died. However, the cause(s) of these abnormalities remain(s) unknown.

CLINICAL PRESENTATION

There are three typical presentations of infants with AOI. The first is the occurrence of apnea during sleep, usually associated with a change in color and tone. Frequently, there is a history of some degree of stimulation that is used by the caretaker to terminate the episode and return the infant to normal breathing, color, and tone. The second presentation is that of an infant who experiences an episode of apnea while awake. Such episodes frequently follow choking or regurgitation and are commonly associated with stiffening, redness, and a frightened look. The mouth is often opened as if trying to breathe. If uninterrupted by caretakers, the event can proceed to cyanosis, limpness, unconsciousness, and central apnea in some infants. Finally, infants may present for an evaluation because of a history of color change during sleep with shallow or irregular breathing or because the caretaker has observed numerous episodes of sleep apnea without a change in tone or color.

843

DIFFERENTIAL DIAGNOSIS

The following diseases must be considered in the differential diagnosis of apnea of infancy: *congenital*—anatomic airway abnormalities, vascular abnormalities causing airway obstruction, congenital heart disease and cardiac arrhythmias; *infectious*—sepsis, meningitis, pneumonia, and RSV infection; *toxic*—botulism, sedative drug usage or overdose; *metabolic*—hypoglycemia, hyponatremia, hypothermia, and some unborn errors of metabolism; *neoplastic*—tumors in or around the airway leading to an obstruction or in the brain causing seizures resulting in apnea; and *other*—gastroesophageal reflux, seizures, hypoxemia, anemia in the preterm infant, and abnormalities in the control of ventilation.

WORK-UP

History

An evaluation of an apneic event should include a meticulous history taken from every person who observed the infant during the event or immediately following the episode (Fig. 202-1). The detailed history is necessary to help the clinician determine the severity and possibly the cause of the episode as judged by the manner of presentation as well as by the type, duration, and appropriateness of the intervention used to terminate the event. A thorough past history and family history should also be obtained.

Physical Examination

A careful physical examination should be performed to determine if signs of partial airway obstruction, congenital anomalies, intercurrent illness, or metabolic or neurologic abnormalities are present.

Laboratory Tests

Laboratory tests should be performed to attempt to identify a cause for the event, based on the history, the physical examination, and the differential diagnosis. Such an evaluation generally includes a complete blood count, differential white count, serum sodium, potassium, chloride, glucose, urea nitrogen, urinalyses, arterial blood gases, chest radiograph, electrocardiogram, electroencephalogram, and a barium esophagram with fluoroscopy. Other studies such as cultures, lumbar puncture, bronchoscopy, and CT scan may be indicated in some cases.

If no cause can be identified by a careful history, physical examination, and the usual laboratory examinations, tests to identify abnormalities in the control of ventilation including polysomnography, pneumogram, studies of ventilatory and arousal responses to hypercarbia and hypoxia are appropriate to consider. This usually necessitates a referral to a center specializing in the evaluation and management of infants with AOI.

MANAGEMENT

Specific treatment is indicated in those infants in whom a cause of the apneic episode has been identified during the evaluation. For those infants who have idiopathic AOI, their treatment approach is based on the infant's gestational and chronologic age as well as his clinical presentation.

Preterm infants who have idiopathic apnea, documented clinically as well as in the laboratory by an abnormal polygraphic or pneumographic recording, are usually treated with theophylline (5 to 7.5 mg/kg/day) given every 6 to 8 hours. A loading dose is generally not used since this often results in irritability, tachycardia, and regurgitation. At 48 hours after the medication has been started, serum peak and trough levels of theophylline are measured and, if these are in the therapeutic range ($\geq$10 μg/ml and <20 μg/ml), a pneumogram is obtained. If this recording is normal and the symptoms have resolved, the infant is discharged on theophylline, increasing the dose/kg weekly for weight gain and liver maturation in order to maintain serum theophylline levels within the therapeutic range. Between 48 and 52 weeks postconceptional age, the infant is readmitted to determine if the apnea has resolved. At this time the medication is discontinued and the infant is studied by a pneumogram or polygraph. The drug is discontinued if the infant remains asymptomatic and the study is normal. If, however, the infant becomes symptomatic or the study is abnormal, theophylline is continued in the therapeutic range for an additional 4 to 8 weeks at which time the medication is again discontinued and the study is repeated.

If the infant improves initially but does not resolve the clinical or laboratory abnormalities during methyxanthine treatment, then he is discharged on the medication in addition to a home monitor when the clinical apnea or bradycardia has resolved. Following discharge, when the clinical and laboratory abnormalities have resolved, the drug is withdrawn

Name _____

HISTORY OF EVENT (leading to evaluation): Please circle features and complete as needed.

Date: _____; Age: _____; # hours after feed: _____

Last Immunization (specify date / type): _____; Medications; _____

Recent illness: _____

OBSERVER	LOCATION	INFANT POSITION	STATE	COLOR	COLOR CHANGE
Parent	Holding infant	Prone	Asleep	Cyanotic	Entire body
MD	Same room	Supine	Awake	Grey	Extremities
RN	Audible distance	Upright	Drowsy	Pale	Face
Other _____	In car	Infant seat	Feeding	Red	Perioral
	Other _____	Other _____	Other _____	Purple	Lips
				Normal	Other _____

BREATHING	TONE	EYES	NOISE	FLUID	HEART RATE
No effort	Limp	Closed	Cough	Milk	Bradycardia @ ____bpm
Shallow	Stiff	Dazed	Choke	Vomitus	Tachycardia @ ____bpm
Struggling	Tonic/clonic	Scared	Stridor	Mucus	Normal
Rapid	Normal	Rolled	Gasp	Blood	Unknown
Normal	Other _____ __	Staring	Cry	None	
Other _____		Normal	None	Other _____	
		Other _____	Other _____		

STIMULATION	DURATION OF EVENT:	ABNORMALITIES FOLLOWING EVENT
None	___ ____ sec / min	Abnormal breathing x _____ min / hrs
Gentle		Color change x _____ min / hrs
Vigorous		Behavior __ _____
MTM: # breaths ____ __		None
CPR: # cycles _____		

EMT/ER Observations:

Figure 202-1. History form that is used as a guide in obtaining a complete history of the apneic event.

gradually while home monitoring is continued until the criteria to discontinue home monitoring are met.

Finally, if no improvement in the clinical or laboratory abnormalities occur during methylxanthine treatment, then the search for a cause of the disorder must be repeated with special emphasis on gastroesophageal reflux, seizure, hypoxemia, anemia, as well as a congenital central hypoventilation syndrome (Ondine's curse).

Full-term neonates (<1 month of age) with *idiopathic* apnea of infancy who have abnormal pneumographic recordings are managed with methylxanthines as outlined for preterm infants. Those full-term neonates who have no pneumographic or polygraphic abnormalities and no explanation for the apneic event are managed as outlined below for the older infant with idiopathic apnea.

The older infants (≥1 month of age) with *idio-pathic* apnea of infancy are routinely discharged with a cardiorespiratory monitor to be used at home because they may not be completely controlled with methylxanthines alone. In addition, medication is recommended based on the following criteria:

1. Medication for a specific abnormality such as gastroesophageal reflux or a seizure disorder
2. Methylxanthines if there are:
   a. Major abnormalities on testing (prolonged apnea > 20 seconds), episodes of prolonged bradycardia (lasting 10 seconds or longer) for which no cause can be found, or marked hypoventilation (average $P_ACO_2 \geq 50$ mm Hg during quiet sleep).
   b. Continued symptoms of apnea or bradycardia.

If methylxanthine is instituted and the infant has

been asymptomatic for 1 month, the medication is gradually discontinued. If signs or symptoms recur, it is reinstituted.

When a decision is made to institute electronic surveillance at home with a cardiorespiratory monitor, the parents are trained to use the equipment and techniques of observation and intervention and infant cardiopulmonary resuscitation as outlined in our handbook (Haight BF, Kelly D, McCabe KC) and recommended by the American Academy of Pediatrics.

During the course of monitoring, the infants and families are followed carefully by our medical, nursing, and social service staff. The use of a monitor at home for idiopathic AOI is associated generally with acceptable stress and family disruption if accompanied by a strong support system. Without such support, home monitoring can be stressful and disruptive to all family members.

During the course of monitoring, the symptoms of apnea often increase initially with the stress of upper respiratory tract infections or sleep deprivation. However, in most infants, the signs and symptoms of AOI resolve usually within 1 to 3 months. For many infants there is no recurrence of symptoms after the initial episode. We, therefore, recommend that monitoring be discontinued when all the following criteria are met:

1. No apnea or bradycardia requiring vigorous stimulation for 3 months (4 months if 12 to 18 months of age and 6 months if older than 18 months of age)
2. No apnea requiring gentle or no stimulation for 2 months
3. Two normal pneumograms recorded at home
4. Normal polygraphic recording if previously abnormal
5. Resolution of physical abnormalities referrable to apnea, such as bradycardia to ocular pressure or nasal occlusion, neck and shoulder hypotonia, or lack of oral breathing to nasal occlusion)

These criteria are reviewed with the parents during each follow-up visit. Using this method, ~ 95% of the parents can comply with the recommendation to discontinue monitoring within 2 weeks of the time that it is made. Increased support by the nursing staff is necessary at that time.

INDICATIONS FOR ADMISSION OR REFERRAL

All infants who have had a episode of apnea accompanied by a color change should be admitted for continual cardiorespiratory monitoring by med-ical personnel trained in infant monitoring and cardiopulmonary resuscitation while the infant is being evaluated for the cause of the event. Infants requiring tests to determine abnormalities of ventilation other than a pneumogram are best referred to centers specialized in the evaluation of AOI. A referral and possibly a transfer is recommended in those infants who are in the high mortality rate groups. These include (1) siblings of SIDS victims who have had at least one episode of sleep apnea that resolved following mouth-to-mouth resuscitation (25% mortality rate) and (2) infants who presented initially with an episode of sleep apnea requiring resuscitation who have had at least one subsequent severe episode of sleep apnea requiring either vigorous stimulation or resuscitation (28% mortality rate). If these infants with severe AOI develop a seizure disorder during the course of home monitoring, their mortality rate is even higher (4:7). Because of these high mortality rates, a referral of such infants to a center specializing in the evaluation and management of infants with apnea of infancy is strongly recommended.

OUTCOME

For many infants who experience an apneic episode, the etiology can be discovered with careful searching. For those with idiopathic AOI, treatment with methylxanthines or home monitoring with appropriate teaching and support is usually successful although, depending on the type and severity of their initial episode, between 30% and 50% will have a subsequent significant sleep apnea episode during home monitoring. Ninety-two percent of infants are well by 12 months of age. However, some infants with severe AOI have died during home monitoring and half of these deaths occurred when intervention was incorrectly performed or at an inopportune time. Meticulous investigation and management of these high risk infants will result hopefully in improved control of the symptoms and a decreased mortality rate.

ANNOTATED BIBLIOGRAPHY

American Academy of Pediatrics Task Force on Prolonged Infantile Apnea: Prolonged Infantile Apnea: 1985. Pediatrics 76:129, 1985 (Official statement of the American Academy on the evaluation and management of infants with apnea.)

Haight BF, Kelly D, McCabe KC: A manual for home monitoring, 1980 (Summarizes the specifics of the training program for the infant's caretakers which is necessary before an infant can be discharged with a monitor.)

Kelly DH, Shannon DC: Sudden infant death syndrome and near sudden infant death syndrome: A review of the literature. 1964 to 1982. Pediatr Clin North Am 29:1241, 1982 (Reviews the epidemiology of SIDS, recent research of the cause of SIDS, and research of the pathophysiology and management of infants with apnea of infancy.)

Kelly DH, Shannon DC: Treatment of apnea and excessive periodic breathing in the full-term infant. Pediatrics 68:183, 1981 (Demonstrates that pneumogram abnormalities in full-term infants normalize with theophylline.)

Kelly DH, Shannon DC, O'Connell K: Care of infants with near miss sudden infant death syndrome. Pediatrics 61:511, 1978 (Describes an approach to the evaluation and management of infants with apnea and the outcome of home monitoring, including four deaths.)

Oren J, Kelly DH, Shannon DC: Identification of a high risk group for sudden infant death syndrome among infants who were resuscitated for sleep apnea. Pediatrics 77:495–499, 1986 (Identifies the characteristics of the infants with AOI who have a high mortality rate (13% to 57%) and suggests methods of managing those infants to decrease mortality.)

Steinschneider A: Prolonged apnea and the sudden infant death syndrome. Clinical and laboratory observations. Pediatrics 50:646, 1972 (Report of the first two cases of sudden and unexplained death during sleep in two infants [siblings] who had apnea.)

Valdes–Dapena MA: Sudden infant death syndrome: A review of the medical literature 1974–1979. Pediatrics 66:597, 1980 (State-of-the-art review of the epidemiology and the current theories and research of the causes of SIDS.)

203
Breath-Holding Spells

PETER T. HEYDEMANN

Breath-holding spells constitute a distinct variety of syncope in early childhood and are the most dramatic benign episodes of childhood. They consist typically of a sudden upset to the child followed by a period of unconsciousness and perhaps convulsive movement. There are cyanotic and pallid varieties, both of which have their highest incidence in the first 2 years of life and are uncommon after the age of 6 years. Such spells have been estimated to occur in nearly 1% of children and mild variations occur in up to 5% of young children. Recurrences of spells are common, but the exact incidence has not been determined.

PATHOPHYSIOLOGY

The pathophysiology of the cyanotic and pallid types of spells differ. Cyanotic spells occur during episodes in which the child cries and then suddenly holds his breath. During crying the Pco_2 is lowered, thus causing cerebral vasoconstriction and a diminished cerebral perfusion. The diminished perfusion is aggravated by the child's Valsalva maneuver, which decreases cardiac stroke volume and may cause reflex bradycardia. As breath-holding continues, progressive hypoxia ensues and the child loses consciousness. A seizure may result if the hypoxia or ischemia is severe. As breathing resumes during the seizure, cerebral hypoxia improves, the seizure ends, and consciousness is restored. It has been shown that prolonged breath-

holding is not due to altered respiratory center chemosensitivity. It is more likely that the "willpower" of the cerebral cortex is able to overcome medullary respiratory drive reflexes.

Most children with pallid spells have abnormally active vagal reflexes that produce severe bradycardia with decreased cardiac output and cerebral perfusion. A sudden scare or mild physical trauma induces the reflex vagal cardiac slowing. The ensuing loss of postural tone and unconsciousness is equivalent to fainting. If diminished cerebral perfusion lasts more than a few seconds a generalized seizure follows. At that point, the heart rate improves, and awareness resumes. The neural circuitry of this presumed limbic-vagal pathway is poorly delineated.

CLINICAL PRESENTATION

The physician is usually presented with the history that a small child has had a spell consisting of sudden brief interruption of normal behavior and consciousness. Cyanotic breath-holding spells are the most common. Nearly all spells are preceded by crying, which is brought on most frequently by anger and frustration; sudden pain, surprise, or fear are the other usual precipitants. Vigorous crying is interrupted within 1 to 2 minutes by the sudden quiet of breath-holding in expiration. The initial reddish facial flush of crying turns into cyanosis which is most prominent on the face. After a few seconds of cyanosis, the child becomes limp. At this point, the spell may resolve or develop into a true anoxic seizure with tonic (opisthotonic) or tonic-clonic movements. As with all convulsions, incontinence may accompany the event and a postictal state lasting minutes to several hours may follow.

Pallid breath-holding spells typically are preceeded by sudden pain or an emotional "startle." The child lets out a quick cry or whimper, becomes quite pale, and loses consciousness and postural tone. If the pulse is monitored, severe bradycardia is noted, with a transient rate as low as 15 beats per minute. Asystole up to 50 seconds has been reported. When the limpness lasts more than a few seconds or the child's head is elevated, a generalized convulsion, which typically lasts less than a minute, may occur and be followed by a postictal state. The child's color returns at the end of the unconsciousness. If the child should begin to rise (or be carried head up) too quickly, the sequence to unconsciousness may recur.

DIFFERENTIAL DIAGNOSIS

Breath-holding spells are one cause of recurrent seizures. The major diagnostic difficulties occur in separating such spells from epilepsy and febrile seizures. In the small group of children with congenital cardiac disease, it is important to distinguish *tet* spells (as seen in tetralogy of Fallot).

Epileptic seizures are provoked uncommonly by emotional or external stimuli. Although small children with epilepsy may suddenly fall and have a seizure, it is important to note if the child was frightened by the fall or sustained an injury immediately before the spell.

When a brief uncomplicated generalized seizure occurs during a febrile illness, the physician usually diagnoses a febrile convulsion. Febrile illnesses probably also reduce the seizure threshold for other types of convulsions, including those from breath-holding spells. In the infant with known or suspected cyanotic heart disease (especially tetralogy of Fallot), paroxysmal attacks of dyspnea and increased cyanosis due to spasm of the right ventricular outflow tract and diminished pulmonary circulation may occur. The onset of a *tet* spell may be spontaneous or may be brought on by crying, feeding, or straining at bowel movement. The spell may cause marked hypoxia and convulsions. It resolves over minutes to hours and should be treated acutely by putting the infant in knee–chest position, giving O_2 and by injecting morphine and bicarbonate. Cor-

rect diagnosis and prompt treatment are critical (see Chap. 189).

WORK-UP

A careful history is the cornerstone of the diagnosis. As with the evaluation of any paroxysmal event, it is important to elicit the details of events that precede the spell (*e.g.*, environmental occurrences, child's actions, or parental actions), the sequence of events during the spell, and the nature of the postspell behavior. A mild trauma, fright, or frustration precedes all breath-holding spells. In the cyanotic type, crying is prominent in contrast to the brief whimper heard in the pallid variety. In the cyanotic type, the cyanosis occurs prior to the seizure, whereas the occasional cyanosis of epilepsy occurs later in the seizure. In the pallid type, a child has often fallen to the ground and then stands or is put over the shoulder by an adult. In minor cyanotic or pallid spells, the child simply becomes limp, but more severe spells include typical of grand mal convulsions.

The standard physical and neurologic examinations are not generally helpful. Most children appear perfectly healthy. Although lethargy may be present, if it is observed immediately after the spell, the physician should check factors that predispose to syncope such as pallor, pulse, blood pressure, fever, and hydration state. With regard to the differential diagnosis of other causes of seizures, the physician should look for signs of neurocutaneous diseases (*e.g.*, hypopigmented macules, Shagreen patches, café-au-lait spots, other nevi); he should also examine optic fundi, palpate the fontanel, measure the head circumference, and evaluate for hepatosplenomegaly.

Laboratory testing may be avoided when a clear picture has emerged from the history and physical examinations. When necessary, blood may be drawn for CBC and simple chemistries (*e.g.*, sodium, BUN, glucose, calcium) to check for anemia and for metabolic causes of seizures. An EEG is a helpful adjunctive test in evaluating for epilepsy; however, the history is more important, and it must be remembered that up to 3% of normal children may have epileptiform abnormalities on EEG. If an EEG is obtained during a breath-holding attack, a high voltage slowing is noted during the hypoxic–ischemic phase. In rare instances (in the differential diagnosis of epilepsy), a CT scan of the brain with infusion is indicated when there are abnormal neurologic findings, an atypical history, or a focal EEG abnormality. Certain experienced physicians will perform an evocative test under ECG monitoring as part of the physical examination: firm gentle ocular compression evokes bradycardia in most children with pallid spells, and a complete spell with convulsion may follow. A good history, however, generally provides a secure enough diagnosis to avoid the ocular compression test.

MANAGEMENT

Cyanotic breath-holding spells are best managed by counseling the caretaker to avoid preventable frustrations and confrontations with the child. In this manner, the crying that precedes the spell will be avoided. If a potential tantrum begins, the caretaker should walk out of sight in an effort to interrupt the child's focus on secondary gain from the caretaker. If a cyanotic spell with seizure occurs, routine seizure advice should be heeded: Keep the child horizontal with the head turned toward the side to avoid pooling of saliva in the posterior pharynx.

Pallid spells should also be managed by attempting to avoid situations that produce sudden frights or minor physical trauma. When the fright or trauma occurs, the child should be kept supine in an effort to prevent exacerbating the cerebral ischemia. This is an effective treatment in many cases. Thus, the susceptible child should not be comforted in the standard parental hug position with the child's head upright at the parent's shoulder. Children who have frequent pallid spells may be treated effectively with vagolytic agents; however, the need for such treatment is rare, and there is no widely established regimen. Atropine sulfate, crushed ¼ or ½ pills of Bellafoline plus phenobarbital (Belladenal), or glycopyrrolate (Robinul), which is not yet approved in children, may be used daily or bid.

PATIENT EDUCATION

The aforementioned counseling measures are important in treating breath-holding spells. In addition, it is imperative to reassure parents that the spells are benign; that they do not predispose to epilepsy; and that they resolve typically in early childhood.

ANNOTATED BIBLIOGRAPHY

Laxdal T, Gomez MR, Reiher J: Cyanotic and pallid syncopal attacks in children (breath-holding spells). Develop Med Child Neurol 11:755–763, 1969 (Descriptive retrospective series of 150 children with prolonged follow-up results.)

Lombroso CT, Lerman P: Breathholding spells (cyanotic and pallid infantile syncope). Pediatrics 39:563–581, 1967 (Large prospective and retrospective study including incidence figures, descriptive findings, and case reports; includes use of the ocular compression test with ECG and EEG monitoring.)

McGee JP, Saidel DH: Individual behavior therapy. In Harrison S, Noshpitz J (eds): Basic Handbook of Child Psychiatry, Vol 3, Chap 5, pp 98–99. New York, Basic Books, 1979 (Gives a brief discussion of behavior modification techniques as applied to tantrums.)

McWilliam RC, Stephenson JBP: Atropine treatment of reflex anoxic seizures. Arch Dis Child 59:473–485, 1984 (Documents success of anticholinergic therapy in pallid spells.)

Stephenson JBP: Reflex anoxic seizures ("white"): Nonepileptic vagal attacks. Arch Dis Child 53:193–200, 1978 (Reviews a British experience in 58 children with pallid breath-holding spells; a good descriptive report with analysis of ocular compression testing.)

204
Colic
MARC WEISSBLUTH

Colic in infants is characterized by spells or paroxysmal attacks of crying, irritability, or fussiness occurring in the evening hours in babies who are clinically healthy. Unfortunately, there is disagreement among researchers and practitioners on almost every clinical feature of colic because there are not objective diagnostic criteria. It would be useful to have measurements from audiotaped crying using voice-activated microphones and videotapes of parent–child interactions in their homes during the day and evening using dim nightlight conditions. These procedures have been performed successfully in other studies but they have not been used for the study of colic. Thus, data regarding infantile colic have been obtained almost exclusively by a reliance on reports from parents.

Obviously, parental anxiety, fatigue, and preconceptions may influence their descriptions of their infants' behavior.

PRESENTATION

Illingworth defined colic as "violent rhythmical, screaming attacks which did not stop when the infants were picked up, and for which no cause, such as underfeeding, could be found." Wessel diagnosed a colicky infant as "one who, otherwise healthy and well-fed, had paroxysms of irritability, fussing or crying lasting for a total of more than 3 hours a day and occurring on more than 3 days in one week . . . and that the paroxysms continued to recur for more than 3 weeks." These pediatricians studied ~150 infants. Their combined results showed that the attacks do not usually occur during the first few days but they are present in about 80% of affected infants by 2 weeks of age. All affected infants have their onset of the spells by 3 weeks of age. About 80% of colicky infants begin their spells between 5 PM to 8 PM and their spells usually end by midnight. An additional 12% of infants experience their spells later in the evening, starting between 7 PM to 10 PM and ending by 2 AM. At 2 months of age, about 50% of colicky infants no longer have these crying spells and by 3 months of age, an additional 30% of infants are free of colic. By about 4 months of age, an additional 10%, or 90% of all previously colicky infants, are free of symptoms. The average duration of the colic spell lasts almost 4 hours. The onset of colic in premature infants is usually delayed and starts near the expected date of delivery regardless of the gestational age at birth.

Some pediatricians view the colicky crying spells as qualitatively different from normal infant crying and they use specific clinical features as diagnostic criteria. For example, colicky infants are diagnosed as such only if they are observed to draw up their legs onto their abdomen or only if they exhibit inconsolability. Most practitioners, however, would agree that crying with the legs drawn up onto the abdomen is not a pathognomonic sign of colic. Inconsolability means that the infant does not become quiet with conventional soothing techniques and may be defined differently by different pediatricians. A pediatrician with a background in temperament research or psychophysiology might describe inconsolability as a within-the-child trait but another pediatrician with a psychodynamic perspective might consider inconsolability from an interaction viewpoint and focus on maternal anxiety as the major contributing factor.

Other pediatricians view colicky crying spells not as qualitatively different from normal crying but only differing from normal infant crying in intensity, duration, or persistence. Data from several studies tend to support this viewpoint because there are no measurable discontinuities in crying behavior between infants who do and do not have colic. For example, for the upper 25% of crying duration in normal babies at age 6 weeks, the mean duration is 3.5 hours which is close to the mean duration of colicky crying spells (3.7 to 3.9 hours). The documented natural history of infant crying regarding its onset, time of occurrence, and cessation parallels that of colic and lends support to the notion that colic represents only an extreme form of normally occurring infant behaviors. Thus, colic and unexplained crying in infants may reflect normal developmental or maturational processes that occur during the first few months. The delayed onset in prematures also supports the view that colic is time-locked to postconceptual age.

During colic spells, the infant is often described as hypertonic because of the stiffening of the entire body, the fists are tightly clenched, and the legs are flexed rigidly over the abdomen. The babies sometimes have uncoordinated jerky movements of their limbs described as batting or flapping of the arms or kicking the legs. At other times the movements are described as writhing, twisting, or turning. These movements are not present at other times and these babies have normal neurologic examinations. Air swallowing occurs during these agitated movements and during the crying spells, and this swallowed air is probably the explanation for the gassiness that is another feature of colicky infants. There is no evidence to suggest that the gassiness in colicky infants is caused by primary gastrointestinal pathology. There is also no strong evidence associating colic with the method of feeding or food allergy.

Another feature of some, but not all, colicky infants is stimulus sensitivity; they appear to be either easily startled or easily awakened. Frequent awakenings at night often occur in these infants. A bothersome feature of colicky infants in general is extreme daytime wakefulness manifested by brief naps or no naps.

DIFFERENTIAL DIAGNOSIS

Most pediatric texts include in their list of possible causes of colic or in their differential diagnosis of colic every organ system or disease known to cause pain or gassiness in infants. When a condition is diagnosed, such as cow's milk protein allergy, then the child has pain or discomfort from that problem, not colic. The term *infantile colic* is usually used when there is no diagnosable medical or surgical problem. If the infant is clinically well on repeated physical examinations and the presentation fits the usual description of colic, then there are only a few alternative diagnostic possibilities. Problems relating to feeding are often mentioned because the gassiness suggests gastrointestinal cramps or pain. Feeding problems are rarely discovered and these can easily be detected by a careful history and repeated weight measurements. Urinary tract infections tend to cause crying and irritability at any time and the pain does not occur with the evening periodicity of colic. Children with urinary tract infections do not usually gain weight well or they may develop fever.

The progressive quality over time of increasingly severe pain, increasing weakness, or increasing listlessness that commonly occurs with organic diseases is notably absent in colicky infants. They appear completely healthy when they are not having their characteristic evening spells.

WORK-UP

A careful history and physical examination are usually sufficient to establish the diagnosis of infantile colic. The physical examination, or repeated examinations, should be considered as a sufficient diagnostic test. Laboratory tests or radiographic examinations, sometimes including hospitalization, are usually unnecessary if the child is gaining weight normally and has a normal physical examination. Tests such as blood counts or urine cultures are sometimes performed on the infant to create the impression of professional thoroughness in order to reduce *parental* anxiety. Under the guise of a laboratory work-up, the physician hopes to better convince the family (and sometimes himself) that there is no organic disease. Thus, after winning their trust and confidence in his professional judgment, the pediatrician can better support the parents as they wait out the 3 or 4 months of colic. However, one potential problem of doing laboratory tests performed with the intent to reduce parental anxiety, rather than based on clinical suspicions, is that a somewhat abnormal result may occur. Obviously, the slightly abnormal test result does not necessarily signify pathology. Nevertheless, one abnormal test could lead to further unneeded tests in a fruitless search to eliminate some uncommon or obscure condition. Another disadvantage in performing laboratory tests is that the performance of the tests themselves or hospitalizing the infant might reinforce the parents' belief that something must be medically wrong with their child. After all, they may think, why else would the doctor do these tests if he did not truly suspect something might be wrong with my baby? With this attitude, the discovery of a few normal results might only cause parents to request additional tests, studies, or consultations.

On the other hand, if the physician does not perform tests, this might lead to heightened anxiety, parental dissatisfaction based on a perception of a lack of thoroughness, and may cause the parents to change pediatricians. There is enormous variability among families and pediatricians in how they handle the stresses caused by a colicky infant. Sensitivity to this variability of how both the parents are affected and how you, the pediatrician, are affected should encourage a highly individualized approach to working up and treating an infant who might have colic.

The method that the physician uses to explain the reason for the tests might make a great difference. Some parents might feel much more relaxed when the physician tells them that he honestly does not think the test will show anything abnormal but that he is going to do it so that they can stop worrying. Other parents might find this approach unacceptable.

I believe that the work-up for colic should usually be based on clinical indications and that an attitude of intellectual honesty in explaining why the physician is doing or not doing laboratory tests is essential to maintain his professional integrity.

MANAGEMENT

The major principle of management is not exactly *what* the physician recommends but *how* he does it. The physician should take the parents' complaint *seriously* and he should perform a *thorough* examination. When he suspects colic, a thorough examination is diagnostic, and also therapeutic, because the thoroughness itself reassures the parents that their child is healthy and is being looked after by someone who really cares. This situation is analogous to carefully examining the child with fever even when you suspect a common cold. The physician should be patient, sympathetically supportive, and appropriately tentative when offering advice regarding remedies of questionable value such as herbal teas or hot water bottles. The way in which the physician presents these therapies is important because overly encouraging home remedies or formula switching may only heighten parental anxiety when each of these items might eventually fail.

If the physician spends extra time in the office or on the phone expressing optimism regarding the health of the child and emphasizing that this stressful period will soon end, this will help the parents maintain their morale. Their increased optimism from your reassurance might not only reduce parental anxiety but it might also cause the parents to handle their baby in a calmer fashion and thus actually reduce the crying. The major error in management is to trivialize the parents' complaint because colic is known to be a transitory condition with no known morbidity or complications.

Parents must be explicitly told that they are not causing the crying. Self-doubt or feelings of inadequacy of parenting skills or failure to nurse well is a topic that should be openly discussed, because every parent blames himself for the infant crying.

TREATMENT AND MANAGEMENT

The three major methods of reducing infant crying are (1) rhythmic rocking motions using swings, cradles, springs on crib casters, automobile rides, rocking chairs, or in parents' arms; (2) encouraging sucking at the breast, bottle, pacifier, wrist, fist, or thumb; and (3) swaddling, bundling, or cuddling. These methods should be encouraged whenever the infant needs to be soothed, and parents need to be told explicitly that the young infant will not become "spoiled" from all this attention. In other words, the child will not learn a crying habit or always expect to be picked up when the parents behave this way during the first 6 weeks.

In order to alleviate unnecessary guilt and prevent misdirected therapies focused on parental psychological factors, parents should be informed that there is no good scientific evidence to suggest that their inexperience, anxiety, or parenting practices are directly causing the colic. Parents should also be told that treatments with sedatives, hypnotics, antiflatulents, antacids, antihistamines, alcohol, or gripe water are no better than a placebo. Antispasmotics are commonly used, but only dicyclomine hydrochloride has been shown to be an effective drug to reduce crying; however, it is no longer used because of questions regarding its safety. Placebo effects commonly occur during the first few weeks after an initial brief period of fussiness subsides, shortly after about 6 weeks of age when the peak of unexplained fussiness or crying is passed, and after 3 to 4 months of age when all unexplained crying or fussiness disappears.

During the first month or so, it is important for the parents to learn to accept and love their baby despite his crying. To maintain their morale, they need to take time off away from their baby by hiring help, even for short periods of time. The pediatrician can help the parents cultivate a watchful waiting attitude until the colic passes. Parents can learn to become sensitive to subtle shifts in their baby's behavior so that they begin to modify their caretaking behaviors as the colic begins to subside.

After about 6 weeks of age, for some mild colicky babies, when the baby begins to exhibit specific social smiling, the baby might benefit from less attention when overly tired. The soothing parental efforts might be so socially pleasurable to the child that he fights sleep to enjoy the parents' company. The end result is fatigue-driven fussiness. However, for severe colicky babies, because they are so irregular regarding sleep/wake transitions, it is difficult for parents to distinguish between colicky crying and fatigue-driven crying until about 3 to 4 months of age. At this age, for all colicky babies, the evening crying spells have diminished and most parents should now be encouraged to give their child less attention when they think that the child is tired and needs to sleep. After 3 to 4 months, most parents are better able to differentiate the child's *need* to sleep from his *desire* to play.

The failure of parents to shift their parenting strategies after about 3 to 4 months of age, in response to the increasing social maturity of the child, often causes severe postcolic sleep problems. Letting the child "cry it out" probably helps no one when the child is under several weeks of age. However, letting the child "learn to sleep" after 3 to 4 months helps produce a calmer, less fussy baby. Parents should be told that they should allow their child to learn the self-soothing skill of falling asleep unassisted and they should be reassured that they are not hurting their child. Learning to be alone to develop self-soothing skills is a developmental healthy habit for the child and pediatricians can guide parents' behavior, which helps or hinders its evolution.

ANNOTATED BIBLIOGRAPHY

Brazelton TB: Crying in infancy. Pediatrics 29:579–588, 1962 (Naturalistic study of infant crying based on parents' reports.)

Illingworth RS: Infantile colic revisited. Arch Dis Child

60:981–985, 1985 (Update from his classic 1954 article and a review of current therapeutic ideas.)

Illingworth RS: Three months' colic. Arch Dis Child 29:167–174, 1954 (Comprehensive review of the literature and a clinical study comparing colicky and noncolicky babies.)

Rebelsky F, Black R: Crying in infancy. J Genetic Psych 121:49–57, 1972 (Infant crying study based on tape recordings.)

Weissbluth M: Crybabies. New York, Berkley, 1983 (Data-based guide for parents and professionals describing how colic relates to normal crying, temperament, and sleep disturbances.)

Weissbluth M: Healthy Sleep Habits, Happy Child. New York, Fawcett Columbine, 1987 (Detailed discussion on postcolic sleep problems.)

Weissbluth M, Christoffel KK, Davis AT: Treatment of infantile colic with dicyclomine hydrochloride. J Pediatr 104:951–955, 1984 (Randomized, placebo-controlled, double blind study regarding colic, temperament, and sleep.)

Wessel MA, Cobb JC, Jackson EB, Harris GS, Detwiller AC: Paroxysmal fussing in infancy sometimes called "colic." Pediatrics 14:421–434, 1954 (Comprehensive description of the clinical features of colic.)

205
Cystic Fibrosis
ALLEN LAPEY

Cystic fibrosis (CF) is the most common lethal genetic disease of white people. Although early recognition and effective therapy have brightened prospects over the past 20 years, the disease continues to cause substantial morbidity and mortality in affected patients.

Inherited as a Mendelian autosomal recessive trait, CF affects ~1 individual in 2000 live births, corresponding to a carrier rate of 5%. The basic defect is unknown and carriers are phenotypically normal. The identification of markers, closely linked to the CF gene, has established that the CF gene resides on the long arm of chromosome 7 near the centromere. Reliable carrier detection and prenatal diagnosis are now available for over 90% of CF families with a living affected offspring. The CF gene will likely be identified within the next several years and the molecular basis of the disorder understood.

PATHOPHYSIOLOGY

Cystic fibrosis is characterized by an increased viscosity of exocrine secretions and an increased salt content of sweat. Defective Cl^- ion transport in CF epithelial cells has been demonstrated and confirmed in several laboratories. This mechanism is likely to result in dehydration of the sol and gel layers lining the bronchial epithelium. This phenomenon is possibly accentuated in viral respiratory illnesses, thus explaining the difficulties with secretions seen with respiratory infections. The same chloride transport defect leads to faulty reabsorption of Na^+ and Cl^- in the sweat duct and elevated sweat electrolytes. This is the basis for the sweat test, which is still considered the most important diagnostic test for CF.

Viscid exocrine secretions underly all the clinical features of CF: pancreatic duct obstruction with achylia and maldigestion; progressive obstructive airways disease beginning with a suppurative bronchiolitis, evolving to chronic bronchitis and ultimately bronchiectasis; chronic sinusitis, often with inflammatory nasal polyps; and various intestinal obstructive phenomena ranging from meconium ileus at birth to recurrent intussusception, intestinal impaction, cholestatic jaundice, and cirrhosis.

CLINICAL PRESENTATION

Over 60% of CF patients are diagnosed in infancy with the characteristic features of failure to thrive secondary to maldigestion as well as the chronic unremitting cough of suppurative bronchiolitis and bronchitis. Yet to be explained is the striking variation in severity. For example, those with normal digestion usually escape detection until adulthood. The more typical presenting features of CF are listed in the box, Presenting Features of Cystic Fibrosis. Given the known variability and at times subtlety of early clinical features, the clinician should maintain a high index of suspicion and obtain a sweat test when indicated. *A child is never too well to have CF.*

Although usually colonized with *Staphylococcus aureus, Hemophilus influenzae*, and eventually *Pseudomonas aeruginosa*, the CF patient is rarely

Presenting Features of Cystic Fibrosis

NEWBORN

Meconium ileus, intestinal atresia
Prolonged neonatal jaundice

INFANT

Failure to thrive
Chronic cough
Recurrent bronchiolitis, hyperinflation, persistent
  infiltrates, atelectasis
Chronic diarrhea, abdominal distention
Persistent vomiting, especially with cough
Chronic hypochloremic alkalosis
Hypovitaminosis A with pseudotumor cerebri

CHILD

Rectal prolapse
Steatorrhea
Nasal polyposis
Clubbing
Hyperinflation, infiltrates, rales, ronchi, and wheeze
Sputum culture: *Staphylococcus aureus* or
  Pseudomonas aeruginosa

ADOLESCENT, ADULT

Sterility in males
Portal hypertension
Growth failure, delayed puberty
Pansinusitis, nasal polyposis
Chronic pulmonary disease

acutely ill with pneumonia or sepsis. Rather, the process is insidious and is typically endobronchial. Unlike the infant or toddler with reactive airway disease who is generally free of cough between episodes of illness, CF results in an unremitting chronic cough, at times with cough-induced emesis, that clears only following prolonged antimicrobial therapy. The ravenous appetite with a large oral intake secondary to pancreatic insufficiency often also leads to an increased cough and emesis.

Airway obstruction is usually reversible early in the course. It is not surprising that patients will appear to have asthma, with symptomatic improvement following theophylline, adrenergic agonist, or steroid therapy. Wheeze, dyspnea, and retractions following respiratory viral infections are as much a part of the clinical spectrum of CF as they are of childhood asthma. In general, however, patients with CF are slower to recover and may require prolonged antibiotic therapy for superimposed bacterial bronchiolitis. The hyperinflation on a chest roentgenogram and physical examination rarely reverses entirely.

At least 15% of patients have normal or ade-

quate pancreatic function. The presentation in this group, as expected, is more subtle, with better growth, normal appetite, and normal bowel function. Chronic or recurrent respiratory symptoms may be the only hints of disease. Even with pancreatic insufficiency and malabsorption, many otherwise healthy CF children maintain normal growth by a voracious appetite with phenomenal caloric intake. Generally, however, malabsorption results in bulky foul stools, a marked increase in gaseous distention and fecal mass with a protuberant abdomen, and a tendency to rectal prolapse. Protein malabsorption, in its extreme, can result in hypoalbuminemia and edema. In addition, there can be hypocarotenemia, vitamin A deficiency with xerophthalmia and pseudotumor cerebri, and hypoprothrombinemia with bruising. Any one or combination of these consequences of pancreatic insufficiency can be present.

The pulmonary features in some patients are sufficiently mild to escape detection in childhood. Patients who are diagnosed in adolescence or adulthood characteristically demonstrate pansinusitis, *S. aureus* or *P. aeruginosa* on sputum culture, and chronic changes on chest film, associated with hyperinflation. On history, there is usually only a cough, which is often productive. Digital clubbing evolves early in the course of bronchiectasis in CF and helps to differentiate such patients from those with asthma. Nasal polyposis is another important clinical feature. The allergic child will rarely demonstrate polyps prior to age 10. In CF, polyps are not unusual early in childhood. Their presence should alert the physician to the possibility of CF and a sweat test should be ordered. Aspermia in the adult male may also be a presenting manifestation of CF.

DIFFERENTIAL DIAGNOSIS

With a respiratory presentation, respiratory syncytial virus (RSV) bronchiolitis, chlamydia pneumonitis, gastroesophageal reflux with aspiration, asthma, ciliary dysmotility, and immune deficiency are frequently considered. RSV is usually epidemic and is diagnosed readily by an analysis of nasal washings. Chlamydia has a typical history of conjunctivitis, onset weeks after birth, eosinophilia, and lack of hyperinflation on chest film. The child with reflux and aspiration may be a spitter; he has an abnormal pH probe or barium swallow study; and he typically responds to positioning, thickened feedings, antacids, and metoclopramide. Ciliary dysmotility is rare; it can be associated with dextrocardia and situs inversus and early on results primarily in rhinosinusitis and serous otitis. Pulmonary symptomatology occurs most often later in the course. These patients are not particularly ill and they thrive. Immune-deficient children suffer from recurrent acute sinopulmonary infections typically due to the encapsulated organisms *S. pneumoniae, H. influenzae* type b, and *Streptococcus hemolyticus*. The infections are acute, with hyperpyrexia and possible septic complications. The pulmonary presentation is not one of dyspnea, cough, and hyperinflation; rather, consolidation with localized changes on an examination and chest film are the rule. Other than tachypnea, symptoms are more apt to be systemic than pulmonary. A prompt response to appropriate antibiotics and laboratory evidence of IgG or IgG-subclass deficiency confirm the diagnosis.

Asthma in early childhood is the pulmonary illness most easily confused with CF; it coexists in many patients. The cough is a helpful differential feature and should be analyzed carefully. The cough of hyperreactive airways is typically tight, nonproductive, and responsive to bronchodilators. The CF cough is unique; it is deep, resonant, and strenuous enough in the extreme to result in rib fractures and cough emesis.

Only 10% of CF patients present with isolated pancreatic insufficiency. In infancy, the only unusual feature is persistent diarrhea. Older patients demonstrate more typical steatorrhea (*i.e.,* frequent, bulky, greasy, foul-smelling stools). The differential diagnosis includes chronic nonspecific diarrhea, gluten-induced enteropathy, intestinal lymphangiectasia, parasitism, and milk protein allergy. Although rare, pancreatic insufficiency not due to CF can be seen in Schwachman–Diamond syndrome and isolated deficiencies in lipase, trypsinogen, and enterokinase.

WORK-UP

The current standard diagnostic test for CF is the sweat test. With rare exceptions, it is abnormal in all CF patients at all times. Sweat chloride values over 60 Meq/L are generally considered diagnostic of CF, with mean values of ~100 Meq/L compared to 20 Meq/L in controls. Unfortunately, although many have been tried, no reliable screening tests are available.

Reliable sweat testing requires a rather laborious procedure known as the quantitative pilocarpine iontophoric test (QPIT). This procedure is required for a definitive diagnosis at all accredited CF centers in the United States. Sweat is stimulated at two sites (forearm) by iontophoresis of a cholinergic drug. The samples are collected on preweighed gauze; they are weighed and the sweat is eluted. Concentrations of sodium, chloride, or both are measured by standard methods. Preferably over 100 mg sweat is collected from each site, because smaller volumes are inadequate for a determination. The testing of the neonate is usually deferred until 1 month of age, when adequate sweat volumes can be reliably obtained.

A positive sweat test in the presence of a positive family history or clinical features of CF establishes the diagnosis. Although other conditions have been reported associated with elevated sweat electrolytes, they are rare. Malnutrition, nephrogenic diabetes insipidus, and adrenal insufficiency are probably the most important entities associated with a mild elevation of sweat electrolytes.

An evaluation of the child suspected as having CF should also include a chest roentograph, a sputum culture, and when indicated, a quantitative 72-hour stool collection for fecal fat. Early chest roentgenographic changes include hyperinflation and increased peribronchial markings that do not clear completely with therapy. There is a predcliction to involvement of the upper lobes, a feature of CF that is yet to be explained. Lobar or segmental atelectasis, in particular involving the right upper or middle lobes, is common in infancy. While the disease progresses, bronchiectasis inevitably develops and is seen on a roentgenogram as parallel bronchial markings (tram lines) extending to the periphery, often associated with hilar adenopathy.

The laboratory assessment of pancreatic function is cumbersome. In most patients, maldigestion and steatorrhea are evident by a history and physical examination. On the other hand, chronic pulmonary suppuration alone can result in inadequate intake, malnutrition, and growth failure. A direct examination of the stool for fat is helpful; however, a positive sudan stain for fat is normal in infants up to 6 months of age. Quantitation of fecal fat on a 72-hour stool collection is still the most reliable means of assessment, assuming an adequate fat intake (3 g/kg/day in infants, 50 to 100 g/day in older children).

TREATMENT AND MANAGEMENT

The therapeutic goals of CF management are the following:

- Prevent bronchial obstruction and control infection.
- Optimize nutrition with adequate caloric intake and replace pancreatic enzymes and fat-soluble vitamins.

- Identify and correct pulmonary and gastroenterologic complications promptly.
- Provide a healthy positive psychosocial climate that will allow the patient and his family to lead as normal a life as possible.

Prevention of Bronchial Obstruction and Infection

Excluding meconium ileus, ~90% of the morbidity and 98% of the mortality in CF relate to pulmonary disease.

The goal is to maintain clean and patent airways. Regular physical activity to stimulate cough is encouraged; it should never be suppressed. Whenever a spontaneous cough does not suffice to clear the airways, physical therapy (which uses gravity), chest percussion, vibration, and voluntary coughing to remove retained secretions are used. If there is clinical or physiologic evidence of reversible airway obstruction, bronchodilators are added, either as an aerosol or as an oral preparation. Patients are followed at frequent intervals and sputum or deep throat specimens are monitored for pathogens, which early in the course are likely to be *S. aureus* and *H. influenzae*. Patients are typically treated with dicloxacillin, erythromycin, sulfisoxazole, trimethaprim–sulfamethoxazole, or cefaclor. Chloramphenicol appears particularly effective for more serious involvement with *S. aureus* or β-lactamase producing strains of Hemophilus. These drugs are unfortunately ineffective against *P. aeruginosa*, which eventually colonizes all but a few patients.

Patients who have an acute exacerbation of lower respiratory disease respond best to hospitalization for high dose intravenous (IV) antibiotic therapy. For *P. aeruginosa*, or if the pathogen is unknown, a β-lactamase-resistant penicillin and aminoglycoside are used. Second generation cephalosporins such as cefuroxime and third generation cephalosporins such as ceftriaxone are highly effective against *S. aureus* and *H. influenzae*. Serum antibiotic levels are monitored as indicated. Treatment is continued until the improvement in chest examination, sputum production, weight gain, and pulmonary function tests reaches a plateau, presumably representing the best achievable therapeutic response. The usual course is 10 to 14 days.

Patients who have established chronic bronchiectasis in a slow decline are often admitted to the hospital for antibiotic administration in an effort to improve their well-being and pulmonary function. Such admissions are now at times replaced by home IV antibiotic therapy.

What is the role of "prophylactic" antibiotic administration in healthy patients with no definable sputum pathogens? There are no long-term controlled studies to answer this question. However, both intuition and what data are available would suggest an accelerated rate of colonization with *P. aeruginosa* in patients thus treated.

Optimal Nutrition

The availability of enteric-coated pancreatic capsules has dramatically improved the nutritional management of CF. Coated enzymes escape gastric breakdown and deliver their product to the small bowel. This has allowed considerable liberalization of the CF diet so that patients can eat with minimum restriction and enjoy the enhanced variety and flavor that dietary fat allows. Nonetheless, caloric intake continues to be deficient in a significant proportion of CF patients, not so much a function of fecal loss than of persistent high basal energy requirement related to the work of breathing and chronic infection. Every effort must be made to increase caloric intake with food that the patient enjoys, rather than with rigid unpalatable supplements.

Infants with CF are generally started on a formula that is predigested (Pregestimil or Portagen) supplemented with medium-chain triglycerides or glucose polymers. Pancreatic enzymes are given with each feeding. The diet is liberalized as tolerated, and parents are given free reign to adjust enzyme dosage depending on the nature of the stool and change in diet. Generally, by 2 years of age, the child is switched over to cow's milk, gradually moving from skim to whole milk.

Fat-soluble vitamins A, D, and E are provided in twice the recommended daily dose, whereas vitamin K is generally supplemented weekly for the first year of life.

INDICATIONS FOR REFERRAL

A list of multiple complications of CF involves every organ system of the body. A thorough discussion is beyond the scope of this presentation. The major pulmonary complications necessitating a referral include atelectasis for aggressive medical management and consideration of bronchoscopy; pneumothorax for tube thoracostomy and possible pleurodysis; massive hemoptysis for close observation and possible bronchial artery embolization; and cor pulmonale. Intestinal complications include meconium ileus, intussusception, rectal prolapse, biliary cirrhosis and portal hypertension, and intestinal impaction with bowel obstruction. The pancreatic complications of diabetes mellitus and acute pancreatitis are common and serious. All of these complications, if recognized and referred, can be corrected or controlled; herein lies the art of the management of CF.

ANNOTATED BIBLIOGRAPHY

Lloyd–Still JD (ed): Textbook of Cystic Fibrosis. Littleton, MA, John Wright PSG, 1983 (Extremely readable, well organized and well documented text that is particularly strong on the historical as well as psychosocial aspects of cystic fibrosis.)

Loening–Bancke VA, Mischler E, Myers MG: A placebo controlled trial of cephalexin therapy in the ambulatory management of patients with cystic fibrosis. J Pediatrics 95:630, 1979 (The best placebo-controlled study of prolonged antibiotic therapy for the CF outpatient.)

Taussig LM (ed): Cystic Fibrosis. New York, Thieme–Stratton, 1984 (Comprehensive text that emphasizes pathophysiology with ample discussion of basic science. The bibliography alone makes this book invaluable.)

206

Acquired Immunodeficiency Syndrome (AIDS) in Children

ANTHONY B. MINNEFOR,
JAMES M. OLESKE, AND
EDWARD M. CONNOR

Given the origins of the acquired immunodeficiency syndrome (AIDS) epidemic in the United States, it seemed unlikely that infants and children would be affected. Once it became apparent that the causative agent could be transmitted by blood products and that women could become infected through intravenous drug abuse (IVDA) and by sexual contact with infected men, the potential for pediatric involvement increased. Indeed, by late 1982, the Centers for Disease Control (CDC) had received reports of infants and children with clinical and laboratory findings compatible with AIDS. Because the natural history of infantile AIDS was not defined and the need to exclude congenital immune deficiency states, the acceptance by CDC of pediatric AIDS as a distinct entity was slow in coming.

It soon became apparent that these infants fulfilled established criteria for the diagnosis of "adult AIDS." Vertical spread from an infected mother to an infant has emerged as the main mode of transmission. Pediatricians may also encounter infected hemophiliacs and other recipients of blood products, as well as those whose route of acquisition is sexual (including sexual abuse). Clinical and laboratory features may vary markedly over what is generally considered the pediatric age group. As with the initial descriptions of other congenital or perinatally acquired infections, the most severe cases of pediatric AIDS were being recognized. It is now clear that a spectrum of clinical expression exists ranging from an asymptomatic carrier state, through the AIDS-related complex (ARC), to the full-blown form of the disease.

PATHOPHYSIOLOGY

There is now incontrovertible evidence that a human retrovirus, designated human immunodeficiency virus (HIV), is the causative agent for AIDS. The virus is trophic for T-lymphocytes, specifically the subpopulation termed *helper cells* (T-helper/inducer, T4). Infection can occur by cell-associated or cell-free virus that attaches to the CD4 antigen that defines T-helper lymphocytes. The virus is typically cytolytic or, under certain circumstances, may integrate as a provirus. Consequently, HIV infection is considered to be chronic and lifelong.

Because of the quantitative depletion of T-helper cells, along with functional defects, these lymphocytes are no longer capable of effectively modulating B-lymphocyte antibody production directed by triggering antigens. Similarly, suppressor T-lymphocytes (cytotoxic, T8) are also no longer regulated in a normal fashion. Thus, the immunologic dysfunction may be profound. Normal humoral immune and specific cytotoxic responses are not possible. Autoantibodies and circulating immune complexes result in tissue injury. This broad defect results in the development of opportunistic infections (OI) and malignancies that characterize AIDS.

Unfortunately, HIV is also clearly neurotropic. The evidence includes detection of HIV genome by in-situ hybridization, intrathecal synthesis of anti-HIV antibodies, the presence of HIV antigen in cerebrospinal fluid, and virus isolation from brain tissue.

Clinical Manifestations of Pediatric HIV Infection

Failure to thrive
Chronic interstitial pneumonitis
Hepatosplenomegaly
Infections
Lymphadenopathy
Recurrent febrile episodes
Recurrent diarrhea
Encephalopathy
Chronic parotid swelling
Skin rashes (eczema-like)
Nephropathy/nephritis
Cardiomyopathy
Hepatitis
Dysmorphic syndrome
Malignancies

CLINICAL PRESENTATION

Since both intrauterine and perinatal acquisition of HIV may occur, newborns may present with features commonly associated with "congenital" infections—namely, toxoplasma, rubella, and cytomegalovirus (TORCH) agents. Low birth weight (often small for gestational age), hepatosplenomegaly, petechiae, and jaundice are frequently seen.

There is a growing appreciation of the diversity of presentations. The onset may be abrupt or slowly progressive. Dysfunction of one organ system may dominate the clinical picture or there may be a combination of problems. The triad of failure to thrive (or wasting syndrome), chronic interstitial pneumonitis, and hepatosplenomegaly is a common presentation. The most frequently encountered clinical manifestations are listed in the box, Clinical Manifestations of Pediatric HIV Infection.

Invasive bacterial infections may be severe and recurrent and may herald the identification of HIV infection. The fevers may be protracted and high grade without an apparent explanation, in part presumably because of a reactivation of latent agents such as cytomegalovirus (CMV), Epstein–Barr virus (EBV), or HIV itself. The immunologic defect is such that multiple pathogens may be present simultaneously at the same or different body sites. Dermatologic lesions occasionally reflect systemic illnesses (*e.g.*, disseminated candidiasis or cryptococcosis) and may be atypical in appearance or progression (*e.g.*, herpes simplex virus [HSV] or varicella-zoster [VZ]).

The lung is the most common site of clinically recognizable infection with *Pneumocystis carinii* and lymphocytic interstitial pneumonias (LIP), the most important causes of morbidity and mortality.

LIP is felt to represent one part of the spectrum of lymphoid hyperplasia seen with HIV infection. The genomes of both EBV and HIV have been identified in sections of lung from children with LIP. The precise role of either agent in LIP is unclear. Less common pulmonary opportunists include CMV, *Mycobacterium avium-intracellulare* (MAI), HSV, and candida.

The gastrointestinal tract is the next common site for an OI, with Candida esophagitis being the most frequent infection. Thrush, although not a classic OI, is nearly universal in AIDS. The more severe the thrush, the greater the likelihood of esophagitis, although one may be present without the other. Cryptosporidiosis is responsible for most of the chronic diarrhea seen in AIDS patients when a specific organism is identified. Gastrointestinal and hepatobiliary disease may also appear as periodic abdominal pain and distention, enterocolitis caused by OI with MAI or CMV, colonic polyps, biliary obstruction, and rarely as Kaposi's sarcoma (KS) or other tumors/malignancies.

The central nervous system (CNS) involvement in pediatric HIV is considered a primary, persistent, and progressive retroviral infection of the brain. It may precede other manifestations of the disease. In older patients, an acute HIV meningoencephalitis with or without seizures may be part of an acute mononucleosis-like illness associated with the recent acquisition of HIV infection. In infants and children, a progressive loss of developmental milestones or an arrest in development is perhaps the commonest early sign. There may be secondary microcephaly. In older children, it may be possible to discern an AIDS dementia comparable to that in the adult. Other features are truncal ataxia with pyramidal tract signs, paraparesis, incontinence, and peripheral neuropathy.

Intrauterine infection is an accepted mode of transmission of HIV, and an HIV embryopathy has apparently been identified. Of the 20 initial patients, investigators have noted growth failure (75%), microcephaly (70%), and other craniofacial abnormalities, ocular hypertelorism (50%), prominent box-like forehead (75%), flat nasal bridge (70%), mild upward or downward obliquity of the eyes (65%), long palpebral fissures with blue sclerae (60%), short nose with flattened columella and well-formed, triangular philtrum (65%), and patulous lips (60%). The children ranged in age from 5 months to 7½ years at the time of the evaluation. An expression of the embryopathy appears variable. It is uncertain how early in life the stigmata can be discerned. They appear to be distinguishable from the fetal alcohol syndrome and ethnic variability.

DIFFERENTIAL DIAGNOSIS

Given the possibility of protean manifestations noted earlier, the differential diagnosis is widely varied depending on the organ system(s) affected. In general, the two most important considerations are congenital immunodeficiency states and congenital infections. The former usually has distinct genetic patterns and diagnostic clinical or laboratory features. The clinical and laboratory abnormalities associated with congenital infections are usually limited to that infection. It is generally possible to exclude the secondary immunodeficiency seen with severe malnutrition, immunosuppressive chemotherapy, and malignancy.

WORK-UP

History

The key element is to establish whether a patient can be considered at risk for HIV infection. A personal or parental history of homosexuality/bisexuality, blood/blood products transfusion, IVDA, and signs and symptoms consistent with HIV infection should be sought. Other risk factors include prostitution and residence in a country where heterosexual transmission of HIV is thought to play a major role (Africa and Haiti). It must be emphasized that HIV-positive mothers need not be ill to transmit the infection to their offspring. Although the data are incomplete, current indications are that about 50% of infants born to seropositive mothers will themselves become infected.

Despite careful histories, the first indication that a pregnancy has been complicated by HIV may be the development of illness in a patient. For perinatal acquisition, most children become ill during the first year of life, although notable exceptions have been observed. Children also seem to have a shorter incubation period than adults following transfusions, ranging from 1 month to 2 years or longer (median, 8 months). Adolescents generally follow a more adult pattern with incubation periods of 5 years or longer common, whatever the route of transmission. The history should emphasize those features of HIV infection outlined the box, Clinical Manifestations of Pediatric HIV Infection.

Physical Examination

The physical findings, although almost never diagnostic, but coupled with a positive history for HIV "exposure," will often trigger an expedited AIDS work-up. Untreated patients almost always have thrush. Lymphadenopathy is nontender and nodes are usually large (greater than 1 cm) and present at two or more noncontiguous sites. Growth and development are generally impaired. Stigmata of the embryopathy should be sought (photos may be a useful adjunct). Children with *P. carinii* pneumonia (PCP) are often febrile, with tachypnea and retractions and they have diminished breath sounds, wheezes, and rhonchi on auscultation. Patients with LIP are less hypoxic than those with PCP and have digital clubbing, parotid enlargements, and generalized lymphadenopathy.

The neurodevelopment status should be assessed. The skin manifestations of invasive infections or KS may be present. The latter are papulonodular, red-purple lesions, but on occasion they can closely resemble pigmented, cystic acne. They may involve any area of the skin (as well as the gastrointestinal tract or other viscera.) Asymptomatic HIV carriers may have no changes discernible on examination.

Laboratory Tests

Viral isolation is not generally available or practical for HIV. Evidence of infection can be determined by screening with an ELISA technique, with positive tests confirmed by Western blot analysis. Paradoxically, antibody positivity to HIV denotes *infection* with the virus and *not* protection as is the case with most other antigen–antibody systems.

The other baseline studies include complete blood count (CBC) with differential, erythrocyte sedimentation rate (ESR), platelet count, quantitative immunoglobulins, T-helper and T-suppressor cell numbers and ratio, chest roentgenogram, and routine urinanalysis. All febrile patients should have blood and other appropriate cultures performed.

A gallium scan can be useful in determining "hot spots" in the lung that are likely to yield a diagnosis if a biopsy is contemplated. Comprehensive stains and cultures for the full range of potential pathogens are mandatory on all surgical specimens. The key laboratory findings in pediatric HIV infection are HIV seropositivity, marked hypergammaglobulinemia, and reduction in T-helper cells with a reversal of the helper/suppressor ratio to less than 1.5. Currently available assays for HIV antibody will not identify infected newborns because of placental transfer of maternal antibody. The latter is usually gone by 12 months of age. Tests are under development for detection of HIV antigen that could cir-

Differences Between Pediatric and Adult HIV Infection

1. Kaposi's sarcoma and B cell lymphoma are rare in children.
2. Hepatitis B infection is less frequent than in adults.
3. Hypergammaglobulinemia is more pronounced in children.
4. Peripheral lymphopenia is uncommon in children.
5. Lymphocytic interstitial pneumonia (LIP) is much more common in children.
6. Some children will have a normal ratio of helper/suppressor T-cells (although quantitatively, T-helper cells are diminished).
7. Serious bacterial sepsis is a major problem in children.
8. Dysmorphic features may be found in some children (embryopathy).
9. Acute mononucleosis-like presentations are rare in children.
10. Progressive neurologic disease secondary to primary HIV CNS infection may be more pronounced in children.
11. Opportunistic infections and tumors of CNS are rare in children.

cumvent this shortcoming and allow for early (perhaps even at birth) diagnosis of infection. The major differences between *adult* and pediatric AIDS are summarized in the box, Differences Between Pediatric and Adult HIV Infection.

TREATMENT AND MANAGEMENT

At present, treatment focuses on supportive therapy and management of the secondary OIs that occur. Details concerning the latter are beyond the scope of this chapter. However, the key elements to be considered are nutritional support and regular infusions of intravenous gammaglobulin (IVGG). Many patients require nasogastric feeding, but if chronic diarrhea is present, parenteral hyperalimentation is accomplished by the placement of central lines (Broviac catheters), if necessary. Despite their hypergammaglobulinemia, functional hypogammaglobulinemia is present. The incidence of bacterial sepsis can be reduced greatly by the use of IVGG in a dose of 400 mg/kg given over several hours and repeated every 3 to 4 weeks. If *allergic* reactions of a mild-to-moderate nature occur, a premedication with age-appropriate doses of aspirin and Benadryl the evening before and again 30 to 60 minutes before infusion is beneficial. Serodiagnostic testing should be obtained before an IVGG program is begun, because antibodies in the preparation will render most results uninterpretable.

Intercurrent bacterial infections are common

and pending culture results, parenteral antibiotics are usually given. Either cefuroxime or cefotaxime (150 mg/kg/day, given IV in three divided doses every 8 hours) has been efficacious empiric treatment. Short courses of prednisone (2 mg/kg/day) are administered for patients with LIP and Po$_2$ of less than 65 torr. Trimethoprim–sulfamethoxasole (TMP–SMX), calculated as 20 mg/kg/day of the TMP component, is given IV in four divided doses every 6 hours for known or suspected PCP. Pentamedine is an alternative for patients who fail to respond in 72 to 96 hours or for those with allergic reactions to TMP–SMX. It is given in a 4 mg/kg/day, single dose by the IV or IM route.

As with other immunocompromised hosts, live vaccines may cause severe morbidity or death. Accordingly, the CDC recommends that none of the following be given to symptomatic HIV patients: MMR, OPV, or BCG. Inactivated polio vaccine (IPV) should be given to all HIV-positive children, along with DPT and *H. influenzae* type b vaccine in accordance with standard schedules. Children older than 6 months of age should receive an annual immunization with inactivated influenza vaccine and those older than 2 years of age, a one-time immunization with pneumococcal vaccine. Postexposure prophylaxis should be given for measles (immune serum globulin) and varicella (VZIG). Except for the routine use of IPV, asymptomatic HIV children are routinely being immunized. Any child residing in a household with HIV-positive individuals should receive IPV. Breast-feeding by HIV-positive women should be prohibited.

INDICATIONS FOR REFERRAL OR ADMISSION

Most symptomatic HIV patients are best treated in consultation with a physician or team experienced in the management of these patients. Social problems often dictate the need for some admissions. In stable children, IVGG is routinely administered on an outpatient basis. Unfortunately, the frequency and severity of opportunistic infections is such that hospitalizations are frequent and prolonged.

No anti-HIV therapy is yet available for routine use in children. An advantage of maintaining a liaison with appropriate subspecialists is the potential use of investigational antiviral agents. Physicians are also advised to follow evolving recommendations concerning household and hospital infection control procedures and policies concerning foster care, preschool, and school attendance for HIV-positive children.

ANNOTATED BIBLIOGRAPHY

Bernstein L, Krieger B, Novick B et al: Bacterial infection in the acquired immunodeficiency syndrome of children. Pediatr Infect Dis 4:472, 1985 (Reviews the type, frequency, and basis for bacterial infections in pediatric HIV infection.)

Calvelli T, Rubenstein A: Intravenous gamma-globulin in infant acquired immunodeficiency syndrome. Pediatr Infect Dis 5:5207, 1986 (Scientific basis of and support for this treatment modality.)

Centers for Disease Control: Classification system for human immunodeficiency virus (HIV) infection in children under 13 years of age. MMWR 36:225, 1987 (Latest, well-referenced scheme to assist in categorizing patients in pediatric age groups.)

Friedland G, Saltzman B, Rogers M et al: Lack of transmission of HTLV-III/LAV infection to household contacts of patients with AIDS or ARC with oral candidiasis. N Engl J Med 314:344, 1986 (Reassuring data concerning the lack of HIV transmission even with close household, nonsexual exposure.)

Goudsmit J, Paul D, Lange J et al: Expression of human immunodeficiency virus antigen (HIV-Ag) in serum and cerebrospinal fluid during acute and chronic infection. Lancet 1:177, 1986 (New methodology to supplement earlier antigen–antibody detection systems.)

Ho D, Rota T, Schooley R et al: Isolation of HTLV-III from cerebrospinal fluid and neural tissues of patients with neurologic syndromes related to the acquired immunodeficiency syndrome. N Engl J Med 313:1493, 1985 (Important article in our understanding of the pathogenesis of CNS infection with HIV.)

Marion R, Wiznia A, Hutcheon G, Rubinstein A: Human T-cell lymphotropic virus type III (HTLV-III) embryopathy. Am J Dis Child 140:638, 1986 (Initial publication dealing with the dysmorphic syndrome. Includes illustration and photo.)

Robert–Guroff M, Oleske J, Connor E et al: Relationship between HTLV-III neutralizing antibody and clinical status of pediatric acquired immunodeficiency syndrome (AIDS) and AIDS-related complex cases. Pediatr Res 21:547, 1987 (Helps to clarify the discrepancy between the ELISA/Western blot antibody system with classic neutralizing antibody techniques.)

Rogers M: AIDS in children: A review of the clinical, epidemiologic and public health aspects. Pediatr Infect Dis 4:230, 1985 (Provides excellent overview of the epidemiology of pediatric AIDS.)

Scott G, Fischl M, Klimas N et al: Mothers of infants with the acquired immunodeficiency syndrome. Evidence for both symptomatic and asymptomatic carriers. JAMA 253:363, 1985 (Retrospective analysis on the risk to infants born of HIV-positive mothers.)

Appendix A
Transfer of Drugs
and Other Chemicals
into Human Breast Milk*

Table 1. Drugs That Are Contraindicated During Breast-Feeding

DRUG	REPORTED SIGN OR SYMPTOM IN INFANT OR EFFECT ON LACTATION
Amethopterin*	Possible immune suppression; unknown effect on growth or association with carcinogenesis
Bromocriptine	Suppresses lactation
Cimetidine†	May suppress gastric acidity in infant, inhibit drug metabolism, and cause CNS stimulation
Clemastine	Drowsiness, irritability, refusal to feed, high-pitched cry, neck stiffness
Cyclophosphamide*	Possible immune suppression; unknown effect on growth or association with carcinogenesis
Ergotamine	Vomiting, diarrhea, convulsions (doses used in migraine medications)
Gold salts	Rash, inflammation of kidney and liver
Methimazole	Potential for interfering with thyroid function
Phenindione	Hemorrhage
Thiouracil	Decreased thyroid function; does not apply to propylthiouracil

* Data not available for other cytotoxic agents.
† Drug is concentrated in breast milk.

Table 2. Drugs That Require Temporary Cessation of Breast-Feeding

DRUG	RECOMMENDED ALTERATION IN BREAST-FEEDING PATTERN
Metronidazole	Discontinue breast-feeding 12–24 hr to allow excretion of dose
Radiopharmaceuticals	Radioactivity present in milk, consult nuclear medicine physician before performing diagnostic study so that radionuclide, which has shortest excretion time in breast milk, can be used; prior to study the mother should pump her breast and store enough milk in freezer for feeding the infant; after study the mother should pump her breast to maintain milk production but discard milk pumped for the required time that radioactivity is present in milk.
Gallium-69 (^{69}Ga)	Radioactivity in milk present for 2 wk
Iodine-125 (^{125}I)	Risk of thyroid cancer; radioactivity in milk present for 12 days
Iodine-131 (^{131}I)	Radioactivity in milk present 2–14 days depending on study.
Radioactive sodium	Radioactivity in milk present 96 hr
Technetium-99m (^{99m}Tc), ^{99m}Tc macroaggregates, ^{99m}Tc O$_4$	Radioactivity in milk present 15 hr to 3 days

* Adapted from Pediatrics 72:375, 1983. Reprinted with permission from The American Academy of Pediatrics.

Table 3.   Maternal Medication Usually Compatible with Breast-Feeding

DRUG	REPORTED SIGN OR SYMPTOM IN INFANT OR EFFECT ON LACTATION
Anesthetics, Sedatives	
Alcohol	Drowsiness, diaphoresis, deep sleep, weakness, decrease in linear growth, abnormal weight gain; maternal ingestion of 1 g/kg daily decrease milk ejection reflex
Barbiturate	None; see antiepileptic drugs
Bromide	Rash, weakness, absence of cry with maternal intake of 5.4 g/day
Chloral hydrate	Sleepiness
Chloroform	None
Halothane	None
Magnesium sulfate	None
Methyprylon	Drowsiness
Secobarbital	None
Anticoagulants	
Bishydroxycoumarin	None
Warfarin	None
Antiepileptics	
Carbamazepine	None
Ethosuximide	None
Phenobarbital	Methemoglobinemia (1 case); decreased responsiveness, decreased weight gain, excessive sleeping if mother's plasma level $\geq$30 μg/mL
Phenytoin	Methemoglobinemia (1 case)
Primidone	None
Thiopental	None
Valproic acid	None
Antihistamines, Decongestants, and Bronchodilators	
Dexbrompheniramine maleate with d-isoephedrine	Crying, poor sleeping patterns, irritability
Diphenhydramine	None
Dyphylline*	None
Iodides	Affects thyroid activity; see miscellaneous iodine
Theophylline	Irritability
Trimeprazine	None
Tripelennamine	None
Antihypertensive and Cardiovascular Drugs	
Atenolol	None
Captopril	None
Digoxin	None
Disopyramide	None
Guanethidine	None
Hydralazine	None
Methyldopa	None
Metoprolol*	None
Nadolol*	None
Propranolol	None
Quinidine	None
Reserpine	Galactorrhea

Table 3. Maternal Medication Usually Compatible with Breast-Feeding *(continued)*

DRUG	REPORTED SIGN OR SYMPTOM IN INFANT OR EFFECT ON LACTATION
Antiinfective Drugs (*All* Antibiotics transfer into breast milk in limited amounts)	
Amantadine	Urinary retention, vomiting, and skin rash
Cefadroxil	None
Cefazolin	None
Cefotaxime	None
Chloramphenicol	None
Chloroquine	None
Clindamycin	None
Ethambutol	None
Isoniazid	None
Nalidixic acid	Hemolysis in infant with glucose-6-phosphate deficiency (G6PD)
Nitrofurantoin	Hemolysis in infant with G6PD
Pyrimethamine	None
Quinine	None
Rifampin	None
Salicylazosulfapyridine (sulfasalazine)	None
Sulfapyridine	Caution in infant with jaundice or G6PD, and ill, stressed, or premature infant
Sulfathiazole	None; nonabsorbable by mother
Sulfisoxazole	Caution in infant with jaundice or G6PD, and ill, stressed, or premature infant
Tetracycline	None; negligible absorption by infant
Trimethoprim	None
Antithyroid Drugs	
Carbimazole	Goiter
Propylthiouracil	None
Cathartics (Drugs that cause abdominal cramping in mother)	Abdominal cramping, colic-like syndrome
Danthron	Increased bowel activity
Diagnostic Agents	
Iodine	Goiter; see miscellaneous, iodine
Iopanoic	None
Metrizamide	None
Diuretics	
Bendroflumethiazide	Suppresses lactation, thrombocytopenia (1 case)
Chlorothiazide	May suppress lactation, therefore avoid prescribing in 1st month of lactation; this may also apply to other thiazides, questionably dose related
Chlorthalidone	Excreted slowly
Methyclothiazide	None
Spironolactone	None
Hormones	
Chlorotrianisene	None
[3]H-norethynodrel	None
19 norsteroid	None
Contraceptive pill with estrogen/progesterone	Breast enlargement, dose related; decrease in milk production and protein content
Estradiol	Withdrawal, vaginal bleeding

Table 3. Maternal Medication Usually Compatible with Breast-Feeding   (*continued*)

DRUG	REPORTED SIGN OR SYMPTOM IN INFANT OR EFFECT ON LACTATION
Muscle Relaxants	
Baclofen	None
Carisoprodol	Drowsiness, intestinal upset
Methocarbamol	None
Narcotics, Non-Narcotic Analgesics, Antiinflammatory Agents	
Acetaminophen	None
Butorphanol	None
Codeine	None
Flufenamic acid	None
Heroin	None
Ibuprofen	None
Indomethacin	Seizure (1 case)
Mefenamic acid	None
Meperidine	None
Methadone	None if mother receiving ≤20 mg/24 hr
Morphine	None
Naproxen	None
Phenylbutazone	None
Prednisolone, prednisone	None
Propoxyphene	None
Salicylates	Metabolic acidosis (dose related); may affect platelet function, rash
Psychotropic Agents	
Antianxiety	
Chlordiazepoxide	Conflicting reports of drowsiness
Clorazepate	
Diazepam	
Meprobamate*	
Oxazepam	
Prazepam*	
Antidepressants	
Amitriptyline	None
Amoxapine	
Desipramine	
Dothiepin	
Imipramine	
Lithium	
Tranylcypromine	
Antipsychotic	
Chlorpromazine	Galactorrhea in adult; drowsiness and lethargy in infant
Haloperidol	None
Mesoridazine	None
Piperacetazine	
Prochlorperazine	
Thioridazine	
Trifluoperazine	
Other	
Marijuana*	Unknown, only 1 report in literature

Table 3.   Maternal Medication Usually Compatible with Breast-Feeding (*continued*)

DRUG	REPORTED SIGN OR SYMPTOM IN INFANT OR EFFECT ON LACTATION
Stimulants	
Amphetamine	Irritability; poor sleeping pattern
Caffeine	Irritability, poor sleeping pattern excreted slowly
Nicotine (excess)	Shock, vomiting, diarrhea, rapid heart rate, restlessness; decreased milk production
Vitamins	
B_1	None
B_{12}	None
D	Increased calcium levels
Folic acid	None
K_1	None
Pyridoxine	None
Riboflavin	None
Thiamin	None
Miscellaneous	
Atropine, scopolamine	None
Bethanechol	Abdominal pain, diarrhea
Diphenoxylate with atropine	None
Iodine (povidone–iodine/vaginal douche)	Elevated iodine levels in breast milk, odor of iodine on infant's skin
Tolbutamide	Jaundice

* Drug is concentrated in breast milk.

Table 4.   Food and Environmental Agents: Effect on Breast-Feeding

AGENT	REPORTED SIGN OR SYMPTOM IN INFANT OR EFFECT ON LACTATION
Aspartame	Caution in patient carrier of phenylketonuria
Bromide (photographic laboratory)	Potential absorption and bromide transfer into milk; see "Anesthetics, Sedatives"
Chlordane	None reported
Chocolate	Irritability or increased bowel activity if excess amounts (16 oz/day) consumed by mother
Cyclamate	None
DDT, benzenehexachlorides, dieldrin, aldrin, hepatachlorepoxide	None
Fava beans	Hemolysis in patient with glucose-6-phosphate deficiency (G6PD)
Fluorides	None
Hexachlorobenzene	Skin rash, diarrhea, vomiting, dark urine, neurotoxicity, death
Hexachlorophene	None; contamination of milk from nipple washing
Lead	Neurotoxicity
Methyl mercury	Affects neurodevelopment
Monosodium glutamate (MSG)	None
Polychlorinated biphenyls and polybrominated biphenyls	Lack of endurance, hypotonia, sullen expressionless facies
Saccharin	None
Tetrachlorethylene (cleaning fluid)	Obstructive jaundice, dark urine
Vegetarian diet	Signs of B_{12} deficiency

Appendix B
Age-Appropriate Toys
LUCINDA LEE KATZ

BIRTH TO 24 MONTHS

Activities that encourage adult–child interaction

Activities that encourage large body movement–reaching, rolling, pulling

Activities that encourage batting, retrieving, mouthing, tracking, watching

Activities that encourage listening, sound making, turn-taking

Activities that encourage problem solving, making relationships between ideas, people, places, and objects

Crib toys: peek-a-boo, crib gyms, rattles, key rings, teethers, busy boxes, mobiles, track and watch, flip fingers, small balls

Stuffed toys: teddy bears, monkeys, and other stuffed animals

Music boxes: Jack-in-the-box, mobiles, merry-go-music, animal wind-up music boxes

Rolling toys: water floating toys, nerf and small rubber balls, flutter-balls, larger balls, plastic see-through toys

Pop-up toys: pop-up animals, Jack-in-the-ball, Jack-in-the-box

Blocks: soft blocks, unit blocks

Push and pull toys: corn poppers, vacuum cleaners, lawn bubbler, clatter-pillar

Pounding toys: pots and pans, peg pounders, hammer boards

Puzzles: large 2–10 piece puzzles

Housekeeping toys: telephones, cash registers, dress-up clothes, dolls

2 TO 5 YEARS

Activities that encourage problem solving

Activities that encourage fantasy play

Activities that encourage child to child, and adult to child interactions

Activities that encourage multiple skill levels (*e.g.*, scribbling an order for lunch, pretend making the food, serving the food to friend)

Activities that encourage observations of cause and effect, logic and order, strategy skills

Blocks; dress-up clothes; water play; sand play; wheel toys; superhero figures; small construction toys; legos; books; pencil–paper–scissor–crayon–markers; dolls; stuffed animals; transformers; puzzles (10–300 pieces); simple board games; simple card games; simple group games; items for pretend play; paints; small collections of cars, animals, fantasy figures

5 TO 12 YEARS

Activities that encourage problem solving, strategy building, and multidimensional thinking

Activities that encourage child–group, child–child, child–adult interactions

Activities that encourage independence

Activities that encourage team, club, group activities

Board games; card games; group games that encourage rituals, rules, and specific roles; collections of baseball cards, stickers, stuffed animals, porcelain animal families, dolls, books, hats, cars; athletics; books; science and math activities; computers; bike riding; skate boards; swimming; skating; instruments; hobbies

12 YEARS TO ADULTHOOD

Activities that encourage depth and breadth of subject matter

Activities that encourage skill acquisition, problem solving, and multidimensional thinking

Activities that encourage more involvement with larger community

Activities that encourage friendship patterns, group activities, developing individual roles

Community service projects; clubs; international and national travel; long and short planned trips; tutoring; sports activities; intergenerational projects; apprenticeship in adult roles or hobbies and interest areas

Appendix C
Age-Appropriate Books
LUCINDA LEE KATZ

BIRTH TO 3 YEARS

Books that encourage listening, singing, talking in preparation for reading

Books that encourage repetition, sentence building, question asking

Stories that encourage making relationships of people, places, ideas, and objects

Nursery rhymes, picture books, easy-to-read books, folk tales, repetition stories, choral-response, songs, poems, finger-plays, conversations, ABC and counting books, animal stories, goodnight books, wordless books

3 TO 5 YEARS

Books that encourage story telling, story dictation, and story dramatization

Books that encourage picture and word reading

Books that encourage building a story line–beginning, middle, end

Books that encourage story and sequence building, rhythm and repetition, logic and order

Same kinds of books as listed in the birth to 3-year period

Books by the following authors (not an exclusive list): Margaret Wise Brown, Brian Wildsmith, Russell Hoban, Arnold Lobel, Merces Mayer, Ezra Jack Keats, Gyo Fujikawa, Pat Hutchins, Tana Hoban, Dr. Seuss, Eric Carle, Robert McCloskey, Maurice Sendak, Tara Yashima, James Marshall, Marie Ets, Gene Zion, Stan and Jan Berenstain, Bernard Walser, John Burningham, John Steptoe, William Steig, Charlotte Zolotow, Anne Mitsumatso, Judith Viorst

5 TO 12 YEARS

Books that encourage oral expression, reading aloud, storytelling

Books that share interest of child—mysteries, jokes and riddles, folk tales, information books, biographies, autobiographies, poetry, special interest areas

Funny stories, adventures, fantasy, supernatural, history, fact and fiction, problems, family tension, mysteries, animal stories, ethnic groups, science–nature–technology, animal and plants, space and weather, magic, poetry, heroes, riddle–jokes–nonsense, anthologies, magazines, comic books

12 YEARS TO ADULTHOOD

Stories that build self-esteem

Stories that build depth and breadth of subject matter

Books that focus on: current interests, raises questions and seeks answers, emotional content, suspense and mysteries, personal problems, relationships, imagination, poetry, writing about trips, hobbies; diaries

Resource for reading and writing: dictionaries, atlases, encyclopedias, almanacs

Appendix D
Child Development Resources
for Parents
LUCINDA LEE KATZ

INFANCY

Brazelton TB: Infants and Mothers. New York, Delacorte, 1969 (Profiles three different types of temperaments in infants, giving parents a sense of the wide range of infant dispositions.)

Caplan F: The First Twelve Months of Life. New York, Bantam, 1978 (Details developmental characteristics of infants month by month.)

Dunn J: Distress and Comfort. Cambridge, MA, Harvard University Press, 1977 (First in the series The Developing Child, edited by Jerome Bruner, Michael Cole, and Barbara Lloyd. Provides good introduction to theories of attachment and separation in the first months of life.)

Greenspan S: The First Feelings. New York, Penguin/Viking, 1985 (Focuses on the parent–infant dyad and the importance of establishing healthy interaction from the beginning.)

Kaye K: The Mental and Social Life of Babies. Chicago, University of Chicago Press, 1982 (Author describes the development of the parent–infant interaction, progressing from the child as an apprentice to the child as an adult.)

Mahler M: The Psychological Birth of the Human Infant. New York, Basic Books, 1975 (Describes the process of separation/individuation that culminates in the psychological birth of a human infant. Traces the symbiotic union through ego identity.)

PRESCHOOL

Brazelton TB: Toddlers and Parents. New York, Dell, 1976 (Profiles of families illuminating the universal struggle for independence and self-mastery by children between the ages of 1 and 3 years.)

Caplan T de F: The Early Childhood Years: Two to Six. New York, GP Putnam, 1983 (Practical information about raising children between the ages of 2 through 6 years. Includes health care, toilet training, major areas of growth and development. Extensive reading lists.)

Fraiberg S: The Magic Years. New York, Scribner, 1959 (Describes the wonder of childhood and the development of imagination.)

Kagan J: The Second Year. Cambridge, MA, Harvard University Press, 1981 (Provides information on the emotional and cognitive changes in the second year of life such as the child's recognition of standards of behavior and of his or her own ability to meet those standards.)

SCHOOL AGE

Best R: We've All Got Scars. Indiana University Press, 1984 (Concentrates on the "informal curriculum" that the schools teach *vs* the academic one. In this "informal curriculum," the boys and girls are seen to learn patterns of behavior and socialization skills that are passed to them depending on their gender. Also discussed is their experiences of an informal sex education from their peers. Interesting insights for all those interested in the socialization and schooling of children.)

Clarke–Stewart A, Koch J: Children: Development Through Adolescence. New York, Wiley, 1983

Kagan J: The Nature of the Child. New York, Basic Books, 1984 (In challenging many long held views of human development, the author argues that early experience does not shape our lives forever; rather, humans have the potential for changing and continually transforming their own experiences.)

ADOLESCENCE

Elkind D: All Grown Up and No Place to Go. New York, Addison–Wesley, 1984 (Book for parents, uses research, case studies, and personal

870

experiences to communicate the situation that today's teenagers face. The book speaks to the "me" generation of parents, giving advice about supporting and raising the adolescent in the computer age.)

Group for the Advancement of Psychiatry: Normal Adolescence. New York, Scribner, 1968 (Compiles the research and perceptions of a group of psychiatrists, psychologists, and an anthropologist who came together in this informative book about adolescents. They discuss adolescence in terms of biologic, cultural, and psychological development. The authors believe that adolescence can be positive and that its conflicts and resolution can be a constructive force in our society.)

Kaplan L: Adolescence: The Farewell to Childhood. New York, Simon and Schuster, 1984 (Author treats the adolescent period with respect, showing it to be a phase that is profoundly complicated. Within the historical context of philosophy, psychology, and literature, the author draws a vivid series of contrasts that characterize the adolescent. She shows us how it is a time of life that has both an ending and a frightening, exciting beginning.)

CHILD CARE–PARENT CARE

Bettelheim B: Dialogues with Mothers. New York, The Free Press of Glencoe, 1962 (This is not a book that gives answers; it helps parents to learn to ask questions of themselves about the type of child they wish to have. By helping parents understand their own expectations in bringing up a child, it enhances the family's chances of being emotionally healthy.)

Christophersen ER: The Baby Owner's Manual. Shawnee Mission, KA, Overland Press, 1984 (What to expect and how to survive the first 30 days of having a baby. This illustrated book also provides expectant parents with practical, basic information to help them in their daily routine, both before and during the first month of childbirth.)

Fraiberg S: Every Child's Birthright: In Defense of Mothering. New York, Bantam, 1977 (Concerned with the love affair that exists between parents and their children. Discusses the treatment that a human infant needs and is entitled to receive from his caregivers. This treatment is seen to be related to the bond that forms between the caretaker and the infant, and the value that our society puts on the act of mothering.)

Kanter CN: And Baby Makes Three: Your Feelings and Needs as New Parents. Minneapolis, Winston Press, 1983 (Book about parenting that focuses not only on the care of the infant, but also on the feelings of the new parent. The author is a psychiatric social worker and her clear style of writing, interwoven with developmental theory, makes this a good book for parents.)

Leach P: Your Baby and Child: From Birth to Age Five. New York, Alfred A. Knopf, 1984 (Developmental approach to the first 5 years of life. Covers the psychological, social, and physical development of the child. The author includes many topics such as feeding, play, and interaction, and emphasizes reading and responding to the child's needs rather than rigidly following rules or generalizations about children.)

McBride AB: The Growth and Development of Mothers. New York, Harper & Row, 1975 (Looks at the process of becoming a mother. Written by a professor of psychiatric nursing who is also a mother of two, this book combines personal experience, case studies and theoretical analysis in an attempt to explain the challenging, ever-changing experience of motherhood.)

Rakowitz E, Rubin GS: Living With Your New Baby. New York, Franklin Watts, 1978 (Provides practical information to help couples deal with the emotional and physiologic changes that occur during the first 3 months after childbirth. It gives a view of prenatal occurrences, including choosing a pediatrician and preparing the home, as well as advice about the legal aspects of parenthood and single parenting.)

Spock B: Baby and Child Care. New York, Pocket, 1975 (Bestseller in the child care field for over 30 years. It is an informative, practical book that gives advice on the psychological and physical care of infants and children. The author covers a wide array of subjects, including childbirth, fathering, nutrition, choosing daycare, and single family homes.)

Stoppard M: Day By Day Baby Care. New York, Ballantine Books, 1983 (Covers every aspect of childcare, from birth through age three. It has easily accessible organization and full illustrations. The author is a physician, a medical educator, and a mother of two herself. This book is an extremely usable and valuable resource for new parents or professionals working with infants.)

CHILD DEVELOPMENT AND INFANT MENTAL HEALTH

The Developing Child Series. Cambridge, MA, Harvard University Press (Applies to all references in this section.)

Bower TGR: The Perceptual World of the Child. 1977 (Traces key elements in the development of perception in the child, concluding that the human perceptual system remains fairly constant throughout life but that our interpretation of the perceptual data changes with growth.)

Clarke–Stewart A: Daycare. 1982 (Practical book based on research exploring the effects of daycare on young children. The author presents information on the United States society and its need for daycare, on the history of daycare, types of daycare currently used, effects of daycare, and hints for parents on making practical daycare decisions.)

deVillier PA, deVillier JG: Early Language. 1979 (Gives a summary of work in the area of early language development, tracing development in the sequence that it appears in the infant. Little information on theories of language development is offered.)

Dunn J: Distress and Comfort. 1977 (Good introduction on the theories of attachment/separation in the first months of life, including a cross-cultural view of attachment and distress, and the long-term consequences of the caregivers' method of handling early distress.)

Farnham–Diggory S: Learning Disabilities. 1978 (Gives definitions and descriptions of learning disabilities. It provides a historical review, describes brain functions, gives statistics and case studies, compares learning disabilities with hyperactivity, and examines the information processing approach to disabilities.)

Garvey C: Children's Talk. 1984 (The major discussions in this book bring together information from several bodies of research that discuss the child's attempt to use language in a social context.)

Garvey C: Play. 1977 (Not an introductory book: this well-written volume covers the definition of play, play in connection with elements in the child's environment, and learning to play. The

reader is advised to have prior experience before reading this book.)

Goodnow J: Children's Drawing. 1977 (Examines research on children's drawing, looking at drawing as a reflection of cognitive development rather than of emotional development.)

Greenfield PM: Mind and Media: The Effects of Television, Video, Games and Computers. 1984 (Using information from an array of disciplines, this book summarizes what television, video games, and computers can and should do. This book shows us that although the medias can be effective tools, they are not a substitute for teaching.)

Kempe CH, Kempe RS: Child Abuse. 1978 (Focuses on the nature and treatment of child abuse and describes the organization of programs that treat child abuse. This book is useful to all those who come into contact with children.)

Macfarlane A: The Psychology of Childbirth. 1977 (Discusses life before birth, psychosocial factors in pregnancy, variations during delivery, the beginning of life, the capabilities of the newborn, research on early bonding, and other issues. This is a good introduction to research on early socialization.)

Parke RD: Fathers. 1981 (Describes new research on the history of fathering, the role of the father, the expectant father, the relationship between father and infant, the role of fathers in socialization and intellectual development, and the issues of job sharing, divorce, and career families.)

Rubin Z: Children's Friendships. 1980 (Describes the development of friendships, beginning with a historical summary and then tracing the development of friendship from the first year through the changes that accompany growing up. The author discusses such issues as what it means to be a friend, what it means to lose a friend, children's division into same sex friendship groups, and friendship patterns across different ages and cultures.)

Schaffer R: Mothering. 1977 (Describes mothering from the various perspectives: (1) the traditional, (2) the writers of practical handbooks for parents, and (3) the last 10 years of research. A good introductory book.)

Stern D: The First Relationship: Infant and Mother. 1977 (Describes the social interaction of the parent–infant dyad during the first 6 months of life. It shows in detail how the interactive nature of the relationship is critically dependent on input and participation from both the parent and the infant. A fascinating and new way to look at infants and their parents.)

COMBINING CAREER AND FAMILY

Brazelton TB: Working Parents. 1986

Curley J, Ladar S, Siegler A et al: The Balancing Act. Chicago, Review Press, 1975 (Composed of the essays of five young professional women who have become mothers for the first time. They are all committed to their work and to their children. They describe their experiences, their successes, and failures at balancing their careers and their home life. An interesting, honest, and helpful account for parents and would-be parents in this career-oriented age.)

Curley J, Ladar S, Siegler A et al: The Balancing Act II. Chicago, Review Press, 1981

Grossman C: Infant care guide for new mothers who are considering returning to a job before the baby is a toddler. In The Robert Hamilton Wallace Infant Care Program, Evanston Hospital, 1984

BREAST-FEEDING

Ewy D, Ewy R: Preparation for Breast-feeding. New York, Dolphin Books, 1975 (Fully explains breast-feeding in a step-by-step coverage of how to prepare and what to expect in the months prior to birth. Comprehensive for parents.)

La Lèche League: The Womanly Art of Breast-feeding. Franklin Park, IL, La Lèche League, 1981 (Fully illustrated, complete manual to breast-feeding based on research and vast practical experience. Written by a worldwide organization that is considered one of the world's foremost authorities on breast-feeding.)

Pryor K: Nursing Your Baby. New York, Pocket, 1972 (Describes the psychological as well as the physical adjustments that a mother must make in order to breast-feed her infant. Gives helpful information, complete with photographs, on day-to-day management of nursing; also reviews current knowledge in the field from a wide variety of disciplines.)

Index

ISBN 0-397-50758-5

90000